# About Pearson

*Pearson is the world's learning company, with presence across 70 countries worldwide. Our unique insights and world-class expertise comes from a long history of working closely with renowned teachers, authors and thought leaders, as a result of which, we have emerged as the preferred choice for millions of teachers and learners across the world.*

*We believe learning opens up opportunities, creates fulfilling careers and hence better lives. We hence collaborate with the best of minds to deliver you classleading products, spread across the Higher Education and Test Preparation spectrum.*

*Superior learning experience and improved outcomes are at the heart of everything we do. This product is the result of one such effort.*

*Your feedback plays a critical role in the evolution of our products and you can contact us -* reachus@pearson.com. *We look forward to it.*

7e

Rajiv Vijay

# OBJECTIVE BIOLOGY *for* NEET 2026

National Eligiblity Cum Entrance Test

## Volume II

Pearson

ISBN: 978-93-6713-661-4

**First Impression**

Published by Pearson India Education Services Pvt. Ltd, CIN: U72200TN2005PTC057128.

Head Office: 1st Floor, Berger Tower, Plot No. C-001A/2, Sector 16B, Noida - 201 301, Uttar Pradesh, India.
Registered Office: Featherlite, 'The Address' 5th Floor, Survey No 203/10B, 200 Ft MMRD Road, Zamin Pallavaram, Chennai – 600 044.
Website: in.pearson.com, Email: companysecretary.india@pearson.com

*Compositor:* Saksham Printographics, Delhi
Printed in India by Rajkamal Electric Press, Kundli, Haryana-131 028.

# Contents

# Preface

*Objective Biology for NEET, Volumes I and II* are the recommended preparatory books for students aspiring to crack the prestigious medical entrance examinations. It provides class-tested material and practice problems which help the aspirants to understand important theories and concepts. The series can also be used as a resource to prepare for Classes XI and XII board examinations based on NCERT.

The series is adhered to the latest pattern of NEET and syllabus aligned with the NMC. The content is developed in accordance with previous years' papers from AIPMT, NEET and other competitive medical entrance examinations. All chapters in this series conform to the pattern laid out in NCERT textbooks. Hence, utmost effort has been made to develop each chapter overview to revise or run through the concepts. Explanatory figures and descriptive tables and mind-maps are added in this edition to strengthen the learning.

The objective of this series is to provide the course material in a structured manner that could help students to go beyond classroom teaching. It also acts as a source of higher learning to strengthen the fundamental and advanced concepts of Biology.

The unique feature of this series is its systematic theory accompanied with detailed diagrams and huge repository of multiple-choice questions with detailed solutions. Practice exercise is further divided into two stages: Practice Exercise Level I (to revise the concepts) and Practice Exercise Level II (to sharpen the concepts). Level II exercises are incorporated with detailed solutions to apply concepts and sharpen the fundamentals. Furthermore, Assertion-Reason, Statement based and Matrix Match Types questions are included as per the latest pattern of NEET examination. Written in lucid language, the series aims to assist students in understanding the concepts without the help of any instructor.

**Salient Features of the Series**

- Structured as per Classes XI and XII syllabi of NCERT and NMC curriculum
- Based on the latest NEET exam pattern
- Includes latest solved NEET (UG) 2025 Question Paper (Botany and Zoology) for exam practice
- Theory incorporated with detailed diagrams for better comprehension
- Practice exercises divided into Level I and Level II to revise and apply the concepts
- Level II practice questions are accompanied with detailed Solutions to sharpen concepts
- Includes Assertion & Reason, Statement- based and Matrix-Match Type questions as per the latest NEET exam pattern
- Previous years' questions with explanatory Solutions embedded in each chapter
- Chapterwise solved NCERT Exemplar questions along with ample number of practice questions
- Mock tests are also provided for self-assessment

As an experienced teacher, I would suggest that before starting any chapter of this series, as a student you should meticulously scan the theory and diagrams of the NCERT textbook and complete minimum three rounds of reading of its chapter.

Careful attempts have been made in making the series error free; however, corrections, suggestions, queries, and criticism of readers will be highly appreciated and are welcome. Any suggestions for added or updated additional readings are always welcome. Students can share their feedback at reachus@pearson.com

**Rajiv Vijay**

# Acknowledgment

The contentment that accompanies the successful completion of my work would remain essentially incomplete if I fail to mention the people whose constant guidance and support has encouraged me.

This series is a result of the enormous effort given by my team members who were always there to support me. I believe that the blessings of my parents (Late Gopal Lal Vijay and Late Suryakanta Vijay) and my grandparents have always played a prime role in making me more focused and determined towards my goal. My wife Shubha Vijay, my brother Jeetu Vijay and all other family members inspired me throughout the preparation of this series.

My sincere thanks to the team of Pearson Education for providing me the platform to serve students. I appreciate their efforts in bringing out this series in such an excellent manner.

Once again special thanks to my wife Shubha Vijay for always being there with me and helping me in ensuring high quality throughout the series.

**Rajiv Vijay**

# About the Author

Dr. Rajiv Vijay has completed his schooling from JNV HURDA, Bhilwara, Rajasthan and qualified for MBBS through PMT in 1997. After completing MBBS in 2003 from Government Medical College, Kota, he established his Medical and Engineering Entrance Coaching Institute in Vadodara (Gujarat) which is today known as RJ VISION Pvt. Ltd.

In his career of 22+ years, he has taught a lot of students and most of them are extremely successful in various reputed pre-medical division of Resonance, Kota. As the head of pre-medical division and HOD of Biology, he nurtured, developed, installed, and supervised the pre-medical division at Kota and all centers across India.

Many of his students have secured excellent ranks in different medical entrance examinations in India and have enrolled in prestigious medical colleges such as AIIMS, SMS Jaipur, KEM Mumbai, AFMC Pune, and JIPMER Puducherry etc. Moreover, many of his students who are using this book have scored perfect marks in biology i.e., 360/360 in the NEET exam. Dr Rajiv Vijay also mentors his students through free video lectures on his youtube page, www.youtube.com/c/drrajiv_vijay.

# About the Examination

The National Eligibility Cum Entrance Test (NEET) is conducted by National Testing Agency (NTA). The merit list of this entrance test is also used by state governments/universities/institutions for admission in the medical and dental colleges against seats under their control.

## NEET (UG) 2025 EXAM PATTERN

- NEET (UG) is carried out in pen-paper mode every year by NTA. Students can take a look at the latest exam pattern before going to the syllabus provided by the NMC. Here is an idea about the exam pattern of NEET 2025.
- As per the exam pattern, the exam paper will be divided into four parts-Physics, Chemistry, Zoology and Botany.
- There will be 180 compulsory Multiple Choice Questions in total (45 questions each in Physics, Chemistry, Botany and Zoology). Each correct question carries 4 marks.
- There will be a negative marking of minus one (–1) mark for each incorrect answer.
- The total duration of the NEET 2025 Exam is 3 hours (180 minutes).

| S. No. | Subjects | No. of Questions | Marks | Duration of Exam |
|---|---|---|---|---|
| 1. | Physics | 45 | 180 | 3 hours (180 minutes) |
| 2. | Chemistry | 45 | 180 | |
| 3. | Botany | 45 | 180 | |
| 4. | Zoology | 45 | 180 | |
| **Total** | | **180** | **720** | |

| MARKING SCHEME FOR NEET (UG) EXAM | |
|---|---|
| **Particulars** | **Marks Allotted** |
| Correct Answer | +4 |
| Incorrect Answer | –1 |
| No answer/Multiple answer | 0 |

MCQ questions comprise the following types:

- Single Choice Questions,
- Statement-based Questions,
- Assertion-Reason Questions,
- Matrix-Match Type Questions,
- Multiple Statement Questions (mainly, true or not true-based statements).

## TIME MANAGEMENT

In order to successfully crack NEET, one must prepare profoundly. Consistent hard work, practice and perseverance are needed to crack this examination. Statistically, NEET is one of the toughest examinations in India. During this examination, one must exercise clinical precision with speed since the average duration to respond to one question is hardly a minute. The aspirants should be conceptually clear in the subject owing to the negative marking in the examination. A better strategy to solve the paper is to go for the easiest first and then the toughest questions.

Regular practice of MCQs will assist the aspirants to assess their preparation for the examination. In a nutshell, hard work, conceptual clarity and self-assessment are the essential ingredients to achieve success in NEET. NCERT texts play an important role in understanding the concepts. All concepts/theories must be referred in a regular manner.

## TIME MANAGEMENT TIPS

**Step 1 (First 30 mins):** In order to solve maximum questions in limited time frame, attempt the easy questions first. You may start from Physics/Chemistry Section, where some problems may be answered by comparing the units of the options.

**Step 2 (Next 60 mins):** For the remaining questions, where dimensional analysis fails, recognize the proper limits of the answer and mark the correct answers.

**Step 3 (Next 60 mins):** In some problems, solution may not be obtained from a simple formula and hence we need to calculate the formula. At that time try cause and result method to solve the problem and use estimation rule.

**Step 4 (Last 30 mins):** Try the difficult questions and revise the complete answer script.

# Detailed Syllabus – Class XII

## Unit I: Reproduction

- Sexual reproduction in flowering plants: Flower structure; Development of male and female gametophytes; Pollination-types, agencies and examples; Outbreeding devices; Pollen-Pistil interaction; Double fertilization; Post fertilization events- Development of endosperm and embryo, Development of seed and formation of fruit; Special modes-apomixis, parthenocarpy, polyembryony; Significance of seed and fruit formation.
- Human Reproduction: Male and female reproductive systems; Microscopic anatomy of testis and ovary; Gametogenesis-spermatogenesis & oogenesis; Menstrual cycle; Fertilisation, embryo development upto blastocyst formation, implantation; Pregnancy and placenta formation (Elementary idea); Parturition (Elementary idea); Lactation (Elementary idea).
- Reproductive health: Need for reproductive health and prevention of sexually transmitted diseases (STD); Birth control-Need and Methods, Contraception and Medical Termination of Pregnancy (MTP); Amniocentesis; Infertility and assisted reproductive technologies – IVF, ZIFT, GIFT (Elementary idea for general awareness).

## Unit II: Genetics and Evolution

- Heredity and variation: Mendelian Inheritance; Deviations from Mendelism-Incomplete dominance, Co-dominance, Multiple alleles and Inheritance of blood groups, Pleiotropy; Elementary idea of polygenic inheritance; Chromosome theory of inheritance; Chromosomes and genes; Sex determination-In humans, birds, honey bee; Linkage and crossing over; Sex linked inheritance-Haemophilia, Colour blindness; Mendelian disorders in humans-Thalassemia; Chromosomal disorders in humans; Down's syndrome, Turner's and Klinefelter's syndromes.
- Molecular basis of Inheritance: Search for genetic material and DNA as genetic material; Structure of DNA and RNA; DNA packaging; DNA replication; Central dogma; Transcription, genetic code, translation; Gene expression and regulation-Lac Operon; Genome and human genome project; DNA finger printing.
- Evolution: Origin of life; Biological evolution and evidences for biological evolution from Paleontology, comparative anatomy, embryology and molecular evidence); Darwin's contribution, Modern Synthetic theory of Evolution; Mechanism of evolution-Variation (Mutation and Recombination) and Natural Selection with examples, types of natural selection; Gene flow and genetic drift; Hardy-Weinberg's principle; Adaptive Radiation; Human evolution.

## Unit III: Biology and Human Welfare

- Health and Disease; Pathogens; parasites causing human diseases (Malaria, Filariasis, Ascariasis, Typhoid, Pneumonia, common cold, Dengue, Chikungunya, amoebiasis, ring worm); Basic concepts of immunology-vaccines; Cancer, HIV and AIDS; Adolescence, drug and alcohol abuse.
- Microbes in human welfare: In household food processing, industrial production, sewage treatment, energy generation and as biocontrol agents and biofertilizers.

## Unit IV: Biotechnology and Its Applications

- Principles and process of Biotechnology: Genetic engineering (Recombinant DNA technology).
- Application of Biotechnology in health and agriculture: Human insulin and vaccine production, gene therapy; Genetically modified organisms-Bt crops; Transgenic Animals; Biosafety issues-Biopiracy and patents.

## Unit V: Ecology and Environment

- Organisms and environment: Habitat and niche; Population and ecological adaptations; Population interactions-mutualism, competition, predation, parasitism; Population attributes-growth, birth rate and death rate, age distribution.
- Ecosystem: Patterns, components; productivity and decomposition; Energy flow; Pyramids of number, biomass, energy.
- Biodiversity and its conservation: Concept of Biodiversity; Patterns of Biodiversity; Importance of Biodiversity; Loss of Biodiversity; Biodiversity conservation; Hotspots, endangered organisms, extinction, Red Data Book, biosphere reserves, National parks and sanctuaries.

# Trend Analysis 2011–2025

| Ch. No | Chapter Name | Number of Question(s) in 2011 | 2012 | 2013 | 2014 | 2015 | 2016 | 2017 | 2018 | 2019 | 2020 | 2021 | 2022 | 2023 | 2024 | 2025 |
|---|---|---|---|---|---|---|---|---|---|---|---|---|---|---|---|---|
| 1 | The Living World | 1 | 0 | 1 | 0 | 0 | 1 | 1 | 1 | 2 | 0 | 1 | 1 | 0 | 0 | 0 |
| 2 | Biological Classification | 8 | 4 | 1 | 6 | 2 | 5 | 4 | 5 | 2 | 1 | 1 | 2 | 0 | 2 | 2 |
| 3 | Plant Kingdom | 1 | 3 | 4 | 4 | 4 | 2 | 3 | 2 | 4 | 4 | 4 | 3 | 3 | 1 | 5 |
| 4 | Animal Kingdom | 3 | 1 | 4 | 4 | 3 | 3 | 3 | 2 | 7 | 4 | 4 | 2 | 4 | 4 | 4 |
| 5 | Morphology of Flowering Plants | 4 | 4 | 2 | 5 | 5 | 5 | 4 | 2 | 5 | 3 | 2 | 3 | 3 | 4 | 3 |
| 6 | Anatomy of Flowering Plants | 4 | 5 | 3 | 2 | 4 | 1 | 2 | 4 | 2 | 2 | 4 | 3 | 3 | 3 | 1 |
| 7 | Structural Organizations in Animals | 3 | 2 | 1 | 2 | 2 | 2 | 2 | 2 | 2 | 3 | 4 | 4 | 4 | 4 | 4 |
| 8 | Cell: The Unit of Life | 4 | 5 | 3 | 4 | 4 | 5 | 4 | 4 | 2 | 2 | 3 | 2 | 2 | 4 | 6 |
| 9 | Biomolecules | 2 | 3 | 4 | 2 | 1 | 3 | 4 | 2 | 4 | 5 | 4 | 4 | 4 | 6 | 3 |
| 10 | Cell Cycle and Cell Division | 1 | 2 | 2 | 3 | 2 | 3 | 2 | 2 | 2 | 4 | 5 | 4 | 6 | 4 | 2 |
| 11 | Transport in Plants | 0 | 0 | 1 | 0 | 1 | 2 | 0 | 1 | 1 | 1 | 2 | 3 | 3 | 0 | 0 |
| 12 | Mineral Nutrition | 4 | 3 | 1 | 1 | 2 | 1 | 2 | 2 | 1 | 2 | 1 | 2 | 2 | 0 | 0 |
| 13 | Photosynthesis in Higher Plants | 2 | 2 | 1 | 1 | 2 | 3 | 2 | 2 | 2 | 2 | 2 | 3 | 3 | 3 | 2 |
| 14 | Respiration in Plants | 0 | 0 | 2 | 1 | 0 | 0 | 1 | 2 | 1 | 1 | 1 | 2 | 2 | 0 | 1 |
| 15 | Plant Growth and Development | 0 | 0 | 2 | 4 | 2 | 1 | 2 | 0 | 1 | 3 | 3 | 3 | 3 | 0 | 2 |
| 16 | Digestion and Absorption | 2 | 1 | 1 | 2 | 2 | 2 | 1 | 2 | 3 | 2 | 2 | 2 | 2 | 0 | 0 |
| 17 | Breathing and Exchange of Gases | 0 | 1 | 2 | 1 | 2 | 2 | 2 | 3 | 2 | 2 | 2 | 2 | 1 | 2 | 1 |
| 18 | Body Fluids and Circulation | 5 | 0 | 1 | 2 | 3 | 1 | 2 | 2 | 1 | 2 | 2 | 2 | 2 | 2 | 1 |
| 19 | Excretory Products and their Elimination | 5 | 1 | 1 | 1 | 2 | 1 | 3 | 2 | 2 | 1 | 0 | 1 | 1 | 2 | 1 |
| 20 | Locomotion and Movement | 0 | 1 | 3 | 1 | 2 | 1 | 3 | 2 | 2 | 1 | 3 | 2 | 2 | 1 | 0 |
| 21 | Neural Control and Coordination | 2 | 3 | 2 | 3 | 2 | 1 | 2 | 3 | 2 | 1 | 0 | 1 | 2 | 2 | 0 |
| 22 | Chemical Coordination and Regulation | 2 | 3 | 3 | 2 | 1 | 3 | 2 | 1 | 4 | 3 | 1 | 1 | 3 | 2 | 3 |
| 23 | Reproduction in Organisms | 1 | 1 | 3 | 0 | 0 | 1 | 2 | 2 | 1 | 0 | 1 | 1 | 0 | 0 | 0 |
| 24 | Sexual Reproduction in Flowering Plants | 5 | 3 | 6 | 3 | 4 | 5 | 3 | 5 | 5 | 2 | 3 | 3 | 3 | 3 | 5 |
| 25 | Human Reproduction | 3 | 4 | 3 | 3 | 3 | 2 | 2 | 4 | 3 | 3 | 3 | 3 | 4 | 5 | 4 |
| 26 | Reproductive Health | 2 | 2 | 3 | 3 | 1 | 2 | 3 | 1 | 2 | 2 | 3 | 2 | 3 | 2 | 1 |

| Ch. No | Chapter Name | Number of Question(s) in 2011 | 2012 | 2013 | 2014 | 2015 | 2016 | 2017 | 2018 | 2019 | 2020 | 2021 | 2022 | 2023 | 2024 | 2025 |
|---|---|---|---|---|---|---|---|---|---|---|---|---|---|---|---|---|
| 27 | Principles of Inheritance and Variations | 4 | 2 | 4 | 4 | 3 | 7 | 4 | 4 | 5 | 4 | 2 | 6 | 5 | 6 | 3 |
| 28 | Molecular Basis of Inheritance | 1 | 4 | 2 | 4 | 6 | 3 | 5 | 4 | 6 | 3 | 9 | 7 | 8 | 6 | 8 |
| 29 | Evolution | 1 | 4 | 4 | 2 | 1 | 3 | 2 | 3 | 2 | 4 | 2 | 2 | 1 | 4 | 1 |
| 30 | Human Health and Disease | 5 | 6 | 2 | 2 | 6 | 4 | 2 | 3 | 3 | 3 | 1 | 2 | 3 | 5 | 5 |
| 31 | Strategies for Enhancement in Food Production | 3 | 2 | 1 | 1 | 2 | 1 | 2 | 0 | 2 | 1 | 4 | 1 | 1 | 0 | 0 |
| 32 | Microbes in Human Welfare | 2 | 7 | 2 | 1 | 0 | 1 | 0 | 1 | 2 | 2 | 1 | 1 | 0 | 1 | 3 |
| 33 | Biotechnology: Principles and Processes | 2 | 5 | 2 | 3 | 0 | 3 | 1 | 1 | 3 | 4 | 5 | 5 | 4 | 7 | 6 |
| 34 | Biotechnology and its Applications | 3 | 1 | 1 | 2 | 3 | 2 | 4 | 4 | 3 | 4 | 6 | 3 | 1 | 2 | 4 |
| 35 | Organisms and Environment | 4 | 0 | 2 | 4 | 2 | 3 | 1 | 3 | 2 | 3 | 5 | 3 | 4 | 2 | 4 |
| 36 | Ecosystem | 2 | 6 | 3 | 1 | 6 | 2 | 3 | 1 | 2 | 2 | 3 | 3 | 2 | 1 | 3 |
| 37 | Biodiversity and its Conservation | 3 | 2 | 1 | 4 | 2 | 2 | 1 | 2 | 3 | 2 | 0 | 3 | 2 | 5 | 2 |
| 38 | Environmental Issues | 4 | 3 | 3 | 2 | 3 | 3 | 4 | 4 | 2 | 2 | 1 | 3 | 4 | 0 | 0 |
| | **Total Questions** | **100** | **100** | **90** | **90** | **90** | **90** | **90** | **90** | **90** | **90** | **100** | **100** | **100** | **100** | **90** |

# NEET (UG) 2025 SOLVED QUESTION PAPER — BIOLOGY

**1.** 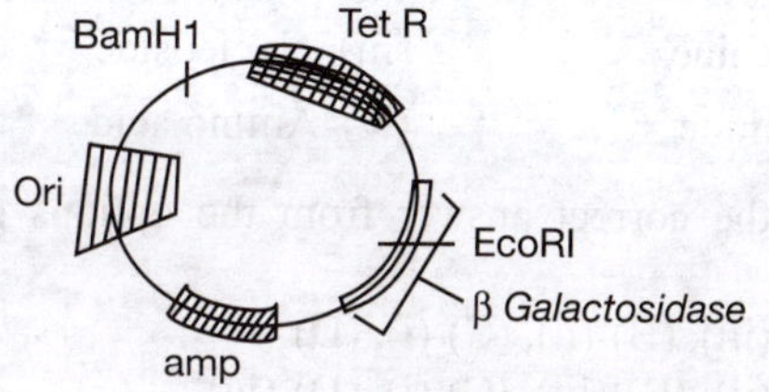


In the above represented plasmid, an alien piece of DNA is inserted at EcoRI site. Which of the following strategies will be chosen to select the recombinant colonies?
(a) White colour colonies will be selected plates can be selected.
(b) Blue color colonies grown on ampicillin plates can be selected.
(c) Using ampicillin & tetracycline containing medium plate.
(d) Blue colour colonies will be selected.

**2.** The Protein portion of enzyme is called:
(a) Apoenzyme (b) Prosthetic group
(c) Cofactor (d) Coenzyme

**3.** Given below are two statements:
**Statement I:** The primary source of energy in an ecosystem is solar energy.
**Statement II:** The rate of production of organic matter during photosynthesis in an ecosystem is called net primary productivity (NPP).
In the light of the above statements, choose the **most appropriate** answer from the options given below:
(a) Statement I is correct but Statement II is incorrect.
(b) Statement I is incorrect but Statement II is correct.
(c) Both Statement I and Statement II are correct.
(d) Both Statement I and Statement II are incorrect.

**4.** Given below are two statements: One is labelled as **Assertion (A)** and the other is labelled as **(Reason) (R)**.
**Assertion (A):** A Typical unfertilized, angiosperm embryo sac at maturity is 8 nucleate and 7 celled.
**Reason (R):** The egg apparatus has polar nuclei.
(a) A is true and R is false.
(b) A is false bur R is true.
(c) Both A and R are true and R is the correct explanation of A.
(d) Both A and R are true but R is NOT the correct explanation of A.

**5.** Neoplastic characteristics of cells refer to:
A. A mass of proliferating cells
B. Rapid growth of cells
C. Invasion and damage to the surrounding tissue
D. Those confined to the original location
Choose the correct answer from the options given below.
(a) A, B, D only (b) B, C, D only
(c) A, B only (d) A, B, C only

**6.** Which one of the following is the characteristic feature of gymnosperms?
(a) Seeds are absent.
(b) Gymnosperms have flowers for reproduction.
(c) Seeds are enclosed in fruits.
(d) Seeds are naked.

**7.** Match List-I with List-II

| List-I | List-II |
|---|---|
| (A) Progesterone | (i) Pars Intermedia |
| (B) Relaxin | (ii) Ovary |
| (C) Melanocyte Stimulating Hormone | (iii) Adrenal Medulla |
| (D) Catecholamines | (iv) Corpus Luteum |

(a) (A)-(ii), (B)-(iv), (C)-(i), (D)-(iii)
(b) (A)-(iii), (B)-(ii), (C)-(iv), (D)-(i)
(c) (A)-(iv), (B)-(ii), (C)-(i), (D)-(iii)
(d) (A)-(iv), (B)-(ii), (C)-(iii), (D)-(i)

**8.** Which chromosome in the human genome has the highest number of genes?
(a) Chromosome 1 (b) Chromosome 10
(c) Chromosome X (d) Chromosome Y

**9.** Which of the following statements about RuBisCO is true?
(a) It is an enzyme involved in the photolysis of water.
(b) It catalyzes the carboxylation of RuBP.
(c) It is active only in the dark.
(d) It has the higher affinity for oxygen than carbon dioxide.

**10.** The first menstruation is called:
(a) Diapause (b) Ovulation
(c) Menopause (d) Menarche

**11.** Which of the following genetically engineered organisms was used by Eli Lilly to prepare human insulin?
(a) Virus (b) Phage
(c) Bacterium (d) Yeast

**12.** Given below are two statements: one is labelled as **Assertion (A)** and the other is labelled as **Reason (R)**.
**Assertion (A):** All vertebrates are chordates but all chordates are not vertebrates.
**Reason (R):** The members of subphylum vertebrata possess notochord during the embryonic period, the notochord is replaced by a cartilaginous or bony vertebral column in adults.
In light of the above statements, choose the correct answer from the options given below:
(a) A is true but R is false.
(b) A is false but R is true.
(c) Both A and R are true and R is the correct explanation of A.
(d) Both A and R are true but R is not the correct explanation of A.

**13.** What is the main function of the spindle fibres during mitosis?
(a) To repair damaged DNA
(b) To regulate cell growth
(c) To separate the chromosomes
(d) To synthesize new DNA

**14.** Match List I with List II:

| List-I | List-II |
|---|---|
| (A) Alfred Hershey and Martha Chase | (i) Streptococcus pneumoniae |
| (B) Euchromatin | (ii) Densely packed and dark-stained |
| (C) Frederick Griffith | (iii) Loosely packed and light-stained |
| (D) Heterochromatin | (iv) DNA as genetic material confirmation from |

Choose the correct answer from the options given below:
(a) (A)-(iv), (B)-(iii), (C)-(i), (D)-(ii)
(b) (A)-(iii), (B)-(ii), (C)-(iv), (D)-(i)
(c) (A)-(ii), (B)-(iv), (C)-(i), (D)-(iii)
(d) (A)-(iv), (B)-(ii), (C)-(i), (D)-(iii)

**15.** Match List I with List II:

| List-I | List-II |
|---|---|
| (A) Adenosine | (i) Nitrogen base |
| (B) Adenylic acid | (ii) Nucleotide |
| (C) Adenine | (iii) Nucleoside |
| (D) Alanine | (iv) Amino acid |

Choose the correct answer from the options given below:
(a) (A)-(iii), (B)-(ii), (C)-(i), (D)-(iv)
(b) (A)-(ii), (B)-(iii), (C)-(i), (D)-(iv)
(c) (A)-(iii), (B)-(iv), (C)-(ii), (D)-(i)
(d) (A)-(iii), (B)-(ii), (C)-(iv), (D)-(i)

**16.** In frog, the Renal portal system is a special venous connection that acts to link:
(a) Kidney and intestine
(b) Kidney and lower part of body
(c) Liver and intestine
(d) Liver and kidney

**17.** Which of the following are the post-transcriptional events in an eukaryotic cell?
A. Transport of pre–mRNA to cytoplasm prior to splicing.
B. Removal of introns and joining of exons.
C. Addition of methyl group at 5' end of hnRNA.
D. Addition of adenine residues at 3' end of hnRNA.
E. Base pairing of two complementary RNAs.
Choose the correct answer from the options given below:
(a) B, C, E only (b) C, D, E only
(c) A, B, C only (d) B, C, D only

**18.** Polymerase chain reaction (PCR) amplifies DNA following the equation.
(a) $2n + 1$ (b) $2N^2$
(c) $N^2$ (d) $2^n$

**19.** Given below are two statements: one is labelled as **Assertion (A)** and the other is labelled as **Reason (R)**.
**Assertion (A):** Both wind and water pollinated flowers are not very colourful and do not produce nectar.
**Reason (R):** The flowers produce enormous amount of pollen grains in wind and water pollinated flowers.

In light of the above statements, choose the correct answer from the options given below:

(a) A is true but R is false
(b) A is false but R is true
(c) Both A and R are true and R is the correct explanation of A
(d) Both A and R are true but R is NOT the correct explanation of A

**20.** Epiphytes that are growing on a mango branch is an example of which of the following?
(a) Predation (b) Amensalism
(c) Commensalism (d) Mutualism

**21.** Find the correct statements:
A. In human pregnancy, the major organ systems are formed at the end of 12 weeks.
B. In human pregnancy, the major organ systems are formed at the end of 8 weeks.
C. In human pregnancy, heart is formed after one month of gestation.
D. In human pregnancy, limbs and digits develop by the end of the second month.
E. In human pregnancy, the appearance of hair is usually observed in the fifth month.

Choose the correct answer from the options given below:
(a) B, C, D and E only (b) A, C, D and E only
(c) A and D only (d) B and C only

**22.** Identify the part of a bio-reactor which is used as a foam breaker from the given figure.

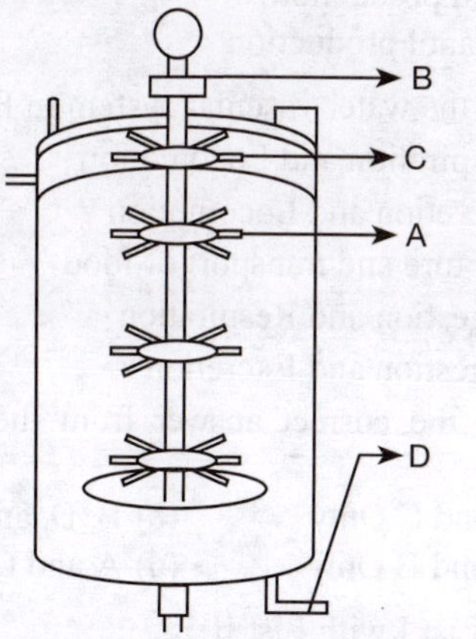


(a) D (b) C
(c) A (d) B

**23.** Frogs respire in water by skin and buccal cavity and on land by skin, buccal cavity and lungs.
Choose the correct answer from the following:
(a) The statement is false for water but true for land.
(b) The statement is false for both the environment.
(c) The statement is true for water but false for land.
(d) The statement is true for both the environment.

**24.** Consider the following statements regarding function of adrenal medullary hormones:
A. It causes pupillary constriction.
B. It is a hyperglycemia hormone.
C. It causes piloerection.
D. It increases strength of heart constriction.

Choose the correct answer from the options given below:
(a) A, C and D only (b) D only
(c) C and D only (d) B, C and D only

**25.** Read the following statements on plant growth and development.
A. Parthenocarpy can be induced by auxins.
B. Plant growth regulators can be involved in promotion as well as inhabitation of growth.
C. Dedifferentiation is a pre-requisite for re-differentiation.
D. Abscisic acid is a plant growth promoter.
E. Apical dominance promotes the growth of lateral buds.

Choose the options with all correct statements.
(a) A, D, E only (b) B, D, E only
(c) A, B, C only (d) A, C, E only

**26.** Which of the following hormones released from the pituitary is actually synthesized in the hypothalamus?
(a) Follicle-stimulating hormone (FSH)
(b) Adrenocorticotropic hormone (ACTH)
(c) Luteinizing hormone (LH)
(d) Anti-diuretic hormone (ADH)

**27.** Which of the following is an example of non-distilled alcoholic beverage produced by yeast?
(a) Beer (b) Rum
(c) Whisky (d) Brandy

**28.** What is the pattern of inheritance for polygenic trait?
(a) Autosomal dominant pattern
(b) X-linked recessive inheritance pattern
(c) Mendelian inheritance pattern
(d) Non-Mendelian inheritance pattern

**29.** Match List I with List II:

| List-I | List-II |
|---|---|
| (A) Head | (i) Enzymes |
| (B) Middle piece | (ii) Sperm motility |
| (C) Acrosome | (iii) Energy |
| (D) Tail | (iv) Genetic material |

Choose the correct answer from the options given below:
(a) (A)-(iii), (B)-(iv), (C)-(ii), (D)-(i)
(b) (A)-(iii), (B)-(ii), (C)-(i), (D)-(iv)
(c) (A)-(iv), (B)-(iii), (C)-(i), (D)-(ii)
(d) (A)-(iv), (B)-(iii), (C)-(ii), (D)-(i)

**30.** Which of the following is an example of a zygomorphic flower?
(a) Pea (b) Chilli
(c) Petunia (d) Datura

**31.** Which of the following organisms *cannot* fix nitrogen?
A. *Azotobacter* B. *Oscillatoria*
C. *Anabaena* D. *Volvox*
E. *Nostoc*
Choose the correct answer from the options given below:
(a) B only (b) E only
(c) A only (d) D only

**32.** Which one of the following is an example of ex-situ conservation?
(a) Zoos and botanical gardens
(b) Protected areas
(c) National Park
(d) Wildlife Sanctuary

**33.** Who is known as the father of Ecology in India?
(a) Ram Udar (b) Birbal Sahni
(c) S.R. Kashyap (d) Ramdeo Misra

**34.** Given below are two statements:
**Statement I:** In the RNA world, RNA is considered the first genetic material evolved to carry out essential life processes. RNA acts as a genetic material and also as a catalyst for some important biochemical reactions in living systems. Being reactive, RNA is unstable.
**Statement II:** DNA evolved from RNA and is a more stable genetic material. Its double helical strands being complementary, resist changes by evolving repairing mechanism.
In light of the above statements, choose the most appropriate answer from the options given below:
(a) Statement I is correct but Statement II is incorrect.
(b) Statement I is incorrect but Statement II is correct.
(c) Both Statement I and Statement II are correct.
(d) Both Statement I and Statement II are incorrect.

**35.** Given below are two statements:
**Statement I:** Transfer RNAs and ribosomal RNA do not interact with mRNA.
**Statement II:** RNA interference (RNAi) takes place in all eukaryotic organisms as a method of cellular defence.
In light of the above statements, choose the most appropriate answer from the options given below:
(a) Statement I is correct but Statement II is incorrect.
(b) Statement I is incorrect but Statement II is correct.
(c) Both Statement I and Statement II are correct.
(d) Both Statement I and Statement II are incorrect.

**36.** Match List I with List II:

| List-I | List-II |
|---|---|
| (A) Heart | (i) Erythropoietin |
| (B) Kidney | (ii) Aldosterone |
| (C) Gastrointestinal tract | (iii) Atrial natriuretic factor |
| (D) Adrenal cortex | (iv) Secretin |

Choose the correct answer from the options given below:
(a) (A)-(i), (B)-(iii), (C)-(iv), (D)-(ii)
(b) (A)-(iii), (B)-(i), (C)-(iv), (D)-(ii)
(c) (A)-(ii), (B)-(i), (C)-(iii), (D)-(iv)
(d) (A)-(iv), (B)-(iii), (C)-(ii), (D)-(i)

**37.** All living members of the class Cyclostomata are:
(a) Symbiotic (b) Ectoparasite
(c) Free living (d) Endoparasite

**38.** Streptokinase produced by bacterium *Streptococcus* is used for:
(a) Liver disease treatment
(b) Removing clots from blood vessels
(c) Curd production
(d) Ethanol production

**39.** Role of the water vascular system in Echinoderms is:
A. Respiration and Locomotion
B. Excretion and Locomotion
C. Capture and transport of food
D. Digestion and Respiration
E. Digestion and Excretion
Choose the correct answer from the options given below:
(a) B and C Only (b) B, D, and E Only
(c) A and B Only (d) A and C Only

**40.** Match List I with List II:

| List-I | List-II |
|---|---|
| (A) Pteridophyte | (i) Salvia |
| (B) Bryophyte | (ii) Ginkgo |
| (C) Angiosperm | (iii) Polytrichum |
| (D) Gymnosperm | (iv) Salvinia |

Choose the correct answer from the options given below:

(a) (A)-(iii), (B)-(iv), (C)-(i), (D)-(ii)
(b) (A)-(iv), (B)-(iii), (C)-(ii), (D)-(i)
(c) (A)-(iii), (B)-(iv), (C)-(ii), (D)-(i)
(d) (A)-(iv), (B)-(iii), (C)-(i), (D)-(ii)

**41.** Which are correct:

A. Compound tomography and magnetic resonance imaging detect cancers of internal organs.
B. Chemotherapeutic drugs are used to kill non-cancerous cells.
C. $\alpha$-interferon activates the cancer patients' immune system and helps in destroying the tumour.
D. Chemotherapeutic drugs are biological response modifiers.
E. In the case of leukaemia blood cell counts are decreased.

Choose the correct answer from the options given below:

(a) C and D only (b) A and C only
(c) B and D only (d) D and E only

**42.** What are the potential drawbacks in the adoption of the IVF method?

A. High fatality risk to mother
B. Expensive instruments and reagents
C. Husband/wife necessary for being donors
D. Less adoption of orphans
E. Not available in India
F. Possibility that the early embryo does not survive

Choose the correct answer from the options given below:

(a) A, B, C, D only (b) A, B, C, E, F only
(c) B, D, F only (d) A, C, D, F only

**43.** Consider the following:

A. The reductive division for the human female gametogenesis starts earlier than that of the male gametogenesis.
B. The gap between the first meiotic division and the second meiotic division is much shorter for males compared to females.
C. The first polar body is associated with the formation of the primary oocyte.
D. Luteinizing Hormone (LH) surge leads to disintegration of the endometrium and onset of menstrual bleeding.

Choose the correct answer from the options given below:

(a) B and D are true (b) B and C are true
(c) A and B are true (d) A and C are true

**44.** In bryophytes, the gemmae help in which one of the following?

(a) Nutrient absorption
(b) Gaseous exchange
(c) Sexual reproduction
(d) Asexual reproduction.

**45.** Given below are two statements: one is labelled as **Assertion (A)** and the other is labelled as **Reason (R)**.

**Assertion (A):** The primary function of the Golgi apparatus is to package the materials made by the endoplasmic reticulum and deliver it to intracellular targets and outside the cell.

**Reason (R):** Vesicle containing materials made by the endoplasmic reticulum fuse with the cis face of the Golgi apparatus, and they are modified and released from the trans face of the Golgi apparatus.

In light of the above statements, choose the correct answer from the options given below:

(a) A is true but R is false
(b) A is false but R is true
(c) Both A and R are true and R is the correct explanation of A
(d) Both A and R are true but R is not the correct explanation of A

**46.** Which one of the following statements refers to Reductionist Biology?

(a) Chemical approach to study and understand living organisms.
(b) Behavioural approach to study and understand living organisms.
(c) Physico-chemical approach to study and understand living organisms.
(d) Physiological approach to study and understand living organisms.

**47.** After maturation, in primary lymphoid organs, the lymphocytes migrate for interaction with antigens to secondary lymphoid organ(s)/tissue(s) like:

A. thymus
B. bone marrow
C. spleen
D. lymph nodes
E. Peyer's patches

Choose the correct answer from the options given below:

(a) E, A, B, only
(b) C, D, E only
(c) B, C, D only
(d) A, B, C only

**48.** Match List I with List II:

| List-I | List-II |
|---|---|
| (A) The Evil Quarter | (i) Cryopreservation |
| (B) Ex situ conservation | (ii) Alien species invasion |
| (C) *Lantana camara* | (iii) Causes of biodiversity losses |
| (D) Dodo | (iv) Extinction |

Choose the option with all correct matches.

(a) (A)-(iii), (B)-(iv), (C)-(ii), (D)-(i)
(b) (A)-(iii), (B)-(ii), (C)-(iv), (D)-(i)
(c) (A)-(iii), (B)-(ii), (C)-(i), (D)-(iv)
(d) (A)-(iii), (B)-(i), (C)-(ii), (D)-(iv)

**49.** How many meiotic and mitotic divisions need to occur for the development of a mature female gametophyte from the megaspore mother cell in an angiosperm plant?

(a) 1 Meiosis and 3 Mitosis
(b) No Meiosis and 2 Mitosis
(c) 2 Meiosis and 3 Mitosis
(d) 1 Meiosis and 2 Mitosis.

**50.** Which of the following types of immunity is present at the time of birth and is a non-specific type of defense in the human body?

(a) Cell-mediated Immunity
(b) Humoral Immunity
(c) Acquired Immunity
(d) Innate Immunity

**51.** Given below are two statements:

**Statement I:** Fig fruit is a non-vegetarian fruit as it has enclosed fig wasps in it.

**Statement II:** Fig wasp and fig tree exhibit mutual relationship as fig wasp completes its life cycle in fig fruit and fig fruit gets pollinated by fig wasp.

In light of the above statements, choose the most appropriate answer from the options given below:

(a) Statement I is correct but Statement II is incorrect.
(b) Statement I is incorrect but Statement II is correct.
(c) Both Statement I and Statement II are correct.
(d) Both Statement I and Statement II are incorrect.

**52.** Given below are two statements: One is labelled as Assertion (A) and the other is labelled as Reason (R)

**Assertion (A):** Cells of the tapetum possess dense cytoplasm and generally have more than one nucleus.

**Reason (R):** Presence of more than one nucleus in the tapetum increases the efficiency of nourishing the developing microspore mother cells.

In light of the above statements, choose the most appropriate answer from the options given below:

(a) A is true and R is false
(b) A is false bur R is true
(c) Both A and R is true and R is the correct explanation of A
(d) Both A and R is true but R is not the correct explanation of A

**53.** From the statements given below, choose the correct option:

A. The eukaryotic ribosomes are 80S and prokaryotic ribosomes are 70S.
B. Each ribosomes has two sub-units.
C. The two sub- units of 80S ribosome are 60S and 40S while that of 70S are 50S and 30S.
D. The two sub-units of 80S ribosome are 60S. and 20S and that of 70S are 50S and 20S.
E. The two sub-units of 80S are 60S and 30S and that of 70S are 50S and 30S.

(a) A, B, E are true
(b) B, D, E are true
(c) A, B, C are true
(d) A, B, D are true

**54.** Which one of the following enzymes contains 'Haem' as the prosthetic group?

(a) Succinate dehydrogenase
(b) Catalase
(c) RuBisCO
(d) Carbonic anhydrase

**55.** What is the name of the blood vessel that carries deoxygenated blood from the body to the heart in a frog?

(a) Pulmonary vein
(b) Vena cave
(c) Aorta
(d) Pulmonary artery

**56.** Given below are the stages in the life cycle of pteridophytes. Arrange the following states in the correct sequence.

A. Prothallus stage
B. Meiosis in spore mother cells
C. Fertilization
D. Formation of archegonia and antheridia in gametophyte.
E. Transfer of antherozoids to the archegonia in the presence of water.

Choose the correct answer from the options given below:

(a) D-E-C-A-B
(b) E-D-C-B-A
(c) B-A-D-E-C
(d) B-A-E-C-D

**57.** The blue and white selectable markers have been developed which differentiate recombinant colonies from non-recombinant colonies on the basis of their ability to produce colour in the presence of a chromomeric substrate.

Given below are two statements about this method:

**Statement I:** The blue coloured colonies have DNA insert in the plasmid and they are identified as recombinant colonies.

**Statement II:** The colonies without blue colour have DNA insert in the plasmid and are identified as recombinant colonies.

In light of the above statements, choose the most appropriate answer from the options given below:

(a) Statement I is correct but Statement II is incorrect.
(b) Statement I is incorrect but Statement II is correct.
(c) Both Statement I and Statement II are correct.
(d) Both Statement I and Statement II are incorrect.

**58.** Which of the following microbes is NOT involved in the preparation of household products?

A. *Aspergillus niger*
B. *Lactobacillus*
C. *Trichoderma polysporum*
D. *Saccharomyces cerevisiae*
E. *Propionibacterium sharmanii*

Choose the correct answer from the options given below:

(a) C and D only (b) C and E only
(c) A and B only (d) A and C only

**59.** Silencing of specific mRNA is possible via RNAi because of

(a) Complementary tRNA
(b) Non-complementary ssRNA
(c) Complementary dsRNA
(d) Inhibitory ssRNA

**60.** The complex II of mitochondrial electron transport chain is also known as

(a) Cytochrome c oxidase
(b) NADH dehydrogenase
(c) Cytochrome $bc_1$
(d) Succinate dehydrogenase

**61.** While trying to find out the characteristic of a newly found animal, a researcher did the histology of an adult animal and observed a cavity with presence of mesodermal tissue towards the body wall but no mesodermal tissue was observed towards the alimentary canal. What could be the possible coelom of that animal?

(a) Schizocoelomate (b) Spongocoelomate
(c) Acoelomate (d) Pseudocoelomate

**62.** Given below are two statements:

**Statement I:** In a floral formula, ⊕ stands for zygomorphic nature of the flower, and $\underline{G}$ stands for inferior ovary.

**Statement II:** In a floral formula, ⊕ stands for actinomorphic nature of the flower and $\underline{G}$ stands for superior ovary.

In light of the above statements, choose the most appropriate answer from the options given below:

(a) Statement I is correct but Statement II is incorrect.
(b) Statement I is incorrect but Statement II is correct.
(c) Both Statement I and Statement II are correct.
(d) Both Statement I and Statement II are incorrect.

**63.** Given below are two statements:

**Statement I:** In ecosystem, these is unidirectional flow of energy of sum from producers to consumers.

**Statement II:** Ecosystems are exempted from 2nd law of thermodynamics.

In light of the above statements, choose the most appropriate answer from the options given below:

(a) Statement I is correct but Statement II is incorrect.
(b) Statement I is incorrect but Statement II is correct.
(c) Both Statement I and Statement II are correct.
(d) Both Statement I and Statement II are incorrect.

**64.** Which of the following is the unit of productivity of an ecosystem?

(a) KCal $m^{-3}$ (b) (KCal $m^{-2}$) $yr^{-1}$
(c) $gm^{-2}$ (d) KCal $m^{-2}$

**65.** With the help of given pedigree, find out the probability for the birth of a child having no disease and being a carrier (has the disease mutation in one allele of the gene) in $F_3$ generation.

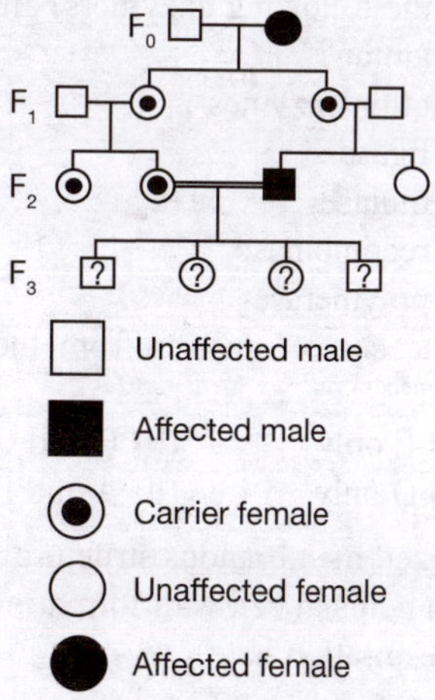


(a) $\frac{1}{8}$ (b) Zero
(c) $\frac{1}{4}$ (d) $\frac{1}{2}$

**66.** In the seeds of cereals, the outer covering of endosperm separates the embryo by a protein rich layer called:

(a) Integument (b) Aleurone layer
(c) Coleoptile (d) Coleorhiza

**67.** Match List I with List II:-

| List-I | List-II |
|---|---|
| (A) Chlorophyll a | (i) Yellow-green |
| (B) Chlorophyll b | (ii) Yellow |
| (C) Xanthophylls | (iii) Blue-green |
| (D) Carotenoids | (iv) Yellow to Yellow-orange |

Choose the correct answer from the options given below:

(a) (A)-(i), (B)-(ii), (C)-(iv), (D)-(iii)
(b) (A)-(i), (B)-(iv), (C)-(iii), (D)-(ii)
(c) (A)-(iii), (B)-(iv), (C)-(ii), (D)-(i)
(d) (A)-(iii), (B)-(i), (C)-(ii), (D)-(iv)

**68.** Who proposed that the genetic code for amino acids should be made up of three nucleotides?

(a) Jacque Monod
(b) Franklin Stahl
(c) George Gamow
(d) Francis Crick

**69.** Histones are enriched with

(a) Phenylalanine & Leucine
(b) Phenylalanine & Arginine
(c) Lysine & Arginine
(d) Leucine & Lysine

**70.** Which of the following enzyme(s) are NOT essential for gene cloning?

A. Restriction enzymes
B. DNA ligase
C. DNA mutase
D. DNA recombinase
E. DNA polymerase

Choose the correct answer from the options given below:

(a) D and E only (b) B and C only
(c) C and D only (d) A and B only.

**71.** A specialized membranous structure in a prokaryotic cell which helps in cell wall formation, DNA replication and respiration is:

(a) Cristae
(b) Endoplasmic Reticulum
(c) Mesosome
(d) Chromatophores.

**72.** Which factor is important for the termination of transcription?

(a) ρ (rho) (b) γ (gamma)
(c) α (alpha) (d) σ (sigma)

**73.** Which of the following statements is correct about the location of the male frog copulatory pad?

(a) Second digit of fore limb
(b) First digit of the fore limb
(c) First and Second digit of fore limb
(d) First digit of hind limb

**74.** Which of the following diagrams is correct with regard to the proximal (P) and distal (D) tubule of the Nephron?

(a)
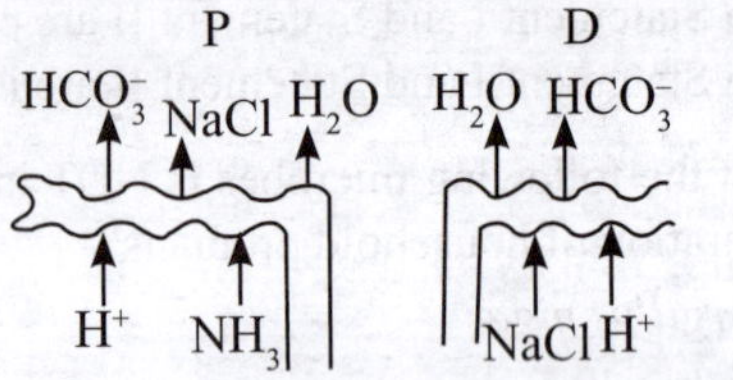


(b)
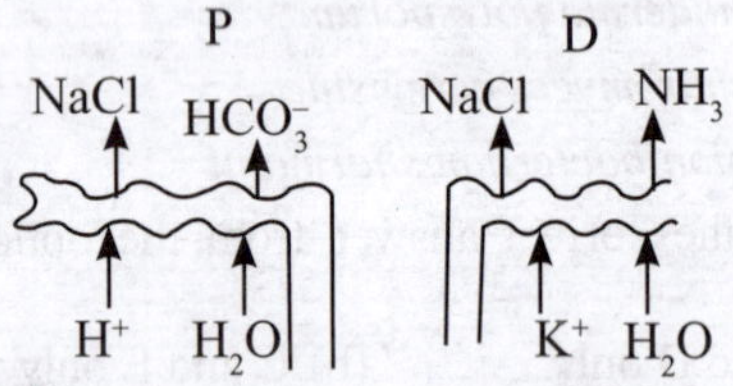


(c)
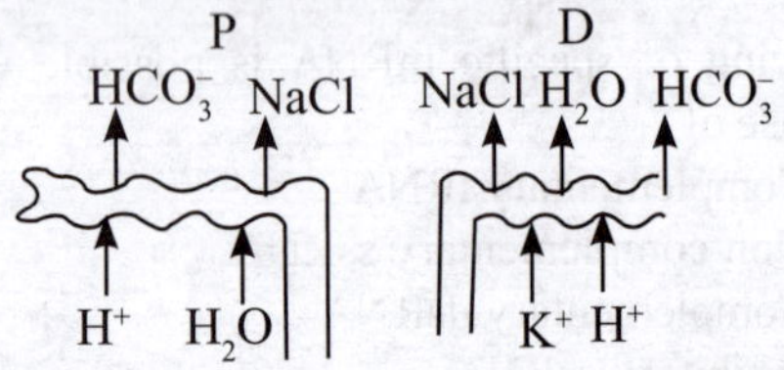


(d)
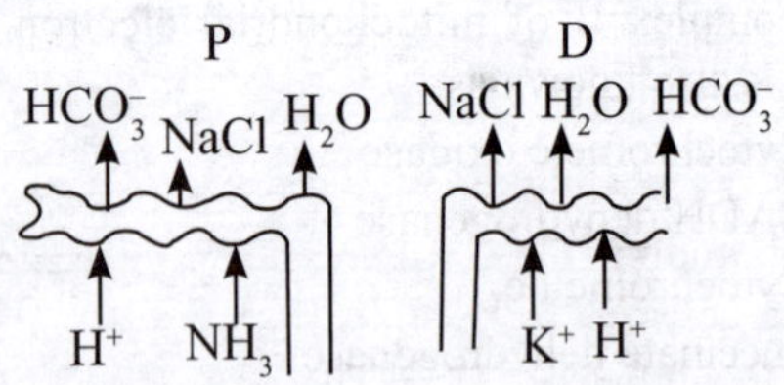


**75.** Identify the statement that is NOT correct.

(a) Antigen binding site is located at C-terminal region of antibody molecules.
(b) Constant region of heavy and light chains is located at C-terminus of antibody molecules.
(c) Each antibody has two light and two heavy chains.
(d) The heavy and light chains are held together by disulfide bonds.

**76.** Match List I with List II:

| List-I | List-II |
|---|---|
| (A) Scutellum | (i) Persistent nucellus |
| (B) Non-albuminous seed | (ii) Cotyledon of monocot seed |
| (C) Epiblast | (iii) Groundnut |
| (D) Perisperm | (iv) Rudimentary cotyledon |

Choose the correct answer from the options given below:

(a) (A)-(iv), (B)-(iii), (C)-(i), (D)-(ii)
(b) (A)-(ii), (B)-(iv), (C)-(iii), (D)-(i)
(c) (A)-(ii), (B)-(iii), (C)-(iv), (D)-(i)
(d) (A)-(iv), (B)-(iii), (C)-(ii), (D)-(iv)

**77.** Find the statement that is NOT correct with regard to the structure of the monocot stem.

(a) Vascular bundles are conjoint and closed.
(b) Phloem parenchyma is absent.
(c) Hypodermis is parenchymatous.
(d) Vascular bundles are scattered.

**78.** Twins are born to a family that lives next door to you. The twins are a boy and a girl. Which of the following must be true?

(a) They were conceived through in vitro fertilization.
(b) They have 75% identical genetic content.
(c) They are monozygotic twins.
(d) They are fraternal twins.

**79.** Sweet potato and potato represent a certain type of evolution. Select the correct combination of terms to explain the evolution.

(a) Homology, convergent
(b) Analogy, divergent
(c) Analogy, convergent
(d) Homology, divergent

**80.** Which one of the following phytohormones promotes nutrient mobilization which helps in the delay of leaf senescence in plants?

(a) Gibberellin (b) Cytokinin
(c) Ethylene (d) Abscisic acid.

**81.** Why can't insulin be given orally to diabetic patients?

(a) Because of structural variation
(b) Its bioavailability will be increased
(c) Human body will elicit strong immune response
(d) It will be digested in Gastro-Intestinal (GI) tract

**82.** Name the class of enzyme that usually catalyze the following reaction:

$$S - G + S^{\neq} \rightarrow S + S^{\neq} - G$$

Where, G $\rightarrow$ a group other than hydrogen
S $\rightarrow$ a substance
$S^{\neq} \rightarrow$ another substance

(a) Transferase (b) Ligase
(c) Hydrolase (d) Lyase

**83.** Given below are two statements:

**Statement I:** The DNA fragments extracted from gel electrophoresis can be used in construction of recombinant DNA.

**Statement II:** Smaller size DNA fragments are observed near anode while larger fragments are found near the wells in an agarose gel.

In light of the above statements, choose the most appropriate answer from the options given below:

(a) Statement I is correct but Statement II is incorrect.
(b) Statement I is incorrect but Statement II is correct.
(c) Both Statement I and Statement II are correct.
(d) Both Statement I and Statement II are incorrect.

**84.** The correct sequence of events in the life cycle of bryophytes is:

A. Fusion of antherozoid with egg.
B. Attachment of gametophyte to substratum.
C. Reduction division to produce haploid spores.
D. Formation of sporophyte.
E. Release of antherozoids into water.

Choose the correct answer from the options given below:

(a) B-E-A-D-C (b) D-E-A-B-C
(c) D-E-A-C-B (d) B-E-A-C-D

**85.** Genes R and Y follow independent assortment. If RRYY produce round yellow seeds and rryy produce wrinkled green seeds, what will be the phenotypic ratio of the $F_2$ generation?

(a) Phenotypic ratio – 9:3:3:1
(b) Phenotypic ratio – 9:7
(c) Phenotypic ratio – 1:2:1
(d) Phenotypic ratio – 3:1

**86.** Each of the following characteristics represents a Kingdom proposed by Whittaker. Arrange the following in increasing order of complexity of body organization.

A. Multicellular heterotrophs with cell wall made of chitin.
B. Heterotrophs with tissue/organ/organ system level of body organization.
C. Prokaryotes with cell wall made of polysaccharides and amino acids.

D. Eukaryotic autotrophs with tissue/organ level of body organization.
E. Eukaryotes with cellular body organization.
(a) A-C-E-D-B (b) C-E-A-B-E
(c) A-C-E-B-D (d) C-E-A-D-B

**87.** Match List – I with List – II.

| List-I | List-II |
|---|---|
| (A) Centromere | (i) Mitochondrion |
| (B) Cilium | (ii) Cell division |
| (C) Cristae | (iii) Cell movement |
| (D) Cell membrane | (iv) Phospholipid Bilayer |

Choose the correct answer from the options given below:
(a) (A)-(iv), (B)-(ii), (C)-(iii), (D)-(i)
(b) (A)-(ii), (B)-(iii), (C)-(i), (D)-(iv)
(c) (A)-(i), (B)-(ii), (C)-(iii), (D)-(iv)
(d) (A)-(ii), (B)-(i), (C)-(iv), (D)-(iii)

**88.** Which one of the following equations represents Verhulst-Pearl Logistic Growth of population?

(a) $\frac{dN}{dt} = rN\left(\frac{N-K}{N}\right)$ (b) $\frac{dN}{dt} = N\left(\frac{r-K}{K}\right)$

(c) $\frac{dN}{dt} = r\left(\frac{K-N}{K}\right)$ (d) $\frac{dN}{dt} = rN\left(\frac{K-N}{K}\right)$

**89.** Match List – I with List – II.

| List-I | List-II |
|---|---|
| (A) Emphysema | (i) Rapid spasms in muscle due to low $Ca^{++}$ in body fluid |
| (B) Angina Pectoris | (ii) Damaged alveolar walls and decreased respiratory surface |
| (C) Glomerulo-nephritis | (iii) Acute chest pain when not enough oxygen is reaching to heart muscle |
| (D) Tetany | (iv) Inflammation of glomeruli of kidney |

Choose the correct answer from the options given below:
(a) (A)-(ii), (B)-(iv), (C)-(iii), (D)-(i)
(b) (A)-(ii), (B)-(iii), (C)-(iv), (D)-(i)
(c) (A)-(iii), (B)-(i), (C)-(iv), (D)-(ii)
(d) (A)-(iii), (B)-(i), (C)-(ii), (D)-(iv)

**90.** Cardiac activities of the heart are regulated by
A. Nodal tissue
B. A special neural centre in the medulla oblongata
C. Adrenal medullary hormones
D. Adrenal cortical hormones
Choose the correct answer from the options given below:
(a) A, C and D Only (b) A, B and D Only
(c) A, B and C Only (d) A, B, C and D

## Answer Keys

| | | | | | | | | | |
|---|---|---|---|---|---|---|---|---|---|
| **1.** (a) | **2.** (a) | **3.** (a) | **4.** (a) | **5.** (d) | **6.** (d) | **7.** (c) | **8.** (a) | **9.** (b) | **10.** (d) |
| **11.** (c) | **12.** (c) | **13.** (c) | **14.** (a) | **15.** (a) | **16.** (b) | **17.** (d) | **18.** (d) | **19.** (d) | **20.** (c) |
| **21.** (b) | **22.** (b) | **23.** (a) | **24.** (d) | **25.** (c) | **26.** (d) | **27.** (a) | **28.** (d) | **29.** (c) | **30.** (a) |
| **31.** (d) | **32.** (a) | **33.** (d) | **34.** (c) | **35.** (b) | **36.** (b) | **37.** (b) | **38.** (b) | **39.** (d) | **40.** (d) |
| **41.** (b) | **42.** (c) | **43.** (c) | **44.** (d) | **45.** (c) | **46.** (c) | **47.** (b) | **48.** (d) | **49.** (a) | **50.** (d) |
| **51.** (d) | **52.** (c) | **53.** (c) | **54.** (b) | **55.** (b) | **56.** (c) | **57.** (b) | **58.** (d) | **59.** (c) | **60.** (d) |
| **61.** (d) | **62.** (b) | **63.** (a) | **64.** (b) | **65.** (c) | **66.** (b) | **67.** (d) | **68.** (c) | **69.** (c) | **70.** (c) |
| **71.** (c) | **72.** (a) | **73.** (b) | **74.** (d) | **75.** (a) | **76.** (c) | **77.** (c) | **78.** (d) | **79.** (c) | **80.** (b) |
| **81.** (d) | **82.** (a) | **83.** (c) | **84.** (a) | **85.** (a) | **86.** (d) | **87.** (b) | **88.** (d) | **89.** (b) | **90.** (c) |

## Hints and Explanations

1. **(a)**
   - The lac Z gene encodes β-galactosidase, the presence of a chromogenic substrate gives blue colour colonies if the plasmid does not have an insert.
   - Insertion of a foreign gene at the EcoRI site within lac Z disrupts its function.
   - Recombinant colonies cannot metabolize X-gal → appear white.
   - Non-recombinant colonies still have a functional lac Z → appear blue.

   So, to identify recombinant colonies, we select white-colored

2. **(a)** Enzymes are composed of one or several polypeptide chains. However, there are a number of cases in which non-protein constituents called cofactors are bound to the enzyme to make the enzyme catalytically active. In these instances, the protein portion of the enzymes is called the apoenzyme. Three kinds of cofactors may be identified: prosthetic groups, co-enzymes and metal ions.

3. **(a)**
   Statement I is correct: Sun is the primary source of energy in ecosystems.
   Gross primary productivity (GPP): total energy fixed by plants.
   Statement II is incorrect.
   Net primary productivity (NPP) = GPP – energy lost in respiration.
   Therefore, NPP is indeed the rate of production of organic matter after respiration.

4. **(a)** The female gametophyte (embryo sac) indeed has 8 nuclei and 7 cells:
   1 egg cell
   2 synergids
   3 antipodals
   1 central cell with 2 polar nuclei
   The egg apparatus = 1 egg cell + 2 synergids (Nn polar nuclei here)
   The polar nuclei are in the central cell, not egg apparatus.
   Thus:
   A is true.
   R is false.

5. **(d)**
   A. A mass of proliferating cell — Correct (neoplasm = abnormal growth)
   B. Rapid growth of cells — Correct (feature of tumours)
   C. Invasion and damage to the surrounding tissue — Correct (malignant neoplasms invade)
   D. Those confined to original location — Incorrect (benign tumours, but neoplasia refers to abnormal uncontrolled growth, not just benign)

6. **(d)** Gymnosperms are plant whose seeds are not enclosed within an ovary (fruit). The seeds are exposed (naked) on cones or similar structures.

7. **(c)**

| | |
|---|---|
| (A) Progesterone | (iv) Corpus Luteum |
| (B) Relaxin | (ii) Ovary |
| (C) Melanocyte Stimulating hormone | (ii) Adrenal Medulla |
| (D) Catecholamines | (iii) Corpus Luteum |

8. **(a)** The chromosome in the human genome with the highest number of genes is chromosome 1. It contains over 2968 genes. And Y has the fewest genes which is 231. Therefore, the answer to the question is: **Chromosome 1**

9. **(b)** RuBisCO(ribulose-1,5-bisphosphate carboxylase/ oxygenase) is an enzyme involved in the first major step of carbon fixation, a process by which atmospheric carbon dioxide is converted by plants and other photosynthetic organisms to energy-rich molecules such as glucose.
   - Water splitting complex associated with PS II involved in the photolysis of water.
   - It is generally active during dark & light period.
   - Its affinity changes with the concentration of oxygen and carbon dioxide.

10. **(d)**
    - Menarche = Onset of first menstruation
    - Menopause = Permanent cessation of menstruation. Occur at the age of approx. 50 years.
    - Ovulation = The process in which egg is released from an ovary.
    - Diapause = A period of suspended development in many zooplanktons.

11. **(c)** Eli Lilly, an American pharmaceutical company, produced recombinant human insulin using **genetically engineered bacteria (E. coli).** The genes encoding the A and B chains of insulin were inserted into

bacterial plasmids, enabling the bacteria to produce human insulin.

**12.** **(c)** Reason (R) correctly explains Assertion (A) because the presence of a notochord (at least during embryonic development) and its subsequent replacement by a vertebral column is what defines vertebrates as a subgroup within chordates.

**13.** **(c)** During mitosis, spindle fibres attach to the centromeres of chromosomes and pull the sister chromatids apart towards opposite poles. This ensures equal distribution of chromosomes to the daughter cells. So, it is used to separate the chromosomes.

**14.** **(a)**

- Hershey & Chase: Unequivocally proved DNA is genetic material (using bacteriophages).
- Euchromatin: Lightly packed, transcriptionally active.
- Frederick Griffith: Discovered bacterial transformation (in Streptococcus pneumoniae).
- Heterochromatin: Densely packed, transcriptionally inactive.

**15.** **(a)**

| | |
|---|---|
| (A) Adenosine | (iii) Nucleoside |
| (B) Adenylic acid | (ii) Nucleotide |
| (C) Adenine | (i) Nitrogen base |
| (D) Alanine | (iv) Amino acid |

**16.** **(b)** In frogs, the renal portal system is a special venous connection that acts to link the kidney and the lower part of the body. Therefore, the correct answer is kidney and lower part of body.

**17.** **(d)**

A. Transport of pre-mRNA to cytoplasm prior to splicing — Incorrect (Splicing happens before transport)

B. Removal of introns and joining of exons — Correct (Splicing)

C. Addition of methyl group at 5' end of hnRNA — Correct (5' Capping)

D. Addition of adenine residues at 3' end of hnRNA — Correct (Polyadenylation)

E. Base pairing of two complementary RNAs — Incorrect (Not part of post-transcriptional modifications but of RNAi mechanism)

**18.** **(d)** PCR is a method used to amplify DNA exponentially. After each cycle, the amount of DNA doubles. So, after n cycles, the amount of DNA is $2^n$ times the original. This exponential amplification is the principle behind PCR.

**19.** **(d)** Both statements are true individually.
But R does not directly explain A; A is due to lack of need to attract pollinators, not because of pollen production.

**20.** **(c)** In commensalism, one organism benefits while the other is neither harmed nor benefited.
Epiphytes (plants like orchids) grow on mango trees for physical support without affecting the mango tree's growth or health.

**21.** **(b)**

A. In human pregnancy, the major organ systems are formed at the end of 12 weeks — Correct

B. Major organ systems are formed at the end of 8 weeks — Incorrect

C. Heart is formed after one month (4 weeks) of gestation — Correct

D. Limbs and digits develop by the end of the second month (~8 weeks) — Correct

E. Appearance of hair is observed in the fifth month — Correct

**22.** **(b)** In a bioreactor, foam formation during fermentation is common due to aeration and agitation.
A foam breaker (foam buster) is installed near the top of the reactor to break foam and avoid overflow or contamination.
In the figure:
A = Impeller (mixes medium)
B = Sparger (introduces air/gas)
C = Foam breaker (top part)
D = Outlet/Drain

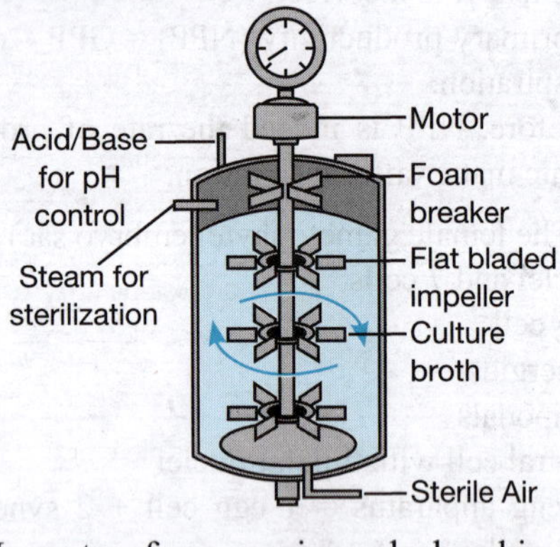


**23.** **(a)** In water, frogs respire only by skin (cutaneous respiration), not buccal cavity.
On land, frogs respire by skin, buccal cavity, and lungs. Thus, the statement is false for water but true for land.

**24.** **(d)** Pupillary constriction is caused by parasympathetic nerves, while adrenaline causes dilation, so A is incorrect.
Increase blood glucose (hyperglycemic effect) → B is correct

The adrenal medulla secretes adrenaline and noradrenaline which cause piloerection (hair stands up) → C is correct

Increase heart contraction strength → D is correct

**25. (c)**

A. True → Auxins induce parthenocarpy (fruit development without fertilization).

B. True → Growth regulators can promote (e.g., auxins, gibberellins) or inhibit (e.g., ABA).

C. True → Cells must dedifferentiate first before they can re-differentiate into new types.

D. False → Abscisic acid is a growth inhibitor, not a promoter.

E. False → Apical dominance suppresses lateral bud growth.

**26. (d)** ADH and oxytocin is synthesized in the hypothalamus but stored and released from the posterior pituitary.

**27. (a)** Beer and wine are made by fermentation by yeast and is not distilled.

Whisky, brandy, and rum are distilled beverages.

**28. (d)** Polygenic inheritance is controlled by two or more genes (multiple genes) influencing a single trait (e.g., skin colour, height).

It does not follow Mendelian ratios (like 3:1 or 9:3:3:1).

Instead, it shows continuous variation and is called a Non-Mendelian inheritance pattern.

**29. (c)** Head → genetic material

Acrosome → enzymes

Middle piece → energy (mitochondria)

Tail → motility

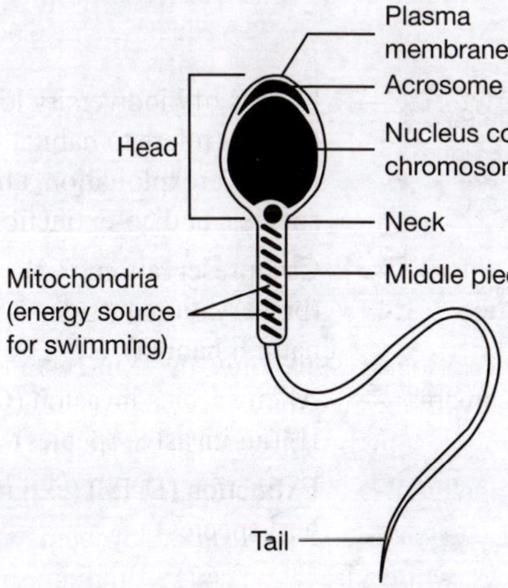


**30. (a)** Zygomorphic = Bilaterally symmetrical (can be divided into two equal halves only in one plane) because of vexillary aestivation

Examples:

Pea, Bean → Zygomorphic

Petunia, Datura, Chilli → Actinomorphic (radial symmetry)

**31. (d)**

- Azotobacter, Oscillatoria, Anabaena, and Nostoc are all capable of nitrogen fixation.
- Volvox is a green alga and does not fix nitrogen.

**32. (a)**

- Ex-situ conservation: conservation outside natural habitats (e.g., zoos, botanical gardens, seed banks).
- In-situ conservation: conservation within natural habitats (e.g., national parks, sanctuaries).

**33. (d)** Ramdeo Misra is called the Father of Indian Ecology for his pioneering research in ecosystem studies, particularly in India.

**34. (c)**

1. Statement I: Correct

According to the RNA world hypothesis, RNA was the first genetic material.

RNA could both store genetic information and catalyze biochemical reactions (ribozymes).

RNA is chemically unstable because of the presence of a 2'-OH group → makes it more reactive and prone to hydrolysis.

2. Statement II: Correct

DNA evolved from RNA later because DNA is more chemically stable (lacks 2'-OH group).

The double-stranded nature of DNA allows repair mechanisms by using one strand as a template.

DNA's stability and repair mechanisms made it a better long-term storage molecule for genetic information.

**35. (b)**

- Statement I is incorrect: tRNA interacts with mRNA during translation (codon-anticodon interaction), and rRNA forms the ribosome which also binds mRNA — both interact with mRNA.
- Statement II is correct: RNAi is a natural mechanism in eukaryotes to silence gene expression, playing a role in cellular defense against viruses.

**36. (b)**

| | |
|---|---|
| (A) Heart | (iii) Atrial natriuretic factor |
| (B) Kidney | (i) Erythropoietin |
| (C) Gastro-intestinal tract | (iv) Secretin |
| (D) Adrenal cortex | (ii) Aldosterone |

**37. (b)** Cyclostomata = Jawless vertebrates (lampreys and hagfish). They are ectoparasites on fishes.

**38. (b)** Streptokinase is an enzyme used as a clot-buster; it dissolves fibrin clots in heart attack and pulmonary embolism patients.

**39. (d)** In echinoderms (like starfish), the water vascular system helps in:
Locomotion and respiration (A)
Capture and transport of food (C)
but not directly in digestion or excretion.

**40. (d)**

| | |
|---|---|
| (A) Pteridophyte | (iv) Salvinia (fern ally, spore-producing |
| (B) Bryophyte | (iii) Polytrichum (a moss) |
| (C) Angiosperm | (i) Salvia (flowering plant) |
| (D) Gymnosperm | (ii) Ginkgo |

**41. (b)**

- A (Correct): CT and MRI are imaging techniques used for detecting tumors and cancers.
- B (Incorrect): Chemotherapeutic drugs are used to target cancerous, not non-cancerous cells.
- C (Correct): α-interferons stimulate the immune system to attack cancer cells.
- D (Incorrect): Biological response modifiers (like interferons) are different from typical chemotherapeutic drugs.
- E (Incorrect): In leukemia, WBC count increases abnormally, not decreases.

**42. (c)**

- B (correct): IVF is a costly procedure requiring expensive tools and technology.
- D (correct): There is a possibility that IVF-conceived children may be orphaned (in case of issues with older parents, etc.).
- F (correct): Embryo implantation may fail or the embryo may not survive, which is a known risk.

Options A, C, and E are incorrect.

- A: IVF doesn't necessarily pose a high fatality risk to the mother.
- C: Donors can be anonymous; husband/wife are not mandatory.
- E: IVF is available in India.

**43. (c)**

A. The reductive division (meiosis I) for female gametogenesis starts earlier than that of males — True (Female meiosis starts during fetal development; male meiosis starts at puberty.)

B. The gap between meiosis I and meiosis II is shorter in males compared to females — True (In males, meiosis happens continuously; in females, it is arrested at certain stages.)

C. The first polar body is associated with formation of primary oocyte — False (The first polar body is formed after the primary oocyte completes meiosis I.)

D. LH surge leads to disintegration of endometrium and onset of menstruation — False (LH surge causes ovulation; progesterone withdrawal causes menstruation.)

**44. (d)** Gemmae are small multicellular structures that detach and develop into new individuals, facilitating asexual reproduction in bryophytes like Marchantia.

**45. (c)** Both A and R are true and R is the correct explanation of A.

**46. (c)** Reductionist Biology is the approach that studies biological systems by breaking them down into their component parts, often studying the chemical and physical processes that underlie biological functions. The concept of physics and chemistry are applied to understand biology Hence, the physico-chemical approach is the correct match.

**47. (b)** The primary lymphoid organs are bone marrow and thymus where immature lymphocytes differentiate into antigen-sensitive lymphocytes. After maturation the lymphocytes migrate to secondary lymphoid organs like spleen, lymph nodes, tonsils, Peyer's patches of small intestine and appendix.

**48. (d)**

| | | |
|---|---|---|
| Evil Quartet | → | Causes of biodiversity loss (A-III) (refers to habitat loss, overexploitation, alien species, and co-extinctions) |
| Ex situ conservation | → | Cryopreservation (B-I) (preservation outside natural habitat) |
| Lantana camara | → | Alien species invasion (C-II) (an invasive species) |
| Dodo | → | Extinction (D-IV) (extinct bird species) |

**49. (a)** Megaspore mother cell (MMC) → undergoes Meiosis (1 division) → produces 4 megaspores (only 1 functional)

Functional megaspore → undergoes 3 mitotic divisions → forms 8-nucleate embryo sac → thus the answer is 1 Meiosis + 3 Mitosis

**50. (d)** Innate immunity is present from birth and provides general, non-specific defense (e.g., skin, mucous membranes, phagocytes).

**51. (d)** Fig fruit is still vegetarian; fig wasps are involved in pollination, but it's not a non-veg fruit.
Fig wasp and fig tree exhibit mutual relationship as fig wasp completes its life cycle in fig fruit and fig fruit gets pollinated by fig wasp. → false because inflorescence get pollinated by fig wasp not fruit.

**52. (c)** The tapetum is a nutritive tissue of anther; its cells are multinucleate and dense.
Multinucleated cells synthesize and supply nutrients/proteins effectively.

**53. (c)** A is correct: Eukaryotic ribosomes = 80S, Prokaryotic = 70S
B is correct: Ribosomes have two subunits
C is correct: 80S = 60S + 40S
D is incorrect: 70S = 50S + 30S, not 60S + 30S
E is incorrect:

**54. (b)** Catalase contains haem (iron-porphyrin) as a prosthetic group. It is tightly bound to enzyme.
It breaks down hydrogen peroxide ($H_2O_2$) into water and oxygen.
Other options:
RuBisCO → contains $Mg^{2+}$ (not haem)
Carbonic anhydrase → contains $Zn^{2+}$ (not haem)
Succinate dehydrogenase → contains FAD (not haem)

**55. (b)** The vena cava is a major vein that carries deoxygenated blood from the body back to the heart, both in humans and frogs. It drains into the right atrium of the heart.

**56. (c)** In pteridophytes, the main plant body is a sporophyte.
The sporangia produce spores by meiosis in spore mother cells.
The spores germinate to give rise to inconspicuous, small but multicellular, free-living, mostly photosynthetic thalloid gametophytes called prothallus.
The gametophytes bear male and female sex organs called antheridia and archegonia, respectively. Water is required for transfer of antherozoids-the male gametes released from the antheridia, to the mouth of archegonium.
Fusion of male gamete with the egg present in the archegonium result in the formation of zygote (Fertilization).

**57. (b)** In blue-white screening, plasmid has lac Z gene coding for β-galactosidase.
If foreign DNA is inserted into lac Z gene, it disrupts the gene → no enzyme → colony stays white → recombinant colony.
If no insert, lac Z gene remains intact → makes β-galactosidase → metabolizes X-gal → blue colonies → non-recombinant.
Thus:
Blue = non-recombinant
White = recombinant

**58. (d)** Aspergillus niger: used in industrial citric acid production (not household food).
Trichoderma polysporum: produces antifungal agents → used in agriculture/medicine.
Lactobacillus: makes curd → household.
Saccharomyces cerevisiae: baking/brewing yeast → household.
Propionibacterium sharmanii: used in Swiss cheese → household.

**59. (c)** RNA interference (RNAi) is mediated by complementary double-stranded RNA (dsRNA).
This binds and degrades target mRNA, silencing it.

**60. (d)** **Complex II** in the mitochondrial electron transport chain is also known as **succinate dehydrogenase**. It is unique because it is the only complex that is involved in both the Krebs cycle (citric acid cycle) and the electron transport chain (ETC). It catalyzes the oxidation of succinate to fumarate and transfers electrons to ubiquinone (coenzyme Q).

**61. (d)** Pseudocoelomate: mesoderm lines body wall but not gut (e.g., Ascaris).
True coelomates have mesoderm around gut and body wall; acoelomates lack coelom.

**62. (b)** In floral formula:
⊕ stands for actinomorphic (radial symmetry), not zygomorphic.
$\bar{G}$ (with line above) = inferior ovary.
$\underline{G}$ (without line) = superior ovary.

**63. (a)**
Statement I: TRUE. Energy flows unidirectional from sun → producers → consumers → decomposers.
Statement II: FALSE. Ecosystems follow the second law of thermodynamics (energy is lost as heat in every transfer).

**64. (b)**
→ Productivity is measured as amount of biomass or energy produced per unit area per unit time.
Standard unit = Kcal $m^{-2}$ $yr^{-1}$ (or g $m^{-2}$ $yr^{-1}$)

**65. (c)** We want probability of child being unaffected + carrier in $F_3$ generation.
Let's analyze step by step:
The symbol for carrier female given diagram is for X-linked recessive disease.
So, cross in $F_2$ generation is
Cross: $X^CX^C \times X^cY$
Offspring possibilities:
$\frac{1}{4} \rightarrow X^CX^C$ A (normal, non-carrier)
$\frac{1}{4} \rightarrow X^CX^c$ (normal and carrier)
$\frac{1}{4} \rightarrow X^cX^c$ (diseased)
$\frac{1}{4} \rightarrow X^cY$ (diseased) therefore, answer is $\frac{1}{4}$

**66. (b)** The Aleurone layer is the outermost layer of the endosperm and is rich in proteins. It separates the endosperm from the embryo.
The other options:
Coleoptile → Protective sheath covering the emerging shoot
Coleorhiza → Protective sheath covering the emerging root
Integument → Becomes seed coat

**67. (d)**

| | |
|---|---|
| (A) Chlorophyll a | (iii) Blue – green |
| (B) Chlorophyll b | (i) Yellow – green |
| (C) Xanthophylls | (ii) Yellow |
| (D) Carotenoids | (iv) Yellow to Yellow – orange |

Chlorophyll a gives a blue-green colour. → A-III
Chlorophyll b gives a yellow-green colour. → B-I
Xanthophylls are yellow pigments. → C-II
Carotenoids range from yellow to orange. → D-IV

**68. (c)** George Gamow proposed that a triplet of nucleotides (codon) codes for one amino acid to cover 20 amino acids using 4 nucleotide bases.

**69. (c)** Histones are rich in basic amino acids (positively charged): → Lysine and Arginine
This helps bind negatively charged DNA

**70. (c)** Essential enzymes in gene cloning:
Restriction enzymes (A) → to cut DNA at specific sites
DNA ligase (B) → to join DNA fragments
DNA polymerase (E) → for amplification (optional but commonly used in PCR)
Not essential:
DNA mutase (C) → used for mutation, not cloning
DNA recombinase (D) → helps recombination, but not mandatory for cloning

**71. (c)** Mesosomes are infoldings of the plasma membrane in prokaryotes (especially bacteria).
Functions of Mesosomes:
Cell wall formation during cell division
DNA replication and distribution to daughter cells
Respiration by providing surface for respiratory enzymes

**72. (a)** Explanation: In prokaryotes, rho factor (ρ) helps in the termination of transcription by dislodging RNA polymerase from the DNA template.

**73. (b)** Male frogs develop a nuptial pad (copulatory pad) on the first digit of the forelimb during the breeding season to grip females.

**74. (d)** In the Proximal Convoluted Tubule (PCT):
Reabsorption of $Na^+$, $HCO_3^-$, and water takes place.
Secretion of $H^+$ and $NH_3$ (ammonia) into the tubular fluid.
In the Distal Convoluted Tubule (DCT):
Reabsorption of $Na^+$, $HCO_3^-$, and water occurs.
Secretion of $K^+$ and $H^+$ into the tubular fluid.
The diagram in option (2) correctly shows:
In PCT: $Na^+$, $HCO_3^-$, and $H_2O$ reabsorbed; $H^+$ and $NH_3$ secreted.
In DCT: $Na^+$, $HCO_3^-$, and $H_2O$ reabsorbed; $K^+$ and $H^+$ secreted.

**75. (a)**
1. Each antibody has 2 light and 2 heavy chains — True
2. Heavy and light chains held by disulfide bonds — True
3. Antigen binding site is located at C-terminal region — False
   → Antigen binding site is at the N-terminal region of variable domains
4. Constant regions are located at C-terminal — True

**76. (c)** Scutellum: Single cotyledon in monocots
Non-albuminous seed: Seed where endosperm is used up (ex: pea)
Epiblast: Rudimentary second cotyledon in monocots
Perisperm: Remnant of nucellus (persists in seeds like black pepper)

**77. (c)** In monocot stems, the hypodermis is made up of sclerenchyma, not parenchyma.

Other options are correct characteristics of monocot stems:

- Vascular bundles are scattered, closed, and conjoint.
- Phloem parenchyma is absent in monocots.

**78.** **(d)** Boy and girl twins = different sexes → they must be dizygotic (fraternal) twins.

Monozygotic twins are genetically identical and same sex.

**79.** **(c)**

→ Both are storage organs but:

Sweet potato = Root modification

Potato = Stem modification

Same function, different origin → Analogy (Convergent evolution)

**80.** **(b)** Cytokinin delays leaf senescence (aging) by promoting nutrient mobilization (called Richmond-Lang effect).

**81.** **(d)** Insulin is a protein hormone. If taken orally, digestive enzymes in the stomach and intestines will break it down, making it ineffective. Therefore, it must be injected to bypass digestion.

**82.** **(a)** This reaction shows the transfer of a functional group (G) from one molecule to another. Enzymes that catalyze such reactions belong to the class Transferases, which are responsible for transferring a group (like methyl, glycosyl, etc.) between molecules.

**83.** **(c)** In gel electrophoresis, smaller fragments migrate faster toward the positive electrode (anode).

DNA fragments obtained from gel electrophoresis are purified and used in rDNA technology.

**84.** **(a)**

- B – The gametophyte attaches to the substratum.
- E – Male gametes (antherozoids) are released into water.
- A – Fertilization occurs; antherozoid fuses with egg.
- D – Formation of a sporophyte (diploid).
- C – Sporophyte undergoes meiosis to produce haploid spores.

This sequence aligns with the bryophyte life cycle, which is gametophyte-dominant.

**85.** **(a)** Cross = RrYy × RrYy (Dihybrid cross)

Phenotypic ratio = 9 (round yellow) : 3 (round green) : 3 (wrinkled yellow) : 1 (wrinkled green)

**86.** **(d)**

A. Multicellular heterotrophs with cell wall made of chitin → Fungi

B. Heterotrophs with tissue/organ/organ system → Animalia

C. Prokaryotes with cell wall made of polysaccharides & amino acids → Monera

D. Eukaryotic autotrophs with tissue/organ level → Plantae

E. Eukaryotes with cellular body organization → Protista

Increasing complexity order: C (Monera) < E (Protista) < A (Fungi) < D (Plantae) < B (Animalia)

**87.** **(b)**

| | |
|---|---|
| (A) Centromere | (ii) Cell division |
| (B) Cilium | (iii) Cell movement |
| (C) Cristae | (i) Mitochondrion |
| (D) Cell membrane | (iv) Phospholipid Bilayer |

Centromere is involved in cell division, specifically the attachment of spindle fibers during mitosis/meiosis.

Cilia are hair-like structures responsible for cell movement.

Cristae are the inner folds of the mitochondrion, where ATP generation happens — hence linked to mitochondrion.

Cell membrane is made up of a phospholipid bilayer.

**88.** **(d)** *Verhulst-Pearl Logistic Growth* and is described by the following equation:

$$\frac{dN}{dt} = rN\left(\frac{K-N}{K}\right)$$

Where N = Population density at time $t$

$r$ = Intrinsic rate of natural increase

K = Carrying capacity

**89.** **(b)** Emphysema: Damage to alveolar walls → reduced respiratory surface.

Angina pectoris: Pain due to reduced oxygen in heart muscles.

Glomerulonephritis: Inflammation of glomeruli (kidney).

Tetany: Spasms from low calcium.

**90. (c)**

A. Nodal tissue: Includes SA node and AV node which generate and conduct electrical impulses in the heart — correct.

B. Medulla oblongata: The cardiovascular center here regulates heartbeat via autonomic nervous system — correct.

C. Adrenal medullary hormones: Epinephrine and norepinephrine increase heart rate — correct.

D. Adrenal cortical hormones: Mainly regulate metabolism and salt balance, not heart activity — incorrect.

# BOTANY

# 1

# Sexual Reproduction in Flowering Plants

## LEARNING OBJECTIVES

- State the structure and function of the floral parts including: Sepal, petal,stamen,carpel.
- State that the pollen grain produces male gamete.
- Outline seed structure and function of following: testa, plumule, radicle, embryo, cotyledon. Explain embryo and food supply (endosperm or seed leaves).
- Outline fruit and seed dispersal and give with examples of wind/water/animal/self dispersal.
- Make reference to non-endospermic seed.
- Outline fruit formation and seedless fruit production.

## Chapter Overview

- All angiosperms perform sexual reproduction and sexual organ of plant is flower. Flower have following parts **(Fig. 1.1)**.

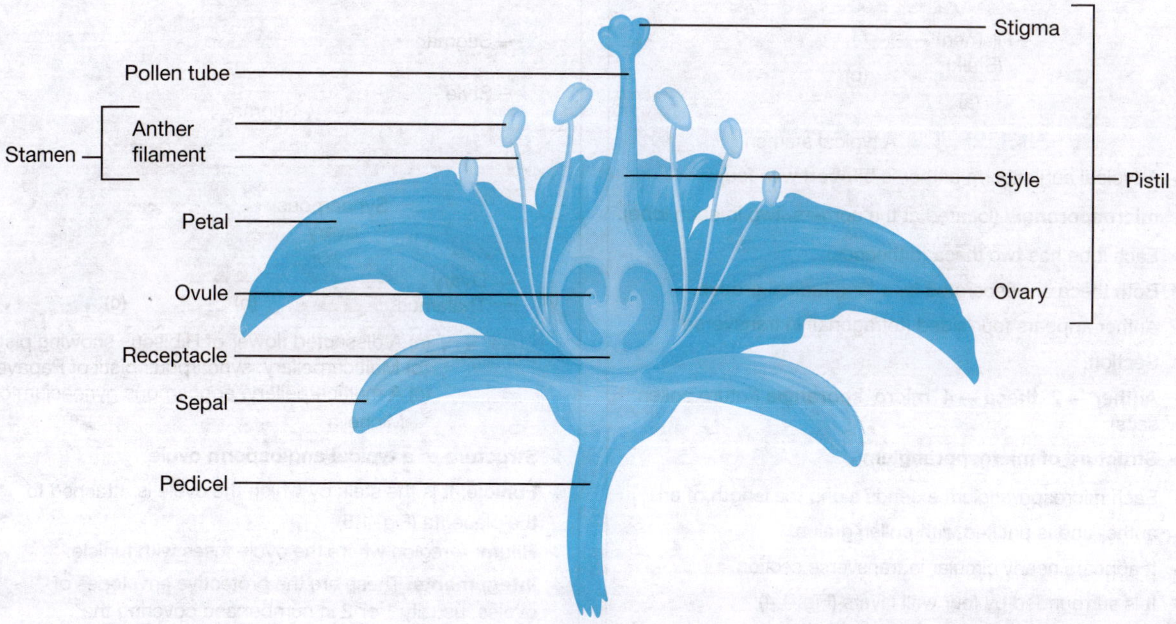


**FIGURE 1.1** Parts of a flower

Refer NCERT Ch 1: Sexual Reproduction in Flowering Plants

## Pre–fertilization: Structures and Events

- Flowers are formed over mature plants in response to hormone induced structural and physiological changes in shoot apices. Shoot apices are transformed into an inflorescence over which primordia develop.
- Two types of reproductive structures are found in flowers:

### Androecium

➢ It consists of a whorl of stamens.

➢ **Stamen = Anther** (bilobed) + **Filament** (long and slender stalk) (Fig. 1.2).

➢ Filament is having two ends:

**(1) Distal end:** attached to the anther

**(2) Proximal end:** attached to the thalamus or the petals of the flower.

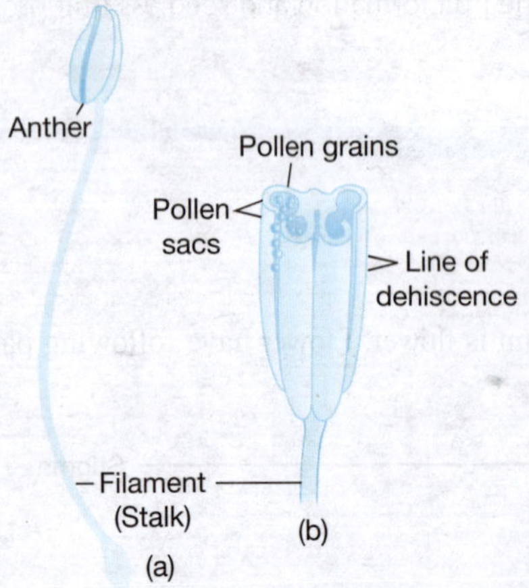


FIGURE. 1.2 A typical stamen

➢ A typical angiosperm anther is **bilobed** with four **microsporangia** (located at the corners, two in each lobe).

➢ Each lobe has two theca (dithecous)

➢ Both theca are separated by a longitudinal groove.

➢ Anther appears four-sided (tetragonal) in transverse Section.

➢ **Anther → 2 theca → 4 micro sporangia** (future pollen sacs).

➢ **Structure of microsporangium**

➢ Each microsporangium extends along the length of an anther and is packed with pollen grains.

➢ It appears nearly circular in transverse section.

➢ It is surrounded by four wall layers (Fig. 1.4):

**(1) Epidermis** (outermost)

**(2) Endothecium**

**(3) Middle layers**

**(4) Tapetum** (innermost)

### Gynoecium

➢ **Gynoecium** (female reproductive part) consists of 1 pistil (**monocarpellary**) or more (**multicarpellary)** (Fig. 1.3).

➢ The pistils are either fused together (**syncarpous**) or may be free (**apocarpous**).

➢ **Pistil:** It consists of three parts (Fig. 1.3):

**(1) Stigma:** Landing platform for pollen grains.

**(2) Style:** Elongated slender part beneath the stigma. (provides passage for the entry and elongation of pollen tube).

**(3) Ovary:** Basal bulged part of the pistil.

➢ Ovarian cavity is known as locule.

➢ The placenta give rise to **megasporangia (or ovules)** which may be:

(1) One (as in **wheat, paddy** and **mango**).

(2) Many (as in **papaya, water melon** and **orchids**).

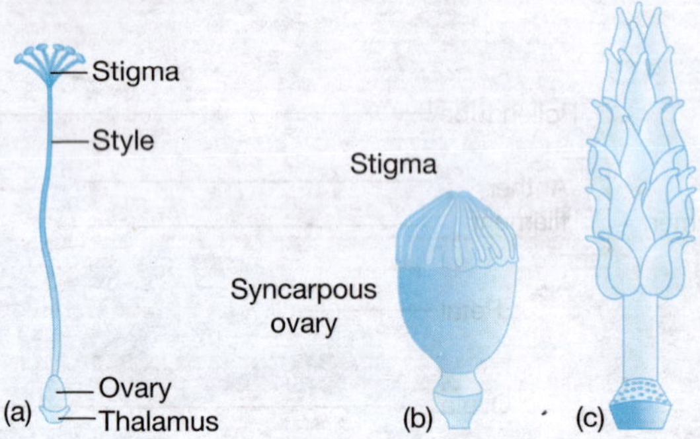


FIGURE. 1.3 (a) A dissected flower of Hibiscus showing pistil; (b) Multicarpellary, syncarpous pistil of Papaver; (c) A multicarpellary, apocarpous gynoecium of Michelia.

➢ **Structure of a typical angiosperm ovule**

➢ **Funicle:** It is the stalk by which the ovule is attached to the placenta (Fig. 1.5).

➢ **Hilum:** A region where the ovule fuses with funicle.

➢ **Integuments:** These are the protective envelopes of ovules, usually 1 or 2 in number and covering the nucellus.

➢ **Mircopyle:** A region that doesn't have covering of integument and provides way for pollen tube to enter the embryo sac.

➢ **Chalaza:** It is the basal part of the ovule just opposite to micropyle.

➢ Functions of outer three wall layers:
(1) Protection
(2) Dehiscence of anther to release the pollen

➢ **Tapetum:** Tapetal cells are usually bi-/multi-nucleated with dense cytoplasm.
**(1) Function:** These give nourishment to the developing pollen grains. It secretes enzymes and hormones.

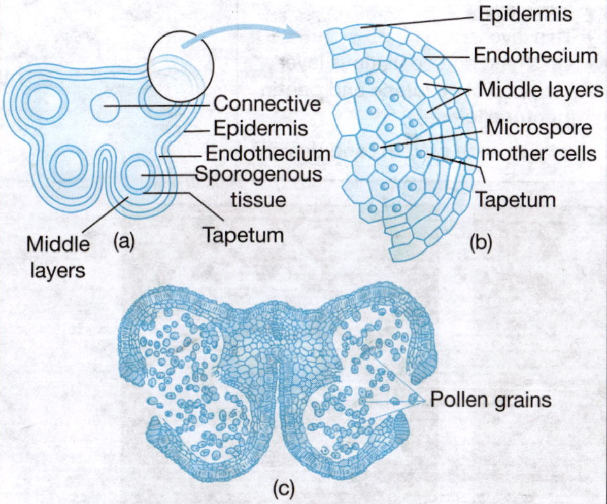


**FIGURE. 1.4** (a) T.S. of young anther
(b) 3-dimensional cut section of an anther
(c) T.S. of anther at the time of dehiscence

➢ **Nucellus**
(1) It represents a mass of cells surrounded by integuments.
(2) Nucellar cells have abundant reserve food.

➢ **Embryo sac (or female gametophyte)**
(1) It is located in the ovule.
(2) It is formed from a megaspore. (usually 1 in nucellus).

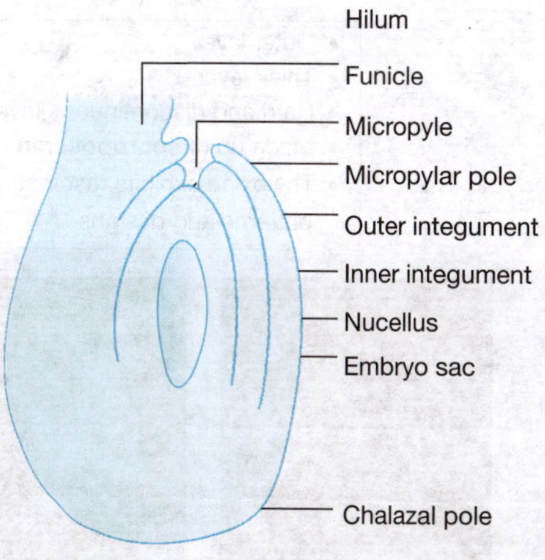


**FIGURE. 1.5** A diagrammatic view of a typical anatropous ovule

## Microsporogenesis

- **Sporogenous tissue:** It is the group of compactly arranged homogenous cells in the centre of each micro sporangium in a young anther. (Surrounded by tapetum).
- Each cell of sporogenous tissue act as Pollen mother cell (PMC/2n) undergo (Meiosis I Process: Microsporogenesis) forms microspore tetrad than when anthers mature and dehydrate, 4 Microspores [Each haploid (n)] are released. Each microspore develops into a pollen grain after (Dehiscence) produce thousands of pollen grains come out of anther.

**Note:**

Tracheophytes, which produce two distinct sizes or sexes, contain microsporangium.

## Megasporogenesis

- A single nucellar cell towards the micropylar region differentiates into **megaspore mother cell (MMC).**
- MMC is a large cell having dense cytoplasm and a prominent nucleus.
- MMC undergo (meiosis) leads formation of 4 megaspores, 3 megaspores degenerate while 1 remains functional. Functional megaspore develops into female gametophyte (embryo sac).
- **Monosporic development:** If the embryo sac develops from a single megaspore.
- **Functional megaspore** undergoes (Mitosis) 2 Nuclei are formed which move to the opposite poles, undergo further (Mitosis) forms 4 nucleated stage, then 8 nucleated stage.
- These mitotic divisions are free nuclear type and cell wall formation occur after attaining the 8-nucleate stage. 6 of the 8 nuclei develop cell wall while the remaining 2 nuclei (called polar nuclei) are enclosed in a common cell wall making a central large cell, situated below the egg apparatus.

## Pollen Grain

- **Shape:** Generally spherical.
- **Size: 25–50 $\mu$** in diameter (Fig. 1.6).

Wall of pollen grain is two layered:

**Exine**

- Outer layer
- Thick layer
- Hard and discontinuous layer
- Made up of **sporopollenin**
- The exine exhibits fascinating patterns and designs

**Intine**

- Inner layer
- Thin layer
- Less hard and continuous layer
- Made up of **cellulose** and **pectin (pectocellulose)**
- It lacks such patterns and designs

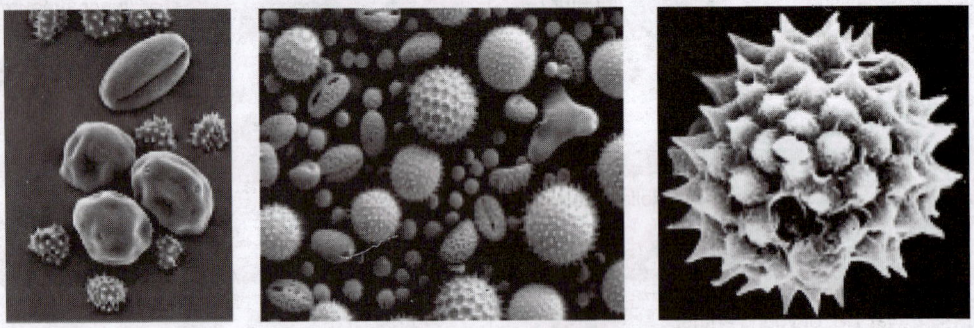

FIGURE 1.6 Scanning electron micrographs of a few pollen grains

## Embryo Sac

**8-nucleated, 7-celled:** It consists of

**(1) Egg apparatus** (3 cells = **2 Synergids + 1 Egg cell**): Towards the micropylar end.

- **Filiform apparatus:** These are the special cellular thickenings in synergids at the micropylar tip. It guides the pollen tubes into the synergid (Fig. 1.7(a) and (b)).

**(2) Antipodals** (3 cells): Towards the chalazal end.

**(3) Large central cell** (1 cell): It possess 2 polar nuclei.

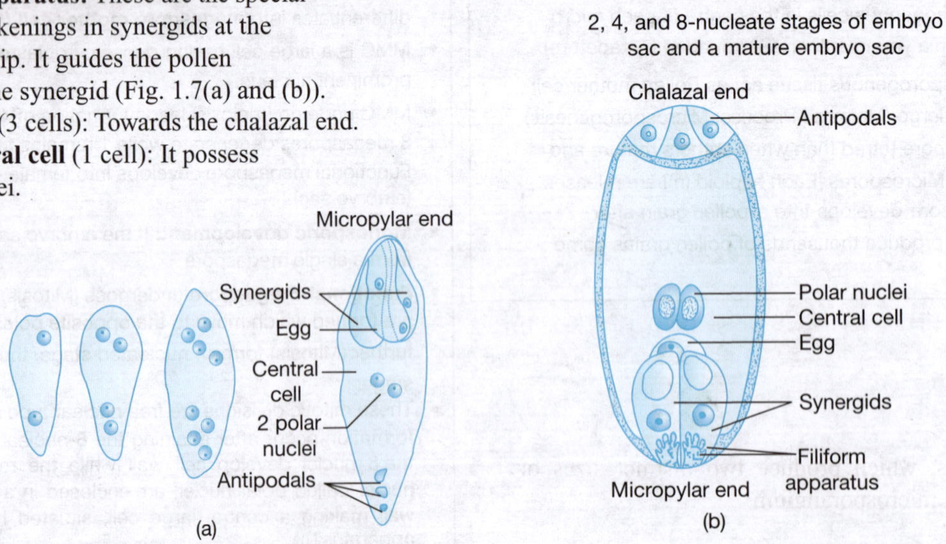


FIGURE 1.7 A diagrammatic representation of the mature embryo sac

## Sporopollenin

(1) Pollen grains are preserved as fossils for very long durations because of sporopollenin in exine.
(2) Few features of sporopollenin:
- One of the most resistant organic materials known.
- It can resist damage from high temperature, strong acids and bases.
- No enzyme is known to degrade sporopollenin.

## Germ Pores

Those prominent apertures in exine of pollen grain where sporopollenin is absent. Function of germ pore: it provides space for emergence of pollen tube.

(1) Structure of pollen grain
(2) Initially the pollen grain is one celled but when the pollen grain matures, it acquires 2–celled stage **(Fig. 1.8)**:

**Mature pollen grain in 2-celled stage**

**Vegetative cell**
- Larger in size
- Generally spherical
- Large irregularly shaped nucleus
- It has abundant food reserve

**Generative cell**
- Small in size and floats in the cytoplasm of the vegetative cell
- Spindle shaped
- Dense cytoplasm and a typical nucleus
- Food reserve is nil

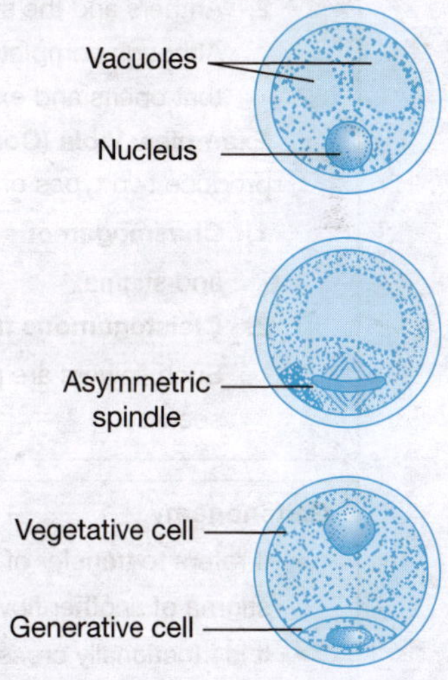


**FIGURE 1.8** 2–celled stage of pollen grain

## Pollen Grain

- **Stage of shedding of pollen grains:** 2-celled stage (in > 60 % of angiosperms).
- In remaining species of angiosperms, generative cell divides mitotically to form 2 male gametes, acquire **3-celled stage** (1 vegetative cell + 2 male gametes) and then are shedded at the same stage.
- Pollen grains of many plants may cause severe allergy in some people, ultimately leading to asthma, bronchitis, etc. Pollen allergy is also caused by ***Parthenium*** or **carrot grass.** It has come into India with imported wheat, as a contaminant but now it has become very common throughout India.
- As the pollen grains are rich in nutrients, in recent years these are used as pollen tablets (a food supplement).
- Athletes and race horses also consume pollen to increase their performance.
- **Viability period of pollen grains:** It is the period during which the pollen remains viable after shedding. Viability period may vary species to species.
  (1) **Upto 30 min.:** In cereals like **rice** and **wheat.**
  (2) **Few months:** In some members of **Rosaceae, Leguminoseae** and **Solanaceae.**
- **Storing of pollen grains:** Pollen grains are stored for years in **liquid nitrogen (–196°C)** and can be used as pollen banks in crop breeding programmes.

## Pollination

- **Pollination:** It refers to the transfer of pollen grains from the anther to the stigma of a pistil.
- Both female and male gametes of angiosperms are non-motile.
- Types of Pollination (depending on the source of pollen):

**Self – pollination**

- No genetic variation occurs

**Autogamy:** It refers to the transfer of pollen grains from anther to stigma of the same flower. Conditions required for autogamy:

1. There should be synchrony in pollen release and stigma receptivity.
2. Anthers and the stigma should lie close to each other.

Although complete autogamy is rare for a normal flower that opens and exposes the anthers and the stigma.

**Examples: Viola (CommonPansy), Oxalis** and **Commelina** produce two types of flowers:

1. **Chasmogamous flowers:** Flowers with exposed anthers and stigma.
2. **Cleistogamous flowers:** Flowers that do not open at all. Such flowers are purely autogamous and produce assured seed-set.

**Geitonogamy**

- It refers to transfer of pollen grains from the anther to the stigma of another flower of the same plant.
- It is functionally cross-pollination (involving a pollinating agent) and genetically autogamy.

**Cross – pollination**

- Genetic variation occurs

**Xenogamy:** It refers to transfer of pollen grains from anther to the stigma of genetically different plant.

Allogamy include both geitonogamy and xenogamy.

**Note:**

Anywhere between 75% and 95% of all flowering plants on the earth need help with pollination.

**Agents of pollination**

- Abiotic agents
  - Wind (Anemophily) E.g. Corn cob, grasses
  - Water (Hydrophily) E.g. Bryophytes, sea grasses
- Biotic agents
  - Animals
    - Entomophily (Insect) E.g. Most of the angiosperms
    - Ornithophily (Bird)
    - Chiropterophily (Bat)
    - Malacophily (Snail)

- Most of the plants use biotic agents for pollination while only a small proportion of plants use abiotic agents.
- Most of water and wind pollinated pollen grains get wasted so to compensate this, flowers produce enormous amount of pollens (in comparison to the number of ovules).

## Types of Pollinations

### Wind

- It is more common in comparison to other abiotic pollinators.
- **Important Features of Wind pollination:**
  (1) Pollen grains are light and non-sticky (for easy transport).
  (2) Stamens are usually well exposed (for easy dispersal).
  (3) Stigma is large and often feathery (for easy trapping of pollen grains).
  (4) Number of ovule per ovary: Usually one.
  (5) Flowers are numerous and are packed into an inflorescence.
  - The tassels of **Corn cob** are the stigma and style which wave in the wind to trap pollen grains.
  - Pollination by wind is common in **Grasses.**

### Water

- It is very rare in flowering plants (limited to only 30 genera, usually monocots).
- **Important Features of Water Pollination:**
  (1) Pollen grains have a mucilaginous covering (protection from getting wet).
  (2) Flowers are not very colourful.
  (3) Flowers do not produce nectar.
  - In lower plant groups like **Algae, bryophytes** and **pteridophytes,** male gametes are usually transported by water.
  - Plants like **Vallisneria** and **Hydrilla** (fresh water).
  - In Vallisneria, long stalk of the female flower reach the surface of water and the pollens from the male flowers are released on the surface of water, then carried passively by water currents.
  - Several **marine sea-grasses such as Zostera.**
  - In Zostera, female flowers are submerged in water. Pollen grains (usually long and ribbon like) are released inside the water, spread passively and some of them reach the stigma.
  - In most of aquatic plants (including **Water hyacinth** and **Water lily**), both male and female flowers emerge above the level of water and pollinated by biotic (insects) or abiotic (wind) means just like most of the land plants.

### Animals

- Common pollinating animal agents are: **Bees** (most common or dominant biotic pollinating agent), butterflies, flies, ants, wasps, moths, birds (specially–sunbirds and humming birds), beetles, bats, lemurs (a primate), arboreal rodents and reptiles (garden lizard, gecko lizard, etc.), etc.
- **Important Features of Animal Pollination:**
  (1) Large and colorful flowers (mostly).Even if the flowers are small, these become conspicuous by arranging themselves into a inflorescence.
  (2) Flowers are usually fragrant.
  (3) Those flowers which are pollinated by **flies** and **beetles,** have a foul odour. Flowers provide nector and pollen grain as **floral rewards** to the animals.
  (4) Pollen grains are usually sticky.
  - **Mechanism:** Animals visit the flowers for the floral rewards → Body of animal gets coated with pollen grains → Animal body when comes in contact with stigma, pollination occurs.
  - Floral reward of providing safe places to lay eggs: It is provided by–
  - Tallest flower of **Amorphophallus** (6 ft.).
  - **Yucca plant:** Yucca plant and a moth species are dependent on each other to complete their life cycles. Moth enters the flower to deposit its eggs in the locule of the ovary and while doing so it pollinates the flower. As the seeds start developing, larvae of the moth come out of the eggs.

## Outbreeding Devices

- Most of the flowering plants produce hermaphrodite or bisexual flowers which may promote self-pollination. But as continued self-pollination results in inbreeding depression, plants have developed many devices to promote cross-pollination. Such devices are known as outbreeding devices.

**Outbreeding Devices**

- (1) In some species, time of **pollen release** and **stigma receptivity** are different, i.e., time is **not synchronized.**
- (2) Anther and stigma are located at different positions in a same flower to avoid the contact between the pollen and stigma.
- (3) **Self-incompatibility:** It is a genetic mechanism by which the pollen grain of same plant (from the same flower or other flowers of the same plant) is prevented from fertilising the ovules by inhibiting pollen germination or pollen tube growth.
- (4) Production of unisexual flowers. Unisexual flowers may be produced on:
  - Same plant **(monoecious plants)**: Example: **Castor, Maize.** This prevents autogamy but not geitonogamy.
  - Different plants **(dioecious plants, Phenomenon Dioecy)**: Example: **Papaya.** This prevents both autogamy and geitonogamy.

## Pollen – Pistil Interaction

- All the events occurring from pollen deposition on the stigma upto the entry of pollen tubes into the ovule are collectively termed as pollen-pistil interaction. It is a dynamic process.
- During pollination, both types of pollen land on stigma—**Compatible pollen** (right type of pollen) or **Incompatible pollen** [wrong type of pollen either from the same plant (**self-incompatible**) or other species].

**Pollen Recognition**

- The ability of pistil to recognisethe type of pollen as compatible or incompatible

**Pollen Promotion or Inhibition**

- **Fate of compatible pollen:** The pollens are accepted by pistil and post–pollination events are initiated.

**Formation of pollen tube**

- Pollen grain germinates on the stigma and produces a pollen tube emerging through one of the **germ pores.**
- All the contents of the pollen grain enter the pollen tube.

**Entry of pollen tube into the ovule**

- Filiform apparatus located at the micropylar part of the synergids guides the entry of pollen tube → Pollen tube enters the micropyle → Pollen tube then enters one of the

*(Continued)*

*(Continued)*

| | | |
|---|---|---|
| • **Fate of incompatible pollen:** Pistil rejects the pollen by preventing either the pollen germination on the stigma or growth of the pollen tube in the style. | • Pollen tube grows through the stigma, style and finally reaches the ovary.<br>• In most of the plants pollen tube initially carries 2 cells–**vegetative cell** and **generative cell** out of which the generative cell later on divides mitotically to form two male gametes.<br>• In those plants, in which the pollen was shed at the 3-celled condition, pollen tubes carry the 2 male gametes from the starting. | synergids through the filiform apparatus. |

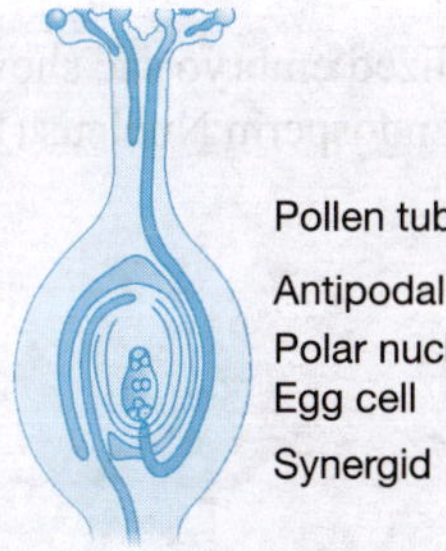


FIGURE. 1.9 Longitudinal section of a flowershowing growth of pollen tube
Pollen grains germinating on the stigma

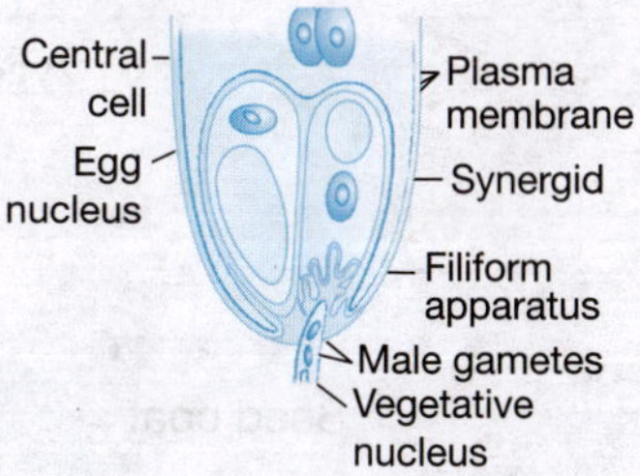


FIGURE. 1.10 Enlarged view of an eggapparatus showing entry of pollentube into a synergid.

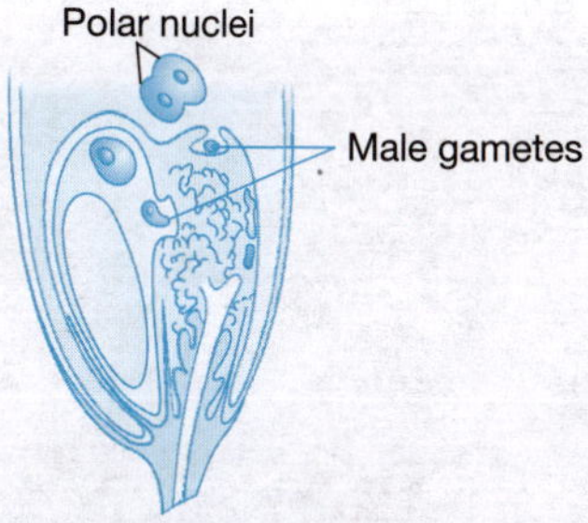


FIGURE. 1.11 Discharge of male gametes into a synergid and the movements of the sperms, one into the egg and the other into the central cell.

- Both steps 1 and 2 is the result of a **continuous dialogue** (mediated by chemicals of the pollen interacting with those of the pistil) between pollen grain and the pistil.

**To Observe Pollen Germination**

- Dust some pollen from flowers (of Pea, Chickpea, Balsam, Vinca and Crotalaria) on a glass slide and add a drop of sugar solution (about 10%). After 15–30 min, if we observe the slide under low power lens of the microscope, we can observe pollen tubes emerging from the pollen grains.

## Artificial Hybridization

- In **artificial hybridization** (one of the major approaches of crop improvement programme), two important processes are involved to ensure that only the desired pollen grains are used for pollination:

**(1) Emasculation [Only if the flower is bisexual]**
Removal of anthers by using a pair of forceps from the bisexual flowers before the anther dehisces. Emasculation is not required in unisexual flowers

**(2) Bagging**
It refers to covering the emasculated flowers with a bag of suitable size (usually made up of butterpaper) to prevent contamination of stigma with unwanted pollens.

- **Process:** Bagging → Bagged flower attains receptivity → Removal of bag and dusting of pollens from male parent on the stigma → Rebagging of flowers → Fruits allowed to develop.

## Double Fertilization

- Pollen tube releases the two male gametes into the cytoplasm of the synergid.
  Male gamete 1 (n) + Egg cell (n) referred as (**Syngamy**) leads to formation of **Zygote (2n)**
  Male gamete 2 (n) + Central cell (2n) called (**Triple Fusion**) leads to formation of **(Fig. 1.12) Primary endosperm nucleus** (**PEN**) (3n) (two nuclei of n each). It forms primary endosperm cell [PEC].
- **Syngamy and triple fusion = Double fertilization**
- Double fertilization is found in flowering plants only. PEC develops into the endosperm while the zygote develops into an embryo.

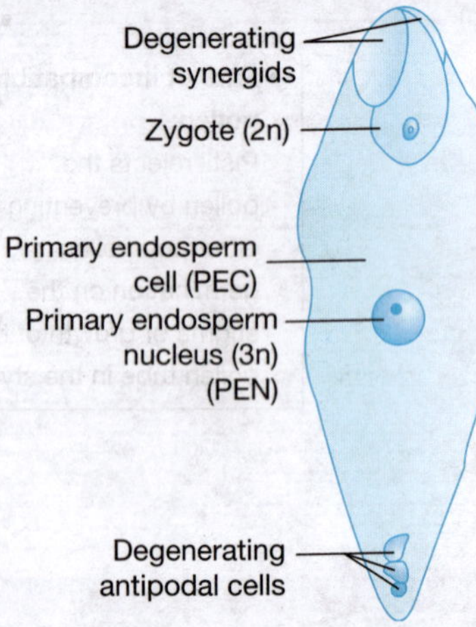


FIGURE 1.12 Fertilized embryo sac showing zygote and Primary Endosperm Nucleus (PEN)

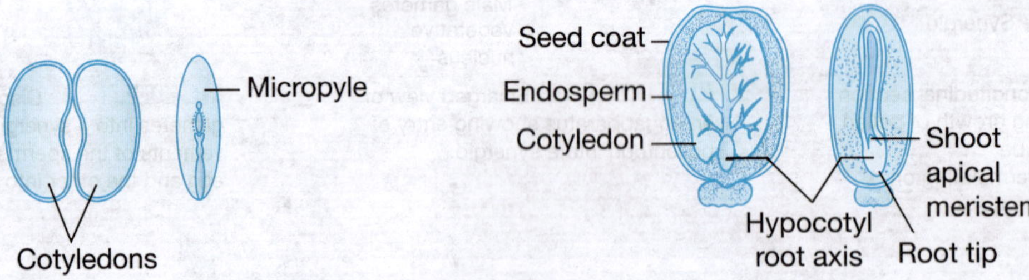


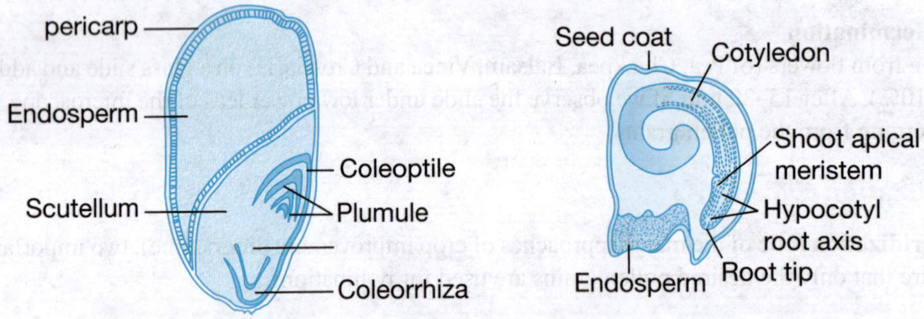


FIGURE 1.13 Structure of some seeds

## Post Fertilization Events

### 1. Endosperm

- Endosperm development precedes embryo development.
- Primary endosperm cell (PEC) divides repeatedly to forms a triploid endosperm tissue which are filled with reserve food materials. This food is utilized by the developing embryo during its growth.
- During typical endosperm development, the PEN undergoes successive free nuclear divisions and give rise to a stage-**free-nuclear endosperm.** This is later on followed by cell wall formation and the endosperm becomes cellular.
- In coconut, water represents the free-nuclear endosperm and the surrounding white kernel represents the cellular endosperm.
- **Fate of Endosperm** during the development of embryo (before seed maturation):
  (1) Endosperm is completely consumed in plants like **Pea, Groundnut, Beans,** etc.
  (2) Endosperm may persist in the mature seed of plants like **Castor** and **Coconut.**

### 2. Embryo

- Embryo develops near to the micropylar end of the embryo sac.
- Usually zygotes start dividing only when some amount of endosperm is formed. This is to ensure the nutrition to the developing embryo.
- Although the seeds of monocots and dicots differ greatly, but their early stages of embryo development (embryogeny) are very similar.
- **Zygote → Proembryo → Globular, heart-shaped and mature embryo.**
- **Structure of a typical dicotyledonous embryo**
- **Dicot embryo = 1 Embryonal axis + 2 Cotyledons**
- **Epicotyl:** It is the portion of embryonal axis above the level of cotyledons. It terminates as plumule or stem tip.
- **Hypocotyl:** It is the cylindrical part of embryonal axis below the level of cotyledons. It terminates in the radicle or root tip.
- The root tip is covered by a root cap.
- Monocot embryos possess only one cotyledon.
- **Scutellum:** It refers to cotyledon of the grass family and is located towards the lateral side of the embryonal axis.
- **Coleorrhiza:** Radical and the root cap (located at the lower end of the embryonal axis) are enclosed in an undifferentiated sheath called coleorrhiza.
- **Coleoptile:** It is a hollow foliar structure in epicotyl which encloses the shoot apex and few leaf primordia.
- **Epiblast:** It is a ruminant of second cotyledon in monocot embryo.

### 3. Maturation of ovule and ovary

- The seed (or fertilised ovule) is the final product of sexual reproduction in angiosperms.
- Seeds are formed inside the fruits.
- **Parts of a typical seed:** Seed coatis), Cotyledon(s) and an embryo axis.
- The cotyledons of embryo are generally thick and swollen structures that performs the storage of food (as in legumes).
- Mature seeds can be classified as (Fig. 1.13) as discussed below:

**(1) Non-albuminous (Ex-albuminous or Non-endospermic) seeds**

Such seeds have no residual endosperm as it is completely consumed during embryo development. Examples: **Pea, Groundnut, Sunflower,** etc.

**(2) Albuminous (Endospermic) seeds**

Endosperm is not completely consumed so some amount is retained.

Examples: **Wheat, Maize, Barley, Castor,** etc.

- **Perisperm:** In some seeds, remnants of nucellus are also persistent which is termed as perisperm.
  Examples: **Black pepper** and **Beet.**
- Initially the embryo may enter a state of inactivity called dormancy during which:

**(1)** Its water content: Reduces (**upto 10 15% moisture** by mass).
General metabolic activity of the embryo slows down.

**(2)** Seeds germinate during favourable conditions (adequate moisture, oxygen and suitable temperature).

Diagramatic representation of embryo development in dicot, a dicot embryo and L.S. of an embryo of grass are shown in the **Fig. 1.14, 1.15. and 1.16**

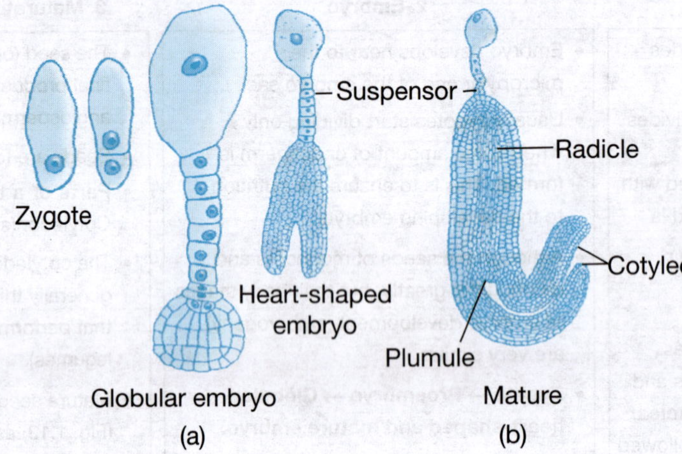


**FIGURE 1.14** Stages in embryo development in a dicot [shown in reduced size as compared to (a)]

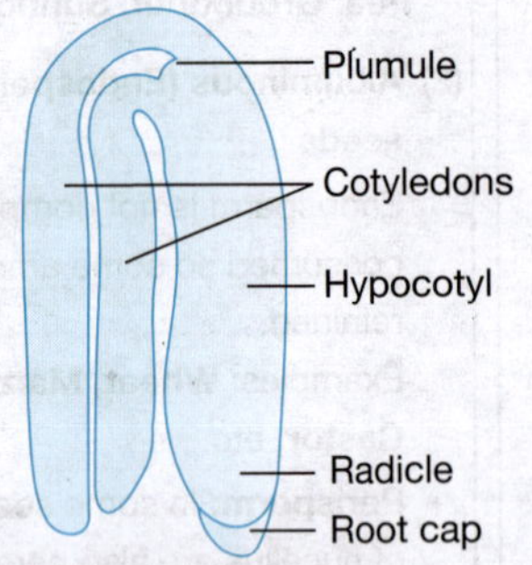


**FIGURE 1.15** A typical dicot embryo

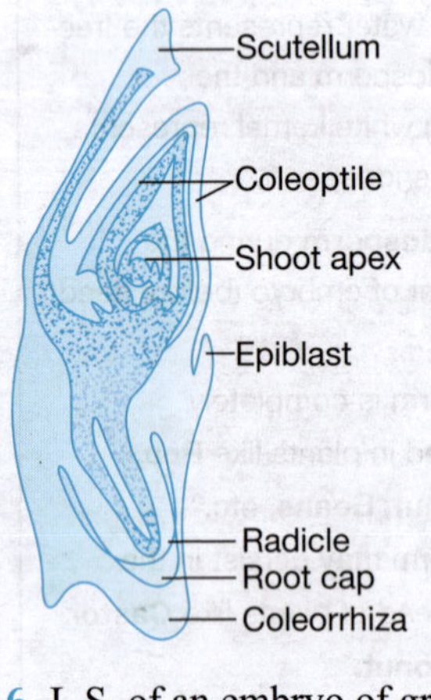


**FIGURE 1.16** L.S. of an embryo of grass

## Fruit

- After fertilization ovary is converted to fruit.
- Fleshy fruits are found in **Guava, Orange** and **Mango.**
- Dry fruits are found in **Groundnut** and **Mustard.**

**True fruits**

- Fruits developing only from the ovary. Examples: **Most of the fruits.**

**False fruits**

- In such fruits, thalamus also contributes to fruit formation (Fig. 1.17). Examples: **Apple, Strawberry, Cashew,** etc.

**Parthenocarpic fruits**

- Fruits developing without fertilization. Example: **Banana.**
- Parthenocarpy can be induced by the application of growth hormones and the resulting fruits are seedless.

Diagrammatic representation of false fruits of apple and strawberry are shown in **Fig. 1.17**.

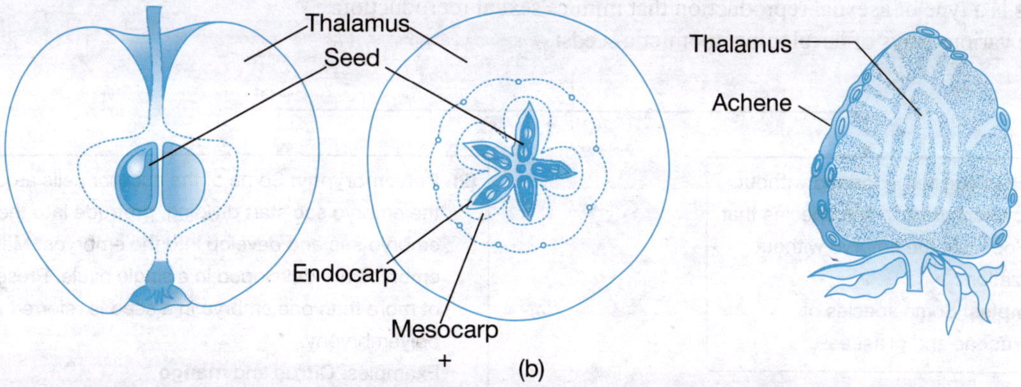


FIGURE 1.17 False fruits of apple and strawberry

## Advantages of Seeds to Angiosperms

(1) Seeds provide better dispersal strategies and help the species to colonise in other areas.
(2) Seeds have food reserves for developing young seedlings.
(3) Hard seed coat provides protection to the developing young embryo.
(4) Because seeds are produced as a result of sexual reproduction, these introduce variations.
(5) In agriculture, dehydration and dormancy of mature seeds are crucial for storage of seeds (for future use to raise the crop in the next season.

- **Viability period of seed** may vary from few months upto several years.
  - Seeds of **Lupine (*Lupinus arcticus*)** excavated from Arctic Tundra germinated after an estimated record of **10,000 years of dormancy.**
  - Seeds of **date palm, *Phoenix dactylifera*** may have viability period of **2000 years.**
- Examples of plants in which the fruits contain very large number of seeds: **Orchids, Ficus,** and parasitic plants like **Orobanche** and **Striga.**

TABLE 1.1 Pre-fertilization and post-fertilization

| Pre-fertilization structure | Post-fertilization Structure |
|---|---|
| Ovule | Seed |
| Ovary | Fruit |
| Integuments of ovules | Tough protective seed coats |
| Micropyle | Small pore in the seed coat (To facilitate the entry of oxygen and water into the seed during germination) |
| Wall of the ovary | Pericarp (wall of fruit) |
| Other floral parts | Degenerate and fall off |

## Apomixis

- Seed formation takes place without fertilization.
- Apomixis is a type of asexual reproduction that mimics sexual reproduction.
- There are various ways of developing apomictic seeds:

**(1)** A diploid egg cell is formed without reduction division in few species that develops into the embryo without fertilization.
**Examples:** Some species of **Asteraceae** and **grasses.**

**(2) Polyembryony:** Some of the nucellar cells around the embryo sac start dividing, protrude into the embryo sac and develop into the embryos. Many embryos are developed in a single ovule. Presence of more than one embryo in a seed is referred to as polyembryony.
Examples: **Citrus** and **mango.**

- **Importance of apomixis in hybrid seed industry**

(a) Use of Hybrid varieties of our food and vegetable crops has tremendously increased productivity but there are some disadvantages:

(i) Hybrid seeds have to be produced every year because the seeds produced by the hybrids if sown, do not maintain hybrid characters in the progeny.

(ii) Production of hybrid seeds is costly.

(b) If these hybrid seeds are made by apomixis, there will be no segregation of characters in the hybrid progeny. Thus the farmers can use the hybrid seeds year after year instead of buying them every year. This proves the importance of apomixis in hybrid seed industry.

# PRACTICE EXERCISES

**Direction:** Read the question carefully and choose the correct option for each.

## Multiple Choice Questions: Level I

### Flower

1. Flowers convey important human feelings such as
   (a) Love and affection (b) Happiness and grief
   (c) Mourning (d) All of these
2. Flowers are considered as objects of
   (a) Aesthetic value
   (b) Ornamental value
   (c) Religious and cultural value
   (d) All of these
3. Biologists consider flowers to be objects of
   (a) Morphological marvels
   (b) Embryological marvels
   (c) Sites of sexual reproduction
   (d) All of these
4. When does plant decides to flower?
   (a) In embryonic development
   (b) During the appearance of flower buds
   (c) Before the actual flower appear on plant
   (d) All the above
5. Identify the parts A to E in this figure.

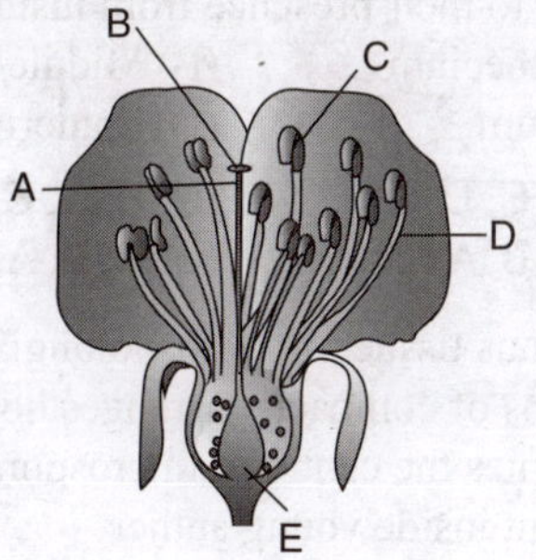


   (a) A: Style, B: Stigma, C: Petal, D: anther, D: Filament, E: Ovary
   (b) A: Stigma, B: Style, C: Anther, D: Filament, E: Ovary
   (c) A: Style, B: Stigma, C: Anther, D: Petal, E: Ovule
   (d) A: Style, B: Stigma, C: Anther, D: Filament, E: Ovary
6. The initiation and development of floral primordium takes place by
   (a) Only by hormonal changes in plant
   (b) Only structural changes in plant
   (c) Changes in seasonal variation
   (d) Both by hormonal and structural changes in plant
7. Whorl of stamens in flower represents
   (a) Gynoecium (b) Androecium
   (c) Calyx (d) Corolla
8. Whorl of carpel in flower represents
   (a) Gynoecium (b) Androecium
   (c) Calyx (d) Corolla
9. Whorl of petals in flower represents
   (a) Gynoecium (b) Androecium
   (c) Calyx (d) Corolla
10. Whorl of sepals in flower represents
   (a) Androecium (b) Gynoecium
   (c) Calyx (d) Corolla

### Male Reproductive Organ

11. Identify A, B, C and D in this figure?

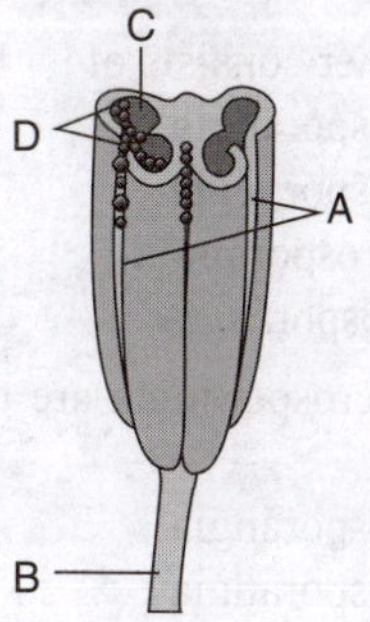


   (a) A: Pollen grains, B: Filament (Stalk), C: Line of dehiscence, D: Pollen sacs
   (b) A: Line of dehiscence, B: Filament (Stalk), C: Pollen sacs, D: Pollen grains
   (c) A: Filament (Stalk), B: Pollen grains, C: Line of dehiscence, D: Pollen sacs
   (d) A: Line of dehiscence, B: Pollen sacs, C: Pollen grains, D: Filament (Stalk)
12. What indicates 'A' in the below figure?

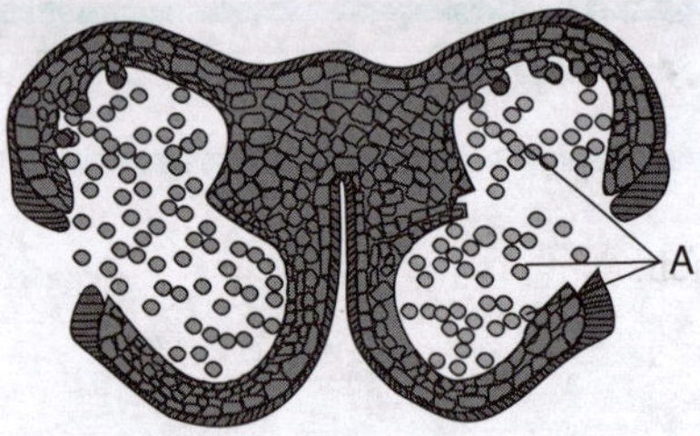


(a) Pollen grains (b) Pollen sacs
(c) Generative cell (d) Vacuoles

**13.** Stamens consists of which of the following parts?
(a) Filament (b) Style, stigma
(c) Anther (d) Both (a) and (c)

**14.** The number and length of stamens in flowers are
(a) Variable in different species.
(b) Same in plants present in similar climatic condition.
(c) Variable and dependent on the amount of hormonal secretion.
(d) Variable in different species and depend on the seasonal variation.

**15.** Typical angiosperm anther is
(a) Unilobed and dithecous
(b) Bilobed and dithecous
(c) May be both (a) and (b)
(d) Bilobed and tetrathecous

**16.** The anther in transverse section appears to be
(a) Diagonal (b) Tetragonal
(c) Unilobed (d) Mosaic

**17.** Tetragonal anther consists of
(a) One microsporangia
(b) Two microsporangia
(c) Three microsporangia
(d) Four microsporangia

**18.** How many microsporangia are there in each lobe of anther?
(a) One microsporangia
(b) Two microsporangia
(c) Three microsporangia
(d) Four microsporangia

**19.** Pollen sacs develop from
(a) Microspore
(b) Microspore mother cell
(c) Microsporangium
(d) Megaspore

**20.** Typical microsporangium appear ______ in transverse section.
(a) Wavy (b) Circular
(c) Oval (d) Irregular

**21.** Which one amongst the given perform the function of protection in typical microsporangium?
(A) Epidermis (B) Endothecium
(C) Tapetum (D) Middle layer
(a) A and B (b) A and C
(c) A and D (d) A, B and D

**22.** Which of the following layer of microsporangium provides nourishment to the developing anther?
(a) Middle layers (b) Tapetum
(c) Endothecium (d) Epidermis

**23.** Function performed by the outer three layers of microsporangium?
(a) Protection to developing pollen
(b) Provides nourishment to developing pollen
(c) Helps in the dehiscence of anther to release pollen
(d) Both (a) and (c)

**24.** The microsporangium cells which posses d ense cytoplasm and have more than one nucleus is the characteristic of
(a) Middle layers (b) Tapetum
(c) Endothecium (d) Epidermis

**25.** In young anther the tissue occupying the centre of each microsporangium is called
(a) Megaspore mother cell
(b) Sporogenous tissue
(c) Parietal tissue
(d) None of these

**26.** Arrange the following layers of microsporangium according to their presence from inside to outside.
(A) Endothecium (B) Middle layer
(C) Tapetum (D) Epidermis
(a) A, B, C, D (b) B, A, C, D
(c) D, C, B, A (d) C, B, A, D

**27.** Sporogenous tissue of microsporangia is
(a) Groups of compactly arranges homogenous cells
(b) Occupies the centre of microsporangium
(c) Present inside young anther
(d) All the above

**28.** Each cell of microspore tetrad is
(a) 2n (b) n
(c) Some n and some 2n (d) 3n

**29.** Which type of cell division occurs in the cell of sporogenous tissue to form microspore?
(a) Reduction division
(b) Equational division
(c) Both (a) and (b)
(d) Amitosis

**30.** Formation of pollen from pollen mother cell is referred to as
(a) Pollenogenesis
(b) Megasporogenesis
(c) Microsporogenesis
(d) Ovulation

**31.** Pollen grains are
(a) Microspore tetrad
(b) Dehydrated microspores
(c) Megaspore tetrad
(d) Pollen mother cells

**32.** Male gametophyte in angiosperm is represented by
(a) Anther (b) Androecium
(c) Microsporangium (d) Pollen grain

**33.** Pollen grains are
(a) Spherical (b) Oval
(c) Generally spherical (d) Irregular

**34.** Diameter of pollen grain is
(a) 20–50 μm (b) 25–50 μm
(c) 30–50 μm (d) 10–50 μm

**35.** Exine of pollen is
(A) Hard outer layer of pollen grain
(B) Most resistant organic matter known.
(C) Layer made up of sporopollenin.
(D) Layer which can withstand high temperature, strong acids and alkali.
(E) Layer which cannot be degraded by any known enzyme.

Which one of the following is correct?
(a) A and B (b) A, B, C and D
(c) A, B, C, D and E (d) A, C and E

**36.** What are the parts A and B in this figure?

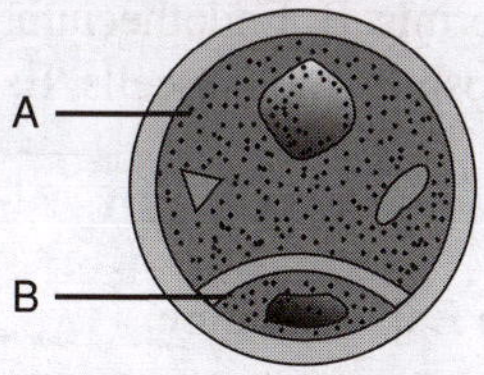


(a) A: Generative cell, B: Vegetative cell
(b) A: Tapetal cell, B: Generative cell
(c) A: Vegetative cell, B: Generative cell
(d) A: Homogenous cell, B: Tapetal cell

**37.** Sporopollenin is
(a) Most resistant organic matter known
(b) Present in exine of pollen grain
(c) Absent in the germ pole of pollen grain
(d) All of these

**38.** Pollen grains can be preserved as fossil because
(a) They vary from species to species
(b) They have variety of architecture
(c) They are made up of sporopollenin
(d) They exhibit a fascinating array of pattern and design

**39.** Which part of pollen exhibit a fascination array of pattern and design?
(a) Intine (b) Exine
(c) Germ pore (d) None of these

**40.** Intine of pollen grain is
(a) Inner layer of pollen grain
(b) A thin and continuous layer
(c) Made up of cellulose and pectin
(d) All of these

**41.** Pollen grains are mature when
(a) It contains vegetative and generative cell
(b) It contains only single haploid cell
(c) Contains two haploid cell
(d) Both (a) and (c)

**42.** Thin and continuous layer of pollen made up of cellulose and pectin
(a) Intine (b) Exine
(c) Germ pore (d) None of these

**43.** Pollen grains are shed in 2 celled stage in
(a) > 90% Angiosperm plant
(b) < 50% Angiosperm plant
(c) > 60% Angiosperm plant
(d) < 40% Angiosperm plant

**44.** Generate cell floats in the cytoplasm of
(a) Vegetative cell (b) Microspore mother cell
(c) Pollen mother cell (d) Megasporangium

**45.** The bigger cell that receives abundant food and has irregularly shaped nucleus is called
(a) Generative cell (b) Vegetative cell
(c) Germ cell (d) Sperm cell

**46.** The spindle-shaped cell with dense cytoplasm and nucleus in pollen grain is called
(a) Vegetative cell (b) Generative cell
(c) Sperm cell (d) Egg cell

**47.** Match the following

| Column – I | Column – II |
|---|---|
| A. Vegetative cell | 1. Sporopollenin |
| B. Generative cell | 2. Spindle-shaped cell |
| C. Exine | 3. Large sized and has abundant food reserve |
| D. Intine | 4. Cellulose and pectin |

(a) A:1, B:2, C:3, D:4
(b) A:4, B:3, C:2, D:1
(c) A:3, B:2, C:1, D:4
(d) A:2, B:1, C:4, D:3

**48.** Male gametes in angiosperms are formed by
(a) Mitotic division in vegetative cell
(b) Meiotic division in pollen mother cell
(c) Meiotic division in vegetative cell
(d) Mitotic division in generative cell

**49.** The pollen grains are shed in 3 celled stage in
(a) > 60% Angiospermic plant
(b) > 70% Angiospermic plant
(c) < 40% Angiospermic plant
(d) < 20% Angiospermic plant

**50.** Which of the following statement is correct?
(A) Pollen grains are shed in 2-celled stage in > 40% plants.
(B) Pollen grains are shed in 3-celled stage in < 60% plant.
(C) Generative cell divides meiotically to form male gametes.
(D) Intine of pollen is made up of sporopollenin.
(a) A, B, C
(b) All are correct
(c) All are wrong
(d) Only C

**51.** The plant which came in India as a contaminant with imported wheat is?
(a) Vinca
(b) Parthenium
(c) Striga
(d) Orobanche

**52.** Pollen grains
(A) Represent gametophytic phase of plant
(B) Can cause severe allergies like asthma and bronchitis
(C) Are rich in nutrient
(D) Are used as food supplements
(E) Are available in form of tables and syrups in market of western countries
(a) Only A is correct
(b) All are correct
(c) All are wrong
(d) Only A, B and C are correct

**53.** Viability of pollen grains depend upon
(a) A particular species
(b) Prevailing temperature
(c) Humidity
(d) All of the above

**54.** Rice pollen grains are viable for
(a) 6.0 mins
(b) 30 mins (approx)
(c) 60 mins (approx)
(d) 40 mins

**55.** Pollens are stored in
(a) Oxygen (–196°C)
(b) Nitrogen (–196°C)
(c) Oxygen (196°C)
(d) Nitrogen (+196°C)

**56.** The below figure represents

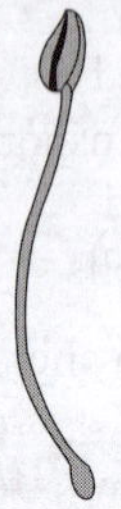

(a) Anther
(b) Typical stamen
(c) Pollen grain
(d) Microsporangium

**57.** What are the parts A, B, C, D and E in the below figure?

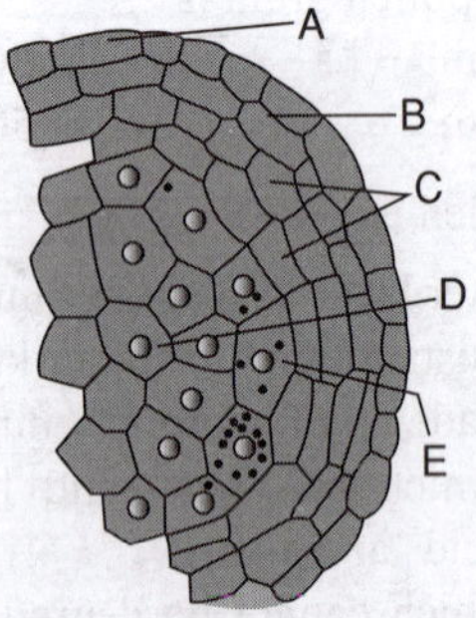


(a) A: Tapetum, B: Middle layers, C: Microspore mother cells, D: Endothecium, E: Epidermis
(b) A: Middle layers, B: Endothecium, C: Tapetum, D: Epidermis, E: Microspore mother cell
(c) A: Endothecium, B: Epidermis, C: Tapetum, D: Endothecium, E: Microspore mother cell
(d) A: Epidermis, B: Endothecium, C: Middle layers, D: Microspore mother cells, E: Tapetum

## Female Reproductive Organ

**58.** Identify A to E in this figure.

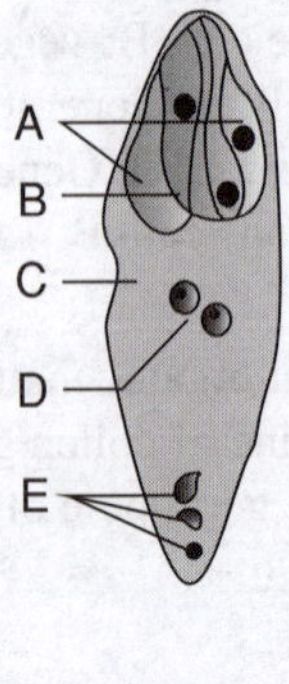

(a) A: Synergids, B: Egg, C: Central cell, D: 2 polar nuclei, E: Antipodals
(b) A: Antipodals, B: Synergids, C: Central cell, D: Egg, E: 2 polar nuclei
(c) A: Synergids, B: Central cell, C: 2 polar nuclei, D: Antipodals, E: Egg
(d) A: Egg, B: 2 polar nuclei, C: Antipodals, D: Central cell, E: Synergids

**59.** Which one of the following is incorrect?
(A) Parthenium or carrot gases causes pollen allergy.
(B) Vegetative cell of pollen has abundant food reserve.
(C) All pollen's cause severe allergies and bronchial afflictions.
(D) Sporopollenin is the most resistant organic matter known.

(a) All are correct (b) A
(c) B (d) C

**60.** Syncarpous condition is referred to as
(a) Gynoecium containing single pistil
(b) More than one pistil fused together
(c) More than one pistil free from one another
(d) Gynoecium containing many pistils

**61.** Landing platform for pollen grains is
(a) Stigma (b) Style
(c) Ovary (d) None of them

**62.** Bulged basal part of pistil is
(a) Stigma (b) Style
(c) Ovary (d) None of these

**63.** Elongated slender part of pistil is
(a) Stigma (b) Style
(c) Ovary (d) None of these

**64.** Megasporangia is referred to as
(a) Ovule (b) Ovary
(c) Gynoecium (d) All of these

**65.** Plants having single ovule in ovary are
(a) Wheat (b) Paddy
(c) Mango (d) All of these

**66.** More than one ovule is found in the ovary of
(a) Wheat (b) Paddy
(c) Papaya (d) None of these

**67.** The stalk attaching ovule to placenta is
(a) Funiculus (b) Hilum
(c) Raphe (d) Chalaza

**68.** The junction between ovule and funiculus is
(a) Placenta (b) Hilum
(c) Raphe (d) Chalaza

**69.** The tips on the ovule where integument are absent are called
(a) Germ pore (b) Micropyle
(c) Both (a) and (b) (d) None of these

**70.** The end opposite to micropyles end is called
(a) Funicle (b) Chalaza
(c) Germ pore (d) Hilum

**71.** The mass of cell present inside the integuments of megasporangium having abundant food reserve is
(a) Ovule (b) Nucellus
(c) Sporogenous cells (d) None of these

**72.** Female gametophyte of angiosperm is referred to as
(a) Megasporangium (b) Megaspore
(c) Embryo sac (d) Nucleus

**73.** Embryo sac is formed by
(a) Reduction division in megaspore
(b) Equational division in megaspore
(c) Reduction division followed by equational division in megaspore mother cell
(d) Both (b) and (c)

**74.** How many embryo sacs are present in an ovule?
(a) One embryo sac
(b) More than one embryo sac
(c) One embryo sac (generally)
(d) Two embryo sacs

**75.** What is functional megaspore referred to as?
(a) The megaspore that degenerates after formation.
(b) The megaspore that only develops in female gametophyte.
(c) The megaspore that undergoes reduction division.
(d) The megaspore that is functionally inactive.

**76.** Identify the parts of A to F in the following figure?

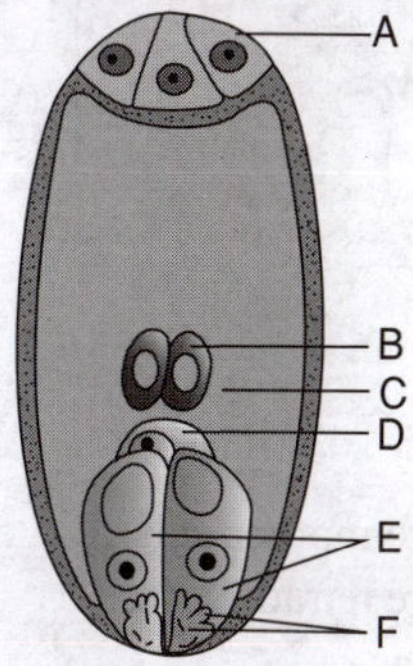


(a) A: Filiform apparatus, B: Polar nuclei, C: Antipodals, D: Synergids, E: Egg, F: Central cell
(b) A: Antipodals, B: Polar nuclei, C: Central cell, D: Egg, E: Synergids, F: Filiform apparatus

(c) A: Antipodals, B: Central cell, C: Polar nuclei, D: Egg, E: Synergids and F: Filiform apparatus
(d) A: Eggs, B: Central cell, C: Filiform apparatus, D: Polar nuclei, E: Antipodals, F: Synergids

**77.** Monosporic development is referred to as
(a) Single megaspore developing in the embryo sac
(b) Single megaspore mother cell undergoing meiosis
(c) Presence of single ovule in ovary
(d) None of them is correct

**78.** What is the ploidy level of nucleus, MMC, functional megaspore and female gametophyte?
(a) 2n, n, 2n, 2n (b) 2n, n, 2n, n
(c) 2n, 2n, n, n (d) n, 2n, n, n

**79.** How many mitotic division takes place for complete development of embryo sac?
(a) 4 (b) 3
(c) 2 (d) 1

**80.** The inside three mitotic division which occurs in the megaspore are
(a) Followed by cytoplasmic division immediately.
(b) Strictly free nuclear not immediately followed by cell wall formation.
(c) Wall formation occurs after the completion of the second mitosis.
(d) Wall formation will never occur.

**81.** Typical female gametophyte is
(a) 7-celled 8 nucleate
(b) 6-celled 8 nucleate
(c) 4-celled 6 nucleate
(d) 5-celled 6 nucleate

**82.** What is 'A' in this figure?

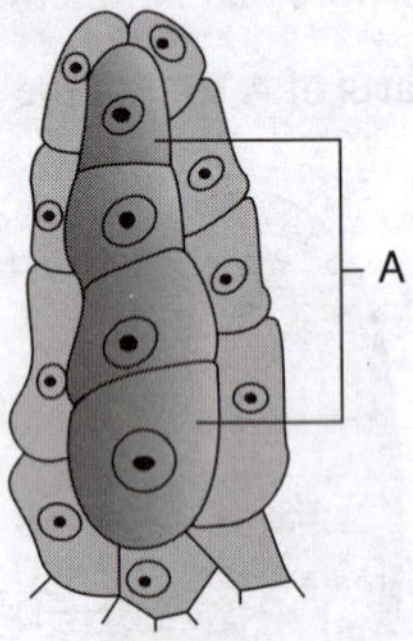


(a) Megaspore mother cell
(b) Megaspore tetrad
(c) Embryo sac
(d) Micropyle

**83.** Egg apparatus consists of
(a) Two synergids (b) Two antipodals
(c) Egg cell (d) Both (a) and (c)

**84.** The cellular thickening at the tip of micropyle is
(a) Synergids (b) Egg apparatus
(c) Filiform apparatus (d) All of these

**85.** The cells located at chalazal ends are called as
(a) Synergids (b) Antipodals
(c) Egg apparatus (d) None of these

**86.** Identify the parts A and B in this figure.

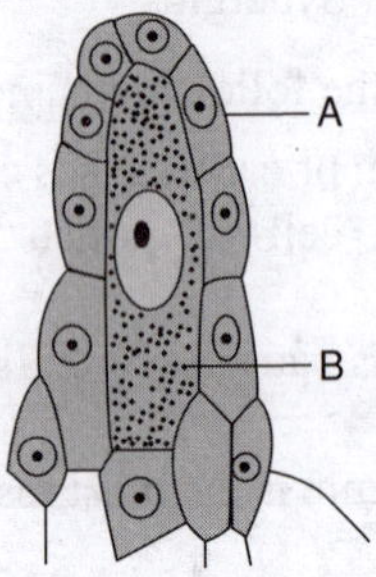


(a) A: Megaspore tetrad, B: Nucleus
(b) A: Central cell, B: Megaspore dyad
(c) A: Nucellus, B: Megaspore mother cell
(d) A: Nucellus, B: Central cell

**87.** The central cell
(a) Contains two haploid nuclei
(b) Has two polar nuclei
(c) Located in the centre of embryo sac
(d) All of these

**88.** The cells in embryo sac located at the micropyles end are
(a) Egg apparatus (b) Only synergid
(c) Antipodal cell (d) Central cell

**89.** The male and female gametes of angiosperm are respectively
(a) Motile, non-motile
(b) Non-motile, motile
(c) Motile, motile
(d) Non-motile, non-motile

**90.** After three mitotic divisions in the functional megaspore, the gametophyte (embryosac)has how many cells.
(a) 7 cells (b) 4 cells
(c) 5 cells (d) 8 cells

**91.** What indicates 'A' in the below figure?

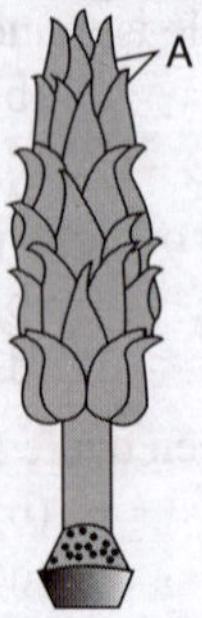

(a) Pericarp (b) Scutellum
(c) Carpels (d) Radicle

**92.** Identify A and B in this figure.

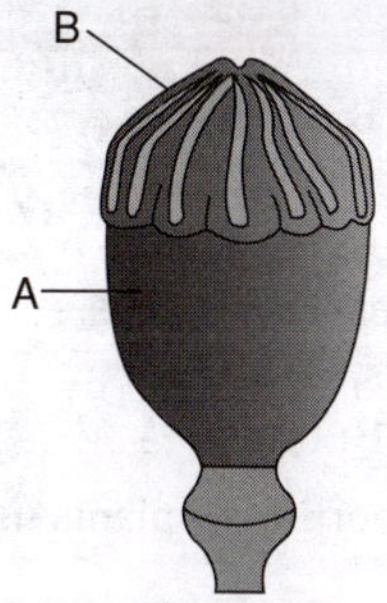


(a) A: Ovary, B: Syncarpous ovary
(b) A: Filament, B: Ovary
(c) A: Stigma, B: Filament
(d) A: Syncarpous ovary, B: Stigma

**93.** What are A, B, C and D in this figure?

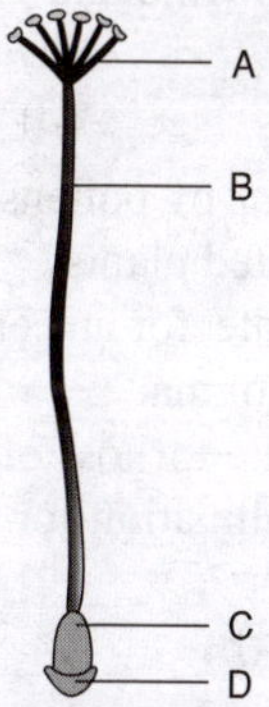


(a) A: Thalamus, B: Style, C: Ovary, D: Stigma
(b) A: Style, B: Ovary, C: Stigma, D: Thalamus
(c) A: Stigma, B: Style, C: Ovary, D: Thalamus
(d) A: Ovary, B: Stigma, C: Thalamus, D: Style

## Pollination

**94.** The below figure represents

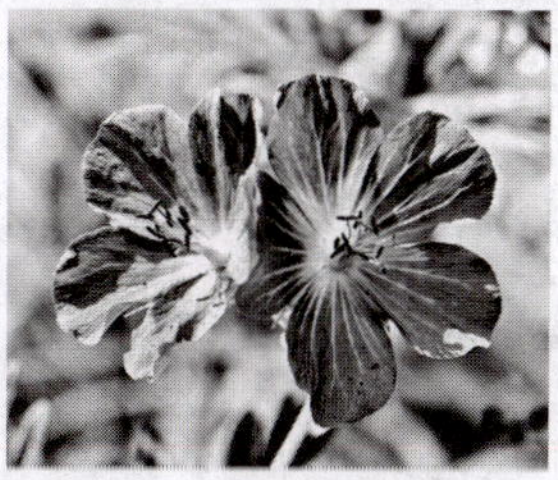

(a) Self-pollinated flowers
(b) Cross-pollinated flowers
(c) Chasmogamous
(d) None of these

**95.** The below figure represents

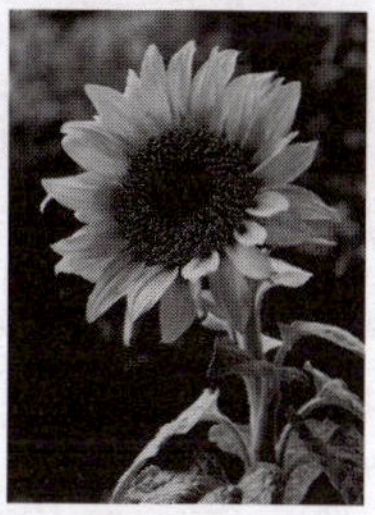

(a) Self-pollinated flowers
(b) Cross-pollinated flowers
(c) Cleistogamous flowers
(d) None of these

**96.** What are A and B in this figure?

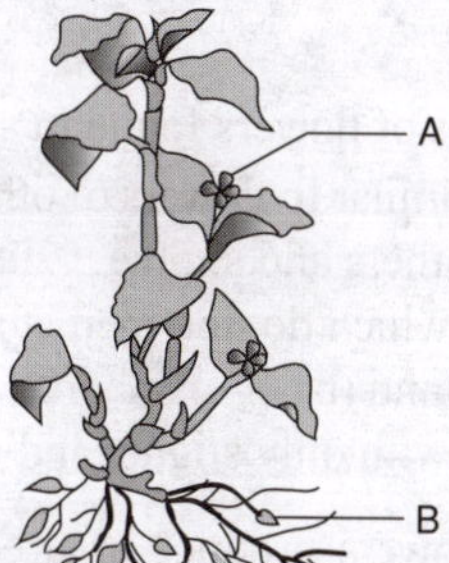


(a) A: Chasmogamous flower, B: Cleistogamous flower
(b) A: Cleistogamous flower, B: Chasmogamous flower
(c) A: Chasmogamous flower, B: Chasmogamous flower
(d) A: Cleistogamous flower, B: Self-pollinated flower

**97.** Pollination is essential in angiosperm plants because
(a) It decreases the time required for fertilization.
(b) Both of the male and female gametes are non-motile and they need to be brought together for fertilization.
(c) It is a useless process
(d) Both (a) and (b)

**98.** Pollination in plants is referred to as
(a) Fusion of male and female gametes.
(b) Transfer of pollen grain to stigma of pistil.
(c) Germination of pollen of stigma.
(d) Production of pollen grew inside the micro-sporangium.

**99.** Autogamy refers to
(a) Transfer of pollen grain to stigma of another flower
(b) Transfer of pollen grain to stigma of same flower
(c) Both (a) and (B)
(d) None of these

**100.** What is observed in a normal flower which opens and exposes the stigma and anther?
(a) Autogamy is absent
(b) Complete autogamy is rare
(c) Always autogamous
(d) Always xenogamous

**101.** Plants which produce two types of flowers are
(a) Viola
(b) Oxalis
(c) Commelina
(d) All of these

**102.** The two types of flowers found in autogamous plant is
(a) Flower similar to flowers of other species with exposed anthers and stigma.
(b) Flowers which do not open at all.
(c) Both (a) and (b)
(d) Flowers with only stigma and no anther.

**103.** ________ flowers produce assured seed set even in the absence of pollinators
(a) Cleistogamous flower
(b) Chasmogamous flowers
(c) Both (a) and (b)
(d) Flowers showing geitonogamy

**104.** A type of cross pollination involving a pollinating agent is genetically similar to autogamy since pollen grain come from same plant, it is called
(a) Xenogamy
(b) Geitonogamy
(c) Autogamy
(d) All of these

**105.** The only type of pollination during which pollination brings genetically different types of pollen grains to stigma
(a) Xenogamy (b) Geitonogamy
(c) Autogamy (d) All of these

**106.** Majority of plants uses which types of pollinating agents?
(a) Biotic
(b) Abiotic
(c) Both (a) and (b)
(d) None of these

**107.** What are A and B in the following figure?

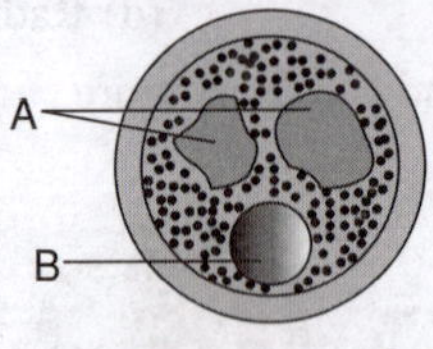


(a) A: Vacuoles, B: Intine
(b) A: Vacuoles, B: Nucleus
(c) A: Nucleus, B: Intine
(d) A: Exine, B: Intine

**108.** ________ proportion of plants uses abiotic agents for pollination.
(a) Major
(b) Most
(c) Small
(d) Can be small or major

**109.** ________ factor is responsible for the contact of pollen with stigma in wind and water pollinated plants.
(a) Luck (b) Chance
(c) Time (d) Temperature

**110.** Enormous amount of pollens are produced in wind and water pollinated plants
(a) To compensate for uncertainties for contact of pollen with stigma.
(b) To compensate for loss of pollen grains.
(c) To ensure pollination for large number of ovules present.
(d) Both (a) and (b)

**111.** Most of the common abiotic pollinating agent for plant is
(a) Anemophily
(b) Hydrophily
(c) Pollination by bees
(d) Pollination by ants

**112.** Light and non-sticky pollen grains are favourable for
(a) Water pollinated plant
(b) Wind pollinated plant
(c) Plants with fatherly sigma
(d) Both (a) and (c)

**113.** Which of the following are true for wind pollinated plants?
(A) Well exposed statements
(B) Large and often feathery stigma
(C) Single ovule in each ovary
(D) Large number of flower packed into an inflorosence
(a) Only A (b) Only B and C
(c) Only C (d) All are correct

**114.** Wind pollinated flowers have
(a) Single ovule in one ovary
(b) More than one ovule in ovary
(c) Been packed into an inflorosence
(d) Both (a) and (c)

**115.** The tassels of corn cob are
(a) Stigma and style
(b) Meant to trap pollen grains in wind
(c) Both (a) and (b)
(d) All are incorrect

**116.** Wind pollination is commonly found in
(a) Large trees (b) Shrubs
(c) Grasses (d) All of these

**117.** Pollination by water is
(a) Rare in flowering plants
(b) Limited to about 30 genera
(c) Most of the genera are monocotyledons
(d) All the above

**118.** Water is the main medium of transport for male gametes of
(a) Algae (b) Bryophytes
(c) Pteridophyte (d) All of these

**119.** The distribution of pteridophytes and bryophytes is limited to some geographical zones only
(a) Because their spores can germinate in only specific kind of soil only.
(b) Because they require water for fertilization.
(c) Because they have only specific pollination which are available in narrow geographical range.
(d) Only some weather conditions permit fruit formation in them.

**120.** Which of the following is incorrect for aquatic plants?
(A) Vallisneria and Hydrilla are fresh water plants pollinated by wind.
(B) Zostera a marine grass uses water as its pollinating agent.
(C) Water hyacinth and water lily are pollinated by insects or wind.
(D) Most of the aquatic plant flowers emerges out of water and are pollinated by wind or insects.
(a) Only B (b) Only A
(c) Only A, B and C (d) All are incorrect

**121.** Which one of the following is correct for aquatic plants?
(a) All aquatic plants use water for pollination.
(b) Not all aquatic plants use water for pollination.
(c) Vallisneria flowers are pollinated by water under the water surface.
(d) All the above

**122.** Which one of the following is correct for Vallisneria?
(A) It grows in fresh water.
(B) Female flowers or pollen grains reach the surface by long stalk.
(C) Male flowers are released on to the surface of water.
(D) Pollen grains are carried passively by water currents.
(a) Only A (b) Only A and B
(c) Only A, B and C (d) A, B, C and D

**123.** In water pollinated species
(A) Pollen grains are long and ribbon like
(B) All pollen grains are protected from getting wet
(C) Flowers are not very colourful
(D) They do not produce nectar
(a) Only A and B are correct
(b) Only A and B are wrong
(c) All are correct
(d) All are wrong

**124.** Amongst the pollinating agent which one is the most dominant?
(a) Butterflies and flies (b) Bees
(c) Beetles and wasps (d) Moths and birds

**125.** Which of the following is correct in reference to animal pollinated plants?
(a) Butterflies, flies, beetles, wasps, ants, moths and bats are common pollinating agents.
(b) Rodents, lizards and primates are also pollinators in some species.
(c) Animal pollinated plants are specifically adapted for particular species.
(d) All the above

**126.** What are the parts A, B, C, D and E in this figure?

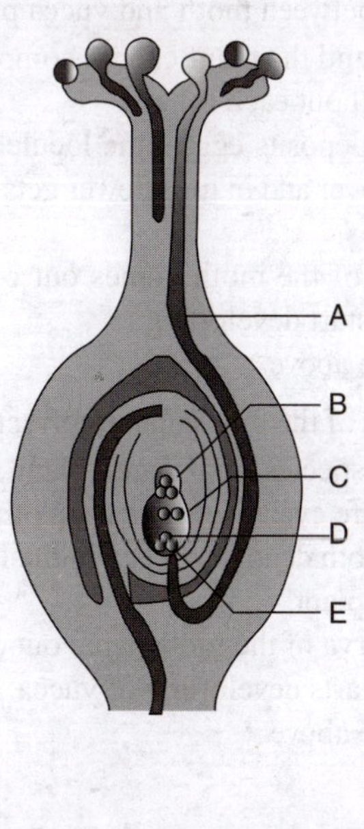

(a) A: Egg cell, B: Synergid, C: Antipodal, D: Polar nuclei, E: Pollen tube
(b) A: Pollen tube, B: Antipodal, C: Polar nuclei, D: Egg cell, E: Synergid
(c) A: Pollen tube, B: Egg cell, C: Polar nuclei, D: Antipodal, E: Synergid
(d) A: Synergid, B: Pollen tube, C: Egg cell, D: Antipodal, E: Polar nuclei

**127.** Insect pollinated plants are
(a) Large and colourful (b) Fragrant
(c) Rich in nectar (d) All of these

**128.** The foul odour secreted by flowers are pollinated by
(a) Flies and beetles (b) Wasps and ants
(c) Birds (d) None of these

**129.** The reward produced by plants to their animal visitors is in the form of
(a) Nectar (b) Pollen grain
(c) Both (a) and (b) (d) None of these

**130.** Which one of the following is correct for animal pollinated plants?
(a) Nectar and pollen grains are usual floral rewards.
(b) To harvest the rewards from the flower, animal come in contact with anther and stigma.
(c) Animal carrying pollen when come in contact with stigma, it brings about pollination.
(d) All the above

**131.** Amorphophallus provide floral rewards in the form of
(a) Providing safe place to lay eggs
(b) Tallest flower
(c) Both (a) and (b)
(d) None of these

**132.** Which of the following is correct for the relationship existence between moth and yucca plant?
(a) Moth and the plant cannot complete their life cycle without each other.
(b) Moth deposits egg in the locule of the ovary and the flower and in turn flower gets pollinated by the moth.
(c) Larva of the moth comes out of the eggs as the seeds start developing.
(d) All the above

**133.** Which one of the following is correct for yucca plant?
(a) Moth species and yucca plant cannot complete their life cycles without each other.
(b) The moth deposits in egg in the locule of ovary of yucca plant.
(c) The larva of the moth came out of the eggs as the seed starts developing of yucca
(d) All the above

**134.** The devices developed by plants to discourage self-pollination include
(A) In some species, the pollen release and receptive stigma are not synchronized.
(B) In some species, the anther and stigma are placed at different positions, so they do not come in contact.
(C) Self-incompatibility
(a) All are correct (b) A and B only
(c) A only (d) B only

**135.** Dioecy is the mechanism for some plants to
(a) Promote autogamy
(b) Promote self-fertilization
(c) Promote cross pollination
(d) All are incorrect

**136.** In Castor and maize plant, flowers are
(a) Unisexual
(b) Both male and female flowers on same plants (monoecious)
(c) Both male and female flowers on different plants
(d) All are incorrect

**137.** Autogamy and geitonogamy is absent in
(a) Papaya (b) Maize
(c) Castor (d) All are correct

**138.** The pollen pistil interaction refers to
(a) Pistil's ability to recognize the pollen
(b) Acceptance of pollen to promote post-pollination events
(c) Both are incorrect
(d) Both (a) and (b) are correct

**139.** The acceptance and rejection by continuous dialogue between pollen grain and pistil mediated by chemical components of pollen and pistil result in
(a) Autogamy (b) Pollen pistil interaction
(c) Geitonogamy (d) Pollination

**140.** During pollen pistil the interaction chemical components are released from
(a) Only pollen
(b) Only pistil
(c) Both pollen and pistil
(d) The ovary

**141.** What happens when the pollen falls on the stigma?
(a) Pollination
(b) Reject of pollen
(c) Only the compatible pollen germinates
(d) Autogamy

**142.** The pore from which the pollen tube germinates
(a) Seed pore (b) Germ pore
(c) Intine (d) Exine

**143.** Which way of pollen to ovary is sequentially correct?
(a) Ovary → Style → Stigma
(b) Style → Stigma → Ovary
(c) Stigma → Ovary → Style
(d) Stigma → Style → Ovary

**144.** During pollination in plants which shed pollens in 2-celled stage, the cells are called as
(a) Two vegetative cell
(b) Two generative cell
(c) Both are correct
(d) One vegetative and one generative cell

**145.** Generative cell in pollen tube divides and forms
(a) One male gamete (b) Two male gamete
(c) Three male gamete (d) Four male gamete

**146.** The plants in which pollen are shed in 3-celled stage contain?
(a) Two male gametes only
(b) A large vegetative cell only
(c) Both (a) and (b)
(d) None of these

**147.** The knowledge of pollen pistil interaction is helpful to plant breeders in which manner?
(a) Manipulating pollen-pistil interaction
(b) To get desired hybrids in incompatible pollination
(c) None of them
(d) Both (a) and (b) are correct

**148.** Which one of the following is correct for artificial hybridization?
(A) Combine desirable characters to produce superior varieties.
(B) Approach towards crop improvement programme.
(C) Desired pollen grains are used for pollination.
(D) Stigma is exposed to receive pollen.
(a) All are correct (b) Only A
(c) Only A and B (d) Only A, B and C

**149.** Artificial hybridization is achieved by
(a) Emasculation (b) Bagging
(c) Both are required (d) None of these

**150.** Emasculation is
(a) Removal of anther from unisexual flowering using a pair of forceps.
(b) Removal of anther from flower bud after its dehisces using a pair of forceps.
(c) Removal of anther from bisexual flower bud before its dehisces using a pair of forceps.
(d) All the above

**151.** Emasculated flowers are covered with a bag of suitable size; the process is referred to as
(a) Emasculation (b) Bagging
(c) Both (a) and (b) (d) None of these

**152.** Why bagging is done in an emasculated flower?
(a) To prevent contamination of its stigma with unwanted pollen.
(b) To pollinate the stigma with required anthers only.
(c) Both (a) and (b)
(d) None of these

**153.** For artificial hybridization purpose which flowers of female plant is emasculated.
(a) Only having pistil (unisexual)
(b) Having both pistil and anthers (bisexual)
(c) Having only anthers (unisexual)
(d) All are correct

**154.** The female parent plants produce unisexual flowers
(a) Do not require emasculation
(b) Requires emasculation
(c) The flowers are bagged during bud stage
(d) Both (a) and (c)

## Fertilization and Post Fertilization Events

**155.** Label A, B, C, D and E in the below Figure?

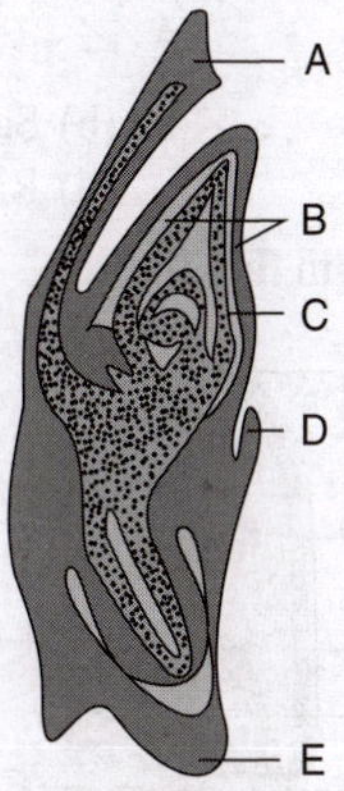


(a) A: Scutellum, B: Coleoptile, C: Shoot apex, D: Epiblast, E: Coleorhiza
(b) A: Radicle, B: shoot apex, C: Shoot apex, D: Epiblast , E:Coleorhiza
(c) A: Scutellum, B: Coleoptile, C: Shoot apex, D: Epiblast, E: Coleorhiza
(d) A: Epiblast, B: Coleoptile, C: Shoot apex, D: Root cap, E: Coleorhiza

**156.** What are parts A to E in this below figure?

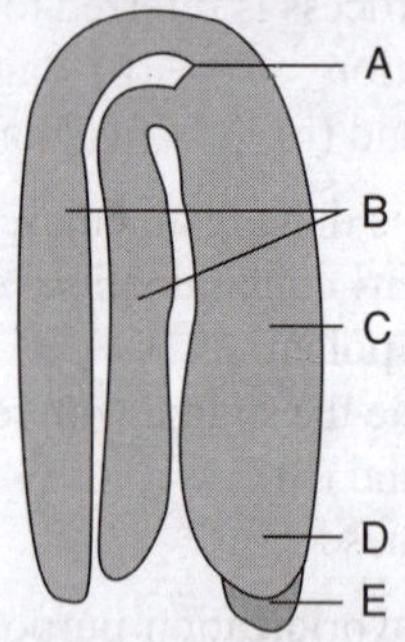


(a) A: Plumule, B: Cotyledons, C: Hypocotyl, D: Radicle, E: Root cap
(b) A: Root cap, B: Hypocotyl, C: Plumule, D: Radicle, E: Cotyledons
(c) A: Cotyledons, B: Root cap, C: Cotyledons, D: Plumule, E: Hypocotyl
(d) A: Plumule, B: Cotyledons, C: Root cap, D: Radicle, E: Hypocotyl

**157.** What represents 'A' in the following figure?

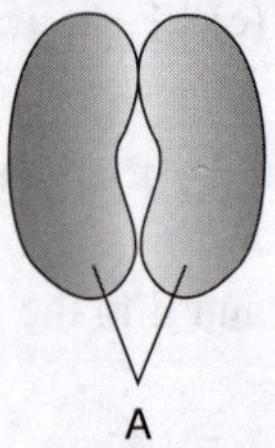


(a) Cotyledons (b) Scutellum
(c) Shoot apex (d) Radicle

**158.** Identify A to G in this figure.

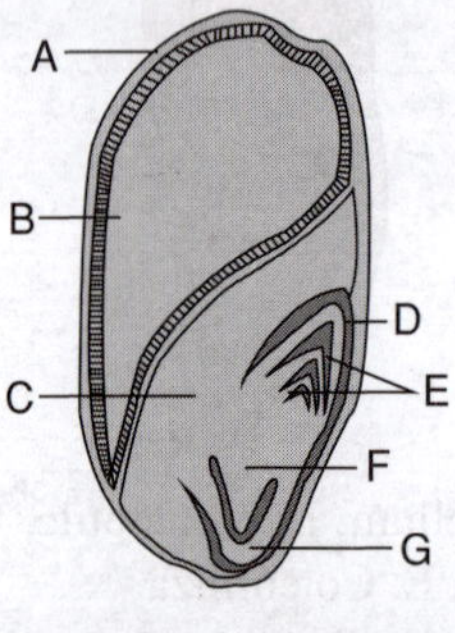


(a) A: Plumule, B: Endosperm, C: Pericarp, D: Radicle, E: Coleorhiza, F: Scutellum,G: Coleoptile
(b) A: Coleorhiza, B: Radicle, C: Endosperm, D: Pericarp, E: Plumule, F: Coleoptile,G: Scutellum
(c) A: Pericarp, B: Scutellum, C: Endosperm, D: Coleoptile, E: Plumule, F: Coleorhiza,G: Radicle
(d) A: Pericarp, B: Endosperm, C: Scutellum, D: Coleoptile, E: Plumule, F: Radicle,G: Coleorhiza

**159.** Identify A and B in this figure.

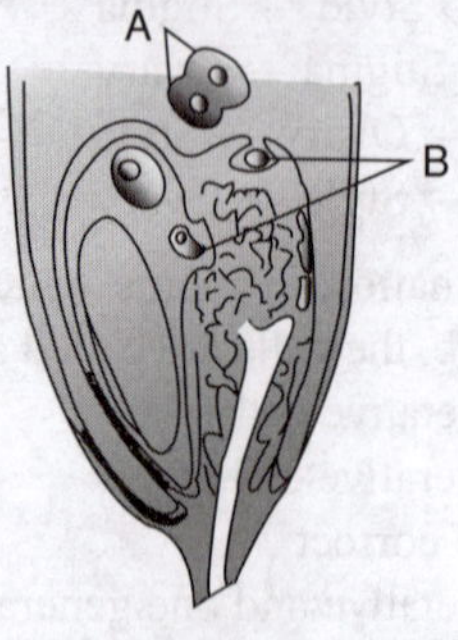


(a) A: Polar nuclei, B: Male gametes
(b) A: Female gametes, B: Polar nuclei
(c) A: Synergid, B: Egg cell
(d) A: Male gametes, B: Synergid

**160.** What indicates A, B, C and D in the below figure?

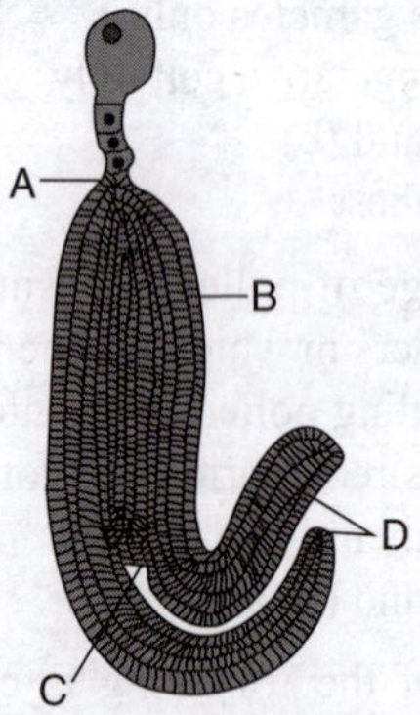


(a) A: Radicle, B: Plumule, C: Cotyledon, D: Suspensor
(b) A: Plumule, B: Suspensor, C: Radicle, D: Cotyledon
(c) A: Suspensor, B: Radicle, C: Plumule, D: Cotyledon
(d) A: Cotyledon, B: Suspensor, C: Cotyledon, D: Radicle

**161.** Seed is
(a) Fertilized ovule
(b) Fertilized endosperm
(c) Modification of integument
(d) Formed from pericarp

**162.** Typical seed consists of
(a) Seed coat (b) Cotyledon
(c) Embryo axis (d) All of these

**163.** All are examples of albuminous seeds except
(a) Wheat (b) Sunflower
(c) Castor (d) Groundnut

**164.** The following figure represents

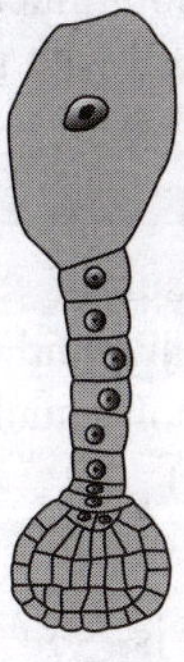

(a) Globular embryo (b) Heart-shaped embryo
(c) Zygote (d) Syngamy

**165.** Persistent nucellus perisperm is found in
(a) Wheat and maize (b) Pea + ground nut
(c) Barley and castor (d) Black paper + bect

**166.** Wheat is the ploidy of perisperm
(a) n (b) 2n
(c) 3n (d) 4n

**167.** Select the total number of albuminous seed from the following.
*Pea, Groundnut, Wheat, Maize, Barely, Castor, Sunflower*
(a) 4 (b) 5
(c) 2 (d) 6

**168.** Mature seed contains how much moisture generally?
(a) 10–15% by mass (b) 5–10% by mass
(c) 25–30% by mass (d) 40% by mass

**169.** Select the false statement from the following.
(a) Persistent nucellus is the perisperm.
(b) Integuments of ovule harden as though protective seed coat.
(c) Micropyle remains as a small pore in seed coat and facilitates the entry of oxygen and water into seed during germination.
(d) General metabolic activity of embryo is high.

**170.** The favourable conditions available for germination are
(a) Adequate moisture
(b) Oxygen
(c) Suitable temperature
(d) All of these

**171.** Example of false fruit
(a) Apple (b) Strawberry
(c) Cashew (d) All of these

**172.** Thalamus takes part in fruit formation in
(a) Guava (b) Orange
(c) Strawberry (d) Mango

**173.** Identify the parts A, B, C and D in this figure.

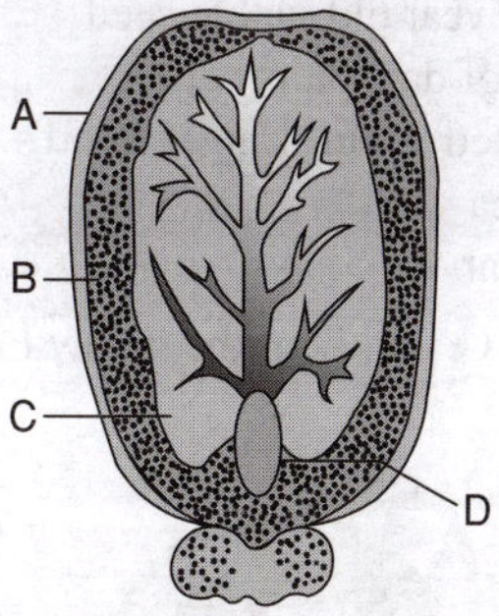


(a) A: Seed coat, B: Endosperm, C: Cotyledon, D: Hypocotyl root axis
(b) A: Cotyledon, B: Seed coat, C: Hypocotyl root axis, D: Endosperm
(c) A: Endosperm, B: Cotyledon, C: Seed coat, D: Hypocotyl root axis
(d) A: Hypocotyl root axis, B: Endosperm, C: Seed coat, D: Cotyledon

**174.** Which of the following is an example of dry fruit?
(a) Groundnut (b) Mustard
(c) Both (a) and (b) (d) Mango

**175.** Fruit develops from
(a) Sepals (b) Petals
(c) Thalamus (d) Ovary

**176.** Fruit developed without fertilization is known as
(a) Parthenocarpy (b) Amphimixis
(c) Apomixis (d) Polyembryony

**177.** Which is true about parthenocarpic fruit?
(a) Seedless
(b) Banana is an example
(c) Can be induced by growth hormones
(d) All of these

**178.** Select the false statement.
(a) Hard seed coat provides protection to young embryo.
(b) Generally seed is the product of sexual reproduction, so they generate new genetic combination leading to variation.
(c) Seeds have better adaptive strategies for dispersal to new habitat and help the species to colonize in other areas.
(d) Pollination and fertilization in angiosperm depend on water.

**179.** Which oldest seed is excavated from Arctic Tundra?
(a) Lupin arcticus
(b) Phoenix dactylitera
(c) Solanum nigrum
(d) Raphanus sativus

**180.** Phoenix dactylifera is
(a) A 2000 year old viable seed
(b) A type of date palm
(c) Excavated from king Herod's palace near the Dead sea
(d) All the above

**181.** Label A, B, C, and D in the below Figure?

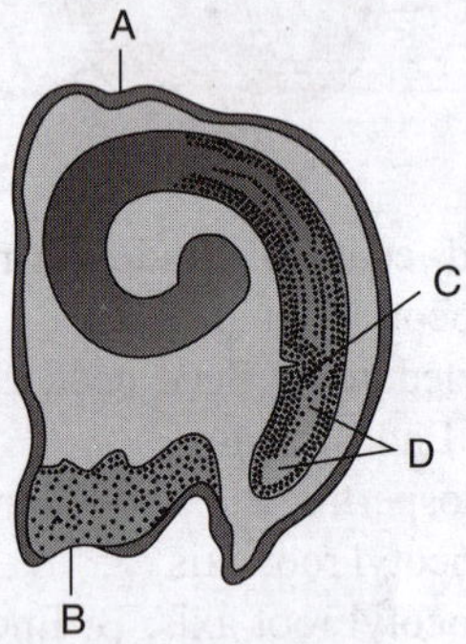


(a) A: seed coat, B: Endosperm, C: Shoot apical meristem, D: Hypocotyl root axis
(b) A: Endosperm, B: seed coat, C: Shoot apical meristem, D: Hypocotyl root axis
(c) A: Endosperm, B: Endosperm, C: Shoot apical meristem, D: Hypocotyl shoot axis
(d) A: seed coat, B: Endosperm, C: apical meristem, D: seed coat

**182.** What indicates 'A' in the following figure?

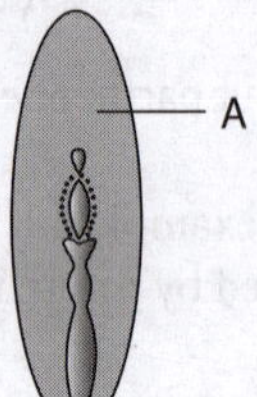


(a) Micropyle (b) Cotyledon
(c) Endosperm (d) Scutellum

**183.** The pollen tube after reaching the ovary enters inside the ovule generally through which part of ovule?
(a) Chalazal end (b) Micropyle end
(c) Any of these (d) Integument of ovule

**184.** The pollen enters one of the synergids through
(a) Micropyles end (b) Filiform apparatus
(c) Integument (d) Both (a) and (b)

**185.** During syngamy
(a) Male gamete fuses with two polar nuclear
(b) Male gamete fuses with egg cell
(c) Both (a) and (b)
(d) None of these

**186.** Primary endosperm nucleus is a result of
(a) Fusion of two polar nuclei with male gamete
(b) Fusion of egg cell with male gamete
(c) Both (a) and (b)
(d) None of these

**187.** Triple fusion is a result of
(a) Fusion of three haploid nuclei
(b) Fusion of two polar nuclei with male gamete
(c) Both (a) and (b)
(d) None of these

**188.** Double fertilization is
(A) Unique to flowering plant
(B) Results in formation of zygote and primary endosperm cell.
(C) A process in which triple fusion and syngamy takes place.
(D) A process in which triple fusion only takes place.
(a) Only A and B (b) Only A, B and C
(c) All are correct (d) Only A

**189.** Triple fusion results in ________ while syngamy results in ________.
(a) Zygote and endosperm
(b) Endosperm and zygote
(c) Both form of zygote
(d) Both fern endosperm

**190.** Endosperm is a product of ________ and embryo is a product of ________.
(a) Triple fusion, syngamy
(b) Syngamy, triple fusion
(c) Syngamy, Syngamy
(d) Triple fusion, Triple fusion

**191.** Post-fertilization events do not include
(A) Formation of primary endosperm cell
(B) Maturation of ovules in seed
(C) Formation of ovary into fruit
(D) Formation of embryo inside seed
(a) Only A (b) Only B
(c) Only C (d) None of these

**192.** Which of the following precedes the other?
(a) Development of embryo before endosperm
(b) Endosperm developing before embryo
(c) Both the development of embryo and endosperm occurs simultaneously
(d) All the above

**193.** Which one of the following is correct for endosperm?
(a) The cells of this tissue are filled with reserve food material.
(b) Used for nutrition of developing embryo.

(c) PEN undergoes nuclear division followed by cytokinesis.
(d) All the above

**194.** Endosperm is earlier ________ and then develops into ________
(a) cellular, nuclear (b) nuclear, cellular
(c) cellular, cellular (d) nuclear, nuclear

**195.** The number of nuclei in free nuclear endosperm before cellularization is
(a) Fixed (b) Varies greatly
(c) Fixed in species (d) None of these

**196.** Coconut water is ________ part of endosperm
(a) Cellular
(b) Free nuclear
(c) Cellular as well as nuclear
(d) Neither cellular nor free nuclear

**197.** White kernel of coconut is which part of endosperm?
(a) Cellular
(b) Free nuclear
(c) Cellular as well as nuclear
(d) Neither cellular nor free nuclear

**198.** Endosperm is completely consumed during seed formation in
(a) Pea, castor and coconut
(b) Castor and coconut
(c) Pea and beans
(d) Groundnut and castor

**199.** Endosperm persist in mature seed of
(a) Pea, castor and coconut
(b) Castor and coconut
(c) Pea and beans
(d) Groundnut and castor

**200.** Development of embryo takes place at
(a) Chalazal end of embryo sac
(b) Micropyle end of embryo sac
(c) Near the integument of embryo sac
(d) All of these

**201.** Zygote divides after the formation of endosperm
(a) To provide assured nutrition to develop the endosperm.
(b) To provide assured nutrition to develop embryo.
(c) None of these
(d) Both (a) and (b)

**202.** The development of embryo in both monocotyledons and dicotyledons
(a) Same
(b) Differ greatly in seed stage
(c) Similar in early stage of development
(d) Both (b) and (c)

**203.** Which of the following is correct?
(a) Proembryo → Mature embryo → Globular embryo
(b) Proembryo → Globular embryo → Mature embryo
(c) Globular embryo → Proembryo → Mature embryo
(d) Mature embryo → Globular embryo → Proembryo

**204.** The portion of embryo above the cotyledon is called ________ and below the cotyledon is called as ________
(a) Epicotyl, hypocotyl (b) Hypocotyl, epicotyl
(c) Plumule, radical (d) Radical and plumule

**205.** Epicotyl terminates into
(a) Stem tip (b) Root tip
(c) Plumule (d) Both (a) and (c)

**206.** Hypocotyl terminates into
(a) Root tip (b) Stem tip
(c) Plumule (d) Both (a) and (c)

**207.** Embryo of monocotyledon possess only
(a) Two cotyledon (b) One cotyledon
(c) Scutellum (d) Both (b) and (c)

**208.** The root cap of monocot is covered in
(a) Coleoptile (b) Coleorhiza
(c) Root tip (d) None of these

**209.** The leaf primordia is enclosed in hollow foliar structure called as
(a) Coleoptile (b) Coleorhiza
(c) Root tip (d) None of these

**210.** Identify A and B in this figure.

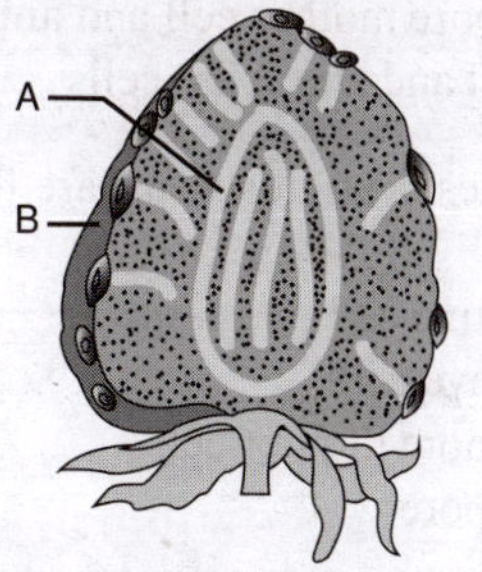


(a) A: Thalamus, B: Endocarp
(b) A: Thalamus, B: Achene
(c) A: Endocarp, B: Mesocarp
(d) A: Mesocarp, B: Endocarp

## Apomixis and Polyembryony

**211.** Apomixis is seen in
(a) Asteraceae (b) Grasses
(c) Both (a) and (b) (d) None of these

**212.** Apomixis means
(a) Fruit without seed
(b) Fruit with seed
(c) Seed without fertilization
(d) Fruit without fertilization

**213.** Polyembryony is
(a) One embryo in one seed
(b) More than one embryo in a seed
(c) More seed in one embryo
(d) Seed development without fertilization

**214.** Polyembryony is seen in
(a) Citrus fruits
(b) Coconut
(c) Date palm
(d) Pineapple

# Multiple Choice Questions: Level II

**215.** Unisexuality of flowers prevents
(a) geitonogamy, but not xenogamy
(b) autogamy and geitonogamy
(c) autogamy, but not geitonogamy
(d) Both geitonogamy and xenogamy

**216.** Which one of the following is resistant to enzyme?
(a) Pollen exine (b) Leaf cuticle
(c) Cork (d) Wood fibre

**217.** What does the filiform apparatus do at the entrance ovule?
(a) It brings about opening of the pollen tube
(b) It guides pollen tube from synergids to egg
(c) It helps in entry of pollen tube into synergids
(d) It prevents entry of more than one pollen tube into embryo sac

**218.** Which one of the following pairs of plant structures has haploid number of chromosomes?
(a) Nucellus and antipodal cells
(b) Egg nucleus and secondary nucleus
(c) Megaspore mother cell and antipodal cells
(d) Egg cell and antipodal cells

**219.** Male gametes in angiosperms are formed by the division of
(a) Generative cell
(b) Vegetative cell
(c) Microspore mother cell
(d) Microspore

**220.** Which one of the following is surrounded by a callose wall?
(a) male gamete
(b) egg
(c) pollen grain
(d) microspore mother cell

**221.** What would be the number of chromosomes in the cells of the aleuron layer in a plant species with 8 chromosomes in its synergids?
(a) 24 (b) 32
(c) 8 (d) 16

**222.** The arrangement of the nuclei in a normal embryo sac in dicot plants is
(a) 3 + 2 +3 (b) 2 + 3 + 3
(c) 3 + 3 +2 (d) 2 + 4 +2

**223.** Why is vivipary an undesirable character for annual crop plants?
(a) It reduces the vigour of the plant.
(b) It adversely affects the fertility of the plant.
(c) The seeds exhibit long dormancy.
(d) The seeds cannot be stored under normal conditions for the next season.

**224.** Formation of gametophyte directly from sporophyte without meiosis is
(a) Apospory (b) Apogamy
(c) Parthenogenesis (d) Amphimixis

**225.** Parthenogenesis is
(a) Development of embryo without fertilization
(b) Development of fruit without fertilization
(c) Development of fruit without hormones
(d) Development of embryo from egg without Fertilization

**226.** Through which cell of the embryo sac does the pollen tube enter the embryo sac?
(a) Egg cell
(b) Persistent synergid
(c) Degenerated synergid
(d) Central cell

**227.** Male gametophyte of angiosperms is shed as
(a) Four-celled pollen grain
(b) Three-celled pollen grain

(c) Microspore mother cell
(d) Anther

**228.** In a flowering plant, archesporium gives rise to
(a) only tapetum and sporogenous cells
(b) only the wall of the sporangium
(c) both wall and the sporogenous cells
(d) wall and the tapetum

**229.** In angiosperms, all the four microspores of tetrad are covered by a layer which is formed by
(a) pectocellulose (b) callose
(c) cellulose (d) sporopollenin

**230.** Which type of association is found in between entomophilous flowers and pollinating agents?
(a) mutualism (b) commensalism
(c) cooperation (d) co-evolution

**231.** What is the direction of micropyle in anatropous ovule?
(a) Upward (b) Downward
(c) Right (d) Left

**232.** In angiosperms, pollen tubes liberate their male gametes into the
(a) central cell (b) antipodal cell
(c) egg cell (d) synergids

**233.** Adventive polyembryony in citrus is due to
(a) Nucellus
(b) Integuments
(c) Zygotic embryo
(d) Fertilized egg

**234.** Anemophily type of pollination is found in
(a) Salvia (b) Bottle brush
(c) Vallisneria (d) Coconut

**235.** Eight nucleate embryo sacs are
(a) always tetrasporic
(b) always monosporic
(c) always bisporic
(d) sometimes monosporic, sometimes bisporic and sometimes tetrasporic

**236.** Double fertilization leading to initiation of endosperm in angiosperms is required for
(a) fusion of one polar nucleus and the second male gamete only
(b) fusion of two polar nuclei and the second male gamete
(c) fusion of four or more polar nuclei and the second male gamete only
(d) all the above kinds of fusion in different angiosperms

**237.** Total number of meiotic division required for forming 100 zygotes/100 grains of wheat is
(a) 100 (b) 75
(c) 125 (d) 50

**238.** The endosperm of gymnosperm is
(a) triploid (b) haploid
(c) diploid (d) polyploidy

**239.** If an angiospermic male plant is diploid and female plant tetraploid, the ploidy level of endosperm will be
(a) haploid (b) triploid
(c) tetraploid (d) pentaploid

**240.** In angiosperms, triple fusion is required for the formation of
(a) embryo (b) endosperm
(c) seed coat (d) fruit wall

**241.** How many pollen grains will be formed after meiotic division in ten microspore mother cells?
(a) 10 (b) 20
(c) 40 (d) 80

**242.** The polyembryony commonly occurs in
(a) Citrus (b) Turmeric
(c) Tomato (d) Potato

**243.** In an angiosperm, how many microspore mother cells are required to produce 100 pollen grains
(a) 25 (b) 50
(c) 75 (d) 100

**244.** One of the most resistant biological materials is
(a) Lignin (b) Hemicellulose
(c) Lignocellulose (d) Sporopollenin

**245.** Fertilization involving carrying of male gametes by the pollen tube is
(a) Porogamy (b) Siphonogamy
(c) Chalazogamy (d) Syngonogamy

**246.** Transfer of pollen to stigma of another flower of the same plant is
(a) Autogamy (b) Allogamy
(c) Xenogamy (d) Geitonogamy

**247.** Chief pollinators of agricultural crops are
(a) Butterflies (b) Bees
(c) Moths (d) Beetles

**248.** Haploid plant cultures are got from
(a) Leaves (b) Root tip
(c) Pollen grain (d) Buds

**249.** Number of meiotic divisions required to produce 200/400 seeds of Pca would be
(a) 200/400 (b) 400/800
(c) 300/600 (d) 250/500

**250.** Double fertilization is characteristic of
(a) Angiosperms
(b) Pteridophytes
(c) Gymnosperms
(d) Bryophytes

**251.** Total number of meiotic division required for forming 100 zygotes/100 grains of wheat is
(a) 100 (b) 75
(c) 125 (d) 50

**252.** Study of formation, growth and development of new individual from an egg is
(a) Apomixis
(b) Embryology
(c) Embryogeny
(d) Cytology

**253.** A population of genetically identical individuals obtained from asexual reproduction is
(a) Callus (b) Clone
(c) Deme (d) Aggregate

**254.** Double fertilization and triple fusion were discovered by
(a) Holfmeister
(b) Nawaschin and Guignard
(c) Leeuwenhoek
(d) Strasburger

**255.** Double fertilization is fusion of:
(a) Two eggs
(b) Two eggs and polar nuclei with pollen nuclei
(c) One male gamete with egg and other with synergid
(d) One male gamete with egg and other with secondary nucleus

**256.** Point the odd one out
(a) Nucellus (b) Embryo sac
(c) Micropyle (d) Pollen grain

**257.** Which of the following pair has haploid structures?
(a) Nucellus and antipodal cells
(b) Antipodal cells and egg cell
(c) Antipodal cells and megaspore mother cell
(d) Nucellus and primary endosperm nucleus

**258.** Embryo sac occurs in
(a) Embryo
(b) Axis part of embryo
(c) Ovule
(d) Endosperm

**259.** Pollination occurs in
(a) Bryophytes and angiosperms
(b) Pteridophytes and angiosperms
(c) Angiosperms and gymnosperms
(d) Angiosperms and fungi

**260.** Entry of pollen tube through micropyle is
(a) Chalazogamy (b) Mesogamy
(c) porogamy (d) Pseudogamy

**261.** Female gametophyte of angiosperms is represented by
(a) Ovule
(b) Megaspore mother cell
(c) Embryo sac
(d) Nucellus

**262.** Male gametophyte of angiosperms/monocots is
(a) Microsporangium
(b) Nucellus
(c) Microspore
(d) Stamen

**263.** A diploid female plant and a tetraploid male plant are crossed. The ploidy of endosperm shall be
(a) Tetraploid
(b) Triploid
(c) Diploid
(d) Pentaploid

**264.** Which is correct?
(a) Gametes are invariably haploid
(b) Spores are invariably haploid
(c) Gametes are generally haploid
(d) Both spores and gametes are invariably haploid

**265.** Generative cell was destroyed by laser but a normal pollen tube was still formed because
(a) vegetative cell is not damaged
(b) contents of killed generative cell stimulate pollen growth
(c) laser beam stimulates growth of pollen tube
(d) the region of emergence of pollen tube is not harmed

**266.** Nucellar embryo is
(a) Amphimictic haploid
(b) Amphimictic diploid
(c) Apomictic haploid
(d) Apomictic diploid

## A & R and Statement-based Questions

### Assertion and Reason Questions

***Direction for questions 267 to 271:*** *Read the* ***assertion*** *and* ***reason*** *carefully to mark the correct option out of the options given below:*

**(a)** **(A)** is **true** but **(R)** is **false**.
**(b)** **(A)** is **false** but **(R)** is **true**.
**(c)** Both **(A)** and **(R)** is **true** and **(R)** is the correct explanation of **(A)**.
**(d)** Both **(A)** and **(R)** is **true** and **(R)** is not the correct explanation of **(A)**.

**267.** **Assertion:** Pollen grains are well preserved as fossils.
**Reason:** Pollen possess sporopollenin.

**268.** **Assertion:** Pollen tablets used as food supplement.
**Reason:** Pollen grains are rich in nutrient.

**269.** **Assertion:** Pollen tube usually enters the ovule through micropyle.
**Reason:** Pollen tube enters in one of synergids through filiform apparatus.

**270.** **Assertion:** Coconuts water is nuclear endosperm.
**Reason:** In initial stage of endosperm development in coconut free nuclear division occur without cytokinesis and cell wall formation.

**271.** **Assertion:** Most zygote divide only after certain amount of endosperm is formed.
**Reason:** This is an adaptation to provide assumed nutrition to the developing embryo.

### Statement-based Questions:

***Direction for questions 272 to 276:*** *These type of questions consist of two statement each, printed as* **Statement-I** *and* **Statement-II**. *While answering such questions, a student is needed to choose any one of the following four responses.*

**(a)** **Statement I** is **correct Statement II** is **incorrect**.
**(b)** **Statement I** is **incorrect Statement II** is **correct**.
**(c)** Both **Statement I** and **Statement II** are **correct**.
**(d)** Both **Statement I** and **Statement II** are **incorrect**.

**272.** **Statement-I:** Pollen tube can germinate on glass slide if we provide 10% sugar solution to pollen grains of *Crotalaria* and balsam.
**Statement-II:** In the grass family, the cotyledon is called scutellum.

**273.** **Statement-I:** Early stage of embryogeny are different in monocots and dicots.
**Statement-II:** The portion of embryonal axis above the level of cotyledon is called plumule.

**274.** **Statement-I:** Physical dialogue occur between pollen grains and pistil during pollen pistil interaction.
**Statement-II:** Removal of anther form flower bud is called as emasculation.

**275.** **Statement-I:** Dioecy is out breeding device.
**Statement-II:** When flowers are small, number of flower are clustered into inflorescence to make them inconspicuous.

**276.** **Statement-I:** Water hyacinth is pollinated by water.
**Statement-II:** Water hyacinth is an aquatic plant.

## Matrix-Match Type Questions

**277.** Identify & match the parts of flower.

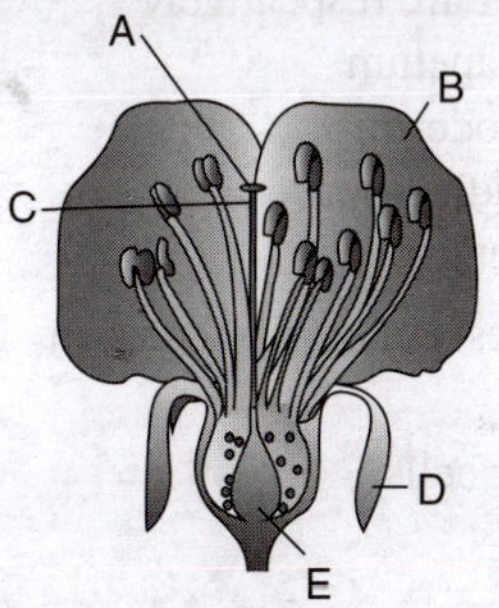


(a) A – Stigma, B – Style, C – Filament, D – Sepal, E – Ovary
(b) A – Stigma, B – Sepal, C – Style, D – Sepal, E – Ovary
(c) A – Style, B – Petal, C – Stigma, D – Sepal, E – Ovary
(d) A – Stigma, B – Petal, C – Style, D – Sepal, E – Ovary

**278.** Arrange the following parts of androecium starting from the smallest to the largest one.
(a) Lobes → Theca → Anther → Stamen
(b) Theca → Lobes → Anther → Stamen
(c) Lobes → Theca → Stamen → Anther
(d) Theca → Lobes → Stamen → Anther

(Note : Question can be asked in reverse order, means largest to smallest)

**279.** Arrange the layers of microsporangium from innermost to outermost layer.
(a) Epidermis, Middle layer, Endothecium, Tapetum
(b) Epidermis, Endothecium, Middle layer, Tapetum
(c) Tapetum, Middle layer, Endothecium, Epidermis
(d) Tapetum, Endothecium, Middle layer, Epidermis

**280.** Match the following:

| List-I | List-II |
|---|---|
| 1. Tapetum | (i) Develop into pollen sac |
| 2. Epidermis | (ii) Contain pollen grains |
| 3. Pollen sac | (iii) Protection and dehiscence of anther |
| 4. Microsporangium | (iv) Nourishes pollen grain |

**The correct matching is :**

| | 1 | 2 | 3 | 4 |
|---|---|---|---|---|
| (a) | (iii) | (iv) | (ii) | (i) |
| (b) | (iv) | (iii) | (i) | (ii) |
| (c) | (ii) | (i) | (iv) | (iii) |
| (d) | (iv) | (iii) | (ii) | (i) |

**281.** Identify the A, B, C, D in following figure.

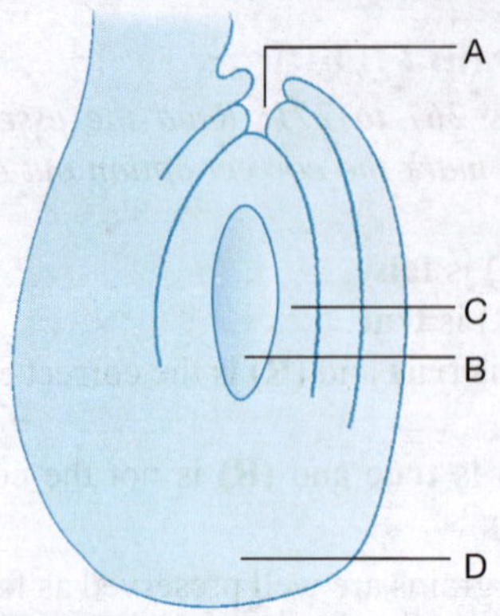


(a) A – Micropyle, B – Embryo sac, C – Nucellus, D – Chalazal pole
(b) A – Chalazal pole, B – Nucellus, C – Embryo sac, D – Micropyle
(c) A – Micropyle, B – Nucellus, C – Embryo sac, D – Chalazal pole
(d) A – Chalazal pole, B – Embryo sac, C – Nucellus, D – Micropyle

## NCERT Exemplar Questions

**1.** Among the terms listed below, those that are not technically correct names for a floral whorl are
i. Androecium ii. Carpel
iii. Corolla iv. Sepal
(a) i and iv (b) iii and iv
(c) ii and iv (d) i and ii

**2.** Embryo sac is to ovule as ________ is to an anther.
(a) Stamen (b) Filament
(c) Pollen grain (d) Androecium

**3.** In a typical complete, bisexual and hypogynous flower the arrangement of floral whorls on the thalamus from the outermost to the innermost is
(a) Calyx, corolla, androecium and gynoecium
(b) Calyx, corolla, gynoecium and androecium
(c) Gynoecium, androecium, corolla and calyx
(d) Androecium, gynoecium, corolla and calyx

**4.** A dicotyledonous plant bears flowers but never produces fruits and seeds. The most probable cause for the above situation is
(a) The plant is dioecious and bears only pistillate flowers
(b) The plant is dioecious and bears both pistillate and staminate flowers
(c) The plant is monoecious.
(d) The plant is dioecious and bears only staminate flowers.

**5.** The outermost and innermost wall layers of microsporangium in an anther are respectively
(a) Endothecium and tapetum
(b) Epidermis and endodermis
(c) Epidermis and middle layer
(d) Epidermis and tapetum

**6.** During microsporogenesis, meiosis occurs in
(a) Endothecium
(b) Microspore mother cells
(c) Microspore tetrads
(d) Pollen grains

**7.** From among the sets of terms given below, identify those that are associated with the gynoecium.
(a) Stigma, ovule, embryo sac, placenta
(b) Thalamus, pistil, style, ovule
(c) Ovule, ovary, embryo sac, tapetum
(d) Ovule, stamen, ovary, embryo sac

**8.** Starting from the innermost part, the correct sequence of parts in an ovule are
(a) Egg, nucellus, embryo sac, integument
(b) Egg, embryo sac, nucellus, integument
(c) Embryo sac, nucellus, integument, egg
(d) Egg, integument, embryo sac, nucellus

**9.** From the statements given below, choose the options that are true for a typical female gametophyte of a flowering plant.
i. It is 8-nucleate and 7-celled at maturity.
ii. It is free-nuclear during the development.
iii. It is situated inside the integument but outside the nucellus.
iv. It has an egg apparatus situated at the chalazal end.

Choose the correct answer from the options given below:
(a) i and v
(b) ii and iii
(c) i and ii
(d) ii and iv

**10.** Autogamy can occur in a chasmogamous flower if
(a) Pollen matures before the maturity of ovule.
(b) Ovules mature before the maturity of pollen.
(c) Both pollen and ovules mature simultaneously.
(d) Both anther and stigma are of equal lengths.

**11.** Choose the correct statement from the following:
(a) Cleistogamous flowers always exhibit autogamy.
(b) Chasmogamous flowers always exhibit geitonogamy.
(c) Cleistogamous flowers exhibit both autogamy and geitonogamy.
(d) Chasmogamous flowers never exhibit autogamy.

**12.** A particular species of plant produces light, non-sticky pollen in large numbers and its stigmas are long and feathery. These modifications facilitate pollination by
(a) Insects (b) Water
(c) Wind (d) Animals

**13.** From among the situations given below, choose the one that prevents both autogamy and geitonogamy.
(a) Monoecious plant bearing unisexual flowers.
(b) Dioecious plant bearing only male or female flowers.
(c) Monoecious plant with bisexual flowers.
(d) Dioecious plant with bisexual flowers.

**14.** In a fertilized embryo sac, the haploid, diploid and triploid structures are
(a) Synergid, zygote and primary endosperm nucleus.
(b) Synergid, antipodal and polar nuclei.
(c) Antipodal, synergid and primary endosperm nucleus.
(d) Synergid, polar nuclei and zygote.

**15.** In an embryo sac, the cells that degenerate after fertilization are
(a) Synergid and primary endosperm nucleus cell
(b) Synergid and antipodal
(c) Antipodal and primary endosperm nucleus cell
(d) Egg and antipodals

**16.** While planning for an artificial hybridization programme involving dioecious plants, which of the following steps would not be relevant?
(a) Bagging of female flower
(b) Dusting of pollen on stigma
(c) Emasculation
(d) Collection of pollen

**17.** In the embryos of a typical dicot and a grass, the true homologous structures are
(a) Coleorhiza and coleoptile
(b) Coleoptile and scutellum
(c) Cotylendons and scutellum
(d) Hypocotyl and radical

**18.** The phenomenon observed in some plants wherein the parts of the sexual apparatus is used for forming embryos without fertilization is called
(a) Parthenocarpy
(b) Apomixis
(c) Vegetative propagation
(d) Sexual reproduction

**19.** In a flower, if the megaspore mother cell forms megaspores without undergoing meiosis and if one of the megaspores develops into an embryo sac, its nuclei would be
(a) Haploid
(b) Diploid
(c) A few haploid and a few diploid
(d) With varying ploidy

**20.** The phenomenon wherein, the ovary develops into a fruit without fertilization is called
(a) Parthenocarpy
(b) Apomixis
(c) Asexual reproduction
(d) Sexual reproduction

## Previous Years' Questions

**1.** Wind pollinated flowers are [AIPMT 2010 PRE]
(a) Small, brightly coloured, producing large number of pollen grains
(b) Small, producing large number of dry pollen grains
(c) Large, producing abundant nectar and pollen
(d) Small, producing nectar and dry pollen

**2.** The scutellum observed in a grain of wheat or maize is comparable to which part of seed in other monocotyledons? [AIPMT 2010 PRE]
(a) Cotyledon
(b) Endosperm
(c) Aleurone layer
(d) Plumule

**3.** Transfer of pollen grains from anther to the stigma of another flower of the same plant is called [AIPMT 2010 PRE]
(a) Xenogamy
(b) Geitonogamy
(c) Karyogamy
(d) Autogamy

**4.** Apomictic embryos in Citrus arise from [AIPMT 2010 PRE]
(a) Synergids
(b) Maternal sporophytic tissue in ovule
(c) Antipodal cells
(d) Diploid egg

**5.** What is common between vegetative reproduction and apomixis? [AIPMT MAINS 2011]
(a) Both are applicable to only dicot plants
(b) Both bypass the flowering phase
(c) Both occur around the year
(d) Both produce progeny identical to the parent

**6.** In angiosperms, functional megaspore develops into: [AIPMT MAINS 2011]
(a) Embryo sac (b) Ovule
(c) Endosperm (d) Pollen sac

**7.** In which one of the following, pollination is autogamous? [AIPMT 2011 PRE]
(a) Xenogamy
(b) Chasmogamy
(c) Cleistogamy
(d) Geitonogamy

**8.** Nucellar polyembryony is reported in species of: [AIPMT 2011 PRE]
(a) Gossypium (b) Triticum
(c) Brassica (d) Citrus

**9.** Wind pollination is common in: [AIPMT 2011 PRE]
(a) Lilies (b) Grasses
(c) Orchids (d) Legumes

**10.** What would be the number of chromosomes of the aleurone cells of a plant with 42 chromosomes in its root tip cells? [AIPMT 2011 PRE]
(a) 63 (b) 84 (c) 21 (d) 42

**11.** Filliform apparatus is a characteristic feature of: [AIPMT 2011 PRE]
(a) Egg (b) Synergid
(c) Zygote (d) Suspensor

**12.** Coconut water and its edible part are equivalent to: [AIPMT PRE 2012]
(a) Endosperm (b) Endocarp
(c) Mesocarp (d) Embryo

**13.** Even in absence of pollinating agents seed, setting is assured in: [AIPMT 2012 PRE]
(a) Commellina (b) Zostera
(c) Salvia (d) Fig

**14.** An organic substance that can withstand environmental extremes and cannot be degraded by any enzyme is: [AIPMT PRE 2012]
(a) Cuticle (b) Sporopollenin
(c) Lignin (d) Cellulose

**15.** The gynoecium consists of many free pistils in flowers of: [AIPMT PRE 2012]
(a) Aloe (b) Tomato
(c) Papaver (d) Michelia

**16.** Which one of the following statements is wrong? [AIPMT MAINS 2012]
(a) Vegetative cell is larger than generative cell
(b) Pollen grains in some plants remain viable for months
(c) Intine is made up of cellulose and pectin
(d) When pollen is shed at two-called stage, double fertilization does not take place

**17.** What is the function of germ pore? [AIPMT MAINS 2012]
(a) Absorption of water for seed germination
(b) Initiation of pollen tube
(c) Release of male gametes
(d) Emergence of radical

**18.** Plants with ovaries having only one or a few ovules are generally pollinated by: [AIPMT MAINS 2012]
(a) Butterflies (b) Birds
(c) Wind (d) Bees

**19.** Both, autogamy and geitonogamy are prevented in [AIPMT PRE 2012]
(a) Papaya (b) Cucumber
(c) Castor (d) Maize

**20.** Perisperm differs from endosperm in: [AIPMT 2013]
(a) Being a haploid tissue
(b) Having no reserve food
(c) Being a diploid tissue
(d) Its formation by fusion of secondary nucleus with several sperms

**21.** Advantage of cleistogamy is: [AIPMT 2013]
(a) Higher genetic variability
(b) More vigorous offspring
(c) No dependence on pollinators
(d) Vivipary

**22.** Which one of the following statements is correct? [AIPMT 2013]
(a) Hard outer layer of pollen is called intine
(b) Sporogenous tissue is haploid
(c) Endothecium produces microspores
(d) Tapetum nourishes the developing pollen

**23.** Non-albuminous seed is produced in: [AIPMT 2014]
(a) Maize (b) Castor
(c) Wheat (d) Pea

**24.** Function of filiform apparatus is to: [AIPMT 2014]
(a) Recognize the suitable pollen at stigma
(b) Stimulate division of generative cell
(c) Produce nectar
(d) Guide the entry of pollen tube

**25.** Pollen tablets are available in the market for: [AIPMT 2014]
(a) In-vitro fertilization
(b) Breeding programmes
(c) Supplementing food
(d) Ex-situ conservation

**26.** Male gametophyte with least number of cells is present in: [AIPMT 2014]
(a) Pteris (b) Funaria
(c) Lilium (d) Pinus

**27.** Geitonogamy involves: [AIPMT 2014]
(a) Fertilization of a flower by the pollen from another flower of the same plant
(b) Fertilization of a flower by the pollen from the same flower
(c) Fertilization of a flower by the pollen from a flower of another plant in the same population
(d) Fertilization of a flower by the pollen from a flower of another plant belonging to a distant population

**28.** In angiosperms, microsporogeneis and megasporogenesis: [RE-AIPMT 2015]
(a) From gametes without further divisions
(b) Involve meiosis
(c) Occur in ovule
(d) Occur in anther

**29.** Filiform apparatus is a characteristic feature of: [RE-AIPMT 2015]
(a) Nucellar embryo
(b) Aleurone cell
(c) Synergids
(d) Generative cell

**30.** Which one of the following fruits is parthenocarpic? [RE-AIPMT 2015]
(a) Apple (b) Jackfruit
(c) Banana (d) Brinjal

**31.** Male gametophyte in angiosperms produces: [RE-AIPMT 2015]

(a) Single sperm and a vegetative cell
(b) Single sperm and two vegetative cells
(c) Three sperms
(d) Two sperms and a vegetative cell

**32.** Which of the following are important floral rewards to animal pollinators? [AIPMT 2015]

(a) Colour and large size of flower
(b) Nectar and pollen grains
(c) Floral fragrance and calcium crystals
(d) Protein pellicle and stigmatic exudates

**33.** Transmission tissue is a characteristic feature of [AIPMT 2015]

(a) Hollow style (b) Solid style
(c) Dry stigma (d) Wet stigma

**34.** Which one of the following statements is not true? [AIPMT 2015]

(a) Pollen grains are rich in nutrients, and they are used in the form on tablets and syrups
(b) Pollen grains of some plants cause severe allergies and bronchial afflications in some people
(c) The flowers pollinated by flies and bats secrete foul odour to attract them
(d) Honey is made by bees by digesting pollen collected from flowers

**35.** Which one of the following may require pollinators, but genetically similar to autogamy? [AIPMT 2015]

(a) Geitonogamy (b) Xenogamy
(c) Apogamy (d) Cleistogamy

**36.** The ovule of an angiosperm is technically equivalent to [NEET 2016 – PHASE II]

(a) Megasporophyll
(b) Megaspore mother cell
(c) Megaspore
(d) Megasporangium

**37.** Pollination in water hyacinth and water lily is brought about by the agency of [NEET 2016 – PHASE II]

(a) Insects or wind (b) Birds
(c) Bats (d) Water

**38.** In majority of angiosperms [NEET 2016 – PHASE II]

(a) There are numerous antipodal cells
(b) Reduction division occurs in the megaspore mother cells
(c) A small central cell is present in the embryo sac
(d) Egg has a filiform apparatus

**39.** Which one of the following generates new genetic combinations leading to variation? [NEET 2016 – PHASE II]

(a) Parthenogenesis
(b) Sexual reproduction
(c) Nucellar polymbryony
(d) Vegetative reproduction

**40.** Which of the following statements is not correct? [NEET 2016 – PHASE I]

(a) Pollen grains of many species can germinate on the stigma of a flower, but only one pollen tube of the same species grows into the style
(b) Insects that consume pollen or nectar without bringing about pollination are called pollen nectar robbers
(c) Pollen germination and pollen tube growth are regulated by chemical components of pollen interacting with those of the pistil
(d) Some reptiles have also been reported as pollinators in some plant species

**41.** Seed formation without fertilization in flowering plants involves the process of: [NEET 2016 – PHASE I]

(a) Sporulation
(b) Budding
(c) Somatic hybridization
(d) Apomixis

**42.** Which one of the following statements is not true? [NEET 2016 – PHASE I]

(a) Tapetum helps in dehiscence of anther
(b) Exine of pollen grains is made up of sporopollenin
(c) Pollen grains of many species cause severe allergies
(d) Stored pollen in liquid nitrogen can be used in crop breeding programmes

**43.** Proximal end of the filament of stamen is attached to the: [NEET 2016 – PHASE I]

(a) Anther (b) Connective
(c) Placenta (d) Thalamus or petal

**44.** The coconut water from tender coconut represents: [NEET 2016 – PHASE I]

(a) Endocarp
(b) Fleshy mesocarp
(c) Free nuclear proembryo
(d) Free nuclear endosperm

**45.** Seed formation without fertilization in flowering plants involves the process of: [NEET 2016 – PHASE I]
(a) Sporulation
(b) Budding
(c) Somatic hybridization
(d) Apomixis

**46.** Choose the correct sequence representing the ploidy of Nucellus; Megaspore mother cell; Megaspore; Egg cell; Zygote; A polar nucleus of embryo sac; Secondary nucleus and primary endosperm nucleus. [NEET Regional 2017]
(a) n; 2n; 2n; n; 2n; n; 2n; and 2n
(b) 2n; 2n; n; 2n; n; 2n; 3n; and 2n
(c) 2n; 2n; n; n; 2n; n; 2n; and 3n
(d) 2n; n; n; 2n; 3n; 2n; n; and 3n

**47.** Continued self-pollination results in: [NEET Regional 2017]
(a) Genetic drift
(b) Heterosis
(c) Inbreeding depression
(d) Polyembryony

**48.** Pollen grains can be stored for years in liquid nitrogen, maintained at temperature [NEET Regional 2017]
(a) – 120°C (b) – 20°C
(c) – 70°C (d) – 196°C

**49.** The hollow foliar structure in a wheat embryo that encloses the shoot apex and a few leaf primordial is called: [NEET Regional 2017]
(a) Coleoptile (b) Coleorrhiza
(c) Epicotyl (d) Hypocotyl

**50.** A dioecious flowering plant prevents both: [NEET 2017]
(a) Autogamy and geitonogamy
(b) Geitonogamy and xenogamy
(c) Cleistogamy and xenogamy
(d) Autogamy and xenogamy

**51.** Flowers which have single ovule in the ovary and are packed into inflorescence are usually pollinated by: [NEET 2017]
(a) Bee (b) Wind
(c) Bat (d) Water

**52.** Functional megaspore in an angiosperm develops into: [NEET 2017]
(a) Endosperm (b) Embryo sac
(c) Embryo (d) Ovule

**53.** Attractants and rewards are required for: [NEET 2017]
(a) Entomophily (b) Hydrophily
(c) Cleistogamy (d) Anemophily

**54.** Which of the following has proved helpful in preserving pollens as fossils? [NEET 2018]
(a) Pollenkitt
(b) Oil content
(c) Cellulosic intine
(d) Sporopollenin

**55.** Which one of the following plants shows very close relationship with a species of moth, where none of the two can complete its life cycle without the other? [NEET 2018]
(a) *Hydrilla* (b) Banana
(c) *Yucca* (d) *Viola*

**56.** Pollen grains can be stored for several years in liquid nitrogen of temperature [NEET 2018]
(a) –120°C (b) –196°C
(c) –80°C (d) –160°C

**57.** Double fertilization is [NEET 2018]
(a) Fusion of two male gametes of a pollen tube with two different eggs
(b) Fusion of two male gametes with one egg
(c) Fusion of one male gamete with two polar nuclei
(d) Syngamy and triple fusion

**58.** Winged pollen grains are present in [NEET 2018]
(a) Mustard (b) Mango
(c) *Cycas* (d) *Pinus*

**59.** What is the fate of the male gametes discharged in the synergid? [NEET 2019]
(a) All fuse with the egg
(b) One fuses with egg, other(s) fuse(s) with synergid nucleus
(c) One fuses with the egg and other fuses with central cell nuclei
(d) One fuses with the egg, other(s) degenerate(s) in the synergid

**60.** Persistent nucellus in the seed is known as: [NEET 2019]
(a) Perisperm (b) Hilum
(c) Tegmen (d) Chalaza

**61.** The body of the ovule is fused within the funicle at: [NEET 2020]
(a) Hilum (b) Micropyle
(c) Nucellus (d) Chalaza

**62.** In water hyacinth and water lily, pollination takes place by: [NEET 2020]
(a) Insects or wind
(b) Water currents only
(c) Wind and water
(d) Insects and water

**63.** The term used for transfer of pollen grains from anthers of one plant to stigma of a different plant which, during pollination, brings genetically different types of pollen grains to stigma, is: [NEET 2021]
(a) Cleistogamy
(b) Xenogamy
(c) Geitonogamy
(d) Chasmogamy

**64.** Atypical angiosperm embryo sac at maturity is: [NEET 2021]
(a) 8-nucleate and 8-celled
(b) 8-nucleate and 7-celled
(c) 7-nucleate and 8-celled
(d) 7-nucleate and 7-celled

**65.** In some members of which of the following pairs of families, pollen grains retain their viability for months after release? [NEET 2021]
(a) Rosaceae : Leguminosae
(b) Poaceae : Rosaceae
(c) Poaceae : Leguminosae
(d) Poaceae : Solanaceae

**66.** Identify the incorrect statement related to pollination. [NEET 2022]
(a) Pollination by wind is more common amongst abiotic pollinations.
(b) Flowers produce foul odours to attract flies and beetles to get pollinated.
(c) Moths and butterflies are the most dominant pollinating agents among insects.
(d) Pollination by water is quite rare in flowering plants.

**67.** Given below are two statements:

**Statement I:** Cleistogamous flowers are invariably autogamous.

**Statement II:** Cleistogamy is disadvantageous as there is no chance for cross pollination.

In the light of the above statements, choose the correct answer from the options given below: [NEET 2022]
(a) Both **Statement I** and **Statement II** are incorrect.
(b) **Statement I** is correct but **Statement II** is incorrect.
(c) **Statement I** is incorrect but **Statement II** is correct.
(d) Both **Statement I** and **Statement II** are correct.

**68.** Which part of the fruit, labelled in the given figure makes it a false fruit? [NEET 2022]

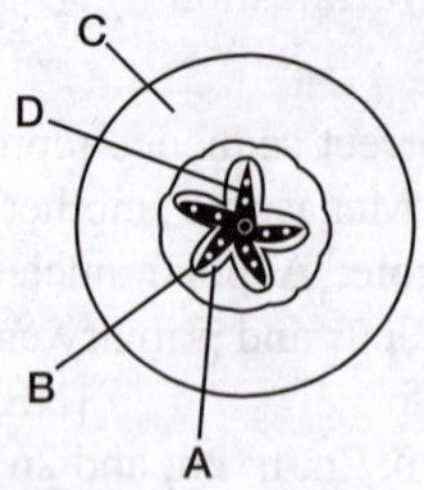


(a) B → Endocarp
(b) C → Thalamus
(c) D → Seed
(d) A → Mesocarp

**69.** What is the function of tassels in the corn cob? [NEET 2023]
(a) To trap pollen grains
(b) To disperse pollen grains
(c) To protect seeds
(d) To attract insects

**70.** Large Colourful fragrant flowers with nectar are seen in: [NEET 2023]
(a) Bird pollinated plants
(b) Bat pollinated plants
(c) Wind pollinated plants
(d) Insect pollinated plants

**71.** In angiosperm , the haploid a, diploid and triploid structures of a fertilized embryo sac sequentially are: [NEET 2023]
(a) Antipodals, synergids, and primary endosperm nucleus
(b) Synergids, Zygote and Primary endosperm nucleus
(c) Synergids, antipodals and Polar nuclei
(d) Synergids, Primary endosperm nucleus and Zygote

**72.** Identify the set of correct statements: [NEET 2024]
A. The flower of *Vallisneria* are colourful and produce nectar.
B. The flowers of waterlily are not pollinated by water.
C. In most of water-pollinated species, the pollen grains are protected from wetting.
D. Pollen grains of some hydrophytes are long and ribbon like

E. In some hydrophytes, the pollen grains are carried passively inside water:

Choose the correct answer from the option given below:

(a) C, D and E only
(b) A, B, C and D only
(c) A, C, D and E only
(d) B, C, D and E only

**73.** Identify the part of the seed from the given figure which is destined to form root when the seed germinates. [NEET 2024]

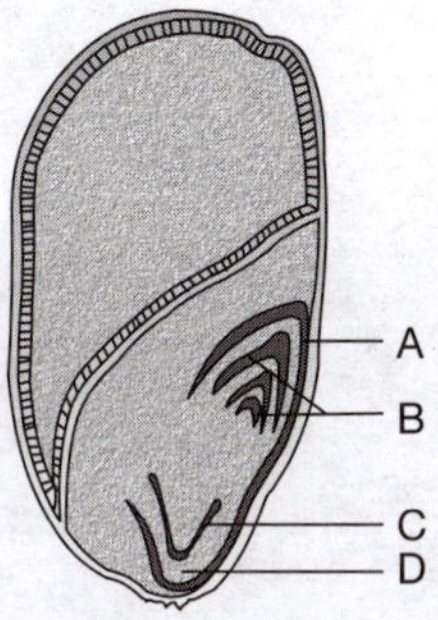


(a) A (b) B
(c) C (d) D

**74.** Identify the correct description about the given figure. [NEET 2024]

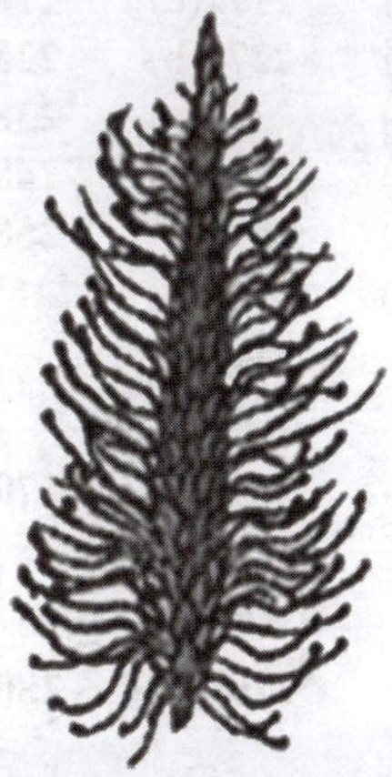

(a) Wind-pollinated plant inflorescence showing flower with well exposed stamens.
(b) Water-pollinated flowers showing stamens with mucilaginous covering.
(c) Cleistogamous flower showing autogamy.
(d) Compact inflorescence showing complete autogamy.

## Answer Key

### Multiple Choice Questions: Level I

| | | | | | | | | | |
|---|---|---|---|---|---|---|---|---|---|
| **1.** (d) | **2.** (d) | **3.** (d) | **4.** (c) | **5.** (d) | **6.** (d) | **7.** (b) | **8.** (a) | **9.** (d) | **10.** (c) |
| **11.** (b) | **12.** (a) | **13.** (d) | **14.** (a) | **15.** (b) | **16.** (b) | **17.** (d) | **18.** (b) | **19.** (c) | **20.** (b) |
| **21.** (d) | **22.** (b) | **23.** (d) | **24.** (b) | **25.** (b) | **26.** (d) | **27.** (d) | **28.** (b) | **29.** (c) | **30.** (c) |
| **31.** (b) | **32.** (d) | **33.** (c) | **34.** (b) | **35.** (c) | **36.** (c) | **37.** (d) | **38.** (c) | **39.** (b) | **40.** (d) |
| **41.** (d) | **42.** (a) | **43.** (c) | **44.** (a) | **45.** (b) | **46.** (b) | **47.** (c) | **48.** (d) | **49.** (c) | **50.** (c) |
| **51.** (b) | **52.** (b) | **53.** (d) | **54.** (b) | **55.** (b) | **56.** (b) | **57.** (d) | **58.** (a) | **59.** (d) | **60.** (b) |
| **61.** (a) | **62.** (c) | **63.** (b) | **64.** (a) | **65.** (d) | **66.** (c) | **67.** (a) | **68.** (b) | **69.** (b) | **70.** (b) |
| **71.** (b) | **72.** (c) | **73.** (d) | **74.** (c) | **75.** (b) | **76.** (b) | **77.** (a) | **78.** (c) | **79.** (b) | **80.** (b) |
| **81.** (a) | **82.** (b) | **83.** (d) | **84.** (c) | **85.** (b) | **86.** (c) | **87.** (d) | **88.** (a) | **89.** (d) | **90.** (a) |
| **91.** (c) | **92.** (d) | **93.** (c) | **94.** (a) | **95.** (b) | **96.** (a) | **97.** (b) | **98.** (b) | **99.** (b) | **100.** (b) |
| **101.** (d) | **102.** (c) | **103.** (a) | **104.** (b) | **105.** (a) | **106.** (a) | **107.** (b) | **108.** (c) | **109.** (b) | **110.** (d) |
| **111.** (a) | **112.** (b) | **113.** (d) | **114.** (d) | **115.** (c) | **116.** (c) | **117.** (d) | **118.** (d) | **119.** (b) | **120.** (b) |
| **121.** (b) | **122.** (d) | **123.** (c) | **124.** (b) | **125.** (d) | **126.** (b) | **127.** (d) | **128.** (a) | **129.** (c) | **130.** (d) |
| **131.** (a) | **132.** (d) | **133.** (d) | **134.** (a) | **135.** (c) | **136.** (b) | **137.** (a) | **138.** (d) | **139.** (b) | **140.** (c) |
| **141.** (c) | **142.** (b) | **143.** (d) | **144.** (d) | **145.** (b) | **146.** (c) | **147.** (d) | **148.** (d) | **149.** (c) | **150.** (c) |
| **151.** (b) | **152.** (c) | **153.** (b) | **154.** (d) | **155.** (a) | **156.** (a) | **157.** (a) | **158.** (d) | **159.** (a) | **160.** (c) |
| **161.** (a) | **162.** (d) | **163.** (d) | **164.** (a) | **165.** (d) | **166.** (b) | **167.** (b) | **168.** (a) | **169.** (d) | **170.** (d) |
| **171.** (d) | **172.** (c) | **173.** (a) | **174.** (c) | **175.** (d) | **176.** (a) | **177.** (d) | **178.** (d) | **179.** (a) | **180.** (d) |
| **181.** (a) | **182.** (a) | **183.** (b) | **184.** (b) | **185.** (b) | **186.** (a) | **187.** (c) | **188.** (b) | **189.** (b) | **190.** (a) |
| **191.** (a) | **192.** (b) | **193.** (d) | **194.** (b) | **195.** (b) | **196.** (b) | **197.** (a) | **198.** (c) | **199.** (b) | **200.** (b) |
| **201.** (b) | **202.** (d) | **203.** (b) | **204.** (a) | **205.** (d) | **206.** (a) | **207.** (b) | **208.** (b) | **209.** (a) | **210.** (b) |
| **211.** (c) | **212.** (c) | **213.** (b) | **214.** (a) | | | | | | |

## Multiple Choice Questions: Level II

| | | | | | | | | | |
|---|---|---|---|---|---|---|---|---|---|
| **215.** (c) | **216.** (a) | **217.** (c) | **218.** (d) | **219.** (a) | **220.** (d) | **221.** (a) | **222.** (a) | **223.** (d) | **224.** (a) |
| **225.** (d) | **226.** (c) | **227.** (b) | **228.** (c) | **229.** (b) | **230.** (a) | **231.** (a) | **232.** (d) | **233.** (a) | **234.** (d) |
| **235.** (b) | **236.** (b) | **237.** (c) | **238.** (b) | **239.** (d) | **240.** (b) | **241.** (c) | **242.** (a) | **243.** (a) | **244.** (d) |
| **245.** (b) | **246.** (d) | **247.** (b) | **248.** (c) | **249.** (d) | **250.** (a) | **251.** (c) | **252.** (b) | **253.** (b) | **254.** (b) |
| **255.** (d) | **256.** (d) | **257.** (b) | **258.** (c) | **259.** (c) | **260.** (c) | **261.** (c) | **262.** (c) | **263.** (a) | **264.** (a) |
| **265.** (a) | **266.** (d) | | | | | | | | |

## A & R and Statement-based Questions

| | | | | | | | | | |
|---|---|---|---|---|---|---|---|---|---|
| **267.** (c) | **268.** (c) | **269.** (d) | **270.** (c) | **271.** (c) | **272.** (c) | **273.** (d) | **274.** (b) | **275.** (a) | **276.** (b) |

## Matrix-Match Type Questions

| | | | | |
|---|---|---|---|---|
| **277.** (d) | **278.** (b) | **279.** (c) | **280.** (d) | **281.** (a) |

## NCERT Exemplar Questions

| | | | | | | | | | |
|---|---|---|---|---|---|---|---|---|---|
| **1.** (c) | **2.** (c) | **3.** (a) | **4.** (d) | **5.** (d) | **6.** (b) | **7.** (a) | **8.** (b) | **9.** (c) | **10.** (c) |
| **11.** (a) | **12.** (c) | **13.** (b) | **14.** (a) | **15.** (b) | **16.** (c) | **17.** (c) | **18.** (b) | **19.** (b) | **20.** (a) |

## Previous Years' Questions

| | | | | | | | | | |
|---|---|---|---|---|---|---|---|---|---|
| **1.** (b) | **2.** (a) | **3.** (b) | **4.** (b) | **5.** (d) | **6.** (a) | **7.** (c) | **8.** (d) | **9.** (b) | **10.** (a) |
| **11.** (b) | **12.** (a) | **13.** (a) | **14.** (b) | **15.** (d) | **16.** (d) | **17.** (b) | **18.** (c) | **19.** (a) | **20.** (c) |
| **21.** (c) | **22.** (d) | **23.** (d) | **24.** (d) | **25.** (c) | **26.** (c) | **27.** (a) | **28.** (b) | **29.** (c) | **30.** (c) |
| **31.** (d) | **32.** (b) | **33.** (b) | **34.** (d) | **35.** (a) | **36.** (d) | **37.** (a) | **38.** (b) | **39.** (b) | **40.** (a) |
| **41.** (d) | **42.** (a) | **43.** (d) | **44.** (d) | **45.** (d) | **46.** (c) | **47.** (c) | **48.** (d) | **49.** (a) | **50.** (a) |
| **51.** (b) | **52.** (b) | **53.** (a) | **54.** (d) | **55.** (c) | **56.** (b) | **57.** (d) | **58.** (d) | **59.** (c) | **60.** (a) |
| **61.** (a) | **62.** (a) | **63.** (b) | **64.** (b) | **65.** (a) | **66.** (c) | **67.** (d) | **68.** (b) | **69.** (a) | **70.** (d) |
| **71.** (b) | **72.** (d) | **73.** (c) | **74.** (a) | | | | | | |

# HINTS AND EXPLANATION

## Multiple Choice Questions: Level II

**215.** Unisexuality of flowers prevents autogamy, but not geitonogamy. In self-fertilization, the male and female gametes are derived from the same individual. Among plants, self-fertilization also called autogamy is common in many cultivated species, e.g., wheat and oats. However, self-fertilization is a form of inbreeding and does not allow for mixing of genetic material; if it occurs over a number of generations, it will result in offspring being less vigorous and productive than those resulting from cross fertilization.

**216.** Pollen grains are generally spherical measuring about 25–50 micrometers in diameter. It has a prominent two-layered wall. The hard outer layer called the **exine** is made up of sporopollenin which is one of the most resistant organic materials known. It can withstand high temperatures and strong acids and alkali. No enzyme that degrades sporopollenin is so far known. Pollen grain exine has prominent apertures called **germ pores** where sporopollenin is absent and pollen tube arises.

**217.** Filiform apparatus present at the micropylar part of the synergids guides the entry of pollen tube.

**218.** Secondary nucleus ,MMC and nucellus are diploid cells.

**219.** Generative cell which is a cell of the male gametophyte or pollen grain in seed plants that divide to give rise directly or indirectly to sperm.

**220.** MMC (megaspore mother cell is surrounded by a callose wall, ovules generally differentiate single MMC in the micropylar region of MMC. It is a large cell containing dense cytoplasm and a prominent nucleus).

**221.** Aleurone is the layer formed by the endospermic tissue in the members of family Graminae, e.g. wheat, rice, maize, etc. Obviously it will be a triploid tissue. Thus, if synergid have 8 chromosomes which are haploid then the aleurone layer must have 24 chromosomes.

**222.** In a dicot plants, general arrangement of nuclei in the embryo sac is that of 3 nuclei in 3 cells of egg apparatus (one egg cell and 2 synergids) at micropylar end and 2 polar nuclei in almost middle region and 3 nuclei in the form of antipodals at the distal end from micropyle towards the nucellus. So, total nuclei is 3 + 2 + 3.

**223.** Vivipary is the condition when seeds germinate on the plant. It is an undesirable character for annual crop plants because germinated seeds cannot be stored under normal conditions for the next season.

**224.** A somatic cell in the nucellus directly forms an unreduced embryo sac and the diploid egg parthenogenetically develops into embryo, i.e. formation of gametophyte from sporophyte without meiosis. It is known as apospory and it is a type of apomixis.

**225.** Parthenogenesis is a method of asexual reproduction, with embryo formation without fertilization, and parthenocarpy involves fruit formation, without seed formation. The plant equivalent of parthenogenesis is apomixis.

**226.** After entering the ovule, the pollen tube is attracted towards the micropylar end of the embryo sac. The attractants are secreted by synergids or help cells. The pollen tube pierces one of the two synergids and bursts open into it. The synergid is simultaneously destroyed.

**227.** In majority of angiosperms, the pollen grains are shed from the anther at bi-celled stage (one generative cell and one vegetative cell) but in some angiosperms the generative cell divides prior to the dehiscence of anther and pollen grains are shed at 3 celled.

**228.** In flowering plants, archesporium cells undergo periclinal (transverse) division to form and outer primary parietal layer and inner sporogenous cells. Primary parietal wall after few more periclinal divisions form anther wall, and sporogenous cells give rise to sporogenous tissue.

**229.** The outermost covering of the pollen grain is made of sporopollenin. Microsopre tetrad ic covered by callose.

**230.** Commensalism is interaction between two individuals in which one is benefitted while the other is unaffected. In mutualism, both individuals are beneficial for each other. The pollinating insect gets nectar from flower and in turn helps in pollination of flowers.

**231.** In orthotropous ovule, micropyle is upward.

**232.** Antipodal cells occur at the chalazal end of the ovule. Synergids are the helping cells.

**233.** The embryos arising from the maternal sporophyte tissues are called adventive embryos. In polyembryonate species, the adventive embryo arises by the proliferation of the nucellus cells.

**234.** Vallisneria exhibits hydrophily. Salvia is pollinated by honey bee. In bottle brush, pollination is carried out by birds.

**235.** Monosporic type - eight nucleated Polygonum type.
Bisporic type - eight nucleated Allium type.
Tetrasporic type - eight nucleated Adoxa type.

**236.** The second full gamete entering the ovary fuses with two haploid polar nuclei to form triploid primary endosperm nucleus which develops into endosperm. The fusion of two male gametes with two different structures (egg and secondary nucleus) in the same female gametophyte is called double fertilization.

**237.** 100 zygotes require 100 pollen grains and 100 embryo sacs. 100 pollen grains are formed from 25 microspore mother cells, while 100 embryo sacs are formed from 100 functional megaspores which in turn are produced by 100 megaspore mother cells since three out of four megaspores degenerate, in each case.

**238.** In gymnosperms, the female gametophyte forming archegonia provides nourishment to the developing embryo. It later gets transformed into food-laden endosperm inside the seed. Endosperm provides nourishment for growth of seed at the time to seed germination. Triploid endosperm occurs in angiosperms.

**239.** The male gamete will be haploid (n). 2 polar nuclei will be diploid (2n). Endosperm is formed by fusion of male gamete with two polar nuclei.

$$\underset{(n)}{\text{Male gamete}} + 2\ \underset{(2n)}{\text{polar}}\ \underset{(2n)}{\text{nuclei}} \rightarrow \underset{(5n)}{\text{Endosperm}}$$

**240.** In angiosperms, one male gamete fuses with the egg resulting in the formation of a diploid zygote. The other male gamete fuses with the two polar nuclei forming the primary endosperm nucleus. This type of fertilization is called double fertilization.

**241.** Each microspore mother cell gives rise to four microspores which develop into pollen grains.

**242.** Polyembryony refers to the formation of more than one embryo within a seed of a flowering plant. E.g., Citrus.

**243.** Each microspore mother cell undergoes meiosis to produced four pollen grains. Thus, 25 microspore mother cells are required to produce 100 pollen grains.

**244.** Sporopollenin is one of the most chemically inert biological polymers. It is a major component of the tough outer (exine) walls of plant spores and pollen grains. It is chemically very stable and is usually well preserved in soils and sediments.

**245.** In angiosperms, the male gametes are carried by the pollen tube; this was discovered by Strasburger in 1884. The process is called Siphonogamy.

**246.** Autogamy = Self-pollination

Geitanogamy - (geiton = neighbour; gamos marriage) i.e. when pollen grains are transferred to the stigma of other flower of the same plant (i.e. neighbouring flower).

Allogamy = Xenogamy – Cross-pollination.

**247.** Pollination by insect is known as Entomophily. Among insects, bees are the most common pollinators which pollinate about 80% of the total insect pollinated flowers.

**248.** All others are diploid. Best method of haploid plant culture is pollen grain culture.

**249.** 200 seeds of pea would be produced from 200 pollen grains and 200 embryo sac. 200 pollen grains will be formed by 50 microspore mother cell while 200 embryo sac will be formed by 200 megaspore mother cell (because 3 will degenerate) so 250/500.

**250.** Double fertilization in a characteristic feature of angiosperms in which one male gamete fuses with egg (called syngamy) and other male gamete fuses with 2 polar nuclei (called triple fusion).

**254.** In angiosperms, one male gamete fuses with the egg to form diploid zygote. The process is called syngamy. The other male gamete fuses with the two polar nuclei to form triploid primary endosperm nucleus. The process is called triple fusion. These two acts together are known as double fertilization. The process was first demonstrated by Nawaschin and Guignard in Fritillaria and Lilium.

**255.** One sperm fertilizes the egg to form the $2n$ zygote, while the other sperm fuses with two polar nuclei to form the $3n$ endosperm. This is called a double fertilization. After fertilization, embryonic development begins.

**256.** They are all found in ovule (Nucellus, Embryo sac and Micropyle) while pollen grain is male gametophyte.

**257.** (a) Nucellus – 2n, antipodal cells – n
(b) Antipodal cells – n, egg cell – n
(c) Antipodal cells – n, megaspore mother cell –2n
(d) Nucellus - 2n primary endosperm nucleus – 3n

**258.** It is a female gametophyte which contains the egg apparatus is present in ovule.

**259.** Pollen grains are found only in Gymnosperms and Angiosperms.

**260.** In porogamy, the tip of pollen tube enters the micropyle, pushes through the nucellar tissue and finally pierces the egg apparatus end of the embryo sac. If pollen tube enters, through chalazal side, it is called chalazogamy and if it enters laterally it is called mesogamy.

**261.** Functional megaspore develops into female gametophyte (embryo sac)

**262.** Microspore is haploid, uninucleate, minute spores produced in large number as a result of meiosis in microspore mother cell inside, the microsporangia. These are the first cell of gametophytic generation in angiosperms.

**263.** Diploid female plant will have 2 polar nuclei (each haploid) with which one male gamete from tetraploid male plant (male gamete of tetraploid plant will be diploid) fuses, making endosperm which is tetraploid.

Male gamete (2n) + 2 polar nuclei (n) → Endosperm (4n)

**264.** Spores are formed in lower plants by mitotic division, and they may be diploid but gametes are always made by meiosis and they are always haploid.

**265.** Each microspore divides by mitotic division making a smaller generative cell and a larger vegetative cell or tube cell. If generative cell in damaged, then the normal pollen tube will be formed because pollen tube is formed by vegetative cell not by generative cell of microspore.

**266.** Substitution of usual sexual reproduction by a form of reproduction which does not include meiosis syngamy is called apomixis. In this technique, embryo in developed by some other tissue without fertilization, e.g., nucellus or integuments or unfertilized egg. Nucellus in a diploid tissue so nucellar embryo is apomictic diploid.

## NCERT Exemplar Questions

**1.**
- There are four floral whorls, viz., calyx, corolla, androecium and gynoecium. Calyx and corolla are accessory organs or non-essential whorl, while androecium and gynoecium are reproductive organs
- Calyx is the outermost whorl of the flower and the members are called sepals.
- Gynoecium is the female reproductive part of the flower and is made up of one or more carpels.

**2.**
- Embryo sac (female gametophyte)
- Ovule (megasporangium)
- Pollen grain (male gametophyte)
- Anther (microsporangium)

**3.** Arrangement of floral whorls on the thalamus from the outermost to the innermost is calyx, corolla, androecium and gynoecium.

**4.** A dicotyledonous plant bears flowers but never produces fruits and seeds because the plant is dioecious and bears only staminate flowers.

**5.** Wall layers of micro sporangium in an anther are:

Epidermis – Endothecium – Middle layers – Tapetum
(Outermost) (Innermost)

**6.** During microsporogenesis, meiosis occurs **in microspore mother** cells.

**7.** Stigma, ovule, embryo sac and placenta are associated with the gynoecium.

**8.** The correct sequence of parts in an ovule are

Egg – embryo sac – nucellus – integument
(Inner) (Outer)

**9.** A typical female gametophyte of a flowering plant is 8-nucleate and 7-celled at maturity and free-nuclear during the development.

**10.** In a normal flower which opens and exposes the anthers and stigma, complete autogamy is rather rare. Autogamy in such flowers requires synchrony in pollen release and stigma receptivity and also the anthers and the stigma should lie close to each other so that self-pollination can occur.

**11.** Cleistogamous flowers are invariably autogamous as there is no chance of cross-pollen landing on the stigma. Cleistogamous flowers produce assured seed set even in the absence of pollinators.

**12.** Pollination by wind is called anemophily. Anemophilous flowers are small, in conspicuous non-scented without bright colours, nectar and fragrance. Wind pollination also requires that the pollen grains are light and non-sticky which is in large numbers and its stigmas are long and feathery.

**13.**
- Autogamy (same flower); geitonogainy (different flowers of same plants; xenogamy (different plant's flower)
- Dioecious plant bearing only male or female flowers prevents both autogamy and geitonogamy.

14. In a fertilized embryo sac, the haploid, diploid and triploid structures are synergid, zygote and primary endosperm nucleus, respectively.

15. In an embryo sac, synergids and antipodals degenerate after fertilization.

**Post-fertilization modifications**

| | |
|---|---|
| **1.** Ovary | Fruit |
| **2.** Ovary wall | Pericarp (fruit wall) |
| **3.** Ovule | Seed |
| **4.** Outer integument | Testa (Outer seed coat) |
| **5.** Inner integument | Tegmen (Inner seed coat) |
| **6.** Secondary nucleus | Endosperm |
| **7.** Egg | Zygote |

16. • Artificial hybridization is one of the major approaches of crop improvement programme. In such crossing experiments, it is important to make sure that only the desired pollen grains are used for pollination and the stigma is protected from contamination (from unwanted pollen). This is achieved by emasculation and bagging techniques.
• Emasculation is relevant in monoecious plants.

17. Cotyledons of the typical dicot embryo are simple structures generally thick and swollen due to storage of food reserves (as in legumes) and embryo of mono cots consists of one large and shield-shaped cotyledon known as scutellum situated towards one side (lateral) of the embryonal axis. E.g.: Grass family, *Sorghum*.

18. • Apomixis is the special mechanism to produce seed without fertilization. It is observed in few flowering plants such as some species of asteraceae and grasses.
• Apomixis is a form of asexual reproduction that mimics sexual reproduction. If a fruit is formed without fertilization of ovary, it is called a parthenocarpic fruit, e.g., banana and grape.

19. In a flower, if the megaspore mother cell forms megaspores without undergoing meiosis and if one of the megaspores develops into an embryo sac, its nuclei would be **diploid.**

20. If a fruit is formed without fertilization of ovary, it is called a parthenocarpic fruit, e.g., banana and grape.

## Previous Years' Questions

1. Pollination taking place by means of wind is known as anemophily, e.g., Zea mays, Cannabis, Pinus.
2. In wheat or maize (family: Poaceae), the scutellum is thought to be a modified cotyledon or seed leaf.
3. Transfer of pollen grains from anther to stigma of another flower of the same plant is called self-pollination. In self-pollination, pollen grains are transferred from anther to the stigma of the same flower or pollen grains are transferred from anther to the stigma of a different flower of the same plant
4. Substitution of usual sexual reproduction by a form of reproduction which does not involve meiosis and syngamy is called apomixis. In citrus, apomictic embryos arise from diploid cells (maternal sporophytic tissue) of the ovule occurring outside the embryo sac.
5. Both vegetative and apomixis are asexual reproduction. The progeny produced are genetically similar to parent and are called clone.
6. In angiosperms, the unit of female gametophyte (embryo sac) is a functional megaspore.
7. Cleistogamy is autogamous pollination. When pollination and fertilization occur in unopened flower bud, it is known as cleistogamy. It ensures self-pollination and prevents cross-pollination.
8. Occurrence of more than one embryo in a seed is referred to as polyembryony. In many citrus and mango varieties, some of the nucellar cells surrounding the embryo sac start dividing, protruding into the embryo sac and develop into embryos in such species where each ovule contains many embryos (nucellar polyembryony).
9. Pollination by wind (anemophily) is more common amongst abiotic pollinations. Wind pollination is quite common in grasses.
10. The outermost cell layer of the endosperm (3n) of seed is called aleurone layer. Since the cells of aleurone layer are triploid, the number of chromosomes would be = 63, as root tip cells (2n) has 42 chromosomes.
11. Filiform apparatus is a finger-like projection of the cell membrane of synergids or help cells at the micropylar end of the ovule. Filiform apparatus is rich in polysaccharides and chemoattracts pollen tube towards micropyle.
12. The coconut water obtained form the tender coconut is nothing but free nuclear endosperm (made up of

thousands of nuclei) and the surrounding white kernel is the cellular endosperm.

**13.** • In plants like **Viola (Common Pansy), Oxalis** and **Commelina** produce two types of flowers:
- **Chasmogamous flowers:** Flowers with exposed anthers and stigma.
- **Cleistogamous flowers:** Flowers that do not open at all. Such flowers are purely autogamous and produce assured seed sets.

**14.** Pollen grains are generally spherical measuring about 25–50 micrometers in diameter. It has a prominent two-layered wall. The hard outer layer called the **exine** is made up of sporopollenin which is one of the most resistant organic material known. It can withstand high temperatures and strong acids and alkali. No enzyme that degrades sporopollenin is so far known. Pollen grain exine has prominent apertures called **germ pores** where sporopollenin is absent and pollen tube arises.

**15.** A multicarpellary, apocarpous gynoecium found in *Michelia*. [Move this to chapter on morphology of flowering plants]

**16.** In remaining species of angiosperms, generative cell divides mitotically to form 2 male gametes, acquire 3-celled stage (1 vegetative cell + 2 male gametes) and then are shedded at the same stage.

**17.** The pollen grain has two layers: outer exine and inner intine. Exine is made up of highly resistant sporopollenin while in tine is pectocellulosic. At certain places where exine is thin or absent is called germpore or germinal furrow. After reaching on stigma, the pollen grain absorbs water and nutrients from the stigmatic secretion through its germ pore. The tube or vegetative cell enlarges. It comes out of the pollen grain through one of the germ pores or germinal furrows to form a pollen tube.

**18.** The transfer of pollen grains from anther to stigma is called pollination. Anemophily is a mode of pollination accomplished through wind, while entomophily is the mode of pollination accomplished by insects like moth, butterflies, wasps, bees, etc.

**19.** Papaya is a dioeicious plant which means male and female flower are present on different plant therefore it prevents both autogamy and geitonogamy.

**20.** Perisperm is a persistent nucellus within seeds. It is not common as nucellus is nutritive tissue which provides nutrition to embryo sac. Nucellus is a diploid tissue. In beet and piper it is persists within seed so it is diploid (2n) while endosperm is a triploid (3n) tissue.

**21.** Cleistogamy means closed flower which are bisexual does not require pollinator however have assured seed set.

**22.** Tapetum is the innermost layer of anther that provides nutrition to developing microspore/pollens.

**23.** In angiosperms, the seed is the final product of sexual reproduction. It is often described as a fertilized ovule. Seeds are formed inside fruits. A seed typically consists of seed coat(s), cotyledon(s) and an embryo axis. The cotyledons of the embryo are simple structures, generally thick and swollen due to storage of food reserves (as in legumes). Mature seeds may be non-albuminous or albuminous.

**24.** Pollen tube grows through tissues of the stigma and style and reaches the ovary. You would recall that in some plants, pollen grains are shed at two-celled condition (a vegetative cell and a generate cell). In such plants, the generative cell divides and forms the two male gametes during the growth of pollen tube in the stigma. In plants which shed pollen in the three-celled condition, pollen tubes carry the two male gametes from the beginning. Pollen tube, after reaching the ovary, enters the ovule through the micropyle and then enters one of the synergids through the filiform apparatus.

**25.** Pollen grains are rich in nutrients. It has become a fashion in recent years to use pollen tablets as food supplements. In Western countries, large number of pollen products in the form of tablets and syrups are available in the market. Pollen consumption has been claimed to increase the performance of athletes and race horses.

**26.** Male gametophyte with least number of cells is present in angiosperm. For example: Lilium.

**27.** Transfer of pollen grains from anther to stigma of another flower of the same plant.

**28.** Each microspore mother cell of anther undergoes meiosis to form microspore tetrad while megaspore mother cell of ovule undergoes meiosis to form megaspore tetrad.

**29.** Filiform apparatus present at the micropylar part of the synergids guides the entry of pollen tube.

**30.** Some species in which fruits develope without fertilization is called parthenocarpic fruit, e.g. Banana.

**31.** • **Stage of shedding of pollen grains:** 2-celled stage (in > 60 % of angiosperms).
- In remaining species of angiosperms, generative cell divides mitotically to form 2 male gametes, acquire **3-celled stage** (1 vegetative cell + 2 male gametes) and then are shedded at the same stage.

**32.** Those flowers which are pollinated by **flies** and **beetles** have a foul odour. Flowers provide nector and pollen grain as **floral rewards** to the animals.

**33.** Style may be hollow or solid. Hollow style has a canal lined by special large cells. Solid style has a special tissue of pectinized thick walls known as transmitting or conducting tissue.

**34.** • Pollen grains of many plants may cause severe allergy in some people, ultimately leading to asthma, bronchitis, etc.

• Pollen allergy is also caused by ***Parthenium*** or **carrot grass.** It has come into India with imported wheat, as a contaminant but now it has become very common throughout India.

• As the pollen grains are rich in nutrients, in recent years, these are used as pollen tablets (a food supplement).

• Athletes and race horses also consume pollen to increase their performance.

**35.** ***Geitonogamy*** – Transfer of pollen grains from anther to stigma of another flower of the same plant. Although geitonogamy is functionally cross-pollinated involving a pollinating agent, genetically it is similar to autogamy since the pollen grains come from the same plant.

**36.** Ovule = Megasporangium.

**37.** • In most of aquatic plants (including **Water hyacinth** and **Water lily**), both male and female flowers emerge above the level of water and are pollinated by biotic (insects) or abiotic (wind) means just like most of the land plants.

**38.** The process of formation of megaspores from the **megaspore mother cell** is called **megasporogenesis.** Ovules generally differentiate a single megaspore mother cell (MMC) in the micropylar region of the nucellus. It is a large cell containing dense cytoplasm and a prominent nucleus. The MMC undergoes meiotic division.

Typical embryo sac of angiosperm consists of

(1) Three antipodal cells

(2) Egg apparatus – one egg cell and two synergids (with filiform apparatus).

**39.** New genetic combination develops after sexual reproduction due to following reasons.

(1) Crossing over during gametes formation.

(2) Chance combination of gametic fusion.

Sexual reproduction involves formation of the male and female gametes, either by the same individual or by different individuals of the opposite sex. These gametes fuse to form the zygote which develops to form a new organism. It is an elaborate, complex and slow process as compared to asexual reproduction. Because of the fusion of male and female gametes, sexual reproduction results in offspring that are not identical to the parents or amongst themselves.

**40.** Pollen grains of many species can germinate on the stigma of a flower, but only one pollen tube of the same species grows into the style because of pollen pistil interaction.

**41.** Seed formation without fertilization in flowering plants involves the process of apomixis.

**42.** It is generally surrounded by four-walled layers, epidermis, endothecium, middle layers and tapetum. The outer three wall layers perform the function of protection and help indehiscence of anther to release the pollen. The innermost wall layer is the tapetum. It nourishes the developing pollen grains. The hard outer layer called the exine is made up of sporopollenin which is one of the most resistant organic material known. Pollen grains of many species cause severe allergies and bronchial afflictions in some people often leading to chronic respiratory disorders and asthma, bronchitis. It is possible to store pollen grains of a large number of species for years in liquid nitrogen (–196°C). Such stored pollen can be used as pollen banks, similar to seed banks, in crop breeding programmes.

**43.** The proximal end of the filament is attached to the thalamus or the petal of the flower.

**44.** Coconut milk represents free-nuclear endosperm where the division of primary endosperm nucleus is not followed by formation of cell walls (cytokinesis) thus all nucleus remain free in liquid form. It is rich in plant hormone cytokinin.

**45.** Seed formation without fertilization in flowering plants involves the process of apomixis.

**46.** Primary endosperm formed by triple fusion therefore its ploidy is 3n.

**47.** Continued self-pollination result in inbreeding depression.

**48.** Pollen grains are stored for years in **liquid nitrogen (–196°C)** and can be used as pollen banks in crop breeding programmes.

**49.** Coleoptile: Sheath enclosing the plumule.

**50.** Production of unisexual flowers. Unisexual flowers may be produced on:

- Same plant (monoecious plants): Example–**Castor, Maize.** This prevents autogamy but not geitonogamy.
- Different plants (dioecious plants, **Phenomenon–Dioecy**): Example, **Papaya.** This prevents both autogamy and geitonogamy.

**51. Pollination by Wind**

- It is more common in comparison to other abiotic pollinators.
- **Important Features of Wind Pollination:**
  (1) Pollen grains are light and non-sticky (for easy transport).
  (2) Stamens are usually well exposed (for easy dispersal).
  (3) Stigma is large and often feathery (for easy trapping of pollen grains).
  (4) Number of ovule per ovary: Usually one.
  (5) Flowers are numerous and are packed into an inflorescence.
- The tassels of **Corn cob** are the stigma and style which wave in the wind to trap pollen grains.
- Pollination by wind is common in **grasses.**

**52.** Functional megaspore develops into female gametophyte (embryo sac).

**53.** Those flowers which are pollinated by **flies** and **beetles** have a foul odour. Flowers provide nector and pollen grain as **floral rewards** to animals.

**54.** The hard outer layer of pollen called the exine is made up of sporopollenin which is one of the most resistant organic material known. It can withstand high temperatures and strong acids and alkali. No enzyme that degrades sporopollenin is so far known. Therefore, pollen grains are well-preserved as fossil because of presence of sporopollenin.

**55.** Species of moth and the plant *Yucca* where both species – moth and the plant – cannot complete their life cycles without each other. The moth deposits its eggs in the locule of the ovary and the flower, in turn, gets pollinated by the moth.

**56.** It is possible to store pollen grains of a large number of species for years in liquid nitrogen (–196°C).

**57.** It involves two types of fusions, **syngamy** (fertilization of male and female gamete ) and **triple fusion** (fusion of one of male gamete with two polar nuclie situated in central cell) take place in an embryo sac; the phenomenon is termed **double fertilization,**

**58.** Winged pollen grains are found in *Pinus*. They involve wind for pollination and are found hundereds of kilometers away from the parent plant after dispersal.

**59.** After entering one of the synergids, the pollen tube releases two male gametes into the cytoplasm of the synergid. One of the male gametes move towards the egg cell and fuses with its nucleus thus completing the **syngamy**. This results in formation of a diploid cell, the **zygote**. The other male gamete moves towards the two polar nuclei located in the central cell and fuses with them to produce a triploid **primary endosperm nucleus** (PEN)

**60.** Occasionally, in some seeds such as black pepper and beet, remnants of nucellus are also persistent. This residual persistent nucellus is the perisperm.

**61.** The attachment point of funicle and body of ovule is known as hilum.

**62.** In majority of aquatic plants, the flowers emerge above the level of water.

These may be pollinated by insects or wind. **eg:** Water hyacinth and water lily.

**63.** Xenogamy :

- Transfer of pollen grains from anther to the stigma of a different plant.
- This is the only type of pollination which during pollination brings genetically different types of pollen grains to the stigma.

**64.** A typical angiospermic embryo sac have:

7 cells - 3 antipodals, 1 central cell,
1 egg cell
2 synergids.

8 nucleated - The central cell has 2 polar nuclei + nucleus of antipodals, egg cell, synergids.

**65.** In members of some plant families like ***Solanaceae, Rosaceae and Leguminosae,*** the pollen grains retain their viability for several months.

**66. Common pollinating animal agents are:** Bees (most common or dominant biotic pollinating agent)

**67.** Some plants such as Viola (common pansy), Oxalis, and Commelina produce two types of flowers – chasmogamous flowers which are similar to flowers of other species with exposed anthers and stigma, and cleistogamous flowers which do not open at all. These flowers are invariably autogamous

Cleistogamous flowers does not open at all. In such flowers autogamy occurs. Lack of cross pollination is a disadvantage of Cleistogamy.

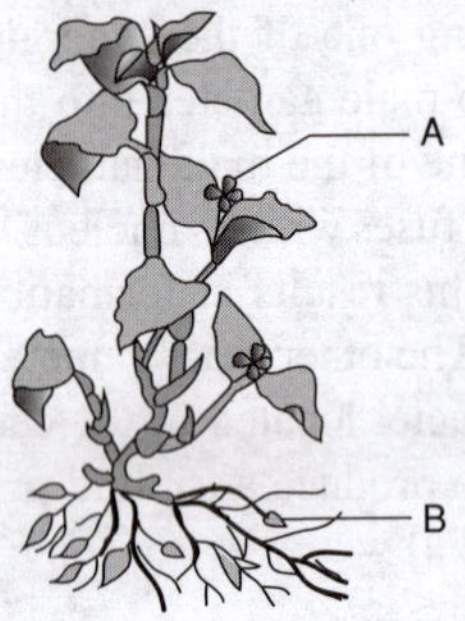


**68.**

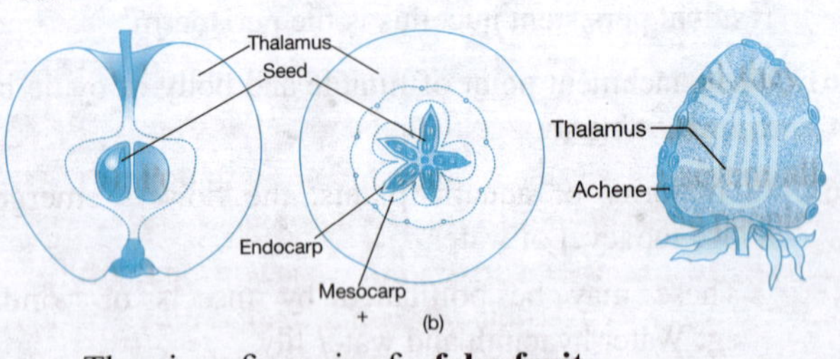


The given figure is of a **false fruit.**

False fruit develops from other floral parts and thalamus along with the development of ovary wall.

**69.** Tassels are female part of flower ,i.e., stigma and style in corn plant which is pollinated by wind pollination. So it waves in wind to trap the pollen grains.

**70.** Large Colourful fragrant flowers with nectar are seen in insect pollinated plants to attract insect for pollination.

**71.** Synergids - haploid (a pair of haploid cells at micropylar end of embryo sac)
Zygote – Diploid (Formed by fusion of male and female gametes which are haploid)
PEN – Triploid (Formed by fusion of 2 polar nuclei and one male gamete)

**72.** Flowers of *Vallisneria* are not colourful and do not produce nectar because they are water-pollinated species. Water lily is pollinated by insect or wind. In water-pollinated species, pollen grains are protected from wetting by a mucilaginous covering.
In some hydrophytes such as *Vallisneria,* pollen grains are carried passively by water current.

**73.** Radicle is destined to form root.
In the given diagram, 'C' represents radicle.

**74.** The given diagram shows a wind pollinated plant showing compact inflorescence and well exposed stamens.

# 2 Principles of Inheritance and Variation

## LEARNING OBJECTIVES

- Understand the mechanism of inheritance
- Understand the difference between dominant and recessive gene
- Discuss how test-cross allows detection of heterozygotes
- How do genes influence traits?
- Explain Mendel's first and second law along with exception to Mendel's law.
- Mutation and brief about heredity disease and pedigree analysis.

## Chapter Overview

- **Inheritance:** It is the process of transferring characters from parents to the progeny and it is the basis of heredity.
- **Variations:** It refers to the degree by which the offsprings differs from the parent.
- **Genetics:** Study of heredity and variation together.
- **Sahiwal cows in Punjab** are well known Indian breeds that have developed from artificial selection and domestication from the wild cows.
- **Pre-mendelian ideas about inheritance-direct transmission of characteristics or blending inheritance:** Different theories were put forward before Mendel to explain the transmission of characters from parents to offsprings. They proposed that the characters of the parents got mixed during transmission to the offspring. Hence, these theories are often **called 'theories of blending inheritance'.** Some of these theories are given below:

1. **Vapour theory:** Greek philosopher **Pythagoras** (500 B.C.) proposed that, during coitus, moist vapours from all parts of a male's body give rise to a similar body in female's womb.
2. **Fluid theory: Aristotle** postulated that, during coitus, the female releases an '*inert*' fluid to which 'life' is given by a *'vitalizing fluid (semen)'* released by male and it considered as 'highly purified blood'.
3. **Particulate theory:** After the invention of microscopes in 17th century, **Graaf, Malpighi** and **Swammerdam** discovered eggs, while **Leeuwenhoek** and **Hamm** discovered spermatozoa. These discoveries took human knowledge from the era of speculation into the era of reality. It was soon realized that gametes, as minute particles formed by male and female parents and unite in sexual reproduction to form new individuals.

- Two different postulates emerged under Particulate Theory. *viz.,*'Preformation Theory' and 'Theory of Continuity of Germplasm'. Under **'Preformation Theory (Encasement Theory)'**, **Hartsoeker** (1694) claimed that he could see, inside a human sperm, a miniature figure of a 'man', the '*homunculus*' **(Fig. 2.1 A)**. **Swammerdam**, **Bonnet** and **Maupertius** held that sex cells (gametes) possess miniature copies, the '*mankins*' **(Fig. 2.1 B and C)** of adult bodies.

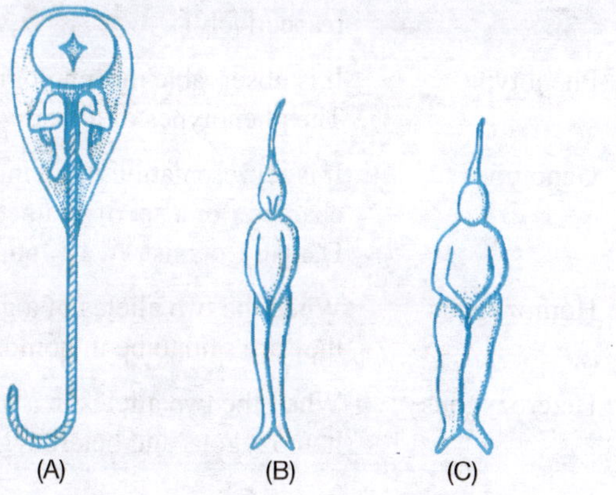


**FIGURE 2.1** "Homunculus" (A) and "Mankins" (B,C)

---
Refer NCERT Ch 4: Principles of Inheritance and Variation

4. **Pangenesis theory:** Proposed by **Charles Darwin** (1868). According to this theory all parts of a living body release in blood their miniature copies called *pangenes* or *gemmules* which collect in gonalds to form gametes.
5. **Theory of Epigenesis:** Preformation theory was however replaced by **Wolff** in 18th century by his **'Theory of Epigenesis'** which postulated that a complex multicellular embryo gradually develops from a single fertilized cell and eventually becomes a baby in later stages of pregnancy.
6. **Weismann theory of germplasm: August Weismann** (1889) suggested the theory of continuity of **germplasm**. He described reproductive cells as germplasm and rest of the body as somatoplasm.

- **Gregor Mendel: Father of Genetics**
  - Gregor Mendel (1822–1884) conducted hybridization experiments on the garden peas (*Pisum sativum*) for 7 years (1856–1863). Mendel published his work in 1865.
  - Mendel selected garden pea (Edible pea, *Pisum sativum*) for his experiments because of the Following reasons:
    1. Large number of true breeding varieties with observable alternative forms for a trait or characters (such as yellow or green seed colour, round or wrinkled seed shape and so on) were available.
    2. Peas are normally self-pollinated (and so self-fertilized) and their corollas completely enclose the reproductive organs until pollination is accomplished. However, pea flowers can be readily cross-pollinated (hybridized) if self-pollination is prevented. This is achieved by removing the anthers (emasculation) before the pollen grains mature, and dusting the stigma of these flowers (female parent) with pollen from the desired plant (male parent).
    3. Pea is an annual plant and gives results within a year.
    4. Large number of seeds are produced by a pea plant that helps in drawing correct conclusions.
    5. Pea plants are easy to cultivate and do not require after care except at the time of pollination.

**TABLE 2.1** Important terms used in inheritance studies

| Terms | Meaning | Examples |
|---|---|---|
| Character | It is the feature of the individual. | Stem height |
| Trait | An inherited character and its detectable variant. | Tall or dwarf |
| Unit factor | A unit of inheritance called gene by modern geneticists. Each gene or factor controls a character. | *D* |
| Allelomorphs or Alleles | It represents at least two alternative forms of a gene or unit factor. Each gene consists of an allelomorphic pair. (Term introduced by **Bateson** in 1906) | *Dd, Dd, Dd* |
| Gene symbol | Each trait is provided a symbol.<br>By one convention the first latter of the mutant trait is chosen to derive the symbol, e.g. *dd* for dwarfness and *Dd* for tallness (this is sometimes referred as tt and *TT* respectively) | |
| Phenotype | It is observable morphological appearance.<br>The phenotypes of an individual are determined by different combinations of alleles | Tall or dwarf |
| Genotype | It is representation of an individual's genetic constitution with respect to a single character or a set of characters. (The term genotype and phenotype introduced by Danish Botanist **W. L. Johannsen** in 1909) | *DD*<br>*Dd*<br>*Dd* |
| Homozygous | When the two alleles of a gene are similar and so two copies of the same allele exist, they are said to be in homozygous. | *DD* or *dd* |
| Heterozygous | When the two alleles in a pair different they are in heterozygous state. (Term homozygous and heterozygous introduced by **Bateson** and **Saunders** in 1902) | Dd |

(*Continued*)

| Terms | Meaning | Examples |
|---|---|---|
| Dominant | An allele that influences the appearance of the phenotype even in the presence of an alternative allele. | *D* |
| Recessive | An allele that influences the appearance of the phenotype only in the presence of another identical allele. | *D* |
| Gene | (Mendel called them factor) In modern sense an inherited factor that determines a biological character of an organism is called gene. (functional unit of hereditary material). | |
| Pseudo allele | Genes having separate but nearby loci and controlling the same trait. | |
| Gene locus | The specific place on a chromosome where a gene is located. | |
| Wild and mutant alleles | An original allele, dominant in expression and wide spread in the population is called wild allele. An allele formed by a mutation in the wild allele, recessive in expression and less common in the population is termed as mutant allele. | |
| Hemizygous | Condition in which only one allele of a pair is present.<br>Hemizygous condition occurs for those genes which are formed on differential parts of *XY* chromosomes.<br>Human males are hemizygous for Haemophilia and red-green colour-blindness.<br>In such hemizygous condition the single recessive allele produces its effect. | |
| Pure-line | Generations of homozygous individuals which produce offsprings of only one type *i.e.,* they breed true for their phenotype and genotype. (The term pure-line was introduced by Danish Botanist **Johannsen**) | |
| Monohybrid, dihybrid and polyhybrid | If only one allelic pair is considered in cross breeding, then it is called monohybrid cross. Similarly, when two allelic pairs are used for crossing, it is called dihybrid cross and when more than two allelic pairs in a cross are called polyhybrid cross. | |
| Reciprocal cross | The reciprocal crosses involve two crosses concerning the same characteristics, but with reversed sexes. | |
| Genome | Total set of genes (DNA instructions) in the haploid set of chromosomes and inherited as unit from parents to offspring is called genome. | |
| Gene pool | All the genotypes of all organisms in a population form the gene pool. | |
| $F_1$ Generation | $F_1$ or first filial (*filus*–son, *filia*–daughter; Bateson, 1905) generation is the generation of hybrids produced from a cross between the genetically different individuals called parents. | |
| $F_2$ Generation (Bateson, 1905) | $F_2$ or second filial generation is the generation of individuals which arises as a result of inbreeding or interbreeding amongst individuals of $F_1$ generation. | |
| Punnett square | It is a checker-board used to show the result of a cross between two organisms; it was devised by geneticist, R.C. Punnett (1927). It depicts both genotypes and phenotypes of the progeny. | |
| Back cross | It is cross which is performed between hybrid and one of its parents. In plant breeding, back cross is performed a few times to increase the traits of that parent. | |
| Out cross | It is cross which is performed between hybrid and dominant parents. | |

(*Continued*)

| Terms | Meaning | Examples |
|---|---|---|
| Test cross | It is a cross to know whether an individual is homozygous or heterozygous for dominant character. The individual is crossed with recessive parent. The ratio will be 50% dominant and 50% recessive in case of hybrid or heterozygous individual. In case of double heterozygote (*e.g.*, *RrYy*) crossed with recessive (*rryy*) the ratio will be 1 : 1 : 1 : 1. Test cross helps to find out genotype of parents. | |
| Self cross/selfing | It is the process of fertilization with pollen or male gametes of the same individual. | |
| Observed Vs expected results | Experimental results confirm to the ones expected through the theory of probability if the size of the sample is small but they tend to approach the latter if the sample size is large. | |
| Hybrid | The organism produced after crossing of two genetically different individuals is called hybrid. | |

## Mendel's Experiments

- Mendel performed experiments is three stages:
  (i) Selection of pure or true breeding parents
  (ii) Hybridization and obtaining $F_1$ generation of plants, (iii) Self-pollination of hybrid plants to raise subsequent generations like $F_2$ $F_3$ and so on,

**(i) Selection of Parents:**

- Mendel selected fourteen pure or true breeding varieties (seven pairs of contrasting forms) of peas as the starting-material for his experiments **(Fig. 2.2)**.

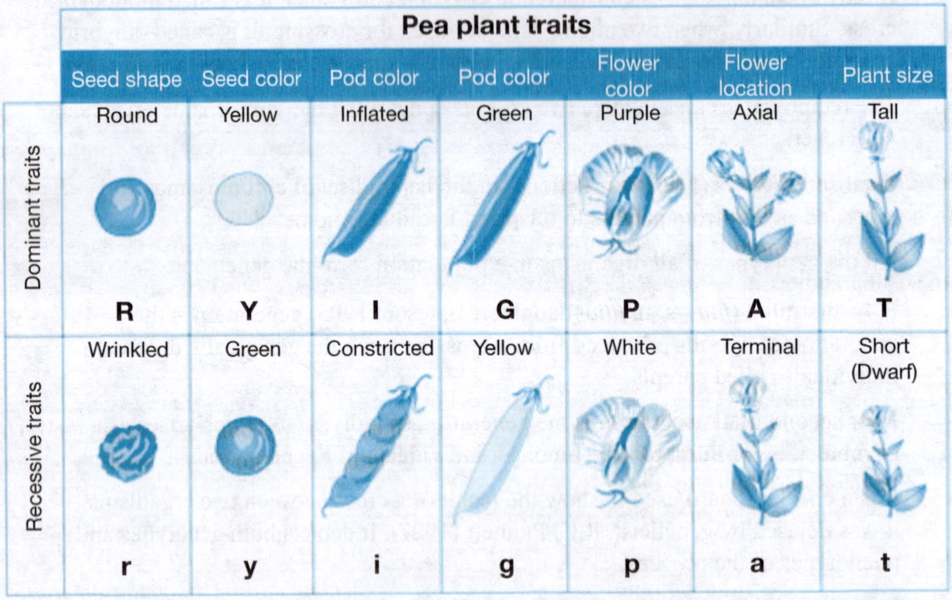


**FIGURE 2.2** Contrasting forms of the seven traits of pea studied by Mendel

- A pure or true breeding variety produces offspring having similar trait on self-pollination or self-breeding. For example, white flowered plant produces white flowered offsprings; purple flowered plant produces purple flowered offspring and so on. Mendel satisfied himself as to true breeding nature of each variety through self-pollination. Any offspring that was not true to the form of the trait was eliminated. True breeding plants formed the **parent** (P) **generation.**

- Mendel employed **seven traits** with easily distinguishable contrasting or alternate forms as shown in. **The traits were seed colour, seed shape, flower colour, pod colour, pod shape, flower position and plant height.**

**(ii) Hybridization for $F_1$ Generation:**

- Mendel hybridized or cross-pollinated plants with alternate forms of a trait. For example, purple flowered and white flowered plants, tall and dwarf plants and so on. He also made reciprocal crosses **(Fig. 2.3)**.
- In such crosses, pollens of one form were dusted over the stigma of the other form and vice versa. For example, pollens from white flowers were used for pollinating emasculated purple flowers and the pollen from purple flowers were deposited on the stigmas of emasculated white flowers.
- The hand pollinated flowers were covered with paper bags to prevent contamination from foreign pollen, and the cross in which two forms of a single trait are brought together or hybridized, is called **monohybrid cross.**

**4.** The hybrid offspring of such a cross is both the seed (the equivalent of an infant) and the plant which grows from the seed (the equivalent of an adult). The hybrid offspring constitutes the next generation and is termed as **first filial** or **$F_1$ generation.**

**5.** Mendel also performed crosses involving alternate forms of two traits. Such crosses are called **dihybrid crosses.** Trihybrid and polyhybrid crosses were performed as well.

**(iii) Self Breeding for $F_2$ and $F_3$ Generations:**

- Mendel allowed the hybrid plants of $F_1$ generation to self-pollinate.
- The resulting seeds, and the plants raised from them constitute the **second filial or $F_2$ generation.** Subsequent generations of the $F_2$, namely $F_3$, $F_4$, etc., were also raised following self-pollination.
- Mendel recorded the number of each type of contrasting form of every generation and analyzed the results.

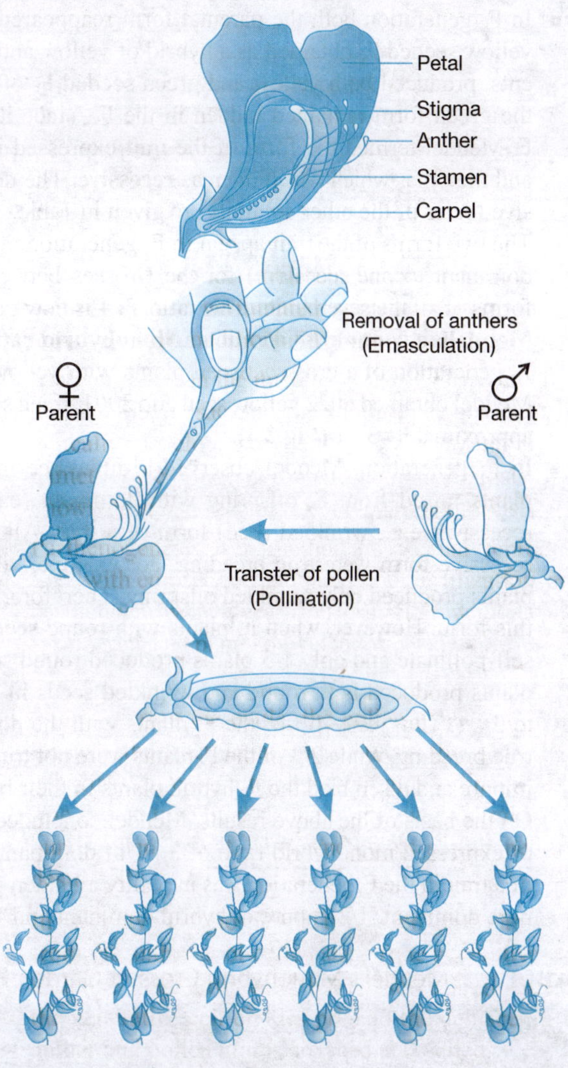


**FIGURE 2.3** Steps in making an artificial hybridization in pea

## Mendel's Findings

- For each of the seven traits examined, Mendel observed that the hybrids or $F_1$ offsprings invariably resembled one parent and not the other. This was true for reciprocal crosses as well.
- For example, a cross between plants with yellow and green seeds gave all yellow seeded $F_1$ offsprings. Similar conditions of the $F_1$ offsprings were observed with regards to the other six traits.

- In $F_2$ generation both the parental form reappeared. For example, the yellow seeded $F_1$ obtained as a hybrid of yellow and green seeded parents, produced both yellow and green seeded $F_2$ offspring. Obviously, the green form remained hidden in the $F_1$, since it reappeared in the $F_2$.Mendel termed the form of the trait expressed in $F_1$ as **dominant** and the other which was hidden as **recessive.** The dominant and recessive forms of the other six traits are given in Table.
- The two forms of the trait appear in $F_2$ generation in ratio of 3: 1 (three dominant to one recessive) for the Crosses between the contrasting forms of all the seven traits. This ratio, 3: 1 is now generally termed the **Mendelian Monohybrid ratio** or **Monohybrid ratio.** For example, in $F_2$ generation of a cross between plants with yellow and green seeds, Mendel obtained 6022 yellow seed and 2001 green seeds. The ratio was approximately 3 : 1 **(Fig 2.4)**.
- In $F_2$ generation, Mendel observed a difference in the behaviour of plants raised from $F_2$ offspring with dominant (e.g., round seed) or recessive (e.g., wrinkled seed) form of a trait. All $F_2$ plants with the recessive form were true breeding. For example, all wrinkled seeded plants produced only wrinkled offspring. Therefore, they were pure for this form. However, when $F_2$ plants with round seeds were allowed to self-pollinate and only 1/3 plants produced round seeds, the other 2/3 plants produced both round and wrinkled seeds in a proportion close to 3 : 1. Thus, only 1/3 of the $F_2$ plants with the dominant form were true breeding, while 2/3 of the $F_2$ plants were not true breeding or were impure and resembled the $F_1$ hybrid plants in their behaviour.
  On the basis of the above results, Mendel concluded that the observed or expressed monohybrid ratio of 3 : 1 of dominant or recessive form of a trait in the $F_1$ generation was in reality a hidden 1 : 2 : 1 ratio of 1/4 pure dominant, 1/2 impure or hybrid dominant and 1/4 pure recessive.

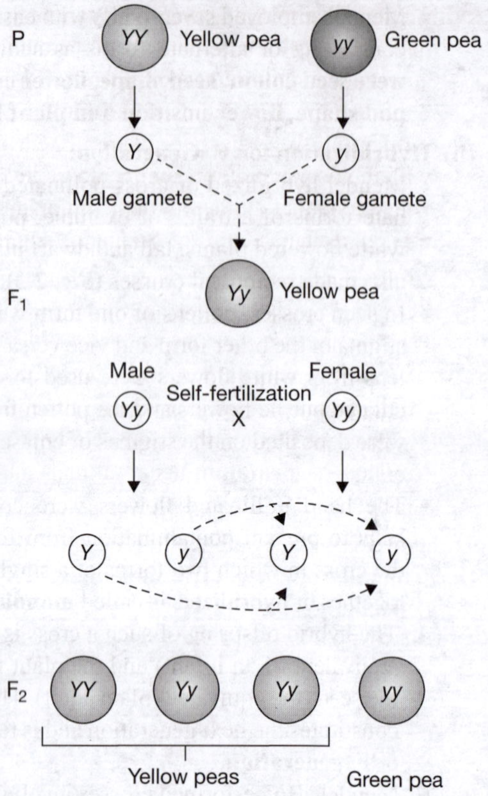


**FIGURE 2.4** A flow chart of a Mendel's monohybrid cross

**TABLE 2.2** Mendel's Monohybrid Cross in Garden Pea (*Pisum sativum*)

| Trait (Parent Forms) | $F_1$ form | $F_2$ Generation Results (Dominant) | (Recessive) | Monohybrid Ratio |
|---|---|---|---|---|
| Seed colour (Yellow × green) | all yellow | 6022 (yellow) | 2001 (green) | 3.01 : 1 |
| Seed shape (round × wrinkled) | all round | 5474(round) | 1850 (wrinkled) | 2.96 : 1 |
| Flower colour (purple × white) | all purple | 705 (purple) | 224 (white) | 3.15 : 1 |
| Pod colour (green × yellow) | all green | 428 (green) | 152 (yellow) | 2.82 : 1 |
| Pod shape (inflated × constricted) | all inflated | 882 (inflated) | 299 (constricted) | 2.95 : 1 |
| Flower position (axial × terminal) | all axial | 651 (axial) | 207 (terminal) | 3.14 : 1 |
| Plant height (tall × dwarf) | all tall | 787 (tall) | 207 (dwarf) | 2.84 : 1 |

- Mendel observed that one of the parental form of a trait was always absent in the $F_1$ hybrid but reappeared unchanged in the $F_2$ generation. This observation conclusively disproved blending inheritance and supported the idea that the inheritance may be **particulate in nature.** If this were so, alternate forms of a trait could retain their identity in the hybrid and re-emerge unchanged in subsequent generations. Therefore, Mendel concluded that what were transmitted from parent to offspring were discrete factors. Each factor contained information about the form of a trait. The factor associated with the form which was expressed in the hybrid ($F_1$) offspring was **dominant,** while the factor associated with the form which remained hidden in the $F_1$ but reappeared in $F_2$ was recessive. Mendel's factor is now recognized as the **'gene'.**
- Mendel explained the 1 : 2 : 1,and he obtained in the $F_2$ generation with the following arguments and conditions:
  **(1)** Each trait of the pea plant is produced by two factors. The factors may be similar or dissimilar. If similar the plant is **'pure'** for the trait. If dissimilar, it is **'impure'** (hybrid) for the trait.
  **(2)** The plant receives one of these factors from the male gamete and the other from the female gamete. The gametes fuse during fertilization to form zygote from which the plant develops.
  **(3)** Each gamete (male or female) has only one factor of the pair. A gamete is therefore **'pure'** for a trait.
  **(4)** The two factors of a pair occur with equal frequency in the male or female gametes.
  **(5)** There is a **random** fusion of male and female gametes to form a zygote.
- Taking symbols A and a for the dominant and recessive forms of the factors for any hypothetical trait, and by using the above arguments and conditions, the 1 : 2 : 1 ratio in $F_2$ generation will be obtained in the following manner.
- **Principles or Laws of Inheritance:** On his work on monohybrid crosses **(Fig. 2.5)**, Mendel succeeded to extract two general principles or laws:

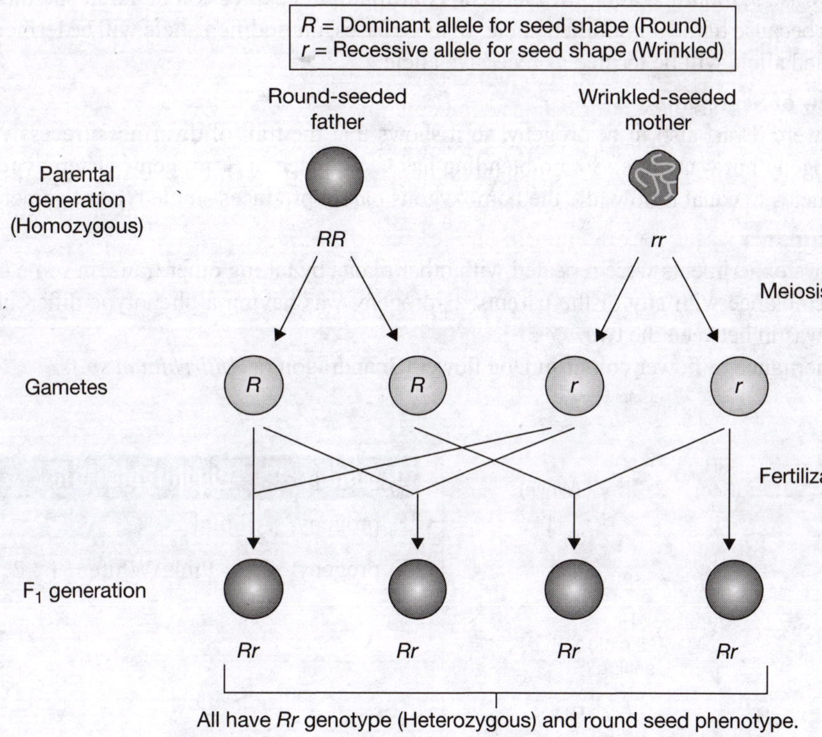


**FIGURE 2.5** A flow chart of a Mendel's monohybrid cross

## A. Principle of Paired Factors:

- The inheritance of each character in an organism is controlled by two determinants called **factors.** In modern terminology, these factors are termed as genes (Johannsen, 1909). The two factors or genes that determine a trait lie on the two homologous chromosomes at the same locus.
- They may represent the same (i.e., homozygous) or alternate (i.e., heterozygous) expression of the same character. The pair of factors or genes representing the same or alternate form of a character are called **alleles** or **allelomorphs.**

**(1) First law: Law of Dominance**

If monohybrid cross is done then only one of the parental character (it will be termed as dominant allele) will be expressed in $F_1$ progeny while both of the parental characters will be expressed in $F_2$ progeny (in ratio of 3 : 1 = Dominant: Recessive). This law states that:

- Factors are discrete units and these control the character.
- Factors remain in pair.
- In heterozygous condition, one of the factors in a pair is able to express itself. It is termed as dominant factor while the other one is termed as recessive.

**Concept of dominance**

- As the organisms are usually diploid, each gene is represented by two alleles.
- In heterozygous condition, one allele is normal but another allele is different from the normal. It has undergone some changes because of which its function or effect has been modified or altered.
  **Example:** A gene is taken which is responsible for the synthesis of an enzyme. Normal allele: Produces normal enzyme.

**Modified allele:**

- Produces case 1: a normal or less efficient enzyme.
- Case 2: non-functional enzyme (same phenotypic effect will not result).
- Case 3: no enzyme (same phenotypic effect will not result).
- In Case 1, same phenotypic effect will result. Such alleles are equivalent and more common.
- In Case 2 and Case 3, modified allele will have no contribution in expression of a trait and the expressed trait will be exclusively because of the unmodified allele. In these cases, unmodified allele will be termed as dominant allele and the modified allele will be termed as recessive allele.

**(2) Second law: Law of Segregation**

As 1/4th plants were dwarf also in $F_2$ progeny, so it shows that the trait of dwarfness (recessive trait) was not expressed in $F_1$ progeny but was there. So, no blending has taken place in $F_1$ progeny. Heterozygous parent produces two types of gametes in equal ratio while the homozygous parent produces single type of gametes.

**Incomplete dominance**

- When the above experiments were repeated with other plants by taking other traits, in some cases $F_1$ progeny did not show resemblance with any of the parents. $F_1$ progeny was having a phenotype different from either of the parent and it was in between the two.
  **Example:** Inheritance of flower colour in Dog flower (Snapdragon or *Antirrhinum sp.*)

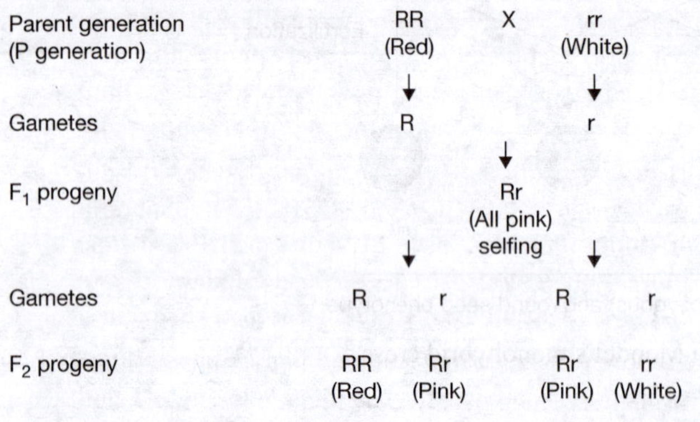


| Result of | Phenotypic ratio | Genotypic ratio |
|---|---|---|
| $F_1$ progeny | All pink | All Rr |
| $F_2$ progeny | Red: Pink: White = 1 : 2 : 1 | RR:Rr:rr = 1 : 2 : 1 |

- **Co-dominance**
  - In a monohybrid cross, if the $F_1$ progeny (or $F_1$ generation) resembles both the parents, it is termed as co-dominance.
    **Example:** ABO blood-group system.
  - Expression of the ABO blood group system is determined by gene I.

- Gene I is responsible for the synthesis of types of sugar polymers (slightly different from each other) that protrude out from the membrane of the RBC.
- Gene I exist in three allelic forms: $I^A$, $I^B$ and i.

**TABLE 2.3** ABO blood group system

| Character | Types of alleles in population (3) | Possible genotypes in an individual (6) | Sugar polymer synthesized | Phenotypic expressions or blood group (4) |
|---|---|---|---|---|
| ABO blood grouping | $I^A$, $I^B$ and i. | $I^A I^A$ | A | A |
| | | $I^A$ i | A | A |
| | | $I^B I^B$ | B | B |
| | | $I^B$ i | B | B |
| | | i i | – | O |
| | | $I^A I^B$ | A and B both | AB |

- Normally in a population, two alleles are found for a gene. But if more than two alleles are there in a population, it is termed as multiple allelism.
- ABO blood group system is an example of multiple allelism, while the blood group AB is an example of co-dominance.
- In blood group AB (heterozygous condition), both A and B sugars are expressed in the membrane of RBC.

- **Pleiotropy**
  - In this case a gene product produces more than one effect.

    **Example:** A gene with two alleles (B and b) in pea seeds control starch synthesis:

    BB: High amount of starch is synthesized → Large sized round starch grains.

    Bb: Lesser amount of starch is synthesized → Intermediate sized round starch grains.

    bb: Least amount of starch is synthesized → Small sized wrinkled starch grains.
  - Above gene is said to be pleiotropic gene, because it possess two phenotypic effects:

    (1) Grain size depending upon the amount of starch synthesis.

    (2) Grain shape (round or wrinkled).
  - If we observe carefully then three types of grain sizes are there, large, intermediate and small. So Bb (heterozygous condition) can be considered as a case of incomplete dominance also.
  - If grain shape is considered, BB and Bb result in round seeds and bb result in wrinkled seeds. So we can say that B is dominant over b.
  - Dominance is not an autonomous feature of a gene or the product that it has information for. Instead it depends upon the gene product and the phenotype expressed.

- **Law of Independent Assortment**
  - Based on various dihybrid crosses. Mendel proposed second set of generalizations in the form of Law of Independent assortment.
  - Law of Independent assortment:

    'In a dihybrid cross, segregation of one pair of alleles (or one pair of characters) is independent of another pair of alleles (or another pair of characters).'
  - According to the above law, all four gametes formed from YyRr (YR, Yr, yR and yr) are in equal proportions (25 % each).

- **Two Gene Interactions (Inter-allelic or Non-allelic Interactions):**
  - In garden pea (*Pisum sativum*), Mendel studied interactions of two alleles of each gene. Such an interaction is called **allelic** or **intra-allelic interaction.** It gives a typical Mendelian 3: 1 in a monohybrid cross and 9: 3: 3: 1 in a dihybrid cross. However, there are cases of interactions between the alleles of different genes located at different location express a trait. Such interaction is termed as **inter-allelic** or **non-allelic interaction.**

- **Example:**
  1. **Complementary genes (9: 7)**
  2. **Supplementary gene (9: 3: 4)**
  3. **Duplicate genes (15: 1)**
  4. **Inhibitory factor (13: 3)**
  5. **Dominant epistasis (12: 3: 1)**
  6. **Recessive epistasis (9: 3: 4)**
  7. **Dominant – Recessive epistasis (13: 3)**

**TABLE 2.4** Some common examples of gene interaction

| S. No. | $F_1$ phenotype (AaBb × AaBb) | $F_2$ genotypes | | | | Phenotypic ratio & explanation |
|---|---|---|---|---|---|---|
| | Example | 9A – B – | 3A – bb | 3 aaB – | 1 aabb | |
| 1 | Coat colour in Mouse | Agouti | Albino | Black | Albino | 9 : 3 : 4<br>Recessive epistasis (Supplementary genes) |
| 2 | Fruit colour in Squash | White | White | Yellow | Green | 12 : 3 : 1<br>Dominant epistasis |
| 3 | Flower colour in Pea | Purple | White | White | White | 9 : 7<br>Complementary genes (both dominant alleles required for a phenotype) |
| 4 | Fruit shape in squash | Disc | Circular | Circular | Long | 9 : 6 : 1<br>New phenotype by either allele |
| 5 | Fruit shape in Shepherd's purse | Triangular | Triangular | Triangular | Ovoid | 15 : 1<br>Either allele separately or together give same phenotype (Duplicate gene) |
| 6 | Feather colour in Fowls | White | White | Coloured | White | 13 : 3<br>Inhibitory gene (one gene inhibits the expression of the other) |

## Polygenic Traits-Quantitative Inheritance

- All the traits studied by Mendel have two alternative forms without any intermediate form in between. The seeds were either round or wrinkled the plant tall or dwarf the flowers purple or white. The traits which have two alternative forms and no intermediate or graded forms are called **qualitative traits.**
- Such traits are controlled by single gene pairs and are therefore, also called **monogenic traits.**
- There are, however, several traits which exhibit continuous gradation between the two extremes. For example, human skin colour can grade from black to white with all intermediate shades.
- **Human height also shows a gradation** from short to tall form. Gradations may be seen many less familiar traits like seed size of beans, grain colour in wheat or cob length in corn. Such traits can be measured in terms of quantity and therefore, are called **quantitative traits.** Both heredity and environment contribute to the expression of quantitative traits (i.e., the production of graded phenotypes).

- The quantitative traits are controlled by additive effects of two or more pairs of genes, and are therefore, also called polygenic traits **(Fig. 2.6)**. The inheritance of quantitative traits or the inheritances in which dominant polygenes have cumulative effect are called quantitative inheritance or polygenic inheritance.
- The quantitative traits are sometimes called **metric traits** because they can be measured in terms of units of size, length, weight or number. Quantitative traits do not show clear differences between individuals and form a spectrum of phenotypes, which blend gradually from one type to another to cause continuous variations. These traits are governed by two or more pairs of non-allelic genes.
- Each dominant allele of the polygenes accounts for a partial expression of the trait or individually produce a certain amount of phenotypic effect. Thus, the presence of more dominant alleles of the polygene makes the trait more prominent.
- The dominant polygenes, which contribute to the expression of the trait are called **contributing alleles,** while the recessive polygenes are known as **non-contributing alleles.** Quantitative inheritance was first studied by **J. Kolreuter (1760)** in case of tobacco and **F. Galton** (1883) in case of human beings.
- **Nilson Ehle (1908)** obtained the first experimental proof of polygenic inheritance in case of **kernel colour in wheat.**
- A common example of quantitative inheritance is seen in the human skin colour.
- The inheritance of **human skin colour** was first studied by **C.B. Davenport (1913).**
- Human skin colour (i.e., quantity of melanin pigment), is believed to be controlled by at least three pairs of polygenes. Each dominant allele contributes to a unit of darkness due to incomplete dominance. Designating the genes *A*, *B* and *C*, the skin shade will vary from a very dark or black in a *AABBCC* individual to very light or white in a *aabbcc* individual. If very dark (*AABBCC*) and very light (*aabbcc*) individuals marry, the offspring or $F_1$ individuals will be heterozygous for all the three genes (*AaBbCc*) and will have an intermediate colour often called **mulatto.**

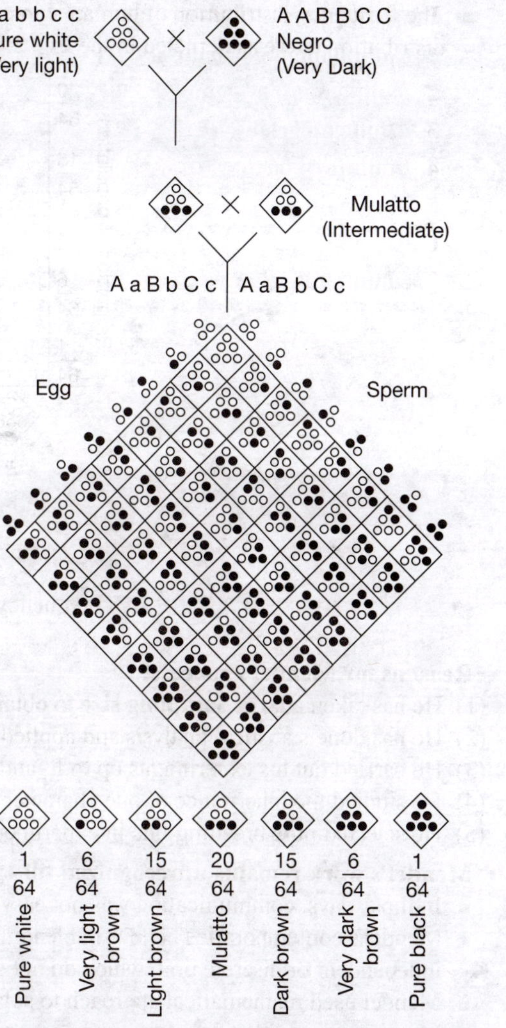


**FIGURE 2.6** A cross showing polygenic (quantitative) inheritance of human skin colour Each dominant gene is represented by a shaded circle and each recessive gene by an unshaded circle for simplicity.

- When two individuals of intermediate colour marry, the skin colour of the children will vary from very dark to very light. A total of eight allele combinations are possible in the gametes of each sex, giving 64 genotype combination in $F_2$ generation attribute into 7 phenotypes.
- The phenotype i.e., skin colour ranges from pure black (*AABBCC*) 1/64 individuals through very dark brown in 6/64 individuals, dark brown in 15/64 individuals, mulatto or intermediate (*AaBbCc*) in 20/64 individuals, light brown in 15/64 individuals very light brown in 6/64 individuals to pure white (*aabbcc*) in 1/64 individuals. The polygenic inheritance can be known from the frequency distribution.
- The number of phenotypes is **3 (1 : 2 : 1)** in case of one pair of polygenes, **5 (1 : 4 : 6 : 4 : 1)** in case of two pairs of polygenes and **7 (1 : 6 : 15 : 20 : 15 : 6 : 1)** when three involved. Thus, we see that the number of intermediate types increase the number of polygenes but the number of parental types remain the same (2 in the above cases).

- The frequency distribution of human skin colour (i.e., for three pairs of polygenes) can be fitted as a bell shaped normal distribution curve as depicted in the **Fig. 2.7**.

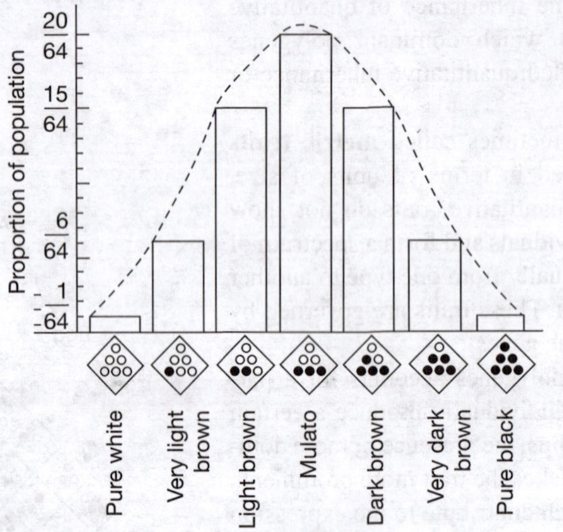


FIGURE 2.7 Frequency distribution of human skin colour in a population.

- **Reasons for Mendel's success?**
  (1) He has taken a **large sampling size** to obtain a higher accuracy (quantitative analysis).
  (2) He has done statistical analysis and applied mathematical logic to extract the results.
  (3) He carried out his experiments up to $F_2$ and $F_3$ generations
  (4) He studied the inheritance of one character at a time.
  (5) He selected pure breeding line in experiments
- **Mendel's work remains unrecognized till 1900. Why?**
  - In those days, communication was not easy and also the work of Mendel was publicized with limited circulation.
  - Mendel's contemporaries believe in blending in heritance while according to Mendel, Mendelian factor (or gene) was an independent or discrete unit, which do not show blending inheritance.
  - Mendel used mathematical approach to solve the biological phenomenon. This was not accepted by many biologists.
  - Mendel was unable to give any physical proof for the existence of Mendelian factors (or genes).
- **Rediscovery of Mendelian work in 1900**
  - **Mendelian work was independently rediscovered by three scientists—Hugo de Vries, Karl Correns and Tshermak.**
  - At that time, it became possible due to the advancements occurred in microscopy that helped them to observe the mechanism of cell division at various stages. This also led to the discovery of chromosomes.
- **Chromosomal theory of inheritance (by Walter Sutton and Theodore Boveri independently in 1902)**
  - Few extracts of the theory were:
    (1) Chromosomes possess genetic material (also the Mendelian factors are responsible for characters).
    (2) Chromosomes occur in pair, i.e., homologous chromosomes (also the Mendelian factors occur in pair).
    (3) Chromosomes are replicated and passed from the parents to the offspring.
    (4) During the formation of gametes, chromosomes segregate independently (also the Mendelian factors segregate independently).
  - Chromosomal theory of inheritance also explains the Mendel's laws.
  - The two alleles of a gene are present on homologous position on homologous chromosomes.
  - Segregation occur at anaphase of meiosis-I.
  - Sutton merged the concept of chromosomal segregation with Mendelian principles and it is called chromosomal theory of inheritance.

- **Experimental verification of Chromosomal theory of inheritance (by Thomas Hunt Morgan and his colleagues)**
  - Thomas Hunt Morgan worked on: *Drosophila melanogaster* (tiny Fruitfly).
  - Movements of chromosomes were the basis of resulting variations during sexual reproduction.
  - Reasons for choosing *Drosophila melanogaster* (tiny Fruitfly) by T.H. Morgan for his experiments:
    (1) These can be easily grown on a simple synthetic medium in laboratory.
    (2) Short life cycle-two weeks.
    (3) Large number of progeny can be produced by single mating.
    (4) Male and female sexes can be easily identified.
    (5) Many contrasting characters are present which can be easily distinguished by using a low power microscope.

## Concept of Linkage and Recombination

- While doing dihybrid experiments on fruitfly, Morgan found that when the genes are present on same chromosome:
  (1) Some genes remain tightly linked with each other and show minimum recombination.
  (2) Other genes remain loosely linked with each other and show higher recombination.
- **Linkage:** It is the tendency of genes to remain together even during the formation of gametes. This is due to the physical association or linkage between the two genes. In such cases, parental gene combinations remain higher than the non-parental gene combinations (recombinants).
- **Recombination:** It is the tendency of generation of non-parental gene combinations. In such cases, non-parental gene combinations (recombinants) remain higher than the parental gene combinations.
- **Example: Both genes which are taken in following cross were X-linked, so XX condition is found in females and XY condition in males. Wild type alleles are dominant.**

**CROSS 1**

| | | | |
|---|---|---|---|
| Parent generation (P generation) | Yellow bodied, white eyed female (yyww) | X | Brown bodied, red eyed male (Wild type) ($y^+$ $w^+$ on X and no allele on Y) |
| | ↓ | | ↓ |
| Gametes | yw (Single type of gametes) | | Gamete with $y^+$ $w^+$ on X or gamete with no allele on Y (Two types of gametes) |
| | | ↓ | |
| $F_1$ progeny | $yy^+$ $ww^+$ (Wild type female) intercrossing | & | yw (Yellow bodied, white eyed male) |
| | | ↓ | |

**$F_2$ progeny**

| Parental type | Recombinant type |
|---|---|
| Male | Male |
| $y^+$ $w^+$ – Wild type | $Y^+$ w – White eyed |
| yw – Yellow bodied, white eyed | y w+ – Yellow bodied |

| Parental type | Recombinant type |
|---|---|
| Female | Female |
| $yy^+$ $ww^+$ – Wild type | $yy^+$ ww – White eyed |
| yyww – Yellow bodied, white eyed | $yyww^+$ – Yellow bodied |
| **98.7%** | **1.3%** |

- Cross 1 indicates very high frequency of linkage between the two genes. Here, parental gene combinations remain higher than the non-parental gene combinations (recombinants).

**CROSS 2**

| | | | |
|---|---|---|---|
| Parent generation (P generation) | White and miniature winged female (wwmm) | X | Wild type ($w^+ m^+$ on X and no allele on Y) |
| | ↓ | | ↓ |
| Gametes | wm (Single type of gametes) | | Gamete with $w^+ m^+$ on X or gamete with no allele on Y (Two types of gametes) |
| | | ↓ | |
| $F_1$ progeny | $ww^+mm^+$ (Wild type female) intercrossing | & | wm (White and miniature winged male) |
| | | ↓ | |

**$F_2$ progeny:**

| Parental type | Recombinant type |
|---|---|
| **Male** | **Male** |
| $w^+ m^+$ - Wild type | $W^+ m$ – Miniature |
| w m - White and miniature winged | w $m^+$ - White |
| **Female** | **Female** |
| $ww^+ rnm^+$ - Wild type | $ww^+ mm$ – Miniature |
| wwmm - White and miniature winged | $wwmm^+$ - White |
| **62.8%** | **37.2%** |

- Cross 2 indicates higher frequency of recombination between the two genes. Here, non-parental gene combinations (recombinants) remain lower than the parental gene combinations.

## Gene Mapping or Genetic Mapping (by Alfred Sturtevant)

- Alfred Sturtevant was student of Morgan.
- He considered the frequency of recombination between the gene pairs on the same chromosome as a measure of the distance between the genes. Thus, he mapped the position of genes on the chromosomes for the first time in 1913.

- **Chromosome Mapping: A step towards a gene map:**
  - A chromosome map is a linear graphic representation of the sequence and relative distances of the various genes present in the chromosomes. A chromosome map is also called a linkage map or **genetic map.**
  - It is similar to linear road map, where the relative distances between different stations are shown without giving the exact mileage. The method of preparing maps of a species is called **chromosome mapping.** The gene mapping exercise requires the setting up of a test cross and the estimation of recombination frequency between the required genes. Chromosome mapping is based on two genetic principles:
    1. The genes are arranged in a linear sequence in the chromosome.
    2. The frequency of crossing over between two genes is directly proportional to the distance between them in the chromosome.
  - Since the frequency of crossing over is used in preparing chromosome maps, the latter are also called **cross over maps.** The frequency of recombination or cross over value (COV) is calculated as follows:

Recombination frequency =

$$\frac{\text{Number of recombinants in test cross}}{\text{Total number of progeny of the test cross}} \times 100 \quad \text{OR} \quad \text{Cross-Over Value (COV)}$$

- The value is generally represented as a per cent of the total population.
- **Map Unit:** A recombination frequency of 0.01 or 1 per cent cross-over or recombination is taken as equivalent to **one map unit distance** now referred to as **one centimorgan** (cM) in the honor of Morgan's contribution. On an average map unit corresponds to physical length of chromosome in which a cross will occur once in fifty meiosis.
- The variation in recombination frequency is governed by the distance between the genes. Closer the two genes less are the chances of crossing over. This is reflected in the lower frequency of recombination and vice versa. In contrast, if the two genes are far apart, crossing over could occur at many points called double or multiple cross overs.
- **Alfred H. Sturtevant** first realized the importance of these proposals and suggested that the frequency of recombination can be used to suggest the relative distance between the genes on the chromosome. Thus, by finding out recombination frequencies between different genes, it could be possible to prepare a map of the linked genes (linkage map).
- To understand, how the frequencies of crossing over between different genes help in chromosome mapping **(Fig. 2.8)**, let us see the following example:
  (a) The region showing the relative location of the genes y, w and m
  (b) Represents the map distance between y and w ; w and m ; and the possibility of placing m to the left or right or y-w
  (c) The actual map derived from the same.

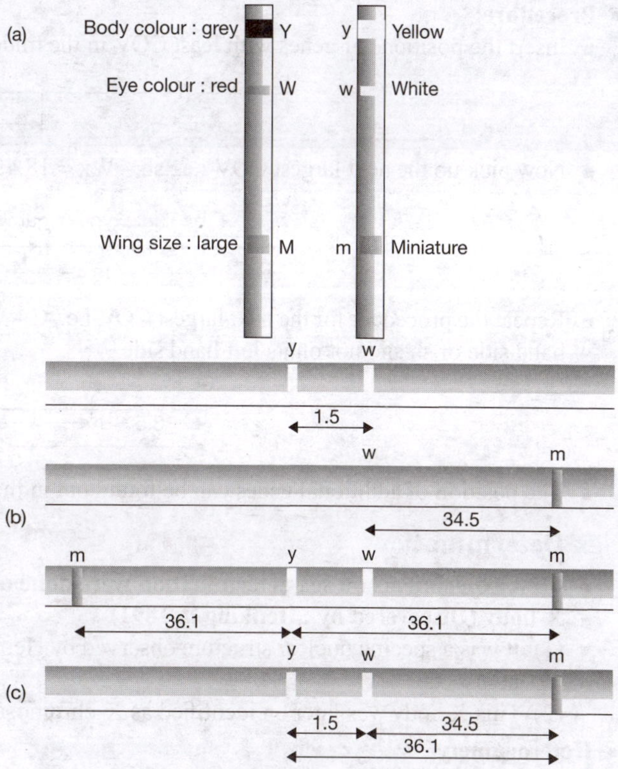


**FIGURE 2.8** A chromosomal map (linkage map) in Drosophila

- In one of the Morgan's study of *Drosophila*, the frequencies of crossing over or recombination between three genes: yellow body (y), white eye (w) and miniature wing (m) were found to be as under:
  - Yellow body - white eye = 1.5%
  - White eye - miniature wing = 34.5%
  - Yellow body - miniature wing = 36.1%
- There could be three possibilities in the order of these genes (i) ywm, (ii) ymw, (iii) wym. Sturtevant suggested that if the genes are linearly arranged, the distances between them should be additive. Based on this, he proposed the map of these genes. Here the map distance between and m is 36.1% unit, which is the sum of the map distances between y and w(1.5% unit) + w and m (34.5% unit) or 1.5% + 34.5% = 36% unit.
- In fact, the value does not add up perfectly because of double cross-over. Different alleles of a gene act as genetic markers that serve as signposts to find out relative positions of other genes along the chromosome.
- These genetic markers on chromosome produce a **genetic map** of that chromosome. Recently most accurate and detailed genetic maps have been constructed by determining the nucleotide sequence of the DNA that makes up each chromosome. **Preparation of Chromosome Maps.** An example is given below to explain the technique of preparing chromosome map. **Example.** In maize, following cross-over values (COV) were obtained.
  Coloured aleurone (C)-shrunken endosperm (sh) = 3.5%
  Shrunken endosperm (sh)-Non-waxy endosperm (Wx) = 18.4%
  Coloured aleurone (C)-Non-waxy endosperm (Wx) = 21.7%.

- **Procedure:**
  - Insert the positions of genes with least COV in the middle of the chromosome drawn as a line i.e., C – sh = 3.5%..

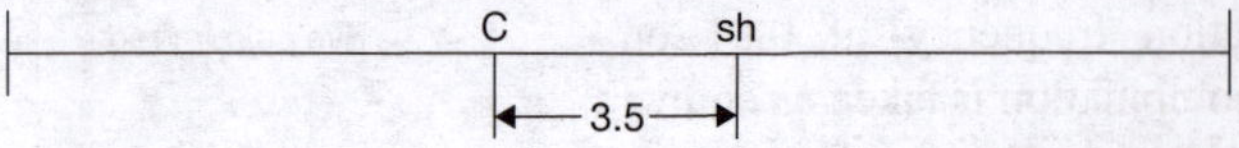


  - Now pick up the next largest COV, i.e., sh – Wx = 18.4%. Insert both positions of Wx of the chromosome relative to sh.

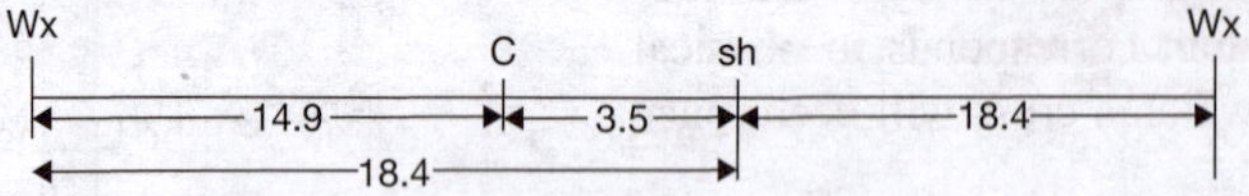


  - Repeat the procedure for the next largest COV, i.e., C – Wx = 21.7%. This indicates that Wx would be located on the right hand side of sh and not on its left hand side.

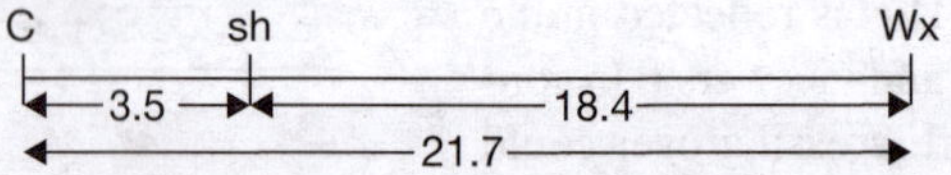


  - The position of additional genes can be found out in the same manner if COV's are available.

## Sex Determination

- **First experiments on sex determination were done on insects.**
- **X-body (Discovered by : Henking in 1891)**

(1) It was a specific nuclear structure observed by Henking in almost 50% of sperms produced during spermatogenesis in insects.

(2) This X body was later on identified as X-chromosome.

- **Heterogamety**
  - It is the production of two different types of gametes, i.e., gametes with two different chromosomal set up.
  - Heterogamety is the feature of either of the sex in a species. It is of two types:

**1. Male heterogamety**

(i) Male produces two types of gametes.

(ii) Male possesses one chromosome less than that of female.

(iii) Male heterogamety is of two types:

**XO type**

It is found in most of insects (e.g., Grasshopper).

Eggs of such insects possess autosomes and one X chromosome while the sperms possess autosomes with or without one X chromosome. As a result of fertilization, male insects (two set of autosomes + XO) and female insects (two set of autosomes + XX) are produced.

**XY type**

It is found in human and many insects.

Eggs of such organisms possess autosomes and one X chromosome while the sperms possess autosomes with X or Y chromosome.

If egg (with X chromosome) is fertilized by:

→ Sperm with X chromosome → Female progeny (XX) is formed

→ Sperm with Y chromosome → Male progeny (XY) is formed

**2. Female heterogamety**

(i) Female produces two types of gametes.

(ii) Female possesses one chromosome less than that of male.

(iii) It is observed in birds.

(iv) Female heterogamety is ZW type.

(v) If the sperm (with X chromosome) fertilizes:

→ Egg with W chromosome → Female progeny (ZW) is formed.

→ Egg with Z chromosome → Male progeny (ZZ) is formed.

- **Sex determination in humans**
  - It is an example of male heterogamety (XY type).

| Human male (44 + XY) | X | Human female (44 + XX) |
|---|---|---|
| ↓ | | ↓ |
| 22 + X or 22 + Y | | 22 + X |
| (Two types of sperms in equal ratio—50% each) | | (All ovum of same type) |

  - If sperm with chromosome make up 22 + X fertilizes the egg, then zygote will be having 44 + XX (develop in a female).
  - If sperm with chromosome make up 22 + Y fertilizes the egg, then zygote will be having 44 + XY (develop in a male).
  - As the two types of sperms are in equal ratio, there are equal chances for a foetus to develop in male or female.
- Sex determination in honey bee: **Haplodiploidy:** (Honey Bee Method). In this sex determination one sex is haploid while other is diploid.
  - Queen Bee picks up all the sperms from a drone during nuplia flight and stores the same in its seminal vesicle. It does not fertilize the eggs, which are to develop into drones or males (arrhenotoky or arrhenotokous parthenogenesis.)
  - Workers and queen bee develop from fertilized eggs and are sexually female.
  - The difference between the workers and queen bee lies in nourishment and hence level of development.
  - Sex determination is progamic in drones and epigamic in females. Drones produce sperms directly without meiosis while queen develops haploid eggs through oogenesis (meiosis). Haplodiploidy also occurs in wasps and ants.
  - It has special characteristic features such as the males produce sperms by mitosis, they do not have father and thus cannot have sons, but have a grandfather and can have grandsons.
- In certain animals and human beings, sex related traits are of three types:

1. **Sex-linked traits:** These are the traits which are determined-by the genes present on the sex chromosomes. All the sex-linked traits present on a sex chromosome are inherited together.
2. **Sex-limited traits:** These are traits which are expressed in a particular sex though their genes also occur in the other sex e.g., milk secretion in mammalian females.
3. **Sex-Influenced traits:** These traits are not due to particular genes but are by products of sex hormones e.g., low pitched voice, beard, moustaches and baldness in human.

## Types of Mutations

Mutations are of two types-Gene mutation and chromosomal mutation.

**A. Gene Mutation:**

- A change in the structure of a gene is called gene mutation'. Mostly, gene mutations involve a change in only single nucleotide or nitrogen base. Therefore, gene mutations are usually called **point mutations.** A mutation involving more than one base pair is termed as gross mutation.
- All types of gene mutations usually occur at the time of DNA replication, when new DNA strand is synthesized. Therefore, It is called **copy error mutation.**
- The smallest portion of a gene that can mutate is called ***muton,*** The smallest *muton* in a gene is a single nucleotide pair of DNA. Gene mutations, though involve very minor changes in DNA, may have far reaching effects in the cell or organism. For example, a single pair of nucleotide causes sickle cell anemia that may prove fatal by the age of 20 years.
- Gene mutations are detected, when they cause a noticeable change in the phenotype of the organisms. They remain undetected, if they do not produce any phenotypic variations. A gene may undergo several point mutations. This gives rise to multiple alleles.
- The mutability or mutation rate differs from gene to gene. Some genes mutate much easily and more often than the others are called **unstable genes,** while those with relatively low mutation rate are known as **stable genes.** The direction of mutation is not predictable. It can occur in every conceivable direction and to any conceivable degree.
- A mutated gene can mutate back to wild type. It is called **back mutation** or **reverse mutation.** Mutations can occur in somatic or germinal cells. Sometimes an organ may possess mutated cells and normal cells, such an organ is called **chimera.** Mutations may be lethal, harmful, neutral or advantageous.

- Most of the mutations are recessive and involve loss of a function. However, a few are dominant ones. Gene mutations may occur naturally and automatically due to internal reasons. They are **spontaneous mutations.** Other is produced by some external factors. They are termed as **induced mutations.**

- **Types of Gene Mutation:**

Gene mutations are of three types-inversions, substitution and frame shift.

**1. Inversion:**

- It is a change in the base sequence of a ***cistron*** in the reverse order caused due to distortion of DNA by a mutagen. The new sequence thus have different *codons* e.g.,

| Alanine | Tyrosine | Leucine |
|---|---|---|
| ...... GCC | TAT | TTG...... |
| | Inversion ↓ | |
| ...... GTT | TAT | CCG ...... |
| Valine | Tyrosine | Proline |

**2. Substitution:** (Replacement)

- It is the replacement of a nitrogenous base by another nitrogenous base or by some derivatives of the nitrogenous base. It is of two types; transition and transversion.

**(i) Transition:**

- It is the replacement of a nitrogen base by another of its type i.e., a purine is replaced by another purine (Adenine ⇌ guanine) while a pyrimidine by another pyrimidine (cytosine ⇌ thymine or uracil). Sometimes, the hydrogen atoms of the base pairs move from one position in purine or pyrimidine to another position. Such rare chemical changes are known as **tautomeric shifts.** The more stable *keto* forms of **T** and **G** and amino forms of A and C may undergo tautomeric shifts to less stable *enol* and *imino* forms respectively, thus changing the base pairing.
- Potential of the bases: The bases exist in their less stable form only for a short period of time.
- However, if such a condition exists during replication of DNA, a mutation is likely to be produced. Thus, **AC** and **GT** base pairing may occur instead of **AT** and **CG** base pairing. These are known as the rare, forbidden or unusual base pairs.

**(ii) Transversion:**

- It is the substitution or replacement of a purine base by a pyrimidine base and vice versa. It would thus involve replacement of **AT** by **TA** and vice versa and also replacement of **CG** by **GC** and vice versa.
- Substitution mutations may result in the synthesis of different protein **(Mis-sense mutation** (e.g., in sickle cell anaemia, *codon* **GAG** changes of **GUG**, replacing **glutamic** acid with **valine**) or much shorter protein, when a *codon* is changed into a chain terminating or non-sense codon **(Non-sense mutation).**

**3. Frame-Shift Mutation (Gibberish Mutations):**

- These are the mutations in which reading of the frame of base sequence shifts laterally either forward direction due to insertion (addition) of one or more nucleotides or in the backward direction due to deletion of one or more nucleotides.
- Therefore, frame shift mutations are of two types-insertion and deletion.

**(i) Insertion.** One or more nucleotides are added in the segment of DNA representing a cistron or gene.

| Tryptophan | Ileucine | Aspergine |
|---|---|---|
| .....ACC | TAT | TTG |
| ↓ | + A | |
| .....AAC | CTA | TTT G....... |
| Leucine | Aspartic acid | Lysine |

**(ii) Deletion.** One or more nucleotides are deleted from a segment of DNA representing a *cistron* or gene.

| Tryptophan | Ileucine | Aspergine |
|---|---|---|
| ........ACC | TAT | TTG |
| ↓ – A | | |
| ........CCT | ATT | TG........ |

**B. Chromosomal Mutation:**

- A change in the structure or number of chromosomes is called chromosomal mutation'. Chromosomal mutations are of two types-Chromosome aberrations and genomic mutations.

**1. Chromosome Aberrations:**

- They are the modifications in the morphology of chromosome. Chromosomal aberration alters the number or position of existing gene in the chromosomes. It causes genes to be lost or move them to new locations on a chromosome.
- It alters the order of genes in a linkage group. Genes in new locations may cause alternations in their expression and those of in the neighborhood.
- Such changes, if they are not lethal can cause profound changes in the phenotype of the organism.
- Chromosomal aberrations may involve changes in single chromosome (intra-chromosomal aberrations) or two chromosomes (interchromosomal aberrations). The aberrations take place in the following four ways.

**(a) Deletion (Deficiency):** A segment of a chromosome separate and is lost. The affected chromosome loses certain genes and become shorter. Deletion in a single chromosome can be known during synapsis of homologous chromosomes, when certain segment of one chromosome remains unpaired or forms loop **(Fig. 2.9).**

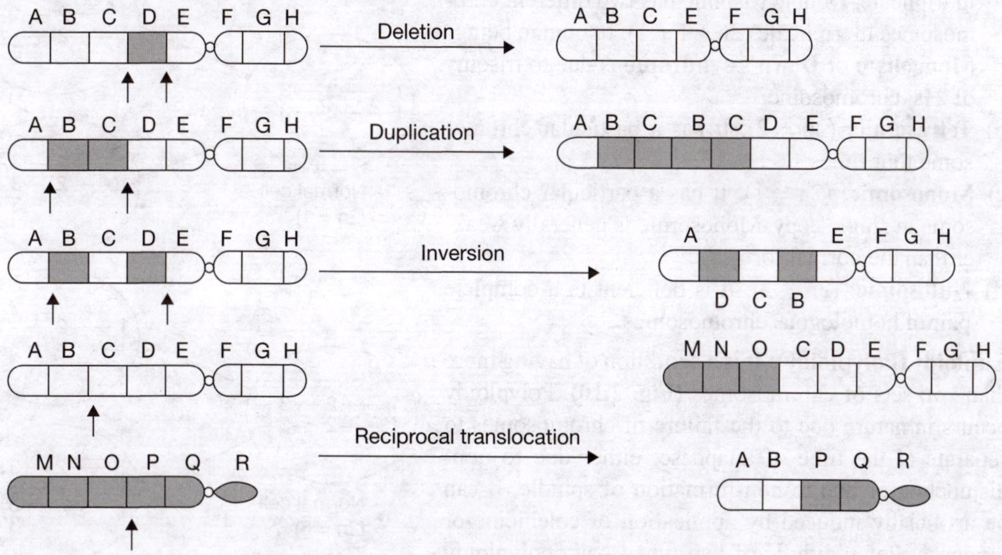


**FIGURE 2.9** Forms of chromosomal mutations

**(b) Duplication:** A fragment of chromosome joins a homologous chromosome, so that a gene or set of genes is represented twice in the same chromosome. If the new segment gets attached adjacent to the region of similar segment the duplication is called **repeat** or **tandem.**

A loop or buckle shall appear in the region of duplication, if synapsis occurs between duplicated and normal chromosome. It helps in evolution.

**(c) Inversion:** A segment of a chromosome separates and rejoins it in an inverted position, Inversion involving centromere is called **pericentric,** while that occurring beyond a centromere is known as **paracentric.** Inversion inhibits the chromosomal synapsis in the region of change. There is reduction in crossing over, and recombination frequencies. Therefore, inversions are often known as **cross-over suppressors.**

A part of a chromosome may be lost or deleted, by duplicated or be inverted. This brings about the loss of genes, duplication of genes or inversion of gene order in a chromosome. A segment of one chromosome may be reciprocally exchanged with a part of another chromosome.

**(d) Translocations:**

- A segment of a chromosome breaks off and joins a non-homologous chromosome. Both the affected chromosomes get modified. The donor suffers deletion and becomes shorter than normal.

- The recipient has an extra set of genes and become longer than normal. Translocation may be reciprocal in which two non-homologous chromosomes exchange segments between them to create new linkage groups in both the chromosome. It helps in evolution
- Reciprocal translocation is also called **Illegitimate crossing over.** Translocation produces imperfect or faulty pairing during meiosis.

**2. Genomic mutations:**

- These mutations involve a change in the number of chromosomes. Genomic mutations are of two types—aneuploidy and euploidy.

**(i) Aneuploidy (Heteroploidy):** It is a condition of having fewer or extra chromosomes than the normal genome number of a species. Aneuploidy commonly arises due to non-disjunction of two chromosomes of homologous pair during meiosis. Such errors produce gametes with particular chromosome either missing or in excess. When these aberrant gametes fuse with normal ones during fertilization, give rise to aneuploidy. An aneuploid condition may bring about profound developmental changes, if it is not already lethal. The important types of aneuploids are as follows:

**(a) Trisomic:** (2n + 1): It has a particular chromosome in triplicate. Double trisomic has two different chromosomes in triplicate (2n + 1 + 1). In human beings **Mongolism** or **Down's syndrome** is due to trisomy of 21st chromosome.

**(b) Tetrasomic:** (2n + 2): It has a particular chromosome four times.

**(c) Monosomic:** (2n – 1): It has a particular chromosome in single copy. Monosomic is generally weaker than the normal form.

**(d) Nullisomic:** (2n – 2): It is deficient in a complete pair of homologous chromosomes.

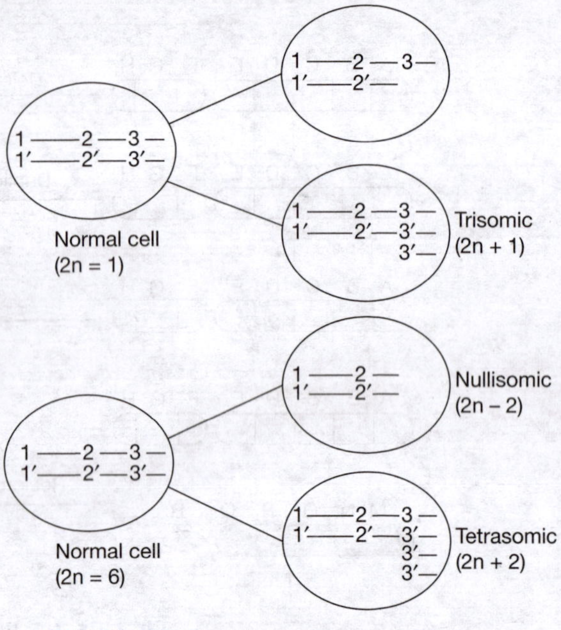


**FIGURE 2.10** The chromosome complements in some aneuploids

**(ii) Euploidy (Polyploidy):** It is a condition of having more than two sets of chromosomes **(Fig. 2.10)**. Polyploidy occurs in nature due to the failure of chromosomes to separate at the time of anaphase, either due to non-disjunction or due to non-formation of spindle. It can be artificially induced by application of colchicine or granosan. Polyploidy is of two types—autopolyploidy and allopolyploidy.

**(a) Autopolyploidy:** It is a condition in which there is present more than two sets of the same genome e.g., Autotriploid (*AAA*) and Autotetraploid (*AAAA*). Some of the economically important plants are autopolyploids e.g., Banana, Grapes, Corn, Marigold, snapdragon etc.

**(b) Allopolyploidy:** It is a condition which develops through hybridization between two species followed by doubling of chromosomes. In allopolyploidy, chromosome sets are derived from two different genomes (e.g., AABB). The common allopolyploids are Wheat, American cotton, Tobacco and Triticale (the first man made cereal) etc.

## Mutagens

- Mutation is a random process often occurring spontaneously with a low frequency. However, mutations may be induced artificially by certain external factors called **mutagens** or **mutagenic agents.**
- Any extracellular physical or chemical factor, which can cause mutations or increase the frequency of mutation, i.e., in organisms, is called mutagen. Mutagens are of three types—radiations, temperature and chemicals.

**1. Radiations:**

- High energy radiations such as X-rays, gamma rays, alpha and beta rays, cosmic rays, ultraviolet rays, etc. have been found to be mutagenic in almost all organisms.
- They cause breaks in the DNA molecule and thus induce mutations. Muller (1927) was the first to induce mutations in Drosophila with the help of X-rays. He found 150 fold increases in the rate of mutation.

**2. Temperature:**

- An increase in temperature increases the rate of mutation. It breaks the hydrogen bonding between the two strands of DNA and hence denatures the latter.
- It disturbs the synthetic processes related with replication and transcription. In rice, low temperature is known to increase-the rate of mutations.

**3. Chemicals:**

- A variety of chemicals act as mutagens. These include nitrous acid, formaldehyde, peroxides, mustard gas, 5-bromo-uracil, acridines etc. Colchicine induce polyploidy by inhibiting the formation of spindle in cell division.

- **Importance of Mutations**
  - Mutations have a manifold importance. They are of great use in the production of new and useful varieties of economically important plants.
  - Likewise mutations are important in the development of useful races of microorganisms and domestic animals. Mutations provide variability among organisms to adapt to the new environment.
  - They are equally important as raw material for evolution.

## Human Genetics

**1. Pedigree analysis:**

- It is the analysis of diagrammatic record of inheritance of particular trait/traits over two or more generations in a family tree **(Fig. 2.11)**. The analysis helps in finding out the possibility of inheritance of a trait in homozygous or heterozygous state in an offspring.

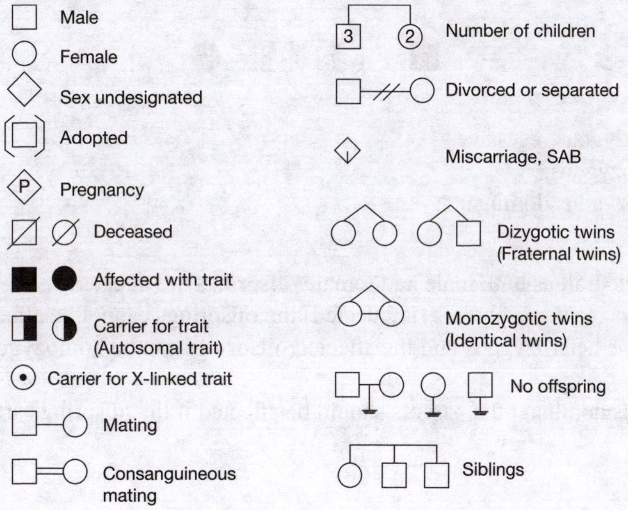


**FIGURE 2.11** Symbols used in human pedigree analysis to study the inheritance of a character

- A family tree or pedigree is drawn up using certain standard symbols. For pedigree analysis, information about the family's history for a particular trait is first collected. Next the expression of the trait is assembled into the family tree.
- For carrying out simple Mendelian analysis involving recessive or dominant allele, certain clues or simple rules are sought from the pedigree. In case of recessive allele, for example, characteristic condition can appear in the progeny of apparently unaffected parents. On the other hand two affected individuals cannot have unaffected child.

- **Importance of Pedigree Analysis:**
  1. Pedigree analysis can help in providing valuable information about the possible genetic makeup of a person for a trait.
  2. It helps genetic counselors to advice couples worried of the possibility of having genetically defective children, when it is known that such a defect 'runs' in their family.

**Problem 1: What type of trait (Autosomal recessive/sex linked/holandric/autosomal dominant) is shown in the following pedigree** (The Heterozygous individuals have not been indicated)

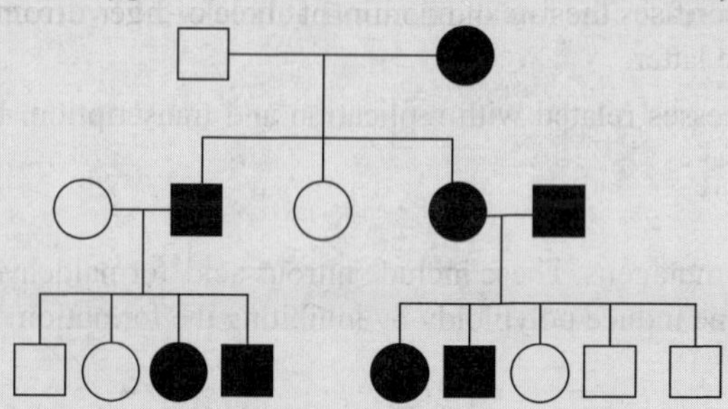

**Sol.:**

1. The trait cannot be holandric as both males and females are affected.
2. It cannot be a sex linked trait because affected male parent cannot have the male offspring, affected.
3. The trait cannot be autosomal recessive also as both the affected (recessive) parents cannot have normal offsprings.
4. The trait shown is autosomal dominant. In such cases the affected parent/parents may produce normal/ affected offsprings.

**Problem 2: Which statement regarding following pedigree is correct?**

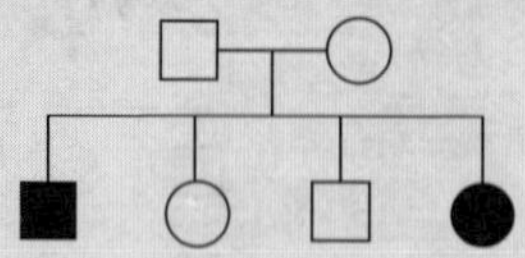

1. The trait is holandric.
2. The parents are homozygous recessive.
3. The parents are heterozygous.
4. The parents are homozygous dominant.

**Sol.:**

1. It cannot be a holandric trait as both male and female offsprings are affected.
2. In case of homozygous recessive parents (unaffected) the offsprings cannot be affected.
3. Both the parents can be heterozygous and the affected offsprings can be homozygous recessive. (Trait autosomal recessive)
4. In case of homozygous dominant the parents should be affected if the offsprings are affected.

2. **Population genetics:**
   - The study of distribution of traits and frequency of gene distribution in the entire population is called population genetics. It utilizes various principles of probability and statistics.
   - For instance, autosomal dominant recessive inheritance in a population can be expressed by **Hardy – Weinberg equation** = ($p^2 + 2pq + q^2 = 1$),
   - Where $p^2$ represents homozygous dominant individuals, $q^2$ represents homozygous recessive individuals, and 2pq represents heterozygous individuals in a population.

- This equation is analogous to monohybrid cross; Aa x Aa, which yields AA + 2Aa + aa (A represents p and a represents q).

  $(p + q)^2 = p^2 + 2pq + q^2 = 1$

  $(A + a)^2 = A^2 + 2Aa + a^2 = 1$
- Thus, the normal frequency of dominant trait will be 2/3 ($p^2 + 2pq$) and that of a recessive trait will be 1/3 ($q^2$) in the population.

- **Problem:** Calculate the frequency of a recessive and dominant allele of a gene from phenotypic study. Select any-of the following:
  **(1)** Tasters (T-) and non-tasters (tt) of the phenyl thiocarbamide (PTC).
  **(2)** Rollers (R-) and non-rollers (rr) of tongue
  **(3)** Free (dominant) and normal (recessive) checks
  **(i)** Ask students of different classes to taste PTC (**phenylthio – caroamide**) papers. Some students will be able to tell that the papers (a drop of PTC can also be used) are bitter while others would find the papers tasteless.
- Take an average of all student studies. Remember Hardy—Weinberg principle (1908) that in a large population the frequency of non-selective recessive allele is equal to square root of the proportion of individuals showing recessive character. Absence of PTC taste is a recessive taste.

  $$\text{Proportion of non – tasters} = \frac{\text{Non – tasters}}{\text{Total}}$$
- Frequency of non-taster gene (t) = square root of proportion of non-tasters. Say 9 out of 100 are non – tasters. Their proportion is 0.09.

  The frequency of non-taster gene $t = \sqrt{0.09} = 0.3$

  Frequency of taster gene (T) = 1 – 0.3 = 0.7

  Proportion of Homozygous tasters = $(0.7)^2 = 0.49$ or 49%

  Proportion of total tasters = 100 – 9 = 91 or 0.91%.

  Proportion of heterozygous tasters = 0.91 – 0.49 = 0.42%

**3. Cell culture:**

- The techniques of culturing human cells in specific media have enabled geneticists to understand biochemical basis of inheritance of number of traits.

**4. Study of twins:**

- There are two types of twins, **identical** or **monozygotic** and **fraternal** (non-identical) or **dizygotic.** The identical twins develop from a single zygote by separation of the two blastomeres after the first cleavage.
- Therefore, they have similar genetic traits, except for rare chance of mutation. Fraternal twins develop from different zygotes. Therefore, they are no more alike than other children born at different times in the same family.
- The two types of twins provide an excellent opportunity to distinguish effect of environment and heredity on the expression of traits. The traits that are similar in the identical twins are considered hereditary, and the features in which they differ are regarded as environmental.
- Such studies have shown that intelligence, diabetes mellitus, feeble mindedness and many others are hereditary traits in man.

**5. Karyotype:**

- It is the chromosome complement of a cell including the description and characteristics of chromosomes.
- Karyotype is often described in the form of an **idiogram,** which is a photograph or diagram of metephasic chromosomes of an organism arranged in homologous pairs in order of their size, except the sex chromosomes that are placed at the end.
- For karyotyping, the cell division of human white blood cells (or some other cells) in culture is arrested using colchicine. The colchicine treated cells are fixed, stained and photographed through microscope.
- The photographs of chromosomes are cut and are systematically arranged according to their size and position of centromere.

## Human Chromosomes

- The correct number of somatic chromosome in human being was determined to the 2n = 46 by **Tjio** and **Levan in 1956. Each cell of human body has 23 pairs of chromosomes.** Out of these, 22 pairs are similar in males and females these are called **autosomes**. The chromosomes of twenty third pair are called **sex chromosomes** or **allosomes.**
- In a human karyotype the homologous chromosomes are paired and classified into seven groups, according to their length and location of centromere. The 22 pairs of autosomes are numbered 1 to 22..
- The sex chromosomes, *XX* or *XY* are not numbered. Individual chromosome pairs in a group, though similar in size, are further differentiated by their banding pattern using special fluorescent dyes, such as Quinacrine mustard or Giesma.
- The banding pattern of a particular chromosome always remains constant for a particular treatment. In this manner, each one of the 22 pairs of autosomes and the sex chromosomes can be visually identified.
- Any defect in any chromosome such as deletion or translocation is identified. Any numerical abnormality such as monosomy (one chromosome less) or trisomy (one chromosome extra) can also be detected.

## Genetic Disorders

Genetic disorders are classified into two types:

- **Mendelian disorders**
  (1) Alteration or mutation occurs in single gene usually.
  (2) These can be dominant or recessive.
  (3) These may be present on autosomes and sex chromosomes.
  (4) These can be traced with pedigree analysis.
  **Examples:** Haemophilia, sickle cell anemia, cystic fibrosis, thalassemia, colour blindness, phenylketonuria, etc.

## Characteristics of Sex – Linked Inheritance

- It is a criss cross inheritance i.e., fathers pass the X-linked allele trait to their daughters, who pass it on to the grandsons.
- Mothers pass the allele of the trait to both sons and daughters.
- Only homozygous females express X linked, recessive trait. She should receive the mutant allele from both her parents.
- Heterozygous females are carriers of X linked recessive trait and they do not express the trait.
- Any male receiving X linked recessive allele from his mother will express the trait as his Y chromosome has No corresponding allele.
- If a recessive X linked gene causes a disorder, then more males than females have the disorder, because the disorder is caused by a single allele in males. Their Y chromosome does not carry any Corresponding allele. In females, the disorder appears only when her mother is a carrier and father also passes the allele of the disorder. Some sex linked disorders in humans are **haemophilia** (bleeder's disease) and **red–green colour blindness.**

  **(i) Haemophilia (Bleeder's Disease):** It is a sex linked disease, in which the patient will continue to bleed even from a minor cut since he or she cannot synthesize **Antihaemophiliac Globulin** or **Factor VIII** (haemophilia – A) or **Plasma Thromboplastin Cofactor** or **Factor IX** (haemophilia – B also called **Christmas disease**) or **Plasma Thromboplastin Antecedent** or **Factor XI** (haemophilia – C) required for normal blood clotting. As a result of continuous bleeding, the patient may die of blood loss.

  - The disease cannot be cured permanently. However, the bleeding can be checked through transfusion of normal blood which provides the vital factors for blood clotting.
  - Nowadays **Antihaemophiliac Globulin** is also available for use in haemophilia – A. Haemophiliais caused by a recessive gene $X^h$, located in the X chromosome.
  - Females have two X chromosomes. For them to be haemophiliac, it is necessary that each X chromosome has a gene for haemophilia ($X^hX^h$). However, such females never born as the combination of these two recessive genes is lethal (fetal). A female having only one gene for haemophilia ($XX^h$) appears normal because its dominant allele in the other X chromosome produces the factor required for normal blood clotting. Such females are called **carriers.**

- In males, a single gene for the defect is able to express itself as the Y chromosome carries no gene for this trait. Hence, haemophilia occurs only in males **(Fig. 2.12)**. Shows the inheritance of haemophilia.

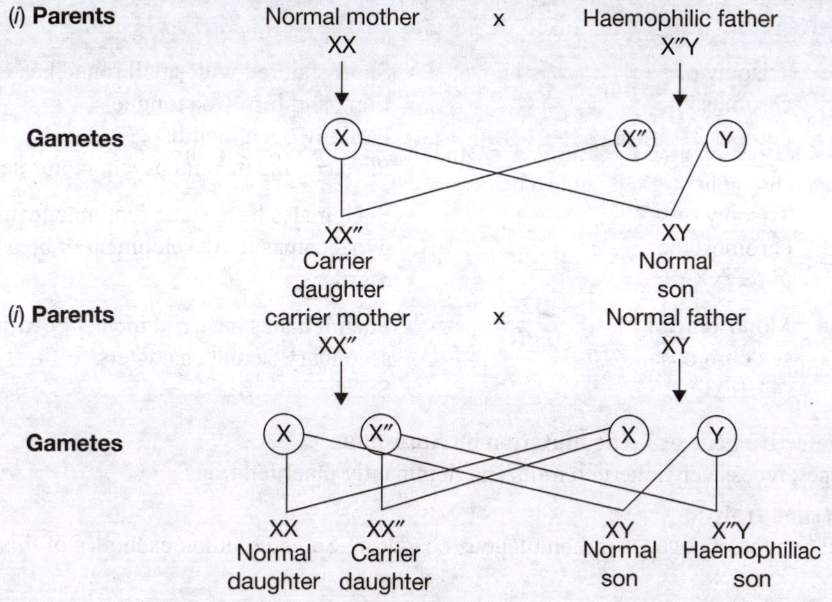


**FIGURE 2.12** Inheritance of haemophilia in humans

- A homozygous normal female (*XX*) and her haemophiliac husband ($X^hY$) will produce normal sons (*XY*) and carrier daughters ($X^hY$). If a carrier woman marries a normal man, half of the sons will be haemophiliac and half of the daughters will be carrier.

**(ii) Colour Blindness (Red Green colour blindness):** Colour blindness is another sex linked disease in which the eye fails to distinguish red and green colors. Both the colors appear grey. The normal gene and its recessive allele are present on the X chromosomes. In females, colour blindness appears only when both the sex chromosomes carry the recessive gene ($X^CX^C$). The females which carry single gene for colour blindness $XX^C$) have normal vision but function as carriers. However, in males the defect appears in the presence of a single recessive gene ($X^CY$), because Y chromosome of males does not carry any gene for colour vision. Thus, this defect is much more common in men than woman. Colour blindness like any other sex linked trait 'shows criss cross inheritance.

- **Chromosomal disorders**
  (1) These occur due to the absence or excess or abnormal arrangement of one or more chromosomes.
  (2) Increase or decrease in number of chromosome (one or more) result from non-disjunction of chromosomes (failure of segregation of chromatids during cell division). This leads to a condition - aneuploidy.
  (3) If after telophase, cytokinesis fails, it leads to increase in whole set of chromosomes. This is termed as polyploidy.
  (4) Polyploidy is commonly seen in plants.

Ongoing research is aimed at understanding the underlying mechanisms of chromosomal disorders and developing potential therapies. For example, researchers are investigating gene editing techniques like CRISPR to correct chromosomal abnormalities.

TABLE 2.5 Chromosomal disorders

| Syndrome | Chromosomal set up | No. of chromosomes | Features |
|---|---|---|---|
| 1. Down's Syndrome (first described by Langdon Down in 1866) | Trisomy of chromosome number 21 | 47 | • Short statured with small round head.<br>• Long and furrowed tongue.<br>• Partially open mouth.<br>• Physical, mental and psychomotor development retarded. |
| 2. Klinefelter's syndrome | Trisomy of sex chromosome (44 + XXY) | 47 | • Such males have some feminine features like gynaecomastia (development of breast), etc.<br>• Sterile. |
| 3. Turner's syndrome | Monosomy of sex chromosome (44 + XO) | 45 | • Such females have rudimentary ovaries and lack other secondary sexual characters.<br>• Sterile. |

- **Disorders due to defective gene or Gene mutation on Autosomes**
  These are of two types, recessively inherited traits and dominantly inherited traits.

**(A) Recessively Inherited traits:**

These are caused by recessive genes in homologous condition. Some common examples of this type of disorders are following:

**(i) Alkaptonuria (Black urine disease):** This disorder is due to a recessive gene and appears only in homozygous recessive individuals. Alkaptonurics excrete alkapton (homogentisic acid) in their urine, which spontaneously combines with oxygen to form a black pigment.

- The pigment causes darkening of cartilages of ears and nose, and blackening of urine. People with dominant allele (both homozygous and heterozygous individuals) excrete normal urine, because their blood contain an enzyme called alkapton oxidize (homogentisate oxidize), which oxidizes alkapton to carbon dioxide and water.
- Alkaptonurics does not produce this enzyme because of the presence of recessive gene in homozygous condition.

**(ii) Phenylketonuria (PKU):** It is an inborn error in metabolism due to a defective recessive gene found on **chromosome twelve**. The homozygous recessive lacks the enzyme phenylalanine oxidase needed to change one amino acid and phenylalanine, to another tyrosine.

- Phenylalanine accumulates in the tissues and some of it changes into phenyl pyruvic acid which damages the brain and causes the reduction of colour of hair and skin. The heterozygous Individuals are normal but carriers.

**(iii) Albinism:** Albinism is characterized by lack of dark pigment **melanin** in the skin, hair and iris. It is caused by the absence of the enzyme tyrosinase which is necessary for the synthesis of the pigment melanin from dihydroxyphenylalanine,

- Albinism is also due to a recessive gene, which is in homozygous condition and blocking the formation of melanin pigment. Albinism by itself is not a disability. However, an albino is susceptible to eye disorders due to damaging effect of bright light.

**(iv) Sickle cell anaemia:** This disorder is caused due to a defective recessive gene can be found on the short arm of **chromosome eleven**. The red blood corpuscles of the affected individuals become elongated and curved under low oxygen tension **(Fig. 2.13)**.

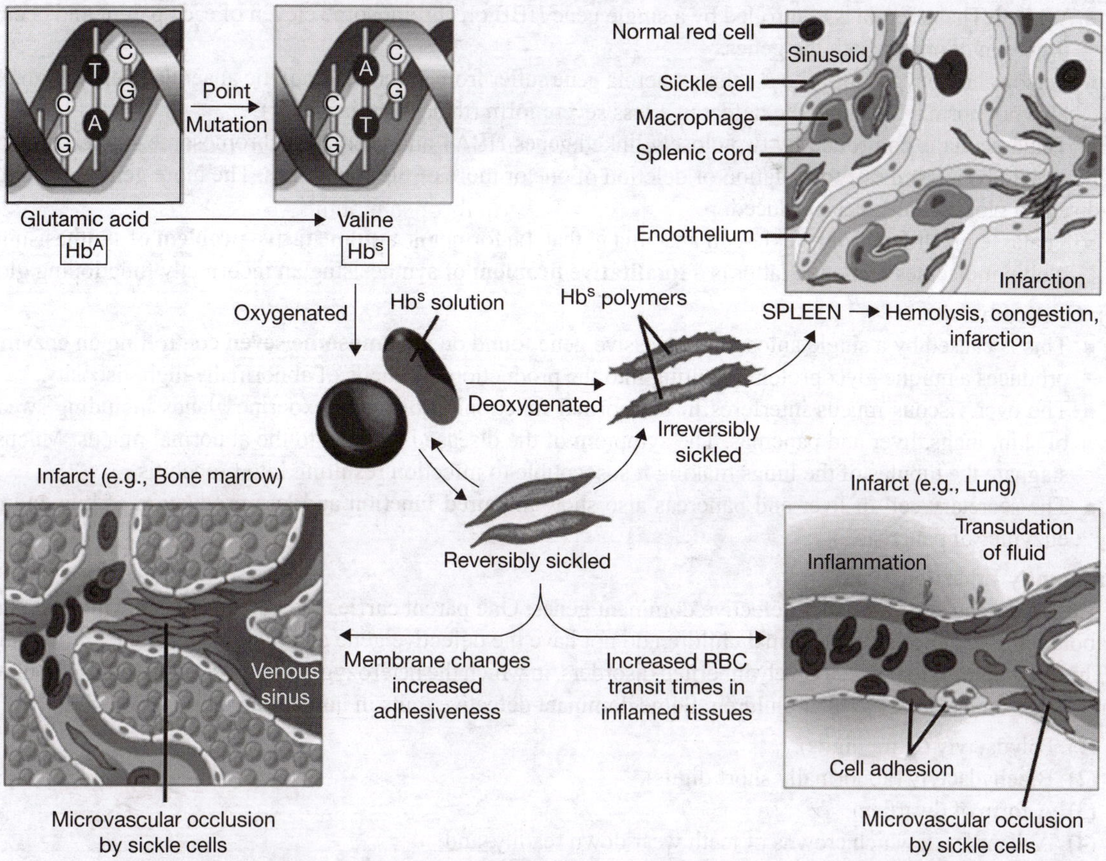


**FIGURE 2.13** Micrograph of the red blood cells and the amino acid composition of the relevant portion of beta-peptide of haemoglobin (a) From a normal individual (b) From an individual with sickle cell anaemia

- The individuals suffer severe tissue damage due to aggregation of RBCs in the venous side of the capillary system under oxygen deficiency. It is known as **sickle cell crisis.**
- The sickled erythrocytes are destroyed more rapidly than the normal ones leading to anaemia. This disease is controlled by a single pair of alleles, $Hb^A$ and $Hb^S$. Recessive homozygotes ($Hb^S/Hb^S$) die early in life due to severe anaemia.
- However, heterozygotes ($Hb^A/Hb^S$) are apparently unaffected, as they carry at least one normal allele. They are carriers of the defective gene and can transmit the same to 50 per cent of their offsprings on an average.
- This defect arises due to substitution of valine for glutamic acid at the sixth position in the $\beta$ chain of globin molecule of haemoglobin. This discovery has provided the direct evidence that genes specify proteins and also established the concept of inherited molecular diseases.

**(v) Thalassaemia:** This is also an autosome-linked recessive blood disease transmitted from parents to the offspring when both the partners are unaffected carrier for the gene (or heterozygous). The defect could be due to either mutation or deletion which ultimately results in reduced rate of synthesis of one of the globin chains (a and b chains) that make up haemoglobin. This causes the formation of abnormal haemoglobin molecules resulting into anaemia which is characteristic of the disease.

- It is characterized by reduced synthesis of either $\alpha$ or $\beta$ chains, likewise designated as $\alpha$- or $\beta$-thalassaemias. $\beta$–thalassaemia was first described by **Cooley,** hence it is also called **Cooley's anaemia** or **thalassaemia major.**
- The reduced synthesis of $\beta$– chain leads to accumulation of $\alpha$ chain which causes damage to the precursors of red blood corpuscles in the bone marrow.

- While b Thalassemia is controlled by a single gene HBB on chromosome eleven of each parent and occurs due to mutation of one or both the genes.
- Persons homozygous for the $\beta-$ thalassaemia gene suffer from severe haemolytic anaemia. Heterozygous persons also not normal but show the defect in a less severe form (thalassaemia minor).
- Thalassemia is controlled by two closely linked genes HBA1 and HBA2 on chromosome sixteen of each parent and it is observed due to mutation or deletion of one or more of the four genes. The more genes affected, the less alpha globin molecules produced.
- Thalassemia differs from sickle-cell anaemia in that the former is a **quantitative problem** of synthesising too few globin molecules while the latter is a **qualitative problem** of synthesising an incorrectly functioning globin.

**(vi) Cystic fibrosis:**

- This is caused by a single autosomal recessive gene found on **chromosome seven** controlling an enzyme, which produces a unique glycoprotein resulting into the production of mucus of abnormally high viscosity.
- The over viscous mucus interferes in the normal functioning of many exocrine glands including sweat glands of skin, lungs, liver and pancreas. The symptom of the disease is related to the abnormal mucus. Mucus usually stagnate the tubules of the lungs making it susceptible to infection resulting into bronchitis.
- The secretary cell of liver and pancreas also show impaired function and less production of bile and digestive enzymes of pancreas.

**(b) Dominantly Inherited Traits:**

- These disorders are caused by defective dominant genes. One parent carries the defective gene which is inherited by about half the children. The normal children do not have the defective gene and their children are all normal.
- This is in contrast to the recessively inherited disorders, in which the heterozygous (carrier) individuals, though normal, may pass on the defect to their children. Some dominant defective traits in humans are
  - **(1)** Polydactyly (extra digits),
  - **(2)** Brachydactyly (abnormally short digits),
  - **(3)** A form of dwarfism,
  - **(4)** A disorder in which crowns of teeth wear down readily, and
  - **(5)** Huntington's chorea (uncontrolled twitching of voluntary muscles and mental deterioration appearing between the ages of 25 to 55).
- All the above mentioned disorders occur due to the mutations of a dominant gene on the autosomes.

**(B) Disorders Due to Defective Gene on Sex Chromosomes:**

- Some genetic disorders are produced by a defective gene on sex chromosomes. These are called sex linked disorders. **Haemophilia, red-green colour blindness,** and **muscular dystrophy** are well known sex linked disorders in humans.
- All these are caused by a recessive gene located on the X chromosome, and affect the males more than the females. The Y chromosome mainly concerned with sex determination. Therefore, genes on the X chromosome in male always express themselves in respective of their dominant and recessive nature. The males are thus, **hemizygous** for these disorders.
- In **muscular dystrophy,** the mutated gene on X chromosome is unable to produce a protein called **dystrophin.** The latter is believed to relay the nerve's signal to the calcium storage in the muscle cell, due to calcium is not released from the muscle cell. As a result, the muscle contraction does not occur at the very first step. Abnormal rise in calcium level in the muscle release an enzyme that destroys actin and myosin. This causes deterioration of muscles at an early age. The victim becomes invalid by the age of 10 and generally dies by the age of 20.

**TABLE 2.6** Some human genetic disorders

| Disorder | Dominant/ Recessive | Autosomal/Sex linked | Symptom | Effect |
|---|---|---|---|---|
| Sickle-cell anaemia | Recessive | Autosomal (Chromosome 11) | Aggregation of erythrocytes, more rapid destruction of erythrocytes leading to anaemia | Abnormal haemoglobin in RBC's |
| Phenylketonuria | Recessive | Autosomal (Chromosome 12) | Failure of brain to develop in infancy and mental retardation | Defective form of enzyme phenylalanine hydroxylase |
| Cystic fibrosis | Recessive | Autosomal (Chromosome 7) | Mucus clogging in lungs, liver and pancreas anomalies | Failure of chloride ion transport mechanism |
| Huntington's disease | Dominant | Autosomal (Chromosome 4) | Gradual degeneration of brain tissue in middle age | Production of an inhibitor of brain cell metabolism |
| Haemophilia A/B/C | Recessive | Sex-linked (X chromosome) | Failure of blood to clot | Defective form of blood clotting factor VIII/IX. |
| Colour blindness | Recessive | Sex-linked (X chromosome) | Failure to discriminate between red and green colour | Defect in either red or/and green cone |

# PRACTICE EXERCISES

**Direction:** Read the question carefully and choose the correct option for each.

## Multiple Choice Questions: Level I

### Mendelian Genetics

**1.** Mendel was born in
(a) 17th century (b) 18th century
(c) 19th century (d) 8th century

**2.** Mendel was the native of
(a) France (b) Sweden (c) India (d) Austria

**3.** Mendel proposed which of the following terms for hereditary units?
(a) Factor (determiner) (b) Genome
(c) Genetic particle (d) None of these

**4.** In genetics, the use of chequer board was done by
(a) Mendel (b) Correns
(c) Punnet (d) Darwin

**5.** In 1900 CE, three biologists independently discovered Mendel's principles. They are
(a) De Vries, Correns and Tschermak
(b) Sutton, Morgan and Bridges
(c) Avery, MacLeod and McCarty
(d) Bateson, Punnet and Bridges

**6.** Which of the following has been used for genetic researches?
(a) Pisum (b) Neurospora
(c) *E. coli* (d) All of these

**7.** Organism of pure line is that which produces individuals of
(a) Dominant characters (b) Recessive characters
(c) Its own characters (d) Intermediate type

**8.** Mendel is famous for his work on
(a) Pisum (b) Drosophila
(c) Neurospora (d) Oenothera

**9.** The main reason for the success of Mendel was
(a) Study of all the characters at the same time
(b) Study of one character at one time
(c) Study of all the plants at the same time
(d) Counting of plants

**10.** The alleles are
(a) A pair of genes governing a specific character such as tallness or dwarfness.
(b) Multiple forms of genes.
(c) Genes governing eye characters.
(d) Genes present in allosomes.

**11.** An allele is said to be dominant if
(a) It is expressed only in heterozygous combination.
(b) It is expressed only in homozygous combination.
(c) It is expressed in both homozygous and heterozygous condition.
(d) It is expressed only in second generation.

**12.** What is the correct sequence of the following events?
1. Formation of the chromosome theory of heredity.
2. Experiments which proved that DNA is the hereditary material.
3. Mendel's laws of inheritance—discovery.
(a) 1, 3 and 2 (b) 1, 2 and 3
(c) 3, 1 and 2 (d) 2, 1 and 3

**13.** When a true breeding pea plant that has yellow seeds is pollinated by a plant that has green seeds, then all the $F_1$ plants have yellow seeds. This means that the allele for yellow is
(a) Heterozygous (b) Dominant
(c) Recessive (d) Lethal

**14.** An organism's genetic constitution is called its
(a) Genotype (b) Phenotype
(c) Holotype (d) None of these

**15.** An organism with two identical alleles for a given trait is
(a) Homozygous (b) Segregating
(c) Dominant (d) A hermaphrodite

**16.** What type of gametes will be formed by genotype RrYy?
(a) RY, Ry, rY, ry (b) RY, Ry, ry, ry
(c) Ry, Ry, Yy, ry (d) Rr, RR, Yy, YY

**17.** Which genotype characterizes an organism that is heterozygous for two genes?
(a) RRYy (b) RrYY
(c) RRYY (d) RrYy

**18.** The dwarfness in plants of $F_2$ generation is
(a) Recessive (b) Dominant
(c) Both (a) and (b) (d) None of these

**19.** When heterozygous tall plants are self-pollinated, then tall and dwarf plants are obtained. This explains
(a) Law of purity of gamete
(b) Law of dominance

(c) Division in spores
(d) Independent assortment

**20.** Mendel's principle of segregation was based on the separation of alleles in the garden pea during
(a) Pollination
(b) Embryonic development
(c) Seed formation
(d) Gamete formation

**21.** Which of the following is the dominant character according to Mendel?
(a) Dwarf plant and yellow fruit
(b) Terminal fruit and wrinkled seed
(c) White testa and yellow pericarp
(d) Green coloured pod and rounded seed

**22.** In Mendelism, the linkage was not observed due to
(a) Mutation
(b) Independent assortment
(c) Synapsis
(d) Crossing over

**23.** Mendel's law of heredity can be explained with the help of
(a) Mitosis
(b) Meiosis
(c) Both mitosis and meiosis
(d) None of these

**24.** A cross between plants having RRYY and rryy composition will yield plants with
(a) Round and yellow seeds
(b) Round and green seeds
(c) Wrinkled and yellow seeds
(d) Wrinkled and green seeds

**25.** The genotype of an individual is Rr Bb. How many different types of gametes will it produce based on the law of independent assortment?
(a) 16 (b) 9 (c) 8 (d) 4

**26.** Which of the following is heterozygous for two pairs of alleles?
(a) TTRR (b) TrRR
(c) ttrr (d) TrtR

**27.** In Mendel's experiment, nature of seed coat, flower colour, position of flower, pod colour, stem height, etc., are referred to as
(a) Alleles (b) Genotypes
(c) Phenotypes (d) All of these

**28.** A cross between a homozygous recessive and a heterozygous plant is called
(a) Monohybrid cross (b) Dihybrid cross
(c) Test cross (d) Back cross

**29.** Cross between $F_1$ plant and recessive female plant is called
(a) Back cross (b) Test cross
(c) Out cross (d) Mutation

**30.** In $F_2$ generation, a phenotypic ratio of 1 : 1 : 1 : 1 exhibits
(a) Back cross (b) Monohybrid test cross
(c) Lethality (d) Dihybrid test cross

**31.** Which of the following depicts the Mendel's dihybrid ratio?
(a) 3 : 1 (b) 9 : 3 : 3 : 1
(c) 9 : 7 (d) 15 : 1

**32.** In dihybrid cross, out of 16 plants obtained in $F_2$ generation, the number of genotypes will be
(a) 4 (b) 9 (c) 16 (d) 12

**33.** Pure homozygous offsprings in a dihybrid cross in the $F_2$ generation will be
(a) $\frac{1}{2}$ (b) $\frac{1}{4}$ (c) $\frac{1}{8}$ (d) $\frac{1}{16}$

**34.** In hybridization, Tt × tt gives rise to the progeny of ratio
(a) 1 : 1 (b) 1 : 2
(c) 2 : 1 (d) 1 : 2 : 1

**35.** Self-pollination between Tt and Tt plants results into the genotype ratio of
(a) 3 : 1 (b) 1 : 2 : 1
(c) 1 : 3 (d) 4 : 0

**36.** Mendel crossed a pure white-flowered recessive pea plant with a dominant pure red-flowered plant. The first generation of hybrids from the cross should show
(a) 50 per cent white-flowered and 50 per cent red-flowered plants
(b) All red-flowered plants
(c) 75 per cent red-flowered and 25 per cent white-flowered plants
(d) All white-flowered plants

**37.** If in a dihybrid cross, Mendel had used two such characters which have linked, he would have faced difficulty in explaining the results on the basis of his
(a) Law of segregation
(b) Law of multiple factor hypothesis
(c) Law of independent assortment
(d) Law of dominance

**38.** From a cross Aa BB × aa BB, which of the following genotypic ratio will be obtained in $F_1$ generation?
(a) 1 Aa BB : 1 aa BB (b) 1 Aa BB : 3 aa BB
(c) 3 Aa BB : 1 aa BB (d) All Aa BB : No aa BB

**39.** A farmer crossed a walnut combed chicken with a single combed one and obtained all walnut combed chickens in F1. The genotype of the parents was
(a) Rr Pp × rr pp (b) RR PP × rr pp
(c) RR pp × rr pp (d) RR Pp × rr pp

**40.** In sweet peas, genes C and P are necessary for colour in flowers. The flowers are white in the absence of either or both the genes. What will be the percentage of coloured flowers in the offspring of the cross Cc pp × cc Pp?
(a) 100% (b) 75%
(c) 25% (d) 50%

**41.** In a monohybrid cross, 120 plants are obtained. The ratio of homozygous and heterozygous will be
(a) 40 : 80 (b) 60 : 60
(c) 20 : 100 (d) 10 : 110

**42.** If Mendel had studied the seven traits using a plant with 12 chromosomes instead of 14, in what way would his interpretation have been different?
(a) He could have mapped the chromosome.
(b) He would have discovered blending or incomplete dominance.
(c) He would not have discovered the law of independent assortment.
(d) He would have discovered sex linkage.

**43.** How many different types of genetically different gametes will be produced by a heterozygous plant having the genotype AABbCc?
(a) 2 (b) 4
(c) 6 (d) 9

**44.** Mendel's law of independent assortment is applicable for
(a) All genes in all organisms
(b) All genes of pea plant only
(c) All linked genes only
(d) All non-linked genes only

**45.** In a plant, red fruit (R) is dominant over yellow fruit (r) and tallness (T) is dominant over shortness (t). If a plant with RRTt genotype is crossed with a plant that is rrtt, then
(a) 75 per cent will be tall with red fruit
(b) All the offspring will be tall with red fruit
(c) 25 per cent will be tall with red fruit
(d) 50 per cent will be tall with red fruit

**46.** When a tall plant with rounded seeds (TTRR) is crossed with a dwarf plant with wrinkled seeds (ttrr), then the generation consists of tall plants with rounded seeds. How many types of gametes a plant would produce?
(a) One (b) Three
(c) Four (d) Eight

**47.** Mendel did his experiment on
(a) Garden pea (*Pisum sativum*)
(b) Snapdragon
(c) Drosophila
(d) Lathyrus odoratus

**48.** How many contrasting traits are chosen by Mendel?
(a) 7 (b) 14
(c) 21 (d) 4

**49.** Mendel conducted an experiment on garden pea for how many years?
(a) 7 (b) 10
(c) 4 (d) 15

**50.** Select the incorrect matching.

| **Characters** | **Dominant trait** | **Recessive trait** |
|---|---|---|
| (a) Seed shape |  Round | 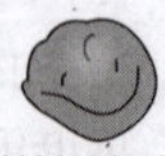 Wrinkled |
| (b) Seed colour |  Yellow |  Green |
| (c) Flower colour |  Violet | 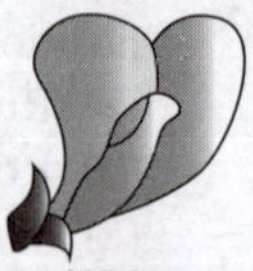 White |
| (d) Pod shape | 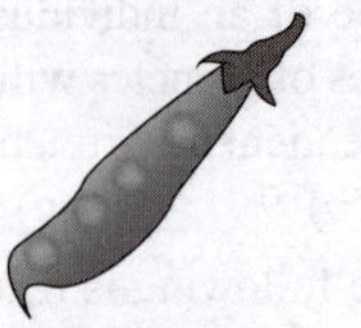 Constricted | 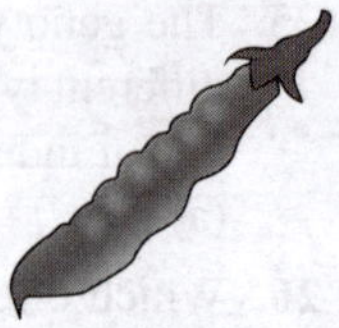 Full |

**51.** Number of character of garden pea flower chosen by Mendel?
(a) 1 (b) 2 (c) 3 (d) 4

**52.** Select the false statement from the following:
(a) Mendel for the first time applied statistical analysis and mathematical logics to problems in biology.
(b) Mendel's experiment had a large sampling size, which gave greater credibility to the data that he collected.

(c) Mendel conducted artificial cross-pollination experiment using true-breeding pea lines.
(d) Mendel selected 16 true-breeding pea plant varieties, as pairs which were similar except for one character with contrasting traits.

**53.** In Mendelian dihybrid cross, how many individuals are homozygous dominant for both the genes in $F_2$ generation?

(a) $\frac{1}{16}$ (b) $\frac{2}{16}$ (c) $\frac{4}{16}$ (d) $\frac{6}{16}$

**54.** In Mendelian dihybrid cross, how many individuals are homozygous recessive for one of the character only in $F_2$ generation?

(a) $\frac{1}{16}$ (b) $\frac{2}{16}$ (c) $\frac{3}{16}$ (d) $\frac{6}{16}$

**55.** In Mendelian dihybrid cross, how many individuals are heterozygous of both the character in $F_2$-generation?

(a) $\frac{1}{16}$ (b) $\frac{2}{16}$ (c) $\frac{3}{16}$ (d) $\frac{4}{16}$

**56.** In Mendelian dihybrid cross, how many of progeny in $F_2$ generation possess genotype rryy?

(a) $\frac{1}{16}$ (b) $\frac{2}{16}$ (c) $\frac{3}{16}$ (d) $\frac{4}{16}$

**57.** How many genotypes are formed in Mendelian dihybrid cross?

(a) 4 (b) 9 (c) 6 (d) 8

**58.** The below diagram shows:

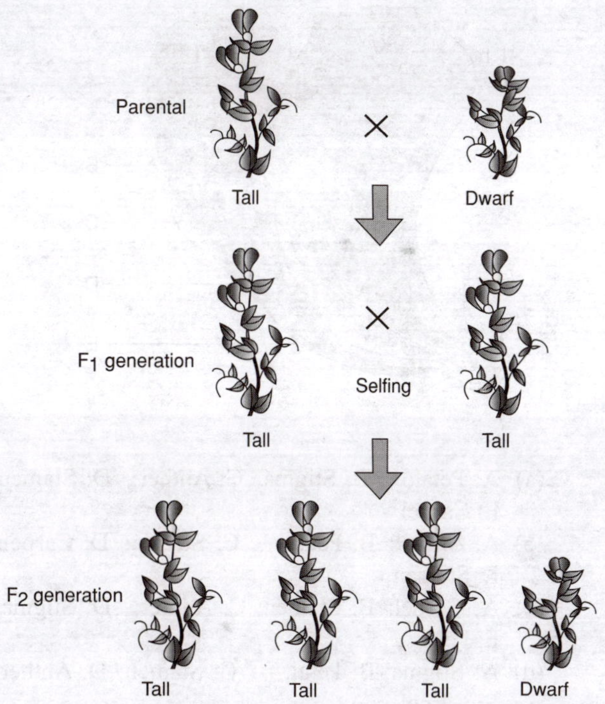


(a) Monohybrid cross
(b) Dihydrid cross
(c) Trihydrid cross
(d) All the above

**59.** The below diagram represents

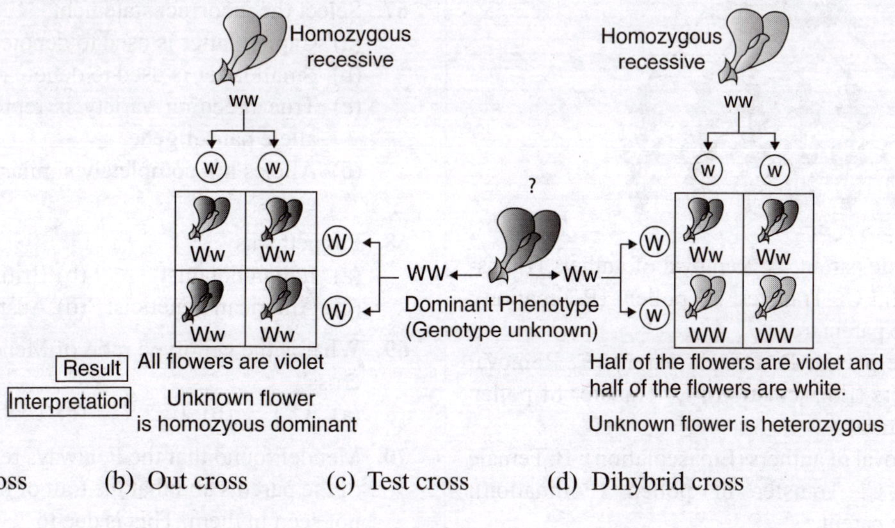


(a) Back cross (b) Out cross (c) Test cross (d) Dihybrid cross

**60.** Identify A to E in this figure.

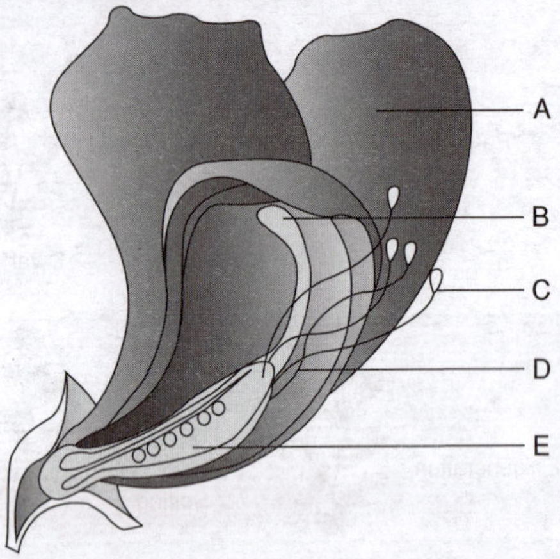


(a) A: Petal; B: Stigma; C: Anther; D: Stamen; E: Carpel
(b) A: Anther; B: Petal; C: Stigma; D: Carpel; E: Stamen
(c) A: Carpel; B: Stamen; C: Anther; D: Stigma; E: Petal
(d) A: Stigma; B: Petal; C: Stamen; D: Anther; E: Carpel

**61.** Identify A, B, C and D in this figure?

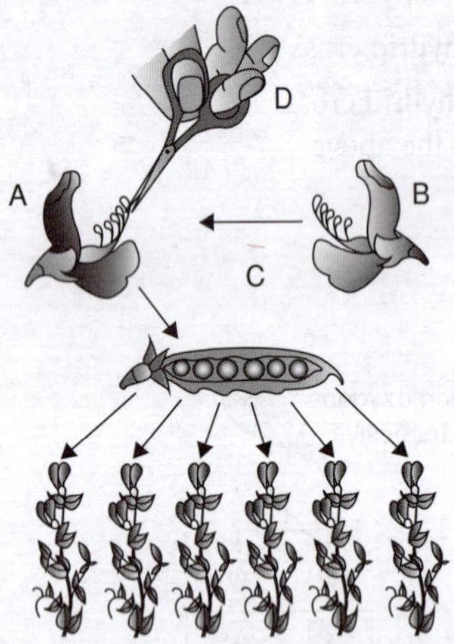


(a) A: Female parent; B: Removal of anthers (Emasculation); C: Transfer of pollen (Pollination); D: Male parent
(b) A: Male parent; B: Female parent; C: Removal of anthers (Emasculation); D: Transfer of pollen (Pollination)
(c) A: Removal of anthers (Emasculation); B: Female parent; C: Transfer of pollen (Pollination); D: Male parent
(d) A: Female parent; B: Male parent; C: Transfer of pollen (Pollination); D: Removal of anthers (Emasculation)

**62.** Why Mendel's work was not recognized till 1900?
(a) His work could not be widely published.
(b) His concept of factor (stable and discrete units that control expression of trait) was not accepted by his contemporaries.
(c) His approach of using mathematics to explain biological phenomenon was totally new and unacceptable by many of the biologists of his time.
(d) All of these

**63.** How many scientists rediscovered mendelism in 1900 independently?
(a) 1 (b) 2 (c) 3 (d) 4

**64.** Mendelian rediscoverers are
(a) De Vries, Holland
(b) Correns, Germany
(c) Von Tschermak, Austria
(d) All of these

**65.** Which result proved that there was no blending in Mendelian Cross?
(a) $Filial_1$ progeny of monohybrid cross
(b) $Filial_2$ progeny of dihybrid cross
(c) $Filial_1$ progeny of dihybrid cross
(d) All of these

**66.** $F_2$ progeny of Mendelian monohybrid cross between tall and dwarf plant is made up of
(a) Tall plant, identical to their parental type
(b) Dwarf plant, identical to their parental type
(c) Plant with intermediate height were produced
(d) Both (a) and (b)

**67.** Select the incorrect statement.
(a) Capital latter is used to denote dominant trait.
(b) Small latter is used to denote recessive trait.
(c) True breeding variety is represented by similar allele pair of gene.
(d) Alleles are completely similar forms of the same genes.

**68.** Punnett was
(a) Italian botanist (b) British geneticist
(c) American geneticist (d) Austrian geneticist

**69.** What is the genotype ratio of Mendelian monohybrid cross?
(a) 3 : 1 (b) 1 : 2 : 1 (c) 1 : 1 (d) 3 : 2

**70.** Mendel found that the $F_1$ always resembled either one of the parents and that the trait of the other parent was not seen in them. This is due to

(a) Segregation (b) Dominance
(c) Partial dominance (d) Unit factor

**71.** In monohybrid cross, the proportion of 3 : 1 explains
(a) Dominance (b) Segregation
(c) Both (a) and (b) (d) Unit factor

**72.** Which of the following was/were applied first time to problems in biology during Mendel's investigations into inheritance?
(a) Statistical analysis
(b) Mathematical logic
(c) Computational devices
(d) Both (a) and (b)

**73.** Mendel proposed how many general rules to consolidate his understanding of inheritance in monohybrid cross?
(a) One
(b) Two
(c) Three
(d) None of the rules, he proposed laws/principles

**74.** In the theoretical explanation of allelic interaction for dominant and recessive forms, the recessive trait is seen due to the production of
(a) Normal or less efficient enzyme
(b) A non-functional enzyme
(c) No enzyme production
(d) Either (b) or (c)

**75.** It is said that Mendel proposed that the factor controlling any character is discrete and independent. This proposition was based on the
(a) Results of $F_3$ generation of a cross.
(b) Observations that the offsprings of a cross made between the plants having two contrasting characters show only one character without any blending.
(c) Self-pollination of $F_1$ offsprings.
(d) Cross-pollination of parental generations.

**76.** Two genes 'A' and 'B' are linked. In a dihybrid cross involving these two genes, the $F_1$ hetero-zygote is crossed with homozygous recessive parental type (aa bb). What would be the ratio of offspring in the next generation?
(a) 1 : 1 : 1 : 1 (b) 9 : 3 : 3 : 1
(c) 3 : 1 (d) 1 : 1

**77.** In the $F_2$ generation of a Mendelian dihybrid cross, the number of phenotypes and genotypes are
(a) phenotypes-4; genotypes-16
(b) phenotypes-9; genotypes-4
(c) phenotypes-4; genotypes-8
(d) phenotypes-4; genotypes-9

**78.** 1 : 1 : 1 : 1 ratio of progenies can be obtained if the plants employed for crossing are
(A) TTRR × ttRR (B) TtRr × ttrr
(C) TtRR × ttrr (D) Ttrr × ttRr

(a) A, C and D (b) A, B, C and D
(c) B and D (d) A and B

**79.** Two allelic genes are located on
(a) The same chromosomes
(b) Two homologous chromosomes
(c) Two non-homologous chromosomes
(d) Any two chromosomes

## Exception to Mendelian Genetics

**80.** In human beings, the colour of skin is controlled by
(a) Multiple alleles (b) Lethal genes
(c) Polygenic effect (d) None of these

**81.** If a certain patient with blood group B requires immediate blood transfusion, the following type can be given to him
(a) O and B (b) O and AB
(c) A and AB (d) B and AB

**82.** The below diagram represents:

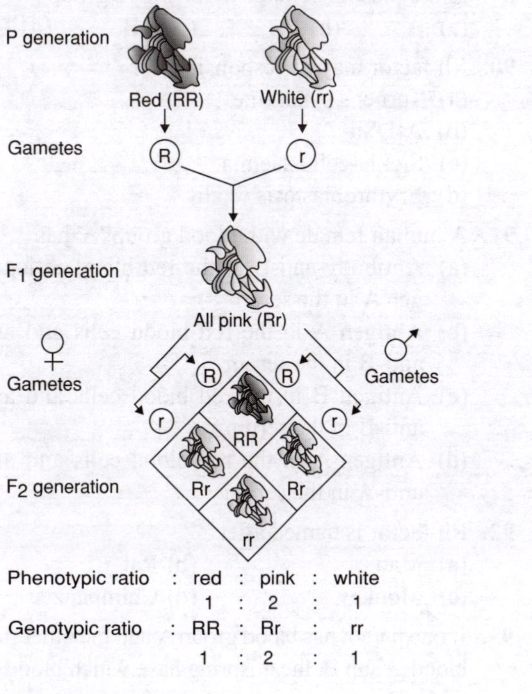


(a) Dominant epistasis
(b) Recessive epistasis
(c) Incomplete dominance
(d) Co-dominance

**83.** In Morgan's experiment, what will be the percentage of recombination in case of body colour and eye colour?
(a) 37.2% (b) 1.3% (c) 98.7% (d) 37.2%

**84.** Inheritance of ABO blood group system is an example of

(a) Multiple allelism (b) Partial dominance
(c) Epistasis (d) Dominance

**85.** Genotype of blood group 'A' will be
(a) $I^AI^A$ (b) $I^BI^B$
(c) $I^AI^A$ or $I^AI^O$ (d) $I^AI^O$

**86.** Blood group 'B' will have alleles
(a) ii (b) $I^AI^A$
(c) $I^BI^B$ (d) $I^AI^B$

**87.** If one parent belongs to 'A' blood group and the other to 'O' blood group, their children possibly represent
(a) A and B groups only
(b) AB only
(c) A and O groups only
(d) All four groups

**88.** If a child has O type of blood group and the father has B type, then the genotype of the father will be
(a) $I^OI^O$ (b) $I^AI^B$ (c) $I^OI^B$ (d) $I^BI^B$

**89.** A person with antigens 'B' in RBC and antibodies 'A' in the plasma belongs to the blood group
(a) A (b) B (c) AB (d) O

**90.** Rh factor may be responsible for
(a) Turner's syndrome
(b) AIDS
(c) Sickle-cell anaemia
(d) Erythroblastosis fetalis

**91.** A human female with blood group 'A' has
(a) Antibody-anti-B in the red blood cells and antigen A in the serum
(b) Antigen A in the red blood cells and antibody-anti-B in the serum
(c) Antigen B in the red blood cells and antibody-anti-B in the serum
(d) Antigen A in the red blood cells and antibody-anti-A in the serum

**92.** Rh factor is named after
(a) Man (b) Rat
(c) Monkey (d) Chimpanzee

**93.** If one parent has blood group A and the other parent has blood group B, the offspring have which blood group?
(a) AB (b) O
(c) BO (d) A, B, AB, O

**94.** Mendel did not recognize the linkage phenomenon in his experiments because
(a) There were many chromosomes to handle.
(b) Characters he studied were located on different chromosomes.
(c) He did not have powerful microscope.
(d) He studied only pure plants.

**95.** Exchange of genetic material between chromatids of homologous chromosomes during meiosis is called
(a) Synapsis (b) Chiasmata
(c) Transformation (d) Crossing over

**96.** In maize, the chromosome number is 2n = 20. The number of linkage groups in it will be
(a) 20 (b) 40 (c) 10 (d) 5

**97.** The map distance between genes A and B is 3 units, between B and C is 10 units and between C and A is 7 units. The order of the genes in a linkage map constructed on the above data would perhaps be
(a) A, B, C (b) A, C, B
(c) B, C, A (d) B, A, C

**98.** Crossing over in diploid organism is responsible for
(a) Dominance of genes
(b) Linkage between genes
(c) Segregation of alleles
(d) Recombination of linked allele

**99.** The percentage of crossing over will be more if
(a) Linked genes are located far apart from each other
(b) Linked genes are located close to each other
(c) Genes are not linked
(d) Genes are located in a different cell

**100.** Linkage was first observed in
(a) Field pea (b) Sweet pea
(c) Pea (d) Grass pea

**101.** Drosophila has four pairs of chromosomes. How many linkage groups does it have?
(a) Eight
(b) Four
(c) One less than the pairs of chromosomes
(d) One more than the pairs of chromosomes

**102.** Linkage in *Drosophila* was first discovered by
(a) Morgan (b) Bateson and Punnett
(c) Sturtevant (d) Bridges

**103.** Number of linkage groups in *Pisum sativum* is
(a) 2 (b) 5 (c) 7 (d) 9

**104.** Who coined the term linkage?
(a) Mendel (b) Tschermak
(c) Sturtevant (d) T. H. Morgan

**105.** Physical association of two genes is known as
(a) Heterozygosis (b) Linkage
(c) Recombination (d) Homozygosis

**106.** Find out the incorrect statement.
(a) Morgan carried out several dihybrid crosses in drosophila to study the genes that were sex linked.
(b) Sturtevant used the frequency of recombination between gene pairs on the same chromosome

as a measure of the distance between genes and mapped their position on chromosome.

(c) Henking gave the term X-body.

(d) Boveri united the knowledge of chromosomal segregation with Mendelian principles and called it the chromosomal theory of inheritance.

**107.** Which cross shows very tight linkage?

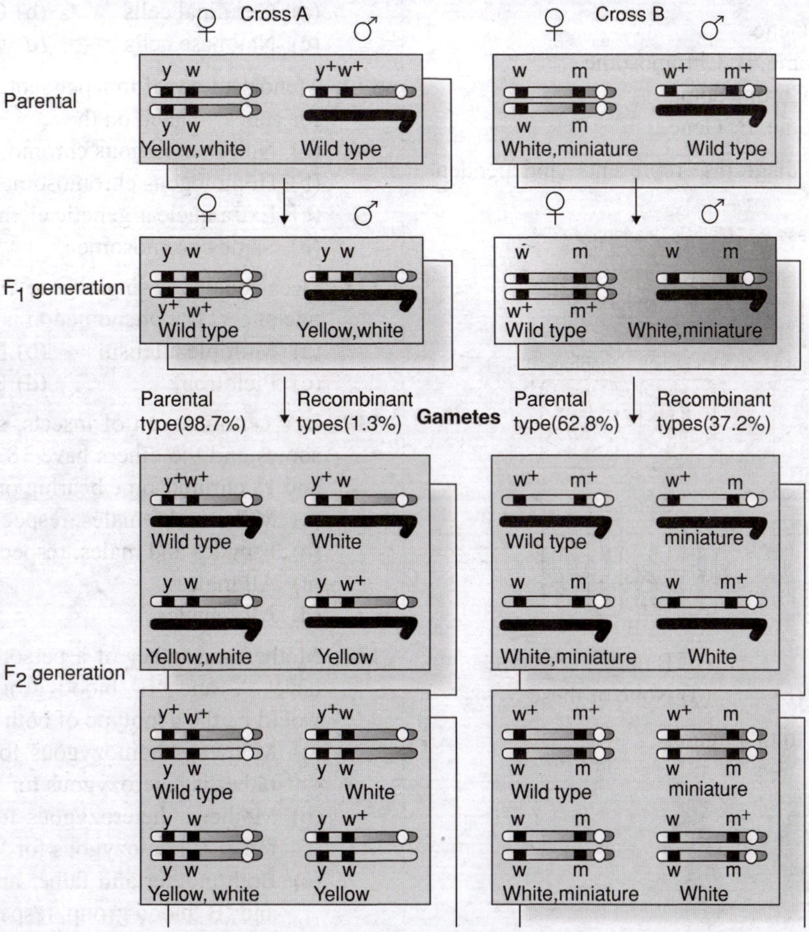


(a) Cross A (b) Cross B (c) Both (a) and (b) (d) None of these

**108.** Why *Drosophila melanogaster* is suitable for the study of genetical variation?

(a) Could be grown on simple synthetic medium in laboratory.

(b) Complete life cycle is 2 weeks and single mating produces a large number of progeny flies.

(c) Clear sexual dimorphism is present and many types of heredity variation can be seen with low power microscope.

(d) All of these

**109.** Who noted that the behaviour of chromosomes was parallel to the behaviour of genes and uses chromosome movement to explain Mendel's law?

(a) T. H. Morgan (b) Hugo de Vries
(c) Sutton and Boveri (d) Beadle and Tatum

**110.** Which of the below column A and B represents genes and chromosomes?

| A | B |
|---|---|
| 1. Occur in pairs. | 1. Occur in pairs. |
| 2. Segregate at the time of gamete formation such that only one of each pair is transmitted to a gamete. | 2. Segregate at the time of gamete formation and only one of each pair is transmitted to a gamete. |

| A | B |
|---|---|
| 3. Independent pairs segregate independently of each other. | 3. One pair segregates independently of another pair. |

(a) A: Gene, B: Gene
(b) A: Chromosome, B: Chromosome
(c) A: Gene, B: Chromosome
(d) A: Chromosome. B; Gene

**111.** Which of the diagrams represents independent assortment?

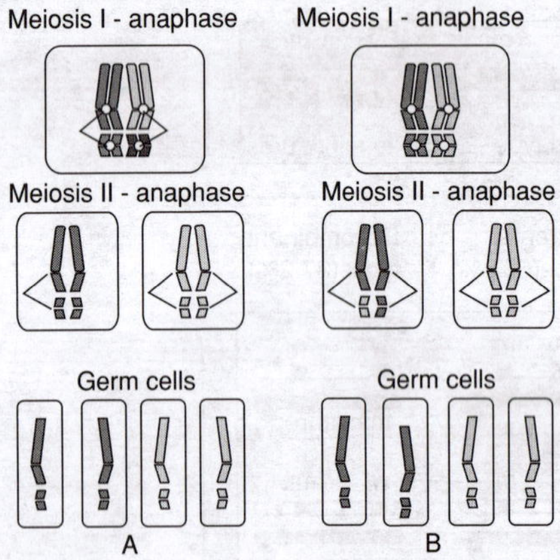


(a) A only (b) B only
(c) Both (a) and (b) (d) None of these

**112.** Identify A and B in this figure.

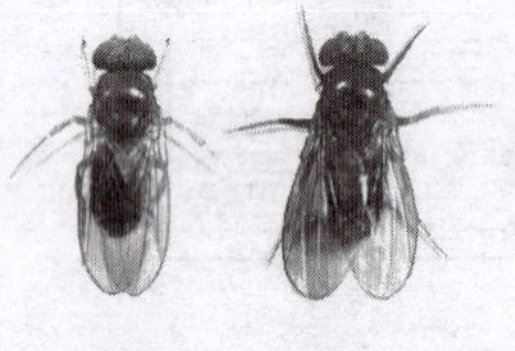

(a) A: Male, B: Female (b) A: Female, B: Male
(c) A: Male, B: Male (d) A: Female, B: Female

**113.** Genes responsible for ABO blood group determines which of the following biomolecules of RBC plasma membrane?
(a) Phospholipid (b) Proteins
(c) Sugars (d) Cholesterols

**114.** The shape of seed depends on starch granules size; so inheritance of seed shape shows _____ relationship, while inheritance of starch grains show ________.
(a) Dominant recessive, codominance
(b) Incomplete dominance, codominance
(c) Dominant-recessive, incomplete dominance
(d) Codominance, incomplete dominance

**115.** If yellow body, white eyed drosophila is crossed with wild brown body red eyes drosophila. Then what would be the frequency of recombinants in $F_1$ generation?
(a) 100% (b) 1.3% (c) 98.7% (d) 0%

**116.** Chromosomal aberrations are commonly observed in
(a) Germinal cells (b) Cancer cells
(c) Nail base cells (d) Gametes

**117.** Mendel's Law of independent assortment holds good for genes situated on the
(a) Non-homologous chromosomes
(b) Homologous chromosomes
(c) Extra nuclear genetic element
(d) Same chromosome

**118.** Occasionally, a single gene may express more than one effect. The phenomenon is called
(a) Multiple allelism (b) Mosaicism
(c) Pleiotropy (d) Polygeny

**119.** In a certain taxon of insects, some have 17 chromosomes and the others have 18 chromosomes. The 17 and 18 chromosome bearing organisms are
(a) Males and females, respectively
(b) Females and males, respectively
(c) All males
(d) All females

**120.** Mother and father of a person with '0' blood group have 'A' and 'B' blood group, respectively. What would be the genotype of both mother and father?
(a) Mother is homozygous for 'A' blood group and father is heterozygous for 'B'.
(b) Mother is heterozygous for 'A' blood group and father is homozygous for 'B'.
(c) Both mother and father are heterozygous for 'A' and 'B' blood group, respectively.
(d) Both mother and father are homozygous for 'A' and 'B' blood group, respectively.

## Sex Determination

**121.** In humans, the chromosomal condition of male is
(a) 44 AA + XO (b) 44 AA + XX
(c) 44 AA + XY (d) 44 AA + XXY

**122.** Cytological observation made in a many number of ________ led to the development of the concept of genetic/chromosomal basis of sex determination
(a) Mammals (b) Birds
(c) Humans (d) Insects

**123.** Who discovered X-body but could not explain its significance?

(a) Mendel (b) Morgan
(c) Henking (d) De vries

**124.** X-body of Henking was
(a) Nucleus (b) Lipid
(c) Chromosome (d) Ribosomes

**125.** X-chromosome is used in the determination of sex; therefore, it is known as
(a) Autosomes (b) Sex chromosomes
(c) Microsomes (d) Oxysomes

**126.** Which type of sex-determination is found in grasshopper?
(a) XO type (b) XY type
(c) ZW type (d) Any of these

**127.** In the number of insects and mammals the type of sex determination is
(a) XO type (b) XY type
(c) ZW type (d) Any of these

**128.** Male is homogametic in
(a) Drosophila (b) Human
(c) Fowl (d) All of these

**129.** How many chromosomes are present in human male?
(a) 22 Pairs + XX (b) 22 Pairs + YY
(c) 22 Pairs + XY (d) 21 Pairs + XY

**130.** The below figure possess which of the following sex chromosomes?

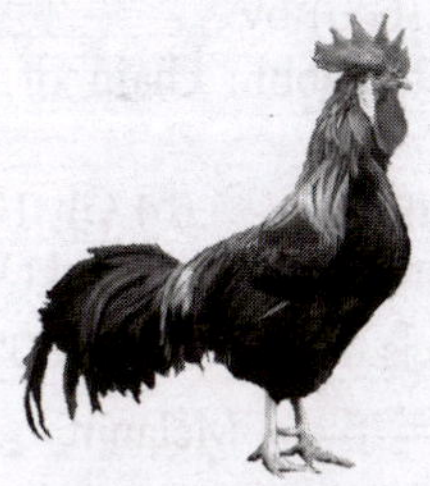

(a) XX (b) XY
(c) ZZ (d) ZW

**131.** The below diagram shows

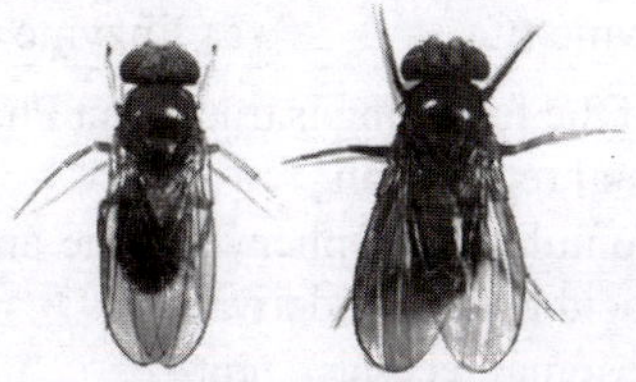

(a) M and F drosophila, respectively
(b) M and F housefly, respectively
(c) F and M drosophila, respectively
(d) F and M housefly, respectively

**132.** Which of the following is responsible for sex of the chicks?
(a) Sperm (b) Egg
(c) Both (a) and (b) (d) None of these

**133.** Find out the correct statement.
(a) Genetic makeup of the egg determines the sex of the child in human.
(b) Genetic makeup of the sperm determines the sex of the child in human.
(c) XO and XY type of sex determination is an example of female heterogamety.
(d) Henking (1891) could trace a specific nuclear structure all through oogenesis of few insects.

**134.** Female heterogamety is found in
(a) Human (b) Drosophila
(c) Chicks (d) All of these

## Mutation and Genetic Disorders

**135.** Failure of segregation of chromatids during cell division cycles results in the gain or loss of a chromosome(s) called
(a) Aneuploidy (b) Polyploidy
(c) Trisomy (d) Nullisomy

**136.** Down's syndrome occurs due to the gain in extra copy of
(a) Chromosome 19
(b) Chromosome 5
(c) Chromosome 21
(d) Chromosome 24

**137.** Turner's syndrome occurs due to the loss of
(a) Chromosome 5
(b) Chromosome 21
(c) Chromosome 'X'
(d) Chromosome 'Y'

**138.** How many sex chromosomes are present in human cell?
(a) 1 pair (b) 2 pairs
(c) 3 pairs (d) 4 pairs

**139.** Gynaecomastia is seen in case of
(a) Down's syndrome (b) Klinefelter's syndrome
(c) Turner's syndrome (d) All of these

**140.** The following features belong to which syndrome?
(A) Furrowed tongue
(B) Palm is broad with characteristic palm crease
(C) Physical, psychomotor and mental retardation
(D) Short statured with small round head
(a) Down's syndrome (b) AIDS
(c) Turner's syndrome (d) Klinefelter's syndrome

**141.** The below diagram shows which type of syndrome?

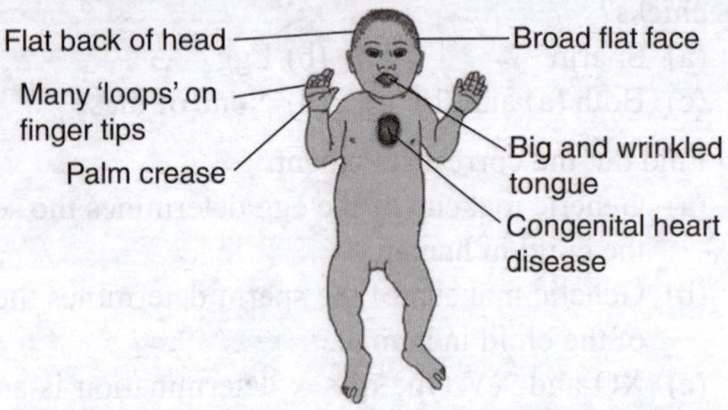


(a) Down's syndrome (b) Cri-du chat syndrome
(c) PKU (d) Turner's syndrome

**142.** Increase in a whole set of chromosome in an organism is known as
(a) Polyploidy (b) Aneuploidy
(c) Trisomy (d) Tetrasomy

**143.** Langdon down described Down's syndrome in which year
(a) 1866 (b) 1890
(c) 1852 (d) 1953

**144.** Which of the following is genetically dominant in man?
(a) Colour blindness (b) Rh positive
(c) Haemophilia (d) Albinism

**145.** Karyotype of Klinefelter's syndrome is
(a) 44 + XXY (b) 44 + XO
(c) 44 + XYY (d) 44 + XXXY

**146.** Which is not a character of Klinefelter's syndrome?
(a) Masculine development
(b) Gynaecomastia
(c) Fertile individual
(d) Sterile individual

**147.** All are characters of Down's syndrome except
(a) Congenital heart disease
(b) Broad flat face
(c) Small and wrinkled tongue
(d) Many 'loops' on finger tips

**148.** Identify the syndrome of diagrams a and b, respectively.

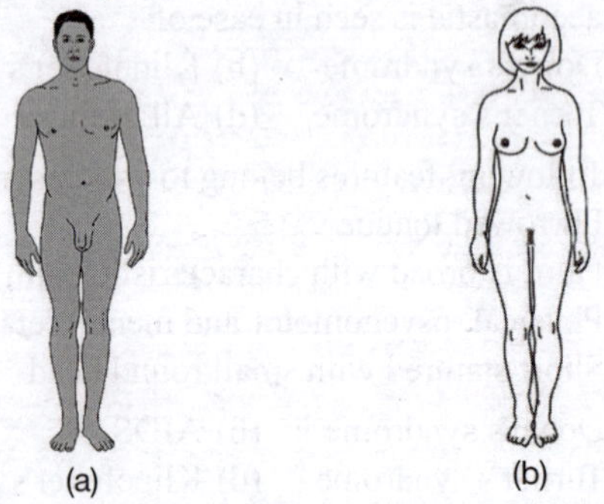


(a) A: Down's syndrome, B: Turner's syndrome
(b) A: Klinefelter's syndrome, B: Turner's syndrome
(c) A: Turner's syndrome, B: Klinefelter syndrome
(d) A: Turner's syndrome, B: Down's syndrome

**149.** Which karyotype present monosomy?
(a) 2n + 1 (b) 2n – 2 (c) 2n – 1 (d) 2n + 2

**150.** Which karyotype represents trisomy?
(a) 2n + 1 (b) 2n – 2 (c) 2n – 1 (d) 2n + 2

**151.** Find out the total number of Mendelian disorder from the following:
*Cystic Fibrosis, Haemophilia, Sickle cell anaemia, Colour blindness, Thalessemia, Phenylketonuria*
(a) 4 (b) 5 (c) 6 (d) 3

**152.** Which of the following is sex-linked recessive disorder?
(a) Myotonic dystrophy (b) Sickle-cell anaemia
(c) Haemophilia (d) Phenylketonuria

**153.** Which of the following is an autosomal dominant trait?
(a) Phenylketonuria (b) Sickle-cell anaemia
(c) Haemophilia (d) Myotonic dystrophy

**154.** Queen Victoria was a carrier of which disease?
(a) Myotonic dystrophy (b) Sickle-cell anaemia
(c) Haemophilia (d) Phenylketonuria

**155.** Sickle cell anaemia is caused by the substitution of Glutamic acid (Glu) by ________ at the sixth position of the beta globin chain of the haemoglobin molecule.
(a) Asn (Aspargine) (b) Gly (Glycine)
(c) Arg (Argenine) (d) Val (Valine)

**156.** Which enzyme is defective in PKU?
(A) DOPA $\xrightarrow{\text{Enzyme(1)}}$ Melanin
(B) Tyrosine $\xrightarrow{\text{Enzyme(2)}}$ Thyroxin
(C) Phenylalanine $\xrightarrow{\text{Enzyme(3)}}$ Tyrosine
(D) Tyrosine $\xrightarrow{\text{Enzyme(4)}}$ Homogentisic acid
(a) Enzyme (A) (b) Enzyme (B)
(c) Enzyme (C) (d) Enzyme (D)

**157.** Which of the following is true about Phenylketonuria?
(a) Mental retardation
(b) Accumulation of phenylalanine and phenylpyruvic acid and other derivatives
(c) Autosomal recessive trait
(d) All the above

**158.** The substitution of amino acid in the globin protein results due to the single bass substitution at the sixth codon of the beta globin gene from.

(a) GAG to GGG (b) CAG to GAG
(c) GAG to GUG (d) GGC to GGA

**159.** Which of the following amino acid is not present in first six amino acids in affected $\beta$-chain of Haemoglobin in sickle cell anaemia?
(a) Val (b) Thr (c) Glu (d) Leu

**160.** Identify A, B and C from the following diagram.

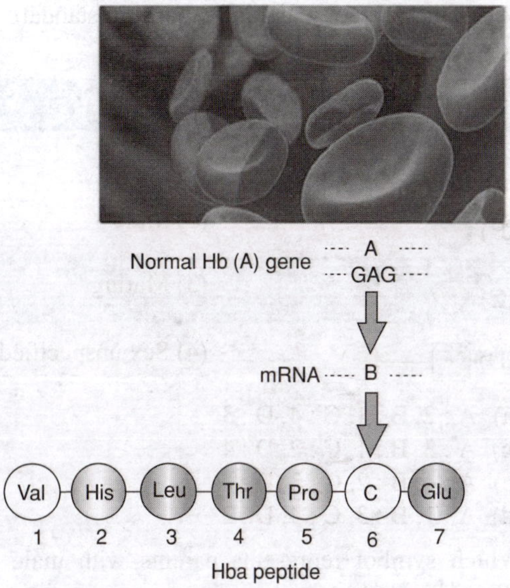


(a) A: CTC; B: GAG; C: Glu
(b) A: GAG; B: CTC; C: Pro
(c) A: CTC; B: GAG; C: Thr
(d) A: CTC; B: GAG; C: Leu

**161.** Identify A, B and C from the following diagram.

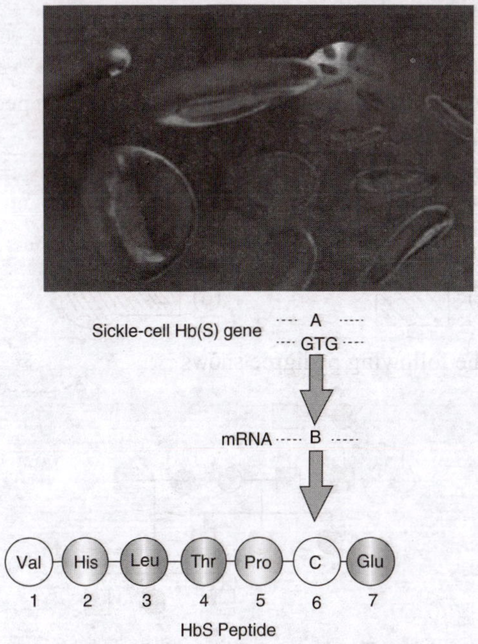


(a) A: CAC; B: GUG; C: Pro
(b) A: CAC; B: GUG; C: Val
(c) A: CTC, B: GUG, C: Leu
(d) A: GAC, B: GUG, C: His

**162.** Name the amino acid which has its 2 molecules present in the first 7 amino acid of $\beta$-chain of haemoglobin.
(a) Val (b) His
(c) Leu (d) Glu

**163.** Probability of which of the following is extremely rare?
(a) Carrier female in haemophilia
(b) Carrier male in haemophilia
(c) Affected male in haemophilia
(d) Affected female in haemophilia

**164.** In hemophilia how many proteins that is a part of the cascade of protein involved in clotting of blood affected?
(a) 1 (b) 2
(c) 3 (d) Multiple/many

**165.** Diseased phenotype in sickle cell anaemia is shown by which of the following genotype?
(a) $Hb^A Hb^A$ (b) $Hb^S Hb^S$
(c) $Hb^A Hb^S$ (d) All of above

**166.** Variation in DNA is due to
(a) Mutation (b) Recombination
(c) Both (a) and (b) (d) None of these

**167.** Alteration in chromosome may be due to
(a) Deletion of a segment of DNA
(b) Addition of segment of DNA
(c) Duplication of segment of DNA
(d) Any of these

**168.** Deletion or insertion of base pairs of DNA causes
(a) Point mutation (b) Frameshift mutation
(c) Transversion (d) All of these

**169.** Find out the correct statement.
(a) UV radiation can cause mutation in organism.
(b) Chromosomal aberration are commonly observed in cancer cells.
(c) Mutation is a phenomenon which results in the alteration of DNA sequences and results in changes in the genotype and the phenotype of an organism.
(d) All the above

**170.** Mutation that arises due to the change in single base pair of DNA is known as
(a) Point mutation (b) Frameshift mutation
(c) Silent mutation (d) Recombination

**171.** A classical example of point mutation is
(a) Haemophilia (b) Sickle cell anaemia
(c) Mongolism (d) Cri-du chat syndrome

**172.** Which of the following disorders is not hereditary?
(a) Haemophilia (b) Cataract
(c) Sickle-cell anaemia (d) Colour blindness

**173.** A pleiotropic gene is one which
(a) Affects one character
(b) Affects more than one characters
(c) Both (a) and (b)
(d) None of these

**174.** Phenylketonuria is a genetic disorder of
(a) Trisomic condition
(b) Monosomic condition
(c) Autosomal dominant gene
(d) Autosomal recessive gene
(e) X-linked

**175.** Which of the following is not X-linked recessive?
(a) Haemophilia-A (b) Colour blindness
(c) BETA-Thalassemia (d) G-6 PD deficiency

**176.** Monosomy and trisomy can be represented as
(a) 2n + 1, 2n + 3 (b) 2n – 1, 2n – 2
(c) 2n, 2n + 1 (d) 2n – 1, 2n + 1

**177.** Which of the following cell cycle event is responsible for polyploidy phenomenon?
(a) Failure of karyokinesis
(b) Failure of cytokinesis
(c) Failure of segregation
(d) Failure of spindle apparatus

**178.** Match the following

| Column – I | Column – II |
|---|---|
| A. Haemophilia | 1. Board palm with characteristic palm creased |
| B. Down's syndrome | 2. Delayed clotting of blood |
| C. Klinefelter's syndrome | 3. Feminine development |
| D. Turner's Syndrome | 4. Rudimentary ovaries |

(a) A : 1; B : 3; C : 2; D : 4
(b) A : 2; B : 1; C : 3; D : 4
(c) A : 4; B : 2; C : 1; D : 3
(d) A : 1; B : 2; C : 3; D : 4

## Pedigree Analysis

**179.** The inheritance pattern of a gene over generations among humans is studied by the pedigree analysis. Character studied in the pedigree analysis is equivalent to
(a) Quantitative trait (b) Mendelian trait
(c) Polygenic trait (d) Maternal trait

**180.** The method for analyzing inheritance pattern of traits in human being is
(a) DNA finger printing (b) Control cross
(c) Pedigree analysis (d) All of these

**181.** The standard symbol used for consanguineous mating in pedigree analysis is
(a) 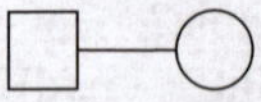 (b) 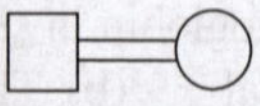
(c) 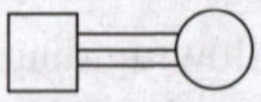 (d) 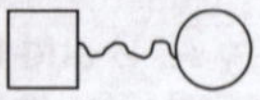

**182.** Select the correct matching regarding standard symbol of pedigree analysis

| Column–I | Column–II |
|---|---|
| (A)  | (1) Female |
| (B)  | (2) Male |
| (C) 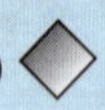 | (3) Mating |
| (D) 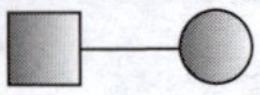 | (4) Sex unspecified |

(a) A : 2, B : 1, C : 4, D : 3
(b) A : 3, B : 1, C : 2, D : 4
(c) A : 1, B : 2, C : 3, D : 4
(d) A : 1, B : 3, C : 4, D : 2

**183.** Which symbol represents parents with male child affected with diseases?
(a) 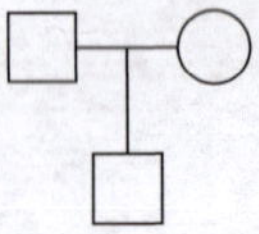 (b) 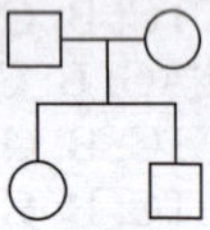
(c) 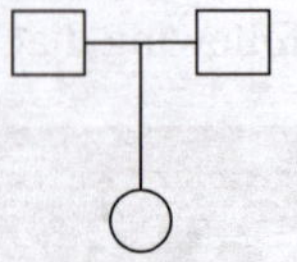 (d) 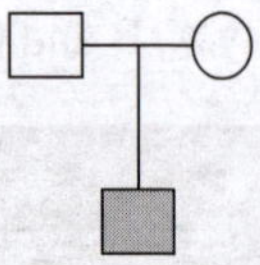

**184.** Which of the following symbol is not used in pedigree analysis?
(a) 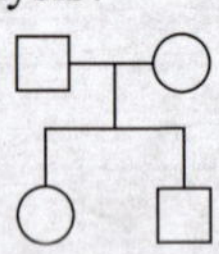 (b) 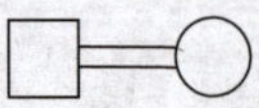
(c) 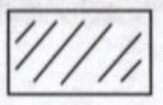 (d) 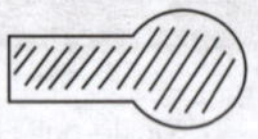

185. The following pedigree shows

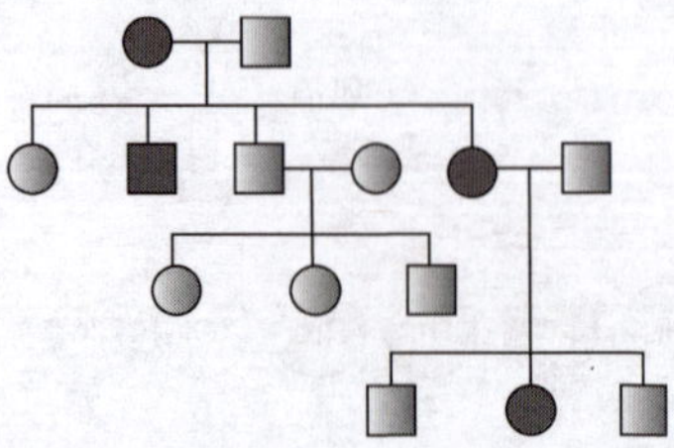

(a) Autosomal dominant trait
(b) Cytoplasmic inheritance
(c) X-linked recessive trait
(d) X-linked dominant trait

**186.** The following pedigree shows

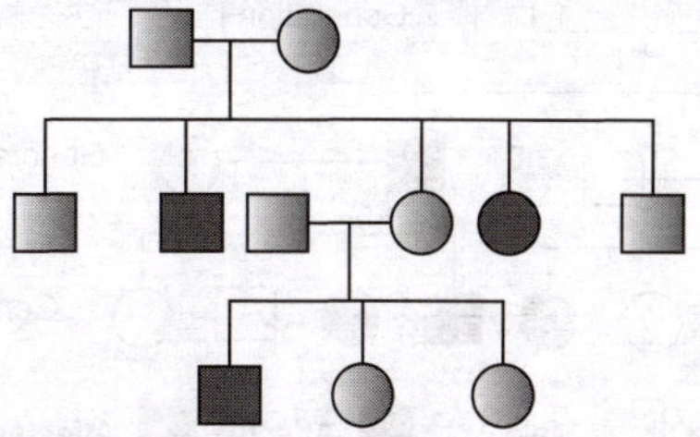

(a) Autosomal dominant trait
(b) Autosomal recessive trait
(c) X-linked recessive trait
(d) X-linked dominant trait

**187.** Given below is a pedigree chart of family with five children. It shows the inheritance of attached ear-lobes as opposed to the free ones. The squares represent the male individuals and circles the female individuals.

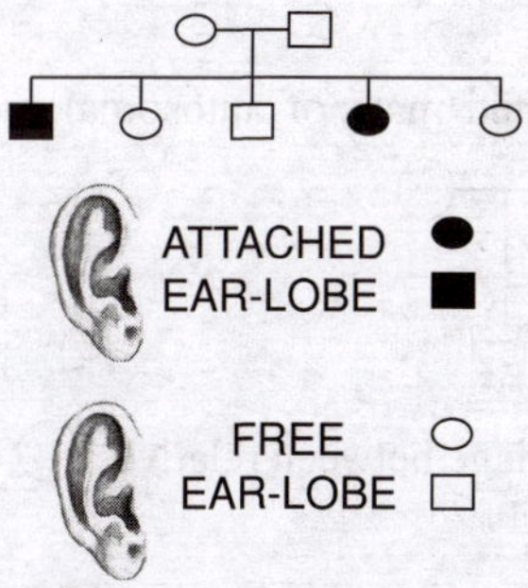


Which one of the following conclusions drawn is correct?
(a) The parents are homozygous recessive.
(b) The trait is Y-linked.
(c) The parents are homozygous dominant.
(d) The parents are heterozygous.

**188.** Predict from the following chart

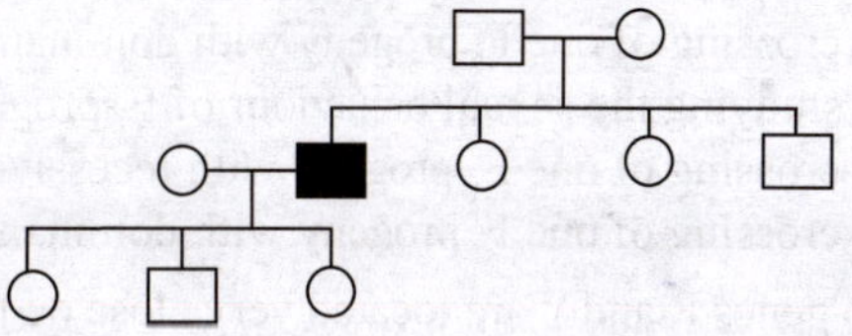

(a) Character is dominant and carried by x chromosome.
(b) Character is carried by y chromosome.
(c) Character is sex-linked recessive.
(d) Character is autosomal recessive.

**189.** The pedigree shows the occurrence of albinism which is a recessive trait. If person 4 is homozygous, the carrier for the trait is

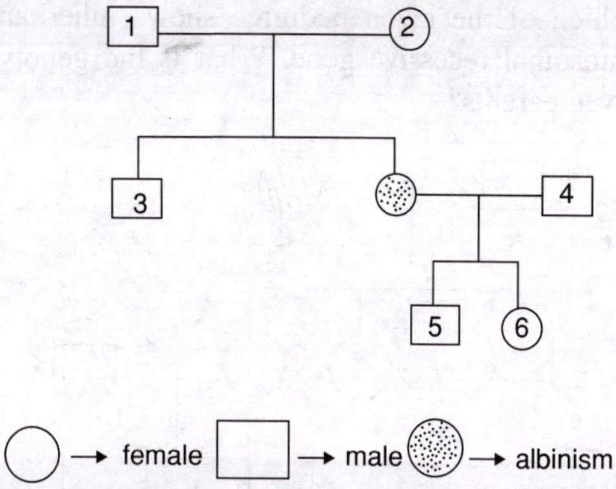


(a) 1, 4, 5 and 6
(b) 5 and 6
(c) 1, 2 and 3
(d) 1, 2, 5 and 6

**190.** This is the pedigree for autosomal recessive disease albinism (aa). What is the probability of II-1 homozygous normal?

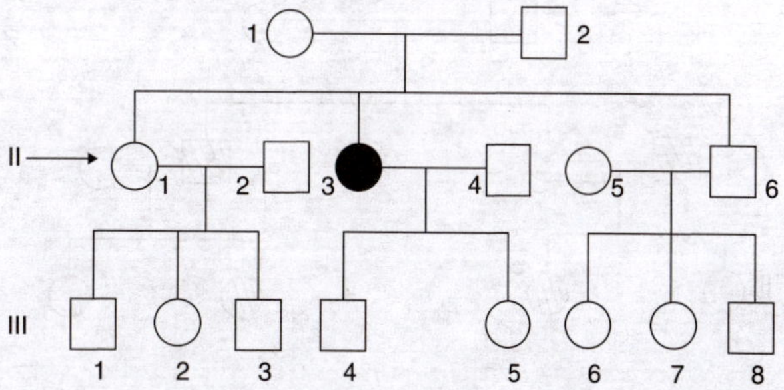


(a) $\frac{1}{3}$ (b) $\frac{1}{2}$ (c) $\frac{2}{3}$ (d) $\frac{1}{4}$

**191.** According to the given pedigree, the trait indicates

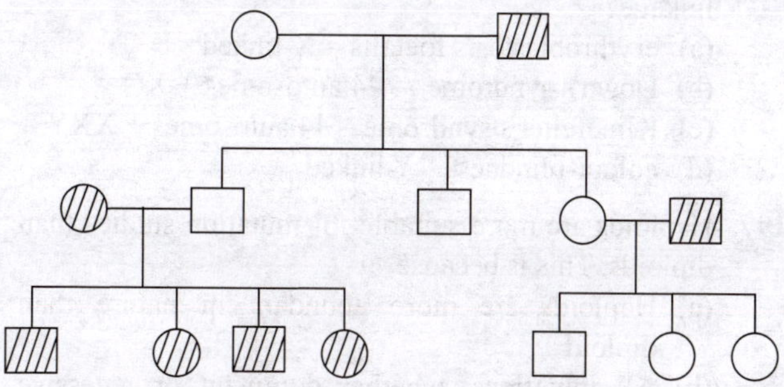

(a) Autosomal recessive □: Normal male
(b) X-linked recessive ▨: Affected male

(c) Maternal imprinting : Normal female
(d) Paternal imprinting : Affected female

**192.** Which of the given pedigree shows inheritance of autosomal recessive gene. What is the genotype of given parents?

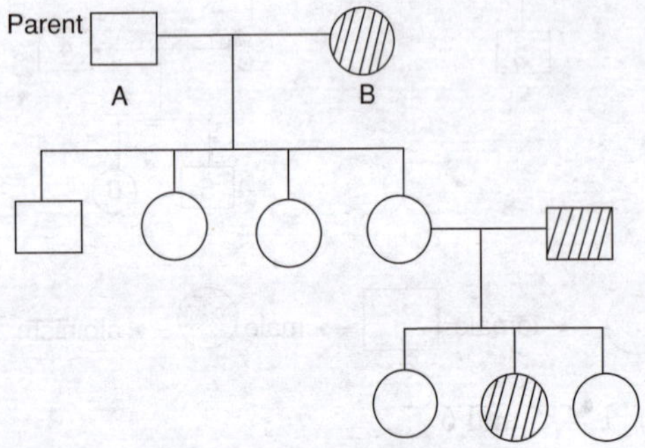


(a) AA, aa (b) Aa, AA
(c) aa, aa (d) Aa, Aa

**193.** A pedigree is shown below for a disease that is autosomal recessive. The genetic makeup of the first generation will be

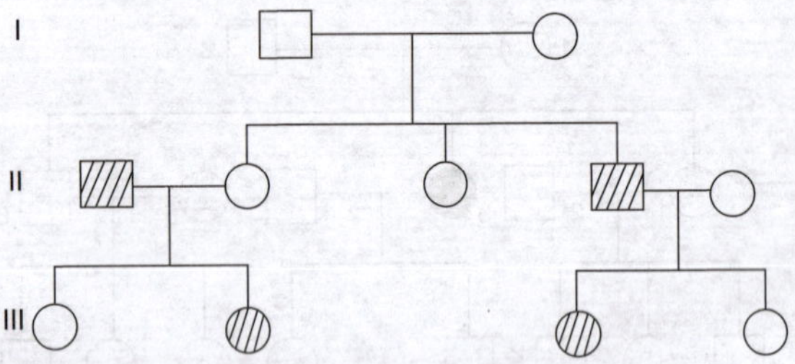


(a) AA, aa (b) Aa, Aa
(c) Aa, aa (d) aa, aa

**194.** A pedigree is shown below for a disease that is autosomal dominant. The genetic makeup of the first generation is

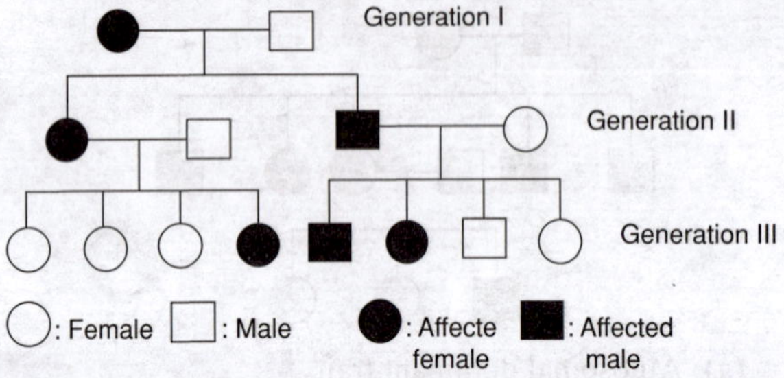


(a) AA, Aa (b) Aa, aa
(c) Aa, AA (d) Aa, Aa

**195.** Which symbol of pedigree is correctly matched?

(a) – Female 

(b) – Affected offspring 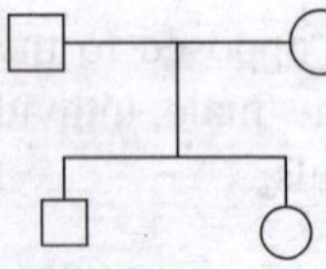

(c) – Affected male of autosomal recessive disease 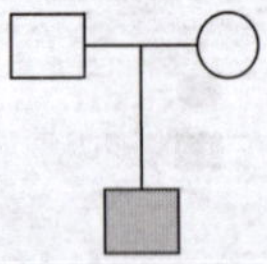

(d) – Marriage between relatives 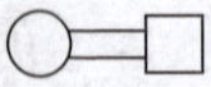

## Multiple Choice Questions: Level II

**196.** Which one of the following conditions in humans is correctly matched with its chromosomal abnormality/linkage?
(a) erythroblastosis foetalis – X-linked
(b) Down's syndrome – 44 autosomes + XO
(c) Klinefelter's syndrome – 44 autosomes + XXY
(d) colour-blindness – Y-linked

**197.** Haploids are more suitable for mutation studies than diploids. This is because
(a) Haploids are more abundant in nature than diploid
(b) All mutations, whether dominant or recessive expressed, are expressed in haploids
(c) Haploids are reproductively more stable than diploids
(d) Mutagens penetrate in haploids more effectively than in diploids

**198.** A common test to find genotype of a hybrid is by
(a) crossing of one $F_2$ progeny with dominant parent
(b) studying the sexual behaviour of $F_1$ progenies
(c) crossing of one $F_1$ progeny with recessive parent
(d) crossing of one $F_2$ progeny with dominant parent

**199.** Two genes R and Y are located very close on the chromosomal linkage map of maize plant. When RRYY and rryy genotypes are hybridized, $F_2$ segregation will show

(a) segregation in expected 9 : 3 : 3 :1 ratio
(b) segregation in 3 : 1 ratio
(c) higher number of parental types
(d) higher number of recombinant types

**200.** In pea plant, yellow seeds are dominant to green. If a heterozygous yellow-seeded plant is crossed with a green-seeded plant, what ration of yellow and green-seeded plants would you expect in $F_1$ generation?
(a) 9 : 1 (b) 1 : 3
(c) 3 : 1 (d) 50 : 50

**201.** Inheritances of skin colour in humans is an example of
(a) point mutation
(b) polygenic inheritance
(c) co-dominance
(d) chromosomal aberration

**202.** A human male produces sperms with genotypes AB, Ab, aB, and ab pertaining to two diallelic characters in equal proportions. What is the corresponding genotype of this person?
(a) AaBB (b) AABb
(c) AABB (d) AaBb

**203.** In Mendel's experiment with garden pea, round seed shape (RR) was dominant over wrinkled seeds (rr), yellow cotyledon (YY) was dominant over green cotyledon (yy). What are the expected phenotypes in the $F_2$ generation of cross RRYY x rryy?
(a) only wrinkled seeds with yellow cotyledons
(b) only wrinkled seeds with green cotyledons
(c) round seeds with yellow cotyledons, and wrinkled seeds with yellow cotyledons
(d) only round seeds with green cotyledons

**204.** Test cross involves
(a) crossing between two $F_1$ hybrids
(b) crossing the $F_1$ hybrid with a double recessive genotype
(c) crossing between two genotypes with dominant trait
(d) crossing between two genotypes with recessive trait

**205.** Phenotype of an organism is the result of
(a) Cytoplasmic effects and nutrition
(b) Environmental changes and sexual dimorphism
(c) Genotype and environment interactions
(d) Mutations and linkages

**206.** How many kinds of gametes will be produced by a plant having the genotype AABbcc?
(a) Four (b) Nine
(c) Two (d) Three

**207.** If a colour-blind woman marries a normal-visioned man, their sons will be
(a) one-half colour-blind and one-half normal
(b) three-fourths colour-blind and one-fourth normal
(c) all colour-blind
(d) all normal-visioned

**208.** Which one of the following is an example of polygenic inheritance?
(a) Production of male honey bee
(b) Pod shape in garden pea
(c) Skin colour in humans
(d) Flower colour in Mirabilis jalapa

**209.** In which mode of inheritance do you expect more maternal influence among the offspring?
(a) Cytoplasmic (b) Y-linked
(c) X-linked (d) Autosomal

**210.** Both sickle cell anaemia and Huntington's chorea are
(a) congenital disorders
(b) pollutant-induced disorders
(c) virus-related diseases
(d) bacteria-related diseases

**211.** Sickle cell anaemia has not been eliminated from the African population, because
(a) it is not a fatal disease
(b) it provides immunity against malaria
(c) it is controlled by dominant genes
(d) it is controlled by recessive genes

**212.** In order to find out the different types of gametes produced by a pea plant having the genotype AaBb, it should be crossed to a plant with the genotype:
(a) AABB (b) AaBb
(c) aabb (d) aaBB

**213.** A woman with normal vision, but whose father was colour-blind, marries a colour-blind man.
Suppose the fourth child of this couple was a boy. This boy
(a) may be colour-blind or may be of normal vision
(b) must be colour-blind
(c) must have normal vision
(d) will be partially colour-blind since he is heterozygous for the colour-blind mutant allele

**214.** With respect to the ABO group, there are four major blood types because this blood group is determined by
(a) three alleles, all of which are recessive
(b) three alleles, of which, two are recessive and the third is dominant
(c) three alleles, of which two are co-dominant and the third is recessive
(d) three alleles, all of which are co-dominant

**215.** Haemophilia is more commonly seen in human males than in human females, because
(a) a greater proportion of girls die in infancy
(b) this disease is due to a Y-linked recessive mutation
(c) this disease is due to an X-linked recessive mutation
(d) this disease is due to an X-linked dominant mutation

**216.** A women with 47 chromosomes due to three copies of chromosome 21 is characterized by:
(a) Super femaleness (b) Triploidy
(c) Turner's syndrome (d) Down's syndrome

**217.** One of the parents of a cross has a mutation in its mitochondria. If that parent is taken as a male. During segregation of $F_2$ progenies that mutation is found in
(a) one-third of the progenies
(b) none of the progenies
(c) all the progenies
(d) fifty per cent of the progenies

**218.** A self-fertilizing trihybrid plant forms
(a) 8 different gametes and 64 different zygotes
(b) 4 different gametes and 16 different zygotes
(c) 8 different gametes and 16 different zygotes
(d) 8 different gametes and 32 different zygotes

**219.** Crossing over that results in genetic recombination in higher organisms occur between
(a) sister chromatids of a bivalent
(b) non-sister chromatids of a bivalent
(c) two daughter nuclei
(d) two different bivalents

**220.** Lack of independent assortment of two genes A and B in fruit fly, Drosophila, is due to
(a) Repulsion (b) Recombination
(c) Linkage (d) Crossing over

**221.** The recessive genes located on X-chromosome in humans are always
(a) Lethal
(b) Sub-lethal
(c) Expressed in males
(d) Expressed in females

**222.** A male human is heterozygous for autosomal genes A and B and is also hemizygous for hemophilic gene h. What proportion of his sperms will be abh?
(a) $\frac{1}{8}$ (b) $\frac{1}{32}$ (c) $\frac{1}{16}$ (d) $\frac{1}{4}$

**223.** A normal woman whose father was colour-blind is married to a normal man. The sons would be
(a) 75% colour-blind (b) 50% colour-blind
(c) all normal (d) all colour-blind

**224.** In Drosophila, the sex is determined by
(a) whether the egg is fertilized or develops parthenogenetically
(b) the ratio of number of X- chromosomes to the sets of autosomes
(c) X and y chromosomes
(d) the ratio of pairs of X- chromosomes to the pairs of autosomes

**225.** The genes controlling the seven pea characters studied by Mendel are now known to be located on how many different chromosomes?
(a) Four (b) Seven
(c) Six (d) Five

**226.** Two crosses between the same pair of genotypes or phenotypes in which the source of the gametes are reversed in one cross is known as
(a) reverse cross (b) test cross
(c) reciprocal cross (d) dihybrid cross

**227.** When a cluster of genes shows linkage behaviour they
(a) induce cell division
(b) do not show a chromosome map
(c) show recombination during meiosis
(d) do not show independent assortment

**228.** Christmas disease is another name for
(a) sleeping sickness (b) haemophilia
(c) hepatitis B (d) Down's syndrome

**229.** Pattern baldness, moustaches and beard in human males are examples of
(a) sex-determining traits
(b) sex-linked traits
(c) sex-limited traits
(d) sex-differentiating traits

**230.** Down's syndrome is caused by an extra copy of chromosome number 21. What percentage of offspring produced by an affected mother and a normal father would be affected by this disorder?
(a) 25% (b) 100%
(c) 75% (d) 50%

**231.** On selfing a plant of $F_1$ generation with genotype 'AABbCC', the genotypic ratio in $F_2$ generation will be
(a) 3 : 1
(b) 1 : 2 : 1
(c) 9 : 3 : 3: 1
(d) 27 : 9 : 9 : 9 :3 : 3 : 3 :1

**232.** There are three genes a, b, c. Percentage of crossing over between a and b is 20%, b and c is 28% and a and c is 8%. What is the sequence of genes on chromosome?
(a) b, a, c (b) a, b, c
(c) a, c, b (d) none of these

**233.** Which of the following is an example of sex-linked disease?
(a) AIDS (b) Colour-blindness
(c) Syphilis (d) Gonorrhoea

**234.** Which of the following is an example of pleiotropic effect?
(a) haemophilia (b) thalassemia
(c) sickle cell anaemia (d) colour-blindness

**235.** A gene is said to be dominant if
(a) it expresses its effect only in homozygous state
(b) it expresses its effect only in heterozygous condition
(c) it expresses its effect both in homozygous and heterozygous conditions
(d) it never expresses its effect in any conditions

**236.** A diseased man marries a normal woman. They have three daughters and five sons. All the daughters were diseased and sons were normal. The gene of this disease is
(a) sex-linked dominant
(b) sex-linked recessive
(c) sex-linked character
(d) autosomal dominant

**237.** Independent assortment of genes does not take place when
(a) Genes are located on homologous chromosomes
(b) Genes are linked and located on same chromosomes
(c) Genes are located on nonhomologous chromosomes
(d) all the above

**238.** When dominant and recessive alleles express together it is called
(a) Co-dominance (b) Dominance
(c) Amphidominace (d) Pseudodominance

**239.** Which one of the following is the most suitable medium for culture of *Drosophila melanogaster*?
(a) Agar agar (b) Ripe banana
(c) Cow dung (d) Moist bread

**240.** Extranuclear inheritance occurs in
(a) Peroxisome and Ribosome
(b) Mitochondria and Chloroplast
(c) Mitochondria and Ribosome
(d) Chloroplast and Lysosome

**241.** A family of five daughters (girls only) is expecting a sixth issue. The chance of it being a son is
(a) Zero (b) 25%
(c) 50% (d) 100%

**242.** A tall true breeding garden pea plant is crossed with a dwarf true breeding garden pea plant. When the F1 plants were selfed the resulting genotypes were in the ratio of:
(a) 1:2:1: Tall homozygous: Tall heterozygous : Dwarf
(b) 1:2:1: Tall heterozygous: Tall homozygous: Dwarf
(c) 3 : 1 : : Tall : Dwarf
(d) 3 : 1 : : Dwarf : Tall

**243.** Probability of four sons to a couple is
(a) $\frac{1}{4}$ (b) $\frac{1}{8}$ (c) $\frac{1}{16}$ (d) $\frac{1}{32}$

**244.** If A and B genes are linked, what shall be genotype of progeny in a cross between AB/ab and ab/ab?
(a) AAbb and aabb (b) AaBb and aabb
(c) AABB and aabb (d) None of these

**245.** In humans, male XXY and female XXX occur due to
(a) Aneuploidy
(b) Euploidy
(c) Autosomal syndrome
(d) None of these

**246.** No. of barr body present in each somatic cell of a female is
(a) 1 (b) 2 (c) 3 (d) 4

**247.** In a certain plant, red fruit (R) is dominant over yellow fruit (R) and tallness (T) is dominant over shortness (t). If a plant with RRTt genotype is crossed with a plant rrtt genotype, what will be the percentage of tall plant percentage of tall plants with red fruits in the progeny?
(a) 50% (b) 100%
(c) 75 % (d) 25 %

**248.** Match the terms in List I with their description in List II and choose the correct option:

| List-I | List-II |
|---|---|
| 1. Dominance | (i) Many genes govern a single character |
| 2. Codominance | (ii) In a heterozygous organism only one allele expresses itself. |
| 3. Pleiotropy | (iii) In a heterozygous organisms both alleles express themselves fully |

| List-I | List-II |
|---|---|
| 4. Polygenic inheritance | (iv) A single gene influences many characters |

**The correct matching is:**

| | 1 | 2 | 3 | 4 |
|---|---|---|---|---|
| (a) | (ii) | (i) | (iv) | (iii) |
| (b) | (ii) | (iii) | (iv) | (i) |
| (c) | (iv) | (i) | (ii) | (iii) |
| (d) | (iv) | (iii) | (i) | (ii) |

**249.** Drosophila flies with XXY genotype are females but in case of humans, such individuals are abnormal males (Klinefelter's syndrome). This indicates that
(a) the Y chromosome has no role in sex determination
(b) in Drosophila, Y chromosome is essential for sex determination
(c) Y chromosome is male determining in humans
(d) Y chromosome is female determining in Drosophila

**250.** Which one pair of the following parents is most likely to get a child who suffers from haemolytic disease of the new-born?
(a) Rh-negative mother and Rh-positive father
(b) Rh-positive mother and Rh-negative father
(c) Rh-negative mother and Rh-negative father
(d) Rh-positive mother and Rh-positive father

**251.** Haploids are able to express both recessive and dominant alleles/mutations, because there are
(a) many alleles for each gene
(b) two alleles for each gene
(c) only one allele for each gene in the individual
(d) only one allele in a gene

**252.** In hybridization, Tt x tt gives rise to the progeny of ratio
(a) 1 : 1 (b) 1: 2 (c) 2:1 (d) 1 : 2 : 1

**253.** One child is haemophilic (sex-linked trait), while its fraternal twin brother is normal. Which one of the following information is most appropriate?
(a) The mother must have been heterozygous
(b) The child is a monozygotic twin
(c) The other child is a female and the father is haemophilic
(d) The haemophilic child is a male

**254.** Red-green colour-blindness in humans is governed by a sex-linked recessive gene. A normal woman whose father was colour-blind marries a colour-blind man. What proportion of their daughters is expected to be colour-blind?
(a) 3/4 (b) 1/2 (c) 1/4 (d) All

**255.** Crossing over in diploid organism is responsible for
(a) Segregation of alleles
(b) Dominance of genes
(c) Linkage between genes
(d) Recombination of linked alleles

**256.** How many genome types are present in a typical green plant cell?
(a) Two (b) Three
(c) More than five (d) More than ten

**257.** If Mendel had studied the 7 traits using a plant with 12 chromosomes instead of 14, in what way would his interpretation have been different?
(a) He would have discovered blending or incomplete dominance
(b) He would not have discovered the law of independent assortment
(c) He would have discovered sex linkage
(d) He could have mapped the chromosome

**258.** How many different types of genetically different gametes will be produced by a heterozygous plant having the genotype AABbCc?
(a) Two (b) Four
(c) Six (d) Nine

**259.** In Down's syndrome, karyotyping has shown that the disorder is associated with trisomy of chromosome number-21 usually due to
(a) non-disjunction during egg-cell formation
(b) non-disjunction during sperm-cell formation
(c) non-disjunction during formation of egg cells and sperm cells
(d) addition of extra chromosome during mitosis of the zygote

**260.** Mental retardation in man associated with sex chromosomal abnormality is usually due to
(a) increase in X complement
(b) moderate increase in Y complement
(c) large increase in Y complement
(d) reduction in X complement

**261.** A woman with two genes for haemophilia and a gene for colour-blindness on one of the 'X' chromosomes marries a normal man. How will the progeny be
(a) Haemophilic and colour-blind daughters
(b) 50% haemophilic, colour-blind sons and 50% haemophilic sons
(c) 50% haemophilic daughters and 50% colour-blind daughters
(d) All sons and daughters haemophilic and colour-blind

**262.** Albinism is known to be due to an autosomal recessive mutation. The first child of a couple with normal skin pigmentation was an albino. What is the probability for their second child towards albinism?
(a) 25% (b) 50%
(c) 75% (d) 100%

**263.** A fruit fly is heterozygous for sex-linked genes. When mated with a normal female fruit fly, the male-specific chromosome will enter egg cells in the proportion of
(a) 1 : 1 (b) 1 : 2
(c) 3 : 1 (d) 7 : 1

**264.** Which of the following contributes to the success of Mendel?
(a) Qualitative analysis of data
(b) Observation of distinct inherited traits
(c) His knowledge of biology
(d) Consideration of one character at one time

**265.** Genetic identity of a human male is determined by
(a) autosomes (b) nucleolus
(c) sex chromosomes (d) cell organelles

**266.** Different mutations referable to the same locus of a chromosome give rise to
(a) multiple alleles (b) pseudoalleles
(c) polygenes (d) oncogenes

**267.** A person with the sex chromosomes XXY suffers from
(a) Down's syndrome
(b) Klinefelter's syndrome
(c) Turner's syndrome
(d) Gynandromorphism

**268.** Alleles that produce independent effects in their heterozygous condition are called
(a) co-dominant alleles
(b) epistatic alleles
(c) complementary alleles
(d) supplementary alleles

**269.** An individual exhibiting both male and female sexual characteristics in the body is known as
(a) hermaphrodite (b) intersex
(c) gynandromorph (d) bisexual

**270.** A man with a certain disease marries a normal woman. They have eight children (3 daughters and 5 sons). All the daughters suffer from their father's disease but none of the sons are affected. Which of the following mode of inheritance do you suggest for this disease?
(a) Sex-linked recessive
(b) Sex-linked dominant
(c) Autosomal dominant
(d) Sex-limited recessive

**271.** If a colourblind woman marries a normal man then what is the probability of their son being colourblind?
(a) 0% (b) 25%
(c) 75% (d) 100%

**272.** Two linked genes a and b show 20% recombination. The individuals of a dihybrid cross between + + / + + x ab/ab shall show gametes
(a) + + 80 : ab : 20
(b) + + 50 : ab : 50
(c) + + 40 : ab 40 : + a 10 : + b : 10
(d) + + 30 : ab 30 : + a 20 : + b : 20

**273.** The most striking example of point mutation is found in a disease called
(a) thalassemia (b) night blindness
(c) Down's syndrome (d) sickle cell anaemia

**274.** A women with albinic father marries an albinic man. The proportion of her progeny is
(a) 2 normal : 1 albinic
(b) All normal
(c) All albinic
(d) 1 normal : 1 albinic

**275.** In a dibhybrid cross AABB x aabb, $F_2$ progeny of AABB, AABb, AaBB and AaBb occurs in the ratio of
(a) 1 : 1: 1 : 1 (b) 9 : 3 : 3 : 1
(c) 1 : 2 : 2 :1 (d) 1 : 2 : 2 :4

**276.** A cross between pure tall pea plant with green pods and dwarf pea plant with yellow pods will produce short $F_2$ plant out of 16
(a) 9 (b) 3
(c) 4 (d) 1

**277.** A child of blood group O cannot have parents of blood groups
(a) AB and AB/O (b) A and B
(c) B and B (d) O and O

**278.** Genes located on Y chromosome are
(a) Mutant genes (b) Sex-linked genes
(c) Autosomal genes (d) Holandric genes

**279.** Mendel studied inheritance of seven pairs of traits in pea which can have 21 possible combination. If you are told that in one of these combinations, independent assortment is not observed in later studies, your reaction will be
(a) Independent assortment principle may be wrong
(b) Mendel might not have studied all the combinations
(c) It is impossible
(d) Later studies may be wrong

**280.** Two dominant nonallelic genes are 50 map units apart. The linkage is
(a) Cis type (b) Trans type
(c) Complete (d) Absent/Incomplete

**281.** Of a normal couple, half the sons are haemophilic while half the daughters are carriers. The gene is located on
(a) X-chromosome of father
(b) Y-chromosome of father
(c) One X-chromosome of mother
(d) Both the X-chromosomes of mother

**282.** If parents have blood groups A and B and both are heterozygous for their respective blood groups then, which blood group can be seen in offsprings?
(a) AB (b) O
(c) A (d) All A, B, AB and O

**283.** Mr. Kapoor has Bb autosomal gene pair and d allele sex-linked. What shall be the proportion of Bd in sperms
(a) Zero (b) 1/2 (c) 1/4 (d) 1/8

**284.** Of both normal parents, the chance of a male child becoming colour-blind is
(a) No
(b) Possible only when all the four grandparents has normal vision
(c) Possible only when father's mother was colour-blind
(d) Possible only when mother's father was colour-blind

**285.** In Down's syndrome of a male child, the sex complement is
(a) XO (b) XY
(c) XX (d) XXY

**286.** Segregation of Mendelian factors (no linkage, no crossing over) occurs during
(a) Anaphase I (b) Anaphase II
(c) Diplotene (d) Metaphase I

**287.** A gene pair hides the effect of another. The phenomenon is
(a) Epistasis (b) Dominance
(c) Mutation (d) None of the above

**288.** A child of O-group has B-group father. The genotype of father will be
(a) $I^oI^o$ (b) $I^BI^B$
(c) $I^AI^B$ (d) $I^BI^O$

**289.** A colour-blind mother and normal father would have
(a) Colour-blind sons and normal/carrier daughters
(b) Colour-blind sons and daughters
(c) All colour-blind
(d) All normal

**290.** When a certain character is inherited only through female parent, it probably represents
(a) Multiple plastid inheritance
(b) Cytoplasmic inheritance
(c) Incomplete dominance
(d) Mendelian nuclear inheritance

**291.** RR (Red) Antirrhinum is crossed with white (WW) one. Offspring RW are pink. This is an example of
(a) Dominant-recessive
(b) Incomplete dominance
(c) Hybrid
(d) Supplementary genes

**292.** Blue eye colour is recessive to brown eye colour. A brown-eyed man whose mother was blue marries a blue-eyed women. The children shall be
(a) Both blue-eyed and brown-eyed 1:1
(b) All brown-eyed
(c) All blue-eyed
(d) Blue-eyed and brown-eyed 3:1

**293.** Mendel's last law is
(a) Segregation
(b) Dominance
(c) Independent assortment
(d) Polygenic inheritance

**294.** First geneticist/father of genetic was
(a) de Vries (b) Mendel
(c) Darwin (d) Morgan

**295.** A man of A-blood group marries a woman of AB blood group. Which type of progeny would indicate that man is heterozygous A?
(a) AB (b) A (c) O (d) B

**296.** A colour-blind girl is rare, because she will be born only when
(a) her mother and maternal grandfather were colour-blind
(b) her father and maternal grandfather were colour-blind
(c) her mother is colour blind and father has normal vision
(d) parents have normal vision but grandparents were colour-blind

**297.** tt mates with Tt. What will be the characteristic of offspring?
(a) 75% recessive (b) 50% recessive
(c) 25% recessive (d) all dominant

**298.** ABO blood group system is due to
(a) Multifactor inheritance
(b) Incomplete dominance
(c) Multiple allelism
(d) Epistasis

**299.** Cross between AaBB and aaBB will form
(a) 1 AaBB :1 aaBB (b) All AaBB
(c) 3 AaBB : 1 aaBB (d) 1 AaBB : 3 aaBB

**300.** Both husband and wife have normal vision though their fathers were colour-blind. The probability of their daughter becoming colour-blind is
(a) 0% (b) 25% (c) 50% (d) 75%

**301.** Which one is a hereditary disease?
(a) Cataract (b) leprosy
(c) Blindness (d) Phenylketonuria

**302.** Haemophilia is more common in male, because it is a
(a) recessive character carried by Y-chromosome
(b) dominant character carried by Y-chromosome
(c) dominant trait carried by X-chromosome
(d) recessive trait carried by X-chromosome

## A & R and Statement-based Questions

### Assertion and Reason Questions

***Direction for questions 303 to 307:** Read the **assertion** and **reason** carefully to mark the correct option out of the options given below:*

**(a)** **(A)** is **true** but **(R)** is **false**.
**(b)** **(A)** is **false** but **(R)** is **true**.
**(c)** Both **(A)** and **(R)** is **true** and **(R)** is the correct explanation of **(A)**.
**(d)** Both **(A)** and **(R)** is **true** and **(R)** is not the correct explanation of **(A)**.

**303. Assertion:** Mendel's work was not recognised till 1900.
**Reason:** His work could not be widely publicised.

**304. Assertion:** Sutton and Boveri explains Mendel law's by chromosomal movement during meiosis.
**Reason:** Behaviour of chromosome is similar to the behaviour of gene.

**305. Assertion:** Gene which code for a pair of contrasting traits are known alleles.
**Reason:** Alleles are slightly different forms of the same gene.

**306. Assertion:** The law of dominance is used to explain the expression of only one of the parental character n a monohybrid cross i.e., in the $F_1$ – generation.
**Reason:** The law of dominance explain the phenotypic ratio of 3 : 1 which is obtained in the $F_2$ – generation.

**307. Assertion:** Deletions & insertions of one or two base pairs of DNA, causes frame–shift mutation.
**Reason:** A classic example of frame–shift mutation is sickle cell anaemia.

### Statement-based Questions:

***Direction for questions 308 to 312:** These types of questions consist of two statement each, printed as **Statement-I** and **Statement-II**. While answering such questions, a student is needed to choose any one of the following four responses.*

**(a)** **Statement I** is **correct Statement II** is **incorrect**.
**(b)** **Statement I** is **incorrect Statement II** is **correct**.
**(c)** Both **Statement I** and **Statement II** are **correct**.
**(d)** Both **Statement I** and **Statement II** are **incorrect**.

**308. Statement-I:** Increase in a whole set of chromosome in an organism is known as polyploidy.
**Statement-II:** Congenital heart disease is commonly seen in case of down's syndrome.

**309. Statement-I:** Change in genetic material is mutation.
**Statement-II:** Sickle cell anaemia is quantitative disorder of haemoglobin.

**310. Statement-I:** Failure of segregation of chromatids during cell division cycle results in gain and loss of a chromosome, called aneuploidy.
**Statement-II:** Aneuploidy is Mendelian disorder.

**311. Statement-I:** Haploid diploid sex-determination is seen in *Drosophila melanogaster.*
**Statement-II:** Y-chromosome is responsible for maleness in human offspring.

**312. Statement-I:** Henking discovered X-body.
**Statement-II:** When single gene have multiple phenotypic effect. It is said to be pleiotropic genes.

## Matrix-Match Type Questions

**313.** Match the following:

| List-I | List-II |
|---|---|
| 1. Dominance | (i) In heterozygote, both alleles express to give phenotype different progeny than parents |
| 2. Codominance | (ii) In heterozygote, only one allele expresses |
| 3. Incomplete dominance | (iii) In heterozygote, both alleles express to themselves fully |

**The correct matching is:**

| | 1 | 2 | 3 |
|---|---|---|---|
| (a) | (ii) | (iii) | (i) |
| (b) | (iii) | (ii) | (i) |
| (c) | (i) | (iii) | (ii) |
| (d) | (ii) | (i) | (iii) |

**314.** Match the following:

| List-I | List-II |
|---|---|
| 1. Flower colour in snapdragon | (i) Dominance |
| 2. Flower colour in Pisum sativum | (ii) Codominance |
| 3. Blood group in humans | (iii) Incomplete dominance |
| 4. Skin colour in humans | (iv) Polygenic inheritance |

**The correct matching is:**

| | 1 | 2 | 3 | 4 |
|---|---|---|---|---|
| (a) | (iii) | (i) | (ii) | (iv) |
| (b) | (iii) | (ii) | (iv) | (i) |
| (c) | (ii) | (iii) | (i) | (iv) |
| (d) | (ii) | (i) | (iii) | (iv) |

**315.** Match the following:

| List-I | List-II |
|---|---|
| 1. Pleiotropy | (i) Many genes control a single character |
| 2. Polygenic inheritance | (ii) Both genes express simultaneously to give intermediate phenotype (character) |
| 3. Incomplete dominance | (iii) A single gene control many characters |
| 4. Codominance | (iv) Both genes express fully to give a character |

**The correct matching is:**

| | 1 | 2 | 3 | 4 |
|---|---|---|---|---|
| (a) | (iii) | (i) | (ii) | (iv) |
| (b) | (iv) | (iii) | (i) | (ii) |
| (c) | (ii) | (i) | (iii) | (iv) |
| (d) | (iii) | (ii) | (i) | (iv) |

**316.** Match the following:

| List-I | List-II |
|---|---|
| 1. Phenylketonuria | (i) Dominance |
| 2. Skin colour in humans | (ii) Polygenic inheritance |
| 3. Flower position in pea plant | (iii) Codominance |
| 4. Blood group in humans | (iv) Pleiotropy |

**The correct matching is:**

| | 1 | 2 | 3 | 4 |
|---|---|---|---|---|
| (a) | (iv) | (ii) | (i) | (iii) |
| (b) | (iv) | (iii) | (i) | (ii) |
| (c) | (ii) | (i) | (iii) | (iv) |
| (d) | (ii) | (iii) | (i) | (iv) |

**317.** Match the following:

| List-I | List-II | List-III |
|---|---|---|
| 1. XO | (i) Birds | X. Male heterogamete |
| 2. XY | (ii) Grasshopper | Y. Female heterogamete |
| 3. ZW | (iii) Drosophila | |

**The correct matching is:**

(a) 1 – (ii) – X, 2 – (iii) – X, 3 – (i) – Y
(b) 1 – (iii) – Y, 2 – (ii) – Y, 3 – (i) – X
(c) 1 – (ii) – X, 2 – (i) – Y, 3 – (iii) – Y
(d) 1 – (i) – X, 2 – (iii) – X, 3 – (ii) – Y

## NCERT Exemplar Questions

1. All genes are located on the same chromosome
   (a) Form different groups depending upon their relative distance.
   (b) Form one linkage group.
   (c) Will not form any linkage groups.
   (d) Form interactive groups that affect the phenotype.
2. Conditions of a karyotype (2n + 1, 2n – 1) and (2n + 2, 2n – 2) are called
   (a) Aneuploidy (b) Polyploidy
   (c) Allopolyploidy (d) Monosomy
3. Distance between the genes and percentage of recombination shows
   (a) A direct relationship
   (b) An inverse relationship
   (c) A parallel relationship
   (d) No relationship
4. If a genetic disease is transferred from a phenotypically normal but carrier female to only some of the male progeny, the disease is
   (a) Autosomal dominant
   (b) Autosomal recessive
   (c) Sex-linked dominant
   (d) Sex-linked recessive
5. In sickle cell anaemia, the glutamic acid is replaced by valine. Which one of the following are triplet codes for valine?
   (a) G G G (b) A A G
   (c) G A A (d) G U G
6. A person having genotype $I^A$ $I^B$ would show the blood group as AB. This is because of
   (a) Pleiotropy
   (b) Co-dominance
   (c) Segregation
   (d) Incomplete dominance
7. ZZ/ZW type of sex determination is seen in
   (a) Platypus (b) Snails
   (c) Cockroach (d) Peacock
8. A cross between two tall plants resulted in offspring having few dwarf plants. What would be the genotypes of both the parents?
   (a) TT and Tt (b) Tt and Tt
   (c) TT and TT (d) Tt and tt
9. In a dihybrid cross, if you get 9 : 3 : 3 : 1 ratio, it denotes that
   (a) The alleles of two genes are interacting with each other.
   (b) It is a multigenic inheritance.
   (c) It is a case of multiple allelism.
   (d) The alleles of two genes are segregating independently.
10. Which of the following will not result in variations among siblings?
    (a) Independent assortment of genes
    (b) Crossing over
    (c) Linkage (d) Mutation
11. Mendel's Law of independent assortment holds good for genes situated on the
    (a) Non-homologous chromosomes
    (b) Homologous chromosomes
    (c) Extra nuclear genetic element
    (d) Same chromosome
12. Occasionally, a single gene may express more than one effect. This phenomenon is called
    (a) Multiple allelism
    (b) Mosaicism
    (c) Pleiotropy
    (d) Polygeny
13. In a certain taxon of insects, some have 17 chromosomes and the others have 18 chromosomes. The 17 and 18 chromosome-bearing organisms are
    (a) Males and females, respectively
    (b) Females and males, respectively
    (c) All males
    (d) All females
14. The inheritance pattern of a gene over generations among humans is studied by the pedigree analysis. Character studied in the pedigree analysis is equivalent to
    (a) Quantitative trait (b) Mendelian trait
    (c) Polygenic trait (d) Maternal trait
15. It is said that Mendel proposed that the factor controlling any character is discrete and independent. His proposition was based on the
    (a) Results of $F_3$ generation of a cross.
    (b) Observations that the offspring of a cross made between the plants having two contrasting characters show only one character without any blending.
    (c) Self-pollination of $F_1$ offsprings.
    (d) Cross pollination of $F_1$ generations with recessive parental.
16. Two genes 'A' and 'B' are linked. In a dihybrid cross involving these two genes, the $F_1$ heterozygote is

crossed with homozygous recessive parental type (aa bb). What would be the ratio of offspring in the next generation?

(a) 1 : 1 : 1 : 1 (b) 9 : 3 : 3 : 1
(c) 3 : 1 (d) 1 : 1

**17.** In the $F_2$ generation of a Mendelian dihybrid cross, the number of phenotypes and genotypes are

(a) Phenotypes-4; genotypes-16
(b) Phenotypes-9; genotypes-4
(c) Phenotypes-4; genotypes-8
(d) Phenotypes-4; genotypes-9

**18.** Mother and father of a person with 'O' blood group have 'A' and 'B' blood group respectively. What would be the genotype of both mother and father?

(a) Mother is homozygous for 'A' blood group and the father is heterozygous for 'B'.
(b) Mother is heterozygous for 'A' blood group and the father is homozygous for 'B'.
(c) Both mother and father are heterozygous for 'A' and 'B' blood group, respectively.
(d) Both mother and father are homozygous for 'A' and 'B' blood group, respectively.

## Previous Years' Questions

**1.** Which one of the following symbols and its representation used in human pedigree analysis is correct? [AIPMT 2010 PRE]

(a) □═○ = Mating between relatives
(b) ○ = Unaffected male
(c) □ = Unaffected female
(d) ◆ = Male affected

**2.** Select the correct statement from the ones given below with respect to dihybrid cross. [AIPMT 2010 PRE]

(a) Tightly linked genes on the same chromosome show higher recombinations
(b) Genes far apart on the same chromosome show very few recombinations
(c) Genes loosely linked on the same chromosome show similar recombinations as the tightly linked ones
(d) Tightly linked genes on the same chromosome show very few recombinations

**3.** ABO blood groups in humans are controlled by gene I. It has three alleles - $1^A$, $I^B$ and i. Since there are three different alleles, six different genotypes are possible. How many phenotypes can occur? [AIPMT 2010 PRE]

(a) Three (b) One
(c) Four (d) Two

**4.** The genotype of a plant showing dominant phenotype can be determined by: [AIPMT 2010 PRE]

(a) Test cross (b) Dihybrid cross
(c) Pedigree analysis (d) Back cross

**5.** Which one of the following cannot be explained on the basis of Mendel's Law of Dominance? [AIPMT 2010 PRE]

(a) The discrete unit controlling a particular character is called a factor
(b) Out of two pair of factors one is dominant, and the other recessive
(c) Alleles do not show any blending and both the characters recover as such in $F_2$ generation
(d) Factors occur in pairs

**6.** Fruit fly Drosophila melanogaster was found to be very suitable for experimental verification of chromosomal theory of inheritance by Morgan and his colleagues because: [AIPMT 2010 MAINS]

(a) it reproduces parthenogenetically
(b) a single mating produces two young fly
(c) smaller female is easily recognizable from larger male
(d) it completes life cycle in about two weeks

**7.** ABO blood grouping is controlled by gene I which has three alleles and show co-dominance. There are six genotypes. How many phenotypes in total are possible? [AIPMT 2010 MAINS]

(a) Six (b) Three
(c) Four (d) Five

**8.** A cross in which an organism showing a dominant phenotype is crossed with the recessive parent in order to know its genotype is called [AIPMT 2010 MAINS]

(a) Monohybrid cross (b) Back cross
(c) Test cross (d) Dihybrid cross

**9.** In antirrhinum, two plants with pink flowers were hybridized. The $F_1$ plants produced red, pink and white flowers in the proportion of 1 red, 2 pink and 1 white. What could be the genotype of two plants used for hybridization. Red flower colour is determined by RR, and white by rr genes. [AIPMT 2010 MAINS]

(a) rrrr (b) RR
(c) Rr (d) rr

**10.** Study the pedigree chart of a certain family given in figure and select the correct conclusion which can be drawn for the character.

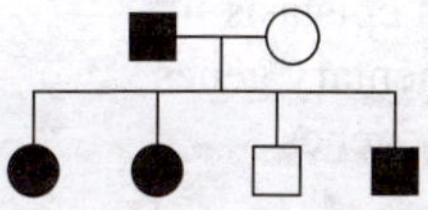

[AIPMT 2010 MAINS]

(a) The female parent is heterozygous
(b) The parents could not have had a normal daughter for this character
(c) The trait under study could not be colour blindness
(d) The male parent is homozygous dominant

**11.** Which one of the following conditions of the zygotic cell would lead to the birth of a normal human female child? [AIPMT 2011 MAINS]

(a) Two X chromosome
(b) Only one Y chromosome
(c) Only one X chromosome
(d) One X and one Y chromosome

**12.** Test cross in plants or in Drosophila involves crossing [AIPMT 2011 MAINS]

(a) Between two genotypes with recessive trait
(b) Between two $F_1$ hybrids
(c) The $F_1$ hybrid with a double recessive genotype
(d) Between two genotypes with dominant trait

**13.** When two unrelated individuals or lines are crossed, the performance of $F_1$ hybrid is often superior to both its parents. This phenomenon is called: [AIPMT 2011 PRE]

(a) Transformation (b) Splicing
(c) Metamorphosis (d) Heterosis

**14.** Which one of the following conditions correctly describes the manner of determining the sex in the given example? [AIPMT 2011 PRE]

(a) XO type of sex chromosomes determine male sex in grasshopper
(b) XO condition in humans, as found in Turner syndrome, determines female sex
(c) Homozygous sex chromosomes (XX) produce male in Drosophila
(d) Homozygous sex chromosomes (ZZ) determine female sex in birds

**15.** $F_2$ generation in a Mendelian cross showed that both genotypic and phenotypic rations are same as 1:2:1. It represents a case of: [AIPMT 2012 PRE]

(a) Co-dominance
(b) Dihybrid cross
(c) Monohybrid cross with complete dominance
(d) Monohybrid cross with incomplete dominance

**16.** A normal-visioned man, whose father was colour-blind, marries a women whose father was also colour-blind. They have their first child, a daughter. What are the chances for this child to be colour-blind? [AIPMT 2012 PRE]

(a) 100% (b) 0%
(c) 25% (d) 50%

**17.** Represented below is the inheritance pattern of certain type of traits in humans. Which one of the following conditions could be an example of this pattern? [AIPMT 2012 MAINS]

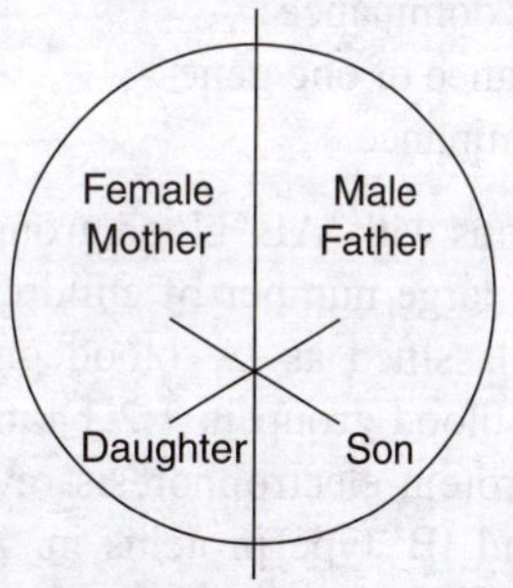


(a) Sickle cell anaemia
(b) Haemophilia
(c) Thalassemia
(d) Phenylketonuria

**18.** A test cross is carried out to: [AIPMT 2012 MAINS]

(a) Predict whether two traits are linked
(b) Assess the number of alleles of a gene
(c) Determine whether two species or varieties will breed successfully
(d) Determine the genotype of a plant at $F_2$

**19.** Which one of the following is a wrong statement regarding mutations? [AIPMT 2012 MAINS]

(a) Cancer cells commonly show chromosomal aberrations.
(b) UV and gamma rays are mutagens.

(c) Change in a single base pair of DNA does not cause mutation.
(d) Deletion and insertion of base pairs cause frame-shift mutations.

**20.** If both parents are carriers for thalassemia, which is an autosomal recessive disorder, what are the chances of pregnancy resulting in the child with diseases? [AIPMT 2013]
(a) No chance (b) 50%
(c) 25% (d) 100%

**21.** The incorrect statement with regard to Haemophilia is: [AIPMT 2013]
(a) It is a sex-linked disease
(b) It is a recessive disease
(c) It is a dominant disease
(d) A single protein involved in the clotting of blood is affected

**22.** Which Mendelian idea is depicted by a cross in which the $F_1$ generation resembles both parents? [AIPMT 2013]
(a) Incomplete dominance
(b) Law of dominance
(c) Inheritance of one gene
(d) Co-dominance

**23.** If two persons with 'AB' blood group marry and have sufficiently large number of children, these children could be classified as 'A' blood group: 'AB' blood group: 'B' blood group in 1:2:1 ratio. Modern technique of protein electrophoresis reveals presence of both 'A' and 'B' type proteins in 'AB' blood group individuals. This is an example of: [AIPMT 2013]
(a) Codominance
(b) Incomplete dominance
(c) Partial dominance
(d) Complete dominance

**24.** Which of the following statements is not true of two genes that shows 50% recombination frequency? [AIPMT 2013]
(a) The genes may be on different chromosomes
(b) The genes are tightly linked
(c) The genes show independent assortment
(d) If the genes are present on the same chromosome, they undergo more than one crossover in every meiosis

**25.** A human female with Turner's syndrome: [AIPMT 2014]
(a) Has 45 chromosomes with XO
(b) Has one additional X chromosome
(c) Exhibits male characters
(d) Is able to produce children with normal husband

**26.** A man whose father was colour-blind marries a woman who had a colour-blind mother and normal father. What percentage of male children of this couple will be colour blind? [AIPMT 2014]
(a) 25% (b) 0%
(c) 50% (d) 75%

**27.** Fruit colour in squash is an example of: [AIPMT 2014]
(a) Recessive epistasis
(b) Dominant epistasis
(c) Complementary genes
(d) Inhibitory genes

**28.** A colour-blind man marries a woman with normal sight who has no history of colour-blindness in her family. What is the probability of their grandson being colour-blind? [RE-AIPMT 2015]
(a) 1 (b) Nil
(c) 0.25 (d) 0.5

**29.** A gene showing codominance has: [RE-AIPMT 2015]
(a) Alleles tightly linked on the same chromosome
(b) Alleles that are recessive to each other
(c) Both alleles independently expressed in the heterozygote
(d) One allele dominant on the other

**30.** A pleiotropic gene: [RE-AIPMT 2015]
(a) Is a gene evolved during pliocene
(b) Controls a trait only in combination with another gene
(c) Controls multiple traits in an individual
(d) Is expressed only in primitive plants

**31.** In his classic experiments on pea plants, Mendel did not use. [RE-AIPMT 2015]
(a) Pod length (b) Seed shape
(c) Flower position (d) Seed colour

**32.** In the following human pedigree, the filled symbols represent the affected individual. Identify the type of given pedigree.

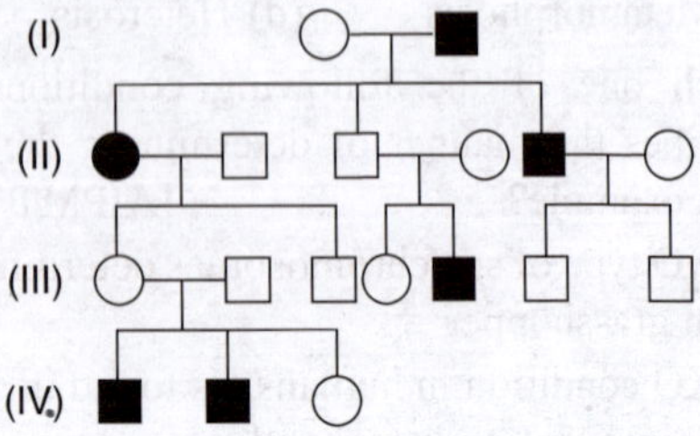


[RE-AIPMT 2015]

(a) X-linked recessive
(b) Autosomal recessive
(c) X-linked dominant
(d) Autosomal dominant

**33.** The term 'linkage' was coined by: [RE-AIPMT 2015]
(a) T. Boveri (b) G. Mendel
(c) W. Sutton (d) T.H. Morgan

**34.** A man with blood group 'A' marries a woman with blood group 'B'. which are all the possible blood groups of their offsprings? [AIPMT 2015]
(a) A and B only
(b) A, B and AB only
(c) A, B, AB and O
(d) O only

**35.** Alleles are: [AIPMT 2015]
(a) Different phenotype
(b) True breeding homozygotes
(c) Different molecular forms of a gene
(d) Heterozygotes

**36.** An abnormal human baby with 'XXX' sex chromosomes was born due to: [AIPMT 2015]
(a) Formation of abnormal sperms in the father
(b) Formation of abnormal ova in the mother
(c) Fusion of two ova and one sperm
(d) Fusion of two sperms and one ovum

**37.** Multiple alleles are present: [AIPMT 2015]
(a) On different chromosomes
(b) At different location of the same chromosome
(c) At the same locus of the chromosome
(d) On non sister chromatids

**38.** The movement of a gene from one linkage group to another is called: [AIPMT 2015]
(a) Inversion (b) Duplication
(c) Translocation (d) Crossing over

**39.** How many pairs by contrasting characters in pea plants was studied by Mendel in his experiments? [AIPMT 2015]
(a) Five (b) Six (c) Eight (d) Seven

**40.** If a colour-blind man marries a woman who is homozygous for normal colour vision, the probability of their son being colour-blind is [NEET 2016 – PHASE II]
(a) 0.5 (b) 0.75 (c) 1 (d) 0

**41.** A true breeding plant is [NEET 2016 – PHASE II]
(a) Produced due to cross-pollination among unrelated plants
(b) Near homozygous and produces offspring of its own kind
(c) Always homozygous recessive in this genetic constitution
(d) One that is able to breed on its own

**42.** The mechanism that causes a gene to move from one linkage group to another is called. [NEET 2016 – PHASE II]
(a) Duplication (b) Translocation
(c) Crossing over (d) Inversion

**43.** A cell at telophase stage is observed by a student in a plant brought from the field. He tells his teacher that this cell is not like other cells at telophase stage. There is no formation of cell plate and thus the cell contains more number of chromosomes as compared to other, dividing cells. This would result in: [NEET 2016 – PHASE I]
(a) Aneuploidy (b) Polyploidy
(c) Somaclonal variation (d) Polyteny

**44.** In a test cross involving $F_1$ dihybrid flies, more parental-type offspring were produced the recombinant-type offspring. This indicates: [NEET 2016 – PHASE I]
(a) Two genes are located on two different chromosomes
(b) Chromosomes failed to separate during meiosis
(c) The two genes are linked and present on the same chromosome
(d) Both the characters are controlled by more than one gene

**45.** Pick out the correct statements:
(A) Haemophilia is a sex-linked recessive disease.
(B) Down's syndrome is due to aneuploiday.
(C) Phenylketonuria is an autosomal recessive gene disorder.
(D) Sickle cell anaemia is an X-linked recessive gene disorder. [NEET 2016 – PHASE I]
(a) A and D are correct
(b) B and D are correct
(c) A, C and D are correct
(d) A, B and C are correct

**46.** Match the terms in Column-I with their description in Column-II and choose the correct option: [NEET 2016 – PHASE I]

| Column – I | Column – II |
|---|---|
| A. Dominance | 1. Many genes govern a single character |
| B. Codominance | 2. In a heterozygous organism, only one allele expresses itself. |
| C. Pleiotropy | 3. In heterozygous organisms, both alleles express themselves fully. |
| D. Polygenic inheritance | 4. A single gene influences many characters. |

(a) A:2, B:1, C:4, D:3 (b) A:2, B:3, C:4, D:1
(c) A:4, B:1, C:2, D:3 (d) A:4, B:3, C:1, D:2

**47.** A tall true breeding garden pea plant is crossed with a dwarf true breeding garden pea plant. When the $F_1$ plants were selfed, the resulting genotypes were in the ratio of: [NEET 2016 – PHASE I]

(a) 1:2:1: Tall homozygous: Tall heterozygous : Dwarf
(b) 1:2:1: Tall heterozygous: Tall homozygous: Dwarf
(c) 3 : 1 :: Tall Dwarf
(d) 3 : 1 : : Dwarf : Tall

**48.** Which of the following most appropriately describes haemophilia? [NEET 2016 – PHASE I]

(a) Recessive gene disorder
(b) X–linked recessive gene disorder
(c) Chromosomal disorder
(d) Dominant gene disorder

**49.** Select the wrong statement : [NEET Regional 2017]

(a) Chromosomal Theory of Inheritance was proposed by Sutton
(b) Law of Dominance and Law of Independent Assortment were proposed by Mendel
(c) Linkage and recombination were discovered by Sutton
(d) Three scientists independently rediscovered Mendel's laws in 1900

**50.** The recessive genes located on X-chromosome in humans are always: [NEET Regional 2017]

(a) sub-lethal
(b) expressed in females
(c) expressed in males
(d) lethal

**51.** Which one of the following is not true for experiments of Mendel on pea? [NEET Regional 2017]

(a) His experiments had large sampling size
(b) He chose characters of two contrasting states
(c) He used true breeding lines
(d) His observations were based on natural, open pollination

**52.** Select the correct option: [NEET Regional 2017]

(a) Klinefelter's syndrome is due to extra X chromosome and results in sterile male.
(b) Phenylketonuria is a X-linked disease and results in accumulation of phenylpyruvic acid.
(c) Down's syndrome is due to triploidy and results in mental retardation.
(d) Turner's syndrome is due to trisomy and results in sterile female.

**53.** Thalassemia and sickle cell anaemia are caused due to a problem in globin molecule synthesis. Select the correct statement [NEET 2017]

(a) Both are due to quantitative defect in globin chain synthesis.
(b) Thalassemia is due to less synthesis of globin molecules.
(c) Sickle cell anaemia is due to quantitative problem of globin molecules.
(d) Both are due to qualitative defect in globin chain synthesis.

**54.** The genotypes of a husband and wife are $I^AI^B$ and $I^Ai$. Among the blood types of their children, how many different genotypes and phenotypes are possible? [NEET 2017]

(a) 3 genotypes; 4 phenotype
(b) 4 genotypes; 3 phenotypes
(c) 4 genotype; 4 phenotypes
(d) 3 genotypes; 3 phenotypes

**55.** Which of the following is the period for Mendel's hybridization experiments? [NEET 2017]

(a) 1840–1850 (b) 1857–1869
(c) 1870–1877 (d) 1856–1863

**56.** Among the following characters, which one was not considered by Mendel in his experiments on pea? [NEET 2017]

(a) Trichomes - Glandular or non-glandular
(b) Seed - Green or Yellow
(c) Pod - Inflated or Constricted
(d) Stem - Tall or Dwarf

**57.** A disease caused by an autosomal primary non-disjunction is: [NEET 2017]

(a) Klinefelter's Syndrome
(b) Turner's Syndrome
(c) Sickle Cell Anaemia
(d) Down's Syndrome

**58.** Select the correct statement [NEET 2018]
(a) Franklin Stahl coined the term 'linkage'
(b) Spliceosomes take part in translation
(c) Punnett square was developed by a British scientist
(d) Transduction was discovered by S. Altman

**59.** Which of the following pairs is wrongly matched? [NEET 2018]
(a) Starch synthesis in pea : Multiple alleles
(b) XO types sex determination : Grasshopper
(c) ABO blood grouping : Co-dominance
(d) T.H. Morgan : Linkage

**60.** Which of the following characteristics represent 'Inheritance of blood groups' in humans?
a. Dominance
b. Co-dominance
c. Multiple allele
d. Incomplete dominance
e. Polygenic inheritance [NEET 2018]

(a) b, c and e (b) b, d and e
(c) a, b and c (d) a, c and e

**61.** A woman has an X-linked condition on one of her X chromosomes. This chromosome can be inherited by [NEET 2018]
(a) Only daughters
(b) Only grandchildren
(c) Only sons
(d) Both sons and daughters

**62.** Select the correct match: [NEET 2018]
(a) Ribozyme - Nucleic acid
(b) T.H. Morgan - Transduction
(c) F2 × Recessive parent - Dihybrid cross
(d) G. Mendel - Transformation

**63.** The frequency of recombination between gene pairs on the same chromosome as a measure of the distance between genes was explained by: [NEET 2019]
(a) Gregor J. Mendel (b) Alfred Sturtevant
(c) Sutton Boveri (d) T. H. Morgan

**64.** In *Antirrhinum* (Snapdragon), a red flower was crossed with a white flower and in $F_1$ generation, pink flowers were obtained. When pink flowers were selfed, the $F_2$ generation showed white, red and pink flowers. Choose the **incorrect** statement from the following. [NEET 2019]
(a) Pink colour in $F_1$ is due to incomplete dominance
(b) Ratio of $F_2$ is $\frac{1}{4}$ (Red) : $\frac{2}{4}$ (Pink) : $\frac{1}{4}$ (White)
(c) Law of segregation does not apply in this experiment
(d) This experiment does not follow the Principle of Dominance

**65.** What is the genetic disorder in which an individual has an overall masculine development, gynaecomastia, and is sterile? [NEET 2019]
(a) Klinefelter's syndrome
(b) Edward syndrome
(c) Down's syndrome
(d) Turner's syndrome

**66.** Select the **incorrect** statement. [NEET 2019]
(a) In male grasshopper, 50% of sperms have no sex chromosome.
(b) In domesticated fowls, sex of progeny depends on the type of sperm rather than egg
(c) Human males have one of their sex chromosome much shorter than the other
(d) Male fruit fly is heterogametic

**67.** What map unit (Centimorgan) is adopted in the construction of genetic maps? [NEET 2019]
(a) A unit of distance between two expressed genes, representing 100% cross over
(b) A unit of distance between genes on chromosome, representing 1% cross over
(c) A unit of distance between genes on chromosome, representing 50% cross over
(d) A unit of distance between two expressed genes, representing 10% cross over

**68.** How many true breeding pea plant varieties did Mendel select as pairs, which were similar except in one character with contrasting traits? [NEET 2020]
(a) 4 (b) 2
(c) 14 (d) 8

**69.** Select the **correct** match : [NEET 2020]

| | | |
|---|---|---|
| (a) Haemophilia | – | Y linked |
| (b) Phenylketonuria | – | Autosomal dominant trait |
| (c) Sickle cell anaemia | – | Autosomal recessive trait, chromosome - II |
| (d) Thalassemia | – | X linked |

**70.** Identify the **wrong** statements with reference to the gene 'I' that controls ABO blood groups. [NEET 2020]
(a) The gene (I) has three alleles.
(b) A person will have only two of the three alleles.
(c) When $I^A$ and $I^B$ are present together, they express same type of sugar.
(d) Allele 'i' does not produce any sugar.

**71.** Experimental verification of the chromosomal theory of inheritance was done by: [NEET 2020]
(a) Mendel (b) Sutton
(c) Boveri (d) Morgan

**72.** The production of gametes by the parents formation of zygotes, the $F_1$ and $F_2$ plants, can be understood from a diagram called [NEET 2021]
(a) Net square (b) Bullet square
(c) Punch square (d) Punnett square

**73.** In a cross between a male and female, both heterozygous for sickle cell anaemia gene, what percentage of the progeny will be diseased? [NEET 2021]
(a) 100% (b) 50%
(c) 75% (d) 25%

**74.** Given below are two statements: [NEET 2022]

**Statement I:** Mendel studied seven pairs of contrasting traits in pea plants and proposed the Laws of Inheritance.

**Statement II:** Seven characters examined by Mendel in his experiment on pea plants were seed shape and colour, flower colour, pod shape and colour, flower position and stem height.

In the light of the above statements, choose the **correct** answer from the options given below:
(a) Both **Statement I** and **Statement II** are incorrect.
(b) **Statement I** is correct but **Statement II** is incorrect.
(c) **Statement I** is incorrect but **Statement II** is correct.
(d) Both **Statement I** and **Statement II** are correct.

**75.** XO type of sex determination can be found in: [NEET 2022]
(a) Birds (b) Grasshoppers
(c) Monkeys (d) *Drosophila*

**76.** Given below are two statements: one is labelled as **Assertion (A)** and the other is labelled as **Reason (R)**.

**Assertion (A):** Mendel's law of Independent assortment does not hold good for the genes that are located closely on the same chromosome. [NEET 2022]

**Reason (R):** Closely located genes assort independently.

In the light of the above statements, choose the **correct answer** from the options given below:
(a) Both **(A)** and **(R)** are correct but **(R)** is not the correct explanation of **(A)**.
(b) **(A)** is correct but **(R)** is not correct.
(c) **(A)** is not correct but **(R)** is correct.
(d) Both **(A)** and **(R)** are correct and **(R)** is the correct explanation of **(A)**.

**77.** Which of the following occurs due to the presence of autosome linked dominant trait? [NEET 2022]
(a) Myotonic dystrophy
(b) Haemophilia
(c) Thalessemia
(d) Sickle cell anaemia

**78.** The recombination frequency between the genes a & c is 5%, b & c is 15%, b & d is 9%, a & b is 20%, c & d is 24% and a & d is 29%. What will be the sequence of these genes on a linear chromosome? [NEET 2022]
(a) d, b, a, c (b) a, b, c, d
(c) a, c, b, d (d) a, d, b, c

**79.** If a colour blind female marries a man whose mother was also colour blind, what are the chances of her progeny having colour blindness? [NEET 2022]
(a) 50% (b) 75%
(c) 100% (d) 25%

**80.** Frequency of recombination between gene pairs on same chromosome as a measure of the distance between genes to map their position on chromosome was used for the first time by: [NEET 2023]
(a) Sutton and Boveri (b) Alfred Sturtevant
(c) Henking (d) Thomas Hunt Morgan

**81.** The phenomenon of Pleiotropism refers to: [NEET 2023]
(a) Presence of two alleles, each of the two genes controlling a single trait.
(b) A single gene affecting multiple phenotypic expression.
(c) More than two genes affecting single character.
(d) Presence of several alleles of a single gene controlling a single crossover.

**82.** Which of the following statements are correct about Klinefelter's Syndrome? [NEET 2023]
A. This disorder was first described by Langdon Down (1866).
B. Such an individual has overall masculine development. However, the feminine development is also expressed.
C. The affected individual is short statured.

D. Physical, psychomotor and mental development is retarded.
E. Such individuals are sterile.

(a) C and D only (b) B and E only
(c) A and E only (d) A and B only

**83.** Broad palm with single palm crease is visible in a person suffering from- [NEET 2023]

(a) Turner's syndrome (b) Klinefelter's syndrome
(c) Thalassemia (d) Down's syndrome

**84.** Which one of the following symbols represents mating between relatives in humans pedigree analysis? [NEET 2023]

(a) 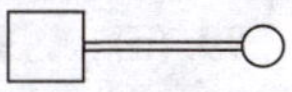

(b) 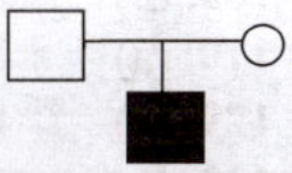

(c) 

(d) 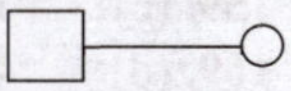

**85.** A pink-flowered Snapdragon plant was crossed with a red-flowered Snapdragon plant. What type of phenotype/s is /are expected in the progeny? [NEET 2024]

(a) Only red-flowered plants
(b) Red flowered as well as pink-flowered plants
(c) Only pink flowered plants
(d) Red, Pink as well as white-flowered plants

**86.** Match List-I with List-II. [NEET 2024]

| List-I | List-II |
|---|---|
| (A) Two or more alternative forms of a gene | (i) Back cross |
| (B) Cross of $F_1$ progeny with homozygous recessive parent | (ii) Ploidy |
| (C) Cross of $F_1$ progeny with any of the parents | (iii) Allele |
| (D) Number of chromosome sets in plant | (iv) Test cross |

Choose the correct answer from the options given below:

(a) (A)-(i), (B)-(ii), (C)-(iii), (D)-(iv)
(b) (A)-(ii), (B)-(i), (C)-(iii), (D)-(iv)
(c) (A)-(iii), (B)-(iv), (C)-(i), (D)-(ii)
(d) (A)-(iv), (B)-(iii), (C)-(ii), (D)-(i)

**87.** In a plant, black seed color (BB/Bb) is dominant over white seed color (bb) In order to find out the genotype of the black seed plant, with which of the following genotype will you cross it? [NEET 2024]

(a) BB (b) bb
(c) Bb (d) BB/Bb

**88.** Which one of the following can be explained on the basis of Mendel's Law of Dominance? [NEET 2024]

A Out of one pair of factors one is dominant and the other is recessive.
B Alleles do not show any expression and both the characters appear as such in $F_2$ generation
C Factors occurs in pairs in normal diploid plants.
D The discrete unit controlling a particular character is called factor.
E The expression of only one of the parental characters is found in a monohybrid cross.

Choose the correct answer from the options given below:

(a) A, B and C only (b) A, C, D and E only
(c) B, C and D only (d) A, B, C, D and E

**89.** Match List-I with List-II: [NEET 2024]

| List-I | List-II |
|---|---|
| (A) Down's syndrome | (i) $11^{th}$ chromosome |
| (B) $\alpha$- Thalassemia | (ii) 'X' chromosome |
| (C) $\beta$-Thalassemia | (iii) $21^{st}$ chromosome |
| (D) Klinefelter's syndrome | (iv) $16^{th}$ chromosome |

Choose the correct answer from the options given below:

(a) (A)-(i), (B)-(ii), (C)-(iii), (D)-(iv)
(b) (A)-(ii), (B)-(iii), (C)-(iv), (D)-(i)
(c) (A)-(iii), (B)-(iv), (C)-(i), (D)-(ii)
(d) (A)-(iv), (B)-(i), (C)-(ii), (D)-(iii)

**90.** As per ABO blood grouping system, the blood group of father is $B^+$, mother is $A^+$ and child is $O^+$. Their respective genotype can be [NEET 2024]

A. $I^Bi$ / $I^Ai$/ii B. $I^BI^B$ / $I^AI^A$ / ii
C. $I^AI^B$ / $iI^A$ / $I^Bi$ D. $I^Ai$ / $I^Bi$ / $I^Ai$
E. $iI^B$ / $iI^A$ / $I^AI^B$

Choose the most appropriate answer from the options given below:

(a) A only (b) B only
(c) C and B only (d) D and E only

## Answer Key

### Multiple Choice Questions: Level I

| | | | | | | | | | |
|---|---|---|---|---|---|---|---|---|---|
| 1. (c) | 2. (d) | 3. (a) | 4. (c) | 5. (a) | 6. (d) | 7. (c) | 8. (a) | 9. (b) | 10. (b) |
| 11. (c) | 12. (c) | 13. (b) | 14. (a) | 15. (a) | 16. (a) | 17. (d) | 18. (a) | 19. (a) | 20. (d) |
| 21. (d) | 22. (b) | 23. (b) | 24. (a) | 25. (d) | 26. (d) | 27. (c) | 28. (c) | 29. (b) | 30. (d) |
| 31. (b) | 32. (b) | 33. (b) | 34. (a) | 35. (b) | 36. (b) | 37. (c) | 38. (a) | 39. (b) | 40. (c) |
| 41. (b) | 42. (c) | 43. (b) | 44. (d) | 45. (d) | 46. (a) | 47. (a) | 48. (b) | 49. (a) | 50. (d) |
| 51. (b) | 52. (d) | 53. (a) | 54. (d) | 55. (d) | 56. (a) | 57. (b) | 58. (a) | 59. (c) | 60. (a) |
| 61. (d) | 62. (d) | 63. (c) | 64. (d) | 65. (d) | 66. (d) | 67. (d) | 68. (b) | 69. (b) | 70. (b) |
| 71. (c) | 72. (d) | 73. (b) | 74. (d) | 75. (b) | 76. (d) | 77. (d) | 78. (c) | 79. (b) | 80. (c) |
| 81. (a) | 82. (c) | 83. (b) | 84. (a) | 85. (c) | 86. (c) | 87. (c) | 88. (c) | 89. (b) | 90. (d) |
| 91. (b) | 92. (c) | 93. (d) | 94. (b) | 95. (d) | 96. (c) | 97. (d) | 98. (d) | 99. (a) | 100. (b) |
| 101. (b) | 102. (a) | 103. (c) | 104. (d) | 105. (b) | 106. (d) | 107. (a) | 108. (d) | 109. (c) | 110. (c) |
| 111. (c) | 112. (a) | 113. (c) | 114. (c) | 115. (d) | 116. (b) | 117. (a) | 118. (c) | 119. (a) | 120. (c) |
| 121. (c) | 122. (d) | 123. (c) | 124. (c) | 125. (b) | 126. (a) | 127. (b) | 128. (c) | 129. (c) | 130. (c) |
| 131. (a) | 132. (b) | 133. (b) | 134. (c) | 135. (a) | 136. (c) | 137. (c) | 138. (a) | 139. (b) | 140. (a) |
| 141. (a) | 142. (a) | 143. (a) | 144. (b) | 145. (a) | 146. (c) | 147. (c) | 148. (b) | 149. (c) | 150. (a) |
| 151. (c) | 152. (c) | 153. (d) | 154. (c) | 155. (d) | 156. (c) | 157. (d) | 158. (c) | 159. (c) | 160. (a) |
| 161. (b) | 162. (d) | 163. (d) | 164. (a) | 165. (b) | 166. (c) | 167. (d) | 168. (b) | 169. (d) | 170. (a) |
| 171. (b) | 172. (b) | 173. (b) | 174. (d) | 175. (c) | 176. (d) | 177. (b) | 178. (b) | 179. (b) | 180. (c) |
| 181. (b) | 182. (a) | 183. (d) | 184. (d) | 185. (a) | 186. (b) | 187. (d) | 188. (d) | 189. (d) | 190. (a) |
| 191. (c) | 192. (a) | 193. (b) | 194. (b) | 195. (d) | | | | | |

### Multiple Choice Questions: Level II

| | | | | | | | | | |
|---|---|---|---|---|---|---|---|---|---|
| 196. (c) | 197. (b) | 198. (c) | 199. (c) | 200. (d) | 201. (b) | 202. (d) | 203. (c) | 204. (b) | 205. (c) |
| 206. (c) | 207. (c) | 208. (c) | 209. (a) | 210. (a) | 211. (b) | 212. (c) | 213. (a) | 214. (c) | 215. (c) |
| 216. (d) | 217. (b) | 218. (a) | 219. (b) | 220. (c) | 221. (c) | 222. (a) | 223. (b) | 224. (b) | 225. (a) |
| 226. (c) | 227. (d) | 228. (b) | 229. (d) | 230. (d) | 231. (b) | 232. (a) | 233. (b) | 234. (c) | 235. (c) |
| 236. (a) | 237. (b) | 238. (a) | 239. (b) | 240. (b) | 241. (c) | 242. (a) | 243. (c) | 244. (b) | 245. (a) |
| 246. (a) | 247. (a) | 248. (b) | 249. (c) | 250. (a) | 251. (c) | 252. (a) | 253. (a) | 254. (b) | 255. (d) |
| 256. (b) | 257. (b) | 258. (b) | 259. (a) | 260. (a) | 261. (b) | 262. (a) | 263. (a) | 264. (d) | 265. (c) |
| 266. (a) | 267. (b) | 268. (a) | 269. (c) | 270. (b) | 271. (d) | 272. (c) | 273. (d) | 274. (d) | 275. (d) |
| 276. (c) | 277. (a) | 278. (d) | 279. (b) | 280. (d) | 281. (c) | 282. (d) | 283. (c) | 284. (d) | 285. (b) |
| 286. (a) | 287. (a) | 288. (d) | 289. (a) | 290. (b) | 291. (b) | 292. (a) | 293. (c) | 294. (b) | 295. (d) |
| 296. (b) | 297. (b) | 298. (c) | 299. (a) | 300. (a) | 301. (d) | 302. (d) | | | |

### A & R and Statement-based Questions

| | | | | | | | | | |
|---|---|---|---|---|---|---|---|---|---|
| 303. (c) | 304. (c) | 305. (c) | 306. (d) | 307. (a) | 308. (c) | 309. (a) | 310. (a) | 311. (b) | 312. (c) |

### Matrix-Match Type Questions

| | | | | |
|---|---|---|---|---|
| 313. (a) | 314. (a) | 315. (a) | 316. (a) | 317. (a) |

### NCERT Exemplar Questions

| | | | | | | | | | |
|---|---|---|---|---|---|---|---|---|---|
| 1. (b) | 2. (a) | 3. (a) | 4. (d) | 5. (d) | 6. (b) | 7. (d) | 8. (b) | 9. (d) | 10. (c) |
| 11. (a) | 12. (c) | 13. (a) | 14. (b) | 15. (b) | 16. (d) | 17. (d) | 18. (c) | | |

## Previous Years' Questions

| | | | | | | | | | |
|---|---|---|---|---|---|---|---|---|---|
| **1.** (a) | **2.** (d) | **3.** (c) | **4.** (a) | **5.** (c) | **6.** (d) | **7.** (c) | **8.** (c) | **9.** (c) | **10.** (a) |
| **11.** (a) | **12.** (c) | **13.** (d) | **14.** (a) | **15.** (d) | **16.** (b) | **17.** (b) | **18.** (d) | **19.** (c) | **20.** (c) |
| **21.** (c) | **22.** (d) | **23.** (a) | **24.** (b) | **25.** (a) | **26.** (c) | **27.** (b) | **28.** (b, c) | **29.** (c) | **30.** (c) |
| **31.** (a) | **32.** (b) | **33.** (d) | **34.** (c) | **35.** (c) | **36.** (b) | **37.** (c) | **38.** (c) | **39.** (d) | **40.** (d) |
| **41.** (b) | **42.** (b) | **43.** (b) | **44.** (c) | **45.** (d) | **46.** (b) | **47.** (a) | **48.** (b) | **49.** (c) | **50.** (c) |
| **51.** (d) | **52.** (a) | **53.** (b) | **54.** (b) | **55.** (d) | **56.** (a) | **57.** (d) | **58.** (c) | **59.** (a) | **60.** (c) |
| **61.** (d) | **62.** (a) | **63.** (b) | **64.** (c) | **65.** (a) | **66.** (b) | **67.** (b) | **68.** (c) | **69.** (c) | **70.** (c) |
| **71.** (d) | **72.** (d) | **73.** (d) | **74.** (d) | **75.** (b) | **76.** (b) | **77.** (a) | **78.** (c) | **79.** (c) | **80.** (b) |
| **81.** (b) | **82.** (b) | **83.** (d) | **84.** (a) | **85.** (b) | **86.** (c) | **87.** (b) | **88.** (b) | **89.** (c) | **90.** (a) |

# HINTS AND EXPLANATION

## Multiple Choice Questions: Level II

**196.** • Klinefelter's syndrome (XXY) is due to extra X chromosome and results in sterile male. Such males have some feminine features like gynaecomastia (development of breast)

- Down's syndrome: It is due to trisomy of chromosome number 21.
- Turner's syndrome: It is due to monosomy of sex chromosome (44 + XO). Such females have rudimentary ovaries and lack other secondary sexual characters. Such females are sterile.
- Colour-blindness is X-linked disorder.
- Erythroblastosis feotalis occur due to antigen antibody reaction.

**197.** Haploid describes organism with a single set of unpaired chromosomes. The haploid number is designated as X. Haploids are more suitable for mutation studies than diploids. This is because all mutations, whether dominant or recessive, are expressed in haploids because they have only one allele.

**198.** Crossing of one $F_1$ progeny with male parent,

RR × rr
(red) ↓ (green)
Rr Rr Rr Rr $F_1$-progeny
Red Red Red Red
♀ ♂
$F_1$-progeny ← (Rr) × RR
↓
RR Rr Rr RR
↓ ↓ ↓ ↓
red (pure) red (dominant) red (dominant) red (pure)

**199.** When the linked genes are situated quite close, the chances of crossing over are highly reduced. Due to this, large number of parental gametes are formed while only few recombinant gametes are formed. This results in higher number of parental types in $F_2$ generation as compared to recombinants.

**200.** Let GG ⇒ homozygous yellow-seeded plant.

gg ⇒ homozygous green

Gg ⇒heterozygous green

According to the question,

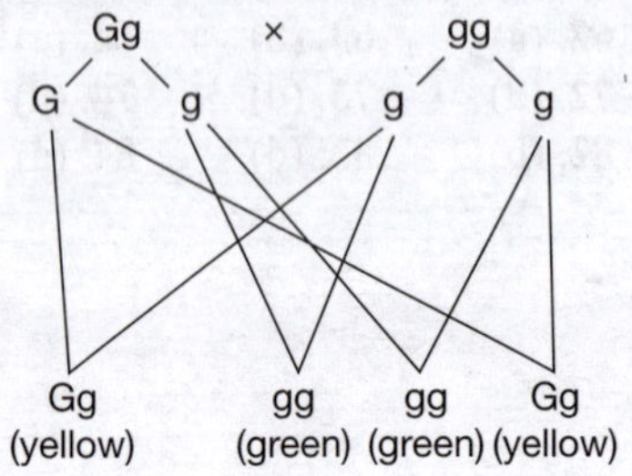


So, the ratio cell be 50 : 50

**201.** Inheritance of skin colour in human is controlled by three genes A, B and C which is polygenic inheritance, other examples are height of human and I.Q. of human.

**202.**

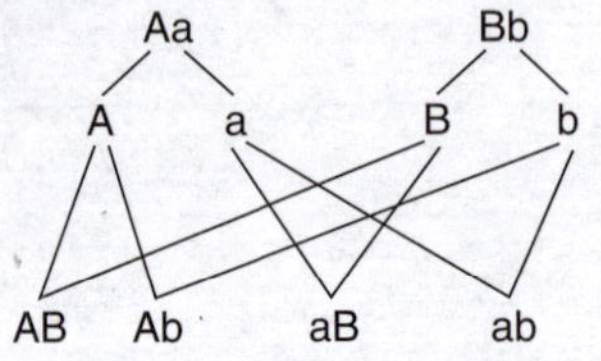


So, the corresponding genotype will be AaBb.

**203.**

P-generation – RRYY (Round seed yellow cotyledon) × rryy (wrinkled seed green cotyledon)
Gametes: (RY) (ry)
↓
F1 generation – RrYy (all heterozygous round seeded and yellow cotyledon)
↓
Selfing

$F_2$ generation →

| ♀ \ ♂ | RY | Ry | rY | ry |
|---|---|---|---|---|
| RY | RRYY Round seed yellow coty. | RRYy Round seed yellow coty. | RrYY Round seed yellow coty. | RrYy Round seed yellow coty. |
| Ry | RRYy Round seed yellow coty. | RRyy Round seed green coty. | RrYy Round seed yellow coty. | Rryy Round seed green coty. |
| rY | RrYY Round seed yellow coty. | RrYy Round seed yellow coty. | rrYY Wrinkled seed yellow coty. | rryy Wrinkled seed yellow coty. |
| ry | RrYy Round seed yellow coty. | Rryy Round seed green coty. | rrYy Wrinkled seed yellow coty. | rryy Wrinkled seed green coty. |

So the ratio of round-seeded with yellow cotyledons: Round-seeded green cotyledons: Wrinkled-seeded yellow cotyledons : Wrinkle-seeded green cotyledons in 9 : 3 : 3 : 1. So, in the $F_2$ generation the round-seeded character remains with yellow cotyledons and wrinkled seeds with yellow cotyledons.

**204.** Test cross is use to find out genotype of tall plants obtained in F2 generation. But it is also cross between F1 hybrid with double recessive genotype.

**205.** Phenotype is the appearance one organism shows while genotype is the gene complement it has from its ancestors. These genes only show their effect in phenotype but environment also plays an important role in this, hence phenotype is a result of genotype and environmental interaction.

**206.** Number of gametes produce = $2^n$, where n is number of heterozygous in given genotype, so here n = 1. It would make only two types of gametes, these are ABc and Abc.

**207.** Colour-blindness in a X-chromosome-linked character. So they'll be having all colour-blind sons and daughters.

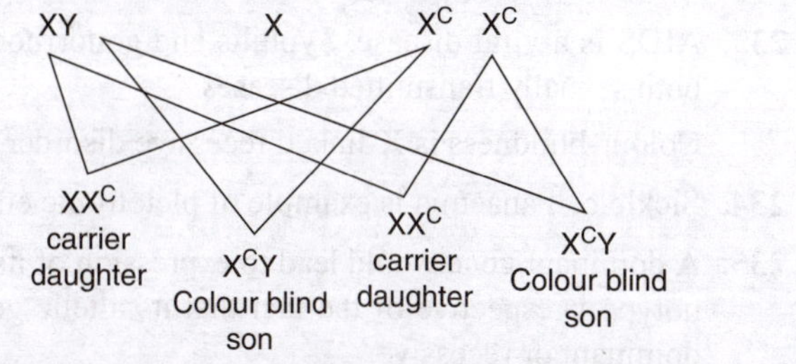


**208.** Skin colour, Height and IQ are example of polygenic inheritance.

**209.** The genes of cytoplasmic characters occur outside the chromosome, in cytoplasm, they inherit their traits like chromosomal genes do. In a zygote formation, the cytoplasm comes from the mother's ova and hence the cytoplasmic characters must come from maternal side and this is the reason why cytoplasmic inheritance is also known as maternal inheritance.

**210.** Sickle cell anaemia is a biochemical disorder in which shape of RBCs become sickle-shaped due to defective haemoglobin. Haemoglobin becomes useless for oxygen transport. Huntington Chorea in a disease in which atrophy of brain occurs resulting in respiratory irregularities, articulation of speech and irregular limbs movements take place. They both are genetic disease present in any person since birth, hence are congenital diseases.

**211.** In sickle cell anaemia, RBCs become sickle-shaped which are not supportive for the growth of malarial parasite Plasmodium, so it provides immunity against malaria.

**212.** In order to find out the gamete or the genotype of an unknown individual, scientists perform a test cross. In test cross, the individual in question is crossed with the homozygous recessive parent. Hence, the answer is aabb.

**213.** Since the woman's father was colour blind. She would be a carrier of the colour-blindness gene. When she marries a colour-blind man. Their progeny could be

| | | | | |
|---|---|---|---|---|
| Parent | $X^CX$ (Carrier woman) | × | $X^CY$ (Colour blind man) | |
| Progeny | $X^CX^C$ | $X^CY$ (Colour blind man) | $XX^C$ (Normal son) | XY |

**214.** Blood group is determined by three alleles: $I^A$, $I^B$, and I. Alleles $I^A$ and $I^B$ are co-dominant. Blood group A is determined by $I^AI^A$ or $I^A$ I. Blood group B is $I^B$ $I^B$ or $I^B$ I. Blood group O is $I^OI^O$. Blood group AB is $I^A$ $I^B$.

**215.** Because it is a X-linked recessive disorder.

**216.** Superfemaleness = XXX (more than 2 'X' chromosomes)

**217.** Mitochondria is an organelle present in the cytoplasm. A zygote receives its cytoplasm from the female parent gamete. Hence, in the given question, $F_2$ progenies do not receive the mitochondrial genome from the male parent and mutation is not passed to progenies.

**218.** A self-fertilizing trihybrid plant forms 8 different gametes and 64 different zygotes. The genotype of trihybrid plant is AaBbCc. Number of gametes formed $= 2^n = 2^3 = 8$
Here n = no. of heterozygosity = 3 in present case.
No. of zygotes formed $= 8^2 = 64$.

**219.** Crossing over occurs between non-sister chromatids of two homologous chromosomes. Homologous chromosomes form bivalent. Crossing over occurs between chromosomes in a nucleus.

**220.** The lack of independent assortment in sweet pea and Drosophila is due to linkage. Linkage is broken down due to crossing over.

**221.** Males have only one X chromosome. Hence, any gene present on the lone X chromosome expresses itself in males. Females have two X chromosomes. The mutant allele must be present on both the X chromosomes to express itself phenotypically. If only one copy of allele is present, then the female only becomes a carrier showing no external manifestation of the gene. Sublethal condition can never arise in males.

**222.** Chance of getting $a = \frac{1}{2}$

Chance of getting $b = \frac{1}{2}$

Chance of getting $h = \frac{1}{2}$

Chance of getting sperms with $abh = \frac{1}{2} \times \frac{1}{2} \times \frac{1}{2} = \frac{1}{8}$

**223.** Normal woman with colour-blind father would be a carrier

Woman ($X^CX$) × Normal man (XY)

| Progeny | $X^CX$ | XX | $X^CY$ | XY |
|---|---|---|---|---|
| | normal but carrier daughter | normal daughter | Colour blind son | normal son |

**224.** Calvin Bridges demonstrated that Drosophila, the sex is determined by ratio of the number of X chromosomes to the sets of autosomes.

**225.** Seven traits were present on 4 chromosomes. But they do not show linkage because of large distances between them on the chromosome.

**226.** Dihybrid cross is made between individual having contrasting tracts in order to study the inheritance of two pairs of alleles. Test cross is a back cross between individual with a dominant trait and its recessive parent to know whether the individual is homozygous or heterozygous for the trait.

**227.** Linkage is the staying together of genes and their en block inheritance from generation to generation. Linked genes do not show independent assortment, since they are present on the same chromosome.

**228.** **Haemophilia-B:** 'Christmas disease' (after the family in which it was first described in detail) results from a defect in Plasma Thromboplastic Component (PTC or Factor IX).

**229.** **(1) Sex-linked traits:** These are the traits which are determined by the genes present on the sex chromosomes. All the sex-linked traits present on a sex chromosome are inherited together.

**(2) Sex-limited traits:** These are traits which are expressed in a particular sex though their genes also occur in the other sex, e.g., milk secretion in mammalian females.

**(3) Sex-influenced traits:** These traits are not due to particular genes but are by-products of sex hormones, e.g., low pitched voice, beard, moustaches and baldness in human.

**230.** 50% of ova will have (n+1) chromosome which would, on fertilization, yield abnormal zygotes (n+1) + (n) = 2n + 1.

**231.**

$F_1$ parent: AABbCC × AABbCC

Gametes: (ABC) (AbC)

| | ABC | AbC |
|---|---|---|
| ABC | AABBCC | AABbCC |
| AbC | AABbCC | AAbbCC |

AABBCC – 1, AABbCC – 2, AAbbCC – 1

Genotypic ratio = 1 : 2 : 1

**232.** a – b = 20%, b – c = 28%, a – c = 8%

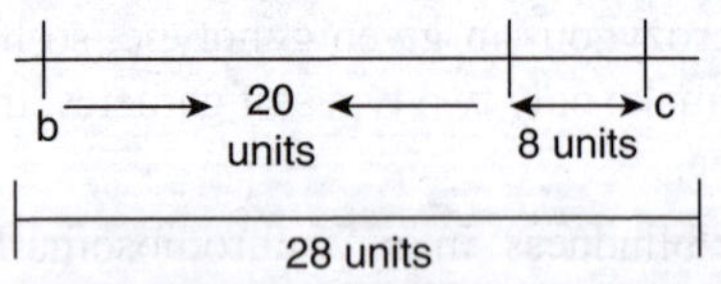


Per cent crossing over between two genes is proportional to the distance between them.

**233.** AIDS is a viral disease. Syphilis and gonorrhoea are both sexually transmitted diseases.

Colour-blindness is X-linked recessive disorder.

**234.** Sickle cell anaemia is example of pleiotropic effect.

**235.** A dominant gene would lead to expression of its phenotype irrespective of the fact that its allelic gene is dominant or recessive.

**236.** Sex-linked disorders follow criss-cross inheritance pattern that affected father passes on to their daughters. The daughters receive one of their X-chromosomes from their fathers.

**237.** Independent assortment of genes takes place only when they are located on separate non-homologous chromosomes. Where two or more than two genes are located on same chromosome, independent assortment will not be possible.

**238.** According to principle of dominance, out of the two factors of alleles representing different traits of a character, only one expresses itself. But when both express themselves, it is co-dominance

**239.** The most suitable culture medium for Drosophila melanogaster is ripe banana.

**240.** In eukaryotic cells, two cytoplasmic organelles, mitochondria and chloroplast of green plants, contain their own genetic materials

**241.** Humans have 22 pairs of autosome and 1 pair of sex chromosomes which are XX in females and XY in males. So, every time the chance of son or daughter is 50:50%.

**242.** It is genotypic ratio of Mendelian monohybrid cross (1 : 2 : 1).

**243.**

Parents: XX × XY

offsprings: XX XX (daughters) XY XY (sons)

probability of son $\frac{2}{4} = \frac{1}{2}$

probability of four son $-\left(\frac{1}{2}\right)^4 = \frac{1}{16}$

**244.**

Parents: AB/ab × ab/ab

Gametes: (AB) (ab) × (ab)

F₁:

| | AB | ab |
|---|---|---|
| ab | AaBb | aabb |

**245.** Aneuploidy is numerical change in the chromosome number in the genome. Euploidy is the phenomenon of having multiple or more than twice the number of genome.

**246.** One bar body is present in each somatic cell of female (XX).

**247.**

Parent: RRTt × rrtt

Gametes: (RT), (Rt), (rt)

Offspring: RrTt (tall with red fruit) Rrtt (tall with yellow fruit)

Ratio = 1 : 1

**248.** Dominance – In a heterozygous organism only one allele expresses itself.

Codominance - In a heterozygous organisms both alleles express themselves fully. E.g., Blood group AB, Flower colour in 4 o'clock plant, dog flower.

Pleiotropy – Multiple phenotypic effect of single gene

Polygenic inheritance – Many genes govern a single character. E.g., Skin colour in human, IQ in human

**249.** In human, Y chromosome bears the androgenic factor or the male-determining factor, whereas in Drosophila, the ratio of sex chromosomes to autosomes is the factor determining sex of the individual.

**250.** Haemolytic disease of the new-born occurs when a $Rh^-$ mother conceives a $Rh^+$ child. Mother's blood starts producing antibodies against the foetal red blood cells.

**251.** In haploid organisms every gene irrespective of dominant or recessive and every mutation find expression because there is only one allele for each gene in individual.

**252.**

Parents: Tt × tt

Gametes: (T) (t) × (t)

Progeny:

| | T | t |
|---|---|---|
| t | Tt | tt |

Ratio = 1 : 1

**253.** The mother must have been a haemophilic carrier ($X^hX$). One of the twins would have inherited the normal X chromosome and the other would have received the X chromosome carrying the gene for haemophilia.

**254.** Normal woman whose father was colour-blind would have received X chromosome from her father → $X^CX^-$ marries a colour-blind man – $X^CY$ → their progeny.

$X^CX$ × $X^CY$

Progeny: $X^CX^C$ Colour blind daughter; $X^CX$ normal daughter; $X^CY$ Colour blind son; XY normal son

**255.** Crossing over involves physical exchange of genetic material between non-sister chromatids of homologous chromosomes. This leads to recombination.

**256.** Three types of genome occur in a typical green plant cell nuclear genome, mitochondrial genome and chloroplast.

**257.** If Mendel studied a plant with 12 chromosomes, he would have encountered linked genes, and hence he would not have arrived at principle of independent assortment.

**258.** Four different types of gametes produced will be ABC, AbC, ABc, Abc.

**259.** It occurs due to non-disjunction during formation of egg cells and sperm cells.

**260.** Mental-retardness is usually found when these are more than two X chromosomes: About 1% of all mentally defective women have one or more extra X chromosomes.

**261.**

| $X^{hc}X^{h}$ | × | XY | h → haemophilia |
|---|---|---|---|
| Female | | Male | c → colour blindness |

| $X^{hc}X$ | $X^{hc}Y$ | $X^{h}X$ | $X^{h}Y$ |
|---|---|---|---|
| daughter (carrier) | haemophilic Colourblind son | daughter (carrier) | haemophilic son |

**262.** A child will be albino only if it is homozygous for albinism genes (since albinism is a recessive character). As parents have normal skin, it means they are heterozygous. As a result of cross between two heterozygous parents, 25% of the children will be homozygous recessive. The nature of the second child is not affected in any way by the nature of the first child because both are independent events.

**263.** In sex determination, the male-specific chromosome will have half as much chance as the other to enter the egg cell. Hence, the proportion will be 1 : 1.

**264.** Gregor Mendel traced inheritance patterns of certain traits in pea plants and showed that they could be described mathematically. Although not all features show these patterns of Mendelian inheritance, his work suggested utility of the application of statistics to the study of inheritance

**265.** Autosomes or sex chromosomes determine the sex of the individual. The rest of the chromosomes are known as autosome. Nucleolus is a cell organelle involved in synthesis of ribosomes.

**266.** Multiple alleles are multiple alternatives or alleles of the same gene which occur in the population of same species.

Polygene is a gene, single dominant allele of which expresses only a unit of trait. Polygenes are genes controlling quantitative inheritances.

Oncogenes are the cancer-causing genes.

**267.** Klinefelter's syndrome (XXY) is due to extra X chromosome and results in sterile male. Such males have some feminine features like gynaecomastia (development of breast)

Gynandromorphism occurs among Drosophila. In such individuals, one half of the body shows male character and the other half shows female characters.

**268.** Epistasis is the suppression of the normal phenotypic expression of the gene by a non-allelic gene. Complimentary genes are two independent genes present on different gene loci which assist each other in expressing a trait. Supplementary genes are two independent genes present on different gene loci, each of which may produce its own trait and interact when present together in dominant state to produce a new trait.

**269.** Hermaphrodite or bisexual refers to an organism having both male and female sex organs. Gynandromorphs are individuals who exhibit both male and female characteristics.

**270.** Daughters receive one X chromosome from the father and one X chromosome from the mother. Since all the daughters suffer from their father's disease, the X chromosome from the father must be carrying a dominant trait.

**271.** (Parents) $X_CX_C$ x XY

Offsprings $X^CX$, $X^CX$, $X^CY$ $X^CY$

↓

100%

Sons are colourblind

**272.** Gene Ab shows 20% recombination which means recombinants out of 100 should be 20. Here recombinants are + a and +b. Therefore, answer is + + 40 : ab 40 : + a 10 : + b : 10

**273.** Sickle cell anaemia (in which nucleotide triplet CTC is changed to CAC) affects the $\beta$-globin chain of haemoglobin. Since these changes occur at a locus or point of a chromosome where specific gene is located, they are called point mutation.

**274.** The women is heterozygous as albinic condition is recessive hence when she marries an albinic man, the offsprings are 50% normal and 50% albinic.

**275.** Genotype is the genetic make-up of an organism. The given 4 genotypes are present in 1 : 2 : 2 : 4 ratio.

**276.** The two factors of each trait arrange or assort at random and are independent of each other in their distribution in the gametes and in the progeny.

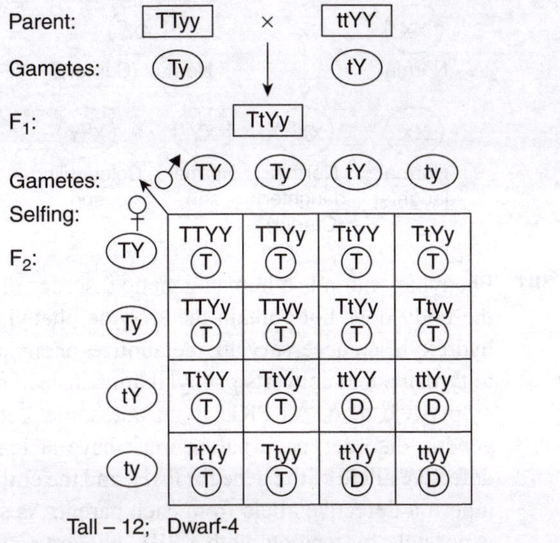


**277.** AB blood group possesses the genotype $I^A$-$I^B$. The alleles $I^A$ and $I^B$ are co-dominant as both express themselves when together in an individual.

**278.** Holandric genes are present on the differential region of Y chromosome. The differential regions carry completely sex-linked genes and they do not undergo crossing over.

**279.** Law of independent assortment is applicable to only those factors or genes which are located on different chromosomes. Probably the characters were present on same chromosome and showed linkage which Mendel might not have studied.

**280.** Chromosome mapping is based on the fact that genes are linearly arranged on the chromosome and frequency of crossing over is directly proportional to the distance between two genes. Dominant genes show cis arrangement. At 50 map units, cis is changed to trans and vice-versa hence no fixed linkage is present.

**281.** Since half the sons are haemophilic the genes for haemophilia is located on X-chromosome of mother

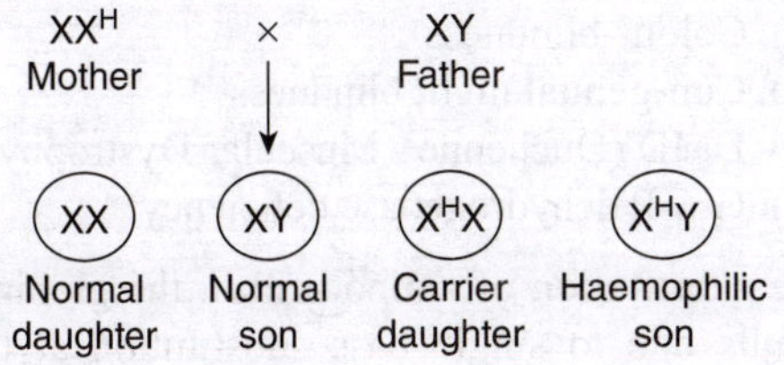


**282.** Parents $I^Ai$ × $I^Bi$
Offsprings $I^AI^B$, $I^Ai$ $I^Bi$, ii
AB A B O

**283.** Genotype of Mr. Kapoor will be Bb hence one-half of the sperms will have Bd.

**284.** On crossing colour-blind woman with a normal man, the sons become colour blind. This is an example of criss-cross inheritance. The genes for colour-blindness are coming from mother's father.

**285.** Down's syndrome is due to trisomy of 21st chromosome and is an autosomal abnormality.

**286.** At anaphase I, actual segregation occurs but two similar alleles occur in the dyad chromosome which separate at Anaphase II.

**287.** Epistasis in the phenomenon of marking or suppressing the phenotypic impression of a gene pair by it non-allelic gene pair which impresses its own effect.

**288.** The genotype of the child would be $I^OI^O$ (recessive). Hence, the genotype of the father can only by $I^BI^O$.

**289.** When a colour-blind woman marries a normal man, the recessive homozygous gene is expressed in sons, whereas the daughters become carriers.

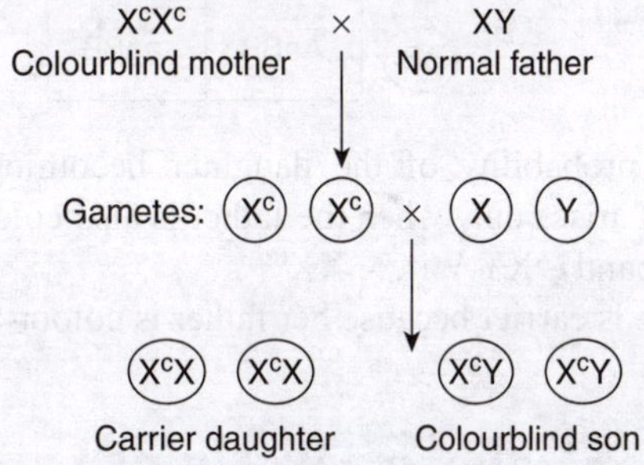


**290.** Plasma genes present in the maternal cytoplasm are transmitted to offspring; hence this type of inheritance is termed as cytoplasmic or maternal inheritance.

**291.** Incomplete dominance is the phenomenon of none of the alleles being dominant with the effect that the hybrid produced by crossing two pure individuals is a mixture between the parents.

**292.** The brown eyed man will have genotype Bb and his wife bb. Hence, Bb x bb= Bb : bb. Hence, ratio is 1 : 1

**293.** According to the Law of Independent Assortment, alleles of different characters located in different pairs of homologous chromosomes are independent of one another in their separation or segregation during gamete formation.

**294.** Gregor Johann Mendel formulated the laws of heredity and is regarded as the father of genetics.

**295.** $I^AI^O$ x $I^AI^B$ gives us the following genotypes $I^AI^A$, $I^OI^B$, $I^AI^B$.

**296.** The genotype of the mother was either $X^C X^C$ or $X^CX$ and that of father $X^CY$ so that the daughter becomes colour-blind.

**297.** On mating tt with Tt, 50% individual offsprings are recessive and 50% inhibit heterozygous dominant characteristics.

**298.** A gene may have more than two alternative forms occupying the same locus on a chromosome such alleles are known as multiple alleles and the phenomenon is turned as multiple allelism. ABO blood group has 3 alleles: la, IA or A, IB or B.

**299.** AaBB x aaBB on crossing gives 50% individuals having genotype AaBB and 50% individuals having genotype aaBB.

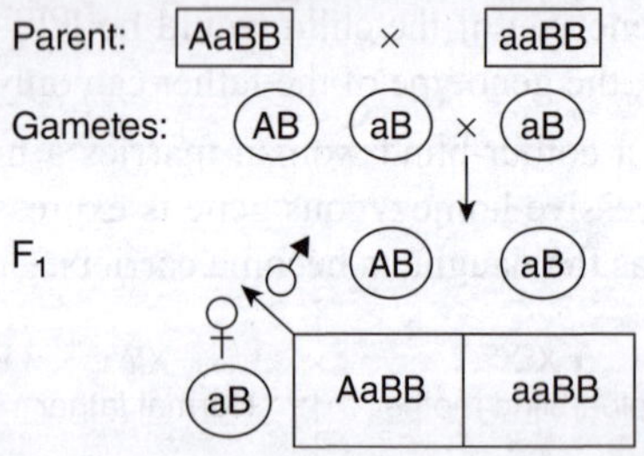


**300.** The probability of the daughter becoming colour-blind arises only when the father is also colour-blind.
Husband – XY Wife – $XX^C$
(wife is carrier because her father is colour-blind)

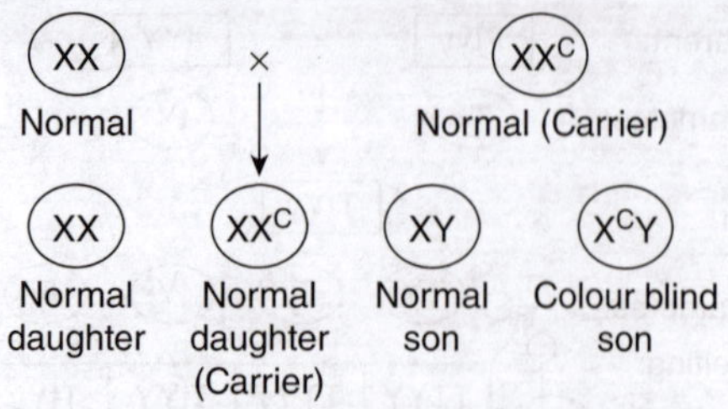


**301.** Phenylketonuria is a human genetic disorder in which the body does not contain the enzyme phenylalanine hydroxylase, necessary to metabolize phenylalanine to tyrosine and converts phenylalanine instead of phenylpyruvic acid. As PKU is an autosomal recessive genetic disorder, each parent must have at least one defective allele of the gene for PAH, and the child must inherit a defective allele from each parent. As such, it is possible for a parent with a PKU phenotype to have a child without PKU if the other parent possesses at least one functional allele of the gene for PAH. A child of two parents with the PKU phenotype will always receive two defective alleles so will always have PKU. The gene for PAH is located on chromosome 12, at location 12q22-q24.

**302.** Haemophilia is a sex-linked recessive trait carried by X chromosome (also known as bleeder's disease).

## NCERT Exemplar Questions

1. **Linkage groups:** A linkage group is a group of linked genes (on the same chromosome) and corresponds to the genome of organism, like human has 23 linkage groups, pea and *Neurospora* has 7 linkage groups, *Drosophila* has 4 linkage groups.
2. Failure of segregation of chromatids during cell division cycle results in gain or loss of a chromosome(s), called aneuploidy. Aneuploidy arises due to non-disjunction of homologous chromosome.
   Aneuploidy is of four types:
   (i) Monosomy = 2n - 1
   (ii) Nullisomy = 2n - 2
   (iii) Trisomy = 2n + 1
   (iv) Tetrasomy = 2n + 2
3. Distance between the genes and percentage of recombination shows direct relationship.
4. *Sex-linked recessive disease:* A genetic disease is transferred from a phenotypically normal but carrier female to only some of the male progeny.
   Examples:
   (i) Haemophilia or Bleeder's disease
   (ii) Colour-blindness
   (iii) Con-genital night blindness
   (iv) DMD (Duchenne's Muscular Dystrophy)
   (v) G-6-P dehydrogenase deficiency
5. The substitution of amino acid in the globin protein results due to single base substitution at the sixth

codon of the betaglobin gene from GAG (Glutamic acid) to GUG (Valine).

**6.**

| Blood group | Genotype | Example |
|---|---|---|
| AB | $I^A I^B$ | Co-dominance |
| A or B | $I^A$ i or $I^B$ i | Dominance |

**7.**

| Type of sex determination | Example |
|---|---|
| ZZ/ZW | Birds (Peacock, etc.) |
| XO type or (XX-XO type) | Insects, grasshopper and cockroach |
| XY type or (XX-XY type) | Human, *Drosophila* and *Melandrium* |

**8.**

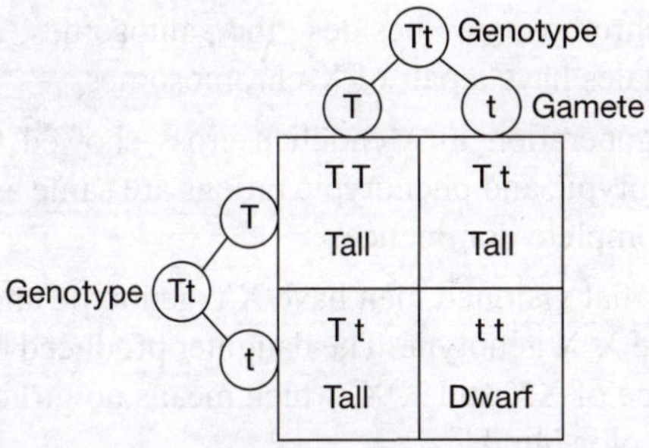


**9.** Based on observations on dihybrid crosses (crosses between plants differing in two traits), Mendel proposed a second set of generalizations that we call Mendel's Law of Independent Assortment. The law states, 'When two pairs of traits are combined in a hybrid, segregation of one pair of characters is independent of the other pair of characters'.

**10.**
- Linkage does not result in variations among siblings.
- A sibling is one or two or more individuals having one or both parents in common. The emotional bond between siblings is often complicated and is influenced by factors such as parental treatment, birth order, personality, and personal experiences outside the family. Identical twins share 100% of their DNA. Full siblings are first-degree relatives and, on average, share 50% of their genes out of those that vary among humans. Half-siblings are second-degree relatives and have, on average, a 25% overlap in their human genetic variation.

**11.** Mendel's Law of independent assortment holds good for genes situated on the homologous chromosomes.

**12.** Occasionally, a single gene may express more than one effect. The phenomenon is called **pleiotropy.**

**13.** The 17 and 18 chromosome-bearing organisms are **males** and **females,** respectively, because it comes under XO-type of sex determination.
Males have only 1 chromosome besides autosomes, whereas females have a pair of X chromosomes besides the autosomes.

**14.** Character studied in the pedigree analysis is equivalent to **Mendelian trait.**

**15.** Mendel proposed that the factor controlling any character is discrete and independent. His proposition was based on the observation that the offspring of a cross made between the plants having two contrasting characters show only one character without any blending.

**16.** Two genes 'A' and 'B' are linked. In a dihybrid cross involving these two genes, $F_1$ heterozygote is crossed with homozygous recessive parental type (aa bb). The ratio of offspring in the next generation will be 1 : 1.

**17.** In the $F_2$ generation of a Mendelian dihybrid cross, the number of phenotypes and genotypes are 4, 9, respectively.

**18.** Genotype of mother – $I^A$ i
Genotype of father – $I^B$ i
Both mother and father are heterozygous for 'A' and 'B' blood group, respectively.

## Previous Years' Questions

**1.** 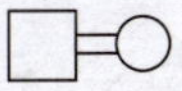 = Mating between relatives

**2.** Recombination is a rearrangement of genes during meiosis so that a gamete contains a haploid genotype with a new gene combination. Morgan and his colleagues found that when genes were grouped on the same chromosome, some genes were very tightly linked (showed very low recombination), while others were loosely linked (showed higher recombination).

**3.** In ABO blood group system, inheritance of grouping is controlled by a single autosomal gene on chromosome 9 with three major alleles A, B and O ($I^A$, $I^B$ and $I^o$). ABO blood group system has at least 6 genotypes.

On the basis of presence or absence of antigens and antibodies, four blood groups (phenotypes) have been differentiated: A, B, AB and O blood groups.

4. In genetics, a test cross, first introduced by Gregor Mendel, is used to determine if an individual exhibiting a dominant trait is homozygous or heterozygous for that trait. More simply, test cross determines the genotype of an individual with a dominant phenotype. In some sources, the test cross is defined as being a type of back cross between the recessive homozygote and $F_1$ generation.

5. Mendel's Law of dominance states that:
   (i) Factors are discrete units and these control the character.
   (ii) Factors remain in pair.
   (iii) In heterozygous condition, one of the factor in a pair is able to express itself. It is termed as dominant factor while the other one is termed as recessive.

6. Reasons for choosing Drosophila melanogaster (tiny Fruitfly) by T.H. Morgan for his experiments:
   (i) These can be easily grown on a simple synthetic medium in laboratory.
   (ii) Short life cycle: two weeks.
   (iii) Large number of progeny can be produced by single mating.
   (iv) Male and female sexes can be easily identified.
   (v) Many contrasting characters are present which can be easily distinguished by using a low power microscope.

7. On the basis of presence or absence of antigens and antibodies, four blood groups (phenotypes) have been differentiated: A, B, AB and O blood groups.

8. When an individual exhibiting a dominant trait is homozygous or heterozygous for that trait. More simply, test cross determines the genotype of an individual with a dominant phenotype. In some sources, the test cross is defined as being a type of back cross between the recessive homozygote and $F_1$ generation.

9.

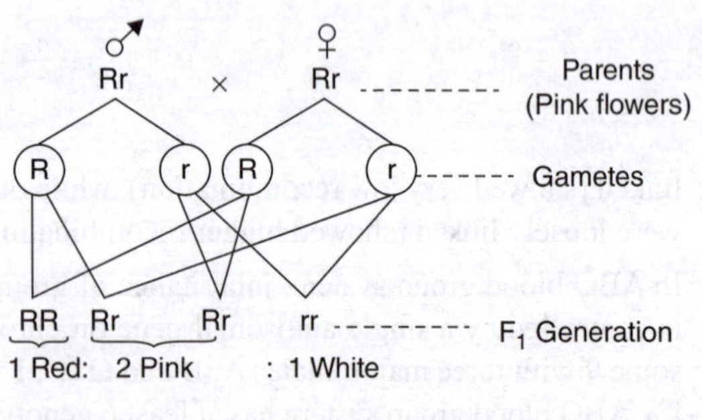


10. The given pedigree chart shows that both the daughters received gene from the parents, while son may be normal or affected. It shows that the female parent is heterozygous.

11. Sex-determining mechanism in case of humans is XY type. Sperms are of two types, one containing X-chromosome and another containing Y-chromosome.

    The ovum is of one type only, i.e., contains X chromosome. Fertilization of ovum with Y-chromosome carrying sperm results into a male offspring.

12. In test cross, genotype of an organism showing dominant phenotype is determined by crossing it with homozygous recessive genotype.

13. The superiority of hybrids over either of the parents (dominant or recessive is called hybrid vigour (G. Shull). Heterosis is equivalent of hybrids vigour.

14. Grasshopper is an example of XO type of sex determination in which the males have only one X-chromosome besides the autosomes, whereas females have a pair of X-chromosomes.

15. $F_2$ generation in Mendelian cross showed that both genotypic and phenotypic rations are same as 1:2:1 in incomplete dominance.

16. Normal visioned man have XY genotype and women have $X^hX$ genotype. The daughter produced have genotype of XX and $X^hX$, which means no girl child will be color-blind.

17. Above case represents criss-cross inheritance and it is shown by X-linked inheritance, e.g. Haemophilia.

18. **Testcross:** It takes place between $F_1$ Generation and recessive parent and it is useful to check the homozygous or heterozygous condition.

19. Change in single base pair of DNA is also a type of mutations called point mutations.

20. Thalassemia is autosomal recessive disease; if both parent are carriers then their genotype will be

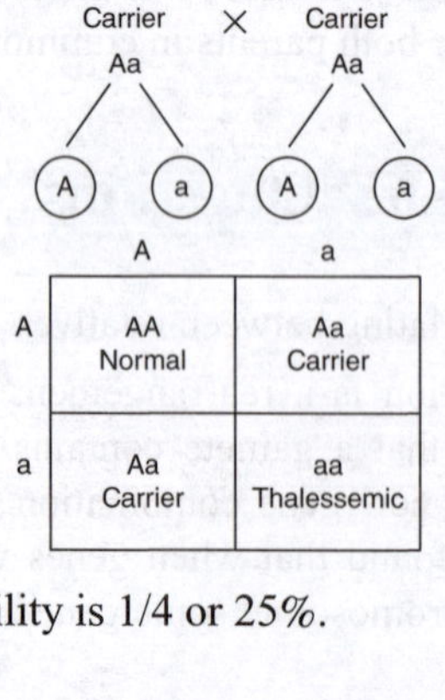


So, probability is 1/4 or 25%.

**21.** Haemophilia is a X-liked recessive disorder. In haemophilia, the blood fails to clot when exposed to air and even a small skin injury results in continuous bleeding which can lead to death from loss of blood. It is also called bleeder's disease, first studied by John Cotto in 1803. The most famous pedigree of haemophilia was discovered by Haldane in the royal families of Europe. The pedigree started from Queen Victoria in the last century. In a patient of haemophilia, blood is deficient due to lack necessary substrate, thromboplastin.
It is of two types:

- **Haemophilia-A:** Characterized by lack of antihaemophilic globulin (Factor VIII). About four-fifths of the cases of haemophilia are of this type.
- **Haemophilia-B:** 'Christmas disease' (after the family in which it was first described in detail) results from a defect in Plasma Thromboplastic Component (PTC or Factor IX).
- **Haemophilia also shows criss-cross inheritance.**

**22.** In codominace, $F_1$ generation resembles both of the parents.

**23.** $I^A$ and $I^B$ present together; they both express their own type of sugar on the surface of RBC is codominance.

**24.** If gene are present on same chromosome and tightly linked, they slow very few recombinant so they show 50% recombinant is wrong statement.

**25.** Turner syndrome is a chromosomal condition that affects the development in females. The most common feature of Turner syndrome is short stature, which become evident by the age of about age 5. An early loss of ovarian function is also very common. The ovaries develop normally at first, but egg cells usually die prematurely and most ovarian tissue degenerates before birth. In other words, the absence of one of the X-chromosome i.e., 45 with XO (or 44 + XO).

**26.** Man with colour-blind; father has Y chromosome from father and women with colour-blind mother may get X chromosome from mother with gene of colour-blindness, therefore, genotype of father is XY and genotype of mother is $XX^h$.
$XY \times XX^h$
Four genotypes can be arrived: XX , $XX^h$, XY and $X^hY$. So 50% of male children are colour-blind.

**27.**

| | |
|---|---|
| Recessive epistasis(9:3:4) | Coat colour in mouse |
| Dominant epistasis (12:3:1) | Fret colour in squash |
| Inhibitory gene (13:3) | Feather colour in fowls |
| Complementary gene (9:7) | Flower colour in pea |

**28. Two solutions are possible.**

XX — Normal woman; $X^cY$ — Colourblind man

| ♀ \ ♂ | $X^c$ | Y |
|---|---|---|
| X | $XX^c$ | XY |
| X | $XX^c$ | XY |

The daughters of this couple will have normal eye sight and if one of the carrier's daughter marries a normal eyed man.

$XX^c$ X XY
Normal women — Colourblind women

| ♀ \ ♂ | X | Y |
|---|---|---|
| X | XX | XY |
| $X^c$ | XX | $X^cY$ |

only 25% grandson will colour-blind

**29.** In co-dominance both the allele express in heterozygote individual. E.g. ABO blood group $I^A$ and $I^B$ are present together. They both express their own types of sugars, this is because of co-dominance.

**30.** Control of multiple traits in an individual by one gene pair is called pleiotropism.

**31.** Pod length was not considered by Mendel in his experiments. For his experiments, Mendel choose seven characters of pea plants which are:

(i) Seed colour (ii) Seed shape
(iii) Flower colour (iv) Pod colour
(v) Pod shape (vi) Flower position and
(vii) Plant height

**32.** In given pedigree shows the autosomal recessive disorder. In this disorder, individual inherit two mutated genes, one from each parent. This disorder is usually passed on by two carriers. Health is rarely affected, but individual have one mutated gene and one normal gene for the condition.

**33.** The term linkage was coined by Morgan. He is also known as father of experimental biology.

**34.** CASE 1 . $I^AI^A \times I^BI^B = I^AI^B$ (AB)
CASE 2. $I^Ai \times I^BI^B = I^Bi$ (B) , $I^AI^B$
CASE 3. $I^Ai \times I^Bi = I^Bi$, $I^AI^B$ ,$I^Ai$(A) , ii (O)
CASE 4. $I^Bi \times I^AI^A = I^Ai$ , $I^AI^B$
Therefore, all type of blood group are possible.

**35.** Genes which code for a pair of contrasting traits are known as **alleles,** i.e., they are slightly different forms of the same gene.

**36.** An abnormal human baby with 'XXX' sex chromosomes was born due to formation of abnormal ova of mother due to non-disjunction of chromosomes.

**37.** More than two alternative forms (alleles) of a gene in a population occupying the same locus on a chromosome or its homologue are known as multiple alleles.

**38.** The movement of a gene from one linkage group to another is called translocation. It is a chromosome abnormality caused by rearrangement of parts between nonhomologous chromosomes.

**39.** Mendel conducted experiment to study genetic variation using pea plant scientifically called as Pisum sativum. He used seven contrasting character of pea plant for his study which includes:

| | |
|---|---|
| 1. Seed shape | 5. Pod shape |
| 2. Seed color | 6. Pod color |
| 3. Flower color | 7. Stem height |
| 4. Flower position | |

**40.** Colour-blindness is sex-linked disorder and the responsible gene for colour-blindness is present on X-chromosome. So it is transmitted from a mother to a child and not from a father to a child.

**41.** True breeding varieties are nearly homozygous and produced by continuous selfing and also produce off-spring of its own kind.

**42.** Translocation: It is separation of a chromosome segment and its union to non-homologous chromosome (two different linkage group).

**43.** Above phenomenon is called polyploidy and induced by colchicine.

**44.** In a test-cross involving $F_1$ dihybrid flies, more parental-type offspring were produced by the recombinant-type offspring. This indicates two genes are linked and present on the same chromosome.

**45. Example of X-linked (sex linked) recessive disorder:**

(i) Haemophilia
(ii) Colour-blindness
(iii) G-6-P deficiency

**Example of autosomal recessive gene disorder:**

| | |
|---|---|
| (i) Sickle-cell anaemia | (iii) Alkaptonuria |
| (ii) Phenyl ketonuria | (iv) Albinism |

**Disease because of chromosomal ploidy:**

(i) Down's syndrome
(ii) Turner's syndrome
(iii) Kleinfelter's syndrome

**46.**
- **Dominance** – In a heterozygous organism, only one allele expresses itself.
- **Codominance** – In a heterozygous organism, both alleles express themselves fully. E.g., Blood group AB, Flower colour in 4 O'clock plant, dog flower.
- **Pleiotropy** – Multiple phenotypic effect of single gene.
- **Polygenic inheritance** – Many genes govern a single character. E.g., Skin colour in human, IQ in human.

**47.** It is genotypic ratio of Mendelian monohybrid cross (1 : 2 : 1).

**48.** Haemophilia is X-linked recessive gene disorder. It is a blood clotting disorder and shows criss-cross inheritance. In this, characters from father are transmitted to daughter and form mother and son.

**49.**
- The phenomenon of linkage was proved and defined by **T.H. Morgan** (1910) on the basis of his breeding experiments in Drosophila melanogaster.
- Mendelian work was independently rediscovered by three scientists: Hugo de Vries, Karl Correns and Tshermak in 1900. Linkage and recombination were discovered by **T.H. Morgan.**

**50.** The recessive genes located on X-chromosome in humans are always expressed in males, because in males hemizygous condition is found for sex chromosome.

**51.** Mendel conducted many artificial pollination/cross-pollination experiments using several true breeding pea lines.

**52.**
- Klinefelter's syndrome (XXY) is due to extra X chromosome and results in sterile male. Such males have some feminine features like gynaecomastia (development of breast).
- Phenyketoneuria is an inborn error of metabolism. It is an autosomal recessive disease. It's gene is present on chromosomal number 12.
- Down's syndrome: It is due to trisomy of chromosome number 21.
- Turner's syndrome: It is due to monosomy of sex chromosome (44 + XO). Such females have rudimentary ovaries and lack other secondary sexual characters. Such females are sterile.

**53.** Thalassemia is a quantitative defect of synthesizing very little globin molecule whereas sickle cell anaemia is a qualitative defect in globin chain synthesis while heamophilia is a quantitative problem of defective functioning of globin molecule.

**54.** Four type of individuals are possible $I^AI^A$ (blood group A), $I^Ai$ (blood group A), $I^AI^B$ (blood group AB), $I^Bi$ (blood group B). Thus, total genotypes are of 4 type and phenotype are of 3 type.

**55.** Gregor Mendel (1822–1884) conducted hybridization experiments on the garden peas (*Pisum sativum*) for 7 years (1856–1863).

**56.** These are seven characters that were chosen by Mendel:

| Characters | Contrasting traits | |
|---|---|---|
| | Dominant | Recessive |
| 1. Stem height | Tall | Dwarf |
| 2. Flower colour | Violet | White |
| 3. Flower position | Axial | Terminal |
| 4. Pod shape | Inflated | Constricted |
| 5. Pod colour | Green | Yellow |
| 6. Seed shape | Round | Wrinkled |
| 7. Seed colour | Yellow | Green |

**57.** Non-disjunction is failure of homologous chromosomes or sister chromatids to separate properly during cell division (aneuploidy). There are three forms of non-disjunction:

(i) Failure in separation of a pair of homologous chromosomes during meiosis-I.

(ii) Failure in separation of sister chromatids during meiosis-II.

(iii) Failure in separation of sister chromatids during mitosis.

**Down's Syndrome (Mongolian idiocy)** is a genetic disorder caused by trisomy in 21[st] pair of autosomes. it occurs due to primary non-disjunction during cell division (meiosis).

**58.** Punnett square was developed by a British geneticist Reginald C. Punnett. Morgan coined the term linkage. Spliceosome takes part in splicing (where introns are removed and exons are joined in a defined order) in transcription of eukaryotes. Transduction was discovered by Zinder and Lederberg in *Salmonella.*

**59.** Starch synthesis in pea seeds is controlled by one gene. It has two alleles (B and b). Therefore, it is not an example of multiple allelism.

**60.** ABO blood grouping in human beings. ABO blood groups are controlled by the gene ***I***. The gene (***I***) has three alleles $I^A$, $I^B$ and ***i***. Because humans are diploid organisms, each person possesses any two of the three ***I*** gene alleles. $I^A$ and $I^B$ are completely dominant over *i*, in other words, when $I^A$ and *i* are present only $I^A$ expresses (because *i* does not produce any sugar), and when $I^B$ and *i* are present $I^B$ expresses. But when $I^A$ and $I^B$ are present together they both express their own types of sugars: this is because of co-dominance.

**61.** This sex-linked recessive disease, which shows its transmission from unaffected carrier female to some of the male progeny.

**62.** There are some nucleic acids that behave like enzymes. These are called ribozymes.

**63.** Alfred Sturtevant used the frequency of recombination between gene pairs on the same chromosome as a measure of distance between genes and 'mapped' their position on the chromosome.

**64.** The inheritance of flower colour in the dog flower (snapdragon or *Antirrhinum sp.*) is a good example to understand incomplete dominance. In a cross between true-breeding red-flowered (RR) and true-breeding white-flowered plants (rr), the $F_1$ (Rr) was pink. When the $F_1$ was self-pollinated, $F_2$ resulted in the following ratio 1 (RR) Red: 2 (Rr) Pink: 1 (rr) White. Here the genotype ratios were exactly as we would expect in any Mendelian monohybrid cross, but the phenotype ratios had changed from the 3:1 dominant : recessive ratio. Law of segregation has no exception.

**65. Klinefelter's Syndrome** is a genetic disorder also caused due to presence of an additional copy of X-chromosome resulting in a karyotype of 47, XXY. Such an individual has overall masculine development, however, the feminine development (development of breast, i.e., Gynaecomastia) is also expressed. Such individuals are sterile.

**66.**
- Grasshopper is an example of XO type of sex determination in which males have only one X-chromosome besides the autosomes, whereas females have a pair of X-chromosomes.
- In many birds, female has a pair of dissimilar chromosomes ZW and male two similar ZZ chromosomes. Therefore in domesticated fowls, sex of progeny depends on the type of egg rather than sperm.
- In human, Y chromosome is shorter than X chromosome.

- In human beings and in *Drosophila,* males have one X and one Y chromosome, whereas females have a pair of X-chromosomes besides autosomes.

**67.** Map unit (Centimorgan) is adopted in construction of genetic maps is a unit of distance between genes on chromosome, representing 1% cross over.

**68.** Mendel selected 14 True breeding plant varieties.

**69.**

| | | |
|---|---|---|
| Phenylketonuria | – | Autosomal recessive disorder |
| Thalassemia | – | Autosomal recessive disorder |
| Haemophilia | – | X linked recessive disorder |
| Sickle cell anaemia | – | Autosomal recessive trait, caused due to mutation in gene present on chromosome no.11 |

**70.** ABO blood groups are controlled by the gene I. The gene I has three alleles $I^A$, $I^B$ and i. The alleles $I^A$ and $I^B$ produce a slightly different form of the sugar while allele i does not produce any sugar. Because humans are diploid organisms, each person can possess at the most any two of the three I gene alleles.

**71.** Experimental verification of the chromosomal theory of inheritance was done by Morgan.

**Note:**

Sutton and Boveri proposed chromosomal theory of inheritance but it was experimentally verified by T.H. Morgan.

**72.**
- The production of gametes by the parents, the formation of the zygotes, the $F_1$ and $F_2$ plants can be understood from a diagram called punnett square.
- It was developed by a British geneticist, Reginald C. Punnett.

**73.** According to given questions;

$Hb^AHb^S \times Hb^AHb^S$ (Parents)

↓

$Hb^SHb^S$, $Hb^AHb^S$, $Hb^AHb^S$, $Hb^AHb^A$ (Progenies)

Total number of affected progenies = 1

∴ Percentage of diseased / affected progenies

$$= \frac{1}{4} \times 100 = 25\%$$

**74.** Gregor J. Mendel, conducted hybridisation experiments on garden peas and **selected 14 true breeding pea plant varieties (seven contrasting traits)**. Contrasting traits studied were smooth or wrinkled seeds, yellow or green seeds, inflated on constricted pods, green or yellow pods, tall or dwarf plants, violet or white flowers and axial or terminal flower positions.

| S.No. | Characters | Contrasting Traits |
|---|---|---|
| (a) | *Stem height* | *Tall/dwarf* |
| (b) | *Flower colour* | *Violet/white* |
| (c) | *Flower position* | *Axial/terminal* |
| (d) | *Pod shape* | *Inflated/constricted* |
| (e) | *Pod colour* | *Green/yellow* |
| (f) | *Seed shape* | *Round/wrinkled* |
| (g) | *Seed colour* | *Yellow/green* |

**75.**

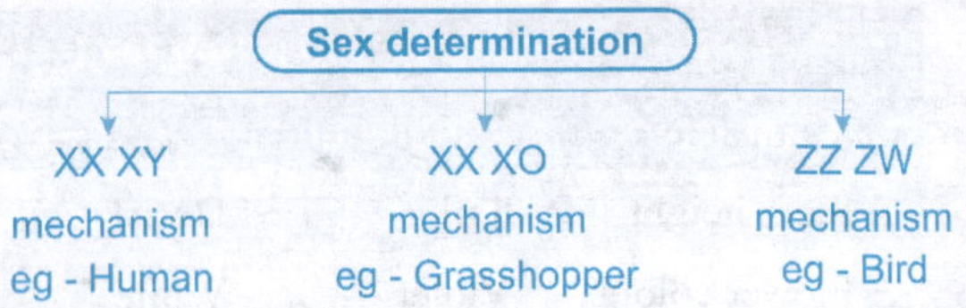


**XO type sex determination-**

It is found in most of insects (e.g., Grasshopper). Eggs of such insects possess autosomes and one X chromosome while the sperms possess autosomes with or without one X chromosome. As a result of fertilization, male insects (two set of autosomes + XO) and female insects (two set of autosomes + XX) are produced.

**76.** Closely located genes do not show independent assortment.

Mendel's law of independent assortment holds good for those genes which are located on different chromosomes.

**77.** **Myotonic dystrophy** is an autosomal dominant disorder i.e. it occurs due to the presence of autosomal linked dominant trait.

**Haemophilia** is a X-linked recessive disorder.

**Thalassemia** is an autosomal recessive disorder.

**Sickle cell anaemia** is an autosomal recessive disorder.

**78.** 1% recombination frequency = 1 centi Morgan

To place the genes on a linear chromosome, decreasing order of recombination frequency will be considered

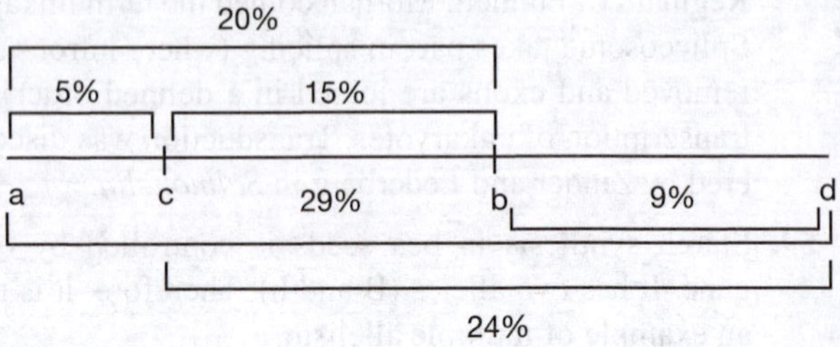

**79.** If mother of man is colourblind, then man will also be colourblind as colour blindness is a X-linked recessive trait and shows criss-cross inheritance.

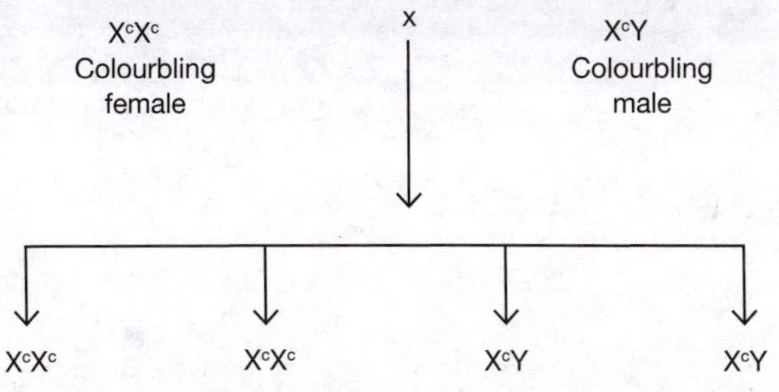


**All progeny are colourblind**

**80.** Frequency of recombination between gene pairs on same chromosome as a measure of the distance between genes to map their position on chromosome was used for the first time by Alfred Sturtevant. The distance between genes is inversely proportional to frequency.

**81.** Pleiotropism refers to a single gene affecting multiple phenotypic expression where many unrelated characters are controlled by one single gene.

**82.** Down syndrome- This disorder was first described by Langdon Down (1866).
The affected individual is short statured.
Physical, psychomotor and mental development is retarded.
Klinefelter's Syndrome- Such an individual has overall masculine development. However, the feminine development is also expressed.
Such individuals are sterile.

**83.** The individual affected with Down's syndrome is short statured with small round head, furrowed tongue and partially open mouth. Palm is broad with characteristic palm crease. Physical, psychomotor and mental development is retarded.

**84.**

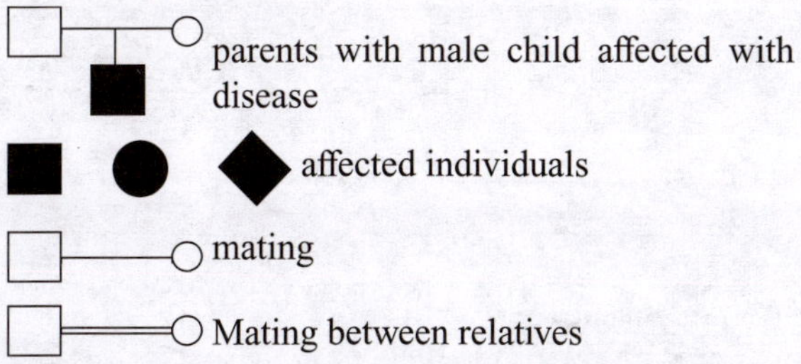


**85.** Pink colour flower in snapdragon have genotype **Rr**
Red-flowered snapdragon have genotype **RR** when they both are crossed.

| ♂ / ♀ | R | R | Phenotype |
|---|---|---|---|
| R | RR | RR | Red : Pink : White |
| r | Rr | Rr | 2 2 0 |

So the progeny that we get are red and pink- flowered plants only.

**86.** A. Two or more alternative forms of gene are called alleles.
B. Cross of $F_1$ progeny with homozygous recessive parent is a test cross.
C. Cross of $F_1$ progeny with any of the parents is a back cross.
D. Number of chromosome sets in plant is called ploidy.

**87.** To determine the genotype of a black seed colour at $F_2$, the black seed from $F_2$ is crossed with the white seed colour. This is called a test cross.
Therefore, to determine the genotype of (BB/Bb) black seed we need to cross them with white seed *i.e.* bb.

**88.** According to Law of Dominance,
(1) Characters are controlled by discrete units called factors
(2) Factors occur in pairs
(3) In a dissimilar pair of factors, one member of the pair dominates (dominant) the other recessive.

The law of dominance is used to explain the expression of only one of the parental characters in a monohybrid cross.
Law of segregation is based on the fact that the alleles do not show any expression and both the characters are recovered as such in $F_2$ generation.

**89.**
- Down's syndrome is due to presence of an additional copy of chromosome number 21, that is trisomy of chromosome number 21
- Klinefelter's syndrome is caused due to presence of an additional copy of X-chromosome.
- $\alpha$-Thalassemia is controlled by two closely-linked genes on chromosome 16 of each parent.
- $\beta$-Thalassemia is controlled by a single gene HBB on chromosome 11 of each parent.

**90.** Genotype of father with blood group $B^+ = I^Bi/iI^D$
Genotype of mother with blood group $A^+ = I^Ai/iI^A$
Genotype of child with blood group $O^+ = ii$
Hence only 'A' is correct.

# Molecular Basis of Inheritance

3

## LEARNING OBJECTIVES

- Understand the mechanism of molecular basis of inheritance
- Understand the concept of central dogma and structure of DNA and nucleotides
- Know more about the various aspect of genetic mutations
- Understand the mechanism, advantages and disadvantages of genetic engineering
- Understand the salient feature of human genome project and also its advantages
- Learn the working of DNA fingerprinting

## Chapter Overview

### Introduction

- Two types of nucleic acid found in living system DNA (deoxyribonucleic acid) and RNA (ribonucleic acid).
- DNA act as genetic material in most of organism.
- RNA can act as genetic material only in some viruses (known as **retrovirus**), however, it can also perform as adapter, structural and sometimes catalytic molecule also.

### DNA

- It is acidic in nature because of presence of phosphate group.
- It was first identified by **Friedrich Meischer** in 1869, he coined the term **'Nuclein'** to it.
- It is long polymer of deoxyribonucleotides. It is double stranded in all organisms except few viruses (**$\phi \times 174$**).
- Length of DNA is defined in terms of number of base pairs or number of nucleotide. It is the characteristic of an organism, i.e., the number of base pairs is specific for a particular species.

  **Examples:**

  (1) **Bacteriophage $\phi \times 174$:** 5386 nucleotides (nucleotides not in pair so its conclusion that genetic material is ssDNA)

  (2) **Bacteriophage Lambda ($\lambda$):** 48,502 base pairs or bp (ds DNA)

  (3) ***Escherichia coli*:** $4.6 \times 10^6$ bp.

  (4) **Human DNA:** $6.6 \times 10^9$ bp ($3.3 \times 10^9$ bp in a haploid content).

### Chemical Composition of Polynucleotide Chain

- DNA and RNA are polynucleotide made up of monomeric unit called nucleotide.
- Nucleotide is composed of Nitrogenous base, Pentose sugar, Phosphate group. Nucleotide is also nucleoside and phosphate group **(joined by Phosphoester linkage formed between 5′ OH of nucleoside sugar with phosphate group).**
- Nucleoside is nitrogen base and pentose sugar joined by **N-glycosidic linkage** (nitrogen base with OH of 1′ C pentose sugar).

Refer NCERT Ch 5: Molecular Basis of Inheritance

- Nitrogenous bases are of two types Purines (Adenine, Guanine) and Pyrimidines (Cytosine, Uracil and Thymine).
- Two nucleotides join together through 3′ to 5′ phosphodiester linkage and form dinucleotide.
- Polynucleotide formed in above manner have free phosphate moiety (functional group) at 5′ –end and free OH moiety (functional group) at 3′ –end.
- **Backbone** of this structure is formed by sugar and phosphate.

**TABLE 3.1** Components of DNA and RNA

| Components of Nucleic acids | DNA | RNA |
|---|---|---|
| **1. Nitrogenous bases** | Purines - Adenine and Guanine | Purines - Adenine and Guanine |
| | Pyrimidines - Cytosine and Thymine | Pyrimidines - Cytosine and Uracil |
| **2. Pentose sugar** | 2′ Deoxyribose sugar (oxygen removed from 2′ of ribose sugar) | Ribose sugar |

**TABLE 3.2** Nucleoside and nucleotide in DNA

| Nucleoside and nucleotide in DNA | | |
|---|---|---|
| Nitrogenous bases | Nucleoside ($N_2$bases + Deoxyribose sugar) | Nucleotide ($N_2$bases + Deoxyribose sugar + Phosphate group) |
| 1. Adenine | Deoxyadenosine | Deoxyadenylic acid or Deoxyadenosine monophosphate (AMP) |
| 2. Guanine | Deoxyguanosine | Deoxyguanylic acid or Deoxyguanosine monophosphate (dGMP) |
| 3. Cytosine | Deoxycytidine | Deoxycytidylic acid or Deoxycytidine monophosphate (dCMP) |
| 4. Thymine | Deoxythymidine | Deoxythymidylic acid or Deoxythymidine monophosphate (dTMP) |

**TABLE 3.3** Nucleoside and nucleotide in RNA

| Nucleoside and nucleotide in RNA | | |
|---|---|---|
| Nitrogenous bases | Nucleoside ($N_2$bases + Ribose sugar) | Nucleotide ($N_2$ bases + Ribose sugar + Phosphate group) |
| 1. Adenine | Adenosine | Adenylic acid or Adenosine monophosphate (AMP) |
| 2. Guanine | Guanosine | Guanylic acid or Guanosine monophosphate (GMP) |
| 3. Cytosine | Cytidine | Cytidylic acid or Cytidine monophosphate (CMP) |
| 4. Uracil | Uridine | Uridylic acid or Uridine monophosphate (UMP) |

## Structure of DNA

- **Double Helix model** for the structure of DNA.
- It was proposed by **James Watson and Francis Crick in 1953**, based on the **X-ray diffraction** data produced by **Maurice Wilkins and Rosalind Franklin**).
- Salient features of the double helix model are following:
  - DNA is made up of two polynucleotide chains with **anti-parallel polarity**, i.e., one with 5′ $\rightarrow$ 3′ polarity while another with 3′ $\rightarrow$ 5′ polarity.
  - Backbone is made up of sugar and phosphate and the nitrogenous bases attached to pentose sugar project inwards from the backbone.
  - Nitrogenous bases on opposite polynucleotide chains are linked by **hydrogen bonds (H-bonds)** and are termed as base pairs (bp). Nitrogenous bases are complementary to each other.
  - A base pair is always formed in between a purine and a pyrimidine.
    **Example:** Adenine is connected with Thymine by two hydrogen bonds.

Cytosine is connected with Guanine by three hydrogen bonds.

- Two polynucleotide chains are coiled in a right handed fashion.
- **Pitch of the helix = 3.4 nm**. Pitch means the length of one coil.
- 10 bp are found per turn. So length between the two base pairs is 0.34 nm.
- As the plane of one base pair overlaps each other, so these contribute to the stability of the DNA helix.

## RNA (Majorly There are Three Type of RNA)

- **t-RNA: the Adapter molecule/s (soluble)- RNA – smallest RNA**
  - **Francis Crick** was first to propose the presence of an adapter molecule which can itself perform two functions: It reads the code and it is linked to amino acids according to the code.
  - Secondary structure of t-RNA (**clover leaf model- 2D structure**): t-RNA possess the following:
    **(1) Anticodon loop:** It has sequence of bases complimentary to the codon.
    **(2) Amino acid acceptor end:** It is the site for binding of amino acids.
    **(3) DHU loop – aminoacyl binding loop**
    **(4) T$\psi$C loop – bind t-RNA with larger subunit of ribosome.**
  - Actual structure of t-RNA: t-RNA looks like **inverted L (3-D structure).**
  - **Initiator t-RNA:** This is the specific t-RNA that initiates the process of translation.
  - There are no t-RNAs to read the stop codons.
- **Ribosome (Structural r-RNAs + Proteins): r-RNA is most abundant RNA found in cell.**
  - It is the cellular factory required for the synthesis of proteins.
  - Composition = Structural RNAs + Proteins (about 80 types).
  - Structure of ribosome in inactive state: It consists of two subunits
    (1) Larger subunit: 50 s in prokaryote and 60 s in eukaryote.
    (2) Smaller subunit: 30 s in prokaryote and 40 s in eukaryote.
  - Process of translation begins when a mRNA is attached to the smaller subunit.
  - Larger subunit possesses two sites and each meant for binding of t-RNA carrying amino acid.
- **mRNA: life span is minimum.**
  - mRNA is formed during transcription and it results in the formation of protein (translation).
  - It is the nucleotide triplet of m-RNA is closed codon.
  - Untranslated regions (UTRs) are required for effective translation. These are those parts of mRNA that are not being translated. These are located before start codon (towards 5′ end) and after stop codon (towards 3′ end).

## Central Dogma

- The proposition of 'double helix' structure of DNA and its simplicity in explaining the genetic implication became revolutionary. Very soon Francis **Crick (1958) proposed the central dogma** in molecular biology, which state that *'the genetic information flows from DNA to RNA and then to protein* **(Fig. 3.1)**.
- The concept of central dogma emphasized that three processes are involved in the flow of information from DNA. These are: (i) Replication (i.e., exact copying or duplication of DNA), (ii) Transcription (*i.e.,* transfer of genetic information from DNA to mRNA), and (iii) Translation (i.e., conversion of genetic information of mRNA in the form of protein).
- Exception to one way flow of information was reported by H. Temin and D. Beltimore (1970) in some viruses.
- They discovered that many tumor viruses contain RNA as genetic material and replicate by first synthesizing a complementary DNA.

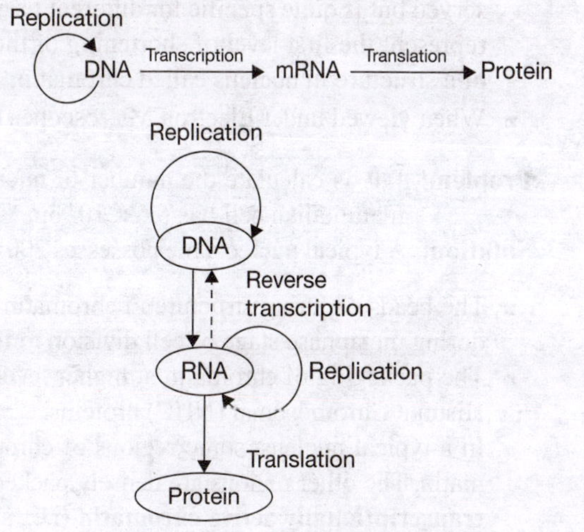


FIGURE 3.1 Central Dogma

This process is called **reverse transcription**. It is carried out by an RNA-dependent DNA polymerase called ***'reverse transcriptase'***.

- These viruses are called retroviruses and include human immunodeficiency virus (HIV) that causes AIDS. This discovery in molecular biology introduced the concept of 'central dogma reverse'.
- It states that the flow of genetic information is not necessarily from DNA to RNA but may be from RNA to DNA also.

## Packaging of DNA Helix

- DNA is a long chain polymer of over a million deoxyribonucleotides (e.g., 3.4 million nucleotide pairs or bp in *Escherichia coli* and 66 million nucleotide pairs or bp in humans).
- The length of DNA in a cell can be calculated by multiplying the number of base pairs with the distance between the two consecutive base pairs (i.e., 0.34 nm or $0.34 \times 10^{-9}$).
- **The DNA of a typical mammalian cell has $6.6 \times 10^9$ bp. Its length will be $6.6 \times 10^9$ bp $\times$ $0.34 \times 10^{-9}$ m/bp.** It comes out to be **approximately 2.2 meters.**
- A length that is far greater than dimension of a typical nucleus, which is approximately $10^{-6}$ m in diameter. Therefore, there must be some special arrangement to accommodate such a long polymer in a cell.

**Problem:** Calculate the number of base pairs in the DNA of *E. coli;* which has a length of 1.36 mm, Length of DNA = 1.36 mm or $1.36 \times 10^6$ nm.

**Solution:** Number Of base pair (bp) = $\mathbf{1.36 \times 10^6/0.34 = 4} \times 10^6$ bp.

- In prokaryotes, such *as E. coli,* there is no well-defined nucleus, still the DNA is not scattered throughout the entire cell. DNA being negatively charged is held with some proteins (such as polyamines) that have '+ve charges in a region termed as 'nucleoid'. The DNA in nucleoid is organized in large loops held by proteins ***(i.e.,* polyamines)**.
- In eukaryotes, the organization of DNA is much more complex. There is a set of positively charged basic proteins called 'histone'.
- A protein acquires charge due to the abundance of amino acid residues with charged side chains. The histone proteins are rich in amino acid residues lysine and arginines. Both the amino acid residues carry positive charges in their side chains.
- There are five types of histone proteins $H_1$, $H_2A$, $H_2B$, $H_3$ and $H_4$. Four of them ($H_2A$, $H_2B$, $H_3$ and $H_4$) occur in pairs to produce 'histone octomer' called nu-body or core. They are one of the most conserved proteins, being similar in different species. Their charged ends (positively) are towards outside.
- The negatively charged DNA is wrapped around positively charged histone octomer almost twice ($1\frac{3}{4}$ turns) to form nucleosome with a diameter about 10 nm.
- DNA connecting the two adjacent nucleosomes is called interbed or linker DNA. It bears $H_1$ **(Fig. 3.2)**. $H_1$ is not conserved but is quite specific for different tissues. A typical nucleosome contains 200 bp of DNA helix. The nucleosomes represent the first level of shortening of the very large strand of DNA. The nucleosomes constitute the repeating unit of a structure in nucleus called chromatin, i.e., thread like stained (coloured) bodies seen in the nucleus.
- When viewed under Electron Microscope (EM), the nucleosomes in **chromatin are 'beads-on-string'.**

**Problem:** Let us calculate the number of nucleosomes in the DNA of a typical mammalian cell. The *DNA* of a typical mammalian cell has $6.6 \times 10^9$ bp.

**Solution:** A typical nucleosome possesses 200 bp. Therefore, the total number of nucleosomes = $6.6 \times 10^9/200 = 3.3 \times 10^7$.

- The beads on string structure in chromatin in packaged to form chromatin fibres, which coiled and condensed further during metaphase stage of cell division to form chromosomes.
- The packaging of chromatin at higher level requires additional set of proteins that are collectively referred to as Non-Histone Chromosomal (NHC) proteins.
- In a typical nucleus, some regions of chromatin are loosely packed and stain light. These regions are termed euchromatin. The other regions are densely packed and stain dark. These regions are called heterochromatin. **Euchromatin is transcriptionally active chromatin** (i.e., synthesizes RNA through the process of transcription), whereas **heterochromatin is inactive.**

Depiction of Nucleosome and Solenoid, Single nucleosome and EM picture – 'Beads-on-string' is shown in **Fig 3.2**.

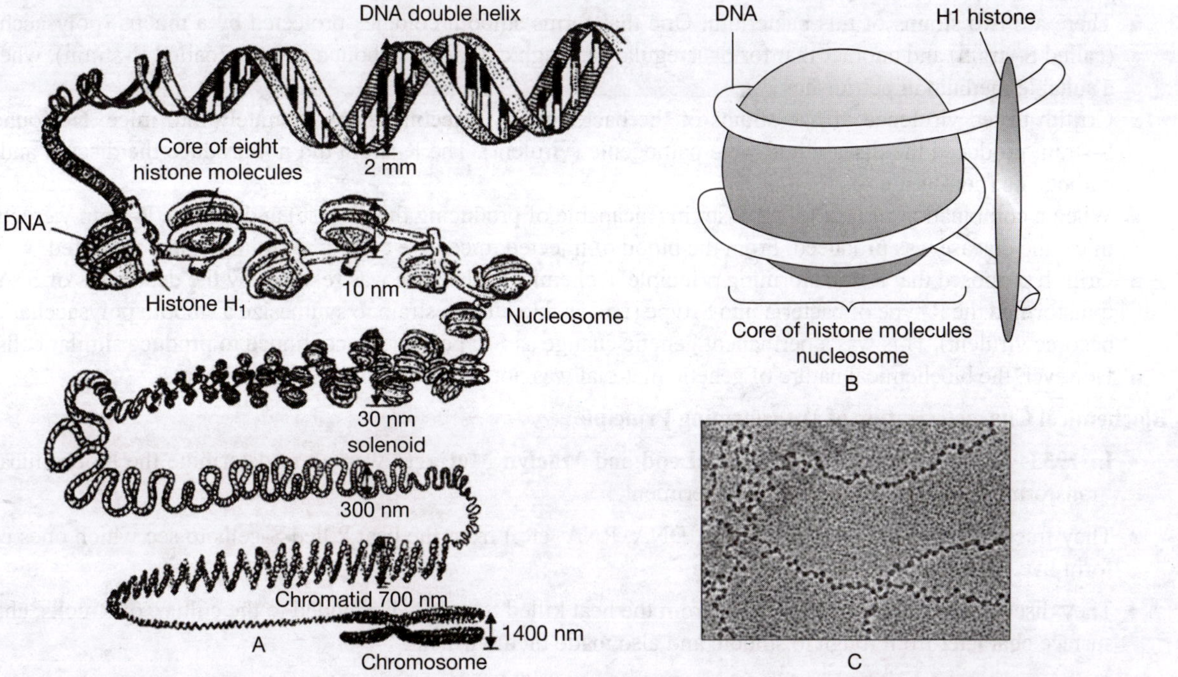


**FIGURE 3.2** A. Nucleosome and Solenoid model of folding and super folding of basic chromatin components to form eukaryotic chromosome. B. Single nucleosome. C. EM picture – 'Beads-on-string'

- **The Search for Genetic Material: Transforming Principle (by Frederick Griffith, 1928) (Fig 3.3)**
  *'Transformation is the change in the genetic constitution of an organism by picking up genes present in the remains of its dead relatives'.*

  ***Or***

  *The phenomenon by which the DNA isolated from one type of cell, when introduced into another type is able to confer some of the properties of the former to the latter is called transformation.*

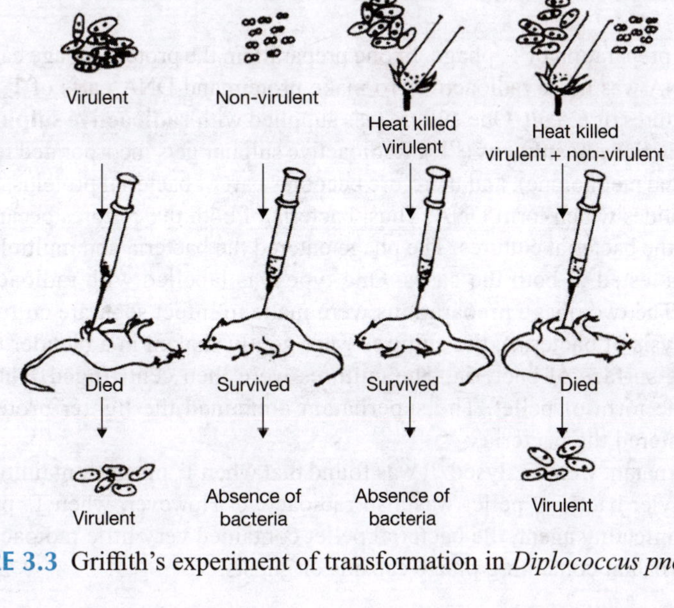


**FIGURE 3.3** Griffith's experiment of transformation in *Diplococcus pneumoniae*

- The process of transformation was first studied by a British-Medical officer, Frederick Griffith (1928) in *Streptococcus pneumoniae (= Diplococcus pnenumoniae),* a bacterium that causes pneumonia in mammals.
- There are two strains of this bacterium. One that forms smooth colonies protected by a mucus (polysaccharide) coat (called S-strain) and another that forms irregular or rough colonies, without a capsule (called R-strain), when grown in a suitable medium in petridishes.
- Griffith tested virulence of two strains of the bacterium by injecting them separately into mice. He found that only S-strain produced the disease and were pathogenic (virulent). The R-strain did not produce the disease and were non-pathogenic (non-virulent).
- When a combination of heat killed S-strain (incapable of producing the disease) and the live R-stain were injected into mice, the disease was produced. From the blood of injected mice, live cells of S-strain could be isolated.
- Griffith proposed that a 'transforming principle' a chemical substance was released by the dead cells of S strain, which transformed the R-type of bacteria into S-type (i.e., enabled the R. strain to synthesize a smooth polysaccharide coat and become virulent). This was a permanent genetic change as S-type bacteria continued to produce similar cells.
- However, the biochemical nature of genetic material was not defined from these experiments.

**Biochemical Characterization of Transforming Principle**

- **In 1933–44, Oswald Avery, Colin MacLeod** and **Maclyn McCarty** worked to determine the biochemical nature of 'transforming principle' in Griffith's experiment.
- They fractionated biochemical (proteins, DNA, RNA, etc.) from the heat killed S-cells to see which ones could transform live R-cells into S-cells.
- They discovered that the DNA isolated from the heat killed S-cells, when added to the culture of R-cells, changed their surface character from rough to smooth and also made them virulent.
- On the contrary, the addition of protein or RNA fraction did not transformed R-cells.
- When the isolated DNA was digested with DNAase, before addition to the culture of R-cells, did not caused transformation. This showed that DNA is the hereditary material.

## The Genetic Material is DNA

- They discovered that the DNA isolated from the heat killed S-cells, when added to the culture of R-cells, changed their surface character from rough to smooth and also made them virulent.
- A non-controversial proof that DNA is the genetic material came from the experiments of Alfred Hershey and Martha Chase (1952).
- They experimented with *Escherichia coli* (a bacterium that occurs as a commensal in human intestine) and $T_2$ phage (a bacteriophage).
- They made two different preparation of $T_2$ phage. In one preparation, the protein (phage capsid) part was made radioactive and in the other, DNA was made radioactive. To make protein and DNA parts of $T_2$ phage radioactive, **Hershey and Chase** grew two cultures of *E. coli.* One culture was supplied with **radioactive sulphur ($^{35}$S)** and the other culture was provided with **radioactive phosphorus ($^{32}$P)**. Radioactive sulphur gets incorporated into sulphur containing amino acids (cystine, cysteine and methionine), and therefore becomes part of bacterial proteins. Radioactive phosphorus gets incorporated into nucleotides which form DNA. Thus, bacteria of both the cultures became labelled. Then, $T_2$ phages were introduced in both the bacterial cultures. The phage entered the bacteria and multiplied.
- The phage progeny was tested in both the cases. One type was labelled with radioactive protein and other type with radioactive DNA. The two phage preparations were made to infect separate cultures of normal *E. coli.* Soon after infection (before lysis of bacteria), the cultures were gently shaken in a blender to remove remains of phage particles sticking to the surface of bacteria. The cultures were then centrifuged. The heavier infected bacterial cells settled down in the form of pellet. The supernatant contained the lighter protein coat of phage capsid or 'ghosts'-that had not entered the bacteria.
- Both the pellet and supernatant were analysed. It was found that when $T_2$ phage containing radioactive DNA was used to infect *E.coli,* the heavier bacterial pellet was also radioactive. However, when $T_2$ phage containing radioactive protein was used as the infecting agent, the bacterial pellet contained very little radioactivity and most of the radioactivity was in the supernatant containing phage capsids or ghosts.

- This experiment indicated that during infection with the virus, it is the DNA that entered into the bacteria. When such bacteria were allowed to grow further, they lysed and new viral particles were released **(Fig 3.4)**. This finding suggests that it is the viral DNA and not protein that contains information for the production of more viral particles and therefore DNA should be the genetic material. However, in some viruses, RNA instead of DNA serves as the genetic material.

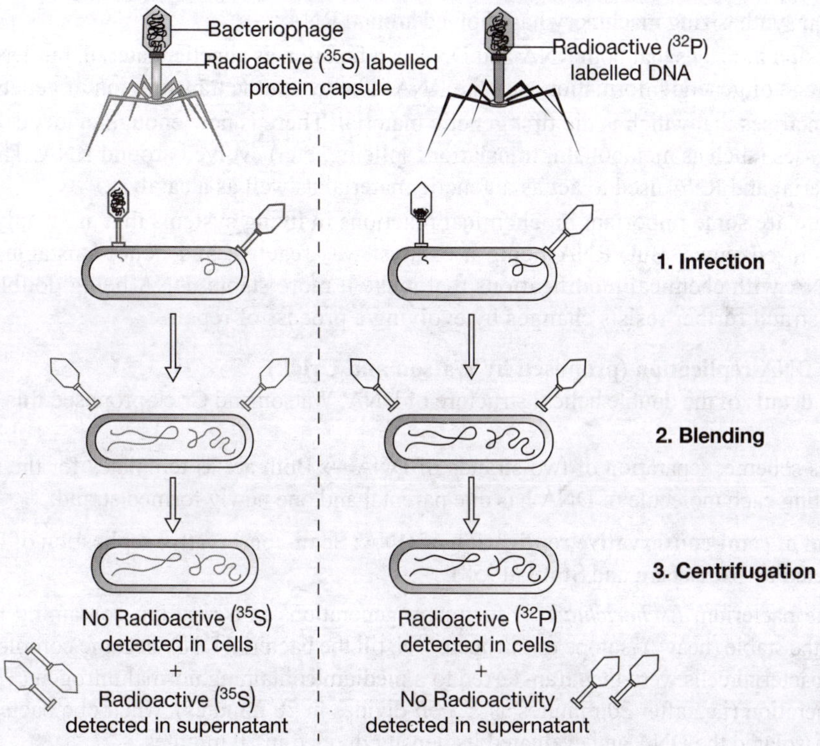


**FIGURE 3.4** The Hershey - Chase experiment

- **Properties of genetic material**
  - The experiment performed by Hershey and Chase unequivocally resolved that DNA acts as genetic material.
  - The differences between chemical structures of the two nucleic acids make DNA as predominant genetic material whereas RNA performs dynamic functions of a messenger and adapter.
  - A molecule must fulfil the following criteria to act as-genetic material.
    1. It should be able to replicate (i.e., produce its replica)
    2. It should chemically and structurally be stable.
    3. It should have the scope of slow changes (mutation) that are required for evolution.
    4. It should be able to express itself in the form of Mendelian characters.
  - Let us examine each of the above requirements one by one. Since there exists the rule of base pairing and complementarity, both the nucleic acids (i.e., DNA and RNA) have the ability to direct their duplications. The other molecules of the living system, such as proteins fail to fulfil the first criteria.
  - The genetic material should be stable enough not to change with different stages of life cycle, age or with change in physiology of the organism. It is quite evident from Griffith's experiment on 'transforming principle', that the heat which killed the bacteria did not destroy some of the properties of genetic material. This can be explained in the light of the fact that the two strands of DNA being complementary, if separated by heating, come together when appropriate conditions are provided.
  - The presence of thymine (present in DNA) at the place of uracil (present in RNA) also confers additional stability to DNA.

- On the other hand 2′-OH group present at every nucleotide in RNA is a reactive group, which makes RNA labile and easily degradable. RNA is also now known to be catalytic, hence reactive. Therefore, DNA is less reactive and structurally more stable as compared to RNA. Hence, among the two nucleic acids, the DNA is a better genetic material.
- Though both DNA and RNA are able to undergo mutation, but RNA being unstable, mutates at a faster rate. This is the reason that the viruses having RNA genome and shorter life span undergoes mutation and evolve faster.
- For the synthesis of proteins, DNA is dependent on RNA, whereas, RNA can directly code for the synthesis of proteins. In fact, the protein synthesizing machinery has evolved around RNA.
- The above discussion indicates that both RNA and DNA can function as genetic material, but DNA being more stable is preferred for storage of genetic information, and the RNA is better for the transmission of genetic information.
- Now the question arises that which is the first genetic material. There is now enough evidence which suggest that essential life processes (such as metabolism, translation, splicing, etc.) evolved around RNA. Therefore, RNA must be first genetic material and RNA used to act as a genetic material as well as a catalyst.
- For instance, there are some important biochemical reactions in living systems that are catalysed by RNA catalysts and not by protein enzymes. But, RNA being a catalyst was reactive and hence unstable. Therefore, DNA has evolved from RNA with chemical modifications that make it more stable. DNA being double stranded and having complementary strand further resists changes by evolving a process of repair.

- **Semi-conservative DNA replication (proposed by Watson and Crick)**
  - While giving the details of the double helical structure of DNA, Watson and Crick proposed this scheme for the replication of DNA.
  - According to this scheme, separation of two strands of DNA → Both act as templates for the synthesis of new DNA strands → Resulting each molecule of DNA has one parental and one newly formed strand.
- **Experimental proof of semi-conservative replication of DNA:** Semi-conservative replication of DNA was proved by the experiments conducted by **Messelson** and **Stahl** (1958).
  1. They grew the bacterium *Escherichia coli* for many generations in a medium containing nitrogen salt ($^{15}NH_4Cl$) labelled with the stable (heavy) isotope of nitrogen- $^{15}N$, till the bacterial DNA became completely labelled **(Fig. 3.5)**.
  2. The labelled bacterial cells were then transferred to a medium containing normal nitrogen ($^{14}N$).
  3. After one generation (i.e., after 20 minutes as *E. coli* divides in 20 minutes), when one bacterial cell had multiplied into two, they isolated the DNA and evaluated its density divided in 20 minutes.
  4. Its density was intermediate between that of heavier $^{15}N$ DNA and lighter $^{14}N$ DNA. This was because during one generation new DNA molecules with one $^{15}N$ old strand and complementary $^{14}N$ new strand were formed. This had an intermediate density between the DNA having $^{15}N$ in both the strands and the DNA having $^{14}N$ in both the strands.
  5. When the daughter cells were allowed to divide again (i.e., after 40 minutes), out of the four second generation cells, the DNA of two cells were found to have intermediate ($^{14}N - ^{15}N$) density and that of the remaining two cells have light ($^{14}N - ^{14}N$) density. In this way at each replication, one strand of parent DNA is conserved in the daughter while the second is freshly synthesized.

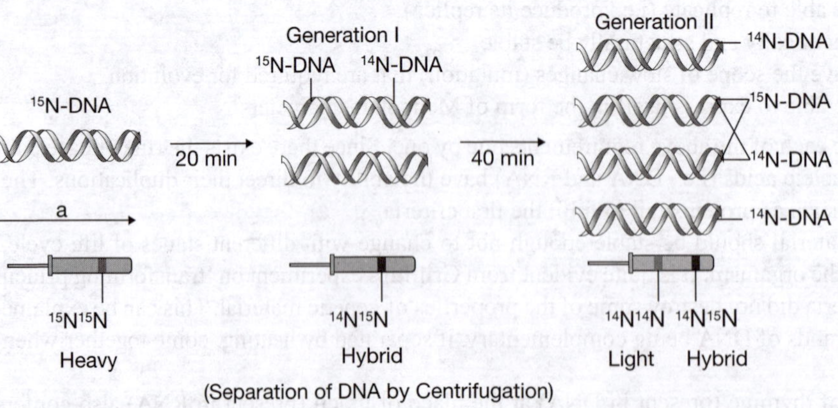


**FIGURE 3.5** Messelson and Stahl's experiment to prove semi-conservative replication of DNA

- To evaluate, the density of DNA of the bacterium-*E. coli,* Masselson and Stahl used **'Cesium Chloride** (CsCl) gradient **centrifugation technique.** A dense solution of CsCl, on centrifugation, at a very high speed (50,000 revolutions per minute) for many hours, form density gradient bands of a solution of lower density at the top that increases gradually towards bottom with highest density.
- If DNAs of different densities are mixed with CsCl solution, these would separate from one another and would form a definite density band in the gradient along with CsCl solution.

## DNA Replication

- This experiment provided evidence for the semi-conservative nature of DNA replication. Just a year before **Messelson and Stahl's experiment, Taylor *et al.,*** (1958) had shown semi-conservative mode of replication at chromosomal level in **root tip cells of *Vicia faba* (fev bean).**
- In process of replication, a set of enzymes is required.
- In prokaryotes like *E. coli,* most important enzyme for replication of DNA is DNA dependent DNA polymerase.
- Number of base pairs in *E. coli* = $4.6 \times 10^6$ bp.
  Time taken by *E.coli* for completion of replication = 18 min. = $18 \times 60$s.

$$\text{Rate of polymerization in } E.coli = \frac{\text{Number of base pairs in } E.coli}{\text{Time taken for completion of replication}} = \frac{4.6\times10^{6}}{18\times60\,\text{s}} = 4260 \text{ bp/s}$$

- Important features of DNA polymerases: These are very fast enzymes and have high degree of accuracy.
- Energetically, replication of DNA is an expensive process.
- Deoxyribonucleotides serve two purposes: These act as substrate for DNA replication. Two terminal phosphates are high energy phosphates which provide energy for the process of polymerization.

- **Mechanism of DNA Replication**
  DNA replication occurs in S-phase of cell cycle.
  - **Initiation of replication**
    (1) Replication of DNA starts at some specific or definite regions. These regions are termed as origin of replication. In *E. coli* there is an origin of replication. In prokaryote there is one ORI and in eukaryote there are multiple ORI. This step is not initiated by DNA polymerases. It requires certain proteins and enzyme helicase, topoisomerase and ssb proteins.
  - **Formation of replication fork**
    (1) This is the separation of the two strands of DNA. This separation results in formation of a replication fork. Unwinding for this process done by helicase enzyme.
  - **Polymerisation**
    (1) The step of polymerisation is mediated by **DNA dependent DNA polymerase.** This enzyme can polymerise in only one direction, i.e., $5' \rightarrow 3'$. For polymerisation we require RNA primer.
    (2) At replication fork, polymerization occur continuously at one strand (template with polarity $3' \rightarrow 5'$) orms leading strand while discontinuously at another strand (template with polarity $5' \rightarrow 3'$) forms lagging strand. The fragments of DNA formed on lagging strand are referred as **Okazaki fragments.**
  - **Joining of discontinuous fragments**
    (1) The discontinuously formed fragments on the template with polarity $5' \rightarrow 3'$ are joined together by the enzyme. **DNA replication is semi discontinuous and bidirectional process.**
    (2) **DNA ligase.**
    During recombinant DNA procedures, vectors provide the origin of replication for the propagation of a piece of DNA. If cell division do not occur after the DNA replication, polyploidy results.

## Transcription

- Transcription is the copying of the genetic information from one strand of DNA into RNA or Synthesis of RNA on DNA strand is termed as transcription. Process of transcription follows the rule of complementarity.
- **During transcription, only one strand of DNA is involved. Why?**

  **Reason 1:** Two strands of DNA are complementary to each other, not identical so these are involved in production of two different proteins. If both strands participate, then a second type of protein will also be formed along with the first type of protein, whether it is required or not by the body.

  **Reason 2:** As the two strands of DNA are complementary to each other, so the resulting RNA will also be complementary to each other. Thus these will pair with each other forming a double stranded RNA. Protein formation will cease in this condition.

- **Transcription Unit**

  In a DNA segment, a transcription unit is defined by three regions (all consists of DNA sequences):

  - **A promoter**

    It is located towards the 5′ ¾ end of the structural gene (upstream) in a coding strand (actually 3′ ¾ end of template strand). It provides the binding site for the RNA polymerase enzyme and the presence of promoter defines the template and coding strands.

  - **A structural gene**

    (1) It is actually flanked or sandwiched between the promoter and terminator.

    (2) **Cistron:** It is a segment of DNA coding for a polypeptide.

    (3) Structural genes are usually **monocistronic** in eukaryotes while **polycistronic** usually in prokaryotes like bacteria.

    (4) Monocistronic structural genes in eukaryotes are said to be **split genes** and are having two types of DNA sequences: **Exons:** These are the coding sequences of DNA which are expressed in mature or processed RNA. These are having introns in between. They are thrown out of nucleus therefore known as exons. **Introns:** These are the non-coding sequences of DNA which are absent in mature or processed RNA.

  - **A terminator**

    (1) It is located towards the 3′ ¾ end of the structural gene (downstream) in a coding strand (actually 5′ ¾ end of template strand).

    (2) It defines the termination or end of the transcription process.

    (3) DNA dependent RNA polymerase enzyme polymerises in only one direction, i.e., 5′ - 3′. So the strand which has polarity 3′ - 5′, will serve as template strand. Another strand which has opposite polarity 5′ - 3′, is termed as coding strand (although it is named so but actually it is not coding anything).

    (4) Base sequence of the coding strand is almost similar to that of the m-RNA except for that thymine will be in place of uracil.

    (5) Some regulatory genes may also be involved in the transcription unit.

### The process of transcription

- In prokaryotes such as bacteria, there is single DNA dependent RNA polymerase that catalyses transcription of all the three types of RNAs.
- The process of transcription involves the following steps **(Fig. 3.6)**:

**(1) *Initiation***

- On specific signal, the RNA polymerase binds to promoter and initiates transcription. The promoter region in the cistron is recognised by sigma (σ) sub unit of the enzyme RNA polymerase in prokaryotes and by many transcription factors in eukaryotes.

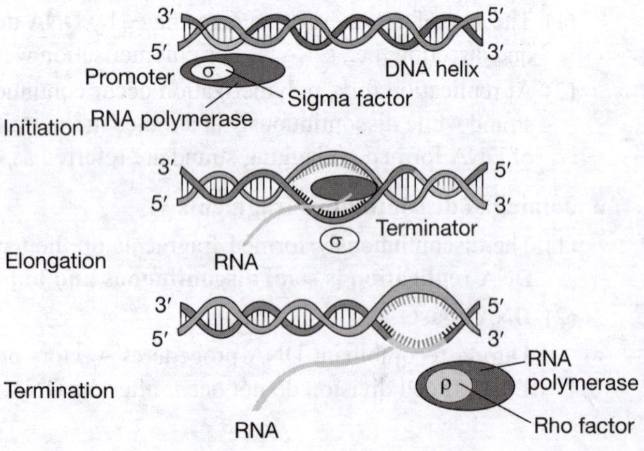


FIGURE 3.6 Process of transcription in Bacteria.

**(2) *Elongation***

- The RNA polymerase uses ribonucleoside triphosphates as substrate and polymerizes in a template dependent manner following the rule of complementarity. RNA polymerase moves along the transcription unit and causes unwinding and opening of the helix and continues the elongation of RNA. The sigma ($\sigma$) factor of the RNA polymerase separates on the initiation of RNA chain. The remaining part of the RNA polymerase, referred as core enzyme moves along the DNA template causing elongation of RNA chain at the rate of some 30 nucleotides per second. Elongation takes place in 5′ - 3′ direction.

**(3) *Termination***

- Once the RNA polymerase reaches to the terminator, the nascent RNA fall off and also the enzyme. A terminator factor-Rho ($\rho$) factor is required for the termination of RNA chain. Unlike the situation in prokaryotes, transcription in eukaryotes occurs within the nucleus and mRNA moves out of the nucleus into the cytoplasm for translation.
- In eukaryotes, there are two additional complexities:
- **There are at least three RNA polymerases in the nucleus (in addition to the RNA polymerase found in the organelles).**

| Type of RNA polymerase found in nucleus of eukaryotes. | They transcribes |
|---|---|
| RNA polymerase I | 28s, 18s and 5.8s |
| RNA polymerase II | Precursor of mRNA (pre-mRNA) or hnRNA (heterogenous nuclear RNA). |
| RNA polymerase III | tRNA, 5s rRNA and sn RNAs (small nuclear RNAs). |

Thus, there is a division of labour in the functioning of the three types of RNA polymerase.

- The second complexity is that the primary transcript contains two types of segments, the non-coding introns or intervening sequences and the coding exons.
- The primary eukaryotic mRNA transcript is much longer and is non-functional. Hence, it is subjected to a process called 'splicing', where the introns are removed and axons are joined in a definite order **(Fig. 3.7)**.

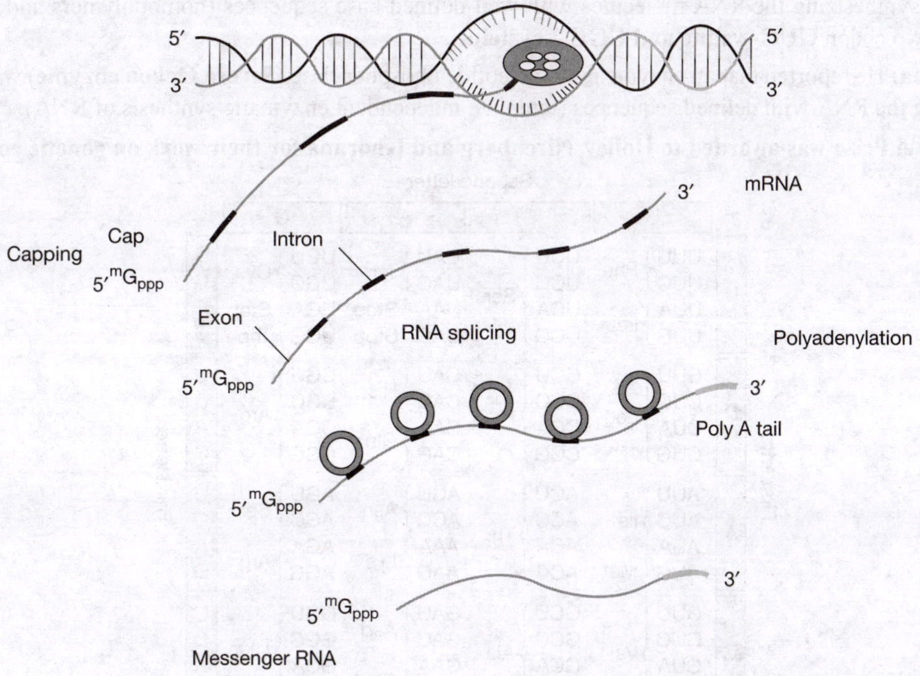


**FIGURE 3.7** Process of transcription in Eukaryotes

- hn RNA (primary mRNA transcript) undergo two additional processing called as 'capping' and 'tailing'. In capping an unusual nucleotide, methyl guanosine triphosphate ($^mG_{ppp}$) is added to the 5′ end of hn RNA. In 'tailing' adenylate residues (200–300) are added (polyadenylation) at 3′-end to hn RNA in a template independent manner (*i.e.* without a template).
- The fully processed mRNA is now called as mRNA, which is transported out of the nucleus for translation.
- Recently the significance of complexity in eukaryotic gene is being studied. It is believed that the split gene arrangement probably represents an ancient feature of the genome. The presence of introns is reminiscent of antiquity, and the process of splicing represents the dominance of 'RNA world'. As such the RNA and RNA dependent processes have assumed more importance in the living system.

## Genetic Code

It was evident that the changes in nucleic acid (genetic material) lead to changes in amino acids in protein. This clearly indicates that during synthesis of proteins, there should be some genetic code that guides the amino acid sequence. **These are sequence of three nucleotide (triplet) in m-RNA.**

- **Contribution of some scientists / geneticists:**
  - **George Gamow:** He was first to propose that the genetic codon is a triplet codon, i.e., a sequence of three nucleotides. He suggested that only four bases code for 20 amino acids. So according to permutation combination:

| If genetic codon is | Maximum no. of possible codons |
|---|---|
| 1. Singlet | $4^1 = 4$ (code for 4 amino acid) |
| 2. Doublet | $4^2 = 16$ (code for 16 amino acid) |
| 3. Triplet | $4^3 = 64$ (code for 20 amino acid) |

    - If the genetic codon is taken to be triplet than maximum number of codon will be 64, which have to cover only 20 amino acids. But actually **61 codon** code for 20 amino acids. Therefore for an amino acid there are average three codons.
  - **Marshall Nirenberg:** He has done the deciphering of genetic code by synthesizing the proteins in cell free systems. The first genetic code decipher was phenylalanine (UUU).
  - **Dr. Har Govind Khurana:** Experimental proof that genetic codon is a triplet codon was given by Dr. Har Govind Khurana by synthesizing the RNA molecules with well-defined base sequences (homopolymers and copolymers). He deciphered two codon **GUG- valine and UGU – cysteine.**
  - **Severo Ochoa:** He reported that an enzyme polynucleotide phosphorylase (**Severo Ochoa enzyme**) was very helpful in polymerizing the RNA with defined sequences (template independent enzymatic synthesis of RNA).
  - **In 1968 Nobel Prize was awarded to Holley, Nirenberg and Khorana for their work on genetic code.**

Second letter

| First letter | U | | C | | A | | G | | Third letter |
|---|---|---|---|---|---|---|---|---|---|
| U | UUU | Phe | UCU | Ser | UAU | Tyr | UGU | Cys | U |
| | UUC | | UCC | | UAC | | UGC | | C |
| | UUA | Leu | UCA | | UAA | Stop | UGA | Stop | A |
| | UUG | | UCG | | UAG | Stop | UGG | Trip | G |
| C | CUU | Leu | CCU | Pro | CAU | His | CGU | Arg | U |
| | CUC | | CCC | | CAC | | CGC | | C |
| | CUA | | CCA | | CAA | Gln | CGA | | A |
| | CUG | | CCG | | CAG | | CGG | | G |
| A | AUU | ile | ACU | Thr | ACU | Asn | AGU | Ser | U |
| | AUC | | ACC | | ACC | | AGC | | C |
| | AUA | | ACA | | AAA | Lys | AGA | Arg | A |
| | AUG | Met | ACG | | AAG | | AGG | | G |
| G | GUU | Val | GCU | Ala | GAU | Asp | GGU | Gly | U |
| | GUC | | GCC | | GAC | | GGC | | C |
| | GUA | | GCA | | GAA | Glu | GGA | | A |
| | GUG | | GCG | | GAG | | GGG | | G |

- **Salient features of Genetic Code**
  - Genetic codon is a triplet.
  - 64 codons are there out of which **61** codons code for amino acids and **three** codons code for nothing. Non-coding codons (**UAA-ochre, UGA-opal and UAG-amber**) are also known as **stop codons/nonsense codon/termination codon**.
  - Genetic codon is **unambiguous or non-ambiguous** and **specific**, i.e., one codon code for only one amino acid only.
  - Single amino acid can be coded by two or more codons. This is **degeneracy/redundancy** of codon. In degenerate codons, generally the first two nitrogen bases are similar while the third one is different. As the third base has no effect on coding, the third position is called **wobble position (Wobble hypothesis: Crick). Only two codons are non-degenerate AUG -methionine and UGG –tryptophan.**
  - In mRNA codon is read in continuous or **contiguous manner**. No punctuations are there in between.
  - Genetic codon is **nearly universal**. **Example:** UUU codes for Phenylalanine (phe) ranging from bacteria to humans. Exceptions are there in mitochondrial codons and in some protozoans.
  - Some codons may perform dual functions. **Example:** AUG codes for Methionine (met) and it act as **initiator codon.**
  - **Codons are collinear, non-overlapping and have polarity.**
- **Mutation and Genetic code**
  - Mutation is the best way to understand the relationship between the genes and DNA.
  - Even a point mutation involving a single base pair change in a gene—it may be **transition** (purine to purine or pyramidine to pyramidine or **transversion** (purine to pyramidine and vice versa) can be understood by mutation. Classical example is **sickle cell anemia** in which change in single base pair in the gene for beta globulin chain result in change in amino acid from **glutamate to valine.**
  - **Point mutation may be of three type :**
    **(i) Silent – if there is no change in amino acid**
    **(ii) Mis-senese – if there is change of amino acid. Example : sickle cell anemia**
    **(iii) Non-sense – if codon is change to non-sense codon.**
  - Insertion or deletion of one or two bases. Reading frame is changed from the point of insertion or deletion.
  - Insertion or deletion of three or its multiple bases. Insert or delete one or more codon. Insert or delete one or more amino acids. Reading frame is shifted from the point onwards. These mutations are termed as frameshift insertion or deletion mutations.
  - Frameshift insertion or deletion mutations provides the genetic basis of proof that the genetic codon is triplet and contiguous in nature.

## Translation

- It is the process of formation of polypeptide chain by polymerisation of amino acids from m-RNA.
- **Steps involved in translation:**

  **(i) Initiation**

  (a) **Activation of amino acids** in presence of ATP.

  (b) **Aminoacylation of t-RNA (or Charging of t-RNA):** In this step charging of amino acids are linked to their cognate t-RNA. It is occur in presence of aminoacyl t-RNA synthetases.

  (c) **Initiation of translation:** Ribosome (smaller subunit) binds to the mRNA at the start codon (AUG) that is recognized by initiator tRNA and this unit bind to larger subunit of ribosome and form initiation complex. It is also an energy consuming process.

  **(ii) Elongation**

  (a) As the ribosome moves from one codon to another on mRNA, more and more aminoacylated t-RNA enter and the peptide bond formation in between the amino acids result in chain elongation it is energctically favored process.

  (b) When the two t-RNAs carrying amino acids are brought together, peptide bond is formed in between. Rate of peptide bond formation can be enhanced by the presence of a catalyst- **peptidyl transferase (23 s rRNA** in bacteria is the enzyme – ribozyme)

  (c) **For every single amino acid incorporated in peptide chain one ATP and two GTP molecules are used.**

**(iii) Termination**

**(a) Termination of translation:** When the ribosome reaches a stop codon **(UAA,UAG and UGA)**, no entry of aminoacylated t-RNA take place. A **release factor** is attached to the stop codon and the whole polypeptide chain is released into the cytoplasm from ribosomes. It is also an energy consuming process.

**(b)** Dissociation factor leads to disassembly of initiation unit. It requires **GTP** as energy.

## Regulation of Gene Expression

Gene regulation is switching off and on of gene depending on cell requirement. Gene regulation is of two types (i) Negative and (ii) Positive. Constitutive genes are those which continuously express themselves in cells.

- **Regulation of gene expression in Eukaryotes**
  - In eukaryotes gene expression can be regulated at following levels:
    (1) At the transcriptional level: during the formation of primary transcript.
    (2) Processing level: regulation of splicing of mRNA.
    (3) Translational level
    (4) During the transport of mRNA from nucleus to the cytoplasm.
  - In general regulation of gene expression is done by the metabolic, physiological or environmental conditions.
- **Regulation of gene expression in Prokaryotes**
  - In prokaryotes gene expression is mainly regulated by the control of the rate of transcriptional initiation.
  - RNA polymerase activity at promoter site is regulated by interaction with accessory proteins to recognize the start sites. Such accessory proteins can activate (activators) or repress (repressors).
  - **Operators:** In many cases, the accessibility of promoter regions of prokaryotic DNA is regulated by the interaction of proteins with DNA sequences termed operators. In most of the operons, operator region is located adjacent to the promoter region. Sequences of the operator bind a repressor protein. Operator and repressor are specific for each operon. **Example:** In lac operon, lac operator is present only in the lac operon and it interacts specifically with lac repressor only.
- **Operon Concept**
  - Lac operon was the first transcriptionally regulated system reported by **Francois Jacob (geneticist) and Jacque Monad (biochemist) in 1961.**
  - In an operon, a group of structural genes is regulated by a common promoter and regulatory genes.
  - Operons are very common in bacteria, e.g., lac operon, trp operon, his operon, val operon, ara operon, etc.
- **Lac operon**
  - In lac operon, lac means 'lactose'.
  - Lac operon consists of
    **(1) Promotor gene:** It is the site for the attachment of RNA polymerase enzyme.
    **(2) Regulator gene:** i (i indicating inhibitor, not inducer). It code for the active repressor protein all the time therefore it is constitutive gene in lac operon.
    **(3) Operator gene (lac operator):** Active repressor protein synthesized by the regulatory gene is attached to the operator and the transcription by RNA polymerase enzyme.
    **(4) Three structural genes (polycistronic)** (z gene, y gene and a gene).

| Structural gene | Enzyme synthesized | Function of enzyme |
|---|---|---|
| z gene | $\beta$-galactosidase | $\beta$-galactosidase results in hydrolysis of the disaccharide, lactose into its monomeric units – galactose and glucose. |
| y gene | Permease | Permease increases the permeability of the cell to $\beta$-galactosides. |
| a gene | Transacetylase | Transfer of acetyl group. |

- As **lactose** regulates the switching on and off of lac operon, so it acts as **inducer (Fig 3.8)**.

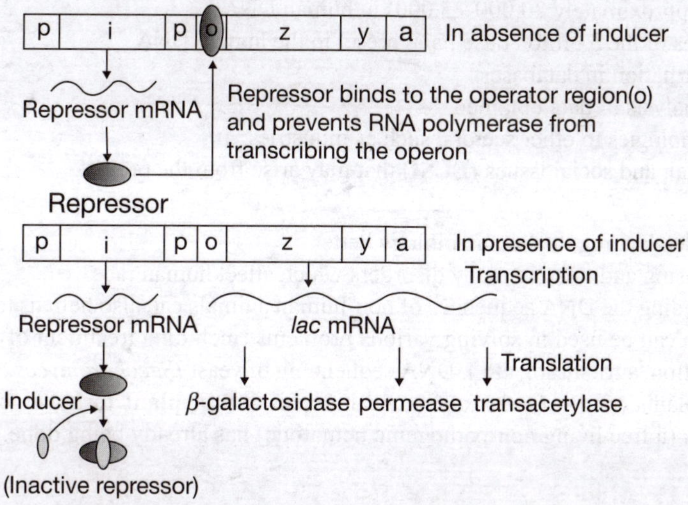


**FIGURE 3.8** Lac Operon

- Lactose is transported into the cells through the action of permease enzyme only when the glucose (preferred carbon source) is absent in the growth medium around the bacteria. Some amount of permease is always there even in the presence of glucose means low level of expression is always present.
- Absence of glucose and presence of an inducer (lactose or allolactose) ® Inducer like lactose enters the bacteria by the action of permease enzyme. Lactose interacts with the repressor and inactivates it. Operator site is free to interact with RNA polymerase and this enzyme access the promotor site. Activation of structural genes to synthesize all the required enzymes.
- Regulation of lac operon is a type of **negative regulation**. **Gratuitous inducers:** There are certain structural analogs of lactose which can induce the lac operon but are not the substrates for the enzyme β-galactosidase. Such substances are known as gratuitous inducers. Isopropylthiogalactoside (IIPTG) is a gratuitous inducer, extensively used for the study of lac operon.
- **The catabolite gene activator protein:** The cells of *E. coli* utilize glucose in preference to lactose; when both of them are present in the medium. After the depletion of glucose in the medium, utilization of lactose starts. This indicates that glucose somehow interferes with the induction of lac operon. This is explained as follows:
- The attachment of RNA polymerase to the promoter site requires the presence of a catabolite gene activator protein (CAP) bound to cyclic AMP. The presence of glucose lowers the intracellular concentration of cAMP by inactivating the enzyme adenylyl cyclase responsible for the synthesis of cAMP. Due to the diminished levels of cAMP, the formation of CAP-cAMP is low. Therefore, the binding of RNA polymerase to DNA (due to the absence of CAP-cAMP) and the transcription are almost negligible in the presence of glucose. Thus, glucose interferes with the expression of lac operon by depleting cAMP levels. Addition of exogenous cAMP is found to initiate the transcription of many inducible operons, including lac operon.
- It is now clear that the presence of CAP-cAMP is essential for the transcription of structural genes of lac operon. Thus, CAP-cAMP acts as a positive regulator for the gene expression. It is, therefore, evident that lac operon is subjected to both positive and negative regulation.

## Human Genome Project (HGP)

- Human Genome Project (HGP) was a mega project of sequencing the complete human genome.
- HGP was **launched in year 1990** and **completed in year 2003** (a 13 year project).
- This project was initially coordinated by the US Department of Energy and National Institute of Health. Initially the Welcome Trust (UK) became a major partner with some contribution from countries like Japan, France, Germany, China, etc.
- HGP is also closely associated with **Bioinformatics** for rapid development of new area of biology.

- **Goals of HGP**
  - Identify all the genes (approximately 20,000-25,000) in human DNA.
  - Determine the sequences of the 3 billion base pairs preset in the human DNA.
  - Store the collected information in databases.
  - Improve the tools for analysis of data obtained.
  - To transfer related technologies to other sectors, such as industries.
  - To solve the ethical, legal, and social issues **(ELSI)** that may arise from the project.
- **Uses of HGP**
  - HGP can help us in understanding the human biology better.
  - It will help us in diagnosing and treating many disorders which affect human race.
  - Knowing and understanding the DNA sequences of non-human animals can also help us to explore the capabilities and potential in them which can be used in solving various problems (including treatment of diseases, energy production, environmental remediation, agriculture, etc.). DNA sequencing of yeast *(Saccharomyces cerevisiae)*, bacteria (*E. coli*), Drosophila (fruitfly), plants (rice – *Oryza sativa*, Arabidopsis – **first plant to have genome sequenced**, etc.) and *Caenorhabditis elegans* (a free living non-pathogenic nematode) has already being done.
- **Methodologies**
  - Two important approaches involved in HGP are:

    (1) **Expressed Sequence Tags (ESTs):** This approach emphasize on identification of all the **genes which are expressed as RNA.**

    (2) **Sequence Annotation:** In this approach, sequencing of whole set of genome (having coding and non-coding sequences) is done. This is followed by indicating the functions of the specific part of genome.
- **Steps of sequencing according to sequence annotation approach.**
  - Isolation of total DNA from a cell and broken this DNA into small fragments (because longer DNA cannot be sequenced due technical issues).
  - Cloning of segments in suitable hosts (**bacteria** and **yeast** are commonly used hosts) by using specific vectors (e.g., **BAC-Bacterial Artificial Chromosome** and **YAC-Yeast Artificial Chromosome**). Cloning leads to amplification of segments after which they can be sequenced easily.
  - Sequencing of fragments is done by the use of **Automated DNA Sequencers**. These work on a method developed by **Frederick Sanger** (he also credit for development of method for sequencing of amino acid in proteins).
  - The sequences thus obtained are arranged on the basis of some overlapping regions present in them. Alignment of sequences is done by the help of computer programs. These sequences are annotated and assigned to a chromosome.
  - Last chromosome to be sequenced was chromosome one (in May 2006). Twenty four chromosomes are sequenced in humans.
  - Assigning the genetic and physical maps on the genome was done by using the information of Polymorphism of restriction endonuclease restriction sites and Microsatellites (some repetitive DNA sequences).
- **Salient features of Human Genome**
  - Numbers of base pairs in human genome are ¾3164.7 million.
  - Size of average gene is 3000 bases.
  - The largest gene in our body is **Duchenne muscular dystrophy** situated on X- chromosome (dystrophin and the size is 2.4 million base pairs).
  - Total number of genes in human genome is about **30,000.**
  - Functions of more >50% of the known genes is still unknown.
  - Almost all (99.9 %) nucleotide bases are exactly the same in all individuals.
  - Less than 2% of the genome codes for proteins.
  - Maximum numbers of genes are found on **chromosome one (2968)** while the minimum number of genes are found on **Y chromosome (231).** The smallest gene is of TDF (testis determining factor) present on Y- Chromosome.
  - A very large portion of the human genome is made up of repeated sequences called satellite DNA. Repeated sequences are the fragments of DNA that repeat themselves many times (even hundred to thousand times). Although these do not have any direct coding functions but they affect the chromosomal structure, dynamics and evolution.

- About **1.4 million** locations have been identified where Single-base DNA differences occur in humans. These are termed as **Single Nucleotide Polymorphism or SNPs (pronounced as 'snips')**. These provide very important information regarding disease-associated sequences and tracing human history.

## DNA Fingerprinting (DNA Typing or DNA Profiling)

- **Alec Jeffery (Father of DNA finger printing)** invented it and **Dr. Lalji (father of Indian finger printing)** started it in India.
- He used a satellite DNA (also termed as **VNTRs-Variable Number Tandem Repeats**) as a probe that was having a degree of polymorphism.
- In earlier used technique, Southern blot hybridization using radio labeled VNTR probe.
- It is a technique of determining nucleotide sequence of certain area of DNA which is unique to each individual.
- 99.9% of the base sequences are exactly same in all individuals, so only 0.1 % of the total base sequences vary in a genome. 0.1% of $3.3 \times 10^9$ bp = $3.3 \times 10^6$ bp (or about $3 \times 10^6$ bp) provide individuality to each human being.
- DNA fingerprinting provides a quick way to compare the DNA sequences of two individuals.
- DNA obtained from a single cell is sufficient to perform DNA fingerprinting.
- PCR (Polymerase chain reaction) enhances the sensitivity of this technique.
- DNA fingerprinting depends upon the identification of differences in **repetitive DNA**. Repetitive DNA is specific sequences in DNA in which a small portion of DNA is repeated many times.
- The DNA is extracted from nuclei of WBCs or spermatozoa or hair follicle cells, skin, bone and saliva.
- By **density gradient centrifugation** bulk DNA is separated a major peak while the repetitive DNA is separated as other small peaks. These small peaks are also referred as **satellite DNA (highly repetitive DNA sequences)**.
- On the basis of base composition (A : T rich or G : C rich), length of segment and the number of repetitive segments, satellite DNA is classified into many categories-**micro satellites** (they are simple sequence repeats with 1-6 base pairs and flanked by conserved sequences), **mini satellites,** etc.
- Some features of **repetitive DNA** sequences:
  (i) Show high degree of polymorphism.
  (ii) Form a large portion of human genome.
  (iii) Do not code for proteins usually.
- Uses of DNA fingerprinting:
  (i) Provide a very useful identification tool in **forensic** applications.
  (ii) Useful in solving paternity/maternity disputes (polymorphisms are also inherited from the parents to their offsprings).
  (iii) Helpful in determining the population and genetic diversities.
  (iv) Individuality.
  (v) Human lineage.
- **DNA polymorphism : Variation at genetic level**
  (i) DNA polymorphism is the basis of both in genetic mapping and DNA fingerprinting. It arises due to mutations. It plays very important role in speciation and evolution.
  (ii) DNA polymorphism refers to an **inheritable mutation** in a population with high frequency.
  (iii) DNA polymorphism can also be known to the **allelic sequence variation** in which more than one allele occur at a locus in human population with a **frequency more than 0.01**.
  (iv) Polymorphisms may range from one nucleotide to large change.
  (v) Mutations can occur in somatic cells **(somatic mutation)** and germ cells **(germinal mutation)** or both, but through germ cell mutations are transmitted to next generation.
  (vi) Mutations are usually occurring with high frequency in non-coding part and recessive; these keep on accumulating and form the basis of variability or polymorphism.

- **VNTR (Variable Number of Tandem Repeats)**
  - VNTRs belong to mini-satellites (a class of satellite DNA). Minisatellite are hypervariable repeat sequences of DNA,11-60 base pairs and flanked by conserved restriction sites.
  - These arranged in many copy numbers that varies from chromosome to chromosome.
  - Size of VNTRs – 0.1 to 20 kb.
- **Process of DNA fingerprint:**
  - Isolation of DNA (DNA from single cell is sufficient for it). Sensitivity of the technique can be increased by PCR.
  - Digestion of isolated DNA by restriction endonucleases **(molecular scissors)** into smaller DNA fragments.
  - Separation of DNA fragments according to size by electrophoresis (AGE—agarose gel electrophoresis or PAGE—polyacrylamide gel electrophoresis).
  - Transferring (or blotting) of separated DNA fragments to synthetic membranes, e.g., nitrocellulose, nylon, etc.
  - Hybridization of DNA fragments using labeled VNTR (Variable Number Tandem Repeats) probe (**Southern blot hybridization**).
  - Now a days STR (Short Tandem Repeats) are used.
  - Detection of hybridised DNA fragments by autoradiography.
  - Autoradiogram gives many bands of different sizes. These bands are in characteristic pattern for an individual DNA which differs from individual to individual in a population except for the monozygotic twins.

# PRACTICE EXERCISES

**Direction:** Read the question carefully and choose the correct option for each.

## Multiple Choice Questions: Level I

### Nucleic Acid (Structure of DNA and RNA)

**1.** What is indicated by 'A' and 'B' in the figure respectively?

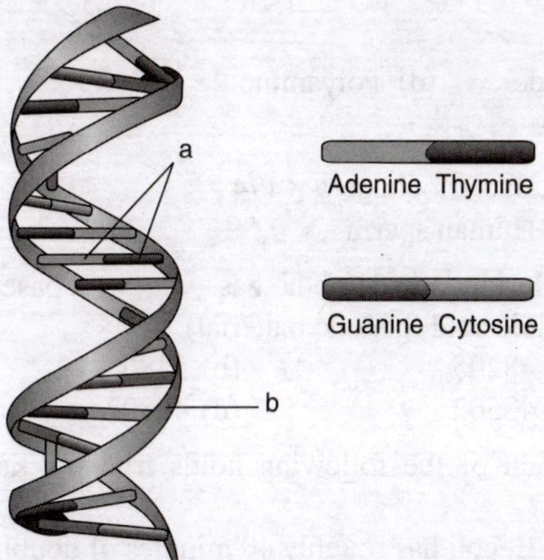


(a) Sugar and Phosphate
(b) Phosphate and Sugar
(c) Base pairs and Sugar phosphate backbone
(d) Sugar and Base pairs

**2.** Type of nucleic acids found in living organism
(a) DNA and Purine
(b) RNA and Cytosine
(c) DNA and RNA
(d) Adenine and Thymine

**3.** Which is act as genetic material in most of organisms?
(a) Deoxyribonucleic acid
(b) Ribonucleic acid
(c) Abscisic acid
(d) Indole butyric acid

**4.** DNA is genetic material in majority of organism but in some viruses which molecule can also act as genetic material?
(a) DNA (b) RNA
(c) m-RNA (d) t-RNA

**5.** Monomeric unit of nucleic acid is
(a) Nucleoside (b) Cytosine
(c) Monosaccharide (d) Nucleotide

**6.** The process of making RNA from DNA is termed as:
(a) Transaction (b) Transformation
(c) Transcription (d) Transduction

**7.** The genetic code:
(a) Is a sequence of nucleotides on rRNA
(b) Determines the sequence of amino acid in proteins
(c) Is sequence of amino acid in polypeptide
(d) Is small segment of tRNA

**8.** The process of protein synthesis in biological systems is termed as:
(a) Transaction (b) Transcription
(c) Translation (d) Transformation

**9.** DNA is a polymer of:
(a) Nucleotides (b) Ribonucleotides
(c) Nucleosides (d) Deoxyribonucleotides

**10.** Most abundant genetic material is
(a) DNA (b) RNA
(c) Protein (d) Carbohydrate

**11.** What is indicated by 'a' and 'b' given in below figure?

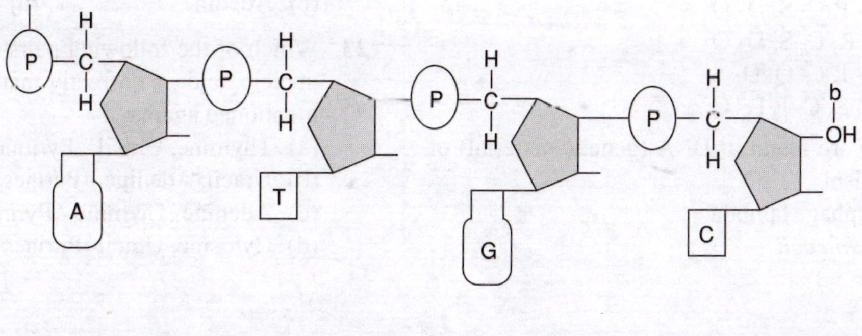

(a) 5′ Phosphate and 3′ Phosphate
(b) 3′ Phosphate and 5′ Hydroxyl
(c) 5′ Phosphate and 3′ Hydroxyl
(d) 3′ Hydroxyl and 5′ Hydroxyl

**12.** Two nucleotides are liked by 3′ – 5′ __________ linkage to form a dinucleotide.
(a) Glycosidic (b) Peptide
(c) Phosphoester (d) Phosphodiester

**13.** What does the figure represent?

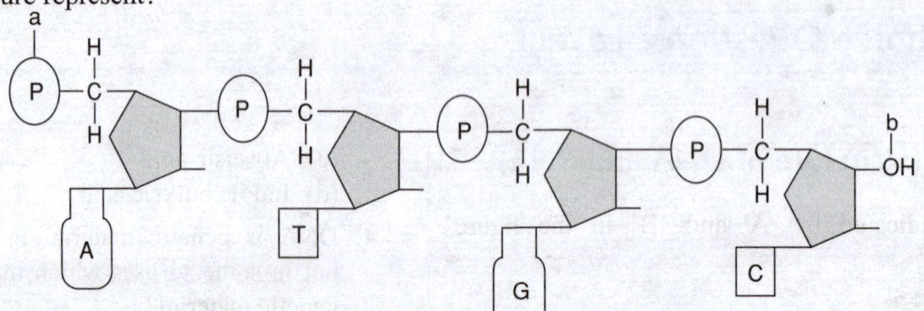


(a) Polysaccharide (b) Polynucleoside (c) Polynucleotide (d) Polyamine

**14.** Base pairs are use to define length of which biomolecule
(a) ss DNA (b) ds DNA
(c) ss RNA (d) Polypeptide

**15.** Genetic material of bacteriophage $\phi \times 174$ contain
(a) 5836 base pairs (b) 5683 nucleotides
(c) 5386 nucleotides (d) 5638 base pairs

**16.** Genetic material of bacteriophage $\phi \times 174$ is
(a) ss DNA (b) ds DNA
(c) ss RNA (d) ds RNA

**17.** Match the column I and column II and choose the correct combination from given option.

| Column I (Name of organism) | Column II (Length of genetic content) |
|---|---|
| **A.** Bacteriophage lambda | **P.** $6.6 \times 10^9$ bp |
| **B.** Diploid human cell(Nucleus) | **Q.** $4.6 \times 10^6$ bp |
| **C.** Bacteriophage $\phi \times 174$ | **R.** 48502 base pairs (bp) |
| **D.** *Escherichia coli* | **S.** 5386 nucleotides |

(a) A- R, B- P, C- S, D- Q
(b) A- P, B- R, C- S, D- Q
(c) A- R, B- P, C- Q, D- S
(d) A- R, B- S, C- P, D- Q

**18.** $4.6 \times 10^6$ bp are found in DNA (genetic material) of which organism
(a) Bacteriophage lambda
(b) *Escherichia coli*
(c) Bacteriophage $\phi \times 174$
(d) Human sperm

**19.** Bacteriophage lambda has ________ base pairs in nucleic acid (genetic material).
(a) 48205 (b) 5386
(c) 48502 (d) 45802

**20.** Which of the following holds true for Escherichia coli?
(a) E. coli has roughly 40 minutes of doubling time
(b) E. coli is a parasite in human digestive tract
(c) E. coli has $4.6 \times 10^9$ bp long genetic material
(d) E. coli has $4.6 \times 10^6$ bp long genetic material

**21.** A nucleotide has the following components:
(a) A phosphate group, Nitrogenous base, A hexose sugar
(b) A phosphorous base, Nitrogenous group, A ribose sugar
(c) A nitrogenous base, phosphate group, A ribose sugar
(d) A nitrogenous base, phosphate group, a hexose sugar

**22.** Which of the following is not a pyrimidine?
(a) Thymine (b) Uracil
(c) Adenine (d) Cytosine

**23.** Which of the following pairs of nitrogenous bases of nucleic acid ,is correctly matched with the category mentioned against it
(a) Thymine, Uracil - Pyrimidines
(b) Uracil, Adenine - Purines
(c) Adenine, Thymine - Pyrimidines
(d) Cytosine, Uracil- Purines

**24.** _______ is present in DNA only and _______ is present in RNA only:
(a) Cytosine, Thymine
(b) Thymine, Uracil
(c) Uracil, Thymine
(d) Thymine, Cytosine

**25.** A nitrogenous base is linked to the OH of 1' C pentose sugar through:
(a) Phosphoester linkage
(b) O-Glycosidic linkage
(c) Phosphodiester linkage
(d) N-Glycosidic linkage

**26.** Which pyrimidine nitrogenous base is common to both DNA and RNA?
(a) Thymine (b) Uracil
(c) Adenine (d) Cytosine

**27.** Which of the following is a nucleoside?
(a) Uridine (b) Guanine
(c) Adenine (d) Cytosine

**28.** In context of genetic material: Base + Sugar →
(a) Nucleotide (b) Nucleoside
(c) Nucleic acid (d) Nuclein

**29.** Nucleoside joins to phosphate group by which linkage
(a) Phosphoester linkage
(b) O-Glycosidic linkage
(c) Phosphodiester linkage
(d) N-Glycosidic linkage

**30.** If a segment of ds DNA contain 40 base pairs. Find out number of Phosphodiester linkage in this segment of DNA
(a) 39 (b) 78 (c) 40 (d) 20

**31.** Number of N-glycosidic linkage found in ssRNA consist of 35 nucleotides.
(a) 36 (b) 35 (c) 34 (d) 32

**32.** DNA is negatively charged because of presence of
(a) Nitrogenous base (b) Hydroxyl group
(c) Phosphate group (d) None of these

**33.** In context of genetic material, nucleotide consists of:
(a) N-base, Ribose sugar, Phosphate group
(b) N-base, Hexose sugar, Phosphate group
(c) Nucleoside + Phosphate
(d) Both (a) and (c)

**34.** Methylated Uracil is
(a) Adenine (b) Thymine
(c) Cytosine (d) Guanine

**35.** Uracil is associated with which sugar?
(a) Generally Deoxyribose
(b) Generally Ribose
(c) Only ribose
(d) Hexose

**36.** 5′- end of ribose sugar in polynucleotide chain bears.
(a) N-base (b) Deoxyribose
(c) Phosphate group (d) Hydroxyl group

**37.** 3′ end of sugar in polynucleotide chain bears:
(a) Phosphate group (b) Hydroxyl group
(c) Methyl group (d) Nitro group

**38.** Select correct matching from the following:
(a) Thymine, Uracil – pentose sugar
(b) Adenosine, Deoxythymidine – Nucleosides used for DNA synthesis
(c) Cytidine ,Uridine – Nucleotides used for RNA synthesis
(d) Deoxyguanosine, Deoxythymidine – Nucleosides used for DNA synthesis

**39.** A nucleoside differs from a nucleotide in not having
(a) Phosphate (b) Sugar
(c) Nitrogen base (d) Phosphate and sugar

**40.** In RNA, every nucleotide residue has an additional _______ group present at _______ position of ribose:
(a) $PO_4^{3-}$, 3′ (b) OH, 3′
(c) OH, 5′ (d) OH, 2'

**41.** Thymine can also be designated as:
(a) 3 - Methyl uracil
(b) 2 - Methyl uracil
(c) 4 - Methyl uracil
(d) 5 - Methyl uracil

**42.** Friedrich Meischer
(a) Identified DNA as a basic substance and named it 'Nucleotide' in 1896
(b) Identified DNA as an acidic substance and named it 'Nuclein' in 1896
(c) Identified DNA as an acidic substance and named it 'Nuclein' in 1869
(d) None of the above

**43.** J.D. Watson and F.H. Crick utilized X-ray diffraction data (to propose double helix model of DNA) produced by
(a) Rosalind Wilkins and Maurice Franklin
(b) Maurice Wilkins and Rosalind Franklin
(c) Sutton and Boveri
(d) Beadle and Tatum

**44.** In which year J.D. Watson and F.H. Crick proposed famous double helical model of DNA?
(a) 1869 (b) 1953
(c) 1935 (d) 1853

**45.** Erwin Chargaff observed that for double stranded DNA
(a) Ratios of Adenine and Cytosine and Thymine and Guanine are constant and equals one
(b) Ratios of Adenine and Thymine and Guanine and Cytosine are constant and equals one
(c) Ratios of Adenine and Guanine and Thymine and Cytosine are constant and equals one
(d) Ratios of Adenine – Guanine and Thymine – Cytosine are constant and equals one

**46.** For ds DNA
(a) A + T/G + C = 1 (b) A + G/T + C = 1
(c) A + C/U + G = 1 (d) A + G/T + U = 1

**47.** Chargaff rule is applicable to
(a) ss DNA (b) ds DNA
(c) ss RNA (d) Protein

**48.** Two strands of DNA are
(a) Supplementary (b) Complementary
(c) Perpendicular (d) Positively charged

**49.** The backbone of DNA double helix consists of:
(a) Sugar-Base
(b) Sugar-Phosphate
(c) Sugar-Hydroxyl group
(d) Sugar-Methyl group

**50.** Anti-parallel polarity is exhibited by:
(a) RNA (b) t-RNA (c) m-RNA (d) DNA

**51.** Which of the following holds true in case of DNA?
(a) A is equal to G
(b) Adenine forms two H-bond with thymine
(c) Adenine forms one π bond with thymine
(d) C is equal to T

**52.** Three H-bonds is exhibited between which DNA bases in double helix structure?
(a) Adenine, Guanine (b) Guanine, Cytosine
(c) Cytosine, Thymine (d) Adenine, Thymine

**53.** Double helix model of B-DNA has a pitch of:
(a) 0.34 nm (b) 3.4 nm
(c) 34 Å (d) Both (b) and (c)

**54.** Length of DNA with 25 base pair is
(a) 85 Å (b) 8.5 Å
(c) 78.2 Å (d) 3.4 Å

**55.** Double helix model of B-DNA proposed by Watson and Crick has how many base pairs in one turn?
(a) 9 (b) 11 (c) 12 (d) 10

**56.** Total number of nitrogen bases are present in one turn of B-DNA.
(a) 6 (b) 24 (c) 20 (d) 10

**57.** Which is responsible for approx uniform distance between two strands of DNA.
(a) Purine comes opposite to purine only.
(b) Pyrimidine comes opposite to pyrimidine.
(c) Purine comes opposite to pyrimidine.
(d) All of these.

**58.** What confers additional stability to double helix model of DNA apart from H-bond?
(a) One base pair provides inductive effect to the other
(b) One base pair is stacked over the other
(c) One base pair is perpendicular to another
(d) One base pair interacts with another base pair via steric hindrance

**59.** The length of human DNA is approximately.
(a) 2.2 meters considering all cells of body
(b) 3.1 meters considering only one cell
(c) 2.2 meters considering only one cell
(d) None of the above

**60.** Hydrolysis of nucleic acid yields
(a) Only sugar
(b) Phosphoric acid only
(c) Nitrogenous base only
(d) All the above

**61.** What is indicated by 'a' in the figure?

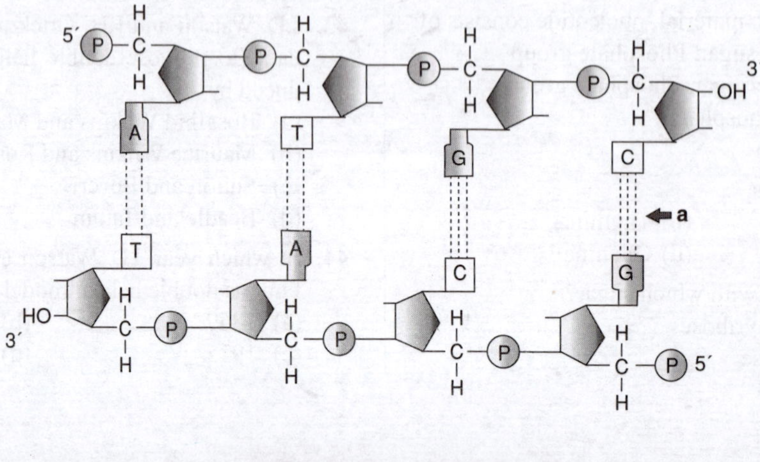

(a) H-bond (b) Ionic bond
(c) Covalent bond (d) Dative bond

**62.** t-RNA attach to larger subunit of ribosomes with the help of which loop-
(a) DHU – loop (b) T Ψ C loop
(c) Anticodon loop (d) Minor loop

**63.** In three dimensional view the molecule of t-RNA is
(a) L-shaped (b) S-shaped
(c) Y-shaped (d) E-shaped

**64.** Which form of RNA has a structure resembling clover leaf?
(a) Rrna (b) hnRNA
(c) mRNA (d) tRNA

**65.** Which of the following is formed in nucleolus
(a) r RNA (b) t RNA
(c) m-RNA (d) DNA

**66.** Correct order of molecular weight is
(a) DNA < r-RNA < t-RNA
(b) DNA < m-RNA < r-RNA
(c) t-RNA < m-RNA < DNA
(d) t-RNA < DNA < m-RNA

**67.** Which is soluble RNA:-
(a) hnRNA (b) rRNA
(c) mRNA (d) tRNA

**68.** Which is correct-
(i) t-RNA has an anticodon loop that has bases complementary to the code
(ii) t-RNA has an amino acid acceptor end
(iii) t-RNA are specific for each amino acid
(iv) For initiation, there is specific t-RNA that is referred to as initiator t-RNA
(v) For termination there is specific t-RNA that is referred to as terminator t-RNA.

(a) (i) and (ii) (b) (i) (ii) and (iii)
(c) (i), (ii), (iii), (iv) (d) (i), (ii), (iii), (iv), (v)

**69.** DNA is a preferred genetic material over RNA due to one of the following reasons:
(a) Bases are arranged linearly in a single strand
(b) Bases show less propensity of mutation
(c) 2' OH group in RNA is more labile
(d) None of the above

**70.** Which was the first genetic material?
(a) DNA (b) RNA
(c) Proteins (d) Polysaccharide

**71.** 2'OH group present at nucleotide of RNA make it
(a) More labile and easily degradable
(b) More stable and easily degradable
(c) Less labile and easily degradable
(d) Less labile and non degradable

**72.** Following are feature of RNA except
(a) RNA mutate at faster rate
(b) High reactivity
(c) Made up of ribonucleotide
(d) It is referred as Griffith's transforming principle

**73.** A molecule that can act as genetic material must fulfill which of the following criteria
(a) Power of duplication
(b) Structural and chemical stability
(c) Scope of slow change and power of expression like Mendelian characters
(d) All of these

**74.** RNA is genetic material in
(a) TMV (b) HIV
(c) QB bacteriophage (d) All of these

**75.** Find out false statement
(a) Viruses having RNA genome and having shorter life span mutate and evolve faster
(b) RNA can easily express the characters
(c) DNA is chemically and structurally more stable.
(d) Protein fulfills the criteria of replication thus act as genetic material.

**76.** Which criteria for substance can be act as genetic material is not fulfilled by protein
(a) Power of duplication
(b) Structural and chemical stability
(c) Scope of slow change(mutation)
(d) Power of expression like Mendelian characters

## Packaging of DNA

**77.** DNA is held together by which proteins in prokaryotes?
(a) Negatively charged proteins
(b) Positively charged proteins
(c) Amphoteric proteins
(d) Histone proteins

**78.** Which statement is true in the context of histone?
(a) They are positively charged acidic proteins
(b) They are positively charged amphoteric protein
(c) They are positively charged basic proteins
(d) They are polysaccharides.

**79.** In a nucleosome, histones are organized in which structure?
(a) Octamer (b) Hexamer
(c) Decamer (d) Septamer

**80.** The initial structure formed at the beginning of coiling of DNA around histones is:

(a) Nuclein (b) Solenoid
(c) Nucleosome (d) Chromatin

**81.** Histones are rich in which amino acid?
(a) Methionine, Arginine
(b) Lysine, Arginine
(c) Lysine, Proline
(d) Methionine, Lysine

**82.** Typical nucleosome consists of how many base pairs:
(a) 190 (b) 200
(c) 300 (d) 310

**83.** E.coli has $4.6 \times 10^6$ bp in its DNA, how many nucleosomes are found in E.coli?
(a) $4.6 \times 10^6$ (b) $2.3 \times 10^5$
(c) $2.3 \times 10^4$ (d) Zero

**84.** Following are found in nucleus of mammalian cell
(a) Ergosomes (b) Nucleoid
(c) Centrosome (d) Nucleosome

**85.** Chromatin is a repeating unit of:
(a) Centromere (b) Nucleoid
(c) Centrosome (d) Nucleosome

**86.** 'Beads - on - string' structure of nucleosome in chromatin can be viewed under
(a) Light microscope
(b) Compound microscope
(c) Confocal Laser microscope
(d) Electron microscope

**87.** 'Beads - on - string' structure in chromatin is packaged to form _______.
(a) Nucleosome
(b) Solenoids
(c) Chromatin fibers
(d) Chromatids

**88.** Chromatin fibers coil and condense at ______ stage of cell division to form ______.
(a) Prophase, Nucleosome
(b) Telophase, Solenoid
(c) Metaphase, Chromosome
(d) Anaphase, Chromatid

**89.** Apart from histones, chromatin at higher level of coiling requires which proteins?
(a) Only sulphur containing proteins
(b) Only aromatic amino acid containing proteins
(c) Non histone chromosomal proteins
(d) Only acidic amino acid containing proteins

**90.** In the nucleus, the region of chromatin which is loosely packed known as:
(a) Heterochromatin (b) Chromatin fibers
(c) Euchromatin (d) Chromosome

**91.** Which is the true about the structure of Heterochromatin?
(a) Loosely packed; Stain light
(b) Loosely packed; Stain dark
(c) Densely packed; Stain light
(d) Densely packed; Stain dark

**92.** Which part of chromatin is transcriptionally active
(a) Heterochromatin (b) Nucleosome
(c) Euchromatin (d) Chromosome

**93.** Which of the following is genetically inert and does not transcribe messenger RNA for protein synthesis
(a) DNA of euchromatin
(b) DNA of heterochromatin
(c) DNA of euchromatin and heterochromatin
(d) None of the above

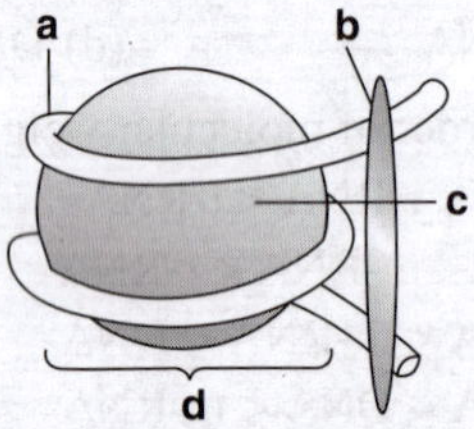


**94.** The above diagram shows an essential biomolecule (C) associated with which cell organelle?
(a) Endoplasmic reticulum
(b) Ribosome
(c) Nucleus
(d) Golgi complex

**95.** What is indicated by A ,B ,C in the above figure given in above question?
(a) RNA, DNA , H1 histone
(b) DNA, H1 histone, Core of Histone molecule
(c) Histone octamer, DNA ,RNA
(d) H1 histone ,RNA ,DNA

**96.** The whole structure indicated in the figure given in question 94 is of _______.
(a) Chromosome (b) Nucleolus
(c) Nucleosome (d) Solenoid

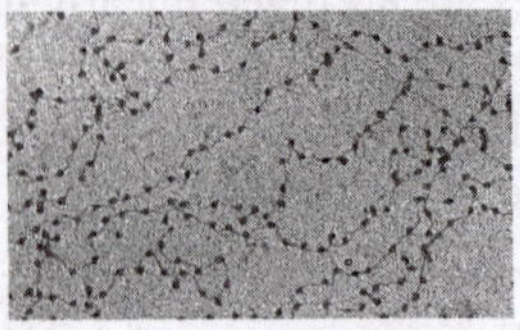

**97.** The above picture in diagram is taken using _______ microscope.
(a) Phase contrast (b) Electron
(c) Bright field (d) Fluorescence

**98.** The picture shown in diagram have characteristic coiling of DNA is known as ______.
(a) Strings-on-beads (b) beads-on-strings
(c) Nano-bead coiling (d) None of the above

## Experiment for DNA as Genetic Material

**99.** Transformation experiments in search of genetic material was performed by:
(a) G.J. Mandel (b) T.H. Morgan
(c) F. Griffith (d) F.H. Crick

**100.** Griffith carried out his experiments in mice using which pathogenic bacterium?
(a) *Haemophilus influenza*
(b) *Corynebacterium diphtheria*
(c) *Streptococcus pneumoniae*
(d) *Yersinia pestis*

**101.** In Griffith's experiment, heat killed S-strain when injected into mice resulted in ______.
(a) Diseased condition only
(b) Death only
(c) Animal survives
(d) Hybrid formation

**102.** The transforming principle in Griffith's experiment was detected:
(a) When live S-strain of S. pneumonia were injected in R stain
(b) When live R-strain of S. pneumonia were injected in S strain
(c) When heat killed R-strain of S. pneumonia were injected in s strain
(d) When heat killed S-strain of S. pneumonia were injected in R strain

**103.** Oswald Avery, Colin MacLeod and Mc Carty (1933–44) worked to determine the ______ nature of 'transforming principle' in Griffith's experiment?
(a) Physical (b) Morphological
(c) Structural (d) Biochemical

**104.** RNA digesting enzymes are commonly known as:
(a) Ribozymes (b) Ribosomes
(c) RNases (d) Ribulose

**105.** What is the difference between DNAs and DNase?
(a) Genetic material–DNA digesting enzyme
(b) DNA digesting enzyme–Genetic material
(c) Protein–Peptide
(d) None of the above

**106.** The experiment which provides unequivocal proof that DNA is genetic material came from the experiment of:
(a) Watson and Crick
(b) Wilkins and Franklin
(c) Hershey and Chase
(d) Avery, MacLeod and Maclyn McCarty

**107.** In the Hershey – Chase experiments the following isotopes were used
(a) $^{32}S$, $^{30}P$ (b) $^{31}S$, $^{29}P$
(c) $^{35}S$, $^{32}P$ (d) $^{34}S$, $^{33}P$

**108.** Hershey – Chase experiment shows following steps chronologically:
(a) Blending, Infection, Centrifugation
(b) Centrifugation, Infection, Blending
(c) Infection, Centrifugation, Blending
(d) Infection, Blending, Centrifugation

**109.** In Hershey – Chase experiment, $^{35}S$ labeled ______ and $^{32}P$ labeled ______ respectively.
(a) Bacteria, DNA (b) DNA, Protein
(c) Protein, DNA (d) DNA, m-RNA

**110.** "It has not escaped our notice that the specific pairing we have postulated immediately suggests a possible copying mechanism for the genetic material." This was a statement of
(a) Wilkins and Franklin
(b) Hershey and Chase
(c) Avery, McLeod, McCarty
(d) Watson and Crick

**111.** Which experiment is shown in the figure?

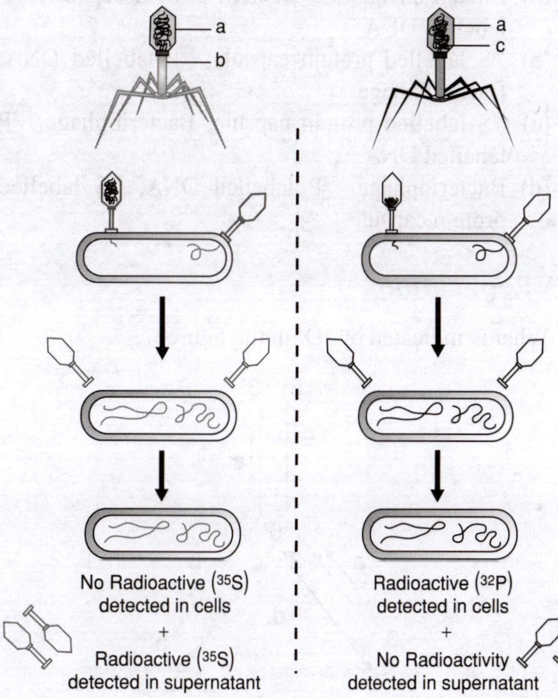

(a) Griffith's experiment
(b) Avery, Mc Leod and Mc Carty
(c) Hershey-Chase experiment
(d) Meselson and Stahl experiment

**112.** What is indicated by A, B and C in the figure?

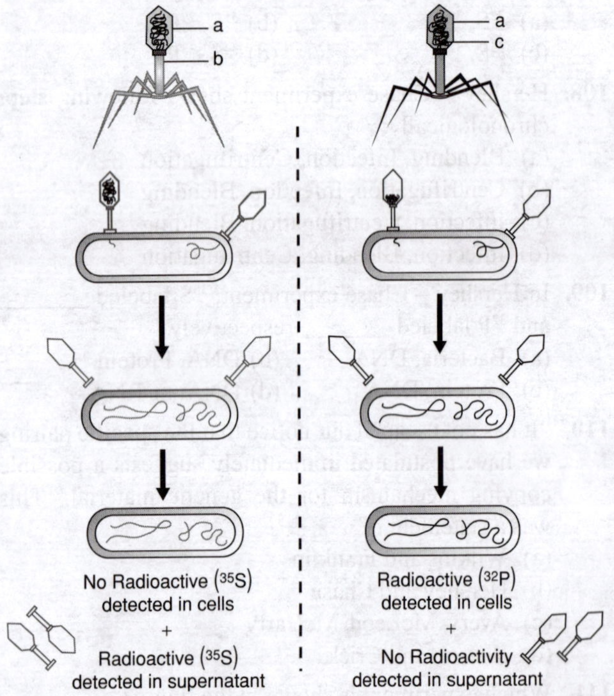


(a) Bacteriophage, $^{35}S$ labelled protein capsule, $^{32}P$ labelled DNA
(b) $^{35}S$ labelled protein capsule, $^{32}P$ labelled DNA, Bacteriophage
(c) $^{35}S$ labelled protein capsule, Bacteriophage, $^{32}P$ labelled DNA
(d) Bacteriophage, $^{32}P$ labelled DNA, $^{35}S$ labelled protein capsule

## DNA Replication

**113.** What is indicated by 'D' in the figure?

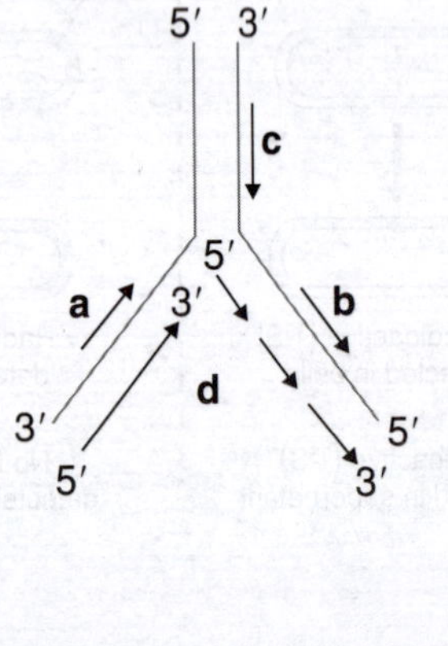


(a) Continuous synthesis
(b) Newly synthesized strands
(c) Template DNA
(d) Parental strand of DNA

**114.** After replication, each DNA molecule has one parental and one newly synthesized strand. This scheme is referred to as:
(a) Fully conservative (b) Mutation
(c) Crossing – over (d) Semi conservative

**115.** Proposed mechanism for DNA replication was
(a) Conservative (b) Semi-conservative
(c) Dispersive (d) All of these

**116.** Semiconservative replication of DNA was demonstrated by:
(a) Meselson and Stahl
(b) Watson and Crick
(c) Hershey and Chase
(d) Wilkins and Franklin

**117.** In Meselson and Stahl experiment, E. coli was grown in a medium containing:
(a) $^{40}KCl$ (b) $^{24}NaCl$
(c) $^{15}NH_4Cl$ (d) CsCl

**118.** In Meselson and Stahl, experiment $^{15}N$ can only be differentiated on basis of:
(a) Radioactivity
(b) Radioactive $t_{1/2}$
(c) Physical observation
(d) Density gradient

**119.** Taylor and his colleagues used which plant to detect distribution of newly synthesized DNA?
(a) Pisum Sativum (b) Mirabilis jalapa
(c) Vicia faba (d) Triticum aestivum

**120.** Taylor and his colleagues used which radioactive probe to detect distribution of newly synthesized DNA in chromosomes:
(a) Thymine (b) Ademine
(c) Guanine (d) Cytosine

**121.** Assuming that 50 heavy (i.e., containing $N^{15}$) DNA molecule replicated twice in a medium containing $N^{14}$, we expect
(a) 100 half heavy and half light and 150 light DNA molecules
(b) 100 half heavy and half light and 100 light DNA molecules
(c) 50 heavy and 150 light DNA molecules
(d) 50 heavy and 100 light DNA molecules

**122.** The enzyme which shows polymerizing activity in 5′ → 3′ direction is:

(a) DNA polymerase III
(b) DNA polymerase II
(c) DNA polymerase I
(d) All of these

**123.** DNA polymerase I is involved in:-
(a) Removal of RNA primer
(b) Filling of gap
(c) Joining of okazaki fragments
(d) Both (a) and (b)

**124.** DNA replication in lagging strand of most of the eukaryotic organisms is:
(a) Conservative and continous
(b) Semi-conservative but discontinuous
(c) Conservative and semi-discontinous
(d) Semi-conservative but continous

**125.** In process of replication deoxyribonucleoside triphosphate
(a) Acting as substrate
(b) Providing energy for polymerization reaction
(c) Acting as an enzyme
(d) Both (a) and (b)

**126.** DNA polymerase is needed for
(a) Replication of DNA
(b) Synthesis of DNA
(c) Elongation of DNA
(d) All of above

**127.** The process of replication of DNA in E. coli requires an enzyme referred to as:
(a) RNA dependent DNA polymerase
(b) RNA polymerase
(c) DNA dependent DNA polymerase
(d) DNA ligase

**128.** E. coli completes replication in approximately
(a) 15 min (b) 20 min
(c) 18 min (d) 40 min

**129.** Generation time in E.coli.is
(a) 15 min (b) 20 min
(c) 18 min (d) 40 min

**130.** Deoxyribonucleotide triphosphate serves dual purpose of _______ and _______ in process of replication of DNA.
(a) Enzyme, Substrate
(b) Catalyst, Substrate
(c) Substrate, Energy provider
(d) Energy, Mutage provider

**131.** The average rate of polymerization process of deoxyribonucleotides in E. coli DNA replication process is:
(a) 2500 bp/s (b) 4295 bp/s
(c) 3000 bp/s (d) 3500 bp/s

**132.** DNA dependent DNA polymerase catalyze polymerization in _______ direction only (in terms of newly synthesized strands)
(a) $5 \rightarrow 3$ (b) $3' \rightarrow 5'$
(c) $5' \rightarrow 3'$ (d) $3 \rightarrow 5$

**133.** Discontinuously synthesized strands of DNA adjacent to _______ DNA template are joined together by _______.
(a) $5' \rightarrow 3'$, DNA endonucleace
(b) $3' \rightarrow 5'$, DNAase
(c) $3' \rightarrow 5'$, DNA ligase
(d) $5' \rightarrow 3'$, DNA ligase

**134.** During which phase of the cell cycle does replication of DNA takes place in eukaryotes?
(a) $G_1$ (b) $G_0$ (c) S (d) $G_2$

**135.** Which experiment is shown in the above figure?

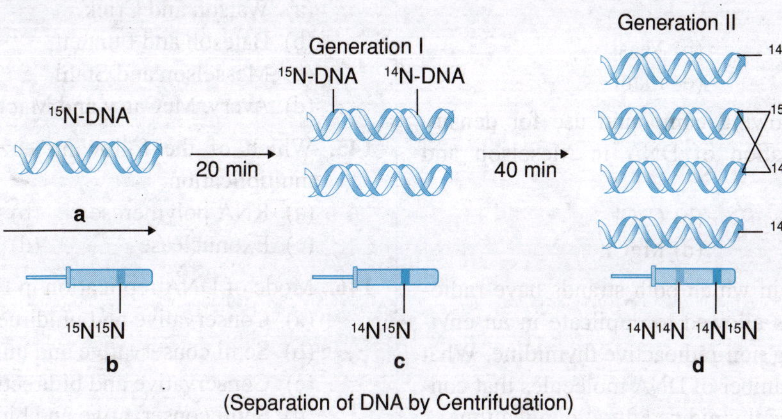

(Separation of DNA by Centrifugation)

(a) Griffith's experiment (1928)
(b) Hershay and Chase experiment (1952)
(c) Meselson and Stahl experiment (1958)
(d) Watson and Crick experiment

**137.** What is indicated by A, B,C and D in the figure?

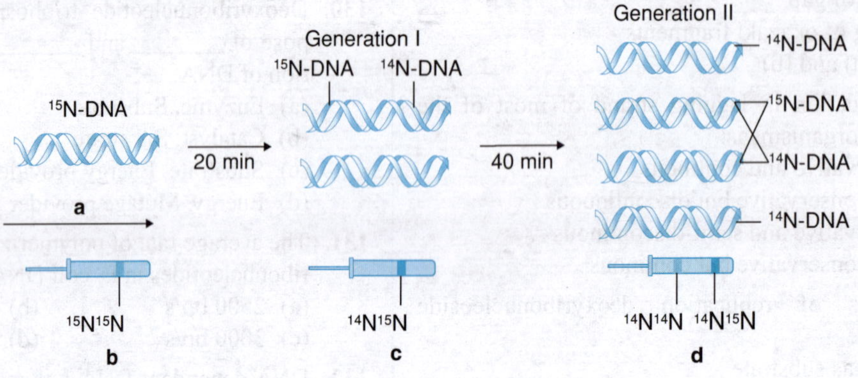

(Separation of DNA by Centrifugation)

(a) Centrifugal force, Heavy, Hybrid and light hybrid
(b) Centripetal force, Heavy, Hybrid and light hybrid
(c) Gravitational force, Heavy, Hybrid and light hybrid
(d) Radioactive force, Heavy, Hybrid and light hybrid

**138.** Following is the sequence of nucleotides of a fragment of DNA molecule.

5′GCCATTG...ACTAAGCATA3′
3′CGGTAAC...TGATTCGTAT5′

The most appropriate primer for replication of the above fragment shall be:
(a) 5′UAUG3′ and 5′GCCA3′
(b) 5′TATG3′ and 5′ACCG3′
(c) 5′GCCU3′ and 5′TATG3′
(d) 5′UGGA3′ and 5′GTAT3′

**139.** DNA replicates semiconservatively was shown first in which organism
(a) Bacteria (b) Yeast
(c) Algae (d) Plant

**140.** Which of the following compound use for density gradient centrifugation of DNA in Meselson and Stahl's experiment
(a) NaCl (b) CsCl
(c) $BeCl_2$ (d) $MgCl_2$

**141.** A DNA molecule in which both strands have radioactive thymidine is allowed to duplicate in an environment containing non-radioactive thymidine. What will be the exact number of DNA molecules that contains the radioactive thymidine after 4 duplications-
(a) One (b) Two
(c) Four (d) Eight

**136.** In Meselson and Stahl's experiment, heavy isotope $^{15}$N was used in the form of
(a) $Na^{15}NO_3$ (b) $^{15}NH_4Cl$
(c) $H^{15}NO_3$ (d) $^{15}NH_4NO_3$

**142.** A bacterium with completely radioactive DNA was allowed to replicate in a non-radioactive medium for three generation what % of the bacteria should contain radioactive DNA
(a) 100 % (b) 50 %
(c) 25 % (d) 12.5 %

**143.** During replication of a bacterial chromosomes DNA synthesis starts from a replication origin site and
(a) RNA primers are not involved
(b) Is facilitated by telomerase
(c) Moves in one direction of the site
(d) Moves in bi-directional way

**144.** Semiconservative replication of DNA was given by
(a) Watson and Crick
(b) Bateson and Punnett
(c) Messelson and Stahl
(d) Avery, McCarty and Macleod

**145.** Which of the following enzyme is used in DNA multiplication
(a) RNA polymerase (b) DNA endonuclease
(c) Exonuclease (d) DNA polymerase

**146.** Mode of DNA replication in E.Coli is
(a) Conservative and unidirectional
(b) Semi conservative and unidirectional
(c) Conservative and bidirectional
(d) Semi conservative and bidirectional

**147.** In DNA replication, the primer is
(a) A small deoxyribonucleotide polymer
(b) A small ribonucleotide polymer
(c) Helix destabilizing protein
(d) Enzyme taking part in joining nucleotides of new strand

**148.** Replication fork is
(a) Large opening of the DNA helix
(b) Small opening of the DNA helix
(c) Tightly coiled part of DNA helix
(d) Loosely coiled part of DNA helix

**149.** Which one statement regarding "Okazaki fragment" is correct
(a) These are double helical fragments of DNA
(b) These are single stranded fragments of DNA
(c) These are fragments of mRNA
(d) These are fragments of tRNA

**150.** Region in E.coli where replication originate is known as
(a) Promoter
(b) Terminator
(c) ORI (origin of replication)
(d) Regulator sequence

**151.** Failure of cell division after DNA replication results in
(a) Aneuploidy (b) Polyploidy
(c) Translocation (d) Duplication

## Central Dogma of Molecular Biology (Flow of Genetic Information: Transcription and Translation) Central Dogma

**152.** Who proposed central dogma in molecular biology.
(a) Francis Crick (b) Frederick Griffith
(c) Hershey and Chase (d) Oswald Avery

**153.** The central dogma of protein synthesis is
(a) DNA $\xrightarrow{\text{Translation}}$ m – RNA $\xrightarrow{\text{Transcription}}$ protein
(b) DNA $\xrightarrow{\text{Transcription}}$ m – RNA $\xrightarrow{\text{Translation}}$ protein
(c) RNA $\xrightarrow{\text{Replication}}$ DNA $\xrightarrow{\text{Transcription}}$ protein
(d) RNA $\xrightarrow{\text{Transcription}}$ m RNA $\xrightarrow{\text{Translation}}$ Protein

**154.** The processes by which mRNA is made by DNA and protein by mRNA are respectively called as
(a) Transcription and translation
(b) Translation and transcription
(c) Synthesis of mRNA and protein
(d) Replication of mRNA and protein

**155.** 'Central Dogma' was proposed by
(a) Crick
(b) Beadle and Tatum
(c) Temin and Baltimore
(d) Klug

**156.** Reverse transcription is shown by?
(a) HIV (b) E. coli
(c) Bacillus subtilis (d) Plasmodium

**157.** Correct representation of centrae dogma is as follows:
(a)
DNA $\xrightarrow{\text{Transcription}}$ mRNA $\xrightarrow{\text{Transformation}}$ Protein
(b)
DNA $\xrightarrow{\text{Transcription}}$ (mRNA) $\xrightarrow{\text{Translation}}$ Proteins
(c)
Replication
(DNA) $\xrightarrow{\text{Transcription}}$ mRNA $\xrightarrow{\text{Transformation}}$ Proteins
(d)
Replication
(DNA) $\xrightarrow{\text{Transcription}}$ mRNA $\xrightarrow{\text{Translation}}$ Proteins

**158.** Which of the unusual metabolic process is shown by viruses?
(a) DNA to RNA (b) RNA to DNA
(c) Proteins to RNA (d) None of these

**159.** RNA $\rightarrow$ DNA is termed as:
(a) Reverse translation
(b) Reverse replication
(c) Reverse transcription
(d) Reverse transformation

## Transcription

**160.** The process of copying genetic information from DNA to RNA is known as:
(a) Translation
(b) Transduction
(c) Transcription
(d) Transformation

**161.** Portion of gene which is transcribed but not translated
(a) Exon (b) Intron
(c) cistron (d) codon

**162.** What is indicated by A,B,C,D,E in below figure?

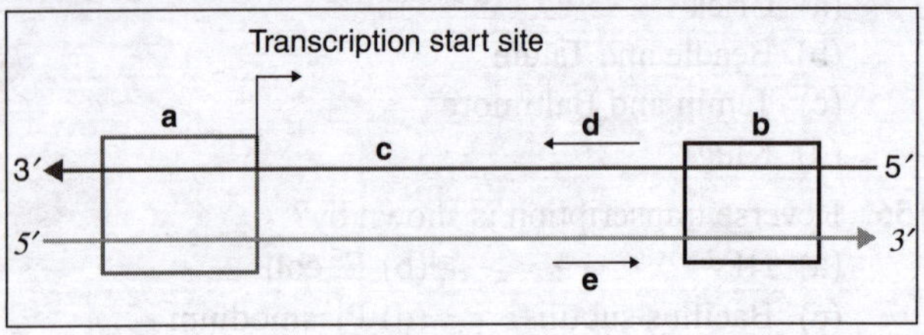


(a) Promoter, Terminator, Structural gene, Template strand ,Coding strand
(b) Promoter, Terminator, Structural gene, Coding strand ,Template strand
(c) Promoter, Terminator, Template strand , Structural gene, Coding strand
(d) Promoter, Template strand ,Terminator, Structural gene, Coding strand

**163.** RNA polymerase bind to which region of DNA to start the process of transcription

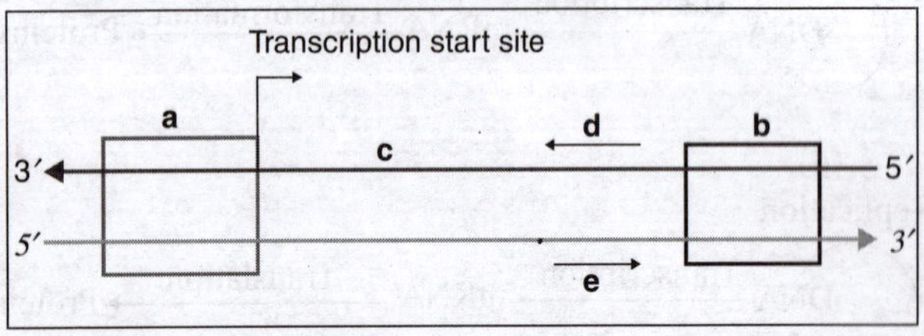


(a) B (b) D (c) A (d) E

**164.** What is indicated by 'A' and 'B' in the figure?

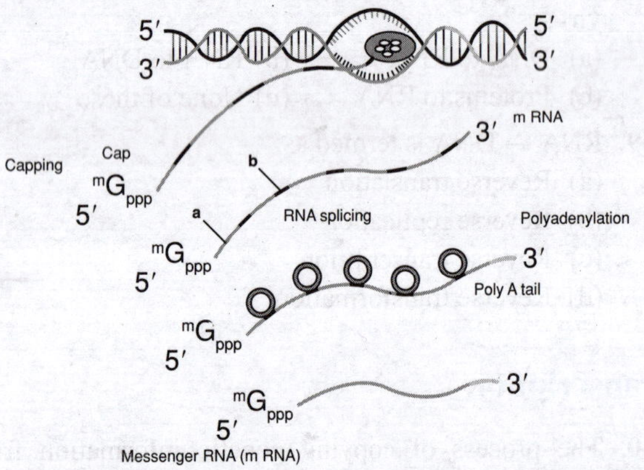


(a) Recon and Muton (b) Cistron and Muton
(c) Introns and Exons (d) Exon and Introns

**165.** In the process of transcription, the strand of DNA with polarity ________ acts as a ________ strand.
(a) $3' \rightarrow 5'$, Coding strand
(b) $3' \rightarrow 5'$, Template strand
(c) $3' \rightarrow 5'$, Sense strand
(d) $5' \rightarrow 3'$, Template strand

**166.** The promoter and ________ flank the structural gene in a transcription unit:
(a) Structure (b) Regulator
(c) Operator (d) Terminator

**167.** A segment of DNA coding for a polypeptide is termed as ________.
(a) Intron (b) Exon
(c) Cistron (d) Muton

**168.** The coding sequences of DNA are known as ________ and the intervening sequences are known as ________ respectively:
(a) Exon, Intron (b) Intron, Exon
(c) Cistron, Exon (d) Exon, Cistron

**169.** The base sequence for a nucleic acid segment is given CAG, AGG, CGA, CCA. From this, it can definitely be concluded that it is a segment of
(a) DNA strand (b) m-RNA strand
(c) t-RNA strand (d) Data not sufficient

**170.** What are the components required for the initiation of transcription in bacteria?
(a) RNA polymerase only
(b) Promoter, RNA polymerase and $\sigma$–factor
(c) RNA polymerase, $\rho$ factor only
(d) $\sigma$ factor only

**171.** $\rho$-factor in the process of transcription in bacteria is also known as:
(a) Initiation factor
(b) Elongation factor
(c) Termination factor
(d) Vital factor

**172.** In bacteria, in context of m-RNA which of the following is not true?
(a) Transcription and translation takes place in different compartment
(b) Post-transcriptional modifications are required
(c) Translation occurs after completion of transcription only
(d) All of these

**173.** Total number of different type of RNA polymerase found in eukaryotes is:
(a) 3 (b) 4
(c) 2 (d) 5

**174.** RNA polymerase II helps in transcription of
(a) t-RNA (b) r-RNA
(c) sn-RNA (d) hn RNA

**175.** RNA polymerase I transcribes ________ in eukaryotes.
(a) t- RNA (b) r- RNA
(c) sn- RNA (d) hn RNA

**176.** In eukaryotes, RNA polymerase III is responsible for synthesis of:
(a) 28 S RNA, 18 S RNA and 5.8 S RNA
(b) t-RNA, hnRNA, r-RNA
(c) t-RNA, 5SRNA, sn RNA
(d) hnRNA, t-RNA, r-RNA

**177.** The intervening sequences in the primary transcript of m-RNA are removed by:
(a) Recombination
(b) Linkage
(c) Capping
(d) Splicing

**178.** Additional post-transcriptional processing like capping and tailing is characteristic to:
(a) r-RNA (b) hnRNA
(c) snRNA (d) t-RNA

**179.** In a post-transcriptional modification, capping adds an unusual nucleotide like:
(a) Guanosine triphosphate
(b) Methyl gunanine triphosphate
(c) Methyl guanosine triphosphate
(d) Adenosine triphosphate

**180.** In a post transcriptional modification called tailing, ______ residues are added at the ______ end of hn-RNA. Respectively:
(a) Adenylate, 5′- end (b) Guanylate, 3′- end
(c) Adenylate, 3′- end (d) Guanylate, 5′- end

**181.** Fully process hn RNA is referred as
(a) m-RNA (b) t-RNA
(c) r-RNA (d) sn RNA

**182.** What is indicated by A, B, D, G and H in figure?

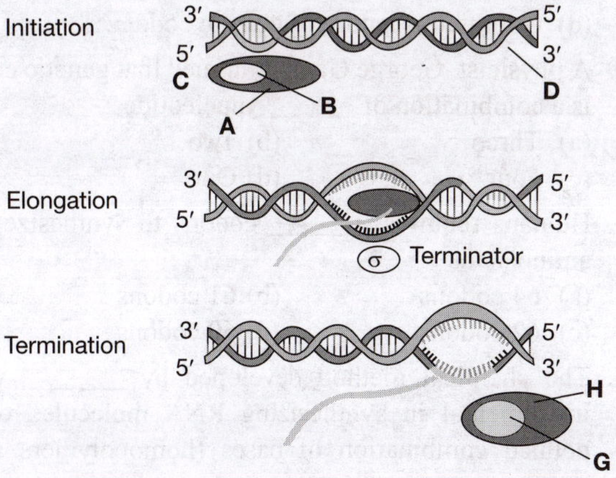


(a) RNA polymerase, Sigma factor, DNA helix
(b) Sigma factor, RNA polymerase, DNA helix Promoter, Terminator
(c) DNA helix, Sigma factor, RNA polymerase RNA, DNA helix
(d) Promoter, Sigma factor, RNA polymerase Promoter, Terminator

**183.** What is indicated by G and H in the figure?

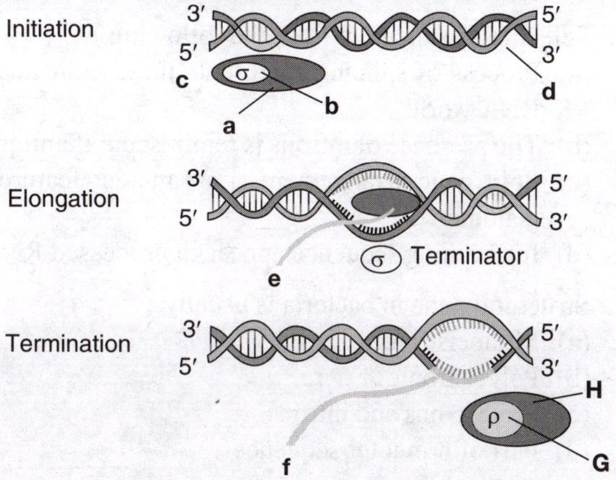


(a) Rho factor and RNA Polymerase
(b) RNA and DNA helix
(c) DNA helix and RNA Polymerase
(d) Promoter and Terminator

**184.** Messenger RNA is produced in
(a) Nucleus
(b) Golgi apparatus
(c) Endoplasmic reticulum
(d) Ribosomes

**185.** Following process takes place in nucleus of eukaryotic cell except
(a) splicing (b) transcription
(c) replication (d) translation

**186.** Select incorrect statement
(a) The DNA sequence coding for t-RNA and r-RNA also defined as gene
(b) Structural gene is eukaryote is mostly monocistronic
(c) DNA dependent RNA polymerase catalyze the polymerization in one direction only
(d) Both the strands of DNA copied during transcription

**187.** Transcription unit is consists of
(a) A Promoter (b) The structural gene
(c) A terminator (d) All of these

**188.** Why both the strands of DNA do not act as template during process of transcription.
(a) Similar m-RNA are formed by both the strand of DNA

(b) Complementary RNAs are synthesized and forms dsRNA and RNA doesn't undergo process of translation.
(c) One segment of DNA code for same proteins
(d) RNA polymerase polymerizes in 5′-3′ direction only.

**189.** Select false statement from the following
(a) Process of splicing represents the dominance of RNA world
(b) The presence of introns is reminiscent if antiquity
(c) Split gene arrangement is an ancient feature of genome
(d) Intervening sequence appear in processed RNA

**190.** Structural gene in bacteria is usually
(a) Monocistronic
(b) Polycistronic
(c) Have exons and introns
(d) Part of promoter sequence

**191.** Find out incorrect statement
(a) Inheritance of character is also affected by promoter and regulator gene
(b) Split gene arrangement is found in eukaryotes
(c) Coding or expressed sequences are known as exons
(d) RNA polymerase II is responsible for transcription of sn RNAs

**192.** The following is a list of events in synthesis of protein from a DNA template.
(i) mRNA attaches to the ribosome.
(ii) The amino acid is attached to the growing polypeptide by a peptide bond.
(iii) mRNA migrates from the nucleus to the cytoplasm.
(iv) An aminoacyl tRNA binds to its specific codon on mRNA.
(v) mRNA is transcribed from its DNA template.

Identify the correct sequence from the following options.
(a) v – iii – i – iv – ii (b) v – ii – i – iii – iv
(c) v – iii – iv – ii – i (d) v – iii – ii – iv – i

**193.** Split gene arrangement is found in
(a) HIV (b) *E.coli*
(c) Yeast (d) *B.thuringienesis*

**194.** Transcription and translation can be couple in
(a) Yeast (b) Chlorella
(c) E.coli (d) Mosquito

**195.** Following are part of post transcriptional modification except
(a) Capping of $^{met}$ GTP at 5′end
(b) Tailing by 200-300 adenylate residues at 3′ end
(c) Above process occur in a template independent manner
(d) exons are removed and introns are joined in defined order during splicing

**196.** The enzyme responsible for transcription is
(a) DNA polymerase-I
(b) RNA polymerase
(c) Reverse transcriptase
(d) DNA polymerase-II

**197.** Transcription of DNA is aided by
(a) RNA polymerase (b) DNA polymerase
(c) Exo nuclease (d) Recombinase

**198.** If the base sequence in DNA is 5′AAAAA 3′ then the base sequence in m-RNA is
(a) 5′ UUUUU 3′ (b) 3′ UUUUU 5′
(c) 5′ AAAAA 3′ (d) 3′ TTTTT 5′

## Genetic Code and Translation and Mutations

**199.** The arrangement of three bases in the genetic code signifies a specific
(a) Protein (b) Amino acid
(c) Plasmid (d) Nucleic acid

**200.** Which of the following bases is absent in the coding dictionary
(a) Uracil (b) Thymine
(c) Cytosine (d) Adenine

**201.** When more than one codon code for the same amino acid, this is called as
(a) Universal nature of genetic code
(b) Redundancy of genetic code
(c) Punctuation in genetic code
(d) Continuous nature of genetic code

**202.** A physicist, George Gamow, argued that genetic code is a combination of ________ nucleotides:
(a) Three (b) Two
(c) Four (d) One

**203.** Humans requires ________ codons to synthesize 20 amino acids
(a) 64 codons (b) 61 codons
(c) 62 codons (d) 60 codons

**204.** The chemical method developed by _______ was instrumental in synthesizing RNA molecules with defined combination of bases (homopolymers and copolymers):
(a) Marshal Nirenberg
(b) George Gamow
(c) Har Gobind Khorana
(d) F.H.C. Crick

**205.** ______ cell–free system for protein synthesis finally helped the genetic code to be deciphered:
(a) George Gamow (b) Marshal Nirenberg
(c) Har Gobind Khorana (d) J.D. Watson

**206.** Some amino acids are coded by more than one codon. Hence the genetic code exhibits:
(a) Specificity (b) Selectivity
(c) Degeneracy (d) Universality

**207.** The codon AUG has dual function as it codes for ______ and also act as a ______ codon.
(a) Phenylalanine, Initiator
(b) Methionine, Terminator
(c) Methionine, Regulator
(d) Methionine, Initiator

**208.** Sickle cell anaemia is a classic example of:
(a) Frame shift mutation
(b) Point mutation
(c) Deletion mutation
(d) Duplication mutation

**209.** In sickle cell anaemia, which amino acid modification occurs in the β-chain of amino acid?
(a) Valine → Glutamate
(b) Threonine → Valine
(c) Tyrosine → Glutamate
(d) Glutamate → Valine

**210.** t-RNA was earlier called
(a) Adapter molecule
(b) Special RNA
(c) Protein carrying RNA
(d) Soluble RNA

**211.** For the initiation of translation process, specific t-RNA involved are known as:
(a) Helper t-RNA (b) Assistor t-RNA
(c) Initiator t-RNA (d) Terminal t-RNA

**212.** The process of polymerization of amino acids to polypeptide is known as:
(a) Transduction (b) Transcription
(c) Translation (d) Transformation

**213.** Charging of t-RNA is also known as:
(a) Acylation (b) Transmination
(c) Amino allylation (d) Amino acylation

**214.** t-RNA for serine bears anticodon______.
(a) AUG (b) UAC (c) UCA (d) UGA

**215.** The structure of t-RNA resembles which leaf?
(a) Olive (b) Neem (c) Clove (d) Clover

**216.** Ribosomes are the cellular factory for synthesis of ______.
(a) Carbohydrates (b) Enzymes
(c) Proteins (d) Lipids

**217A.** Which amino acid is indicated by 'A' and 'B' in the figure?

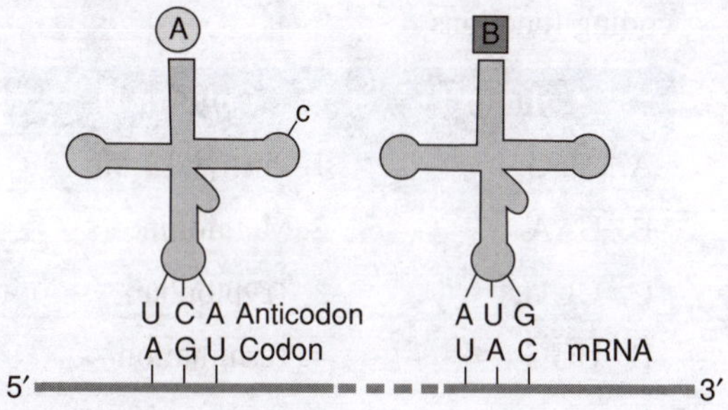


(a) Threonine and Serine
(b) Serine and Tyrosine
(c) Tyrosine and Methionine
(d) Methionine and Tyrosine

**217B.** Identify A, B , C in below diagram

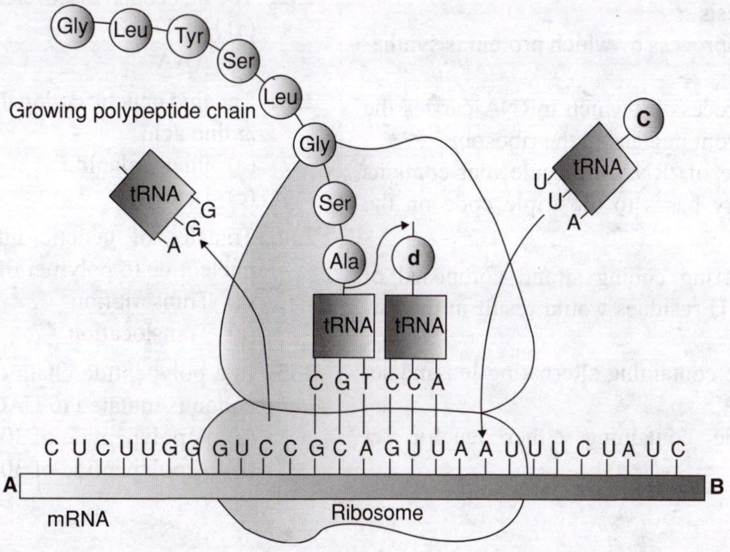

(a) 3′, Asn and 5′ (b) 3′, 5′ and Asn
(c) 5′, 3′ and Asn (d) Asn, 3′ and 5′

**218.** Ribozyme in bacteria is _______ rRNA
(a) 30 S (b) 32 S
(c) 23 S (d) 21 S

**219.** Additional sequences on mRNA referred to as _______ are not translated
(a) Variable number tandem repeats
(b) Non coding sequence
(c) Untranscribed regions
(d) Untranslated regions

**220.** Wobble hypothesis was given by
(a) R. W. Holley (b) H. G. Khorana
(c) M. Nirenberg (d) F. H. C. Crick

**221.** Which one of the following codons codes for the same information as UGC
(a) UGU (b) UGA
(c) UAG (d) UGG

**222.** Identify the correct match between the codons and coding functions

| Column I | Column II |
|---|---|
| A. AUG | 1. Phenylalanine |
| B. UAA | 2. Methionine |
| C. UUU | 3. Tryptophan |
| D. UGG | 4. Termination |

(a) A-I, B-4, C-2, D-3
(b) A-2, B-4, C-1, D-3
(c) A-4, B-3, C-2, D-1
(d) A-4, B-1, C-3, D-2

**223.** Which one of the following pairs is correctly matched
(a) Ribosomal RNA-carries aminoacids to the site of protein synthesis
(b) Transcription-process by which protein is synthesized
(c) Translation-process by which mRNA carries the information from nucleus to the ribosome
(d) Anticodon-site of *t*RNA molecule that contains complementary bases to the triple code on the mRNA

**224.** A naturally occurring coding strand composed of alternating C and U residues would result in the formation of
(a) A polypeptide containing alternating leu and ser residues
(b) A polypeptide containing either leu or ser residues
(c) A polypeptide containing only leu residues
(d) A polypeptide containing only ser residues

**225.** Which one of the following pairs is correctly matched with regard to the codon and the amino acid coded by it
(a) UUA-Valine (b) AAA-Lysine
(c) AUG-Cysteine (d) CCC-Alanine

**226.** Code of m – RNA and proteins are
(a) Coplanar (b) Colinear
(c) Nonlinear (d) Irregular

**227.** Following are the features of genetic code except
(a) Degeneracy or redundancy
(b) Unambiguous or specific
(c) Nearly universal
(d) There is punctuation in reading of genetic codon

**228.** Codon (on m- RNA) and anticodon(on t-RNA) for Methionine amino acid is
(a) AUG and GUG (b) AUG and UAC
(c) UAC and AUG (d) AUG and UGG

**229.** Following amino acids coded by only non-degenerate codon.
(a) Leu and Ile (b) Val and Tyr
(c) Met and Trp (d) Asp and Asn

**230.** Select the correct matching between amino acid and number of codon use to code each amino acid
(a) Ser, Leu and Arg – 6 codon
(b) Gly and Asn – 4 codon
(c) Ile and Glu – 3 codon
(d) Gln and Pro – 4 codon

**231.** One codon code for only one amino acid mean codons are
(a) Universal (b) Redundant
(c) Unambiguous (d) Degenerate

**232.** The first codon discovered by Nirenberg and Mathii was
(a) UUU (b) GGG
(c) AAA (d) CCC

**233.** The first genetic codon deciphered was code for which amino acid
(a) Phenylalanine (b) Methionine
(c) Leucine (d) Tyrosine

**234.** Transfer of genetic information from polymer of nucleotide to polymer of amino acid is referred as
(a) Transcription (b) Splicing
(c) Translocation (d) Translation

**235.** In a polypeptide chain of 300 amino acid, if the 30$^{th}$ codon is mutated to UAG, then
(a) A polypeptide of 300 amino acid is formed
(b) A polypeptide of 30 amino acid is formed

(c) A polypeptide of 29 amino acid is formed
(d) Process of translation will stop

**236.** Following is the sequence of amino acids coded by an m-RNA. Predict the nucleotide sequence in m-RNA

Met-Phe-Phe-Phe-Phe-Phe-Phe

(a) AUGUUCUUCUUCUUCUUCUUC
(b) AUGUUCUUUUUCUUUUUCUUU
(c) AUGUUCUUCUUUUUUUUUUUU
(d) Any of the above is possible

**237.** Which two properties of genetic code is learnt from above question?
(a) Degeneracy and universality
(b) Specificity and degeneracy
(c) Redundancy and ambiguous
(d) Reading punctuation and universality

**238.** The codons causing chain termination are
(a) UUG, UAA, UGA (b) GAG, AAU, AGC
(c) AGG, CAG, UGA (d) UAG, UGA, UAA

**239.** Starting or initiation codon is
(a) UUU (b) UAG (c) AUG (d) UGG

**240.** Given below is the m-RNA

5′- AUG CUA UAC UUU UAG CCAUGC UAA-3′

How many amino acids will be present in polypeptide chain corresponding to above m-RNA
(a) 7 (b) 4 (c) 6 (d) 3

**241.** If genetic code is quadruplet instead of triplet, how many codons are possible?
(a) 16 (b) 64 (c) 256 (d) 255

**242.** Number of initiation and stop codon out of 64 codons are
(a) 3 and 1 (b) 1 and 3
(c) 2 and 3 (d) 3 and 2

**243.** A DNA strand is directly involved in the synthesis of all the following except
(a) t- RNA and r- RNA (b) DNA
(c) m-RNA (d) Protein

**244.** Select incorrect matching
(a) Severo Ochoa enzyme – Polynucleotide phosphorylase
(b) Marshall Nirenberg – Cell free protein synthesis
(c) Deletion mutation – Sickle cell anemia
(d) Har Gobind Khorana – RNA synthesis of defined base combination

**245.** How many t-RNA exist for stop codon?
(a)
(b) 2
(c) 3
(d) There is no t-RNA for stop codon.

**246.** Select incorrect statement for t-RNA
(a) anticodon loop of t-RNA posses base complementary to codon
(b) amino acid acceptor end is 3′ end of t-RNA
(c) secondary structure has clover – leaf shape.
(d) 3-D shape of t - RNA is look like 'T'

**247.** If radioactive amino acid is introduced in cell which is actively involved in protein synthesis. The radioactivity first appear in
(a) Ribosome on which process of translation occur
(b) m-RNA which involve in process of translation
(c) t-RNA act as adaptor molecule
(d) Polypeptide formed in process of translation

**248.** Where UTRs are situated in m-RNA
(a) towards 3′ end only
(b) towards 5′end only
(c) between starting and stop codon
(d) at 5′end before start codon and at 3′end after stop codon

**249.** Genes express their character by forming
(a) Enzymes (b) Carbohydrates
(c) Fats (d) Vitamins

**250.** Genetic codes are
(a) Similar in mtDNA, virusus, bacteria and eukaryotes
(b) Different in viruses and bacteria
(c) Different in mtDNA
(d) Different in mtDNA and bacteria

**251.** In bacteria, which of the following plays a structural and catalytic role in translation process?
(a) m-RNA (b) r-RNA
(c) t-RNA (d) DNA

**252.** Which of the following processes is catalyzed by enzyme?
(a) Delinking of larger and smaller subunit of ribosomes
(b) Linking of amino acids into polypeptide chain in a ribosome
(c) Making complementary copies of short piece of RNA
(d) Making c-DNA from m-RNA

**253.** Find out incorrect statement
(a) Termination of translation done by binding of release factor to stop codon
(b) Formation of peptide bond during translation is energetically favored reaction.
(c) UTRs are required for effective translation process
(d) The ribosome consists of functional RNAs and many different proteins

**254.** Following sequence of RNA, when translated will form a protein molecule of ________ amino acids.
5′GCUCGCAUGCCAGAUGUCUUCGUCCUUUA GUUUAUUAGA 3′
(a) 3 (b) 7 (c) 6 (d) 9

## Regulation of Gene Expression (Lac Operon)

**255.** What is indicated by m, r and q in the below figure?

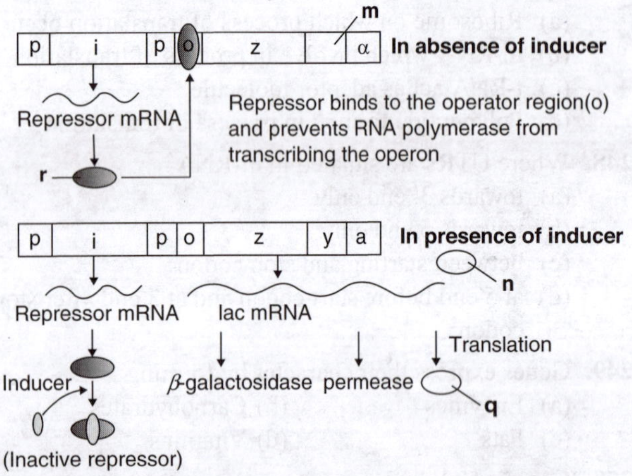


(a) y – gene, repressor protein and transacetylase
(b) repressor protein, y- gene and transacetylase
(c) b – gene, repressor protein and transacetylase
(d) Regulator gene, repressor protein and transacetylase

**256.** Which is act as inducer in lac operon
(a) Glucose (b) Galactose
(c) Lactose (d) Sucrose

**257.** In Lac operon, Lac stands for :
(a) Lactic acid (b) Lactobacillus
(c) Lactamide (d) Lactose

**258.** Lac operon was elucidated by:
(a) Watson and Crick
(b) Jacob (geneticist) and Monod (Biochemist)
(c) Johansson
(d) Friedrich Meischer

**259.** In Eukaryotes, one of the following mechanisms is not correct in terms of regulation of gene expression?
(a) Transcriptional level
(b) Splicing level
(c) Transport of mRNA from cytoplasm to nucleus
(d) Translational level

**260.** β-galactosidase is synthesized by E. coli to catalyze hydrolysis of ______ into ______ and glucose
(a) Galactose, Lactose (b) Galactose, Glucose
(c) Lactose, Galactose (d) Maltose, Galactose

**261.** Gene regulation in eukaryote could be exerted at
(a) Transcriptional level (b) Splicing level
(c) Translational level (d) All of these

**262.** A polycistronic structural gene is regulated by a common promoter and regulator gene in bacteria and such arrangement of gene is commonly termed as:
(a) Codon (b) Operon
(c) Genetic code (d) None

**263.** Regulatory gene in lac operon represented as "i" gene, here "i" derived from
(a) Inducer (b) Inhibitor
(c) Innovation (d) Initiator

**264.** Out of the 3 structural genes z, y and a, the gene (s) which codes for lactose permease is:
(a) z (b) a
(c) y (d) Both (b) and (c)

**265.** Repressor protein in lac operon concept binds to which gene?
(a) d (b) i (c) o (d) z

**266.** In lac operon, the inducer binds to ________ to initiate synthesis of enzymes responsible for lactose metabolism
(a) i gene (b) Repressor
(c) o gene (d) z gene

**267.** Gene regulation is controlled by following conditions
(a) Metabolic (b) Physiological
(c) Environmental (d) Any or all of these

**268.** Generally regulation of lac operon by repressor is referred to as ________ regulation:
(a) Positive (b) Negative
(c) Feedback (d) Both (b) and (c)

**269.** Predominate method for control of gene expression in prokaryote is
(a) Transcriptional rate
(b) Translational rate
(c) Splicing rate
(d) Translocation of m-RNA

**270.** Lac operon consist of
(a) One regulator gene and one structural gene
(b) One regulator gene and two structural gene
(c) One regulator gene and three structural gene
(d) Two regulator gene and one structural gene

**271.** Find out the correct sequence of structural gene in lac operon
(a) y, a, z (b) z, y, a (c) a, y, z (d) y, z, a

**272.** Repressor protein binds sequences of which gene
(a) Operator (b) Regulator
(c) Promoter (d) Structural

**273.** Substrate for beta-galactosidase is
(a) Sucrose (b) Lactose
(c) Glucose (d) Fructose

**274.** Select incorrect statement from the following
(a) Very low level of expression of lac operon always present in bacterial cell.
(b) lac operator is present in all operon
(c) Lactose regulate switching on and off of the lac operon
(d) Coordinated regulation of expression of several genes are required for development and differentiation of embryo

**275.** Constitutive gene in lac operon is
(a) i - gene (b) z - gene
(c) y - gene (d) a – gene

**276.** If there is point mutation (mis-sense) in z-gene which enzyme will not synthesized when transcription proceed in lac operon
(a) beta- galactosidase (b) lactose permease
(c) Transacetylase (d) All of these

**277.** If there is point mutation (non-sense) in y-gene which enzyme will synthesized when transcription proceed in lac operon
(a) beta- galactosidase (b) lactose permease
(c) Transacetylase (d) All of these

**278.** Gratuitous inducer for lac operon is
(a) Lactose
(b) Allolactose
(c) Glucose
(d) IPTG(isopropyle thio galactoside)

**279.** Select incorrect matching
(a) Operator gene – Directly controls the synthesis of m-RNA over structural gene
(b) Regulator gene – Produces repressor protein
(c) Promoter gene – Site for initial binding of RNA polymerase
(d) Structural gene – Gene synthesizes r-RNA

**280.** Which is not true for Operon model
(a) Regulator gene (b) Promotor gene
(c) Repressor gene (d) Operator gene

**281.** Functioning of structural genes is controlled by
(a) Operator (b) Promoter
(c) Ligase (d) Regulatory gene

**282.** In the lactose operon of *Escherichia coli*, what is the function of promoter
(a) Binding of Gyrase enzyme
(b) Binding of RNA polymerase
(c) Codes for RNA polymerase
(d) Processing of messenger RNA

**283.** Operon is
(a) A set of closely linked genes regulating a metabolic pathways in prokaryotes
(b) The sequence of three nitrogen bases determining a single amino acid
(c) The sequence of nitrogen bases in *m*RNA which codes for a single amino acid
(d) A gene responsible for switching on or off other genes

**284.** In the lac operon, the structural genes are switched off when
(a) Repressor binds to operator
(b) Repressor binds to promotor
(c) Repressor binds to regular
(d) Repressor binds to inducer

**285.** The rate of transcription in lac operon is maximum when
(a) Lactose is maximum in medium and Glucose is minimum in cell
(b) Lactose is minimum in medium and Glucose is maximum in cell
(c) Lactose is maximum in medium and Glucose is maximum in cell
(d) Lactose is minimum in medium and Glucose is minimum in cell

## HGP (Human Genomic Project)

**286.** What is indicated in the figure?

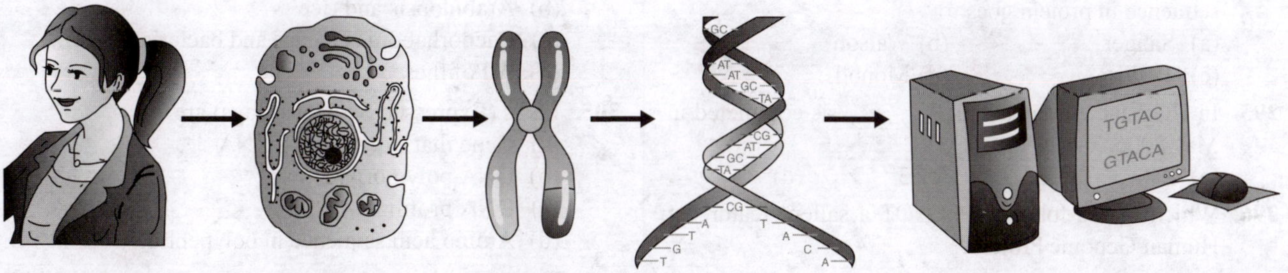

(a) Criminal/Suspect identification
(b) Human genome project
(c) Recombinant DNA technology
(d) Development of Bioinformatics

**287.** Considering cost of sequencing 1 bp to be US 3$ then the approximate cost of HGP (Human Genome Project) would come out to be ______ US $.
(a) 3 billion (b) 9 million
(c) 9 billion (d) 3 million

**288.** Human Genome project was a __X__ year long project starting from __Y__ to __Z__
(a) X = 13, Y = 1980, X = 1993
(b) X = 12, Y = 1990, Z = 2002
(c) X = 13, Y = 1990, Z = 2003
(d) X = 14, Y = 1990, Z = 2004

**289.** ELSI strands for:
(a) Ethical, Logical and Society Issues
(b) Ethical, Legal and Society Issues
(c) Ethical, Logical and Social Issues
(d) Ethical, Legal and Social Issues

**290.** Caenorhabditis elegans is a free-living non-pathogenic ______.
(a) Annelid (b) Nematode
(c) Crustocean (d) Mammal

**291.** Expressed sequence tags (ESTs) is an approach practiced in ______
(a) DNA fingerprinting (b) DNA sequencing
(c) DNA replicating (d) DNA transformation

**292.** Sequencing the whole genome of an organism into coding and non-coding sequences is termed as:
(a) Sequence determination
(b) Sequence detection
(c) Sequence annotation
(d) Sequence completion

**293.** BAC, a vector used in biotechnology for cloning, stands for:
(a) Bacterial Actual Chromosome
(b) Bacterial Artificial Chromosome
(c) Bacterial Annoted Chromosome
(d) None of the above

**294.** The credit for developing a method for determination of nucleotide sequence in DNA as well as amino acid sequence in protein goes to:
(a) Sanger (b) Watson
(c) Taylor (d) Monod

**295.** In HGP, the chromosome ______ was completed in May 2006.
(a) 2 (b) 1 (c) 3 (d) 4

**296.** Which of the following is NOT a salient feature of Human Genome Project?
(a) The human genome contains 3614.7 million nucleotide bases
(b) Less than 2% genome codes for proteins
(c) Over 50% of the genes discovered are yet to the investigated regarding their functions
(d) Chromosome Y has fewest genes

**297.** Under HGP, scientists have located 1.4 million locations where difference in single DNA base exists. It is termed as:
(a) Microsatellites
(b) Single nucleotide polymorphism
(c) Poly morphonucleaur regions
(d) Sequential nucleotide polymorphism

**298.** Under HGP, the largest known human gene was of:
(a) Somatotrophin (b) Dystrophin
(c) Lactrophin (d) Somatostain

**299.** HGP was closely associated with the rapid development of ______.
(a) Chemo informatics
(b) Modern genetics
(c) Pharmaco informatics
(d) Bioinformatics

**300.** HGP launched in which year
(a) 1990 (b) 1995
(c) 1997 (d) 2003

**301.** HGP was started under coordination of
(a) U.S. department of energy
(b) National institute of Health (U.S.)
(c) Wellcome trust (U.K.)
(d) Both (a) and (b)

**302.** DNA of following plant is sequenced
(a) Drosophila
(b) Arabidopsis
(c) Caenorhabditis elegans
(d) Yeast

**303.** Genome of which plant was sequenced first
(a) Wheat (b) Arabidopsis thaliana
(c) Rice (d) Yeast

**304.** DNA of which non-human model organism is sequenced
(a) Drosophila and Yeast
(b) Arabidopsis and rice
(c) Caenorhabditis elegans and bacteria (E. coli.)
(d) All of these

**305.** ESTs (Expressed Sequence Tags) are
(a) Gene that expressed as RNA
(b) DNA polymorphism
(c) DNA profiling
(d) Amino acid sequence in polypeptide

**306.** Following is not a part of DNA sequencing procedure
(a) Fragmentation of DNA
(b) Amplification of fragment of DNA
(c) Automated DNA sequencer
(d) Western blotting

**307.** Commonly used vector for amplification of human gene
(a) Plasmid (b) BAC and YAC
(c) Bacteriophage (d) Ti plasmid

**308.** How many chromosome of human are sequenced
(a) 22 autosomes only
(b) X chromosome only
(c) Y chromosome only
(d) 22 autosomes and X and Y Chromosomes

**309.** RFLP is useful in
(a) Gene mapping (b) DNA profiling
(c) Genetic analysis (d) All of these

**310.** Number of genes found in chromosomes -1 and Y-chromosome are
(a) 2986 and 213 respectively
(b) 2968 and 231 respectively
(c) 2968 and 321 respectively
(d) 2986 and 123 respectively

**311.** Larger portion of human genome is consist of
(a) Exons
(b) Coding sequences
(c) Repeated sequences
(d) All of these

**312.** Largest human gene dystrophin consists of
(a) 2.4 million bp (b) 1.4 million bp
(c) 3000 bp (d) 4.2 million bp

**313.** The approximate gene contained in genome of Rajiv sir
(a) 30,000 (b) 80,000
(c) 1,40,000 (d) 20,000

**314.** Following are feature of human genome select correct one.
(i) Average gene size in human is 3000 bp
(ii) less than 2% genome code for protein.
(iii) Repetitive sequence repeated many times
(iv) chromosome -1 has most genes.
(v) dystrophin is present on X-chromosomes and is largest human gene.
(vi) almost 99.9 % nucleotide babes are same in all individuals.
(a) i,ii,iii (b) all except v
(c) ii,vi and iv (d) All are correct

**315.** Select incorrect matching
(a) ESTs – Expressed sequence tags
(b) HGP – Human Genome Project
(c) YAC – Yeast Artificial Chromosome
(d) STR – Sub tandem Repeat

**316.** Number of genes found in Y – chromosome of human
(a) 3000 (b) 2968
(c) 231 (d) 300

**317.** Maximum number of gene, largest gene and minimum number of gene are respectively found on which human chromosomes
(a) $1^{st}$, Y and X (b) X, $1^{st}$ and Y
(c) $1^{st}$, $2^{nd}$ and X (d) $1^{st}$, X and Y

## DNA Fingerprinting/DNA Profiling/ DNA Typing

**318.** The two allele of a chromosome differ in
(a) Nucleotide sequence
(b) Copy number of VNTR
(c) Copy number of STR
(d) All of these

**319.** STR belongs to which class of satellite DNA
(a) Mini-satellite (b) Micro-satellite
(c) Both of these (d) None of these

**320.** DNA fingerprinting is based on the principle of identifying ______ sequences of DNA:
(a) Cistron (b) Variable
(c) Exons (d) Repetitive

**321.** Variations at genetic level in nucleotides is termed as:
(a) Allotropy (b) Polymorphism
(c) Isomerism (d) Tautomerism

**322.** Satellite DNA is classified on the basis of following criteria
(a) Base composition
(b) Length of segment
(c) Number of repetitive unit.
(d) All of these

**323.** Repetitive DNA are separated from bulk genomic DNA by process of
(a) Elution
(b) Density gradient centrifugation
(c) PCR
(d) Blotting

**324.** Quick way of comparing DNA of two individual is
(a) DNA profiling (b) Western blotting
(c) Blending (d) PCR

**325.** Which one of the following pairs of terms/names mean one and the same thing
(a) Gene pool- Genome
(b) Codon - Gene
(c) Cistron –Triplet
(d) DNA fingerprinting-DNA profiling

**326.** If inheritable mutation is observed in a population at high frequency it is termed as:
(a) DNA mutation
(b) DNA isomerism
(c) DNA polymorphism
(d) None

**327.** DNA polymorphism mainly arises due to
(a) Recombination (b) Random mating
(c) Mutation (d) Replication

**328.** The technique of_______was found by Alec Jeffrey's:
(a) DNA culture (b) DNA modification
(c) DNA mutation (d) DNA fingerprinting

**329.** Which of the following sequence of human genome shows high degree of polymorphism
(a) Exons (b) Bulk genomic DNA
(c) Repetitive DNA (d) Cistron

**330.** Allelic sequence variation can be described as DNA polymorphism if more than one allele at a locus occur in human population with a frequency greater than
(a) 0.001 (b) 0.01
(c) 0.0001 (d) 0.00001

**331.** A well known technique to amplify a small portion of DNA is termed as
(a) PCR (b) VNTR
(c) UTR (d) EST

**332.** VNTRs vary in size of _______ to_______.
(a) 0.1 to 20 bases
(b) 0.1 to 20 kilobases
(c) 0.1 to 20 hectobases
(d) 0.1 to 20 decabses

**333.** Quick way of comparing DNA of two individual is
(a) DNA profiling (b) Western blotting
(c) Blending (d) PCR

**334.** DNA fingerprinting of which of the following is exactly same
(a) Dizygotic twins (b) Monozygotic twins
(c) Siblings (d) Cousin brother

**335.** In DNA fingerprinting, the hybridised strands are detected by:
(a) Radiometery (b) Radioscopy
(c) Auto radiography (d) Scintillation counter

**336.** Following are the features of satellite DNA except
(a) Form large portion of human genome
(b) Generally do not code for protein
(c) Show high degree of polymorphism
(d) Forms m-RNA code for protein

**337.** What is the first step in the Southern Blot technique
(a) Denaturation of DNA on the gel for hybridization with specific probe
(b) Production of a group of genetically identical cells
(c) Digestion of DNA by restriction enzyme
(d) Isolation of DNA from a nucleated cell such as the one from the scene of crime

**338.** Initially in DNA fingerprinting which probe was used
(a) STR (b) VNTR
(c) Mini-satellite (d) Micro-satellite

**339.** VNTR belongs to which class of satellite DNA
(a) Mini-satellite
(b) Micro-satellite
(c) Both of these
(d) None of these

**340.** The sensitivity of DNA fingerprinting increased by
(a) Blending (b) PCR
(c) Centrifugation (d) Autoradiography

**341.** Arrange the following procedure in correct order to perform southern blotting
(i) separation of DNA fragments by gel electrophoresis
(ii) isolation of DNA
(iii) hybridization using labeled VNTR probe
(iv) digestion of DNA by restriction enzyme
(v) transferring of separated DNA to nitrocellulose or nylon membranes
(vi) detection of hybridized DNA fragments by autoradiogrphy
(a) i, ii, iii, iv, v, vi (b) ii, iv, i, v, iii, vi
(c) ii, i, iv, v, iii, vi (d) vi, i, ii, iv, iii, v

**342.** The technique DNA fingerprinting is used in all except
(a) Forensic science
(b) Determination of population genetic diversity
(c) Biogas production
(d) Paternity dispute

**343.** Which cells of given individual show same degree of polymorphism
(a) Skin cells and cells found in saliva
(b) Hair follicle cell and sperm
(c) blood cells and bone cells
(d) All of these

**344.** How many base sequence in genome of two humans are same
(a) 99% only (b) 98% only
(c) 50% only (d) 99.9%

**345.** During separation of DNA by density gradient centrifugation major peak is formed by
(a) Mini-satellite (b) Micro-satellite
(c) Bulk DNA (d) VNTR

**346.** Probability of inheritable mutation is higher in non coding sequence of DNA because
(a) It will not affect reproductive ability of individual.
(b) It will be selected by nature
(c) It will always shows expression
(d) All of these

**347.** Sequence of DNA show which kind of polymorphism
(a) VNTR (b) RFLP
(c) SNPs (snips) (d) All of these

**348.** Select correct matching
(a) Southern blotting – detect DNA
(b) Northern blotting – detect RNA
(c) Western blotting – detect Protein
(d) All of these

**349.** The transfer of protein from electrophoretic gel to nitrocellulose membrane is known as
(a) Transferase (b) Northern blotting
(c) Western blotting (d) Southern blotting

**350.** Which of the following technique is used in analyzing RFLP
(1) Methylation (2) Electrophoresis
(3) Restriction digestion (4) Lipofection
(a) 1 and 2 (b) 2 and 3
(c) 3 and 4 (d) 2 and 4

**351.** Find out incorrect statement
(a) DNA fingerprinting is the basis of paternity testing in case of dispute
(b) DNA polymorphism is low frequency inheritable mutation observed in population.
(c) In Southern blot hybridization radiolabelled VNTR is used as probe.
(d) DNA from single cell is sufficient to perform DNA profiling because of PCR.

**352.** DNA fingerprinting was developed by
(a) Kary Mullis (b) Alec Jeffreys
(c) Dr Lal ji singh (d) M.S. swaminathan

**353.** Steps not involved in DNA profiling
(a) Restriction exonuclease digestion
(b) Electrophoresis
(c) Hybridization by DNA(VNTR) probe
(d) Autoradiography

**354.** Select incorrect matching
(a) VNTR – Variable Number of Tandem Repeats
(b) RFLP – Restriction Fragment Length Polymorphism
(c) SNPs (snips)- Single nucleoside Polymorphism
(d) PCR – Polymerase Chain Reaction

**355.** Synthetic membrane is used in Southern blotting is made from
(a) Nitrocellulose
(b) Nylon
(c) Copper ferrocyanide
(d) Either (a) or (b)

**356.** DNA fingerprinting was developed by
(a) Prof. Alec Jeffrey (b) Arber and Smith
(c) Barbara McClintock (d) Jacob and Monod

**357.** DNA fingerprinting needs
(a) Suitable restriction enzyme
(b) DNA probe
(c) Facilities for gel electrophoresis and southern blotting
(d) All the above

**358.** DNA probe is used in
(a) Gel electrophoresis
(b) Western blot
(c) DNA profiling technique
(d), Interferon synthesis

**359.** During DNA fingerprinting, DNA probes helps in
(a) Gel electrophoresis (b) Southern blotting
(c) Autoradiography (d) None of these

**360.** The method of DNA fingerprinting involves the use of
(a) Restriction enzyme
(b) Taq polymerase
(c) Oligonucleotide primers
(d) All of these

## Multiple Choice Questions: Level II

**361.** What is not true for genetic code?
(a) it is nearly universal
(b) it is degenerative
(c) it is unambiguous
(d) a codon in mRNA is read in a non-contiguous fashion

**362.** Removal of introns and joining the exons in defined order in a transcription unit is called
(a) tailing (b) transformation
(c) capping (d) splicing

**363.** Semi-conservative replication of DNA was first demonstrated in
(a) *Escherichia coli*
(b) *Streptococcus pneumoniae*
(c) *Salmonella typhimurium*
(d) *Drosophila melanogaster*

**364.** Whose experiments cracked the DNA and discovered unequivocally that a genetic code is a 'triplet'?
(a) Hershey and Chase
(b) Morgan and Sturtevent
(c) Beadle and Tatum
(d) Nirenberg and Mathaei

**365.** Point mutation involves
(a) change in single base pair
(b) duplication
(c) deletion
(d) insertion

**366.** In the DNA molecule,
(a) the proportion of adenine in relation to thymine varies with the organism
(b) there are two strands which run anti-parallel one in $5' \rightarrow 3'$ direction and other in $3' \rightarrow 5'$
(c) the total amount of purine nucleotides and pyrimidine nucleotides is not always equal
(d) there are two strands which run parallel in the $5' \rightarrow 3'$ direction

**367.** Which one of the following pairs of codons is correctly matched with their function or the signal for the particular amino acid?
(a) AUG, ACG – start/methionine
(b) UUA, UCA – leucine
(c) GUU, GCU – alanine
(d) UAG, UGA – stop

**368.** The length of DNA molecule greatly exceeds the dimensions of the nucleus in eukaryotic cells. How is this DNA accommodated?
(a) supercoiling in nucleosomes
(b) DNase digestion
(c) through elimination of repetitive DNA
(d) deletion of non-essential genes

**369.** Proteins synthesis in an animal cell takes place
(a) only in the cytoplasm
(b) in the nucleolus as well as in cytoplasm
(c) in cytoplasm as well as in mitochondria
(d) only on ribosomes attached to the nuclear envelope

**370.** A sequential expression of a set of human genes
(a) messenger RNA (b) DNA sequence
(c) ribosome (d) transfer RNA

**371.** During transcription, RNA polymerase holoenzyme binds to a gene promoter and assumes a saddle-like structure, what is its DNA-binding sequence?
(a) AATT (b) CACC
(c) TATA (d) TTAA

**372.** One-gene-one-enzyme relationship was established for the first time in
(a) *Salmonella typhimurium*
(b) *Escherichia coli*
(c) *Diplococcus pneumonia*
(d) *Neuropora crassa*

**373.** Molecular basis of organ differentiation depends on the modulation in transcription by
(a) Ribosome
(b) Transcription factor
(c) Anticodon
(d) RNA polymerase

**374.** Telomere repetitive DNA sequences control the function of eukaryotic chromosomes because they
(a) are RNA transcription initiators
(b) help chromosome pairing
(c) prevent chromosome loss
(d) act as replicons

**375.** Amino acid sequence, in protein synthesis is decided by the sequence of
(a) mRNA (b) cDNA
(c) tRNA (d) rRNA

**376.** The salivary gland chromosomes in the dipteran larvae are useful in gene mapping, because
(a) there are fused
(b) these are much longer in size
(c) these are easy to stain
(d) They have endo-reduplicated chromosomes

**377.** E.coli cells with a mutated z gene of the lac operon cannot grow in medium containing only lactose as the source of energy, because
(a) the lac operon is constitutively active in these cells
(b) they cannot synthesize functional beta-galactosidase
(c) in the presence of glucose, *E. coli* cells do not utilize lactose
(d) they cannot transport lactose from the medium into the cell

**378.** Which one of the following makes use of RNA as a template to synthesize DNA?
(a) DNA polymerase
(b) RNA polymerase
(c) Reverse trancriptase
(d) DNA-dependant RNA polymerase

**379.** Telomerase is an enzyme which is a
(a) simple protein (b) RNA
(c) ribonucleoprotein (d) repetitive DNA

**380.** Which of the following is generally used for induced mutagenesis in crop plants?
(a) X-rays
(b) UV (260 nm)
(c) Gama rays (from cobalt 60)
(d) Alpha particles

**381.** After mutation at a genetic locus, the character of an organism changes due to the change in
(a) protein structure
(b) DNA replication
(c) protein synthesis pattern
(d) RNA transcription pattern

**382.** The following ratio is generally constant for a given species:
(a) A + G / C + T (b) T + C / G + A
(c) G + C / A + T (d) A + C / T + G

**383.** The telomeres of eukaryotic chromosomes consist of short sequences of
(a) Thymine-rich repeats
(b) Cytosine-rich repeats
(c) Adenine-rich repeats
(d) Guanine-rich repeats

**384.** During replication of a bacterial chromosome DNA synthesis starts from a replication origin site and
(a) RNA primers are involved
(b) is facilitated by telomerase
(c) moves in one direction of the site
(d) moves in bi-directional way

**385.** Radioactive thymidine when added to the medium surrounding living mammalian cells gets incorporated into newly synthesized DNA. Which of the following types of chromatin is expected to become radioactive if cells are exposed to radioactive thymidine as soon as they enter the S-phase?
(a) Heterochromatin
(b) Euchromatin
(c) Both heterochromatin and euchromatin
(d) Neither hetrochromatin nor euchromatin but only the nucleolus

**386.** DNA fingerprinting refers to
(a) Molecular analysis of profiles of DNA samples
(b) Analysis of DNA samples using imprinting devices
(c) Techniques used for molecular analysis of different specimens of DNA
(d) Techniques used for identification of fingerprints of individuals

**387.** In a mutational event, when adenine is replaced by guanine, it is a case of
(a) Frame shift mutation
(b) Transcription
(c) Transition
(d) Transvertion

**388.** What does "lac" refers to in what we call the lac operon?
(a) The number 1,00,000
(b) Lactose
(c) Lactase
(d) Lac insect

**389.** During transcription, the DNA site at which RNA polymerase binds is called
(a) enhancer (b) promoter
(c) regulator (d) receptor

**390.** Which proteins are packed into a bacterial chromosome?
(a) histones (b) basic proteins
(c) acidic proteins (d) actin

**391.** Which one of the following triplet codes is correctly matched with its specificity for an amino acid in protein synthesis or as 'start' or 'stop' codon?
(a) UAC – Tyrosine (b) UGC Start
(c) UUU – Stop (d) UGU – Leucine

**392.** What would happen if in a gene encoding a polypeptide of 50 amino acids, 25th codon (UAU) is mutated to UAA?
(a) A polypeptide of 25 amino acids will be formed
(b) A polypeptide of 24 amino acids will be formed
(c) Two polypeptides of 24 and 25 amino acids will be formed
(d) A polypeptide of 49 amino acids will be formed

**393.** In the genetic code dictionary, how many codons are used to code for all the 20 essential amino acids?
(a) 60 (b) 20 (c) 64 (d) 61

**394.** Degeneration of a genetic code is attributed to the
(a) third member of a codon
(b) first member of a codon
(c) second member of a codon
(d) entire codon

**395.** Genetic map is one that
(a) shows the distribution of various species in a region
(b) establishes sites of the genes on a chromosome
(c) establishes the various stages in gene evolution
(d) shows the stages during the cell division

**396.** DNA synthesis can be specifically measured by estimating incorporation of radio labelled

(a) uracil (b) adenine
(c) thymidine (d) deoxyribose sugar

**397.** In E.coli during lactose metabolism repressor binds to
(a) regulator gene (b) operator gene
(c) structural gene (d) promoter gene

**398.** Out of 64 codons, 61 codons code for 20 types of amino acid. It is called
(a) degeneracy of genetic code
(b) overlapping of gene
(c) wobbling of codon
(d) universality of codons

**399.** Jacob and Monod studied lactose metabolism in E.coli and proposed operon concept. Operon concept is applicable for
(a) all prokaryotes
(b) all prokaryotes and some eukaryotes
(c) all prokaryotes and all eukaryotes
(d) all prokaryotes and some protozoans

**400.** Transformation experiment was first performed on which bacteria?
(a) E.coli
(b) Diplococcus Pneumoniae
(c) Salmonella
(d) Pasteurella pestis

**401.** If the DNA percentage of thymine is 20% then what will be the percentage of guanine?
(a) 20% (b) 40% (c) 30% (d) 60%

**402.** Export part of m-RNAs have code for
(a) protein (b) lipid
(c) carbohydrate (d) phospholipid

**403.** The RNA that picks up specific amino acids from the amino acid pool in the cytoplasm to ribosome during protein synthesis is called
(a) mRNA (b) tRNA
(c) rRNA (d) carrier RNA

**404.** Which of the following reunites the exon segments after RNA splicing?
(a) RNA polymerase (b) RNA primase
(c) RNA ligase (d) RNA proteases

**405.** Nucleus of a donor embryonal cell/somatic cell is transferred to an enucleated egg cell. Then after the formation of organism, what shall be true?
(a) Organism will have extranuclear genes of the donor cell
(b) Organism will have extranuclear genes of recipient cell
(c) Organism will have extranuclear genes of both donor and recipient cell
(d) Organism will have nuclear genes of recipient

**406.** Which is not consistent with double helical structure of DNA?
(a) A = T, C ≡ G
(b) Density of DNA decreases on heating
(c) A + T/C + G is not constant
(d) Both A and B

**407.** In which direction is m-RNA synthesized on DNA template?
(a) $5' \rightarrow 3'$ (b) $3' \rightarrow 5'$
(c) Both (a) and (b) (d) Any

**408.** Gene and cistron words are sometimes used synonymously because
(a) One cistron contains many genes
(b) One gene contains many cistrons
(c) One gene contains one cistron
(d) One gene contains no cistron

**409.** A mutant strain of $T_4$ – Bacteriophage, R-II, fails to lyse the E. coli, but when two strains of $R\text{-}II^r$ and $R\text{-}II^y$ are mixed then they lyse the *E. coli*. What may be the possible reason?
(a) Bacteriophage transform in wild
(b) It is not mutated
(c) Both strains have similar cistrons
(d) Both strains have different cistrons

**410.** Protein synthesis occurs
(a) on ribosomes present in cytosol as well in mitochondria
(b) only on ribosomes attached to the nuclear envelope and endoplasmic reticulum
(c) only on the ribosomes present in cytosol
(d) on ribosomes present in the nucleolus as well as cytoplasm

**411.** In DNA, when AGCT occurs, their association is as per which of the following pairs?
(a) AG-CT (b) AC-GT
(c) AT-GC (d) All of these

**412.** Pneumococcus experiment proves that
(a) DNA is the genetic material
(b) Bacteria undergoes binary fission
(c) Bacteria does not reproduce sexually
(d) RNA sometime controls production of DNA and proteins

**413.** Genetic code consists of
(a) Adenine and guanine
(b) Cytosine and uracil
(c) Cytosine and guanine
(d) All the above

**414.** How many base pairs are found in one genome of man?
(a) $7 \times 10^4$ (b) $28 \times 10^7$
(c) $3 \times 10^9$ (d) $4 \times 10^9$

**415.** The eukaryotic genome differs from the prokaryotic genome, because
(a) genes in the former case are organized into operons
(b) DNA is complexed with histones in prokaryotes
(c) repetitive sequences are present in eukaryotes
(d) the DNA is circular and single stranded in prokaryotes

**416.** DNA elements which can switch their position are called
(a) Exons (b) Introns
(c) Cistrons (d) Transposons

**417.** DNA replication is
(a) Conservative and discontinuous
(b) Semiconservative and semi-discontinuous
(c) Semiconservative and discontinuous
(d) Conservative

**418.** In the genetic dictionary, there are 64 codons as
(a) 64 amino acids are to be coded
(b) 64 types of tRNAs are present
(c) There are 44 non-sense codons and 20 sense codons
(d) Genetic code is triplet

**419.** Three codons causing chain termination are
(a) TAG, TAA, TGA (b) GAT, AAT, AGT
(c) AGT, TAG, UGA (d) UAG, UGA, UAA

**420.** A mutation at one base of the first codon, of a gene, produces a non-functional protein. Such a mutation is called
(a) nonsense mutation (b) missense mutation
(c) frameshift mutation (d) reverse mutation

**421.** If a completely radioactive double-stranded DNA molecule undergoes two rounds of replication in a non-radioactive medium, what will be the radioactive status of the four resulting molecules?
(a) Half the number contains no radioactivity
(b) All four still contain radioactivity
(c) Three out of four contain radioactivity
(d) Radioactivity is lost from all four

**422.** An octamer of 4 histones complexed with DNA forms
(a) Endosome (b) Nucleosome
(c) Mesosome (d) Centromere

**423.** In eukaryotes, after transcription of mRNA, some of its nucleotides are removed before it is translated into polypeptide. The nucleotides which are removed from mRNA are called
(a) exons (b) upstream sequences
(c) unusual bases (d) introns

**424.** Okazaki fragments are seen during
(a) transcription (b) translation
(c) replication (d) transduction

**425.** The basis for DNA fingerprinting is
(a) occurrence of restriction fragment length polymorphism (RFLP)
(b) phenotypic differences between individuals
(c) availability of cloned DNA
(d) knowledge of human karyotype

**426.** Wide type E. Coli cells are growing in normal medium with glucose. They are transferred to a medium containing only lactose as sugar. Which of the following changes takes place?
(a) the lac operon is repressed
(b) all operons are induced
(c) the lac operon is induced
(d) E coli cells stop dividing

**427.** Experimental material in the study of DNA replication has been
(a) *Escherichia coli* (b) *Neurospora crassa*
(c) *Pneumococcus* (d) *Drosophila melanogaster*

**428.** An environmental agent, which triggers transcription from an operon, is a
(a) regulator (b) inducer
(c) depressor (d) controlling element

**429.** The lac operon is an example of
(a) arabinose operon (b) inducible operon
(c) repressible operon (d) overlapping genes

**430.** Anticodon is an unpaired triplet of bases in an exposed position of
(a) mRNA (b) rRNA
(c) tRNA (d) sRNA

**431.** Polytene chromosomes were discovered for the first time in
(a) Drosophila (b) Chironomus
(c) Musca nebula (d) Musca domestica

**432.** Protein helping in opening of DNA double helix in the form of replication fork is
(a) DNA gyrase (b) DNA polymerase I
(c) DNA ligase (d) DNA topoisomerase

**433.** Which is not involved in protein synthesis?
(a) Transcription (b) Initiation
(c) Elongation (d) Termination

**434.** DNA template sequence of CTGATAGC is transcribed over mRNA as
(a) GUCTUTCG (b) GACUAUCG
(c) GAUTATUG (d) UACTATCU

**435.** The number of the base substitution possible in amino acid codons is
(a) 261 (b) 264 (c) 535 (d) 549

**436.** Nucleosome core is made of
(a) $H_1$, $H_2A$, $H_2B$ and $H_3$
(b) $H_1$, $H_2A$, $H_2B$, $H_4$
(c) $H_1$, $H_2A$, $H_2B$, $H_3$ and $H_4$
(d) $H_2A$, $H_2B$, $H_3$ and $H_4$

**437.** Nucleotide arrangement in DNA can be seen by
(a) X-ray diffraction (b) Electron microscope
(c) Ultracentrifuge (d) Light microscope

**438.** A DNA with unequal nitrogen bases would most probably be
(a) Single stranded (b) Double stranded
(c) Triple stranded (d) Four stranded

**439.** During DNA replication, strands separate by
(a) DNA polymerase (b) Topoisomerase
(c) Unwindase/Helicase (d) Gyrase

**440.** The transforming principle of Pneumococus as found out by Avery, MacLeod and McCarty was
(a) mRNA (b) DNA
(c) Protein (d) Polysaccharide

**441.** *Escherichia coli* fully labelled with $^{15}N$ is allowed to grow in $^{14}N$ medium. The two strands of DNA molecule of the first generation bacteria have
(a) Different density and do not resemble parent DNA
(b) Different density but resemble parent DNA
(c) Same density and resemble parent DNA
(d) Same density but do not resemble parent DNA

**442.** Khorana first deciphered the triplet codons of
(a) Serine and isoleucine
(b) Cysteine and valine
(c) Tyrosine and tryptophan
(d) Phenylalanine and methionine

# A & R and Statement-based Questions

## Assertion and Reason Questions

***Direction for questions 443 to 447:** Read the **assertion** and **reason** carefully to mark the correct option out of the options given below:*

**(a)** **(A)** is **true** but **(R)** is **false**.
**(b)** **(A)** is **false** but **(R)** is **true**.
**(c)** Both **(A)** and **(R)** is **true** and **(R)** is the correct explanation of **(A)**.
**(d)** Both **(A)** and **(R)** is **true** and **(R)** is not the correct explanation of **(A)**.

**443. Assertion:** RNA act as the genetic material in most of the organisms.
**Reason:** DNA is chemically & structurally a stable molecule has power of replication.

**444. Assertion:** RNA is genetic material in QB bacteriophage.
**Reason:** Bacteriophage is type of bacteria which is divided by fission.

**445. Assertion:** There is uniform distance between two strands of DNA.
**Reason:** Two strand of DNA are antiparallel.

**446. Assertion:** Monocistronic structural gene is found mostly in eukaryotes.
**Reason:** Polycistronic structural gene is found mostly in bacteria.

**447. Assertion:** Genetic codes are degenerate.
**Reason:** Some amino acids are coded by more than one codon.

## Statement-based Questions:

***Direction for questions 448 to 452:** These type of questions consist of two statement each, printed as **Statement-I** and **Statement-II**. While answering such questions, a student is needed to choose any one of the following four responses.*

**(a)** **Statement I** is **correct Statement II** is **incorrect**.
**(b)** **Statement I** is **incorrect Statement II** is **correct**.
**(c)** Both **Statement I** and **Statement II** are **correct**.
**(d)** Both **Statement I** and **Statement II** are **incorrect**.

**448. Statement-I:** AUG has dual nature.
**Statement-II:** Polynucleotide phosphorylase enzyme is Severo Ochoa enzyme.

**449. Statement-I:** Sanger developed method for sequencing of amino acid in protein.
**Statement-II:** Y-chromosome in human have least number of genes.

**450. Statement-I:** Ribozyme is protein enzyme help in process of transcription.
**Statement-II:** Semiconservative replication of DNA is based on complementary hydrogen bonding.

**451. Statement-I:** Coding sequences are introns.
**Statement-II:** Translation is a process evolved around RNA, indicating that life began around RNA.

**452. Statement-I:** Lac operon is the prototype operon in bacteria.

**Statement-II:** Functional RNA in eukaryotes is produced by splicing.

## Matrix-Match Type Questions

**453.** Match the following:

| List-I (Organism) | List-II (DNA Size) |
|---|---|
| 1. Bacteriophage φ × 174 | (i) 48502 bp |
| 2. Bacteriophage lambda | (ii) $3.3 \times 10^9$ bp |
| 3. E.coli | (iii) 5386 base |
| 4. Haploid human DNA | (iv) $4.6 \times 10^6$ bp |

**The correct matching is:**

| | 1 | 2 | 3 | 4 |
|---|---|---|---|---|
| (a) | (iii) | (i) | (iv) | (ii) |
| (b) | (iii) | (iv) | (i) | (ii) |
| (c) | (ii) | (iv) | (iii) | (i) |
| (d) | (iii) | (i) | (ii) | (iv) |

**454.** Match the following:

| List-I (Molecule) | List-II (Bond) |
|---|---|
| 1. Nucleoside | (i) 3-5 phosphodiester bond |
| 2. Nucleotide | (ii) N-glycosidic bond |
| 3. Dinucleotide | (iii) Phosphoester bond |

**The correct matching is:**

| | 1 | 2 | 3 |
|---|---|---|---|
| (a) | (ii) | (iii) | (i) |
| (b) | (iii) | (ii) | (i) |
| (c) | (i) | (ii) | (iii) |
| (d) | (ii) | (i) | (iii) |

**455.** Match the following:

| List-I (Scientist) | List-II (Discovery) |
|---|---|
| 1. Watson & Crick | (i) Ratio between A – T & G – C is constant & value of constant is 1 |
| 2. Wilkins & Franklin | (ii) Base pairing between 2 strands of DNA |
| 3. Chargaff | (iii) X-ray diffraction data of DNA |

**The correct matching is:**

| | 1 | 2 | 3 |
|---|---|---|---|
| (a) | (ii) | (iii) | (i) |
| (b) | (iii) | (ii) | (i) |
| (c) | (ii) | (i) | (iii) |
| (d) | (iii) | (i) | (ii) |

**456.** Match the following:

| List-I | List-II |
|---|---|
| 1. Histone | (i) DNA wrapped around basic proteins |
| 2. Nucleosome | (ii) Positive charged basic proteins |
| 3. Euchromatin | (iii) Densly packed & darkly stained |
| 4. Heterochromatin | (iv) Loosely packed & lightly stained |

**The correct matching is:**

| | 1 | 2 | 3 | 4 |
|---|---|---|---|---|
| (a) | (ii) | (i) | (iv) | (iii) |
| (b) | (iii) | (iv) | (i) | (ii) |
| (c) | (iv) | (ii) | (iii) | (i) |
| (d) | (i) | (iii) | (ii) | (iv) |

**457.** Match the following:

| List-I (Scientist) | List-II (Work Done) |
|---|---|
| 1. F. Griffith | (i) Biochemical characterisation of transforming material |
| 2. Avery, MacLeod, McCarty | (ii) Confirmation of transforming material as DNA |
| 3. Hershey & Chase | (iii) Discovery of Transforming material |

**The correct matching is:**

| | 1 | 2 | 3 |
|---|---|---|---|
| (a) | (iii) | (i) | (ii) |
| (b) | (ii) | (iii) | (i) |
| (c) | (i) | (iii) | (ii) |
| (d) | (iii) | (ii) | (i) |

## NCERT Exemplar Questions

1. In a DNA strand the nucleotides are linked together by
   (a) Glycosidic bonds (b) Phosphodiester bonds
   (c) Peptide bonds (d) Hydrogen bonds
2. A nucleoside differs from a nucleotide. It lacks the
   (a) Base (b) Sugar
   (c) Phosphate group (d) Hydroxyl group
3. Both deoxyribose and ribose belong to a class of sugars called
   (a) Trioses (b) Hexoses
   (c) Pentoses (d) Polysaccharides
4. The fact that a purine base always pairs through hydrogen bonds with a pyrimidine base in the DNA double helix leads to ______________.
   (a) The antiparallel nature
   (b) The semiconservative nature
   (c) Uniform width throughout DNA
   (d) Uniform length in all DNA
5. The net electric charge on DNA and histones is
   (a) Both positive
   (b) Both negative
   (c) Negative and positive, respectively
   (d) Zero
6. The promoter site and the terminator site for transcription are located at
   (a) 3′ (downstream) end and 5′ (upstream) end, respectively of the transcription unit.
   (b) 5′ (upstream) end and 3′ (downstream) end, respectively of the transcription unit.
   (c) The 5′ (upstream) end
   (d) The 3′ (downstream) end
7. Which of the following statements is the most appropriate for sickle cell anaemia?
   (a) It cannot be treated with iron supplements
   (b) It is a molecular disease
   (c) It confers resistance to acquiring malaria
   (d) All of the above
8. Which of the following is true with respect to AUG?
   (a) It codes for methionine only
   (b) It is an initiation codon
   (c) It codes for methionine in both prokaryotes and eukaryotes
   (d) All of the above
9. The first genetic material could be
   (a) Protein (b) Carbohydrates
   (c) DNA (d) RNA
10. With regard to mature mRNA in eukaryotes:
    (a) Exons and introns do not appear in the mature RNA.
    (b) Exons appear but introns do not appear in the mature RNA.
    (c) Introns appear but exons do not appear in the mature RNA.
    (d) Both exons and introns appear in the mature RNA.
11. The human chromosome with the highest and least number of genes in them are respectively
    (a) Chromosome 21 and Y
    (b) Chromosome 1 and X
    (c) Chromosome 1 and Y
    (d) Chromosome X and Y
12. Who amongst the following scientists had no contribution in the development of the double helix model for the structure of DNA?
    (a) Rosalind Franklin
    (b) Maurice Wilkins
    (c) Erwin Chargaff
    (d) Meselson and Stahl
13. DNA is a polymer of nucleotides which are linked to each other by 3′ – 5′ phosphodiester bond. To prevent polymerization of nucleotides, which of the following modifications would you choose?
    (a) Replace purine with pyrimidines.
    (b) Remove/replace 3′ OH group in deoxyribose.
    (c) Remove/replace 2′ OH group with some other group in deoxyribose.
    (d) Both 'b' and 'c'.
14. Discontinuous synthesis of DNA occurs in one strand, because
    (a) DNA molecule being synthesized is very long.
    (b) DNA dependent DNA polymerase catalyses polymerization only in one direction (5′ → 3′).
    (c) It is a more efficient process.
    (d) DNA ligase joins the short stretches of DNA.
15. Which of the following steps in transcription is catalyzed by RNA polymerase?
    (a) Initiation (b) Elongation
    (c) Termination (d) All of the above
16. Control of gene expression in prokaryotes takes place at the level of
    (a) DNA-replication (b) Transcription
    (c) Translation (d) None of the above

**17.** Which of the following statements is correct about the role of regulatory proteins in transcription in prokaryotes?
(a) They only increase expression.
(b) They only decrease expression.
(c) They interact with RNA polymerase but do not affect the expression.
(d) They can act both as activators and as repressors.

**18.** Which was the last human chromosome to be completely sequenced?
(a) Chromosome 1 (b) Chromosome 11
(c) Chromosome 21 (d) Chromosome x

**19.** Which of the following are the functions of RNA?
(a) It is a carrier of genetic information from DNA to ribosomes synthesizing polypeptides.
(b) It carries amino acids to ribosomes.
(c) It is a constituent component of ribosomes.
(d) All of the above

**20.** While analysing the DNA of an organism, a total number of 5386 nucleotides were found out of which the proportion of different bases were:
Adenine = 29%, Guanine = 17%, Cytosine = 32%, Thymine = 17%, considering the Chargaff's rule it can be concluded that
(a) It is a double stranded circular DNA
(b) It is a single stranded DNA
(c) It is a double stranded linear DNA
(d) No conclusion can be drawn

**21.** In some viruses, DNA is synthesized by using RNA as template. Such a DNA is called
(a) A - DNA (b) B-DNA
(c) c DNA (d) r DNA

**22.** If Meselson and Stahl's experiment is continued for four generations in bacteria, the ratio of $^{15}N/^{15}N$ : $^{15}N/^{14}N$ : $^{14}N/^{14}N$ containing DNA in the fourth generation would be
(a) 1 : 1 : 0 (b) 1 : 4 : 0
(c) 0 : 1 : 3 (d) 0 : 1 : 7

**23.** If the sequence of nitrogen bases of the coding strand of DNA in a transcription unit is 5′ - A T G A A T G – 3′, The sequence of bases in its RNA transcript would be
(a) 5′-AUGAAUG-3′ (b) 5′-UACUUAC-3′
(c) 5′-CAUUCAU-3′ (d) 5′-GUAAGUA-3′

**24.** The RNA polymerase holoenzyme transcribes
(a) The promoter, structural gene and the terminator region.
(b) The promoter and the terminator region.
(c) The structural gene and the terminator region.
(d) The structural gene only.

**25.** If the base sequence of a codon in mRNA is 5′-AUG-3′, the sequence of tRNA pairing with it must be
(a) 5′ - UAC - 3′ (b) 5′ - CAU - 3′
(c) 5′-AUG-3′ (d) 5′-GUA-3′

**26.** The amino acid attaches to the tRNA at its
(a) 5′-end (b) 3′-end
(c) Anti codon site (d) DHU loop

**27.** To initiate translation, the mRNA first binds to
(a) The smaller ribosomal sub-unit
(b) The larger ribosomal sub-unit
(c) The whole ribosome
(d) No such specificity exists

**28.** In E. coli, the lac operon gets switched on when
(a) Lactose is present and it binds to the repressor.
(b) Repressor binds to operator.
(c) RNA polymerase binds to the operator.
(d) Lactose is present and it binds to RNA polymerase.

## Previous Years' Questions

**1.** Which one of the following does not follow the central dogma of molecular biology? [AIPMT 2010 PRE]
(a) Pea (b) Mucor
(c) Chlamydomonas (d) HIV

**2.** Satellite DNA is a useful tool in: [AIPMT 2010 PRE]
(a) Organ transplantation (b) Sex determination
(c) Forensic science (d) Genetic engineering

**3.** The one aspect which is not a salient feature of genetic code is its being: [AIPMT 2010 PRE]
(a) Degenerate (b) Ambiguous
(c) Universal (d) Specific

**4.** Select two statements out of the four (1–4) given below about lac operon. [AIPMT 2010 PRE]
(1) Glucose or galactose may bind with the repressor and inactivate it
(2) In the absence of lactose, the repressor binds with the operator region
(3) The z-gene codes for permease

(4) This was elucidated by Francois Jacob and Jacques Monod

The correct statements are

(a) (3) and (3) (b) (1) and (3)
(c) (2) and (4) (d) (1) and (2)

**5.** The 3 –5′ phosphodiester linkages inside a polynucleotide chain serve to join [AIPMT 2010 MAINS]

(a) One DNA strand with the other DNA strand
(b) One nucleoside with another nucleoside
(c) One nucleotide with another nucleotide
(d) One nitrogenous base with pentose sugar

**6.** The lac operon consists of [AIPMT 2010 MAINS]

(a) Four regulatory genes only
(b) One regulatory gene and three structural genes
(c) Two regulatory genes and two structural genes
(d) Three regulatory genes and three structural genes

**7.** Which one of the following statements about the particular entity is true? [AIPMT 2010 MAINS]

(a) Centromere is found in animal cells, which produces aster during cell division
(b) The gene for producing insulin is present in every body cell
(c) Nucleosome is formed of nucleotides
(d) DNA consists a core of eight histones

**8.** In eukaryotic cell transcription, RNA splicing and RNA capping take place inside the [AIPMT 2010 MAINS]

(a) Ribosomes (b) Nucleus
(c) Dictyosomes (d) ER

**9.** Which one of the following does not follow the central dogma of molecular biology? [AIPMT PRE 2010]

(a) Pea (b) Mucor
(c) Chlamydomonas (d) HIV

**10.** In history of biology, human genome project led to the development of: [AIPMT 2011 MAINS]

(a) Biotechnology
(b) Biomonitoring
(c) Bioinformatics
(d) Biosystematics

**11.** The unequivocal proof of DNA as the genetic material came from the studies on: [AIPMT 2011 MAINS]

(a) Bacterium (b) Fungus
(c) Viroid (d) Bacterial virus

**12.** Which one of the following also acts as a catalyst in a bacterial cell? [AIPMT 2011 PRE]

(a) sn RNA (b) hn RNA
(c) 23 S rRNA (d) 5 S rRNA

**13.** What are those structures that appear as 'beads-on-string' in chromosomes when viewed under electron microscope? [AIPMT 2011 PRE]

(a) Nucleotides (b) Nucleosomes
(c) Base pairs (d) Genes

**14.** Removal of introns and joining of exons in a defined order during transcription is called: [AIPMT 2012 PRE]

(a) Looping (b) Inducing
(c) Slicing (d) Splicing

**15.** If one strand of DNA has the nitrogenous base sequence as ATCTG, what would be the complementary RNA strand sequence? [AIPMT 2012 PRE]

(a) TTAGU (b) UAGAC
(c) AACTG (d) ATCGU

**16.** A single strand of nucleic acid tagged with a radioactive molecule is called: [AIPMT 2012 PRE]

(a) Vector (b) Selectable market
(c) Plasmid (d) Probe

**17.** Which one of the following is not a part of transcription unit in DNA? [AIPMT 2012 PRE]

(a) The inducer (b) A terminator
(c) A promoter (d) The structural gene

**18.** PCR and Restriction Fragment Length Polymorphism are methods for: [AIPMT 2012 PRE]

(a) Study of enzymes (b) Genetic transformation
(c) DNA sequencing (d) Genetic fingerprinting

**19.** Removal of RNA polymerase III from nucleoplasm will affect the synthesis of: [AIPMT 2012 PRE]

(a) t RNA (b) hn RNA
(c) m RNA (d) r RNA

**20.** What is it that forms the basis of DNA fingerprinting? [AIPMT 2012 MAINS]

(a) The relative difference in the DNA occurrence in blood, skin and saliva
(b) The relative amount of DNA in the ridges and grooves of the fingerprints
(c) Satellite DNA occurring as highly repeated short DNA segments
(d) The relative proportions of purines and pyrimidines in DNA

**21.** Read the following four statements (A–D): [AIPMT 2012 MAINS]

(A) In transcription, adenosine pairs with uracil
(B) Regulation of lac operon by repressor is referred to as positive regulation
(C) The human genome has approximately 50,000 genes
(D) Haemophilia is a sex-linked recessive disease

How many of the above statements are right?

(a) 3 (b) 4 (c) 1 (d) 2

**22.** Which enzyme/s will be produced in a cell in which there is a nonsense mutation in the lac Y gene? [AIPMT 2013]

(a) β-galactosidase
(b) Lactose permease
(c) Transacetylase
(d) Lactose permease and transacetylase

**23.** The diagram shows an important concept in the genetic implication of DNA. Fill in the blanks A to C [AIPMT 2013]

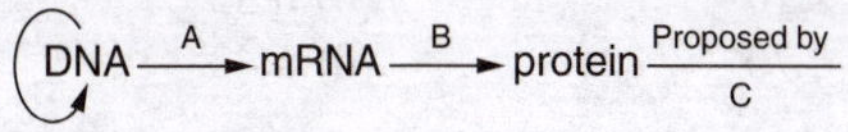


(a) A: transcription B: protein C: James Watson
(b) A: translation B: transcription C: Erevin Chargaff
(c) A: transcription B: translation C: Francis Crick
(d) A: translation B: Extension C: Rosalind Franklin

**24.** Commonly used vectors for human genome sequencing are: [AIPMT 2014]

(a) T – DNA (b) BAC and YAC
(c) Expression Vectors (d) T/Cloning Vectors

**25.** Select the correct option: (A: Direction RNA synthesis, B: Direction of reading of the template DNA strand) [AIPMT 2014]

(a) 5′ ----- 3′ 3′ ----- 5′
(b) 3′ ----- 5′ 5′ ------ 3′
(c) 5′ ----- 3′ 5′ ------ 3′
(d) 3′ ----- 5′ 3′ ------ 5′

**26.** An analysis of chromosomal DNA using the southern hybridization technique does not use [AIPMT 2014]

(a) Electrophoresis (b) Blotting
(c) Autoradiography (d) PCR

**27.** Transformation was discovered by [AIPMT 2014]

(a) Meselson and Stahl (b) Hershey and Chase
(c) Griffith (d) Watson and Crick

**28.** Which one of the following is wrongly matched? [AIPMT 2014]

(a) Transcription – Writing information from DNA to t-RNA
(b) Translation – Using information in m-RNA to make protein
(c) Repressor protein – Binds to operator to stop enzyme synthesis
(d) Operon – Structural genes, operator and promoter

**29.** Satellite DNA is important because it: [RE-AIPMT 2015]

(a) shows high degree of polymorphism in population and also the same degree of polymorphism in an individual, which is heritable from parents to children
(b) does not code for proteins and is same in all members of the population
(c) codes for enzymes needed for DNA repletion
(d) codes for proteins needed in cell cycle

**30.** Balbiani rings are sites of [RE-AIPMT 2015]

(a) Nucleotide synthesis
(b) Polysaccharide synthesis
(c) RNA and protein synthesis
(d) Lipid synthesis

**31.** Identify the correct order of organization of genetic material from largest to smallest: [RE-AIPMT 2015]

(a) Genome, chromosome, nucleotide, gene
(b) Genome, chromosome, gene, nucleotide
(c) Chromosome, genome, nucleotide, gene
(d) Chromosome, gene, genome, nucleotide

**32.** Which one of the following is not applicable to RNA? [RE-AIPMT 2015]

(a) 5′ phosphoryl and 3′hydroxyl ends
(b) Heterocyclic nitrogeneous bases
(c) Chargaff's rule
(d) Complementary base pairing

**33.** In sea urchin DNA, which is double stranded, 17% of the bases were shown to be cytosine. The percentages of the other three bases expected to be present in this DNA are : [AIPMT 2015]

(a) G 34%, A 24.5%, T 24.5%
(b) G 17%, A 16.5%, T 32.5%
(c) G 17%, A 33%, T 33%
(d) G 8.5%, A 50%, T 24.5%

**34.** Gene regulation governing lactose operon of E. coli that involves lac I gene product is: [AIPMT 2015]

(a) Positive and inducible because it can be induced by lactose
(b) Negative and inducible because repressor protein prevents transcription

(c) Negative and repressible because repressor protein prevents transcription
(d) Feedback inhibition because excess of β galactosidase can switch off transcription

**35.** DNA-dependent RNA polymerase catalyses transcription on one strand of the DNA which is called the…… [NEET 2016] PHASE II]
(a) Coding strand
(b) Alpha strand
(c) Antistrand
(d) Template strand

**36.** A molecule that can act as a genetic material must fulfil the traits given below, except [NEET 2016 – PHASE II]
(a) It should be able to generate its replica
(b) It should be unstable structurally and chemically
(c) It should provide scope for slow changes that are required for evolution
(d) It should be able to express itself in the form of Mendelian characters

**37.** Which of the following rRNAs acts a structural RNA as well as ribozyme in bacteria? [NEET 2016 – PHASE II]
(a) 18 S rRNA
(b) 23 S rRNA
(c) 5.8 S rRNA
(d) 5 S rRNA

**38.** The equivalent of a structural gene is [NEET 2016 – PHASE II]
(a) Cistron (b) Operon
(c) Recon (d) Muton

**39.** Which one of the following is a starter codon? [NEET 2016 – PHASE I]
(a) AUG (b) UGA
(c) UAA (d) UAG

**40.** Which of the following is not required for any of the techniques of DNA fingerprinting available at present? [NEET 2016 – PHASE I]
(a) Polymerase chain reaction
(b) Zinc figure analysis
(c) Restriction enzymes
(d) DNA – DNA hybridization

**41.** Which of the following is required as inducer(s) for the expression of Lac operon? [NEET 2016 – PHASE I]
(a) Glucose (b) Galactose
(c) Lactose (d) Lactose and galactose

**42.** Taylor conducted experiments to prove semi-conservative mode of chromosome replication on [NEET 2016 – PHASE II]
(a) *Vicia faba*
(b) *Drosphila melanogaster*
(c) *E. coli*
(d) *Vinca rosea*

**43.** Select the wrong statement: [NEET Regional 2017]
(a) DNA stores genetic information
(b) There is now enough evidence that essential process like metabolism, translation and splicing evolve around RNA
(c) DNA may act as a catalyst
(d) RNA can splice itself and is also able to act as a catalyst

**44.** If the ratio of (T+C) / (A+G) in one strand of DNA is 1.43, same ratio in the complementary strand is: [NEET Regional 2017]
(a) 2.10 (b) 0.35
(c) 0.70 (d) 1.43

**45.** A couple claimed in court that a child belonged to them. Their claim can be true if the DNA fingerprint of the child shows: [NEET Regional 2017]
(a) 50% bands similar to father and 50% similar to mother DNA fingerprint pattern.
(b) 100% similarity to both the parents DNA fingerprint as both contribute equally to zygote formation.
(c) 100% similarity to mothers DNA print because of maternal inheritance.
(d) 100% similarity to fathers DNA print due to large number of mitochondria in sperm.

**46.** The technique of DNA fingerprinting is superior to conventional fingerprinting because it can: [NEET Regional 2017]
(a) be generated more rapidly and is inexpensive
(b) generate unique fingerprints for each finger
(c) compare the whole DNA sequence of two individuals
(d) differentiate between polymorphic DNA sequences among individuals

**47.** Consider the following statements and choose the correct option: [NEET Regional 2017]
(a) Six codons do not code for any amino acid.
(b) Codon is read in m-RNA in a contiguous fashion.
(c) Three codons function as stop codons
(d) The initiator codon AUG codes for methionine.

**Option:**
(a) (a) is wrong
(b) (a), (b) and (d) are wrong
(c) (a), (b) and (c) are wrong
(d) (b), (c) and (d) are wrong

**48.** If there are 999 bases in an RNA that codes for a protein with 333 amino acid, and the base at position 901 is deleted such that the length of the RNA becomes 998 bases, how many codons will be altered? [NEET 2017]
(a) 11 (b) 33 (c) 333 (d) 1

**49.** Which of the following RNAs should be most abundant in animal cell? [NEET 2017]
(a) t - RNA (b) m - RNA
(c) mi - RNA (d) r - RNA

**50.** Spliceosomes are not found in cells of: [NEET 2017]
(a) Fungi (b) Animals
(c) Bacteria (d) Plants

**51.** The final proof for DNA as the genetic material came from the experiments of: [NEET 2017]
(a) Hershey and Chase
(b) Avery, McLeod and McCarty
(c) Hargobind Khorana
(d) Griffith

**52.** During DNA replication, Okazaki fragments are used to elongate: [NEET 2017]
(a) The lagging strand towards replication fork.
(b) The leading strand away from replication fork.
(c) The lagging strand away from replication fork.
(d) The leading strand towards replication fork.

**53.** The association of histone H1 with a nucleosome indicates: [NEET 2017]
(a) DNA replication is occurring
(b) DNA is condensed into a Chromatin Fibre.
(c) DNA double helix is exposed.
(d) Transcription is occurring.

**54.** The experimental proof for semiconservative replication of DNA was first shown in a [NEET 2018]
(a) Fungus (b) Plant
(b) Bacterium (d) Virus

**55.** Select the correct match: [NEET 2018]
(a) Alec Jeffreys - *Streptococcus pneumoniae*
(b) Matthew Meselson and F. Stahl - *Pisum sativum*
(c) Alfred Hershey and Martha Chase - TMV
(d) Francois Jacob and Jacques Monod - *Lac operon*

**56.** All of the following are part of an operon except [NEET 2018]
(a) An operator (b) An enhancer
(c) Structural genes (d) A promoter

**57.** AGGTATCGCAT is a sequence form of the coding strand of a gene. What will be the corresponding sequence of the transcribed mRNA? [NEET 2018]
(a) AGGUAUCGCAU
(b) ACCUAUGCGAU
(c) UGGTUTCGCAT
(d) UCCAUAGCGUA

**58.** Expressed Sequence Tags (ESTs) refers to: [NEET 2019]
(a) Polypeptide expression
(b) DNA polymorphism
(c) Novel DNA sequences
(d) Genes expressed as RNA

**59.** Match the following genes of the Lac operon with their respective products:

| | |
|---|---|
| (1) i gene | (i) β-galactosidase |
| (2) z gene | (ii) Permease |
| (3) a gene | (iii) Repressor |
| (4) y gene | (iv) Transacetylase |

[NEET 2019]

Select the **correct** option,

| | (1) | (2) | (3) | (4) |
|---|---|---|---|---|
| (a) | (iii) | (i) | (ii) | (iv) |
| (b) | (iii) | (i) | (iv) | (ii) |
| (c) | (iii) | (iv) | (i) | (ii) |
| (d) | (i) | (iii) | (ii) | (iv) |

**60.** Which of the following features of genetic code does allow bacteria to produce human insulin by recombinant DNA technology? [NEET 2019]
(a) Genetic code is redundant
(b) Genetic code is nearly universal
(c) Genetic code is specific
(d) Genetic code is not ambiguous

**61.** Under which of the following conditions will there be no change in the reading frame of following mRNA?
5′ AACAGCGGUGCUAUU 3′ [NEET 2019]
(a) Deletion of G from 5th position
(b) Insertion of A and G at 4th and 5th positions, respectively
(c) Deletion of GGU from 7th, 8th and 9th positions
(d) Insertion of G at 5th position

**62.** The first phase of translation is: [NEET 2020]
(a) Binding of mRNA to ribosome
(b) Recognition of DNA molecule
(c) Aminoacylation of tRNA
(d) Recogniton of an anticodon

**63.** Name of enzyme that facilitates opening of DNA helix during transcription. [NEET 2020]
(a) DNA ligase (b) DNA helicase
(c) DNA polymerase (d) RNA polymerase

**64.** If the distance between two consecutive base pairs is 0.34 nm and the total number of base pairs of a DNA double helix in a typical mammalian cell is $6.6 \times 10^9$ bp, then the length of the DNA is approximately: [NEET 2020]
(a) 2.0 meters (b) 2.5 meters
(c) 2.2 meters (d) 2.7 meters

**65.** Complete the flow chart on central dogma.
(a) ↻DNA $\xrightarrow{(b)}$ mRNA $\xrightarrow{(c)}$ (d)
[NEET 2021]
(a) (a)-Transduction; (b)-Translation; (c)-Replication; (d)-Protein
(b) (a)-Replication; (b)-Transcription; (c)-Transduction; (d)-Protein
(c) (a)-Translation;( b)-Replication; (c)-Transcription; (d)-Transduction
(d) (a)-Replication; (b)-Transcription; (c)-Translation; (d)-Protein

**66.** What is the role of RNA polymerase III in the process of transcription in eukaryotes? [NEET 2021]
(a) Transcribes only snRNAs
(b) Transcribes rRNAs (28S, 18S and 5.8S)
(c) Transcribes tRNA, bs rRNA and snRNA
(d) Transcribes precursor of mRNA

**67.** DNA fingerprinting involves identifying differences in some specific regions in DNA sequence, called as: [NEET 2021]
(a) Polymorphic DNA
(b) Satellite DNA
(c) Repetitive DNA
(d) Single nucleotides

**68.** Identify the **correct** statement. [NEET 2021]
(a) Spit gene arrangement is characteristic of prokaryotes.
(b) In capping, methyl guanosine triphosphate is added to the 3' end of hnRNA.
(c) RNA polymerase binds with Rho factor to terminate the process of transcription in bacteria.
(d) The coding strand in a transcription unit is copied to an mRNA.

**69.** Which is the "Only enzyme" that has "Capability to catalyse Initiation, Elongation and Termination in the process of transcription in prokaryotes?[NEET 2021]
(a) DNase
(b) DNA dependent DNA polymerase
(c) DNA dependent RNA polymerase
(d) DNA Ligase

**70.** If Adenine makes 30% of the DNA molecule, what will be the percentage of Thymine, Guanine and Cytosine in it? [NEET 2021]
(a) T : 20; G : 25; C : 25
(b) T : 20; G : 30; C : 20
(c) T : 20; G : 20; C : 30
(d) T : 30; G : 20; C : 20

**71.** Which of the following RNAs is not required for the synthesis of protein? [NEET 2021]
(a) siRNA (b) mRNA
(c) tRNA (d) rRNA

**72.** Which one of the following statements about Histones is wrong? [NEET 2021]
(a) Histones carry positive charge in the side chain.
(b) Histones are organized to form a unit of 8 molecules.
(c) The pH of histones is slightly acidic.
(d) Histones are rich in amino acids Lysine and Arginine.

**73.** **Statement I :** The codon 'AUG' codes for methionine and phenyalanine.
**Statement II :** 'AAA' and 'AAG' both codons code for the amino acid lysine.
In the light of the above statements, choose the **correct** answer from the options given below.
[NEET 2021]
(a) Statement I is incorrect but Statement II is true.
(b) Both Statement I and Statement II are true.
(c) Both Statement I and Statement II are false.
(d) Statement I is correct but Statement II is false

**74.** Read the following statements and choose the set of correct statements: [NEET 2022]
(A) Euchromatin is transcriptionally active.
(B) Heterochromatin is transcriptionally active.
(C) Histone octomer is wrapped by negatively charged DNA in nucleosome.
(D) Histones are rich in lysine and arginine.
(E) A typical nucleosome contains 400 bp of DNA helix.
Choose the **correct answer** from the options given below:
(a) (A), (C), (D) only (b) (B), (E) only
(c) (A), (C), (E) only (d) (B), (D), (E) only

**75.** DNA polymorphism forms the basis of: [NEET 2022]
(a) DNA finger printing
(b) Both genetic mapping and DNA finger printing
(c) Translation
(d) Genetic mapping

**76.** The process of translation of mRNA to proteins begins as soon as: [NEET 2022]
(a) The larger subunit of ribosome encounters mRNA.
(b) Both the subunits join together to bind with mRNA.
(c) The tRNA is activated and the larger subunit of ribosome encounters mRNA.
(d) The small subunit of ribosome encounters mRNA.

**77.** If a geneticist uses the blind approach for sequencing the whole genome of an organism, followed by assignment of function to different segments, the methodology adopted by him is called as: [NEET 2022]
(a) Gene mapping
(b) Expressed sequence tags
(c) Bioinformatics
(d) Sequence annotation

**78.** In an *E.coli* strain, *i* gene gets mutated and its product can not bind the inducer molecule. If growth medium is provided with lactose, what will be the outcome? [NEET 2022]
(a) *z, y, a* genes will be transcribed
(b) *z, y, a* genes will not be translated
(c) RNA polymerase will bind the promoter region
(d) Only *z* gene will get transcribed

**79.** If the length of a DNA molecule is 1.1 metres, what will be the approximate number of base pairs? [NEET 2022]
(a) $6.6 \times 10^9$ bp (b) $3.3 \times 10^6$ bp
(c) $6.6 \times 10^6$ bp (d) $3.3 \times 10^9$ bp

**80.** Ten *E.coli* cells with $^{15}N$ - ds DNA are incubated in medium containing $^{14}N$ nucleotide. After 60 minutes, how many *E.coli* cells will have DNA totally free from $^{15}N$? [NEET 2022]
(a) 40 cells (b) 60 cells
(c) 80 cells (d) 20 cells

**81.** Unequivocal proof that DNA is the genetic material was first proposed by: [NEET 2023]
(a) Alfred Hershey and Martha Chase
(b) Avery, Macleoid and McCarthy
(c) Wilkins and Franklin
(d) Frederick Griffith

**82.** What is the role of RNA polymerase III in the process of transcription in Eukaryotes? [NEET 2023]
(a) Transcription of t RNA, 5s rRNA and snRNA
(b) Transcription of precursor of mRNA
(c) Transcription of only snRNAs
(d) Transcription of rRNAs (28S,18S and 5.8 S)

**83.** Expressed sequence Tags (ESTs) refers to: [NEET 2023]
(a) All genes that are expressed as proteins.
(b) All genes whether expressed or unexpressed.
(c) Certain important expressed genes
(d) All genes that are expressed as RNA

**84.** How many different proteins does the ribosome consist of? [NEET 2023]
(a) 60 (b) 40
(c) 20 (d) 80

**85.** Match List I with List II. [NEET 2023]

| List I | List II |
|---|---|
| A. Gene 'a' | I. β - galactosidase |
| B. Gene 'y' | II. Transacetylase |
| C. Gene 'i' | III. Permease |
| D. Gene 'z' | IV. Repressor protein |

Choose the correct answer from the options given below:
(a) A - II, B - III, C - IV, D - I
(b) A - III, B - IV, C - I, D - II
(c) A - III, B - I, C - IV, D - II
(d) A - II, B - I, C - IV, D - III

**86.** Given below are two statements: [NEET 2023]
**Statements I:** RNA mutates at a faster rate
**Statements II:** Viruses having RNA genome and shorter life span mutate and evolve faster. In the light of the above statements, choose the correct answer from the options given below:
(a) Both Statement I and Statement II are false
(b) Statement I is true but Statement II is False
(c) Statement I is false but Statement II is true
(d) Both Statement I and Statement II are true

**87.** Given below are two statements: [NEET 2023]
**Statement I:** In prokaryotes, the positively charged DNA is held with some negatively charged proteins in a region called nucleoid.
**Statement II:** In eukaryotes, the negatively charged DNA is wrapped around the positively charged histone octamer to form nucleosome.

(a) Both Statement I and Statement II are false.
(b) Statement I is true but Statement II is false.
(c) Statement I is false but Statement II is true.
(d) Both Statement I and Statement II are true.

**88.** Which of the following is the sequence on corresponding coding strand, if the sequence on mRNA formed is as follows: [NEET 2023]
5' AUCGAUCGAUCGAUCGAUCGAUCGAUCG 3'
(a) 3' UAGCUAGCUAGCUAGCUAGCUAGCUAG C 5'
(b) 5' ATCGATCGATCGATCGATCGATCGATCG 3'
(c) 3' ATCGATCGATCGATCGATCGATCGATCG 5'
(d) 5' UAGCUAGCUAGCUAGCUAGCUAGCUAG C 3'

**89.** The lactose present in the growth medium of bacteria is transported to the cell by the action of: [NEET 2024]
(a) $\beta$-galactosidase (b) Acetylase
(c) Permease (d) Polymerase

**90.** A transcription unit in DNA is defined primarily by the three regions in DNA and these are with respect to upstream and downstream end: [NEET 2024]
(a) Repressor, Operator gene, Structural gene
(b) Structural gene, Transposons, Operator gene
(c) Inducer, Repressor, Structural gene
(d) Promotor, Structural gene, Terminator

**91.** Which of the following statements is correct regarding the process of replication in *E.coli*? [NEET 2024]
(a) The DNA dependent DNA polymerase catalyses polymerization in one direction that is $3' \to 5'$
(b) The DNA dependent RNA polymerase catalyses polymerization in one direction, that is $5' \to 3'$
(c) The DNA dependent DNA polymerase catalyses polymerization in $5' \to 3'$ as well as $3' \to 5'$ direction.
(d) The DNA dependent DNA polymerases catalyses polymerizations in $5' \to 3'$ direction.

**92.** Match List-I with List-II [NEET 2024]

| List-I | List-II |
|---|---|
| (A) Frederick Griffith | (i) Genetic code |
| (B) Francois Jacob & Jacque Monod | (ii) Semi-conservative mode of DNA replication |
| (C) Har Gobind Khorana | (iii) Transformation |
| (D) Meselson & Stahl | (iv) Lac operon |

Choose the correct answer from the option given beow:
(a) (A)-(iii), (B)-(ii), (C)-(i), (D)-(iv)
(b) (A)-(iii), (B)-(iv), (C)-(i), (D)-(ii)
(c) (A)-(ii), (B)-(iii), (C)-(iv), (D)-(i)
(d) (A)-(iv), (B)-(i), (C)-(ii),(D)-(iii)

**93.** Which one is the correct product of DNA dependent RNA polymerase to the given template? [NEET 2024]
3′TACATGGCAATATCCATTCA5′
(a) 5′AUGUACCGUUUAUAGGUAAGU3′
(b) 5′AUGUACCGUUUAUAGGUAAGU3′
(c) 5′AUGUAAAGUUUAUAGGUAAGU3′
(d) 5′ATGTACCGTTTATAGGTAAGT3′

**94.** Match List-I with List-II. [NEET 2024]

| List-I | List-II |
|---|---|
| (A) RNA polymerase III | (i) snRNPs |
| (B) Termination of transcription | (ii) Promotor |
| (C) Splicing of Exons | (iii) Rho factor |
| (D) TATA box | (iv) SnRNAs, tRNA |

Choose the correct answer from the options given below:
(a) (A)-(iii), B- IV, (C)-(i), (D)-(iii)
(b) (A)-(iii), B- II, (C)-(iv), (D)-(i)
(c) (A)-(iii), B- IV, (C)-(i), (D)-(ii)
(d) (A)-(iv), B- III, (C)-(i), (D)-(ii)

## Answer Key

### Multiple Choice Questions: Level I

| | | | | | | | | | |
|---|---|---|---|---|---|---|---|---|---|
| **1.** (c) | **2.** (c) | **3.** (a) | **4.** (b) | **5.** (d) | **6.** (c) | **7.** (b) | **8.** (c) | **9.** (d) | **10.** (a) |
| **11.** (c) | **12.** (d) | **13.** (c) | **14.** (b) | **15.** (c) | **16.** (a) | **17.** (a) | **18.** (b) | **19.** (c) | **20.** (d) |
| **21.** (c) | **22.** (c) | **23.** (a) | **24.** (b) | **25.** (d) | **26.** (d) | **27.** (a) | **28.** (b) | **29.** (a) | **30.** (b) |
| **31.** (b) | **32.** (c) | **33.** (d) | **34.** (b) | **35.** (c) | **36.** (c) | **37.** (b) | **38.** (d) | **39.** (a) | **40.** (d) |
| **41.** (d) | **42.** (c) | **43.** (b) | **44.** (b) | **45.** (b) | **46.** (b) | **47.** (b) | **48.** (b) | **49.** (b) | **50.** (d) |
| **51.** (b) | **52.** (b) | **53.** (d) | **54.** (a) | **55.** (d) | **56.** (c) | **57.** (c) | **58.** (b) | **59.** (c) | **60.** (d) |
| **61.** (a) | **62.** (b) | **63.** (a) | **64.** (d) | **65.** (a) | **66.** (c) | **67.** (d) | **68.** (c) | **69.** (c) | **70.** (b) |
| **71.** (a) | **72.** (d) | **73.** (d) | **74.** (d) | **75.** (d) | **76.** (a) | **77.** (b) | **78.** (c) | **79.** (a) | **80.** (c) |
| **81.** (b) | **82.** (b) | **83.** (d) | **84.** (d) | **85.** (d) | **86.** (d) | **87.** (c) | **88.** (c) | **89.** (c) | **90.** (c) |
| **91.** (d) | **92.** (c) | **93.** (b) | **94.** (c) | **95.** (b) | **96.** (c) | **97.** (b) | **98.** (b) | **99.** (c) | **100.** (c) |
| **101.** (c) | **102.** (d) | **103.** (d) | **104.** (c) | **105.** (a) | **106.** (c) | **107.** (c) | **108.** (d) | **109.** (c) | **110.** (d) |
| **111.** (c) | **112.** (a) | **113.** (b) | **114.** (d) | **115.** (d) | **116.** (a) | **117.** (c) | **118.** (d) | **119.** (c) | **120.** (a) |
| **121.** (b) | **122.** (d) | **123.** (d) | **124.** (b) | **125.** (d) | **126.** (d) | **127.** (c) | **128.** (c) | **129.** (b) | **130.** (c) |
| **131.** (b) | **132.** (c) | **133.** (d) | **134.** (c) | **135.** (c) | **136.** (b) | **137.** (c) | **138.** (a) | **139.** (a) | **140.** (b) |
| **141.** (b) | **142.** (c) | **143.** (d) | **144.** (a) | **145.** (d) | **146.** (d) | **147.** (b) | **148.** (b) | **149.** (b) | **150.** (c) |
| **151.** (b) | **152.** (a) | **153.** (b) | **154.** (a) | **155.** (a) | **156.** (a) | **157.** (d) | **158.** (b) | **159.** (c) | **160.** (c) |
| **161.** (b) | **162.** (a) | **163.** (c) | **164.** (d) | **165.** (b) | **166.** (d) | **167.** (c) | **168.** (a) | **169.** (d) | **170.** (b) |
| **171.** (c) | **172.** (d) | **173.** (b) | **174.** (d) | **175.** (b) | **176.** (c) | **177.** (d) | **178.** (b) | **179.** (c) | **180.** (c) |
| **181.** (a) | **182.** (a) | **183.** (a) | **184.** (a) | **185.** (d) | **186.** (d) | **187.** (d) | **188.** (b) | **189.** (d) | **190.** (b) |
| **191.** (d) | **192.** (a) | **193.** (c) | **194.** (c) | **195.** (d) | **196.** (b) | **197.** (a) | **198.** (c) | **199.** (b) | **200.** (b) |
| **201.** (b) | **202.** (a) | **203.** (b) | **204.** (c) | **205.** (b) | **206.** (c) | **207.** (d) | **208.** (b) | **209.** (d) | **210.** (d) |
| **211.** (c) | **212.** (c) | **213.** (d) | **214.** (c) | **215.** (d) | **216.** (c) | **217A.** (b) | **217B.** (c) | **218.** (c) | **219.** (d) |
| **220.** (d) | **221.** (a) | **222.** (b) | **223.** (d) | **224.** (a) | **225.** (b) | **226.** (b) | **227.** (d) | **228.** (b) | **229.** (c) |
| **230.** (a) | **231.** (c) | **232.** (a) | **233.** (a) | **234.** (d) | **235.** (c) | **236.** (d) | **237.** (b) | **238.** (d) | **239.** (c) |
| **240.** (b) | **241.** (c) | **242.** (b) | **243.** (d) | **244.** (c) | **245.** (d) | **246.** (d) | **247.** (c) | **248.** (d) | **249.** (a) |
| **250.** (c) | **251.** (b) | **252.** (b) | **253.** (d) | **254.** (b) | **255.** (a) | **256.** (c) | **257.** (d) | **258.** (b) | **259.** (c) |
| **260.** (c) | **261.** (d) | **262.** (b) | **263.** (b) | **264.** (c) | **265.** (c) | **266.** (b) | **267.** (d) | **268.** (b) | **269.** (a) |
| **270.** (c) | **271.** (b) | **272.** (a) | **273.** (b) | **274.** (b) | **275.** (a) | **276.** (a) | **277.** (a) | **278.** (d) | **279.** (d) |
| **280.** (c) | **281.** (a) | **282.** (b) | **283.** (a) | **284.** (a) | **285.** (a) | **286.** (b) | **287.** (c) | **288.** (c) | **289.** (d) |
| **290.** (b) | **291.** (b) | **292.** (c) | **293.** (b) | **294.** (a) | **295.** (b) | **296.** (a) | **297.** (b) | **298.** (b) | **299.** (d) |
| **300.** (a) | **301.** (d) | **302.** (b) | **303.** (b) | **304.** (d) | **305.** (a) | **306.** (d) | **307.** (b) | **308.** (d) | **309.** (d) |
| **310.** (b) | **311.** (c) | **312.** (a) | **313.** (a) | **314.** (d) | **315.** (d) | **316.** (c) | **317.** (d) | **318.** (d) | **319.** (b) |
| **320.** (d) | **321.** (b) | **322.** (d) | **323.** (b) | **324.** (a) | **325.** (d) | **326.** (c) | **327.** (c) | **328.** (d) | **329.** (c) |
| **330.** (b) | **331.** (a) | **332.** (b) | **333.** (a) | **334.** (b) | **335.** (c) | **336.** (d) | **337.** (d) | **338.** (b) | **339.** (a) |
| **340.** (b) | **341.** (b) | **342.** (c) | **343.** (d) | **344.** (d) | **345.** (c) | **346.** (a) | **347.** (d) | **348.** (d) | **349.** (c) |
| **350.** (b) | **351.** (b) | **352.** (b) | **353.** (a) | **354.** (c) | **355.** (d) | **356.** (a) | **357.** (d) | **358.** (c) | **359.** (c) |
| **360.** (a) | | | | | | | | | |

### Multiple Choice Questions: Level II

| | | | | | | | | | |
|---|---|---|---|---|---|---|---|---|---|
| **361.** (d) | **362.** (d) | **363.** (a) | **364.** (d) | **365.** (a) | **366.** (b) | **367.** (d) | **368.** (a) | **369.** (c) | **370.** (b) |
| **371.** (c) | **372.** (d) | **373.** (d) | **374.** (c) | **375.** (a) | **376.** (d) | **377.** (b) | **378.** (c) | **379.** (c) | **380.** (c) |
| **381.** (a) | **382.** (c) | **383.** (d) | **384.** (d) | **385.** (b) | **386.** (a) | **387.** (c) | **388.** (b) | **389.** (b) | **390.** (b) |
| **391.** (a) | **392.** (b) | **393.** (d) | **394.** (a) | **395.** (b) | **396.** (c) | **397.** (b) | **398.** (a) | **399.** (b) | **400.** (b) |
| **401.** (c) | **402.** (a) | **403.** (b) | **404.** (c) | **405.** (b) | **406.** (c) | **407.** (a) | **408.** (c) | **409.** (d) | **410.** (a) |
| **411.** (c) | **412.** (a) | **413.** (d) | **414.** (c) | **415.** (c) | **416.** (d) | **417.** (b) | **418.** (d) | **419.** (d) | **420.** (b) |

| | | | | | | | | | |
|---|---|---|---|---|---|---|---|---|---|
| **421.** (a) | **422.** (b) | **423.** (d) | **424.** (c) | **425.** (a) | **426.** (c) | **427.** (a) | **428.** (b) | **429.** (b) | **430.** (c) |
| **431.** (b) | **432.** (a) | **433.** (a) | **434.** (b) | **435.** (d) | **436.** (d) | **437.** (a) | **438.** (a) | **439.** (c) | **440.** (b) |
| **441.** (a) | **442.** (b) | | | | | | | | |

## A & R and Statement-based Questions

| | | | | | | | | | |
|---|---|---|---|---|---|---|---|---|---|
| **443.** (b) | **444.** (a) | **445.** (d) | **446.** (d) | **447.** (c) | **448.** (c) | **449.** (c) | **450.** (d) | **451.** (b) | **452.** (c) |

## Matrix-Match Type Questions

| | | | | |
|---|---|---|---|---|
| **453.** (a) | **454.** (a) | **455.** (a) | **456.** (a) | **457.** (a) |

## NCERT Exemplar Questions

| | | | | | | | | | |
|---|---|---|---|---|---|---|---|---|---|
| **1.** (b) | **2.** (c) | **3.** (c) | **4.** (c) | **5.** (c) | **6.** (b) | **7.** (d) | **8.** (d) | **9.** (d) | **10.** (b) |
| **11.** (c) | **12.** (d) | **13.** (b) | **14.** (b) | **15.** (b) | **16.** (b) | **17.** (d) | **18.** (a) | **19.** (d) | **20.** (b) |
| **21.** (c) | **22.** (d) | **23.** (a) | **24.** (d) | **25.** (b) | **26.** (b) | **27.** (a) | **28.** (a) | | |

## Previous Years' Questions

| | | | | | | | | | |
|---|---|---|---|---|---|---|---|---|---|
| **1.** (d) | **2.** (c) | **3.** (b) | **4.** (c) | **5.** (c) | **6.** (b) | **7.** (b) | **8.** (b) | **9.** (d) | **10.** (c) |
| **11.** (d) | **12.** (c) | **13.** (b) | **14.** (d) | **15.** (b) | **16.** (d) | **17.** (a) | **18.** (d) | **19.** (a) | **20.** (c) |
| **21.** (d) | **22.** (a) | **23.** (c) | **24.** (b) | **25.** (a) | **26.** (d) | **27.** (c) | **28.** (d) | **29.** (a) | **30.** (c) |
| **31.** (b) | **32.** (c) | **33.** (c) | **34.** (b) | **35.** (d) | **36.** (b) | **37.** (b) | **38.** (a) | **39.** (a) | **40.** (b) |
| **41.** (c) | **42.** (a) | **43.** (c) | **44.** (c) | **45.** (a) | **46.** (d) | **47.** (a) | **48.** (b) | **49.** (d) | **50.** (c) |
| **51.** (a) | **52.** (c) | **53.** (b) | **54.** (c) | **55.** (d) | **56.** (b) | **57.** (a) | **58.** (d) | **59.** (b) | **60.** (b) |
| **61.** (c) | **62.** (c) | **63.** (d) | **64.** (c) | **65.** (d) | **66.** (c) | **67.** (c) | **68.** (c) | **69.** (c) | **70.** (d) |
| **71.** (a) | **72.** (c) | **73.** (a) | **74.** (a) | **75.** (b) | **76.** (d) | **77.** (d) | **78.** (b) | **79.** (d) | **80.** (b) |
| **81.** (a) | **82.** (a) | **83.** (d) | **84.** (d) | **85.** (d) | **86.** (d) | **87.** (c) | **88.** (b) | **89.** (c) | **90.** (d) |
| **91.** (d) | **92.** (b) | **93.** (a) | **94.** (a) | | | | | | |

# HINTS AND EXPLANATION

## Multiple Choice Questions: Level II

**361.** **(1)** Genetic codon is **unambiguous** and **specific**, i.e., one codon code for only one amino acid.

**(2)** Single amino acid can be coded by two or more codons. This is **degeneracy** of codon.

**(3)** In mRNA codon is read in continuous or **contiguous manner**. No punctuations are there in between.

**(4)** Genetic codon is **nearly universal**. Exceptions are there in mitochondrial codons and in some protozoans.

**362.** It is the process of splicing that occurs in nucleus of eukaryotic cell.

**363.** It is first studied by Messelson and Stahl (1958) in *Escherichia coli.*

**364.** Nirenberg and Mathaei (1961) experimentally proved that a single amino acid is determined by a sequence of three nitrogen bases. The sequence of three nitrogen bases determining a single amino acid is called a triplet code. Nirenberg and Mathaei experiments cracked the DNA and discovered unequivocally that a genetic code is a triplet.

**365.** A point mutation is a simple change in one base of the gene sequence. This is equivalent to changing one letter in a sentence.

**366.** In the DNA molecule, there are two strands which run antiparallel one in 5′-3′ direction and other in 3′-5′ direction. The two chains are held together by hydrogen bonds between their bases. Adenine (A), A purine of one chain is exactly opposite to thymine (T), a pyramidine of the other chain. Similarly, cytosine (C), a pyrimidine lies opposite guanine (G), a purine.

**367.** 64 codons are there out of which **61** codons code for amino acids and **3** codons do not code for any amino acid. Non-coding codons (UAA, UGA and UAG) are also known as **stop codons**.

**368.** The nucleosome model explains the packaging of histone proteins and DNA in the chromatin material which forms the chromosome.

**369.** Protein synthesis in animal cell takes place on RER and ribosomes freely present in cytoplasm. It also takes place in mitochondria as it also contain ribosomes.

**370.** A sequential expression of a set of human genes is the DNA sequence. Because gene is the functional part of DNA sequence.

**371.** It is TATA box.

**372.** It was given by Geneticists George W. Beadle and E. L. Tatum, which states that each gene in an organism controls production of a specific enzyme. It is these enzymes that catalyse the reactions that lead to the phenotype of the organism.

**373.** The process of formation of protein sequence from DNA strand is called transcription which requires RNA polymerase. RNA polymerases are of 3-types in eukaryotes:

(i) RNA polymerase – I
(ii) RNA polymerase – II
(iii) RNA polymerase – III

**374.** Telomere has repetitive DNA sequence rich in 'G'. They along with telomerase enzyme prevent chromosome loss from terminal part.

**375.** mRNA is synthesized by the DNA according to body requirements. This mRNA molecule comes out from the nucleus to bind which ribosomes for protein synthesis tRNA bring the specific amino-acids present in the cytosol, according to the template of mRNA codons so the sequence of amino-acids in a polypeptide chain of protein is decided by mRNA.

**376.** They are formed by endo-reduplicated chromosomes also known as Polytene chromosomes reported by Balbiani.

**377.** Operons are segments of genetic material which function as regulated unit or units that can be switched on and switched off. An operon consists of one to several structural genes (Three in lac operon). These are genes which produce mRNAs for forming polypeptides/proteins/enzymes. Z (produces enzyme β galactosidase for splitting lactose into glucose and galactose). Y (produces enzyme galactoside permease required in entry of lactose). A (produces enzyme thiogalactoside trans acetylase). The three structural genes of the operon produce a single polycistronic mRNA.

**378.** Reverse transcriptase (RNA-dependent DNA polymerase) is present in some retroviruses, e.g. HIV. HIV contains 2 reverse transcriptase and 2 RNA molecules.

**379.** Telomerase is a ribonucleoprotein which synthesizes the rich strand of telomers in DNA. Telomerase is an enzyme that adds specific DNA sequence repeats (TTAGGG in all vertebrates) to the 3′ end of DNA strands in the telomere regions, which are found at the ends of eukaryotic chromosomes. The telomeres contain condensed DNA material, giving stability to the chromosomes. The enzyme is a reverse transcriptase that carries its own RNA molecule, which is used as a template when it elongates telomeres, which are shortened after each replication cycle. Telomerase was discovered by Carol W. Greider in 1984.

**380.** Gamma rays (y) from cobalt 60 are generally used for induced mutagenesis in crop plants because it has high energy.

**381.** Changes in genetic locus, changes the gene and in turn the amino acid it codes for. This alters the nature of protein synthesized which produces change in the organism. DNA replication is not affected neither the method of protein synthesis. Synthesis of RNA over DNA template is called transcription.

**382.** As Adenine (A) combines with Thymine (T) and Guanine (G) combines with Cytosine (C),

A = T, C = G

So, G + C / A + T or A + T / G + C is generally constant for a given species.

**383.** Telomeres have been shown to have unique structures that include short nucleotide sequences present as tandemly repeated units. In eukaryotes the telomeres terminate with a single-stranded DNA (12–16 nucleotides long) rich in guanine.

**384.** Replication begins at the Ori origin of replication and proceeds on both sides from the Ori. Unidirectional replication is rare. RNA primers are involved in both prokaryotes and eukaryotes.

**385.** Heterochromatin is a specialized chromosome material which remains tightly coiled and stains darkly in interphase. Euchromatin is that portion of the chromosome that stains with low intensity and uncoils during interphase.

**386.** It also refer to as molecular analysis of profile of DNA Sample (DNA profiling)

**387.**

| | | |
|---|---|---|
| **Gene mutation (copy error mutation or** | **Tautomerism** | Because of chemical mutagen, rearrangement of electrons and protons occur that results in purine–purine and pyrimidine–pyrimidine interactions. |
| **Point mutation or genetic mutation)** | **Substitutions (replacement)** | **Transition** – Replacement of purine by purine or pyrimidine by pyrimidine.<br>**Transversion** – Replacement of pyrimidine by purine (vice-versa).<br>**Frameshift** – Deletion of nitrogenous base (backward shift) or addition of nitrogenous base (forward shift). |
| **Chromosomal mutation** | **Morphological changes** | **Delection** – a part of chromosome or a group of genes is deleted.<br>**Duplication** – a part of chromosome or a group of genes is repeated.<br>**Translocation** – (a) simple translocation – segment of one chromosome is transferred to another non-homologous chromosome. (b) Reciprocal translocation – segments are exchanged between the two non-homologous chromosomes.<br>**Inversion** – a part of chromosome is inverted. |

**388.** Lactose operon in *E.coli* is a catabolic pathway in which the structural genes remain switched off unless the inducer (Lactose) is present in the medium.

**389.** Regulator is a gene which forms a biochemical for suppressing the activity of operator gene. Promoter is the gene which provides the point of attachment to RNA polymerase required for transcription of structural genes.

**390.** In bacteria, the chromosome or nucleoid is a naked double stranded DNA. The bacterial DNA is folded with the help of RNAs forming a supercoiled circular complex. The coiling is stabilized with the help of non-histonic polyamines and a number of positively changed ions. Eukaryotic DNA is associated with histone proteins that are helpful in its coiling to form chromatin fibres.

**391.** AUG is the initiating codon. UCG codes for serine, UUU codes for phenylalan, UGU codes for cysteine.

**392.** UAA is the stop codon. Therefore, at 25th amino acid the synthesis of polypeptide stops. So, a polypeptide of 24 amino acid is formed.

**393.** Out of total of 64 codons, 3 codons do not make any sense. Hence, only 61 codons are used in the formation of the 20 essential amino acids (polypeptides).

**394.** According to the Wobble hypothesis, tRNA anticodon has the ability to wobble at its 5′ end by pairing with even non-complementary base of mRNA codon. It corresponds to third base degeneracy of the codons.

**395.** Genetic mapping helps in studying the architecture of chromosomes and of the entire genome.

**396.** Thymidine is used to assess the rate of DNA synthesis, since thymine is unique to DNA.

**397.** Regulator gene forms a biochemical for suppressing the activity of operator gene. Promoter gene is the gene which provides point of attachment to RNA polymerase required for transcription of structural genes. Structural genes are genes which transcribe mRNA for polypeptide synthesis.

**398.** Out of 64 codons, only 3 signify stop codons. There are more than one codon for most of the amino acids, the genetic code is non-overlapping. Three successive nucleotides or bases code for only one amino acid wobbling refers to the third base degeneracy.

**399.** Gene regulation of eukaryotes is complex as compared to that of prokaryotes.

**400.** In 1928, Frederick Griffith, in a series of experiments with *Streptococcus pneumoniae* (bacterium responsible for pneumonia), witnessed a miraculous transformation in the bacteria.

**401.** According to Chargaff's rule, the ratio of purine bases to pyrimidine bases is equal A = T, C = G If T is 20% then A is 20% and C and G are 30%.

**402.** Exons are the coding part of mRNA code for protein.

**403.** mRNA or messenger RNA brings coded information from DNA to form polypeptides. rRNA or ribosomal RNA occurs inside ribosomes and is involved in protein synthesis.

**404.** RNA polymerase synthesizes new RNA strand. RNA primase forms the primer.

**405.** Extranuclear genes are present in the mitochondria and chloroplast.

**406.** The base ratio A + T / C+G may vary from one species to another. The base ratio is constant for a given species.

**407.** The enzyme polymerase can synthesize the bases only in $5' \rightarrow 3'$ direction.

**408.** Cistron is the segment of DNA which specifies synthesis of a polypeptide.

**409.** In case of single mutant strain, the enzyme required to lyse the *E.coli* is not synthesized. When cistron of two bacteriophages are mixed to form two different enzymes which act together and thus can lyse the *E.coli* bacterium.

**410.** Ribosomes are the sites of protein synthesis. Mitochondria being a semiautonomous organelle has its own protein synthesizing machinery.

**411.** In DNA, adenine always pairs with thymine, and guanine always pairs with cytosine, this is called complementary base pairing.

**412.** Griffith's experiment with Pneumococcus proves that DNA is the genetic material.

**413.** Genetic code is the relationship of amino acid sequence in a polypeptide chain of protein and base sequence of RNA. It includes adenine, guanine, cytosine and uracil.

**414.** The number of base pairs (bp) found in one genome of man is $3 \times 10^9$.

**415.** DNA is complexed with histones in eukaryotes.

**416.** Transposons are sequences of DNA that can move around to different positions within the genome of a single cell, a process called transposition. In the process, they can cause mutations and change the amount of DNA in the genome. Transposons are also called 'jumping genes' or 'mobile genetic elements'. Discovered by Barbara McClintock.

**417.** In semi-conservative replication of DNA in each replica one half is the old strand and the other half is a new strand synthesized over it. In this case, one strand forms continuously and another strand forms discontinuously, therefore, replication is considered to be semiconservative and semi-discontinuous.

**418.** Genetic code is triplet. There are 64 codons which code for 20 amino acids: In a triplet code of 64 codons there is an excess of 44 codons and therefore more than one codon codes for same amino acid

**419.** Termination codons are stop signals which when encountered cause termination of polypeptide synthesis. They are UAA (ochre), UAG (amber) and UGA (opal). Codons are determined by the sequence of bases on DNA. Thymine is not present on RNA.

**420.** A mutation bringing about early stoppage of polypeptide formation is called nonsense mutation. Frame shift mutation is a type of gene mutation where the reading of codons is changed due to insertion or deletion of nucleotides.

**421.** DNA replication is semiconservative, i.e. at each replication, one of the parental strands is retained and a new daughter strand is obtained. Thus, only half of the parental DNA molecule is carried to the next generation.

**422.** Nucleosomes are oblate spherical structure having an octamer of four histone proteins (constituting 2 molecules of each type).

**423.** Eukaryote RNAs contain non-coding intervening segments called introns. The process of removal of introns through cutting and joining the essential coding sequences (exons) is called splicing.

**424.** Replication of DNA is discontinuous over the lagging strand over which only small stretches of DNAase built due to opposite running of DNA template. The small stretches of DNA are called okazaki fragments.

**425.** Basis for DNA fingerprinting is RFLP.

**426.** If *Escherichia coli,* bacteria grow in normal glucose medium and when transferred to a medium containing lactose, then the lac operon is induced.

**427.** Messelson and Stahl (1958) raised Escherichia coli on ammonium chloride ($^{15}NH_4Cl$) having isotope of nitrogen for several generations to study semi-conservative replication of DNA.

**428.** The inducer is an environmental agent, which triggers transcription from an operon.

**429.** The lac operon consists of a promoter gene, an operator gene and structural genes. There are three structural genes designated as z, y and a, which code for the enzymes β-galactosidase, lac permease and transacetylase, respectively. It is an example of inducible operon.

**430.** tRNA works as an adaptor molecules for carrying amino acid to the mRNA template during 'protein synthesis'. It bears anticodon and recognizes the specific codon on mRNA

**431.** The polytene chromosomes were discovered for the first time in salivary gland of Chironomus larva.

**432.** DNA gyrase participates in the unwinding of DNA helix during replication.

**433.** Trascription is process of formation of m-RNA from DNA. Protein synthesis (translation) involves initiation, elongation, termination.

**434.** During transcription, from the DNA template complementary m-RNA is formed and thymine is replaced by uracil.

**435.** Codons are 64 in number. Each codon possess 3 bases, each of which can undergo transition and transversion ($61 \times 3^2 = 549$)

**436.** The four histone proteins constituting the core of nucleosome are H2A, H2B, H3, H4.

**437.** In 1953, Wilkins obtained very fine X-ray diffraction pictures of dNA from which Watson and Crick developed the double helix model of DNA.

**438.** A single strand of DNA would not possess complementary base pairs. Hence, nitrogenous bases are unequal in number.

**439.** Unwindase or helicase takes part in separation of two DNA strands. In prokaryotes, helicase or unwindase is assisted by gyrase in this function.

**440.** The transforming chemical discovered by Griffith in his experiments with *Pneumococcus* was confirmed as DNA by Avery, Mcleod and McCarty

**441.** After one generation in $^{14}N$ medium DNA of bacteria settled at a level intermediate between heavy and light bands due to semi-conservative DNA replication

**442.** Hargovind Khurana (Nobel Prize in 1968) deciphered the copolymers of repetitive nucleotides.

e.g., ACACACACACA……… in which ACA codes of threonine and CAC codes for histidine. CUCUCUCUCUCU……… in which CUC codes for leusine and UCU codes for serine.

## NCERT Exemplar Questions

**1.** In a DNA strand, the nucleotides are linked together by Phosphodiester bonds.

**2.** Nucleoside = Base + sugar

Nucleotide = Base + sugar + phosphate group

**3.** Both deoxyribose and ribose belong to a pentoses class of sugars.

**4.** A purine base always paired through hydrogen bonds with a pyrimidine base leads to, in the DNA double helix, uniform width throughout DNA.

5. The net electric charge on DNA and histones is negative and positive, respectively.
6. The promoter site and the terminator site for transcription are located at 5′ (upstream) end and 3′ (downstream) end, respectively, of the transcription unit.
7. *Sickle cell anaemia:* It is a molecular disease, autosomal recessive disorder and an example of pleiotropy. It cannot be treated with iron supplements and it confers resistance to acquiring malaria.
8. AUG-It codes for methionine only in both prokaryotes and eukaryotes, it is also an initiation codon.
9. The first genetic material could be RNA but ideal genetic material is DNA.
10. In eukaryotes, exons appear but introns do not appear in the mature RNA.
11. • Chromosome 1 has 2968 genes (highest)
    • Chromosome Y has 231 genes (lowest)
12. **Meselson** and **Stahl** give the experimental proof of semiconservative DNA replication. He had no contribution to the development of the douple helix model for the structure of DNA.
13. DNA is a polymer of nucleotides which are linked to each other by 3′-5′ phosphodiester bond. Remove/replace 3′OH group in deoxyribose, to prevent polymerization of nucleotides.
14. Discontinuous synthesis of DNA occurs in one strand, because DNA-dependent DNA polymerase catalyses polymerization only in one direction (5′ → 3′).
15. Elongation step in transcription is catalysed by RNA polymerase.
16. Control of gene expression takes place at the level of transcription.
17. Regulatory proteins are accessory proteins that interact with RNA polymerase and affect its role in transcription. They can act both as activators and as repressors.
18. The human genome project was completed in 2003. The sequence of chromosome 1 was completed only in May 2006.
19. Functions of mRNA:
    • Carrier of genetic information from DNA to ribosomes synthesizing polypeptides.
    • Carrier of amino acids to ribosomes.
    • Constituent component of ribosomes.
20. In the DNA of an organism, a total number of 5386 nucleotides were found, out of which the proportion of different bases were: Adenine = 29%, Guanine = 17%, Cytosine = 32%, Thymine = 17%. Considering the Chargaff's rule, it can be concluded that it is a single stranded DNA.
21. In some viruses, DNA is synthesized by using RNA as template. Such a DNA is called c-DNA (Complementary DNA).
22. • If Meselson and Stahl's experiment is continued for four generations in bacteria, the ratio of $15_N/15_N:15_N/14_N : 14_N/14_N$ containing DNA in the fourth generation would be 0 : 1 : 7.
    • After third generation (60 min.), bacteria contains *25%* hybrid ($N^{15}N^{14}$) in 1 : 3 ratio.
    • After 4th generation (80 min.), bacteria contains 12:5% hybrid and *87.5%* light DNA in 1 : 7 ratio.
23. Coding strand: 5′ - A T G AA T G - 3′

    Template strand: 3′ - T ACT T A C - 5′

    ↓

    RNA transcript: 5′ - AUG AA U G - 3′
24. The RNA polymerase holoenzyme transcribes the structural gene only.
25. Base sequence of a codon in mRNA is 5′-AUG-3′, the sequence of tRNA pairing with it must be complementary, i.e., 3′ - UAC – 5′.
26. The amino acid attaches to the tRNA at its 3′ end.
27. To initiate translation, the mRNA first binds to the smaller ribosomal subunit.
28. In *E.coli,* the lac operon gets switched on when lactose is present and it binds to the repressor.

## Previous Years' Questions

1. The central dogma of proteins synthesis is expressed as.

DNA —Replication→ DNA —Transcription→ RNA —Translation→ Proteins

Temin described the present of an enzyme, i.e., reverse transcriptase or RNA-dependent DNA polymerase, which controls e synthesis of DNA from a single strand of RNA. **D Baltimore** also described the presence of that enzyme in RNA tumour viruses. The presence of this enzyme changed the central dogma of protein synthesis into central dogma reverse.

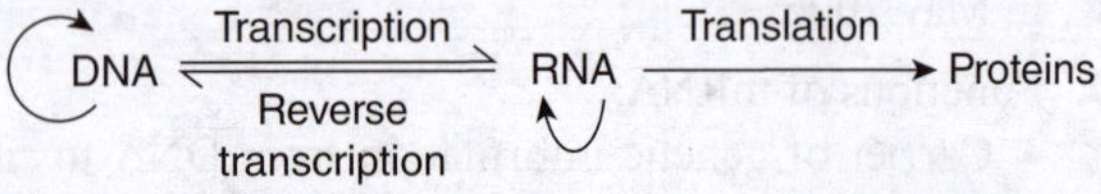


2. Britten and his co-workers (1966–1968) demonstrated that many vertebrate DNAs reassociate, especially if broken into smaller pieces. This observation gave rise to the hypothesis that certain short sequences of bases are repeated hundred or more times in such DNAs. Such DNAs are called repetitive or satellite DNAs. All eukaryotes except years contain satellite DNA. Satellite DNA regions like VNTR/RFLP are the basis of DNA finger printing (forensic science).

3. Genetic code is non ambiguous. There is no ambiguity for a particular codon. A particular codon will always code for the same amino acid, where ever it is found.

4. In prokaryotes, a hypothesis was given in 1961 to explain protein synthesis regulation. This hypothesis was given by F Jacob and J Monod, and for this he was awarded Nobel Prize in 1965, the hypothesis was known as Operon Model.
The operator gene is the segment of DNA, which exercise control over transcriptions. In the absence of lactose, the repressor binds with the operator gene.

5. Phosphodiester bond forms when two nucleotide combine together.

6. Lac operon is the operon that regulates lactose metabolism in the bacterium *E.coli*. Its form was first ostulated in 1961 to explain the control of Beta- galactosidase synthesis. Lac operon system or inducile operon system consists of regulator gene (i) promoter gene, (p) operator gene (o) three structural gene (z, y and a), repressor protein and inducer.

7. The gene for producing insulin is present in everybody cell. Because all cells are derived from zygote but they are transcriptionally active in pancreas only.

8. In eukaryotic cell transcription, RNA splicing and RNA capping, tailing take place inside the nucleus of cell.

9. HIV is a virus.

10. Human Genome Project (HGP) was closely associated with rapid development of a new area in biology called bioinformatics, the science of collecting and analysing complex biological data such as genetic codes.

11. The unequivocal (leaving no doubt; unambiguous) proof that DNA is the genetic material came from the experiments of Alfred Hershey and Martha Chase. They worked with viruses that infect bacteria called bacteriophages.

12. 23 S rRNA in bacteria is the enzyme ribozyme for formation of peptide bond. 23 S rRNA is found in large sub-unit (70 S) of ribosome of bacteria.

13. Nucleosome is sub-microscopic sub-unit of chromatin which is formed by wrapping of DNA over a core of histone proteins. The term was coined by Oudet et. al, (1975). It is a oblate structure with length of 10 nm and thickness of 5–5.7 nm. Its core is called nu-body. The latter is formed of four pairs of histone molecules: $H_2A$, $H_2B$, $H_3$ and $H_4$. DNA makes 1.75 turns over the octamer to form a nucleosome. Two adjacent nucleosomes are connected by a short segment of unbound DNA called linker DNA. A fifth type of histone called $H_1$ is attached over the linker DNA. Nucleosomes appear as 'beads-on-string' in the chromosomes under electron microscope.

14. The primary transcript from a typical eukaryotic gene contains introns as well as exons. During RNA splicing, introns are removed and exons are joined in a defined order, to produce functional RNA.

15. Complementary RNA is UAGAC.

16. Radiolabelled single strand of nucleic acid is called probe.

17.

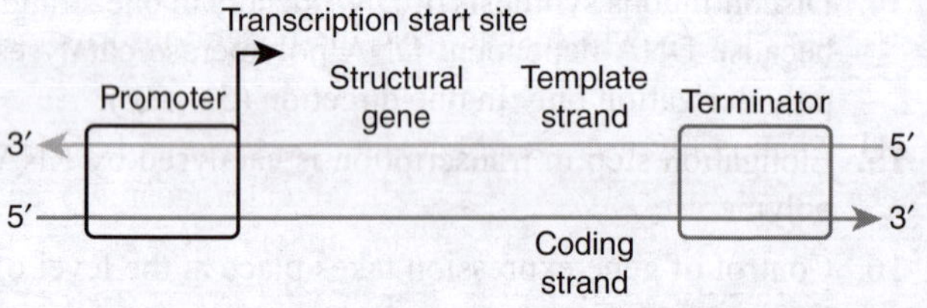


Schematic structure of a transcription unit

18. The hypervariable regions of DNA have Variable Number of Tandem repeats (VNTRs) of short nucleotide sequences which are specific for each individual (except for monozygotic twins). Variations also occur due to mutations, small deletions or insertions. Therefore, DNA cut by a particular endonuclease will have different lengths in different persons. This phenomenon is called Restriction Fragment Length Polymorphism. It is the basis of genetic (or DNA) fingerprinting and is useful in identifying individuals from their semen, blood or tissues or any other DNA sample and resolution of parent hood disputes. Polymerase Chain Reaction (PCR) is also useful in genetic fingerprinting as it can amplify the DNA sample even if available in a very small amount.

**19.** There are at least three RNA polymerases in the nucleus (in addition to the RNA polymerase found in the organelles). There is a clear-cut division of labour. The RNA polymerase I transcribes **rRNAs**(28S, 18S, and 5.8S), whereas the RNA polymerase III is responsible for transcription of **tRNA, 5srRNA** and **snRNAs (small nuclear RNAs)**. The RNA polymerase II transcribes precursor of mRNA, the **heterogeneous nuclear RNA (hnRNA)**.

**20.** DNA fingerprint is individual - specific DNA identification which is made possible by the finding that no two people are likely to have the same of copies of repetitive DNA sequences of regions. Chromosomes of every human cells contains short, highly repeated DNA sequence called mini-satellite scattered throughout.

**21.** Regulation of lac operon by repressor is referred to as negative regulation.

Human genome has approximately 30000 genes.

**22.**

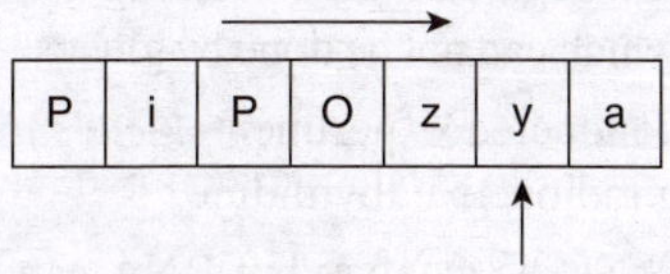


Non-sense mutation take place here then y and a gene will not transcribe thus only β-galactosidase gene (z-gene) will transcribe.

**23.** Francis Crick proposed the central dogma in molecular biology which states that the genetic information flow from DNA → RNA → Protein.

**24.** Commonly used vector for human genome sequencing is **BAC** (bacterial artificial chromosomes) and **YAC** (yeast artificial chromosomes).

**25.**

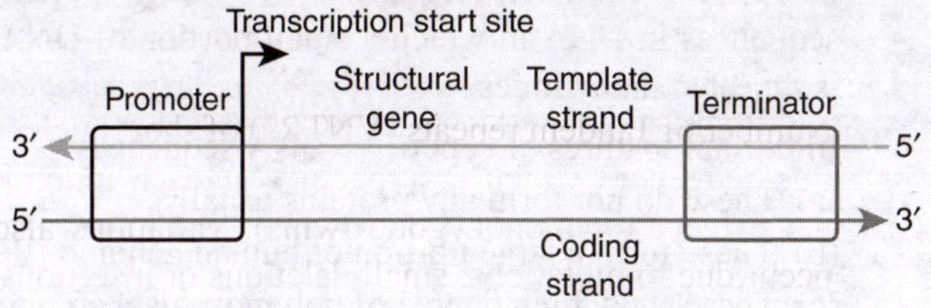


**26.** Southern hybridization is a technique used in molecular biology for detection of a specific DNA sequence in DNA samples in which excepting PCR we use all three methods such as electrophoresis, blotting and autoradiography. Because PCR is the method used for amplification of DNA sample. In vitro clonal propagation is characterized by PCR and RAPD.

**27.** In 1928, Frederick Griffith, in a series of experiments with *Streptococcus pneumoniae* (bacterium responsible for pneumonia), witnessed a miraculous transformation in bacteria. During the course of his experiment, a living organism (bacteria) had changed in physical form.

**28.** **Operon** is a group of genes controlling a particular expression in prokaryotes (e.g. E. coli). It consists of regulator gene, promoter gene, operator gene and structural gene. It is found in all prokaryotes.

**29.** DNA fingerprinting involves identifying differences in some specific regions in DNA sequence called **repetitive DNA**, because in these sequences a small stretch of DNA is repeated many times. These repetitive DNAs are separated from bulk genomic DNA as different peaks during density gradient centrifugation. The bulk DNA forms a major peak and the other small peaks are referred to as **satellite DNA**. Depending on base composition (A : T rich or G:C rich), length of segment and number of repetitive units, the satellite DNA is classified into many categories, such as micro-satellites, mini-satellites, etc. These sequences normally do not code for any proteins, but they form a large portion of human genome. These sequence show high degree of polymorphism and form the basis of DNA fingerprinting.

**30.** **Polytene chromosome:**

**(1)** Polytene chromosome was described by Kollar (1882) and was first reported by Balbiani (1881) in the salivary gland cells of chironomus larva. They are found in salivary glands of insects (*Drosophila*) and called salivary gland chromosomes. These are reported in endosperm cells of embryo sac by Malik and Singh (1979). Length of this chromosome may be up to 2000μ*m*.

**(2)** The chromosome is formed by somatic pairs between homologous chromosomes and repeated replication or endomitosis of chromonemata. These are attached to chromocentre. It has pericentromeric heterochromatin.

**(3)** Polytene chromosomes show large number of various sized intensity bands when stained. The lighter area between dark bands are called interbands. They have puffs bearing *Balbiani rings*.

**(4)** Balbani rings produce number of *m*-RNAs, which may remain stored temporarily in puffs and are temporary structures.

**(5)** These are also occur in Malpighian tubules, rectum, gut, foot pads, fat bodies, ovarian nurse cells, etc.

**31.** Organization of genetic material from smallest to largest.

Nucleotide →gene→ chromosome→ genome

**32.** Erwin Chargaff in 1949 proposed Chargaffs rules regarding the composition of bases in DNA as follows:

**(i)** Total amount of purine nucleotides always equals the total amount of pyrimidine nucleotides i.e. (A) + (G) = (T) + (C).

**(ii)** The proportion of A is equal to T and also proportion of G is equal to C, but amount of (A)+(T) is not necessarily equal to (G) + (C). Therefore, (A) = (T) : (G) = (C). But $\frac{A+T}{G+C}$ = varies with the organism. Chargaff's rule is not applicable to RNA.

**33.** The proportion of A is equal to T and also proportion of G is equal to C. So if A = 17% , T = 17% therefore total is 34%. Rest is 66% G = 33% and C = 33%.

**34.** Regulation of lac operon is a type of **negative regulation** because product of regulator gene will lead to inhibition of process of transcription and lactose regulates the switching on and off of lac operon, so it acts as inducer.

**35.** The strand of DNA on which RNA polymerase binds to perform transcription is called **template strand** also known as **antisense strand/non-coding strand.**

**36.** Criteria for a molecule to act as genetic material:

(a) It should be able to replicate.

(b) It should be chemically and structurally stable so that it may resist any change due to changing environment or age or physiology of an organism.

(c) It should slowly undergo mutations as mutations are very important source of evolution.

(d) It should be able to express itself in the form of Mendelian characters.

**37.** Bacterial cells use their 23 srRNA as an enzyme during protein synthesis. This is the only non-proteinaceous enzyme known so far.

**38.** Cistron is the functional unit of DNA molecule. It codes for a particular gene product equivalent to structural gene.

**39.** AUG is the start codon. It also codes for amino acid called methionine which is the first amino acid in a polypeptide chain. UAA, UAG and UGA are stop codons and are meant for termination of polypeptide chain during protein synthesis.

**40.** The technique of DNA fingerprinting was initially developed by Alec Jeffreys. It included

(i) isolation of DNA

(ii) digestion of DNA by restriction endonucleases

(iii) separation of DNA fragments by electrophoresis

(iv) transferring (blotting) of separated DNA fragments to synthetic membranes, such as nitrocellulose or nylon,

(v) hybridization using labelled VNTR probe

(vi) detection of hybridized DNA fragments by autoradiography.

The sensitivity of the technique has been increased by use of polymerase chain reaction

**Zinc finger analysis:** The factor TFIIIA requires zinc for its activity. On analysis, it was revealed that each TFIIIA contains zinc ions as a repeating coordinated complex. This complex is formed by the closely spaced amino acids cysteine and cysteine, followed by a histidine–histidine pair. In some instances, His-His is replaced by a second Cys-Cys pair.

The zinc fingers bind to the major groove of DNA and lie on the face of the DNA. This bonding makes a contact with 5 bp of DNA. The steroid hormone receptor transcription factors use zinc finger motifs to bind to DNA.

**41.** Lac operon becomes active only after inducing lactose as it is a substrate for the enzyme beta- galactosidase and it also regulates the switching on and off of the operon which can not be done by glucose and galactose.

**42.** Taylor conducted experiment *Vicia faba* (faa beans) by using radioactive thymidine.

**43.** DNA not act as catalyst but RNA can; These RNAs are said to be ribozymes.

**44.** If the ratio of (T+C) / (A+G) in one strand of DNA is 1.43 then ratio of same for other strand is 0.07. Because A=G and T=C for complementarity.

**45.** Half of our chromosomes coming from mother and half of from father in sexual reproduction, therefore, 50% of siblings DNA resemble the father and 50% the mother.

**46. Basis of DNA fingerprinting:** DNA fingerprinting depends upon the identification of differences in **repetitive DNA**. Repetitive DNA are specific sequences in DNA in which a small portion of DNA is repeated many times.

Important features of **repetitive DNA** sequences:

(a) These do not form any proteins usually.

(b) These form a large portion of human genome.

(c) These show high degree of polymorphism among individuals which becomes the basis of DNA fingerprinting.

**47. Salient features of Genetic Code:**

**(1)** Genetic codon is a triplet codon.

**(2)** 64 codons are there out of which **61** codons code for amino acids and **3** codons do not code for any amino acid. Non-coding codons (UAA, UGA and UAG) are also known as **stop codons**.

**(3)** Genetic codon is **unambiguous** and **specific**, i.e., one codon code for only one amino acid.

**(4)** Single aminoacid can be coded by two or more codons. This is **degeneracy** of codon.

**(5)** In mRNA codon is read in continuous or **contiguous manner**. No punctuations are there in between.

**(6)** Genetic codon is **nearly universal**. Exceptions are there in mitochondrial codons and in some protozoans.

**(7)** Some codons may perform dual functions. **Example:** AUG codes for Methionine (met) and it act as **initiator codon.**

**48.** Addition or Deletion of any neucleotide from RNA causes frameshift mutation. Deletion of one neucleotide at the position of 901 affect the reading of all the codons after its deletion. Codon is triplet means three nitrogen base code for one aminoacid so if 901 base is deleted, total 33 codons will get altered.

**49.** • **rRNA:** It is most abundant RNA (70–80%) found in cells.
- Transfer RNA (t RNA) forms 15% of total RNA present in cell.
- **m RNA:** It is a long RNA constituting 2–5% of the total RNA content.

**50.** **Splicing** is done in eukaryotic mRNA. During this process, the introns are removed and the exons are joined together to form a processed or functional mRNA. Therefore, this process does not occur in prokaryote, that is, bacteria.

**51.** The final proof that DNA is the genetic material came from the experiments of Alfred Hershey and Martha Chase (1952). Griffith's experiment proved the existance of genetic material while Avery, MacLeod and Mcarty worked to determine the biochemical nature of transforming principle.

**52.** During DNA replication, Okazaki fragments are used to elongate the lagging strand away from the replication fork.

**53.** The association of $H_1$ histone with nucleosome indicates that DNA remains in its condensed form. Concept Enhancer In eukaryotes, DNA packaging is carried out with the help of histone proteins. Nucleosome is the unit of compaction. Its core insists of four pairs of histones. The linker DNA, consisting of $H_1$ histone connects two adjacent nucleosomes. They together constitute chromatosome. It gives rise to a chromatin fibre after further condensation.

**54.** It is now proven that DNA replicates semiconservatively. It was shown first in *Escherichia coli* **(a bacterium)** and subsequently in higher organisms, such as plants and human cells.

**55.** The elucidation of the lac operon was also a result of close association between a geneticist, Francois Jacob and a biochemist Jacque Monod. Alfred Hershey and Martha Chase unequivocally proved that DNA is a genetic material. They worked with viruses that infect bacteria called bacteriophages. The technique of **DNA Fingerprinting** was initially developed **Alec Jeffeys**. Meselson and Stahl experimentally proved that DNA replicates semiconservatively. It was shown first in ***Escherichia coli*** **(a bacterium).**

**56.** Enhancer sequences are present in eukaryotes. Operon concept is for prokaryotes.

**57.** All the reference point while defining a transcription unit is made with coding strand. If coding strand is given then m- RNA formed by it by replacing thymine with uracil, therefore, answer is AGGUAUCGCAU.

**58.** The methods for HGP involved two major approaches. One approach focused on identifying all the **genes that are expressed as RNA (referred to as Expressed Sequence Tags (ESTs)**. The other took the blind approach of simply sequencing the whole set of genome that contained all the coding and non-coding sequence and later assigning different regions in the sequence with functions (a term referred to as Sequence Annotation).

**59.** The *i* gene codes for the repressor of the *lac* operon. The *z* gene codes for beta-galactosidase (b-gal), which is primarily responsible for hydrolysis of disaccharide, lactose into its monomeric units, galactose and glucose. The *y* gene codes for permease, which increases permeability of the cell to b-galactosides. The *a* gene encodes a transacetylase.

**60.** (i) The codon is triplet. 61 codons code for aminoacids and 3 codons do not code for any aminoacids, hence they function as stop codons.

(ii) Some aminoacids are coded by more than one codon, hence the code is **degenerativee** (redundant).

(iii) The codon is read in mRNA in a contiguous fashion. There are no punctuations.

(iv) The code is nearly **universal**: for example, from bacteria to human, UUU would code for Phenylalanine (phe). Some exceptions to this rule have been found in mitochondrial codons and in some protozoans.

(v) AUG has dual functions. It codes for Methionine (met), and it also acts as an **initiator** codon.

(vi) UAA, UAG, UGA are stop terminator codons.

**61.** Insertion or deletion of three or its multiple bases insert or delete in one or multiple codon hence one or multiple amino acids and reading frame remains unaltered from that point onwards.

**62.** The first phase of translation involves activation of amino acid in the presence of ATP and linked to their cognate tRNA – a process commonly called as charging of tRNA or aminoacylation of tRNA.

**63.** RNA polymerase facilitates opening of DNA helix during transcription.

**64.** Length of DNA = $[0.34 \times 10^{-9}]$ m $\times 6.6 \times 10^9$ bp = 2.2 m

Distance between 2 base pair in DNA helix = 0.34 nm $= 0.34 \times 10^{-9}$ m

Total number of base pair = $6.6 \times 10^9$ bp

**65.** Francis Crick proposed the Central dogma in molecular biology, which states that the genetic information flows from DNA → RNA → Protein.

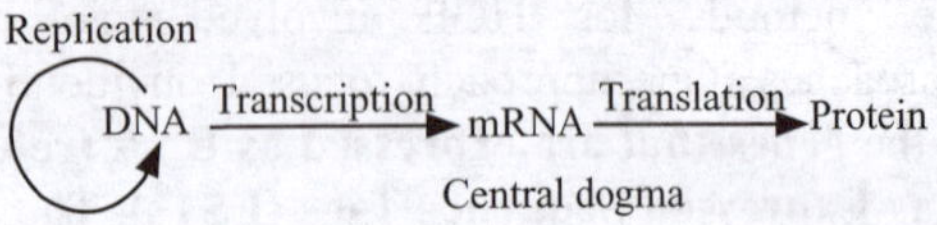


Central dogma

**66.**

| | |
|---|---|
| RNA polymerase I | Transcribes 5.8S, 18S and 28S rRNA. |
| RNA polymerase II | Transcribes hnRNA which is precursor of mRNA |
| RNA polymerase III | Transcribes tRNA, ScRNA, 5S rRNA and SnRNA. |

**67.** DNA fingerprinting involves identifying differences in some specific regions in DNA sequence called as repetitive DNA.

**68.**
- Split gene arrangement is characteristic of eukaryotes.
- In capping, 5-methyl guanosine triphosphate is added at 5' end of hnRNA.
- At 3' end poly-A tail is added.
- The non coding or template strand is copied to an mRNA. RNA polymerase associate with ρ factor (Rho factor) and it alters the specificity of the RNA polymerase to terminate the processes.

**69.** In prokaryotes, the DNA dependent RNA polymerase is a holoenzyme that is made of polypeptides. It is responsible for initiation, elongation and termination during transcription.

**70.** According to Chargaff's rule, for a double stranded DNA,

[A] = [T]

∵ [A] = 30% ⇒ [T] = 30%

Since [C] = [G]

∴ 100 – [A - T]

= 100 – [30 + 30]

= 100 – 60 = 40%

And C – G = 20% each

[A] = 30%

[T] = 30%

[G] = 20%

[C] = 20%

**71.** siRNA – siRNA are small interfering RNA also called silencing RNA. It is a class of double-stranded RNA, non-coding RNA molecules.

**72.** Histones are rich in basic amino acids residue lysine and arginine with charged side chain.

There are five types of histone proteins i.e., $H_1$, $H_2A$, $H_2B$, $H_3$ and $H_4$. Four of them occur in pairs to produce a unit of 8 molecules (histone octamer)

The pH of histones is basic.

**73.** **AUG has dual functions,** it codes for methionine. It also acts as initiator codon.

AUG does not code for phenylalanine.

**74.** Packaging in Eukaryotes

**Histone octamer + DNA → Nucleosome → Chromatin → Chromatin fibre → Chromosome**

**Histone octamer:** It is made up of 8 molecules of histone proteins. Histone proteins are positively charged basic proteins. These proteins are rich in basic amino acids like lysine and arginine. Both of these amino acids possess positive charges in their side chains.

**Nucleosome:** DNA (negatively charged) wraps the positively charged histone octamer. In a nucleosome, about 200 bp are present in DNA.

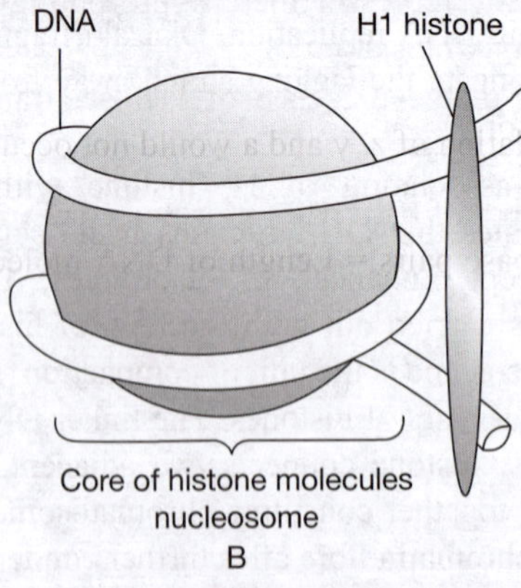


Arrangement of chromatin material in a nucleus occur is two ways:

(a) **Loosely packed chromatin or euchromatin:** It stains light and transcriptionally active.

(b) **Densely packed chromatin or heterochromatin:** It stains dark and transcriptionally inactive.

**75.** Polymorphism in DNA sequence is the basis of **Genetic mapping** of human genome as well as of **DNA fingerprinting**.

**76.** When the **small subunit** of ribosome encounters an mRNA, the process of translation of the mRNA to protein begins. This process is followed by the binding of bigger/larger subunit. t-RNA is activated by the addition of amino acid prior to the attachment of ribosome, in the first phase.

**77.** **Sequence Annotation-** It is blind approach of sequencing the whole set of genome that contained all the coding and non-coding sequences and later assigning different regions in the sequence with functions is called **sequence annotation.**

**Bioinformatics:** It is science of collecting and analysing complex biological data.

**ESTs:** Approach used for HGP emphasizing on identification of all the genes which are expressed as RNA.

**GENE Mapping:** It is determination and graphic representation of position or loci of gene on a chromosome.

**78.** As the product of 'i' gene binds with the operator region and blocks the transcription and translation of z, y and a genes.

It's product is prevented from binding to the operator by attaching it with the inducer. As the inducer can now no more capable of binding with the repressor, thus, in all the cases, operator always gets attached with the repressor thereby preventing the transcription and translation of z, y and a.

Even in the presence of lactose, transcription and translation of z, y and a would not occur.

**79.** Number of base pairs × distance between 2 consecutive base pairs = Length of DNA molecule × 0.34 × $10^{-9}$ m = 1.1 m

$$x = \frac{1.1}{0.3 \times 10^{-9}}$$

$$= 3.6 \times 10^{9}$$

$$= 3.3 \times 10^{9}\ \text{bp}$$

**80.** From 10 parent *E.coli* cells

1st generation

$^{15}N$ containing 10 cells —20 mins→ 20 cells (all hybrid) $^{15}N$–$^{14}N$

2nd generation

20 cells (Hybrid) —20 mins→ 40 cells → 20 cells all hybrid $^{15}N$–$^{14}N$; 20 cells with $^{14}N$

3rd generation

40 cells (20 cells hybrid + 20 $^{14}N$ containing cells) —20 mins→ 20 $^{14}N$ containing cells + 20 hybrid and 40 $^{14}N$ containing cells

Therefore, after 60 minutes, 60 *E.coli* cells will have DNA totally free from $^{15}N$.

**81.** Unequivocal proof that DNA is the genetic material was first proposed by Alfred Hershey and Martha Chase with experiment using bacteriophge.

**82.** RNA polymerase III DNA to synthesize tRNA, 5S rRNA and snRNA in Eukaryotes.

**83.** ESTs are genes which are expressed as mRNA for proteins synthesis. These are used in human genome project foe gene mapping.

**84.** The cellular factory responsible for synthesising proteins is the ribosome. The ribosome consists of structural RNAs and about 80 different proteins.

**85.**

| | |
|---|---|
| Gene 'a' | Transacetylase |
| Gene 'y' | Permease |
| Gene 'i' | Repressor protein |
| Gene 'z' | β - galactosidase |

**86.** Both the statements are correct.

**87.** In prokaryotes, the negatively charged DNA is held with positively charged proteins in nucleoid.

**88.** 5' ATCGATCGATCGATCGATCGATCGATCG 3'

**89.** The *y* gene *lac* operon codes for permease enzyme, which increases the permeability of cell to *β*-galactosides.

So, the lactose present in the growth medium of bacteria is transported into the cell by the action of permease.

**90.** A transcription unit of DNA is defined primarily by the three regions in the DNA:

(i) A promoter

(ii) The structural gene

(iii) A terminator

The promoter is said to be located towards 5′-end (upstream) of the structural gene (the reference is made with respect to the polarity of coding strand) The terminator is located towards 3′-end (downstream) of the coding strand.

**91.** In Prokaryotes, like *E.coli* during replication, the DNA dependent DNA polymerase catalyse polymerization only in one direction, that is 5′ → 3′. Even RNA polymerase also shows polymerisation in 5′ → 3′.

**92.** Frederick Griffith series of experiment witness miraculous transformation in the bacteria (*Pneumococcus*)

The elucidation of *Lac* operon was a result of a close association between geneticist, Francois Jacob and a biochemist, Jacques Monod.

Meselson and Stahl gave semi-conservative mode of DNA replication by preforming experiment on *E. Coli.* Har Gobind Khorana developed chemical method to define combination of bases in genetic code.

**93.** Template DNA is:

3′TACATGGCAAATATCCATTCA5′

5′AUGUACCGUUUAUAGGUAAGU3′ m-RNA

**94.**
- RNA polymerase III codes for snRNAs, tRNA and 5s rRNA in eukaryotes.
- Splicing of exons is performed by snRNPs.
- TATA box is present in promoter region of transcription unit.
- Rho factor is responsible for termination of transcription whereas sigma factor is responsible for initiation of transcription.

4

# Microbes in Human Welfare

## LEARNING OBJECTIVES

- Understand the microbes and application of microbiology in wider aspects.
- Discuss how microbes serve as source of food.
- Learn how source of food in household products (industrial products)
- Explain how microbes act in waste-water treatment and also helps in the production of biogas.
- Describe microbes act as biocontrol agent
- Explain role of microbes as biofertilizers

## Chapter Overview

### Microbes in Household Products

- Micro-organisms like *Lactobacillus* and others which are commonly called **Lactic Acid Bacteria (LAB)** are when added to milk, produce acids. These acids coagulate and partially digest the milk proteins.
- Nutritionally curd is improved because of addition of Vitamin $B_{12}$. These also prevent the diseases of stomach caused by the microbes.
- For making **bread**, the dough is fermented by **baker's yeast** (***Saccharomyces cerevisiae*** **= budding yeast**).
- **Toddy** (a traditional drink in South India) is prepared from fermented sap from Palms.
- Batter for idli and dosa is also fermented by bacteria.
- **Swiss cheese:** Prepared by the action of *Propionibacterium sharmanii*. It possesses large holes due to production of high amount of $CO_2$.
- **Roquefort cheese:** A specific fungi is grown on it to ripen it. This also adds a specific flavour to it.

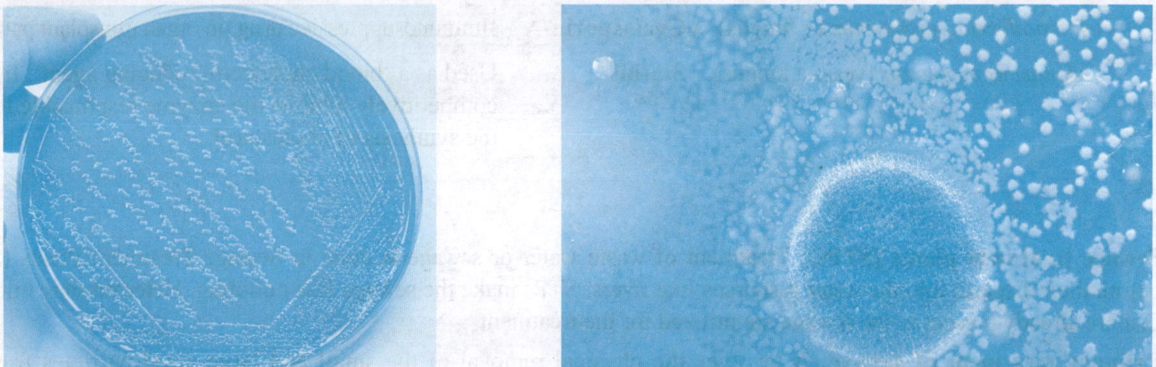

(a) (b)

FIGURE 4.1 (a) Colonies of bacteria growing in a petri dish; (b) Fungal colony growing in a petri dish

Refer NCERT Ch 8: Microbes in Human Welfare

## Microbes in Industrial Products

- **Brewer's yeast (*Saccharomyces cerevisiae*):** (It is the same that is used for making bread) Various types of fermented beverages are prepared by the action of microbes specially yeast. Ferment malted cereals and fruit juices are used to produce ethanol. **Wine and beer are prepared without distillation. Rum, brandy and whisky are produced with distillation.**
- **Antibiotics:** These are chemicals which are produced by some microbes and can kill or retard the growth of other microbes (pathogenic). **Example: Penicillin** was discovered by **Alexander Fleming**. It was the first antibiotic to be discovered.
- **Discovery of Penicillin:** Alexander Fleming observed that *Staphylococci* bacteria was unable to grow around the mould that has grown in one of his unwashed culture plates. He later found that it was because of a chemical produced by the fungus. He gave the term Penicillin to the chemical after the mould *Penicillium notatum*. Full potential of penicillin as an antibiotic was later established by **Ernst Chain** and **Howard Florey**.
- In World War II, penicillin was extensively used to treat the wounded American soldiers. In 1945, **Fleming, Chain** and **Florey** were awarded Nobel Prize for their contribution. Many diseases like plague, whooping cough, diphtheria, leprosy are treated with antibiotics.
- Chemicals, Enzymes and other Bioactive Molecules are also produced using microbes.
- Microbes are also used to produce enzymes:
  (1) **Lipases:** Commercially used in detergents and laundry to remove oily stains from the clothes.
  (2) **Pectinases and proteases:** These enzymes are utilized for making the bottled fruit juices clearer in comparison to homemade fruit juices.

**TABLE 4.1** Different microbes and their product in industry

| S. No. | Microbes | Product | Use of Product |
|---|---|---|---|
| 1. | *Aspergillus niger* (a fungus) | **Citric acid** | Industrial use |
| 2. | *Acetobacter aceti* (a bacterium) | **Acetic acid** | Industrial use |
| 3. | *Clostridium butylicum* (a bacterium) | **Butyric acid** | Industrial use |
| 4. | Lactobacillus (a bacterium) | **Lactic acid** | Industrial use |
| 5. | *Saccharomyces cerevisiae* (yeast-a fungus) | **Ethanol** | Alcoholic beverages |
| 6. | Streptococcus (a bacterium) | **Streptokinase** | Used as 'clot buster' for removal of clots in blood vessels that have resulted in myocardial infarction. |
| 7. | *Trichoderma polysporum* (a fungus) | **Cyclosporin-A** | 'Immunosuppressive drug' in organ transplant patients. |
| 8. | *Monascus purpureus* (yeast-a fungus) | **Statins** | Used as a 'blood cholesterol reducing agent'. It competitively inhibits the enzyme responsible for the synthesis of cholesterol. |

## Microbes in Sewage Treatment

- **Sewage treatment plants (STPs):** Treatment of waste water or sewage is done in Sewage Treatment Plants (STPs) before their disposal into the water resources like rivers. STPs make the sewage less polluting. Heterotrophic microbes that are already present in the sewage are utilized for the treatment.
- **Primary treatment of sewage:** It involves the physical removal of the small and large sized particles from the sewage. Processes involved: **Filtration:** Floating debris is removed by sequential filtration. **Sedimentation:** Grit (soil and small pebbles) is removed by sedimentation in **primary settling tank**. All solids that settle or sediment are collectively termed as **primary sludge** while the supernatant is termed as **effluent**.

- **Secondary treatment or biological treatment of sewage:**
  **(a)** Primary effluent is passed into large aeration tanks in which constant agitation and pumping of air is there → Growth of micro-organisms (especially aerobic) is promoted → Floes (large masses of bacteria along with fungal filaments to appear like a mesh-like network) are formed → These microbes take oxygen during their growth (thus decreasing the BOD) and decompose or consume major organic part of the effluent.
  **(b)** Once the BOD is significantly decreased, effluent is transferred to a large settling tank → Bacterial flocs settle here, which are termed as activated sludge. A small part of the activated sludge is transferred back into the aeration tank to act as inoculum.
  **(c)** Major part of the activated sludge is pumped into the anaerobic sludge digesters which are large tanks having anaerobic bacteria → these anaerobic bacteria digest the bacteria and fungi present in the sludge → in this process of digestion, various gases are produced in the form of a mixture—**methane, hydrogen sulphide and carbon dioxide.** These gases are collectively termed as **biogas (Fig 4.2).**

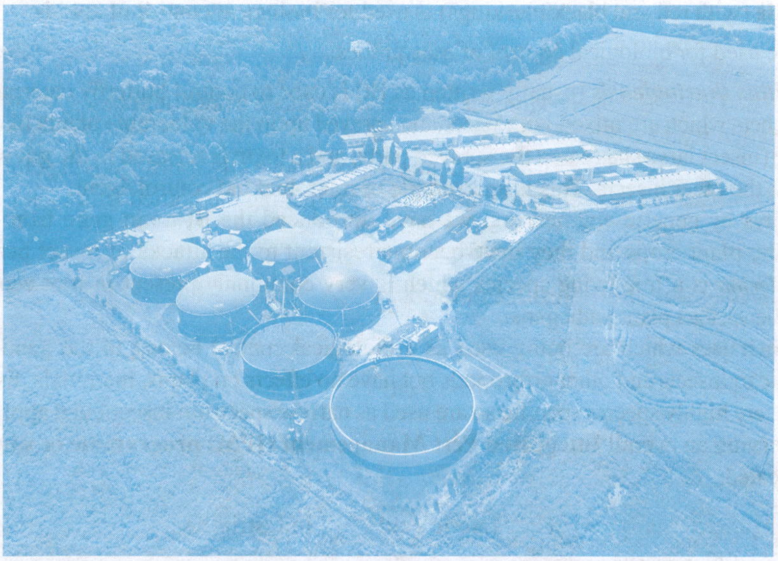

FIGURE 4.2 A typical biogas plant

The effluent obtained after the secondary treatment is usually released into the natural water resources like rivers and streams.

- **BOD (Biological Oxygen Demand):** It is the amount of oxygen that would be consumed by bacteria, if **all organic matter** in one litre of water is oxidized. BOD is measure of organic pollution in water. More the value of BOD more is the polluting potential. During secondary treatment, sewage is treated until the BOD is significantly reduced.
- **Ganga Action Plan** and **Yamuna Action Plan:** These plans were initiated by **The Ministry of Environment and Forests** to protect the major rivers of our country from pollution. Their aim is to build large number of sewage treatment plants (STPs) to treat the sewage before their disposal into the rivers.

## Microbes in Biogas Production

- **Biogas production:** Various microbes produce different types of gaseous end products during their growth and metabolism. **(a)** $CO_2$ is produced during fermentation of dough, production of beverages and cheese making **(b)** Methane ($CH_4$) is predominantly produced along with $CO_2$ and $H_2$ when methanogens (bacteria) grow on cellulosic material.
- **Methanogens (Archaebacteria):** Methanogens refer to group of bacteria that anaerobically grow on cellulosic material and produce methane on large scale along with $CO_2$ and $H_2$. **Example:** *Methanobacterium.*
- Methanogens are commonly found in: Anaerobic sludge digester tanks during sewage treatment. **Rumen (a part of stomach) of cattle** in which these digest celluloses and help in nutrition. This is the reason, why the dung of the cattle is rich in bacteria. Gobar (cow dunk) is used for production of biogas (also known as **gobar gas**).

- The technology for biogas production was developed by Indian Agricultural Research Institute (IARI) and Khadi and Village Industries Commission (KVIC).
- Biowastes and slurry of dung is added in a concrete tank (Digester) which is 10–15 ft. deep.

## Microbes as Biocontrol Agent

- **Biocontrol:** It refers to the use of biological methods for controlling plant diseases and pests.
- **Biological control of pest and diseases:** Instead of using chemicals (pesticides or insecticides), there is a method of controlling pests in agriculture which is based on natural predation.
- **Benefits of biological farming or control:** It reduces the use of toxic chemicals in the field. Beneficial predatory and parasitic insects which depend upon such insects are not eradicated. More biodiversity of a landscape or ecosystem more is its stability.
- The **Ladybird beetle** (with red and black markings) is used for biological control of aphids.
- The **Dragonflies** are used for biological control of mosquitoes.
- The bacteria – ***Bacillus thuringiensis*** (usually written as Bt) is used to control butterfly caterpillars. These are available in spore form in sachets which are mixed with water and sprayed upon the vulnerable plants like brassica and fruit trees. After the caterpillar (insect larva) has eaten the sprayed parts, and a toxin is released in the gut which kills the larva. This toxin does not affect the other insects. This is an example of microbial bio control agent.
- **Bt cotton:** Nowadays by genetic engineering, we have introduced the Bt toxin gene from the bacteria – *Bacillus thuringiensis* into the plant crops and they have become resistant to the attacks of insect pests.
- A fungus – *Trichoderma* is a free-living species which is very commonly present in root ecosystems and is found to effectively control the various plant pathogens.
- Most of the **Baculoviruses** which are being used as a biological control belong to the genus *Nucleopolyhedrovirus*. These are pathogenic to insects and other arthropods but have no effects on plants, mammals, fishes, birds and even non-target insects. These are highly species specific so are used as narrow spectrum insecticidal applications. This is specially required for a conserving an overall **Integrated Pest Management (IPM) programme** or when an ecologically sensitive area is being treated.

## Microbes as Bio-Fertilizers

- **Biofertilizers**: Biofertilizers are organisms that enrich the nutrient quality of the soil. These include mainly bacteria, fungi and cyanobacteria.
- **Rhizobium** is found symbiotically in the root nodules of leguminous plants where it performs $N_2$ fixation.
- *Azotobacter* and *Azospirillum* are free living nitrogen which is fixing bacteria.
- Fungi like those belonging to the genus *Glomus* **(AM fungi)** form **endomycorrhiza** with roots of higher plants. They are obligate symbiont. Fungal partner absorbs phosphorus from the soil and provide it to the plant. In addition, plants also receive other benefits - Resistance to root-borne pathogens, tolerance to salinity and drought and increased growth and development of plants.
- **Cyanobacteria** like *Anabaena* **(symbiotic association with Azolla),** *Nostoc* and *Oscillatoria* fix atmospheric nitrogen. In paddy fields, cyanobacteria serve as an important biofertilizers. Some organic matter is also added by the cyanobacteria which further increases the fertility of the soil.
- *Schizosaccharomyces pombe* is also known as **fission yeast**.

# PRACTICE EXERCISES

**Direction:** Read the question carefully and choose the correct option for each.

## Multiple Choice Questions: Level I

### Various Microbes

1. Choose the correct option with regard to statement A and B.
   A: Microbes are present everywhere on earth.
   B: They cannot live in thermal vents where temperature is as high as 100°C.
   (a) Statement A is correct and B is incorrect
   (b) Statements A and B are correct
   (c) Statement A is incorrect but B is correct
   (d) Statements A and B are incorrect

2. Prions are ________ infectious agents.
   (a) Lipidic (b) Sugar containing
   (c) Proteinaceous (d) Poison containing

3. Microbes after growth on a nutritive medium forms ________.
   (a) Group (b) Colonies (c) Species (d) Family

**Figure given for questions 4 and 5.**

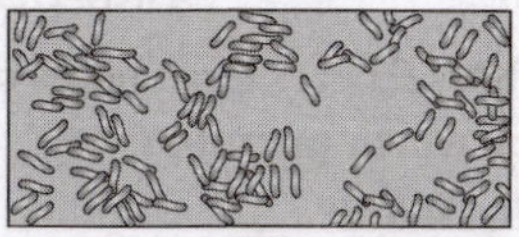
(a)

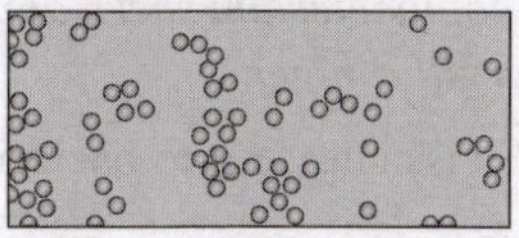
(b)

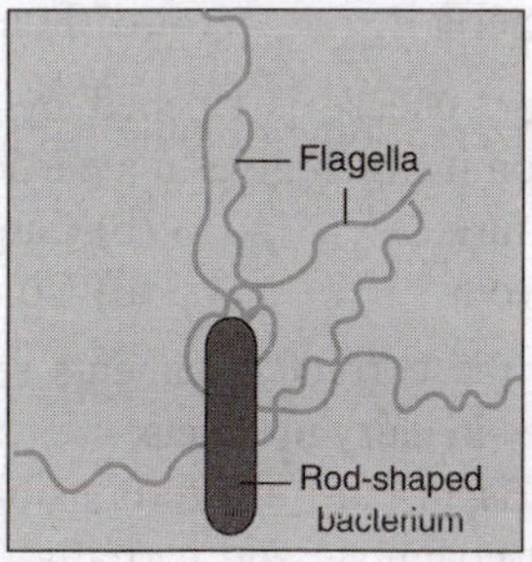

(c)

4. The bacteria shown in figure (a) and (b) are at which level of magnification?
   (a) 150X (b) 1500X
   (c) 15000X (d) 1.5 lacX

5. The rod shaped bacteria showing flagella is magnified at ________.
   (a) $5 \times 10^3$X (b) $5 \times 10^4$X
   (c) $1.5 \times 10^3$X (d) $15 \times 10^4$X

6. Label a and b in the below figure:

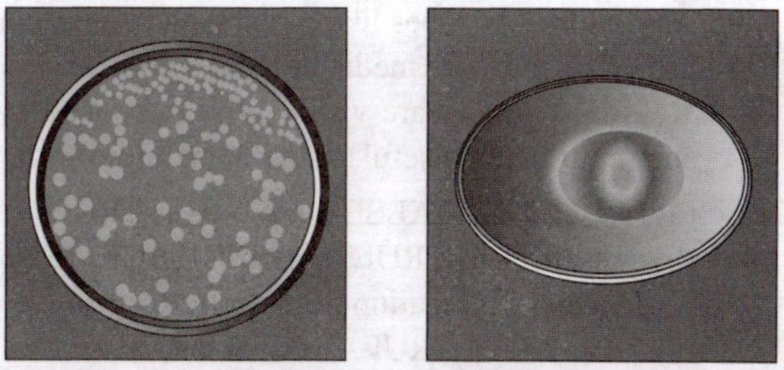
(a) (b)

   (a) Bacterial colony, Fungal colony
   (b) Viral colony, Bacterial colony
   (c) Fungal colony, Viral colony
   (d) Bacterial colony, Viral colony

7. Label Figure (a), (b), (c) and p, q, r, s, t and u in the Figure (a):

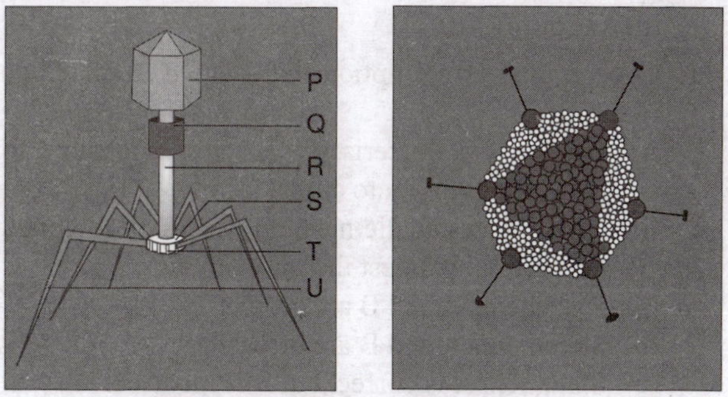

(a) (b)

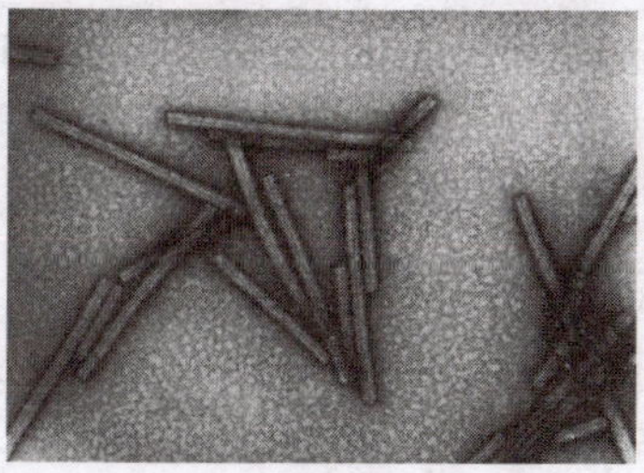
(c)

(a) (a)- Bacteriophage, (b)-Adenovirus (c)-TMV
(b) (a)- Bacteriophage, (b)-Adenovirus (c)-Rhinovirus
(c) (a)- Rhinovirus, (b)-Adenovirus (c)-TMV
(d) (a)- Bacteriophage, (b)-Rhinovirus (c)-TMV

**8.** **Assertion:** Microbes can be harmful to human beings.

**Reason:** They cause a large number of diseases in plants, animals and also in humans.

(a) Assertion is FALSE but reason is TRUE
(b) Assertion is TRUE, reason is TRUE; reason is a correct explanation for assertion.
(c) Assertion is TRUE, reason is TRUE; reason is not a correct explanation for assertion
(d) Assertion is TRUE, reason is FALSE

**9.** **Assertion:** Microbes like bacteria and many fungi are grown on nutritive media to form colonies.

**Reason:** colonies are visible with the naked eye and such cultures are useful in studies on micro-organisms.

(a) Assertion is FALSE but reason is TRUE
(b) Assertion is TRUE, reason is TRUE; reason is a correct explanation for assertion.
(c) Assertion is TRUE, reason is TRUE; reason is not a correct explanation for assertion
(d) Assertion is TRUE, reason is FALSE

## Microbes in Household Products

**10.** ____ is/are responsible for converting milk into curd.
(a) Lactobacillus only
(b) *Lactobacillus* and other microbes
(c) Microbes other than lactobacillus
(d) (a) or (c)

**11.** Choose the correct option with regard to statement A and B.

A: Lactic Acid Bacteria (LAB) are responsible for converting milk into curd.

B: LAB creates acidic medium necessary to coagulate and fully digest the milk proteins.

(a) Statements A and B are correct
(b) Statements A and B are incorrect.
(c) Statement A is correct but B is incorrect
(d) Statement B is correct and A is incorrect

**12.** If someone wants to make curd from milk, a small amount of curd is added to fresh milk. The small amount of curd containing millions of LAB is known as
(a) Accelerator (b) Promoter
(c) Inoculum (d) Germ

**13.** To prevent curd from getting sour, which parameter should be essentially controlled?
(a) Quantity of milk
(b) Amount of LAB added initially
(c) Temperature of the surrounding
(d) Amount of $O_2$ in surrounding air

**14.** Which vitamin is synthesized by LAB?
(a) Vitamin $B_2$ (b) Vitamin $B_6$
(c) Vitamin $B_5$ (d) Vitamin $B_{12}$

**15.** The puffed-up dough of dosa and idli is due to ______.
(a) Fermentation by bacteria and production of $O_2$.
(b) Hydrolysis by bacteria and production of $CO_2$.
(c) Fermentation by bacteria and production of $CO_2$.
(d) Hydrolysis by bacteria and production of $O_2$.

**16.** Which microbe helps us in the preparation of bread?
(a) Bacteria (b) Yeast
(c) Fungi (d) Algae

**17.** Baker's yeast is __________.
(a) *Saccharomyces cariocanus*
(b) *Saccharomyces florentinus*
(c) *Saccharomyces cerevisiae*
(d) *Saccharomyces spencerorum*

**18.** __________ is a traditional drink of south India.
(a) Wine (b) Toddy
(c) Tequila (d) Rum

**19.** The traditional drink of south India is made by fermenting sap from __________ tree.
(a) Eucalyptus (b) Coconut
(c) Palm (d) Date

**20.** 'Swiss cheese' bears large holes due to the production of $CO_2$ by which microbe?
(a) *Lactobacillus*
(b) *Saccharomyces cerevisiae*
(c) *Propionibacterium shermanii*
(d) *Aspergillus niger*

**21.** Just as, Swiss cheese it to bacteria, Roquefort cheese is to ________.
(a) Algae (b) Yeast
(c) Bacteria (d) Fungi

**22.** Roquefort cheese is ripened by growing a specific fungus on it which gives it a particular __________.
(a) Texture (b) Large holes
(c) Flavour (d) Colour

**23.** Choose the correct statements regarding the use of microbes in dairy products:

A. LABs in curd are responsible to produce acids that coagulate and partially digest the milk proteins.

B. Lactic acid bacteria improve nutritional quality of curd by increasing vitamin D3.

C. Fermentation by microbes is not involved in the production of cheese.
D. The 'Roquefort cheese' are ripened by growing a specific fungi on them, which gives them a porous texture.

Choose the correct answer from the options given below:

(a) A, B and D only
(b) A, B, C and D only
(c) A only
(d) B, C and D only

**24.** Choose the correct statements about the use of microbes in the fermentation industry:

A. Bacteria and fungi are used to impart particular texture, taste and flavor to cheese.
B. Microbes are used to produce industrial products like lactic acid, acetic acid and alcohol.
C. Certain dishes such as *idli* and *dosa*, are made from dough fermented by microbes.
D. The dough, which is used to make bread, is fermented by yeast called *Saccharomyces cerevisiae.*

Choose the correct answer from the options given below:

(a) A, B and D only
(b) A, B, C and D only
(c) A only
(d) B, C and D only

**Direction for Q25-29:** Choose the correct option:

(a) Assertion is FALSE but reason is TRUE
(b) Assertion is TRUE, reason is TRUE; reason is a correct explanation for assertion.
(c) Assertion is TRUE, reason is TRUE; reason is not a correct explanation for assertion
(d) Assertion is TRUE, reason is FALSE

**25. Assertion:** LABs improve the nutritional quality of curd by increasing vitamin $B_{12}$.
**Reason:** LABs play very beneficial role in checking disease causing microbes.

**26. Assertion:** LABs grow in milk and convert it to curd.
**Reason:** During growth, the LAB produce acids that coagulate and partially digest the milk proteins.

**27. Assertion:** The dough, used for making foods such as dosa and idli is fermented by yeast.
**Reason:** The dough used for making bread, is fermented using baker's yeast (Saccharomyces cerevisiae).

**28. Assertion:** The 'Roquefort cheese' has a particular flavour.
**Reason:** it is ripened by growing a specific bacteria on them.

**29. Assertion:** Swiss cheese is specialised in having large holes in it.
**Reason:** The large holes in 'Swiss cheese' are due to production of a large amount of $O_2$ by a bacterium named Propionibacterium sharmanii.

## Microbes in Industrial Products

**30.** Vessels for growing microbes on industrial scale are known as ________.

(a) Incubators (b) Sterilizers
(c) Fermenters (d) Microbial vessels

**31.** Alcoholic beverages are produced by microbial fermentation of

(a) Malted cereals (b) Fruit juices
(c) Vegetable juices (d) Both (a) and (b)

**32.** Brewer's Yeast is

(a) *Saccharomyces cariocanus*
(b) *Saccharomyces florentinus*
(c) *Saccharomyces cerevisiae*
(d) *Saccharomyces spencerorum*

**33.** ________ is the alcoholic beverage obtained without distillation.

(a) Whiskey (b) Brandy
(c) Wine (d) Rum

**34.** Point the odd one out.

(a) Rum (b) Beer
(c) Whiskey (d) Brandy

**35.** 'Antibiotics' literally means

(a) Protecting life (b) Against life
(c) Healing life (d) Accelerating life

**36.** Penicillin was discovered by ________.

(a) Edward Jenner (b) Louis Pasteur
(c) Alexander Fleming (d) Howard Florey

**37.** Penicillin was discovered by chance as the organism producing it retarded the growth of ________.

(a) *Lactobacilli* (b) *Staphylococci*
(c) *Streptococci* (d) *E. Coli*

**38.** The name penicillin was given after the mould _____.

(a) *Penicillium notatum*
(b) *Penicillium chrysogenum*
(c) *Penicillium candidum*
(d) *Penicillium glaucum*

**39.** The full potential as an effective antibiotic in the context of penicillin was studied by ________.

(a) Sutton and Boveri (b) Chain and Florey
(c) Watson and Crick (d) Edward Jenner

**40.** Penicillin was extensively used during which war?
(a) World War I (b) World War II
(c) Both (a) and (b) (d) Cold War

**41.** '*Gal ghotu*' is a common name for which disease?
(a) Whooping cough (b) Diphtheria
(c) Plague (d) Leprosy

**42.** '*Kusht rog*' is a common name for which disease?
(a) Dermatitis (b) Plague
(c) Leprosy (d) Whooping cough

**43.** Citric acid is produced by ________.
(a) *Aspergillus niger*
(b) *Saccharomyces cerevisiae*
(c) *Lactobacillus*
(d) *Clostridium butylicum*

**44.** *Acetobacter aceti* essentially produces ________.
(a) Citric acid (b) Acetic acid
(c) Butyric acid (d) Lactic acid

**45.** Which microbe produces butyric acid?
(a) *Sachharomyces cerevisiae*
(b) *Clostridium butylicum*
(c) *Aspergillus niger*
(d) *Propionibacterium shermanii*

**46.** A bacterium which is a rich source of lactic acid is ________.
(a) *Lactobacillus* (b) *Aspergillus*
(c) *Clostridium* (d) *Saccharomyces*

**47.** Which enzyme produced by microbes is an important ingredient in detergent formulations?
(a) Urease (b) Lipase
(c) Pectinase (d) Cleansase

**48.** The fruit juices available commercially are clearer than ones which are homemade. Which ingredient is added in commercially available fruit juices?
(a) Lipase and protease
(b) Pectinase and hydrolase
(c) Pectinase and protease
(d) Hydrolase and protease

**49.** Which enzyme is known as '*clot-buster*'?
(a) Protease (b) Thrombokinase
(c) Streptokinase (d) Hydrolase

**50.** '*Clot-buster*' is produced by which microbe?
(a) *Staphylococcus* (b) *Streptococcus*
(c) *Penicillium* (d) *Aspergillus*

**51.** The enzyme streptokinase is used medicinally to
(a) Check growth of microbes in body fluids
(b) Remove blood clots from the blood vessels
(c) Weaken walls of blood vessels
(d) Create blood clots in blood vessels

**52.** Which drugs are often administered before and after organ transplant procedure?
(a) Immunomodulators (b) Immunosuppressants
(c) Vaccination (d) Anabolic steroids

**53.** Which drug is generally administered at the time of organ-transplant procedure?
(a) Actinomycin-D (b) Bleomycin
(c) Cyclosporin-A (d) Paclitaxel

**54.** Cyclosporine-A is produced by fungus ________.
(a) *Trichoderma polysporum*
(b) *Penicillium notatum*
(c) *Micromonospora*
(d) *Aspergillus niger*

**55.** What is shown in this figure?

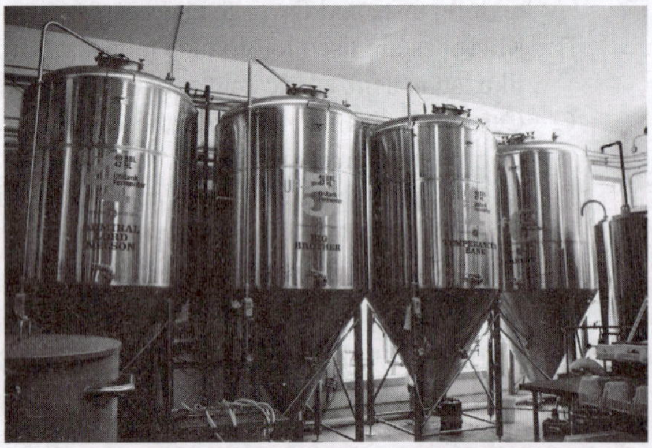

(a) Biogas plant (b) Sewage treatment plant
(c) Fermentors (d) Distillation apparatus

**56.** What is shown in the figure?

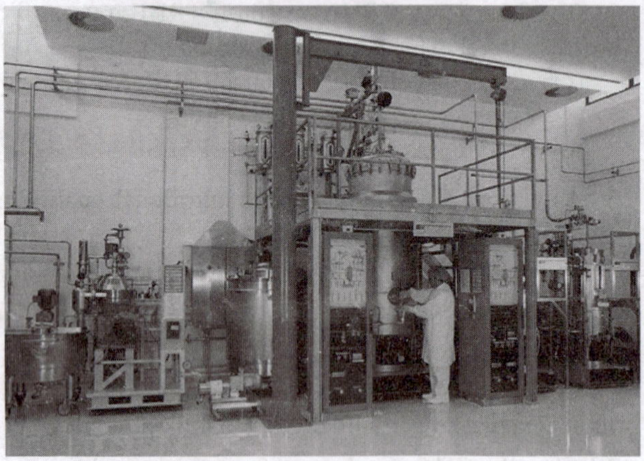

(a) Transmission electron microscope
(b) Fermentation plant
(c) Sewage treatment
(d) Large Hadron Collider

**57.** Blood cholesterol lowering agents are known as ________.

(a) Steroids (b) Statins
(c) Lipolytics (d) Diuretics

**58.** *Monascus purpureus* is a commercial source of ________.
(a) Antibiotics (b) Statins
(c) Pectinase (d) Ethanol

**59.** The mechanism of action of statins is ________.
(a) Allosteric inhibition of enzyme is responsible for the synthesis of cholesterol.
(b) Competitive inhibition of enzyme is responsible for the synthesis of cholesterol.
(c) Irreversible inhibition of enzyme is responsible for the synthesis of cholesterol.
(d) None of the above

**60.** Which of the following statements are correct regarding the role of microbes in the production of antibiotics?
A. Penicillin is produced by the fungus Aspergillus.
B. Streptomycin is produced by the bacterium Streptomyces.
C. Penicillin inhibits growth of Streptococcus.
D. Microbes produce antibiotics as a defence mechanism against other microorganisms.

Choose the correct answer from the options given below:
(a) A, B and D only
(b) A, B, C and D only
(c) A only
(d) B, C and D only

**61.** Which of the following statements are correct regarding the role of microbes in the production of antibiotics?
A. Microbes play a significant role in the synthesis of enzymes used in detergents.
B. Statin acts by competitively inhibiting the enzyme responsible for synthesis of cholesterol.
C. the bottled juices are clarified by the use of pectinases and chitinase.
D. Streptokinase used as a 'clot buster' is produced by the bacterium Staphylococcus .

Choose the correct answer from the options given below:
(a) A, B and D only
(b) A, B, C and D only
(c) A and B only
(d) A and D only

**Direction for Q62–69:** Choose the correct option:
(a) Assertion is FALSE but reason is TRUE
(b) Assertion is TRUE, reason is TRUE; reason is a correct explanation for assertion.
(c) Assertion is TRUE, reason is TRUE; reason is not a correct explanation for assertion
(d) Assertion is TRUE, reason is FALSE

**62. Assertion:** Saccharomyces cerevisiae is commonly called brewer's yeast.
**Reason:** It is used for fermenting malted cereals and fruit juices, to produce butanol.

**63 Assertion:** Different types of alcoholic drinks are obtained depending on the type of processing of raw material.
**Reason:** Wine and beer are produced without distillation whereas whisky, brandy and rum are produced by distillation of the fermented broth.

**64. Assertion:** Lipases are used in detergent formulations
**Reason:** Lipases are helpful in removing oily stains from the laundry.

**65. Assertion:** Bottled fruit juices bought from the market are clearer as compared to those made at home.
**Reason:** The bottled juices are clarified by the use of pectinases and cellulases.

**66. Assertion:** Streptokinase is used in patients who have undergone myocardial infaction leading to heart attack.
**Reason:** Genetically modified Streptokinase is used to lower blood pressure in patients.

**67. Assertion:** Streptokinase is called as a 'clot buster'
**Reason:** It removes clots from the blood vessels

**68. Assertion:** Cyclosporin A is used in treatment of organ-transplant patients
**Reason:** It is an immunosuppressive agent produced by the fungus Trichoderma polysporum

**69. Assertion:** Statins produced by Monascus purpureus have been commercialised as blood-cholesterol lowering agents
**Reason:** Statins act by competitively inhibiting the enzyme responsible for synthesis of cholesterol.

## Microbes in Sewage Treatment

**70.** The major portion of waste water in cities and towns is ________.
(a) Household waste (b) Industrial waste
(c) Human excreta (d) Both (a) and (b)

**71.** Municipal waste water is also known as ________.
(a) Drainage (b) Sewage
(c) Spillage (d) Gutter

**72.** Sewage is treated in ________.
(a) STD (b) STP
(c) SPT (d) SDT

**73.** STP stands for
(a) Sequential Topographical Projection
(b) Standard Test Procedure
(c) Sewage Treatment Plant
(d) None of these

**74.** Which microbes help in sewage treatment?
(a) Autotrophic (b) Heterotrophic
(c) Symbiotic (d) Chemoautotrophic

**75.** Sewage water treatment is done in how many stages?
(a) 1 (b) 3 (c) 2 (d) 4

**76.** Primary treatment of sewage waste involves which processes?
(a) Filtration and incubation
(b) Sedimentation and decantation
(c) Filtration and sedimentation
(d) Sedimentation and microbial proliferation

**77.** In sewage treatment plant, primary treatment involving removal of floating debris is done by
(a) Vacuum filtration (b) Pressure filtration
(c) Sequential filtration (d) Sedimentation

**78.** In primary treatment of sewage water, removal of grit involves which process?
(a) Decantation (b) Picking
(c) Filtration (d) Sedimentation

**79.** In primary treatment of sewage water, after sedimentation, the solids that settle form ________.
(a) Activated sludge (b) Primary sludge
(c) Secondary sludge (d) Both (a) and (c)

**80.** The supernatant left after sedimentation of sewage water during primary treatment is known as
(a) Affluent (b) Flocs
(c) Sludge (d) Effluent

**81.** Which of the following is transferred from primary setting tank to another tank for secondary treatment?
(a) Grit (b) Sludge
(c) Effluent (d) Floc

**82.** The secondary treatment of sewage waste is also known as ________.
(a) Chemical treatment (b) Physical treatment
(c) Biological treatment (d) Detoxification

**83.** Which of the following is used in secondary treatment of sewage water?
(a) Fermentation tanks
(b) Digester tanks
(c) Detoxification tanks
(d) Aeration tanks

**84.** What kind of microbes is present in 'flocs' formed during secondary treatment of sewage?
(a) Aerobic (b) Anaerobic
(c) Symbiotic (d) Aero tolerant

**85.** In context of secondary treatment of sewage, 'flocs' is associated with which microbes?
(a) Bacteria and algae
(b) Algae and fungus
(c) Fungi and bacteria
(d) Fungi and lichen

**86.** What is BOD?
(a) Bacterial Oxygen Demand
(b) Biological Organic Debris
(c) Biochemical Organic Demand
(d) Biochemical Oxygen Demand

**87.** The 'flocs' present in large aeration tanks causes ________ in BOD.
(a) Decrease (b) Increase
(c) No change (d) Either (a) or (b)

**88.** BOD can be defined as
(a) Amount of $CO_2$ consumed if all the inorganic matter in one litre of water is oxidized by bacteria.
(b) Amount of $O_2$ consumed if all the organic matter in one decilitre of water is reduced by bacteria.
(c) Amount of $O_2$ consumed if all the organic matter in one litre of water is oxidized by bacteria.
(d) Amount of $O_2$ consumed if all the inorganic matter in one litre of water is oxidized by bacteria.

**89.** BOD is the measure of ________ in water.
(a) Organic matter (b) Inorganic matter
(c) Bacterial load (d) Toxicity

**90.** BOD ________ polluting potential of waste water.
**(a)Is not proportional to**
(b) Is directly proportional to
(c) Is inversely proportional to
(d) None of these

**91.** Once BOD from the sewage is reduced significantly, the 'flocs' are allowed to sediment and it is known as ________.
(a) Primary sludge (b) Secondary sludge
(c) Activated sludge (d) Inactivated sludge

**92.** The figure shows:

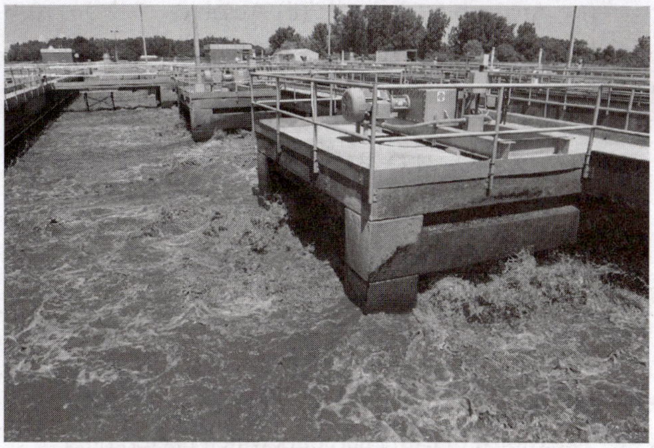

(a) Primary treatment (b) Activated sludge
(c) Secondary treatment (d) Flocs

**93.** This image is an aerial view of a ________.

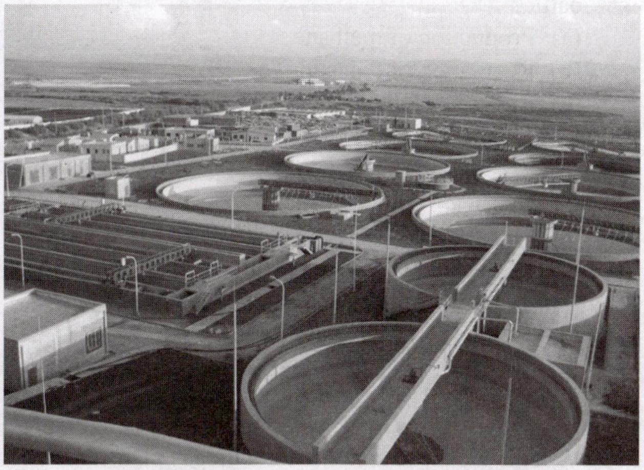

(a) Nuclear reactor (b) Sewage plant
(c) Biogas plant (d) Fermentation plant

**94.** The remaining major part of activated sludge is pumped into large tanks called ________.
(a) Aerobic fermenters
(b) Anaerobic fermenters
(c) Aerobic Sludge digesters
(d) Anaerobic sludge digesters

**95.** In an anaerobic sludge digester, anaerobically digesting bacteria digest which microbes?
(a) Fungi (b) Bacteria
(c) Algae (d) Both (a) and (b)

**96.** In an anaerobic sludge digester, during the digestion process, mixture of gases like ________ are produced.
(a) $CH_4$, $H_2O$, $O_2$ (b) $C_2H_6$, $H_2S$, $CO_2$
(c) $CH_4$, $H_2O_2$, $CO_2$ (d) $CH_4$, $H_2S$, $CO_2$

**97.** The gases that evolve from anaerobic sludge digester constitute ________.
(a) Natural gas (b) Biogas
(c) Water gas (d) None of these

**98.** After secondary treatment, the effluent is released into
(a) Digester tank
(b) Filtration unit
(c) Water bodies
(d) Chemical treatment unit

**99.** Which ministry has initiated Ganga Action Plan and Yamuna Action Plan?
(a) Ministry of Chemicals and Fertilizers
(b) Ministry of Health and Family Welfare
(c) Ministry of Community Health and Diseases
(d) Ministry of Environment and Forest

## Sewage Management

**100.** Which of the following are applications of microbes in waste management?
A. Methanogenic bacteria in the decomposition of organic waste.
B. Use of bacteria and fungi in aerobic treatment of sewage
C. Anaerobic digestion of activated sludge
D. Microbes playing a role in biogas production

Choose the correct answer from the options given below:
(a) A, B and D only
(b) B, C and D only
(c) A and C only
(d) A, B, C and D only

**101.** Which of the following statements are correct regarding the use of microbes in the treatment of industrial effluents?
A. Treatment of waste water is done by the heterotrophic microbes naturally present in the sewage.
B. The major part of the activated sludge is treated with anaerobic bacteria in anaerobic sludge digesters.
C. The biological treatment of effluent involves first with anaerobic microbes and then aerobic microbes.
D. Flocs are masses of bacteria associated with plant cell filaments to form mesh like structures.

Choose the correct answer from the options given below:
(a) A and B only
(b) A, B, and C only
(c) A and D only
(d) B, C and D only

**Direction for Q102–107:** Choose the correct option:

(a) Assertion is FALSE but reason is TRUE
(b) Assertion is TRUE, reason is TRUE; reason is a correct explanation for assertion.
(c) Assertion is TRUE, reason is TRUE; reason is not a correct explanation for assertion
(d) Assertion is TRUE, reason is FALSE

**102. Assertion:** Before disposal, sewage is treated in sewage treatment plants (STPs).
**Reason:** sewage contains large amounts of organic matter and microbes.

**103. Assertion:** Primary treatment steps basically involve filtration and sedimentation.
**Reason:** Sequential filtration removes floating debris and sedimentation removes the grit (soil and small pebbles).

**104 Assertion:** In sewage treatment, the primary effluent is constantly agitated mechanically and air is pumped into it.
**Reason:** This allows vigorous growth of useful aerobic microbes into flocs.

**105. Assertion:** Secondary treatment of sewage significantly reduces the BOD of the effluent.
**Reason:** Microbes growing in effluent consume the major part of the organic matter present in the effluent.

**106. Assertion:** The greater the BOD of waste water, more is its polluting potential
**Reason:** BOD is an indirect measure of the organic matter present in the water

**107. Assertion:** A small part of the activated sludge is pumped back into the aeration tank
**Reason:** It serves as the inoculum which starts growth of microbes.

## Microbes in Production of Biogas

**108.** Which gas is the main constituent of biogas?
(a) $H_2S$ (b) $CH_4$ (c) $C_2H_6$ (d) $C_3H_8$

**109.** The gas produced as end-product during growth and metabolism of microbes depends on
(a) Nature of microbe and substrate
(b) Nature of digester tank and microbe
(c) Nature of microbe only
(d) Oxygen levels in the digester tank

**110.** Methanogens produce certain gases by growing on cellulosic material. What kind of organisms are they?
(a) Fungi (b) Algae
(c) Bacteria (d) Lichen

**111.** Methanogens are ________ microbes.
(a) Anaerobic (b) Aerobic
(c) Microaerophiles (d) Aerotobront

**112.** Methanogens produces which gases amongst the following list of gases?
$CH_4$, $O_2$, $CO_2$, $H_2O_2$, $H_2S$, $H_2$
(a) $CH_4$, $H_2O_2$, $H_2$ (b) $H_2S$, $H_2$, $CO_2$
(c) $CH_4$, $H_2$, $CO_2$ (d) $H_2S$, $H_2O_2$, $CO_2$

**113.** The most commonly found methanogens in anaerobic sludge is ________.
(a) Ethanobacterium (b) Methanobacterium
(c) Cyanobacterium (d) Both (b) and (c)

**114.** The rumen of cattle harbours which bacteria?
(a) Methanogens (b) Cyanobacteria
(c) Cellulogens (d) Ethanogens

**115.** What is the role of bacteria present in the rumen of cattle?
(a) Production of methane
(b) Regulation of digestion
(c) Breakdown of cellulose
(d) Synthesis of polysaccharides

**116.** Gobar gas is the same as ________.
(a) Water gas (b) Biogas
(c) Natural gas (d) None of these

**117.** The depth of concrete tank, a part of biogas plant, ranges from ________ to ________.
(a) 10–15 feet (b) 10–15 metre
(c) 15–20 feet (d) 15–20 metre

**118.** What is the input material for a biogas plant?
(a) Bio wastes (b) Slurry of dung
(c) Industrial waste (d) Both (a) and (b)

**119.** A ________ is placed over the slurry in biogas plant.
(a) Gas holder (b) Floating cover
(c) Digester (d) Gas filter

**120.** The spent slurry in a biogas plant is used as ________.
(a) Pesticide (b) Fertilizer
(c) Insecticide (d) Herbicide

**121.** Apart from cooking, biogas is generally used in rural areas for ________.
(a) Mechanical work
(b) Lighting
(c) Chemical transformation
(d) None of these

**122.** Which institutes have actively participated in the development of technology for biogas production? IARI, IIT, IISC, KVIM, KVIC.
(a) IIT and KVIM (b) IISC and KVIC
(c) KVIC and IARI (d) IARI and KVIM

**123.** IARI stands for
(a) Indian Aviation Research Institute
(b) Indian Aerospace Research Institute
(c) Indian Atomic Research Institute
(d) Indian Agricultural Research Institute

**124.** Label P, R, S, T and U in the below diagram:

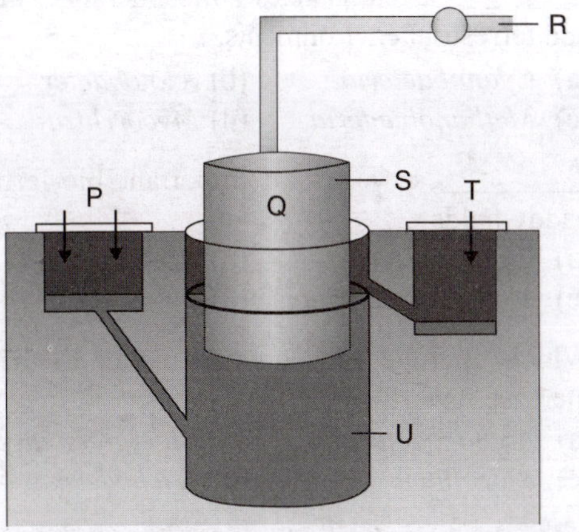


(a) P: water and dung R: Gas S: Gas Holder T: Sludge U: Digester
(b) P: water and dung R: Gas holder S: Gas T: Sludge U: Digester
(c) P: water R: Gas S: Gas Holder T: Sludge U: dung
(d) P: water and dung R: Gas S: Gas Holder T: Sludge U: Water collector

**125.** Methanogens are commonly found in ________ during sewage treatment.
(a) primary Sludge
(b) anaerobic sludge
(c) activated sludge
(d) flocs

**126.** Which of the following statements are true regarding the use of microbes in biogas production?
A. Methanogens are essential for the production of methane in biogas.
B. Bacteria involved in biogas production thrive only in aerobic conditions.
C. Biogas contains primarily carbon dioxide and oxygen.
D. Biogas production is not influenced by the types of microbes involved.

Choose the correct answer from the options given below:
(a) A only
(b) A, B, C and D only
(c) A, B and D only
(d) B, C and D only

**127.** **Statement 1:** Microbes in biogas production thrive in aerobic conditions.
**Statement 2:** Methanogens are essential for the production of methane in anaerobic conditions.
Choose the correct answer from the options given below.
(a) Statement I is incorrect but statement II is correct
(b) Both Statements I and II are correct
(c) Both Statements I and II are incorrect
(d) Statement I is correct but statement II is incorrect

**Direction for Q128–131:** Choose the correct option:
(a) Assertion is FALSE but reason is TRUE
(b) Assertion is TRUE, reason is TRUE; reason is a correct explanation for assertion.
(c) Assertion is TRUE, reason is TRUE; reason is not a correct explanation for assertion
(d) Assertion is TRUE, reason is FALSE

**128.** **Assertion:** $CO_2$ is produced as main gas during production of beverages, while methane is predominant gas produced anaerobically using cellulosic materials.
**Reason:** The type of the gas produced depends upon the microbes and the organic substrates they utilise.

**129.** **Assertion:** Methanogenic bacteria are present in the rumen of cattle.
**Reason:** In rumen, methanogenic bacteria help in the breakdown of cellulose and play an important role in the nutrition of cattle.

**130.** **Assertion:** Dung can be used for generation of biogas, commonly called gobar gas.
**Reason:** The excreta (dung) of cattle, commonly called gobar, is rich in methanogenic bacteria.

**131.** **Assertion:** In biogas plant, a floating cover is placed over the slurry.
**Reason:** The cover keeps on rising as the gas is produced in the tank due to the microbial activity

## Microbes as Biocontrol Agents and as Biofertilizers

**132.** 'Bt' spores are mixed with ________ and sprayed on vulnerable plants.
(a) Only alcohol (b) Any organic solvent
(c) Only water (d) Any aqueous solvent

**133.** _________ are free living bacteria which fix atmospheric nitrogen in soil.
(a) Azobacterium (b) Acetobacterium
(c) Azotobacter (d) Azabacterium

**134.** Biocontrol refers to
(a) Indiscriminate use of microbes for human welfare
(b) Use of microbes to control plant diseases
(c) Use of microbes to control cattle diseases
(d) Both (b) and (c)

**135.** A beetle with 'red and black' markings is known as _________.
(a) Dragonfly (b) Ladybird
(c) Clever Wasp (d) Queen Ant

**136.** Dragonflies are useful to get rid of _________.
(a) Ladybird (b) Aphids
(c) Mosquitoes (d) Both (b) and (c)

**137.** Butterfly caterpillars can be controlled by use of the microbe _________.
(a) *Bacillus stearothermophilus*
(b) *Bacillus thuringiensis*
(c) *Bacillus chemophilus*
(d) *Bacillus terminates*

**138.** 'Bt' is available in sachets as dried _________.
(a) Spores (b) Capsules
(c) Seeds (d) Both (a) and (b)

**139.** Scientists have introduced _________ gene into plants to impart resistance to insect pests.
(a) Ct gene (b) Bt gene
(c) Tt gene (d) Mt gene

**140.** Which fungus is used in plants to provide control against pests?
(a) *Aspergillus* (b) *Trichoderma*
(c) *Trichophyton* (d) *Rhizopus*

**141.** _________ are the pathogens that attack insects and other arthropods.
(a) *Rhinovirus* (b) *Baculovirus*
(c) *Ranikhet Virus* (d) *Bean Virus*

**142.** Baculovirus belongs to the genus
(a) *Retrohedro Virus*
(b) *Nucleohedero-Virus*
(c) *Nucleopolyhedro Virus*
(d) *Polyhedral Virus*

**143.** IPM stands for
(a) Indian Pollution Management
(b) Institute of Pest Management
(c) Integrated Pest Management
(d) Institute of Pollution Management

**144.** Root nodules of leguminous plants bear which microbe?
(a) *Rhizopus* (b) *Rhino virus*
(c) *Rhizome* (d) *Rhizobium*

**145.** Fungi which form symbiotic associations with plants are _________.
(a) *Rhizobium* (b) *Mycorrhiza*
(c) *Azospirillum* (d) *Oscillatoria*

**146.** Mycorrhiza formed by genus glomus absorbs _________ from soil and passes it to the plant.
(a) K (b) P (c) Fe (d) Mg

**147.** _________ bacteria fixes atmospheric $N_2$ in aquatic and terrestrial environments.
(a) *Cyanobacteria* (b) *Azotobacter*
(c) *Methanobacteria* (d) *Mycorrhiza*

**148.** _________ serve as an important bio-fertilizer in paddy fields.
(a) *Cyanobacteria* (b) *Azotobacter*
(c) *Methanobacterium* (d) *Mycorrhiza*

**149.** Which microbe adds organic matter to the soil to increase its fertility?
(a) *Archaebacteria* (b) *Blue-green algae*
(c) *Rhizobium* (d) *Trichoderma*

**150.** **Assertion:** In organic farming, the eradication of the creatures that are often described as pests is not only possible, but also undesirable.
**Reason:** Without Pests, the beneficial predatory and parasitic insects which depend upon them as food or hosts would not be able to survive.
(a) Assertion is FALSE but reason is TRUE
(b) Assertion is TRUE, reason is TRUE; reason is a correct explanation for assertion.
(c) Assertion is TRUE, reason is TRUE; reason is not a correct explanation for assertion
(d) Assertion is TRUE, reason is FALSE

**151.** **Assertion:** Trichoderma is used as a biological control for use in the treatment of plant disease .
**Reason:** Trichoderma are very common in the leaf ecosystems and are effective biocontrol agents of several plant pathogens
(a) Assertion is FALSE but reason is TRUE
(b) Assertion is TRUE, reason is TRUE; reason is a correct explanation for assertion.
(c) Assertion is TRUE, reason is TRUE; reason is not a correct explanation for assertion
(d) Assertion is TRUE, reason is FALSE

**152. Assertion:** The majority of baculoviruses are used as biological control agents.

**Reason:** These viruses are excellent candidates for species-specific, wide spectrum insecticidal applications

(a) Assertion is FALSE but reason is TRUE
(b) Assertion is TRUE, reason is TRUE; reason is a correct explanation for assertion.
(c) Assertion is TRUE, reason is TRUE; reason is not a correct explanation for assertion
(d) Assertion is TRUE, reason is FALSE.

**153. Assertion:** Baculoviruses help in conserving beneficial insects and aid in an overall integrated pest management (IPM) programme

**Reason:** Baculoviruses have been shown to have no negative impacts on plants, mammals, birds, fish or even on non-target insects.

(a) Assertion is FALSE but reason is TRUE
(b) Assertion is TRUE, reason is TRUE; reason is a correct explanation for assertion.
(c) Assertion is TRUE, reason is TRUE; reason is not a correct explanation for assertion
(d) Assertion is TRUE, reason is FALSE

**154.** Select the correct statements about biocontrol agents:

A. The Ladybird and Dragonflies are useful to get rid of mosquitoes and aphids, respectively.
B. The bacteria Bacillus thuringiensis is used in order to control butterfly caterpillars.
C. Trichoderma species used as biocontrol agents are symbiotic fungi that are very common in the root ecosystems.
D. The majority of baculoviruses used as biological control agents are in the genus Nucleopolyhydroxyvirus.

Choose the correct answer from the options given below:

(a) A, B and D only
(b) C and D only
(c) A, B and C only
(d) B only

**155.** Select the correct statements about biofertilizers:

A. Biofertilisers are organisms that enrich the nutrient quality of the soil.
B. Cyanobacteria are autotrophic microbes widely distributed in aquatic and terrestrial environments
C. The main sources are bacteria, fungi and cyanobacteria.
D. Rhizobium can fix atmospheric nitrogen while free-living in the soil.

Choose the correct answer from the options given below:

(a) A, B and D only
(b) A, C and D only
(c) A, B and C only
(d) B and C only

**156.** Select the correct statements about biofertilizers:

A. Fungi form symbiotic associations with plants, called Lichens.
B. The genus Glomus is predominantly observed to form mycorrhiza.
C. The fungal symbiont in the associations absorbs potassium from soil and passes it to the plant.
D. The important biofertiliser in paddy fields are cyanobacteria.

Choose the correct answer from the options given below:

(a) B and D only
(b) A, C and D only
(c) A and D only
(d) B and C only

**157.** Which of the following statements are true regarding the use of microbes in agriculture?

A. Mycorrhizal fungi establish mutualistic associations with plant roots, enhancing nutrient absorption.
B. Pathogenic bacteria are intentionally used to improve crop yields.
C. Nitrogen-fixing bacteria in legume root nodules contribute to soil fertility.
D. Microbes play no role in the decomposition of organic matter in the soil.

Choose the correct answer from the options given below:

(a) A, B and D only
(b) A and C only
(c) A, C and D only
(d) B, C and D only

**158. Statement 1:** Mycorrhizal fungi establish parasitic associations with plant roots.

**Statement 2:** Mycorrhizal associations enhance nutrient absorption by plant roots.

Choose the correct answer from the options given below.

(a) Statement I is incorrect but statement II is correct
(b) Both Statements I and II are correct
(c) Both Statements I and II are incorrect
(d) Statement I is correct but statement II is incorrect

**159. Statement 1:** Activated sludge process involves the use of microbes in industrial effluent treatment.

**Statement 2:** Microbes can be used to kill harmful pests, a process called as biocontrol.

Choose the correct answer from the options given below.

(a) Statement I is incorrect but statement II is correct
(b) Both Statements I and II are correct
(c) Both Statements I and II are incorrect
(d) Statement I is correct but statement II is incorrect

**Direction for Q160–163:** Choose the correct option:

(a) Assertion is FALSE but reason is TRUE
(b) Assertion is TRUE, reason is TRUE; reason is a correct explanation for assertion.
(c) Assertion is TRUE, reason is TRUE; reason is not a correct explanation for assertion
(d) Assertion is TRUE, reason is FALSE

**160.** **Assertion:** The nodules on the roots of leguminous plants are formed by the symbiotic association of Rhizobium.
**Reason:** These bacteria fix atmospheric nitrogen into organic forms, which is used by the plant as nutrient.

**161.** **Assertion:** Azospirillum and Azotobacter enrich the nitrogen content of the soil.
**Reason:** Azospirillum and Azotobacter can fix atmospheric nitrogen during their symbiotic association with plants

**162.** **Assertion:** Mycorrhiza is symbiotic associations of Fungi with plants.
**Reason:** The fungal symbiont in these associations absorbs phosphorus from soil and passes it to the plant.

**163.** **Assertion:** In paddy fields, cyanobacteria serve as an important biofertiliser.
**Reason:** Cyanobacteria can fix atmospheric nitrogen

## Multiple Choice Questions: Level II

**164.** Which one of the following pairs is wrongly matched?
(a) alcohol - nitrogenase
(b) fruit juice - pectinase
(c) textile - amylase
(d) detergents - lipase

**165.** Which of the following is not used as a biopesticide?
(a) *Trichoderma harzianum*
(b) nuclear polyhedrosis virus (NPV)
(c) *Xanthomonas campestris*
(d) *Bacillus thuringiensis*

**166.** *Trichoderma harzianum* has proved to be a useful micro-organism for
(a) Gene transfer in higher plants
(b) Biological control of soil-borne plant pathogens
(c) Bioremediation of contaminated soils
(d) Reclamation of wastelands

**167.** Method of controlling pests relying on natural predation, rather than on chemicals is called
(a) competition (b) predation
(c) biological control (d) physiological control

**168.** Modern detergents contain enzyme preparations of
(a) thermoacidophiles
(b) thermophiles
(c) acidophiles
(d) alkaliphiles

**169.** Probiotics are
(a) cancer-inducing microbes
(b) new kind of food allergens
(c) live microbial food supplement
(d) safe antibiotics

**170.** Which one of the following pairs is wrongly matched?
(a) yeast - ethanol
(b) streptomycetes - antibiotic
(c) coliforms - vinegar
(d) methanogens - gobar gas

**171.** *Bacillus thuringiensis* (Bt) strains have been used for designing novel:
(a) Biofertilizers
(b) Bio-metallurgical techniques
(c) Bio-mineralization processes
(d) Bioinsecticidal plants

**172.** Which of the following is pair of bio-fertilizer?
(a) *Azolla* and BGA
(b) *Nostoc* and legumes
(c) *Rhizobium* and grasses
(d) *Salmonella* and *E. coli*

**173.** Which one of the following is non-symbiotic biofertilizer?
(a) Azotobacter (b) Anabaena
(c) Rhizobium (d) VAM

**174.** One of the major difficulties in the biological control of insects/pests is the
(a) practical difficulty of introducing the predator to specific areas.
(b) method is less effective as compared to the use of insecticides.
(c) predator does not always survive when transferred to a new environment.
(d) the predator develops a preference to other diets and may become a pest itself.

**175.** A sewage treatment process, in which a portion of the decomposer bacteria present in the waste is recycled into the beginning of the process is called
(a) Primary treatment
(b) Activated sludge treatment
(c) Tertiary treatment
(d) Cyclic treatment

**176.** Gobar gas contains mainly
(a) $CH_4 + CO_2$ (b) $CH_4 + O_2$
(c) $CO_2 + H_2$ (d) $CO_2 + SO_2$

## A & R and Statement-based Questions

### Assertion and Reason Questions

***Direction for questions 177 to 181:** Read the **assertion** and **reason** carefully to mark the correct option out of the options given below:*

**(a)** **(A)** is **true** but **(R)** is **false**.
**(b)** **(A)** is **false** but **(R)** is **true**.
**(c)** Both **(A)** and **(R)** is **true** and **(R)** is the correct explanation of **(A)**.
**(d)** Both **(A)** and **(R)** is **true** and **(R)** is not the correct explanation of **(A)**.

**177. Assertion:** Swiss cheese contain large holes.
**Reason:** It is produced by using *Propionibacterium sharmanii.*

**178. Assertion:** BGA increase fertility of soil.
**Reason:** BGA add organic matter to the soil.

**179. Assertion:** Azospirillum and azotobacter are used as biofertilizer.
**Reason:** They can enhance soil fertility by increasing nitrogen content of soil.

**180. Assertion:** Natural predation is better method than use of chemicals to control pests.
**Reason:** It decrease dependence of human on toxic chemicals and pesticides.

**181. Assertion:** Methanogen have important role in nutrition of cattle.
**Reason:** These bacteria help in digestion of cellulose.

### Statement-based Questions:

***Direction for questions 182 to 186:** These type of questions consist of two statement each, printed as **Statement-I** and **Statement-II**. While answering such questions, a student is needed to choose any one of the following four responses.*

**(a)** **Statement I** is **correct Statement II** is **incorrect**.
**(b)** **Statement I** is **incorrect Statement II** is **correct**.
**(c)** Both **Statement I** and **Statement II** are **correct**.
**(d)** Both **Statement I** and **Statement II** are **incorrect**.

**182. Statement-I:** Sediment in settling tank is called activated sludge.
**Statement-II:** Bacterial flocs are present in activated sludge.

**183. Statement-I:** Streptokinase is used to treat patient undergone myocardial infarction leading to heart attack.
**Statement-II:** Yeast is used for commercial production of cyclosporin A.

**184. Statement-I:** Saccharomyces cerevisiae commonly known as Brewer's bacteria.
**Statement-II:** Wine and Beer are prepared without distillation.

**185. Statement-I:** Bt-cotton is resistant to certain fungus attack.
**Statement-II:** Bt-cotton contain toxic gene in their cell itself.

**186. Statement-I:** Baculovirus are excellent for species specific, broad spectrum insecticidal applications.
**Statement-II:** They shown to have negative effect on plant, mammals, birds & fishes.

## Matrix-Match Type Questions

**187.** Match the following:

| List-I (Product) | List-II (Microbes Used) |
|---|---|
| 1. Curd | (i) *Propionibacterium sharmanii* |
| 2. Bread | (ii) *Lactobacillus* |
| 3. Cheese | (iii) *Saccharomyces cerevisiae* |

**The correct matching is:**

| | 1 | 2 | 3 |
|---|---|---|---|
| (a) | (ii) | (iii) | (i) |
| (b) | (i) | (iii) | (ii) |
| (c) | (iii) | (i) | (ii) |
| (d) | (ii) | (i) | (iii) |

**188.** Match the following:

| List-I (Microbes) | List-II (Product) | List-III |
|---|---|---|
| 1. *S. cerevisiae* | (i) Citric acid | Y. Yeast |
| 2. *Aspergillus niger* | (ii) Statin | Z. Fungus |
| 3. *Penicillium notatum* | (iii) Cyclosporin A | |
| 4. *Trichoderma polysporum* | (iv) Penicillin | |
| 5. *Monascus purpereus* | (v) Ethanol | |

**The correct matching is:**

(a) 1 – (v) – Y, 2 – (i) – Z, 3 – (iv) – Z, 4 – (iii) – Z, 5 – (ii) – Y
(b) 1 – (iii) – Y, 2 – (i) – Z, 3 – (iv) – Z, 4 – (v) – Z, 5 – (ii) – Y
(c) 1 – (v) – Y, 2 – (i) – Z, 3 – (ii) – Z, 4 – (iii) – Z, 5 – (iv) – Y
(d) 1 – (ii) – Y, 2 – (v) – Z, 3 – (iv) – Z, 4 – (iii) – Z, 5 – (i) – Y

**189.** Match the following:

| List-I (Microbes) | List-II (Product) |
|---|---|
| 1. *Methanobacterium sp.* | (i) Fermented Beverages |
| 2. *Penicillium sp.* | (ii) Statin |
| 3. *Saccharomyces sp.* | (iii) Biogas |
| 4. *Monascus sp.* | (iv) Antibiotic |

**The correct matching is:**

| | 1 | 2 | 3 | 4 |
|---|---|---|---|---|
| (a) | (iii) | (iv) | (i) | (ii) |
| (b) | (iv) | (iii) | (i) | (ii) |
| (c) | (i) | (iv) | (iii) | (ii) |
| (d) | (ii) | (i) | (iv) | (iii) |

**190.** Match the following:

| List-I (Crop) | List-II (Insect Resistance) |
|---|---|
| 1. Curd production | (i) *Methanobacterium sp.* |
| 2. Bread production | (ii) *Bacillus thuringiensis* |
| 3. Biogas production | (iii) *Nostoc sp.* |
| 4. Biocontrol agents | (iv) *Lactobacillus sp.* |
| 5. Biofertilisers | (v) *Saccharomyces sp.* |

**The correct matching is:**

| | 1 | 2 | 3 | 4 | 5 |
|---|---|---|---|---|---|
| (a) | (iv) | (v) | (i) | (ii) | (iii) |
| (b) | (iv) | (v) | (ii) | (i) | (iii) |
| (c) | (i) | (iv) | (v) | (ii) | (iii) |
| (d) | (ii) | (iii) | (i) | (v) | (iv) |

**191.** Match the following:

| List-I (Microbes) | List-II (Byproducts) |
|---|---|
| 1. *Clostridium sp.* | (i) $C_6H_8O_7$ |
| 2. *Methanobacterium sp.* | (ii) $C_3H_6O_3$ |
| 3. *Acetobacter sp.* | (iii) $CH_4$ |
| 4. *Aspergillus sp.* | (iv) $C_4H_8O_2$ |
| 5. *Lactobacillus sp.* | (v) $CH_3COOH$ ($C_2H_4O_2$) |

**The correct matching is:**

| | 1 | 2 | 3 | 4 | 5 |
|---|---|---|---|---|---|
| (a) | (iv) | (iii) | (v) | (i) | (ii) |
| (b) | (iii) | (ii) | (iv) | (i) | (v) |
| (c) | (i) | (iv) | (v) | (ii) | (iii) |
| (d) | (ii) | (iii) | (i) | (v) | (iv) |

## NCERT Exemplar Questions

**1.** The vitamin whose content increases following the conversion of milk into curd by lactic acid bacteria is
(a) Vitamin C (b) Vitamin D
(c) Vitamin $B_{12}$ (d) Vitamin E

**2.** Wastewater treatment generates a large quantity of sludge, which can be treated by:
(a) Anaerobic Digesters (b) Flock
(c) Chemicals (d) Oxidation pond

**3.** Methanogenic bacteria are not found in
(a) Rumen of cattle
(b) Gobar gas plant
(c) Bottom of water-logged paddy fields
(d) Activated sludge

**4.** Match the following list of bacteria and their commercially important products.

| Bacterium | Product |
|---|---|
| (i) *Aspergillus niger* | (A) Lactic acid |
| (ii) *Acetobacter aceti* | (B) Butyric acid |
| (iii) *Clostridium butylicum* | (C) Acetic acid |
| (iv) *Lactobacillus* | (D) Citric acid |

Choose the correct match:
(a) i-B, ii-C, iii-D, iv-A (b) i-B, ii-D, iii-C, iv-A
(c) i-D, ii-C, iii-B, iv-A (d) i-D, ii-A, iii-C, iv-B

**5.** Match the following list of bioactive substances and their roles:

| Bioactive Substance | Role |
|---|---|
| (i) Statin | (A) Removal of oil stains |
| (ii) Cyclosporin A | (B) Removal of clots from blood vessels |
| (iii) Streptokinase | (C) Lowering of blood cholesterol |
| (iv) Lipase | (D) Immunosuppressive agent |

Choose the correct match:
(a) i-B, ii-C, iii-A, iv-D (b) i-D, ii-B, iii-A, iv-C
(c) i-D, ii-A, iii-B, iv-C (d) i-C, ii-D, iii-B, iv-A

**6.** The primary treatment of waste water involves the removal of
(a) Dissolved impurities (b) Stable particles
(c) Toxic substances (d) Harmful bacteria

**7.** BOD of waste water is estimated by measuring the amount of
(a) Total organic matter
(b) Biodegradable organic matter
(c) Oxygen evolution
(d) Oxygen consumption

**8.** Which one of the following alcoholic drinks is produced without distillation?
(a) Wine (b) Whisky
(c) Rum (d) Brandy

**9.** The technology of biogas production from cow dung was developed in India largely due to the efforts of
(a) Gas Authority of India
(b) Oil and Natural Gas Commission
(c) Indian Agricultural Research Institute & Khadi and Village Industries Commission
(d) Indian Oil Corporation

**10.** The free-living fungus *Trichoderma* can be used for
(a) Killing insects
(b) Biological control of plant diseases
(c) Controlling butterfly caterpillars
(d) Producing antibiotics

**11.** What would happen if oxygen availability to the activated sludge flocs is reduced?
(a) It will slow down the rate of degradation of organic matter.
(b) The centre of flocs will become anoxic, which would cause the death of bacteria and eventually breakage of flocs.
(c) Flocs would increase in size as anaerobic bacteria would grow around flocs.
(d) Protozoa would grow in large numbers.

**12.** Mycorrhiza does not help the host plant in
(a) Enhancing its phosphorus uptake capacity
(b) Increasing its tolerance to drought
(c) Enhancing its resistance to root pathogens
(d) Increasing its resistance to insects

13. Which one of the following is not a nitrogen fixing organism?
(a) *Anabaena* (b) *Nostoc*
(c) *Azotobacter* (d) *Pseudomonas*

14. Big holes in Swiss cheese are made by a
(a) Machine
(b) Bacterium that produces methane gas.
(c) Bacterium producing a large amount of carbon dioxide.
(d) Fungus that releases lot of gases during its metabolic activities.

15. The residue left after methane production from cattle dung is
(a) Burnt
(b) Buried in landfills
(c) Used as manure
(d) Used in civil construction

16. Methanogens do not produce
(a) Oxygen (b) Methane
(c) Hydrogen sulphide (d) Carbon dioxide

17. Activated sludge should have the ability to settle quickly so that it can
(a) Be rapidly pumped back from sedimentation tank to aeration tank.
(b) Absorb pathogenic bacteria present in waste water while sinking to the bottom of the settling tank.
(c) Supernatant be discarded and settled matter be anaerobically digested
(d) Absorb colloidal organic matter.

18. Match the items in 'Column-A' and 'Column-B' and choose the correct answer.

| Column-A | Column-B |
|---|---|
| (i) Lady bird | (A) *Methanobacterium* |
| (ii) Mycorrhiza | (B) *Trichoderma* |
| (iii) Biological control | (C) Aphids |
| (iv) Biogas | (D) *Glomus* |

The correct answer is
(a) i-B, ii-D, iii-C, iv-A
(b) i-C, ii-D, iii-B, iv-A
(c) i-D, ii-A, iii-B, iv-C
(d) i -C, ii-B, iii-A, iv-D

19. Rising of dough is due to
(a) Multiplication of yeast
(b) Production of $CO_2$
(c) Emulsification
(d) Hydrolysis of wheat flour starch into sugars

## Previous Years' Questions

1. Which one of the following is not used in organic farming? [AIPMT 2010 PRE]
(a) Glomus (b) Earthworm
(c) Oscillatoria (d) Snail

2. A common biocontrol agent for control of plant diseases is [AIPMT 2010 PRE]
(a) Baculovirus (b) Bacillus thuringiensis
(c) Glomus (d) Trichoderma

3. Select the correct statement from the following [AIPMT 2010 PRE]
(a) Biogas is produced by the activity of aerobic bacteria on animal waste
(b) Methanobacterium is an aerobic bacterium found in rumen of cattle
(c) Biogas, commonly called gobar gas, is pure methane
(d) Activated sludge-sediment in settlement tank of sewage treatment plant is a right source of aerobic bacteria

4. An example of endomycorrhiza is: [AIPMT 2010 MAINS]
(a) *Nostoc* (b) *Glomus*
(c) *Agaricus* (d) *Rhizobium*

5. When domestic sewage mixes with river water [AIPMT 2010 MAINS]
(a) Small animals like rats will die after drinking river water
(b) The increased microbial activity releases micronutrients such as iron
(c) The increased microbial activity uses up dissolved oxygen
(d) The river water is still suitable for drinking as impurities are only about 0.1%

6. Ethanol is commercially produced through a particular species of [AIPMT 2011 PRE]
(a) *Clostridium*
(b) *Trichoderma*
(c) *Aspergillus*
(d) *Saccharomyces*

**7.** The most common substrate used in distilleries for the production of ethanol is: [AIPMT 2011 PRE]
(a) Soya meal (b) Ground gram
(c) Molasses (d) Corn meal

**8.** Which one of the following is not a biofertilizer? [AIPMT 2011 PRE]
(a) *Rhizobium* (b) *Nostoc*
(c) *Mycorrhiza* (d) *Agrobacterium*

**9.** Secondary sewage treatment is mainly a: [AIPMT 2011 PRE]
(a) Mechanical process (b) Chemical process
(c) Biological process (d) Physical process

**10.** Continuous addition of sugars in 'fed batch' fermentation is done to: [AIPMT 2011 PRE]
(a) Obtain antibiotics (b) Purify enzymes
(c) Degrade sewage (d) Produce methane

**11.** Which one of the following helps in absorption of phosphorus from soil by plants? [AIPMT 2011 PRE]
(a) *Rhizobium* (b) *Frankia*
(c) *Anabaena* (d) *Glomus*

**12.** Which of the following is mainly produced by the activity of anaerobic bacteria on sewage? [AIPMT 2011 PRE]
(a) Propane (b) Mustard gas
(c) Marsh gas (d) Laughing gas

**13.** Which one of the following is a wrong matching of a microbe and its industrial product, while the remaining three are correct? [AIPMT 2011 MAINS]
(a) Yeast – statins
(b) Acetobacter aceti – acetic acid
(c) Clostridium butylicum – lactic acid
(d) Aspergillus niger – citric acid

**14.** Read the following statement having two blanks (A and B). "A drug used for A patients is obtained from a species of the organism B.
The one correct option for the two blanks is [AIPMT 2011 MAINS]

| | A | B |
|---|---|---|
| (a) | Heart | *Penicillium* |
| (b) | Organ-tranplant | *Trichoderma* |
| (c) | Swine flu | *Monascus* |
| (d) | AIDS | *Pseudomonas* |

**15.** Which one of the following is an example of carrying out biological control of pests/diseases using microbes? [AIPMT 2012 PRE]
(a) Trichoderma sp. against certain plant pathogens
(b) Nucleopolyhedorvirus against white rust in Brassica
(c) Bt-cotton to increase cotton yield
(d) Lady bird beetal against aphids in mustard

**16.** A nitrogen-fixing microbe associated with Azolla in rice field is: [AIPMT 2012 PRE]
(a) Spirulina (b) Anabaena
(c) Frankia (d) Tolypothrix

**17.** Yeast is used on the production of: [AIPMT 2012 PRE]
(a) Citric acid and lactic acid
(b) Lipase and pectinase
(c) Bread and beer
(d) Cheese and butter

**18.** Which of the following microbes forms symbiotic association with plants and helps them in their nutrition? [AIPMT 2012 PRE]
(a) *Azotobacter* (b) *Aspergillus*
(c) *Glomus* (d) *Trichoderma*

**19.** A patient brought to a hospital with myocardial infarction is normally immediately given: [AIPMT 2012 PRE]
(a) Penicillin (b) Streptokinase
(c) Cyclosporin-A (d) Statins

**20.** *Monascus purpureus* is yeast used commercially in the production of; [AIPMT 2012 PRE]
(a) Ethanol
(b) Streptokinase for removing clots from the blood vessels
(c) Citric acid
(d) Blood cholesterol lowering statins

**21.** The domestic sewage in large cities: [AIPMT 2012 MAINS]
(a) Is processed by aerobic and then anaerobic bacteria in the secondary treatment in Sewage Treatment Plant (STPs)
(b) When treated in STPs, it does not really require the aeration stop as the sewage contains adequate oxygen
(c) Has very high amounts of suspended solids and dissolved salts
(d) Has a high BOD as it contains both aerobic and anaerobic bacteria

**22.** Read the following four statements (A-D):
(A) Colostrum is recommended for the new-born because it is rich in antigen
(B) Chikengunya is caused by a gram negative bacterium.

(C) Tissue culture has proved useful in obtaining virus-free plants.

(D) Beer is manufactured by distillation of fermented grape juice [AIPMT 2012 MAINS]

How many of the above statements are wrong

(a) Three (b) Four
(c) One (d) Two

**23.** In gobar gas, the maximum amount is that of: [AIPMT 2012 MAINS]

(a) Methane (b) Propane
(c) Carbon dioxide (d) Butane

**24.** During sewage treatment, biogases are produced which include: [AIPMT 2013]

(a) Methane, hydrogen sulphide, carbon dioxide
(b) Methane, oxygen, hydrogen sulphide
(c) Hydrogen sulphide, methane, sulphur dioxide
(d) Hydrogen sulphide, nitrogen, methane

**25.** Which of the following are likely to be present in deep sea water? [AIPMT 2013]

(a) Archaebacteria (b) Eubacteria
(c) Blue–green algae (d) Saprophytic fungi

**26.** A good producer of citric acid is: [AIPMT 2013]

(a) Aspergillus (b) Pseudomonas
(c) Clostridium (d) Saccharomyces

**27.** What gases are produced in anaerobic sludge digesters? [AIPMT 2014]

(a) Methane and $CO_2$ only
(b) Methane, Hydrogen Sulphide and $CO_2$
(c) Methane, Hydrogen Sulphide and $O_2$
(d) Hydrogen Sulphide and $CO_2$

**28.** Match the following list of microbes and their importance: [RE-AIPMT 2015]

| | |
|---|---|
| A. *Sacharomyces cerevisiae* | 1. production of immunosuppressive agents |
| B. *Monoscus purpueus* | 2. ripening of Swiss cheese |
| C. *Trichoderma polysporum* | 3. Commercial production of ethanol |
| D. *Propionibacterium sharmanii* | 4. Production of blood-cholesterol lowering agents |

(a) A:4, B:3, C:2, D:1 (b) A:4, B:2, C:1, D:3
(c) A:3, B:1, C:4, D:2 (d) A:3, B:4, C:1, D:2

**29.** High value of BOD (Biochemical Oxygen Demand) indicates that: [AIPMT 2015]

(a) Water is pure
(b) Water is highly polluted
(c) Water is less polluted
(d) Consumption of organic matter in the water is higher by the microbes

**30.** Match Column–I with Column–II and select the correct options using the codes given below: [NEET 2016 – PHASE II]

| Column–I | Column–II |
|---|---|
| (A) Citric acid | (1) Trichoderma |
| (B) Cyclosporine A | (2) Clostridium |
| (C) Statins | (3) Aspergillus |
| (D) Butyric acid | (4) Monascus |

(a) A:3, B:1, C:4, D:2
(b) A:1, B:4, C:2, D:3
(c) A:3, B:4, C:1, D:2
(d) A:3, B:1, C:2, D:4

**31.** Which of the following is wrongly matched in the given option?

[A: Microbe, B: Product, C: Application] [NEET 2016 – PHASE I]

(a) A: *Trichderma polysporum*, B: Cyclosporin A, C: Immunosuppressive drug
(b) A: *Monascus purpureus*, B: Statins,C: Lowering of blood cholesterol
(c) A: *Streptococcus*, B: Streptockinase,C: Removal of clot from blood vessel
(d) A: *Clostridium butylicum*, B: Lipase,C: Removal of oil stains

**32.** Which of the following in sewage treatment removes suspended solids? [NEET 2017]

(a) Secondary treatment
(b) Primary treatment
(c) Sludge treatment
(d) Tertiary treatment

**33.** Which of the following is correctly matched for the product produced by them? [NEET 2017]

(a) *Methanobacterium*: Lactic acid
(b) *Penicillium notatum*: Acetic acid
(c) *Sacchromyces cerevisiae*: Ethanol
(d) *acetobacter acetii*: Antibiotics

**34.** Which of the following is a commercial blood cholesterol lowering agent? [NEET 2019]

(a) Statin (b) Streptokinase
(c) Lipases (d) Cyclosporin A

**35.** Select the **correct** group of biocontrol agents. [NEET 2019]

(a) *Trichoderma, Baculovirus, Bacillus thuringiensis*
(b) *Oscillatoria, Rhizobium, Trichoderma*
(c) *Nostoc, Azospirillium, Nucleopolyhedrovirus*
(d) *Bacillus thuringiensis*, Tobacco mosaic virus, Aphids

**36.** Match the following organisms with the products they produce:

| | |
|---|---|
| (A) *Lactobacillus* | (i) Cheese |
| (B) *Saccharomyces cerevisiae* | (ii) Curd |
| (C) *Aspergillus niger* | (iii) Citric Acid |
| (D) *Acetobacter aceti* | (iv) Bread |
| | (v) Acetic Acid |

[NEET 2019]

Select the **correct** option.

| | (A) | (B) | (C) | (D) |
|---|---|---|---|---|
| (a) | (ii) | (iv) | (iii) | (v) |
| (b) | (iii) | (iv) | (v) | (i) |
| (c) | (ii) | (i) | (iii) | (v) |
| (d) | (ii) | (iv) | (v) | (iii) |

**37.** Which of the following can be used as a biocontrol agent in the treatment of plant disease? [NEET 2019]

(a) *Chlorella* (b) *Anabaena*
(c) *Lactobacillus* (d) *Trichoderma*

**38.** Match the following columns and select the **correct** option : [NEET 2020]

| Column – I | Column – II |
|---|---|
| (A) *Clostridium butylicum* | (i) Cyclosporin-A |
| (B) *Trichoderma polysporum* | (ii) Butyric Acid |
| (C) *Monascus purpureus* | (iii) Citric Acid |
| (D) *Aspergillus niger* | (iv) Blood cholesterol lowering agent |

| | (A) | (B) | (C) | (D) |
|---|---|---|---|---|
| (a) | (iii) | (iv) | (ii) | (i) |
| (b) | (ii) | (i) | (iv) | (iii) |
| (c) | (i) | (ii) | (iv) | (iii) |
| (d) | (iv) | (iii) | (ii) | (i) |

**39.** Which of the following is put into anaerobic sludge digester for further sewage treatment? [NEET 2020]

(a) Primary sludge
(b) Floating debris
(c) Effluents of primary treatment
(d) Activated sludge

**40.** Match the following: [NEET 2021]

| List-I | List-II |
|---|---|
| 1. *Aspergillus niger* | (i) Acetic acid |
| 2. *Acetobacter aceti* | (ii) Lactic acid |
| 3. *Clostridium butylicum* | (iii) Citric acid |
| 4. *Lacto bacillus* | (iv) Butyric acid |

**The correct matching is:**

| | 1 | 2 | 3 | 4 |
|---|---|---|---|---|
| (a) | (iv) | (ii) | (i) | (iii) |
| (b) | (iii) | (i) | (iv) | (ii) |
| (c) | (i) | (ii) | (iii) | (iv) |
| (d) | (ii) | (iii) | (i) | (iv) |

**41.** Identify the microorganism which is responsible for the production of an immunosuppressive molecule cyclosporin A: [NEET 2022]

(a) *Clostridium butylicum*
(b) *Aspergillus niger*
(c) *Streptococcus cerevisiae*
(d) *Trichoderma polysporum*

**42.** Match List-I with List-II [NEET 2024]

| List-I | List-II |
|---|---|
| (A) *Clostridium butylicum* | (i) Ethanol |
| (B) *Saccharomyces cerevisiae* | (ii) *Streptokinase* |
| (C) *Trichoderma polysporum* | (iii) Butyric acid |
| (D) *Streptococcus sp.* | (iv) Cyclosporin-A |

Choose the correct answer from the option given below:

(a) (A)-(iii), (B)-(i), (C)-(ii), (D)-(iv)
(b) (A)-(ii), (B)-(iv), (C)-(iii), (D)-(i)
(c) (A)-(iii), (B)-(i), (C)-(iv), (D)-(ii)
(d) (A)-(iv), (B)-(i), (C)-(iii), (D)-(ii)

## Answer Key

### Multiple Choice Questions: Level I

| | | | | | | | | | |
|---|---|---|---|---|---|---|---|---|---|
| **1.** (a) | **2.** (c) | **3.** (b) | **4.** (b) | **5.** (b) | **6.** (a) | **7.** (a) | **8.** (b) | **9.** (b) | **10.** (b) |
| **11.** (c) | **12.** (c) | **13.** (c) | **14.** (d) | **15.** (c) | **16.** (b) | **17.** (c) | **18.** (b) | **19.** (c) | **20.** (c) |
| **21.** (d) | **22.** (c) | **23.** (c) | **24.** (b) | **25.** (c) | **26.** (b) | **27.** (a) | **28.** (d) | **29.** (d) | **30.** (c) |
| **31.** (d) | **32.** (c) | **33.** (c) | **34.** (b) | **35.** (b) | **36.** (c) | **37.** (b) | **38.** (a) | **39.** (b) | **40.** (b) |
| **41.** (b) | **42.** (c) | **43.** (a) | **44.** (b) | **45.** (b) | **46.** (a) | **47.** (b) | **48.** (c) | **49.** (c) | **50.** (b) |
| **51.** (b) | **52.** (b) | **53.** (c) | **54.** (a) | **55.** (c) | **56.** (b) | **57.** (b) | **58.** (b) | **59.** (b) | **60.** (d) |
| **61.** (c) | **62.** (d) | **63.** (b) | **64.** (b) | **65.** (d) | **66.** (d) | **67.** (b) | **68.** (b) | **69.** (b) | **70.** (c) |
| **71.** (b) | **72.** (b) | **73.** (c) | **74.** (b) | **75.** (c) | **76.** (c) | **77.** (c) | **78.** (d) | **79.** (b) | **80.** (d) |
| **81.** (c) | **82.** (c) | **83.** (d) | **84.** (a) | **85.** (c) | **86.** (d) | **87.** (a) | **88.** (c) | **89.** (a) | **90.** (b) |
| **91.** (c) | **92.** (c) | **93.** (b) | **94.** (d) | **95.** (d) | **96.** (d) | **97.** (b) | **98.** (c) | **99.** (d) | **100.** (d) |
| **101.** (a) | **102.** (b) | **103.** (b) | **104.** (b) | **105.** (b) | **106.** (b) | **107.** (b) | **108.** (b) | **109.** (a) | **110.** (c) |
| **111.** (a) | **112.** (c) | **113.** (b) | **114.** (a) | **115.** (c) | **116.** (b) | **117.** (a) | **118.** (d) | **119.** (b) | **120.** (b) |
| **121.** (b) | **122.** (c) | **123.** (d) | **124.** (a) | **125.** (b) | **126.** (a) | **127.** (a) | **128.** (b) | **129.** (b) | **130.** (b) |
| **131.** (b) | **132.** (c) | **133.** (c) | **134.** (b) | **135.** (b) | **136.** (c) | **137.** (b) | **138.** (a) | **139.** (b) | **140.** (b) |
| **141.** (b) | **142.** (c) | **143.** (c) | **144.** (d) | **145.** (b) | **146.** (b) | **147.** (a) | **148.** (a) | **149.** (b) | **150.** (b) |
| **151.** (d) | **152.** (d) | **153.** (b) | **154.** (d) | **155.** (c) | **156.** (a) | **157.** (b) | **158.** (a) | **159.** (b) | **160.** (b) |
| **161.** (d) | **162.** (b) | **163.** (b) | | | | | | | |

### Multiple Choice Questions: Level II

| | | | | | | | | | |
|---|---|---|---|---|---|---|---|---|---|
| **164.** (a) | **165.** (c) | **166.** (b) | **167.** (c) | **168.** (d) | **169.** (c) | **170.** (c) | **171.** (d) | **172.** (a) | **173.** (a) |
| **174.** (d) | **175.** (b) | **176.** (a) | | | | | | | |

### A & R and Statement-based Questions

| | | | | | | | | | |
|---|---|---|---|---|---|---|---|---|---|
| **177.** (c) | **178.** (c) | **179.** (c) | **180.** (c) | **181.** (c) | **182.** (c) | **183.** (a) | **184.** (b) | **185.** (d) | **186.** (d) |

### Matrix-Match Type Questions

| | | | | |
|---|---|---|---|---|
| **187.** (a) | **188.** (a) | **189.** (a) | **190.** (a) | **191.** (a) |

### NCERT Exemplar Questions

| | | | | | | | | | |
|---|---|---|---|---|---|---|---|---|---|
| **1.** (c) | **2.** (a) | **3.** (d) | **4.** (c) | **5.** (d) | **6.** (b) | **7.** (d) | **8.** (a) | **9.** (c) | **10.** (b) |
| **11.** (b) | **12.** (d) | **13.** (d) | **14.** (c) | **15.** (c) | **16.** (a) | **17.** (a) | **18.** (b) | **19.** (b) | |

### Previous Years' Questions

| | | | | | | | | | |
|---|---|---|---|---|---|---|---|---|---|
| **1.** (d) | **2.** (d) | **3.** (d) | **4.** (b) | **5.** (c) | **6.** (d) | **7.** (c) | **8.** (d) | **9.** (c) | **10.** (b) |
| **11.** (d) | **12.** (c) | **13.** (c) | **14.** (b) | **15.** (c) | **16.** (b) | **17.** (c) | **18.** (c) | **19.** (b) | **20.** (d) |
| **21.** (a) | **22.** (a) | **23.** (a) | **24.** (a) | **25.** (a) | **26.** (a) | **27.** (b) | **28.** (d) | **29.** (b) | **30.** (a) |
| **31.** (d) | **32.** (b) | **33.** (c) | **34.** (a) | **35.** (a) | **36.** (a) | **37.** (d) | **38.** (b) | **39.** (d) | **40.** (b) |
| **41.** (d) | **42.** (c) | | | | | | | | |

# HINTS AND EXPLANATION

## Multiple Choice Questions: Level II

**164.** Alcohol and Nitrogenase pair is wrongly matched. Nitrogenase helps in nitrogen fixation.

**165.** *Xanthomonas campestris* is not used as a biopesticide, *Xanthomonas campestris* is a plant pathogen that causes black rot in cotton plants.

**166.** ***Trichoderma harzianum***:

- It is fungus that is also used as a fungicide.
- It is used for foliar application, seed treatment and soil treatment for controlling various fungal diseases caused by Botrytis, Fusarium and Penicillium species.

**167.** Suppression of reproduction of one type of organism by utilizing some features of its biology or physiology to destroy it or by use of another organism is known as biological control.

**168.** Modern detergent contains enzymes preparations of alkaliphiles. Alkaliphiles live in alkaline environments like soda lakes or alkaline soil. The pH level in alkaline substances is from about 9 to 11 on the pH scale. The alkaliphiles keep an alkaline level of about 9 pH inside the cells, but the environment has a higher level of alkalinity. Alkaliphiles can keep the right pH level by pumping in the right pH level by pumping in hydrogen ions in out at the right rate.

**169.** Probiotics are defined as live microorganisms, including Lactobacillus species, Bifidobacterium species and yeasts that may beneficially affect the host upon ingestion by improving the balance of the intestinal micro flora. The dietary use of live microorganisms has a long history.

**170.** **Coliform bacteria** are defined as rod-shaped Gram-negative non-spore forming and motile or non-motile bacteria which can ferment lactose with the production of acid and gas when incubated at 35–37°C. They are a commonly used indicator of sanitary quality of foods and water. Coliforms can be found in aquatic environment, in soil and on vegetation; they are universally present in large numbers in the feces of warm-blooded animals. Whilst coliforms themselves are not normally causes of serious illness, they are easy to culture, and their presence is used to indicate that other pathogenic organisms of fecal origin may be present.

**171.** Bt cotton, a transgenic crop variety has been introduced in India. The Bt cotton variety contains a foreign gene obtained from *Bacillus thuringiensis*. This bacterial gene protects cotton from the bollwarm, a major pest of cotton.

**172.** Azolla and BGA are biofertilizers.

**173.** **Free-living Nitrogen-fixing bacteria:** Some bacteria like *Azotobacter* (aerobic), *Clostridium* (anaerobic), *Rhodospirillum*, *Chromatium* (photosynthetic bacteria) are free living nitrogen-fixing bacteria of soil, which increase fertility of soil and hence yield of crop plants.

**174.** Biological control refers to the use of living organisms like natural predators and parasites to reduce pest population and control diseases. However, they may become pest as they can develop a preference to other diets.

**175.** Primary treatment involves removal of grit and larger pieces of organic matter. In secondary treatment, the organic matter is decomposed with the help of microbes. Tertiary treatment is undertaken where the water should be recycled. It involves precipitation, filtration and aeration. Inactivated sludge treatment a portion of the waste containing decomposers (Bacteria) is returned to the aerator.

**176.** Gobar gas contains mainly $CH_4 + CO_2$.

## NCERT Exemplar Questions

1. The **vitamin $B_{12}$** content increases following the conversion of milk into curd by lactic acid bacteria (LAB).
2. Wastewater treatment generates a large quantity of sludge, which can be treated by **anaerobic sludge digesters.**
3. Methanogenic bacteria are found in **rumen of cattle, gobar gas plant** and **bottom** of water-logged **paddy fields.**
4.

| | |
|---|---|
| (i) *Aspergillus niger* | (D) Citric acid |
| (ii) *Acetobacter aceti* | (C) Acetic acid |
| (ii) *Clostridium butylicum* | (B) Butyric acid |
| (iv) *Lactobacillus* | (A) Lactic acid |

5.

| | |
|---|---|
| (i) Statin | (C) Lowering of blood cholesterol |
| (ii) Cyclosporine | (D) Immuno-suppressive agent |
| (ii) Streptokinase | (B) Removal of clots from blood vessels |

6. 1° treatments basically involves physical removal of particles from sewage through:
   (i) Filtration and (ii) Sedimentation
   These are removed in stages:
   (i) Initially floating debris is removed by sequential filtration.
   (ii) Then the grit (soil and pebbles) are removed by sedimentation
7. BOD of waste water is estimated by measuring the amount of oxygen consumption.
8. **Wine** and **beer** are produced **without distillation.** Whisky, brandy and rum are produced by distillation.
9. The technology of biogas production from cow dung was developed in India largely due to the efforts of Indian Agricultural Research Institute and Khadi and Village Industries Commission.
10. The free-living fungus *Trichoderma* can be used for biological control of plant diseases.
11. If oxygen availability to activated sludge floes is reduced, the center of floes will become anoxic, which would cause death of bacteria and eventually breakage of floes.
12. Mycorrhiza helps the host plant in enhancing its phosphorus uptake capacity, increasing its tolerance to drought and enhancing its resistance to root pathogens.
13. *Anabaena, Nostoc* and *Azotobacter* are the cyanobacteria. All are nitrogen-fixing organism.
14. Large holes in Swiss cheese are due to production of large amount of $CO_2$ by a bacterium named *Proponibacterium sharmanii.*
15. • Thus, gobar (excreta/dung) of cattle is rich in these bacteria. Dung can be used for generation of biogas, commonly called gobar gas.
    • The residue left after methane production from cattle dung is used as manure.
16. Methanogens are obligate anaerobes, which produce methane, hydrogen sulphide and carbon dioxide but do not produce oxygen.
17. Activated sludge should have the ability to settle quickly so that it can be rapidly pumped back from sedimentation tank to aeration tank.
18.

| | |
|---|---|
| i. Lady bird | A. *Aphids* |
| ii. Mycorrhiza | B. *Glomus* |
| iii. Biological control | C. *Trichoderma* |
| iv. Biogas | D. *Methanobacterium* |

## Previous Years' Questions

1. Except snail, all these are used in organic farming
   Glomus - Endomycorrhiza
   Oscillatoria - BGA
   Earthworm - Vermicompost
2. Trichoderma is a genus of fungi that is present in all soils, where they are the most prevalent culturable fungi. Many species in this genus can be characterized as opportunistic avirulent plant symbionts. Several strains of Trichoderma have been developed as biocontrol agents against fungal diseases of plants. The various mechanisms include antibiosis, parasitism, inducing host-plant resistance and competition. Most biocontrol agents are from the species *T. harzianum, T. viride and T. hamatum.* The biocontrol agent

generally grows in its natural habitat on the root surface and so affects root disease in particular but can also be effective against foliar disease.

3. Activated sludge is a process dealing with the treatment of sewage and industrial wastewaters. Atmospheric air or pure oxygen is introduced to a mixture of primary treated or screened sewage (or industrial waste water) combined with organisms to develop a biological floc, which reduces the organic content of the sewage. Sediment in settlement tanks of sewage treatment plant is a rich source used as inoculum in secondary treatment or biological treatment stage of sewage treatment.

4. • Nostoc is a blue–green algae capable of fixing nitrogen.
   • Glomus is associated with endomycorrhiza. Agaricus or mushroom is an edible fungus of class Basidiomycetes.
   • Rhizobium is a symbiotic nitrogen-fixing bacterium found in the root nodules of leguminous plants.

5. Domestic sewage consists of a lot of degradable organic matter. When this sewage is released into river water, it will result in an increase of Biochemical Oxygen Demand (BOD) and decrease in the amount of dissolved oxygen due to decomposing activity of microbes.

6. *Saccharomyces cerevisiae* is used for fermenting malted cereals and fruit juices to produce ethanol commercially.

7. Molasses is a viscous by-product of the processing of sugarcane, grapes or sugar beets in sugar. It is the most common substrate used in distilleries for the production of ethanol. It can be used as the base material for fermentation into rum.

8. Agrobacterium is a Gram negative bacterium that causes tumours in plants. It is well known for its ability to transfer DNA between itself and plants, and for this reason, it has become an important tool for genetic engineering. *A. tumefaciens* causes crown-gall disease in plants. It has Ti-plasmid.

   **Biofertilizers:** They are organisms which bring about nutrient enrichment of the soil. Some of the important biofertilizers are **Blue green algae (Cyanobacteria), Bacteria and Fungi.**

9. In secondary or biological treatment of municipal waste rich in sewage, the organic matter is decomposed with the help of microbes. Decomposition of organic matter occurs by one of the three methods: water hyacinth pod, trickling filter method and activated sludge method. After decomposition, the treated water is sterilized through chlorination.

10. A fed batch is a biotechnological batch process which is based on feeding of a growth-limiting nutrient substrate to a culture. Continuous addition of sugars in fed batch fermentation is done to purify enzymes.

11. Glomus is a genus of arbuscular mycorrhizal (AM) fungi. It helps in nutrient uptake mainly the absorption of phosphorus.

12. Anaerobic bacteria digest the bacteria and the fungi in the sludge and produce a mixture of gases such as methane (marsh gas), hydrogen sulphide and carbon dioxide.

13. Microbes are used for commercial and industrial production of certain chemicals like organic acids, alcohols and enzymes. Examples of acid producers are *Aspergillus niger* (a fungus) of citric acid, *Acetobacter aceti* (a bacterium) of acetic acid; *Clostridium butylicum* (a bacterium) of butyric acid and Lactobacillus (a bacterium) of lactic acid.

14. A bioactive molecule, cyclosprin A, that is used as an immunosuppressive agent in organ-transparent patients is produced by the fungus – Trichoderma polysporus

15. **Examples of Biological Control:**

    **(1)** Ladybird beetle (with red and black markings) is used for biological control of aphids.

    **(2)** Dragonflies are used for biological control of mosquitoes.

    **(3)** The bacteria *Bacillus thuringiensis* (usually written as Bt) is used to control butterfly caterpillars. These are available in spore form in sachets which are mixed with water and sprayed upon vulnerable plants like brassicas and fruit trees. After the caterpillar (insect larva) has eaten the sprayed parts, a toxin is released in the gut which kills the larva. This toxins do not affect the other insects. This is an example of microbial biocontrol agent.

    **(4)** **Bt cotton:** Nowadays by genetic engineering, we have introduced the Bt toxin gene from the bacteria Bacillus thuringiensis into the plant crops and they have become resistant to attacks of insect/pests.

**(5)** A fungus Trichoderma is a free living species which is very commonly present in root ecosystems and is found to effectively control the various plant pathogens.

**(6)** Most of the Baculoviruses which are being used as biological control belong to the genus Nucleopolyhedrovirus. These are pathogenic to insects and other arthropods but have no effects on plants, mammals, fishes, birds and even non-target insects. These are highly species specific so are used as narrow spectrum insecticidal applications.

**16.** *Azolla-Anabaena* symbiotic system is the main biofertilizer which is inoculated in rice fields in South-Eastern Asia, which is found to increase yield up to 50%

**17.** **Brewer's yeast** (*Saccharomyces cerevisiae*): It is used for making bread ferment malted cereals and fruit juices to produce ethanol. Wine and beer are prepared without distillation. Rum, brandy and whisky are produced with distillation.

**18.** Fungi like those belonging to the genus Glomus form mycorrhiza with roots of higher plants. Fungal partner absorbs phosphorus from the soil and provide it to the plant.

**19.** Streptokinase (SK), a protein secreted by several species of streptococci can bind and activate human plasminogen. It is used as an effective and inexpensive thrombolysis medication in some cases of myocardial infarction and pulmonary embolism.

**20.** *Monascus purpureus* is a yeast used in the production of statins which are blood cholesterol lowering agents.

**21.** Mechanism of secondary treatment in Sewage Treatment Plant (STPs) = Biological process.

- Primary effluent is passed into large aeration tanks in which there is constant agitation and pumping of air → Growth of micro-organisms **(specially aerobic)** is promoted → Flocs (large masses of bacteria along with fungal filaments to appear like a mesh-like network) are formed → These microbes take oxygen during their growth (thus increasing the BOD) and decompose or consume major organic part of the effluent.
- Once the BOD is significantly decreased, effluent is transferred to a large settling tank → Bacterial flocs settle here, which are termed as activated sludge.
- A small part of the activated sludge is transferred back into the aeration tank to act as inoculums.
- Major part of the activated sludge is pumped into the **anaerobic sludge** digesters which are large tanks having anaerobic bacteria → These anaerobic bacteria digest the bacteria and fungi present in the sludge → In this process of digestion, various gases are produced in the form of a mixture – methane, hydrogen sulphide and carbon dioxide. These gases are collectively termed as biogas.

**22.**
- Colostrum is recommended for the new-born because it contains less fat.
- Chikungunya is caused by a virus.
- Tissue culture has proved useful in obtaining virus-free plants.
- Wine and beer are prepared without distillation.

**23.** In gobar gas, maximum amount of methane is produced by methanogenic bacteria

**24.** During sewage treatment in secondary treatment, the biogas is produced in an aerotric sludge digester have anaerobic bacteria which produce gases like $CO_2$, $H_2S$, $CH_4$.

**25.** In deep sea water, no light will reach the archaebacteria like sulphur methanomonas are present and their nutritional category is chemoautotrophs or chemosyntheic bacteria.

**26.** A good producer of citric acid is *Aspergillus niger* (a fungus). Clostridium produces butyric acid, *Saccharomyces cerevisiae* is used for bread baking fermenting malted cereals and fruit juices to produce ethanol. Pseudomonas (a bacterium) is used in Vitamin $B_{12}$ production.

**27.** Anaerobic digestion is a bacterial process that breaks down organic material within the waste in the absence of oxygen. Municipal sewage treatment facilities also use sludge digesters. In anaerobic sludge digesters, bacteria produce a vital mixture of gases like methane, hydrogen, sulphide and carbon dioxide.

**28.**

| Microbes | Product | Use of Product |
|---|---|---|
| *Aspergillus niger* (a fungus) | **Citric acid** | Industrial use |
| *Acetobacter aceti* (a bacterium) | **Acetic acid** | Industrial use |
| *Clostridium butylicum* (a bacterium) | **Butyric acid** | Industrial use |
| *Lactobacilus* (a bacterium) | **Lactic acid** | Industrial use |
| *Saccharomyces cerevisiae* (yeast-a fungus) | **Alcohol (Ethanol)** | Alcoholic beverages |
| *Streptococcus* (a bacterium) | **Streptokinase** | Used as **'clot buster'** for removal of clots in blood vessels that have resulted in myocardial infarction. |
| *Trichoderma polysporum* (a fungus) | **Cyclosporin A** | 'Immunosuppressive drug' in organ transplant patients. |
| *Monascus purpureus* (yeast-a fungus) | **Statins** | Used as a 'blood cholesterol reducing agent'. It competitively inhibits the enzyme responsible for the synthesis of cholesterol. |

**29.** The greater the BOD of waste water, more is its polluting potential.

**30.** Refer to solution 33.

**31.**

| Microbes | Product | Use of Product |
|---|---|---|
| *Clostridium butylicum* (a bacterium) | Butyric acid | Industrial use |

**32. Sewage Treatment:**

Sewage pollution can be prevented by treating sewage before passing into water course, in **sewage** or **effluent treatment plant (ETP).** It involves three steps:

**(a) Primary Treatment. Larger and suspended particles are removed by simple physical methods** such as shredding, churning, floatation, screening and sedimentation.

**(b) Secondary Treatment.** The organic matter is decomposed through sewage fungus by either **trickling filter method** (passing through thick bed of gravel) or **activated sludge method** (aeration/oxidation tanks). It results in release of $CO_2$ and formation of **sludge** or **biosolid.** The sludge is continuously aerated for further oxidation.

**(c) Tertiary Treatment.** The turbidity in waste water caused by the presence of nutrients (nitrates, phosphates, etc.), dissolved organic matter, metal or pathogens, etc. is removed by physico-chemical process. This step involves chemical oxidation of waste water by strong oxidizing agents, such as chlorine gas, perchlorate salts, ozone gas and irradiation with UV rays to kill pathogens. After tertiary treatment, the waste water can be discharged into natural waters or used for irrigation.

**33.**

| Microbes | Product | Use of Product |
|---|---|---|
| *Saccharomyces cerevisiae* (yeast-a fungus) | Alcohol (Ethanol) | Alcoholic beverages |

**34.** Statins produced by the yeast *Monascus purpureus* have been commercialized as blood-cholesterol lowering agents. It acts by competitively inhibiting the enzyme responsible for synthesis of cholesterol.

**35.**
- An example of microbial biocontrol agents that can be introduced in order to control butterfly caterpillars is the bacteria *Bacillus thuringiensis* (often written as *Bt* ).
- Baculoviruses are pathogens that attack insects and other arthropods. Majority of baculoviruses used as biological control agents are in the genus *Nucleopolyhedrovirus.*
- *Trichoderma* species are free-living fungi that are very common in root ecosystems. They are effective biocontrol agents of several plant pathogens.

**36.** • Micro-organisms such as *Lactobacillus* and others commonly called lactic acid bacteria (LAB) grow in milk and convert it to curd.
• Yeast *Saccharomyces cerevisiae* is used for bread-making.
• *Aspergillus niger* (a fungus) of citric acid, *Acetobacter aceti* (a bacterium) of acetic acid;
• Large holes in 'Swiss cheese' are due to production of a large amount of $CO_2$ by a bacterium named *Propionibacterium sharmanii*.

**37.** *Trichoderma* species are free-living fungi that are common in the root ecosystems. They are effective biocontrol agents of several plant pathogens.

**38.**

| Column - I | Column - II |
|---|---|
| (A) *Clostridium butylicum* | (ii) Butyric Acid |
| (B) *Trichoderma polysporum* | (i) Cyclosporine-A |
| (C) *Monascus purpureus* | (iv) Blood cholesterol lowering agent |
| (D) *Aspergillus niger* | (iii) Citric Acid |

**39.** The sediment in settlement tank is called activated sludge.

A small part of the activated sludge is pumped back into aeration tank.

Remaining major part of the sludge is pumped into large tank called anaerobic sludge digesters.

**40.**

| | |
|---|---|
| *Aspergillus niger* | Aspergillus niger is involved in production of citric acid. |
| *Acetobacter aceti* | Acetobacter aceti is involved in production of acetic acid. |
| *Clostridium butylicum* | Clostridium butylicum is involved in production of butyric acid. |
| *Lacto bacillus* | Lactobacillus is involved in the production of lactic acid. |

**41.** Bioactive molecule, cyclosporin A, that is used as an immunosuppressive agent in organ transplant patients, is produced by the fungus, Trichoderma polysporum.

**42.** A. *Clostridium butylicum* — Butyric acid
B. *Saccharomyces cerevisiae* — Ethanol
C. *Trichoderma polysporum* — Cyclosporin-A
D. *Streptococcus sp.* — Streptokinase

# 5

# Organisms and Populations

**LEARNING OBJECTIVES**

- Understand the concepts of habitat and niche
- Discuss how different organisms are adapted in different environmental conditions
- Understand about population, its growth and its attributes

## Chapter Overview

- The term ecology was coined by **Ernst Hackel**.
- **Autecology/Species Ecology:** The study of reciprocal relationship between every stage of development of population/species and its environment.
- **Four levels of biological organization** in ecology are: (a) Organism (b) Population (c) Community and (d) Biomes.
- A **habitat** is characterized by both abiotic (physico-chemical components like temperature, water, light, soil, etc.) and biotic components (pathogens, predators, parasites, competitors, etc.).
- **Temperature**: It is considered as the most ecologically relevant environmental factor.
- **Eurythermal:** Only few organisms can tolerate wide range of temperatures and such organisms are termed as eurythermal.
- **Stenothermal:** Most of the organisms can tolerate only a narrow range of temperatures and these are termed as stenothermal.
- **Water**: It is another most important ecologically important factor. **Salt concentration** (measured as ***salinity in parts per thousand)*** in given resources: Inland waters: < 5, In the sea water: 30 to 35 Hypersaline lagoons: > 100.
- **Euryhaline:** Organisms tolerant to wide range of salinities.
- **Stenohaline:** Organisms tolerant to a narrow of salinities.
- **Light**: Sunlight regulate the diurnal and seasonal rhythms in animals and affect timing of their foraging, reproductive and migratory activities. As sun is the source of light and temperature both, so the light and temperature of that area are interlinked. Sunlight is absent in the deep part of oceans (> 500 m).
- **Soil**: Important characteristics of the soil that determine the percolation and water holding capacity of the soils are soil composition, grain size and aggregation. **Edaphic factor** are related to soil.
- **Responses to abiotic factors are regulation, conform, migration and suspension.**
- In varying external environmental conditions, organisms try to maintain the constancy of its internal environment by a process called **homeostasis**.
- **Regulation** (Thermoregulation and osmoregulation): These organisms are able to maintain homeostasis by mostly physiological means which ensures constant body temperature, constant osmotic concentration, etc. **Examples:** All birds are mammals and very few lower vertebrates and invertebrate species.
- **Evolutionary 'success'** of mammals is large due to their ability of thermoregulation so that they can thrive in Antarctica or in the Sahara desert.
- **Thermoregulation** is energetically expensive for many organisms, especially small animals, like shrews and humming birds (**larger surface area relative to their volume)** that tend to lose body heat very fast. This is the main reason why very small animals are rarely found in Polar regions.

Refer NCERT Ch 11: Organisms and Population

- **Conform:** In these organisms, body temperature changes with the ambient temperature or the osmotic concentration of the body fluids change with ambient water osmotic concentration (in aquatic animals) **Examples:** Majority (99 per cent) of animals, nearly all plants.
- **Migration:** It refers to the temporary movement away from the stressful habitat to a relatively favorable area and again return when stressful period is over. **Examples:** During winter many animals specially birds, perform long-distance migrations to more hospitable areas. Thousands of migratory birds come from Siberia and other extremely cold northern regions during every winter to the famous **Keoladeo National Park (Bharatpur)** in Rajasthan.
- **Suspend:** Suspension is done by reducing their metabolic activity and going in a state of 'dormancy'.
  **(a)** Thick-walled spores formed in various bacteria, fungi and lower plants.
  **(b)** Seeds and some other vegetative reproductive structures formed in higher plants to overcome the period of stress.
  **(c)** Hibernation during winter and Aestivation during summer. Examples: Some snails and fishes.
- **Diapause (a stage of suspended development)** in many zooplankton species in lakes and ponds.

**Adaptations:**

- To survive in extreme environments, organisms acquire various adaptations which may be morphological, physiological or behavioural. Many adaptations have evolved over a long evolutionary time and are genetically fixed.
- Even in the absence of water, Kangaroo rat in North American deserts can meet all its water requirements from its internal fat oxidation in which water is produced as a by-product. Also, it can concentrate its urine.
- Presence of thick cuticle on the leaf surface of many desert plants. Stomata may be arranged in deep pits (sunken) to minimize transpiration. Stomata remain closed during daytime due to a special photosynthetic pathway (CAM) in them.
- In plants like Opuntia, leaves are reduced to spines while the function of the photosynthesis is done by the flattened stems **(Cladode).**
- **Allen's rule:** In colder climates, mammals generally have shorter ears and limbs to minimize heat loss.
- Presence of blubber in the polar seas aquatic mammals like seals which act as an insulator to reduce heat loss of body.
- At very high altitudes (>3,500m Rohtang Pass near Manali and Leh), **altitude sickness** is observed which is symptoms like-nausea, fatigue and heart palpitations. This is basically due to oxygen debt. But, gradually we get acclimatized (RBC production increases, binding affinity of hemoglobin decreases and breathing rate increases) and stop experiencing altitude sickness.
- Due to some special adaptations, certain microbes (archaebacteria) flourish in hot springs and deep sea hydrothermal vents where temperatures exceed 100°C.
- Many fish in Antarctic waters can survive at below zero temperature. They contain extra solute like glycerol and anti-freezing proteins in their body fluids
- Many marine invertebrates and fish live at great depth. Organism living in extreme environment shows a fascinating array of biochemical adaptation.
- Lizard basks in the sun and absorbs heat when their body temperature becomes low.
- Some species hide in the burrows in the soil to hide and escape from the above-ground heat.

**Populations:**

- Majority of individuals of any species live in groups, interbreed, share or compete for similar resources and constitute a population. Population ecology is an important aspect of ecology which links ecology to population genetics and evolution. Population attributes are following: **(1) Birth rate (Natality) (2) Death rate (Mortality) (3) Sex ratio (4) Age pyramid (5) Population size**

  **Question1:**
  Number of lotus plants in pond last year = 20
  Number of new lotus plants added by reproduction = 8

  Total number of lotus plants in pond = 28
  Birth rate = 8/20 = 0.4 individual per lotus per year.

  **Question 2:**
  Number of fruit flies in a laboratory population = 40
  Number of fruit flies died during a week = 4
  Death rate in the population = 4/40 = 0.1 individual per fruit fly per week.

- **Age pyramid**: It is the structure which is obtained when age distribution (per centage individuals of a given age or age group) is plotted for the population. There are three types of age pyramids on the basis of shape that reflect the growth status of the population whether it is,
  **1.** Growing : when pre- reproductive individual are more than reproductive individuals (upright triangle)
  **2.** Stable : when pre- reproductive individual are almost equal to reproductive individuals (bell shape)
  **3.** Declining : when pre- reproductive individual are less than reproductive individuals (urn shape)
- Indirect measures are also used sometimes to estimate population sizes. Example: The number of tigers in our national parks and tiger reserves is often counted on the basis of pug marks and fecal pellets.
- Usually, births and deaths are the most important factors that affect the population density while the other two factors become important only under special instances. Example: **In a newly colonized habitat, immigration may contribute more in comparison to birth rates.**
- **Population Growth (Formula):** $N_{t+1} = N_t + [(B + I) - (D + E)]$
  where,
  **$N_{t+1}$: Population after time t**
  **$N_t$: Initial Population**
  **B: Natality = Number of births during time t in the population**
  **I: Immigration** = Number of individuals of the same species that have entered the habitat during time t
  **D: Mortality** = Number of deaths during time t in the population
  **E: Emigration** = Number of individuals of the same species that have left the habitat during time t
- **Growth Models**

| Exponential (or geometric) Growth | Logistic (or Verhulst–Pearl Logistic) Growth |
|---|---|
| Resource (food and space) availability is unlimited | Resource availability is limited |
| Rate of change of population<br>$\frac{dN}{dT} = (b-d) \times N$<br>$\frac{dN}{dT} = rN \quad [Let\ (b-d) = r]$<br>$N$ = Size of a population<br>$b$ = Per capita birth rate,<br>$d$ = Per capita death rate<br>$r$ = Intrinsic rate of natural increases | Rate of change of population,<br>$\frac{dN}{dT} = \frac{rN(K-N)}{K}$<br>$N$ = Population density at time t<br>$r$ = Intrinsic rate of natural increase<br>$K$ = Carrying capacity |
| **J–shaped curve** is obtained when we plot N in relation to time. | **Sigmoid–shaped curve** is obtained when we plot N in relation to time. |
| **Phases:**<br>1. Lag phase (initially)<br>2. Phase of acceleration | **Phases:**<br>1. Lag phase (initially)<br>2. Phase of acceleration/deceleration<br>3. Asymptote phase |
| Population density grow beyond the carrying capacity (K) | Population density reaches the carrying capacity (K) (during Asymptote phase) |
| Less realistic | More realistic |
| No population of any species in nature has at its disposal unlimited resources to permit exponential growth. | Natural populations follow Logistic growth. |
| **Example:** Paramecium undergoing binary fission and doubling in numbers everyday (provided food and space remain unlimited) | **Example:** Human population in India for the last hundred years. |

- Value of r for Norway rat = 0.015, Flour beetle = 0.12 and Human population in India in 1981 = 0.0205) **e** = the base of natural logarithms (2.71828)
- Darwin also observed while working on his theory of natural selection then if the resources are unlimited than each species grow with enormous potential.
- Nature's carrying capacity (K): It refers to the maximum number of individuals which can be supported by the resources of a given habitat. Beyond it, further growth is not possible.

- **Life History Variation:** During evolution, populations tend to maximize their reproductive fitness (or Darwinian fitness or High r value) in the habitat in which they live. Organisms tend to follow different but-most efficient reproductive strategy according to their environment.
  - Organisms breeding only once in their life: Pacific salmon fish and Bamboo.
  - Organisms breeding many times during their life: Most birds and mammals.
  - Organisms producing many small-sized offspring **(r- selected species):** Oysters and Pelagic fishes.
  - Organisms producing a small number of large-sized offspring **(k- selected species):** Birds and Mammals
- **r- selected species:** These species that emphasize high growth rates, typically exploits less crowded niches and produce many offsprings, each of which has relatively low probability of surviving to adulthood. **(i.e., high r and low k ).**
- **k- selected species:** They possess relatively stable population and tend to produce relatively low number offspring.
- **Interspecific interactions:** These are interactions in the populations of two different species which could be beneficial, detrimental or neutral to one of the species or both.
- **Predation (+ -):** It is an interaction between members of two species in which member of one species capture, kill and eat up member of other species. All consumers in ecological prospect are predators.
  - Role of predator

    **1.** Act as conduits for energy transfer between the trophic levels.

    **2.** Check on prey populations.

    **3.** Biological control of an exotic, invasive and widespread species.

    (1) The Prickly pear cactus was introduced in Australia in 1920, spreads rapidly and control after introduction of its natural predator-Cactus-feeding Moth.

    (2) Biological control methods are also used in agricultural pest control and are based on the ability of predator to regulate prey population.

    **4.** Maintain species diversity

    (1) Predators reduce the intensity of competition among competing prey species and help in maintaining species diversity in a community.

    Example: In a field experiment done in rocky intertidal communities of American Pacific Coast, removal of starfish Pisaster (an important predator) resulted in extinction of more than ten species of invertebrates due to increased interspecific competition.
  - If a predator is too efficient/overexploits its prey, then it may result in extinction of the prey followed by extinction of predator itself. So the predators in nature are 'prudent'.
- **Defense mechanism** evolve in prey species of animals to reduce impact of predation:
  - Some species of insects and frogs are cryptically-coloured (camouflaged) to avoid being detected easily by the predator.
  - **Monarch butterfly** is highly distasteful to the predator (bird) because of a special chemical in its body which is acquired by it during its caterpillar stage by feeding on a poisonous weed.
  - Most common morphological mean of defense in plants: Thorns. **Examples: Acacia, Cactus, etc.**
  - Many plants produce toxic chemicals that make the herbivore sick or even it kills following ingestion. **Example:** Calotropis (a weed) growing in fields, produces highly poisonous cardiac glycosides. So the cattle or goats avoid browsing on it.
  - Various chemicals that are commercially extracted from the plants (opium, nicotine, caffeine, quinine, strychnine, etc.) are actually produced by them as a chemical defense against herbivores.

- **Competition(- -):** Interaction in which both species suffer.
  - According to Darwin, interspecific competition is also a potent force in organic evolution.
  - It is general belief that 'Competition occurs when closely related species compete for the same resources that are limiting.
    1. Totally unrelated species could also compete for the same resource. **Example:** Visiting Flamingoes and resident Fishes, in some shallow South American lakes compete for the zooplankton (common food).
    2. Resources always need not be limiting for competition to occur. **Example:** In **interference competition,** the feeding efficiency of one species might be reduced due to the presence of another species even if the resources (food and space) are abundant.
- In competition, fitness of one species (measured in terms of its 'r' - intrinsic rate of increase) is significantly lowered in the presence of another species.
- **Gause's Competitive Exclusion Principle:** If the resources are limited, two closely related species competing for the same resources cannot co-exist indefinitely and the competitively inferior species have to be eliminated. **Example:** Within a decade after introduction of goats in Galapagos Islands, Abingdon tortoise became extinct due to the greater browsing efficiency of the goats.
- **Competitive release:** Because of the presence of a competitively superior species, distribution of a species is restricted to a small geographical area. This distributional range is dramatically increased if the competing species is experimentally removed.
- **Connell's elegant field experiments**
  It showed that on the rocky sea coasts of Scotland, barnacle Balanus (larger and competitively superior) dominates the intertidal area and excludes the Chathamalus (smaller barnacle) from that area. Barnacles are marine crustacean.
- Generally, herbivores and plants are affected more adversely by competition in comparison to carnivores.
- **Resource partitioning:** Sometimes the competing species may co-exist by avoiding competition by choosing different times for feeding or different foraging patterns. **Example: MacArthur** showed that five closely related species of **warblers (small birds)** if living on the same tree avoid competition and co-exist due to behavioral differences in their foraging activities.
- **Parasitism(+ -) :**
  - Many parasites are host-specific, i.e., these can parasitize only a single species of host.
  - Parasitism is also an example of co-evolution.
  - Special adaptations of the parasites:
    1. Unnecessary sense organs are lost.
    2. Presence of organs of attachment, eg. adhesive organs /suckers.
    3. Loss of digestive system or ill developed digestive system.
    4. High reproductive capacity and highly developed reproductive system.
  - Parasites may involve one or two intermediate hosts or vectors.
    1. Liver fluke has two intermediate hosts: A snail and a fish.
    2. Malarial parasite (Plasmodium): Human and Mosquito (vector).
  - Parasites may reduce the survival, growth and reproduction of the host and reduce its population density. Host might become physically weak.
  - Parasites may be classified as:
    1. **Ectoparasites: (i)** Lice on humans **(ii)** Ticks on dogs **(iii)** Ectoparasitic copepods (small crustaceans) on many marine fishes, and **(iv)** Cuscuta (parasitic plant) growing on hedge plants.
    2. **Endoparasites:** These are live inside the host and their life cycles are more complex because of their extreme specialization.
  - Female mosquito is not considered as a parasite as mosquito needs our blood for reproduction, and not for nutrition.
  - **Brood parasitism in birds** (Fascinating example of parasitism) parasitic bird lays its eggs in the nest of host and the host incubates them. During evolution, the eggs of the parasitic bird (**Cuckoo or Koel**) have evolved to resemble the host's (**Crow's**) egg in size and color to reduce the chances their detection.

- **Commensalism (+ 0):**
  - This interaction in which one species benefits and the other is neither harmed nor benefited
  - Examples:
    1. An orchid plant growing as an epiphyte on a mango branch.
    2. Barnacles growing on the back of a whale.
    3. Cattle egret and grazing cattle (classic example of commensalism). As the cattle move, insects flush out from the vegetation that would be otherwise difficult for the egrets to find.
    4. Sea anemone and the clown fish. Fish gets protection from predators due to stinging tentacles of sea anemone.
- **Mutualism( ++):**
  - This interaction gives benefit to both the interacting organisms.
  - Mutualists are examples of co-evolution.
  - Examples of mutualism.
    1. Lichens : Relationship between a fungus (mycobiont) and photosynthesizing algae (phycobiont) or cyanobacteria. They are very good pollution indicators ($SO_2$ gas). They don't grow in polluted area.
    2. Mycorrhizae (associations between fungi and roots of higher plants). Fungi help the plant in the absorption of nutrients, it act as substitute for root hairs while the plant provides energy-yielding carbohydrates to the fungi.
    3. Pollination of plants by animals (Most spectacular and evolutionarily fascinating example).
       (i) Fig tree (Ficus) and Wasp : A fig species can be pollinated only by its 'partner' gall wasps species and not by other species. Female wasp uses the fruit as an egg laying (oviposition) site and developing seeds within fruit used for nourishing its larvae.
       (ii) Orchids possess various floral patterns to attract the right pollinator insect (bees and bumblebees). All orchids do not offer rewards. Some orchids like Mediterranean orchid- Ophrys, uses 'sexual deceit' to get pollinated. One of the petals bears a resemblance to the female bee in size, colour and markings. Male bee does pollination by **pseudo copulation.**
       (iii) *Yucca and Pronuba moth*
- In predation, parasitism and commensalism, interacting species live closely with each other.
- **Amensalism** is an interaction in which one species is neither harmed nor benefitted, while another species is harmed. **Example:** Penicillium does not allow growth of staphylococcus bacterium and inhibition of growth achieved by secretion of chemicals called allochemics.
- **Cuscuta:** holoparasitic plant has lost its chlorophyll and leaves in course of evolution.
- 25 per cent of total insects are *phytophagous.*
- **Ecological Niche:** Odum has called habitat an address and niche as profession of a species. No two species occupy same niche and niche support single species.
- Permafrost (Snow laden) polar regions.

# PRACTICE EXERCISES

**Direction:** Read the question carefully and choose the correct option for each.

## Multiple Choice Questions: Level I

### Ecology

**1.** _____ is Known as the Father of Ecology in India.
(a) Varghese Kurein (b) Amartya Sen
(c) Ramdeo Misra (d) Hargobind Khurana

**2.** Ecology is a subject which studies the interactions among organisms and _____.
(a) Amongst the organism and its chemical environment
(b) Between the organism and its physical environment
(c) Amongst the organism and its habitat
(d) Between the organism and its biosphere

**3.** Basically, ecology is concerned with how many levels of biological organizations?
(a) 3 (b) 4 (c) 5 (d) 7

**4.** The levels of biological organization in ecology are –
(a) Cell, Organism, Community, Biosphere
(b) Organisms, Family, Communities, Biomes
(c) Species, Populations, Communities, biomes
(d) Organisms, Populations, Communities, biomes

**5.** Ecology at the level of an individual organism is essentiallly a _____.
(a) Systemic ecology
(b) Somatic ecology
(c) Physiological ecology
(d) Physical ecology

**6.** Which important life process is considered at organism level of ecology?
(a) Respiration (b) Immunity
(c) Reproduction (d) Homeostasis

**7.** How does seasonal variation take place on earth?
(a) Rotation of other planet
(b) Rotation around sun
(c) Rotation of moon around earth
(d) Both (a) and (b)

**8.** The factors responsible for causing annual variation in the intensity and duration of temperature are _____.
(a) Rotation of venus in solar system
(b) Rotation of earth around sun
(c) Tilt in axis of earth
(d) Both (b) and (c)

**9.** Precipitation due to annual variation in seasons includes
(a) Rain (b) Snow
(c) Dew (d) Both (a) and (b)

**10.** Precipitation is an important factor for the formation of major biome such as
(a) Rain forest (b) Tundra
(c) Desert (d) All of the above

**11.** **A:** Regional and local variations occurs with each habitat
**B:** It causes formation of a wide variety of biomes
(a) A is true and B is also true
(b) A is false but B is true
(c) A is true but B is false
(d) A is false and B is also false

**12.** Rain-soaked forest occurs in which state of India?
(a) Assam (b) Meghalaya
(c) Arunachal Pradesh (d) Nagaland

**13.** Just as sand: desert : :_____ : Polar regions
(a) Ice (b) Snow
(c) Permafrost (d) Silt

**14.** Which part of human body is a unique habitat for hundreds of species of microbes?
(a) Mouth (b) Urinary bladder
(c) Intestine (d) Spleen

**15.** Each organism have defined range of condition it can tolerate, various resources it can utilise and distinct functional role in that habitat all these together form
(a) Ecotone (b) Biome
(c) Niche (d) Biodiversity

**16.** Through the process of natural selection animal adapted to optimize following
(a) Locomotion and movement
(b) Survival and reproduction

(c) Nervous system
(d) Excretory system

**17.** Following are major biome of India
(a) Tropical rain forest
(b) Deciduous forest
(c) Desert and Sea coast
(d) All of these

**18.** Following places or organ can act as habitat
(a) Thermal spring (b) Compost pits
(c) Intestine (d) All of these

**19. Assertion:** Temperature is the most ecologically relevant environmental factor.
**Reason:** Temperature affects the kinetics of enzymes and through it the basal metabolism, activity and other physiological functions of the organism.
(a) (A) is false but (R) is true
(b) Both (A) and (R) are true and (R) is the correct explanation of (A)
(c) Both (A) and (R) are true but (R) is not the correct explanation of (A)
(d) (A) is true but (R) is false.

**20.** Read following sentences.
**Statement I:** The levels of thermal tolerance of different species determine to a large extent their geographical distribution.
**Statement II:** the gradually increasing average global temperatures will change the distributional range of some species in ecosystem.
(a) Statement I is incorrect but statement II is true.
(b) Both Statements I and II are true
(c) Both Statements I and II are false
(d) Statement I is correct but statement II is false

**21. Assertion:** Many freshwater animals cannot live for long in sea water and vice versa
**Reason:** The change in their environment would cause organisms to face the osmotic problems.
(a) (A) is false but (R) is true
(b) Both (A) and (R) are true and (R) is the correct explanation of (A)
(c) Both (A) and (R) are true but (R) is not the correct explanation of (A)
(d) (A) is true but (R) is false.

**Direction for Q22–28:** Choose the correct option:
(a) Statement I is incorrect but statement II is true.
(b) Both Statements I and II are true
(c) Both Statements I and II are false
(d) Statement I is correct but statement II is false

**22.** Read following sentences.
**Statement I:** The productivity and distribution of plants is heavily dependent on water.
**Statement II:** organisms living in oceans, lakes and rivers should not face any water-related problems

**23.** Read following sentences.
**Statement I:** Many plants are dependent on sunlight to meet their photoperiodic requirement for flowering.
**Statement II:** Animals use the diurnal and seasonal variations in light intensity and duration as cues for timing their foraging, reproductive and migratory activities.

**24.** Read following sentences.
**Statement I:** The availability of light on land is closely linked with that of temperature
**Statement II:** All the colour components of the visible spectrum are available for marine plants living at different depths of the ocean.

**25.** Read following sentences.
**Statement I:** Various soil characteristics along with parameters such as pH, mineral composition and topography determine to a large extent the vegetation in any area.
**Statement II:** in the aquatic environment, the sediment-characteristics often determine the type of benthic animals that can thrive there.

**26.** Read following sentences.
**Statement I:** All birds and mammals species are indeed capable of thermoregulation and osmoregulation.
**Statement II:** the success of mammals is largely due to their ability to maintain a constant body temperature
(a) Statement I is incorrect but statement II is true.
(b) Both Statements I and II are true
(c) Both Statements I and II are false
(d) Statement I is correct but statement II is false

**27.** Read following sentences.
**Statement I:** Plants show some mechanisms to maintain internal temperatures.
**Statement II:** some animal species have evolved adaptations to avoid unfavourable conditions in space or in time

**28.** Read following sentences.
**Statement I:** Ecology is concerned with three levels of biological organisation- populations, communities and biomes.

**Statement II:** Ecology is the study of the relationships of living organisms with the abiotic and biotic components of their environment.

**Direction for Q29–32:** Choose the correct option:

(a) (A) is false but (R) is true
(b) Both (A) and (R) are true and (R) is the correct explanation of (A)
(c) Both (A) and (R) are true but (R) is not the correct explanation of (A)
(d) (A) is true but (R) is false.

**29.** **Assertion:** small animals have to expend much energy to generate body heat through metabolism.
**Reason:** small animals have a larger surface area relative to their volume and they tend to lose body heat very fast in colder environment.

**30.** **Assertion:** regulators are capable of homeostasis in the face of changing external environment
**Reason:** regulators are able to maintain a constant internal environment which contributes to optimal performance,

**31.** **Assertion:** Some species show migration, aestivation, hibernation and diapause.
**Reason:** These are evolved adaptations to avoid unfavourable conditions in space.

**32.** **Assertion:** the kangaroo rat in North American deserts can survive in the absence of an external source of water.
**Reason:** the kangaroo rat is capable of meeting all its water requirements through its internal protein oxidation in which water is a by product

**33.** Read following sentences.
**Statement I:** migration temporarily to a less stressful habitat is a behavioural adaptation.
**Statement II:** Many adaptations have evolved over a long evolutionary time and are genetically fixed.
(a) Statement I is incorrect but statement II is true.
(b) Both Statements I and II are true
(c) Both Statements I and II are false
(d) Statement I is correct but statement II is false

**34.** Select set of correct statements:
(A) Regional and local variations within each biome lead to the formation of a wide variety of habitats.
(B) Human intestine is a unique habitat for hundreds of species of microbes.
(C) the physico-chemical (abiotic) components alone can characterise the habitat of an organism completely.
(D) over a period of time, the organism had through natural selection, evolved adaptations to optimise its survival and reproduction in its habitat.
(a) A, B and D (b) A, B and C
(c) B, C and D (d) B and D only

**35.** Adaptations shown by desert plants are:
(A) a thick cuticle on their leaf surfaces
(B) their stomata arranged in deep pits
(C) a special photosynthetic pathway (CAM)
(D) their stomata to remain closed during day time
(E) leaves are reduced to spines
(a) A, B and E
(b) A, B and C
(c) B, C and E
(d) A, B, C, D and E

**36.** Some desert plants like Opuntia, have spines instead of leaves. Their photosynthetic function is taken over by
(a) the roots (b) the stems
(c) the flowers (d) the buds

**37.** **Assertion:** seals in polar seas have a thick layer of protein called blubber below their Skin.
**Reason:** blubber acts as an insulator and reduces loss of body heat.
(a) (A) is false but (R) is true
(b) Both (A) and (R) are true and (R) is the correct explanation of (A)
(c) Both (A) and (R) are true but (R) is not the correct explanation of (A)
(d) (A) is true but (R) is false.

**38.** **Assertion:** Humans experience altitude sickness at high altitude place to which body gets gradually acclimatised
**Reason:** The body compensates low oxygen availability by increasing red blood cell production, increasing the binding affinity of hemoglobin and by increasing breathing rate.
(a) (A) is false but (R) is true
(b) Both (A) and (R) are true and (R) is the correct explanation of (A)
(c) Both (A) and (R) are true but (R) is not the correct explanation of (A)
(d) (A) is true but (R) is false.

**39.** **Assertion:** Mammals from hotter climates generally have shorter ears and limbs
**Reason:** This is an adaptation to minimise heat loss.
(a) (A) is false but (R) is true
(b) Both (A) and (R) are true and (R) is the correct explanation of (A)
(c) Both (A) and (R) are true but (R) is not the correct explanation of (A)
(d) (A) is true but (R) is false.

## Abiotic Factors

**40.** The key elements which lead to much variation in the physical and chemical conditions of different habitat are enlisted below:

**Temperature, Wind, Water, light, Soil, Humidity, UV rays**

(a) 5 (b) 6 (c) 4 (d) 3

**41.** A habitat of an organism constitutes _______.
(a) Abiotic components
(b) Biotic components
(c) Symbiotic compounds
(d) Both (a) and (b)

**42.** The organisms through natural selection have evolved _______ to optimize its survival and reproduction in its habitat.
(a) Camouflage
(b) Adaptations
(c) Specialized Physiology
(d) Higher reproduction rate

**43.** In tropical deserts, the temperature goes _______.
(a) > 40°C (b) > 60°C
(c) > 50°C (d) >70°C

**44.** Which of the following is most important ecological environmental factor
(a) Temperature (b) Water
(c) Soil (d) Air

**45.** Habitats such as thermal springs and deep-sea hydrothermal vents have average temperature exceeding _______.
(a) 100°C (b) 150°C
(c) 80°C (d) 1000°C

**46.** _______ trees cannot grow in temperate countries.
(a) Banana (b) Mango
(c) Oranges (d) Peaches

**47.** Mango cannot grow in countries like _______.
(a) Canada (b) Germany
(c) Africa (d) Both (a) and (b)

**48.** _______ are not found in Kerala forests.
(a) Snakes (b) Snow leopards
(c) Elephants (d) Monkeys

**49.** _______ fish is rarely caught beyond tropical latitudes in ocean.
(a) Salmon (b) Shark
(c) Tuna (d) Pomphret

**50.** Which of the following is most commonly affected by temperature of habitat?
(a) Hormones
(b) Enzymes
(c) Inflammatory mediators
(d) Neurotransmitters

**51.** The organisms which can tolerate and thrive in a wide range of temperature are called as _______.
(a) Stenothermal (b) Homiotherm
(c) Eurythermal (d) Poikilotherm

**52.** Example of eurythermal organisms are
(a) All reptiles
(b) All amphibians
(c) Most mammals and birds
(d) All fishes

**53.** The organisms which thrive in a very narrow range of temperatures are known as _______.
(a) Stenothermal (b) Poikilotherm
(c) Homiotherm (d) Eurythermal

**54.** Example of stenothermal organisms are
(a) Lizard (b) Amphibians
(c) Nearly all plants (d) All of these

**55.** The level of thermal tolerance of different species determines the extent of _______.
(a) Survival
(b) Geographical distribution
(c) Morphology
(d) Biodiversity

**56.** Life originated on earth first in
(a) Air (b) Land
(c) Water (d) All of the above

**57.** Special modifications with respect of _______ make it possible for an organism to survive in desert.
(a) Water (b) High temperature
(c) Sand (d) Less abundance plants

**58.** For aquatic organisms _______ of water becomes important.
(a) Quantity (b) Quality
(c) Conductivity (d) Specific gravity

**59.** The salt concentration is measured as salinity in parts per _______.
(a) Billion (b) Million
(c) Hundred (d) Thousand

**60.** The salinity of inland waters is less than _______.
(a) 3 (b) 4
(c) 5 (d) 2

**61.** The salinity of sea water is ______.
(a) > 100 (b) 30 – 35
(c) 60 – 80 (d) 10 – 15

**62.** The salinity of a hyper saline lagoon is
(a) Upto $10^3$ (b) > $10^3$
(c) Upto $10^2$ (d) > $10^2$

**63.** The organisms which are tolerant of a wide range of salinities are
(a) Salinotrophs (b) Euryhaline
(c) Salinosomes (d) Stenohaline

**64.** The organisms which are restricted to a narrow range of salinity are known as
(a) Salinosomes (b) Salinotolerants
(c) Duryhaline (d) Stenohaline

**65.** Fresh water animals cannot live for long in sea water because they would face problems of:
(a) Vapor pressure (b) Purity
(c) Omolarity (d) Thermal change

**66. Assertion:** Photosynthesis is an essential life process of plants
**Reason:** Small plants growing in forest are adapted to other process than photosynthesis because they are over shadowed by tall canopied trees.
(a) A is true and R is also true
(b) R is true and A is false
(c) A is true but R is false
(d) Both A and R are false

**67.** For many animals, light is an important factors which regulates ______ variations..
(a) Nocturnal (b) Diurnal
(c) Urinal (d) Crepuscular

**68.** The activities of animals like foraging, reproductive and migratory depend on
(a) Temperature (b) Water
(c) Light (d) Air

**69.** Marine organisms, which live at a depth > 500 m, receive solar energy in which form?
(a) Different rays from visible spectrum
(b) UV radiations
(c) Cosmic rays
(d) Infra-Red radiations

**70.** The factors which affect percolation and water holding capacity of soil are
(a) Soil composition (b) Grain size
(c) Aggregation (d) All of the above

**71.** Vegetation in any area depend on
(a) pH of soil (b) Mineral composition
(c) Topography (d) All of the above

**72.** The ______ characteristics often determine the type of benthic animals than can thrive there
(a) Composition (b) Sediment
(c) Grain size (d) Water holding capacity

**73.** Which of the natural habitat on earth that is inhabited just by a single species
(a) Hot vents (b) Forest
(c) Polar region (d) None of these

**74.** Select Correct matching for below diagram:

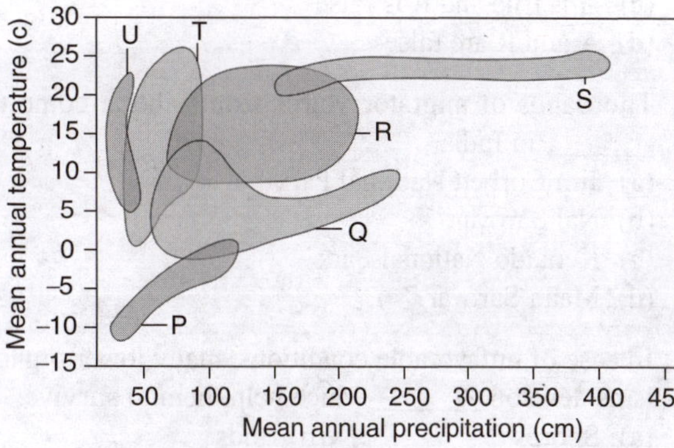


(a) P: Desert, Q: Tropical forest, R: Temperate forest, S: Coniferous forest
(b) P: Grassland, Q: Temperate forest, R: Desert, S: Article and Alpine tundra
(c) P: Article and Alpine tundra, Q: Coniferous forest, R: Temperate forest, S: Tropical forest
(d) P: Coniferous forest, Q: Grassland, R: Desert, S: Tropical forest

## Response to Abiotic Factor

**75.** The process to maintain internal environment of an organism constant is called:
(a) Equilibrium (b) Organostasis
(c) Homeostasis (d) Apoptosis

**76.** The 'success' of mammals is due to
(a) Presence of mammary glands
(b) Efficient osmoregulation
(c) Efficient Thermoregulation
(d) Efficient magnetoception

**77.** 'Shivering' during cold is beneficial for mammals. It helps to
(a) Decrease body temperature
(b) Increase body temperature
(c) No change in body temperature
(d) None of the above

**78.** Which is the most effective way to get relief from high temperature?
(a) Oil secretion increases
(b) Frequent urination
(c) High water intake
(d) Profuse sweating

**79.** **Assertion:** Due to changes in seasons, temperature also changes.

**Reason:** To cope up with this, plants can regulate internal body temperature
(a) A is true and R is also true
(b) A is false but R is true
(c) A is true and R is false
(d) A and R are false

**80.** Thousands of migratory birds from Siberia come to _______ in India.
(a) Jim Corbett National Park
(b) Nal Sarovar
(c) Keolado National Park
(d) Maan Sarovar

**81.** In case of unfavorable conditions, many lower organisms develop _______ which help them to survive.
(a) Spores (b) Buds
(c) Gametes (d) Clones

**82.** In higher plants _______ helps to tide over periods of stress
(a) Roots (b) Fruits
(c) Seeds (d) Stem

**83.** Higher plants survive stressful conditions by reducing their _______ activity.
(a) Reproductive (b) Metabolic
(c) Growth (d) Morphogenetic

**84.** Bears undergo a period of _______ to escape stress during winter.
(a) Hibernation (b) Aestivation
(c) Sedation (d) Metamorphosis

**85.** Snails and fish undergo aestivation to avoid summer related problems of heat and _______.
(a) Hygroscopicity (b) Dessication
(c) Efflorescence (d) Starvation

**86.** Under unfavorable conditions, many species of zooplankton which lives in small water bodies are known to enter _______.
(a) Diapause (b) Metapause
(c) Neopause (d) Monopause

**87.** Diapause is a stage of _______.
(a) Perpetual development
(b) Intermittent development
(c) Suspended development
(d) Sequential development

**88.** The figure given below is a diagrammatic representation of response of organisms to abiotic factors. What do (A), (B) and (C) represent respectively?

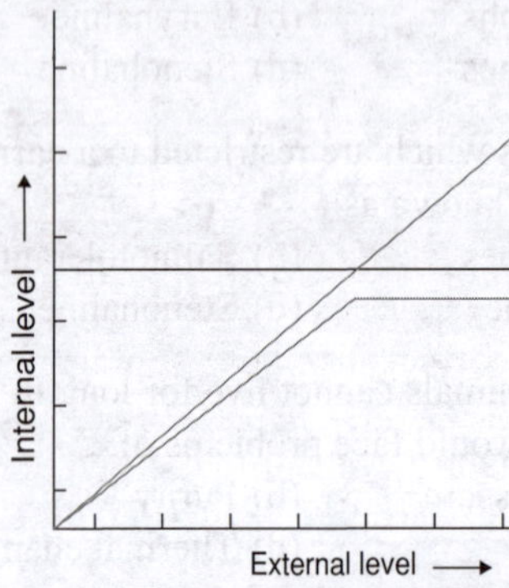


(a) A: Conformers, B: Partial regulaters, C: Regulaters
(b) A: Partial regulaters, B: Conformers, C: Regulaters
(c) A: Regulaters, B: Partial regulaters, C: Conformers
(d) A: Conformers, B: Regulaters, C: Partial regulaters

## Adaptation

**89.** _______ is any attribute of an organism that enables the organism to survive and reproduce in its habitat.
(a) Mutation (b) Evolution
(c) Adaptation (d) Conformation

**90.** Adaption includes _______ attribute of an organism.
(a) Behavioural (b) Physiological
(c) Morphological (d) All of the above

**91.** Many adaptations of an organism have evolved over a long duration of evolution and are _______.
(a) Genetically unstable
(b) Genetically fixed
(c) Genetically disadvantageous
(d) Genetically extemperaneous

**92.** _______ in North American deserts is capable of meeting all its water requirements through its internal biochemical process.
(a) Llama (b) Coyote
(c) Kangaroo rat (d) Weasel

**93.** By which biochemical process, kangaroo rat meets its water requirement?

(a) Reduction of fats
(b) Oxidation of proteins
(c) Reduction of proteins
(d) Oxidation of fats

**94.** Water molecule is a byproduct in which of the following process?
(a) Reduction of fats
(b) Oxidation of proteins
(c) Reduction of proteins
(d) Oxidation of fats

**95.** Desert animals have the capability of forming _______ urine.
(a) Hypotonic (b) Isosmotic
(c) Concentrated (d) Dilute

**96.** Select the incorrect statement from the following options:
(a) Desert plants have thick cuticle on their leaves.
(b) Stomata are arranged superficially in desert plant.
(c) Minimum loss of water through fat oxidation in desert animal.
(d) Special photosynthetic pathway occurs in desert plants.

**97.** An important feature regarding CAM pathway in desert plants
(a) Enables stomata to increase the number of chloroplasts.
(b) Enables stomata to remain open during any time.
(c) Enables stomata to remain closed during day time.
(d) Enables stomata to open during rainy weather.

**98.** Some desert plants like _______ have no leaves.
(a) Meuhlenbeckia (b) Opuntia
(c) Nephrolepis (d) All of the above

**99.** Photosynthetic function in opuntia is performed by _______.
(a) Roots (b) Flowers
(c) Fruits (d) Stems

**100.** In opuntia, leaves are reduced to _______
(a) Thorns (b) Prickles
(c) Spines (d) Buds

**101.** Allen's rule is with respect to _______
(a) Reptiles (b) Mammals
(c) Aves (d) Amphibia

**102.** Mammals from colder climates generally have _______ ears and limbs to minimize heat loss.
(a) Reduced (b) Shorter
(c) Longer (d) Wider

**103.** Aquatic mammals in polar seas have a thick layer of fat known as _______
(a) Blubber (b) Flubber
(c) Rubber (d) Stubber

**104.** A thick layer of fat under skin in aquatic mammals essentially act as _______.
(a) Food reservoir (b) Insulator
(c) Conductor (d) Heat generator

**105.** Visiting a place like Leh and Mansarovar gives you an uncomfortable feeling. This is referred to as _______.
(a) Motion Sickness (b) Altitude Sickness
(c) Acrophobia (d) All of the above

**106.** With the increase in altitude of a place _______.
(a) Atmospheric pressure decreases
(b) Atmospheric pressure increases
(c) Atmospheric pressure remain constant
(d) Either (a) or (b)

**107.** The symptoms of altitude sickness are
(a) Nausea (b) Heart palpitations
(c) Fatigue (d) All of the above

**108.** How acclimatization occurs in case of altitude sickness?
(a) Decrease RBC production
(b) Increase RBC production
(c) Increase rate of breathing
(d) Both (b) and (c)

**109.** Which bacteria can flourish in hot springs and deep sea hydrothermal vents?
(a) Cyanobacteria (b) Archaebacteria
(c) Actinobacteria (d) Acidobacteria

**110.** Many fish thrive in Antarctic water where the temperature is _______.
(a) Always above zero
(b) Always above 4°C
(c) Always below zero
(d) Sometimes below zero

**111.** How much pressure is experienced by marine invertebrates and fishes living at the great depths in oceans?
(a) < 100 times that of normal atmospheric pressure
(b) < 100 times that of hydrostatic pressure
(c) > 100 times that of hydrostatic pressure
(d) > 100 times that of normal atmospheric pressure

**112.** Which of the following animals lack the physiological ability to deal with high temperature in their habitat?

(a) Giant frilled lizard (b) Desert lizard
(c) Kangaroo rat (d) Weasel

**113.** What adaptation desert lizard shows to deal with high temperature?
(a) Bask in sun when body temperature drops
(b) Move in shade when body temperature drops
(c) Bask in sun when ambient temperature drops.
(d) Move in shade when ambient temperature drops.

**114.** The main reason behind building burrows in soil by burrowing animals is ______.
(a) To escape from predators.
(b) To derive nutrition parts of plants from underground.
(c) The mode of evolution chose burrows as a specific habitat.
(d) To hide and escape from the above-ground heat.

**115.** Diapause is
(a) Adaptation to terrestrial life.
(b) Stage of suspended development seen in unfavourable conditions in many zooplankton species in lakes and ponds.
(c) Method of migration from stressful habitat to a more hospitable are.
(d) It is a type of Symbiosis.

## Population (Attributes & Growth)

**116.** Which of the following is not a population attribute?
(a) Majority of them live in groups in a well-defined geographical location.
(b) Share or compete for similar resources.
(c) Potentially interbreed
(d) Single individuals of any species cannot live in isolation.

**117.** Individuals resulting from asexual reproduction are also considered ______ while performing ecological studies.
(a) Biome
(b) Ecosystem
(c) Population
(d) Species

**118.** As teakwood: Forest tracts, ________: Wetland.
(a) Latus (b) Rats
(c) Squirrels (d) Cormorants

**119.** To evolve certain desired traits, natural selection should operate at ______ level.
(a) Species (b) Biome
(c) Population (d) Genus

**120.** Population ecology is a bridge between evolution and ______.
(a) Population morphology
(b) Population genetics
(c) Population proteomics
(d) Population variation

**121.** After poaching 3 lions in certain forest of Gujarat, only 15 are left in a year. Determine death rate per capita.
(a) 5.000 (b) 0.200
(c) 0.166 (d) 0.800

**122.** The population size of Siberian cranes at Bharatpur wetlands in any year is ______.
(a) <10 (b) <100
(c) <1000 (d) <5

**123.** Population size in any given habitat is also known as ______.
(a) Population cluster
(b) Population explosion
(c) Population abundance
(d) Population density

**124.** Tiger census in our national parks and tigers reserves is done by counting
(a) Tiger cubs (b) Tiger pug marks
(c) Tiger fecal pellets (d) Both (b) and (c)

**125.** Natality refers to
(a) No. of births in a given geographical area.
(b) No. of births in a given time period.
(c) No. of births under influence of given environmental factor.
(d) No. of deaths in a given time period.

**126.** Select incorrect matching
(a) Natality : Number of births during a given period in the population that are added to initial density.
(b) Immigration : Number of individuals of the same species that have come into habitat from elsewhere during given time period.
(c) Mortality : Number of individual of population who left the habitat and gone elsewhere during given time period.
(d) Adaptation: It is any attribute of an organism that enables the organism to survive and reproduce in its habitat.

**127.** Identify the correct equation for population density at time t + 1
(a) $N = N_t + [(D+I) - (B+E)]$
(b) $N = N_t + [(B+I) - (D+E)]$
(c) $N_{t+1} = N_t + [(B+D) - (I+E)]$
(d) $N_{t+1} = N_t + [(B+I) - (D+E)]$

**128.** If a new habitat is just being colonized then which of the following option do you think would have a greater contribution towards population density?
(a) Mortality (b) Natality
(c) Immigration (d) Emigration

**129.** While developing theory of natural selection, Darwin observed that each species can realize fully its innate potential to grow in number provided in a particular habitat ______.
(a) Favorable environmental conditions are prevalent.
(b) Absence of natural disasters like floods and famine.
(c) Availability of unlimited resources.
(d) Development of mutation in certain species.

**130.** Study the following equation in context of population growth and choose the correct option
dN/dt = (b - d) x N
Substituting r in place of b – d then
dN/dt = rN
Here 'r' is known as _____
(a) Extrinsic rate of natural decrease
(b) Intrinsic rate of natural decrease
(c) Intrinsic rate of natural increase
(d) Extrinsic rate of natural increase

**131.** The r value for Norway rat, flour beetle and human population (in 1981) is _______.
(a) 0.15, 0.12, 0.0205 (b) 0.0015, 0.0205, 0.12
(c) 0.015, 0.12, 0.0205 (d) 1.5, 0.012, 0.0502

**132.** Any species growing exponentially under ______ resource conditions can reach massive population densities in a short time span
(a) Limited (b) Unlimited
(c) Essential (d) Non-essential

**133. Assertion (A)**: A particular species in nature can achieve exponential growth.
**Reason (R):** Availability of unlimited resources makes it possible.
(a) A is true but R is incorrect
(b) R is correct and A is incorrect
(c) Both A and R are incorrect
(d) Both A and R are correct

**134.** Carrying capacity K means _______
(a) Organism's capability of maximum reproduction.
(b) Nature's limit for supporting maximum growth of a species.
(c) Nature's limit for supporting maximum number of species.
(d) Organism's capability to withstand environmental odds.

**135.** If a population grows in a habitat with limited resources, then following phases of achievement are observed-
(a) Lag → Acceleration → Deceleration → Asymptote
(b) Log → Deceleration → Acceleration → Asymptote
(c) Log → Acceleration → Deceleration → Asymptote
(d) Lag → Acceleration → Asymptote → Deceleration

**136.** The sigmoid curve of population growth is also known as
(a) Wagner-Nelson logistic growth
(b) Lineweaver-Burk logistic growth
(c) Verhulst-Pearl logistic growth
(d) Darwin's logistic growth

**137.** Which of the following equation correctly describes sigmoid growth curve?
(a) $dN/dt = rN\left(\frac{K-N}{r}\right)$ (b) $dN/dt = rN\left(\frac{K-N}{t}\right)$
(c) $dN/dt = N\left(\frac{K-N}{N}\right)$ (d) $dN/dt = rN\left(\frac{K-N}{K}\right)$

**138.** The reproductive fitness of a population in a certain habitat is also termed as _______
(a) Verhulst's fitness (b) Darwin's fitness
(c) Lamarkian fitness (d) Huxley's fitness

**139.** In order to achieve maximum population in a habitat, which of the following is correct?
(a) High *r* value
(b) Low *r* value
(c) Independent of *r* value
(d) Optimum *r* value

**140.** The organism breeding only once in its lifetime is _______
(a) Atlantic tuna fish
(b) Indian pomphret fish
(c) Pacific salmon fish
(d) Arctic whale

**141.** Amongst plants, select the correct option which breeds only once in lifetime.
(a) Banyan (b) Bamboo
(c) Oak (d) Pine

**142.** _______ is a more meaningful measure of population size.
(a) Natality (b) Mortality
(c) Biomass (d) Resources consumed

**143.** Pick out the essential resources for a population in a given habitat from the following

**Food, Water, Air, Space**

(a) Food and water (b) Food and Space
(c) Air and Space (d) Water and Space

**144.** Following breeds many times during their lifetime except

(a) Birds (b) Mammals
(c) Amphibians (d) Pacific salmon fish

**145.** Which of the following produce large number of small sized offspring

(a) Oyster (b) Pelagic fishes
(c) Mammals (d) Both (a) and (b)

**146.** Populations evolve to maximize their

(a) Health fitness (b) Body fitness
(c) Mental fitness (d) Reproductive fitness

**147.** What type of human population is represented by the adjacent pyramid?

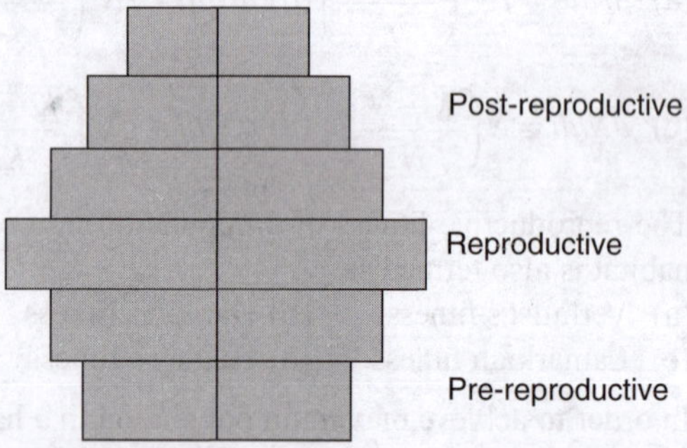


(a) Expanding population
(b) Vanishing population
(c) Stable population
(d) Declining population

**Question from 148 to 152 based on following graph**

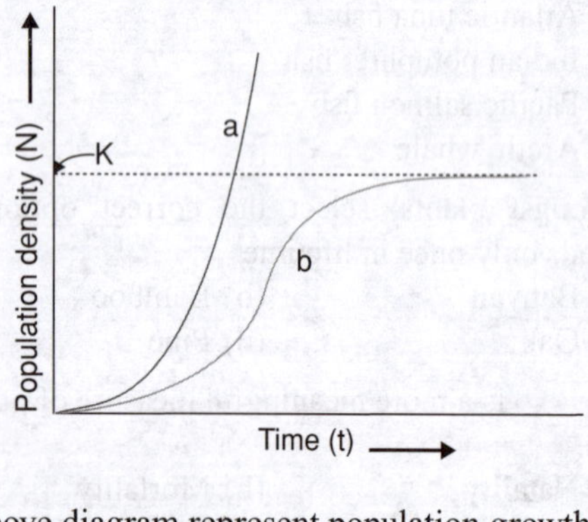


Above diagram represent population growth curve

**148.** Graph 'a' represented by formula:

(a) $\frac{dN}{dt} = rN$ (b) $\frac{dN}{dt} = N$
(c) $\frac{dN}{dt} = rN\left(\frac{K-N}{K}\right)$ (d) $\frac{dN}{dt} = N\left(\frac{K-N}{K}\right)$

**149.** Graph b represented by formula

(a) $\frac{dN}{dt} = rN$ (b) $\frac{dN}{dt} = N$
(c) $\frac{dN}{dt} = rN\left(\frac{K-N}{K}\right)$ (d) $\frac{dN}{dt} = N\left(\frac{K-N}{K}\right)$

**150.** What is the meaning of K in graph

(a) Intrinsic rate of natural increase
(b) Population density at time zero
(c) carrying capacity
(d) Population density after time t

**151.** Plot b is known as

(a) Exponential growth curve
(b) Logistic growth curve
(c) *Verhulst-Pearl Logistic Growth curve*
(d) Both (b) and (c)

**152.** Which of the growth curve is considered a more realistic one

(a) Curve a (b) Curve b
(c) Both (a) and (b) (d) None of these

**153.** Norway rate grow exponentially and its r value is 0.015. How much time it will take to double its population

(a) ln2/0.015 (b) ln3/0.015
(c) ln4/0.015 (d) log2/0.015

**154.** Identify the A, B, C and D in this figure?

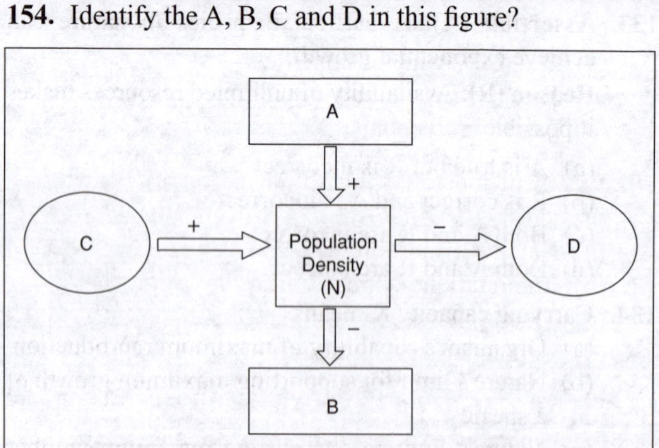


(a) A: Immigration (I), B: Emigration (E), C: Natality (B), D: Mortality (D)

(b) A: Natality (B), B: immigration (I), C: Mortality (D), D: Emigration (E)
(c) A: Mortality (D), B: Emigration (E), C: Natality (B), D: Immigration (I)
(d) A: Mortality (D), B: Natality (B), C: Emigration (E), D: Immigration (I)

**155.** Identify A, B and C in below figure of age pyramid for human population?

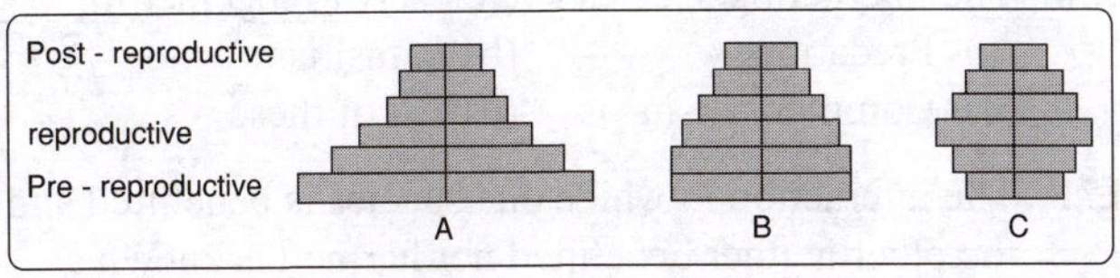


(a) A: Declining, B: Stable, C: Expanding
(b) A: Stable, B: Expanding, C: Declining
(c) A: Expanding, B: Stable, C: Declining
(d) A: Stable, B: Declining, C: Expanding

**156.** Most important factors influencing population density under normal conditions:
(a) Birth rate, Immigration
(b) Emigration, Immigration
(c) Death rate, Birth rate
(d) Death rate, Emigration

**157.** A population has more young individuals compared to the older individuals. What would be the status of the population after some years?
(a) It will decline
(b) It will stabilize
(c) It will increase
(d) It will first decline and then stabilize

**158.** What parameters are used for tiger census in our country's national parks and sanctuaries?
(a) Pug marks only
(b) Pug marks and faecal pellets
(c) Faecal pellets only
(d) Actual head counts

**159.** Which of the following would necessarily decrease the density of a population in a given habitat?
(a) Natality > mortality
(b) Immigration > emigration
(c) Mortality and emigration
(d) Natality and immigration

**160.** A protozoan reproduces by binary fission. What will be the number of protozoans in its population after six generations?
(a) 128 (b) 24
(c) 64 (d) 32

**161.** Select set of correct statements:
(A) individuals of species living in groups in an area, competing for similar resources, potentially interbreeding, constitute a population.
(B) a group of individuals resulting from only sexual reproduction is considered a population
(C) natural selection operates to evolve the desired traits at the individual level.
(D) Population ecology links ecology to population genetics and evolution.
(a) B and D (b) A and D
(c) B, C and D (d) C and D

**162.** Read following sentences.
**Statement I:** A population possesses specific characteristics that distinguish it from an individual organism.
**Statement II:** The size of the population reveals about its status in the habitat.
(a) Statement I is incorrect but statement II is true.
(b) Both Statements I and II are true
(c) Both Statements I and II are false
(d) Statement I is correct but statement II is false

**163.** Read following sentences.
**Statement I:** population density is always measured in numbers only.
**Statement II:** The size of a population for any species is a static parameter.
(a) Statement I is incorrect but statement II is true.
(b) Both Statements I and II are true
(c) Both Statements I and II are false
(d) Statement I is correct but statement II is false

**164. Assertion:** Natality contributes to an increase in population density
**Reason:** Natality refers to the number of births during a given period in the population that are added to the initial density.
(a) (A) is false but (R) is true
(b) Both (A) and (R) are true and (R) is the correct explanation of (A)
(c) Both (A) and (R) are true but (R) is not the correct explanation of (A)
(d) (A) is true but (R) is false.

**165.** Read following sentences.
**Statement I:** In the initial colonization of a new habitat, immigration may play a more substantial role in contributing to population growth than birth rates.
**Statement II:** In a population birth and death rates refer to per capita births and deaths, respectively.
(a) Statement I is incorrect but statement II is true.
(b) Both Statements I and II are true

(c) Both Statements I and II are false
(d) Statement I is correct but statement II is false

**166.** Read following sentences.

**Statement I:** The availability of resources is crucial for the unrestricted expansion of a population.
**Statement II:** 'intrinsic rate of natural increase' is a very important parameter chosen for assessing impacts of any biotic or abiotic factor on population growth.

(a) Statement I is incorrect but statement II is true.
(b) Both Statements I and II are true
(c) Both Statements I and II are false
(d) Statement I is correct but statement II is false

**167.** **Assertion:** There is competition between individuals for limited resources.
**Reason:** unlimited resources to permit exponential growth are not available to any population in nature.

(a) (A) is false but (R) is true
(b) Both (A) and (R) are true and (R) is the correct explanation of (A)
(c) Both (A) and (R) are true but (R) is not the correct explanation of (A)
(d) (A) is true but (R) is false.

**168.** Read following sentences.

**Statement I:** Populations undergo evolutionary processes to enhance their reproductive fitness within their specific habitat.
**Statement II:** Organisms' life history traits have evolved in response to the limitations imposed by both abiotic and biotic components of their habitat.

(a) Statement I is incorrect but statement II is true.
(b) Both Statements I and II are true
(c) Both Statements I and II are false
(d) Statement I is correct but statement II is false

## Species Interaction

**169.** Fill in the blanks A, B, C, and D respectively

| Species A | Species B | None of interaction |
|---|---|---|
| + | + | Mutualism |
| – | – | A |
| + | – | B |
| + | – | Parasitism |
| + | 0 | C |
| – | 0 | D |

(+) Beneficial (–) detrimental (0) Neutral

(a) A: Commensalism, B: Predation, C: Amensalism, D: Competition
(b) A: Predation, B: Parasitism, C: Commensalism, D: Amensalism
(c) A: Competition, B: Predation, C: Commensalism, D: Amensalism
(d) A: Competition, B: Predation, C: Amensalism, D: Commensalism

**170.** The interacting species live closely to together in
(a) Predation (b) Parasitism
(c) Commensalism (d) All of these

**171.** The interaction in which one species is benefitted and the other neither benefitted nor harmed is known as
(a) Predation (b) Parasitism
(c) Commensalism (d) Amensalism

**172.** The interaction which is beneficial to one species and detrimental to other is known as
(a) Predation (b) Parasitism
(c) Commensalism (d) Both (a) and (b)

**173.** The interaction which is beneficial to both species
(a) Predation (b) Parasitism
(c) Commensalism (d) Mutualism

**174.** The interaction which is detrimental to both species
(a) Predation (b) Parasitism
(c) Commensalism (d) Competition

## Predation

**175.** Nearly ________% of all insects is known to be phytophagous
(a) 25% (b) 35% (c) 45% (d) 10%

**176.** Thorns are the most common morphological means of defense in
(a) Acacia (b) Cactus
(c) Calotropis (d) Both (a) and (b)

**177.** Which of the following weed plant produce cardiac glycosides (highly poisonous material)
(a) Acacia (b) Cactus
(c) Calotropis (d) All of the above

**178.** Which of the following substance are produced by plants as defense against grazers and browsers (count number)?

**Nicotine, Caffeine, Quinine, Strychnine, Opium**

(a) 2 (b) 3
(c) 4 (d) 5

**179.** In a field experiment, when all the starfish were removed from an enclosed intertidal area more than

___A___ species of invertebrates becomes extinct within a year, because of ___B___ completion.
(a) A – 10, B-Intra specific
(b) A – 10, B-Inter specific
(c) A – 20, B-Intra specific
(d) A – 20, B-Inter specific

**180.** Following is true about predators.
(a) They keep prey population under control.
(b) They may help in maintaining species diversity in a community by reducing the intensity of competition among competing prey species.
(c) They are prudent in nature.
(d) All of above.

**181.** Which butterfly is highly distasteful to its predator bird because of a species chemical present in its body?
(a) Apis mellifera (b) Viceroy
(c) Monarch (d) Apis indica

**182.** True about predation
(a) It is method to transfer energy across various trophic levels.
(b) It helps in keeping control over prey population.
(c) It helps in maintaining species diversity in a community.
(d) All of these.

**183.** Biological control methods in agriculture pest control is mainly based on which biological interaction
(a) Predation (b) Parasitism
(c) Commensalism (d) Mutualism

**184.** The prickly pear cactus introduced into Australia caused havoc by rapid spreading in rangeland, finally this cactus brought under control by
(a) Predator moth
(b) Predator butterfly
(c) Predator deer
(d) Predator helminth

**185.** Predators are prudent in nature because
(a) It overexploit its prey
(b) It is too efficient in predation
(c) They do not over exploit their prey
(d) All of these

**186.** Following example best represent the maintenance of species diversity by predation.
(a) Spreading of cactus in rangeland of Australia.
(b) Removal of *Pisaster* fishes from rocky intertidal communities of the American Pacific Coast in field experiment lead to extinction of more than 10 invertebrate species within a year.
(c) Exclusion of Cathamalus by Balanus in intertidal area in Connell's elegant field experiment.
(d) All of these.

**187.** Cryptical coloration to camouflage is found in
(a) Some insect species (b) Frogs
(c) Both of these (d) None of these

**188.** Monarch butterfly is highly distasteful because of chemical which acquired by butterfly in which stage of its life cycle by feeding on poisonous weed
(a) Adult (b) Caterpillar
(c) Pupa (d) Nymph

**189.** Development of thorns in Acacia is ______means of defense
(a) Physiological (b) Behavioral
(c) Morphological (d) None of these

## Competition

**190.** Who propose competitive exclusion principle?
(a) Gause (b) Robert May
(c) Darwin (d) Von Humbolt

**191.** Abingdon tortoise in Galapagos Islands became extinct within a decade after _____ were introduced on the island, because of the greater browsing efficiency of introduced animal.
(a) Cow (b) Buffaloes
(c) Goat (d) Camel

**192.** A species whose distribution is restricted to a small geographical area because of the presence of a competitive superior species is found to expand its distributional range dramatically when the competing species is experimentally removed. This phenomenon is known as
(a) Competitive exclusion
(b) Competitive release
(c) Interference competition
(d) Resource partitioning

**193.** Who showed that five closely related species of warblers living on the same tree were able to avoid competition and co-exist due to behavioral differences in their forging activities?
(a) Connell (b) Mc Arthur
(c) Gause (d) Darwin

**194.** In general, which of the following appears to be more adversely affected by competition?
(a) Herbivores (b) Plants
(c) Carnivores (d) Both (a) and (b)

**195.** Gause's competitive exclusion principle states that
(a) Two unrelated species competing for the same resources cannot co-exist indefinitely and competitively inferior one will eliminated eventually.
(b) Two closely related species competing for the same resources cannot co-exist indefinitely and competitively inferior one will eliminated eventually.
(c) Two unrelated species competing for the same resources can co-exist indefinitely and can grow together.
(d) Two closely related species competing for the same resources can co-exist indefinitely and can grow together.

**196.** Connell's elegant field experiments showed that on rocky sea coasts of Scotland, the larger and competitively superior barnacle _______ dominates the intertidal area, and exclude smaller barnacle _______ from that zone
(a) Chathamalus, Balanus
(b) Balanus, Balanus
(c) Chathamalus, chhathamalus
(d) Balanus, Chathamalus

**197.** According to Darwin which competition is a potent force of in organic evolution?
(a) Inter specific (b) Intra specific
(c) Both (a) and (b) (d) None of these

**198.** In some shallow South American lakes, which of the following compete for the same food that is zooplanktons of lake?
(a) Visiting flamingoes (b) Resident fishes
(c) Both (a) and (b) (d) None of these

**199.** Find out true statement
(a) Totally unrelated species could also compete for the same resources.
(b) Resources need not to be limiting for competition to occur.
(c) In interference competition, feed efficiency of one species might be reduced due to the interfering and inhibitory presence of the other species, even if resources are abundant.
(d) All are true.

**200.** Select set of correct statements regarding competition:
(A) Interspecific competition is a potent force in organic evolution.
(B) Totally unrelated species could also compete for the same resource.
(C) Resources need not be limiting for competition to occur;
(D) Competition is a process in which the fitness of one species is significantly lower in the presence of another species.
(a) A, B and D (b) A, B and C
(c) B, C and D (d) A, B, C and D

**201.** Read following sentences.
**Statement I:** The Abingdon tortoise in Galapagos Islands became extinct within a decade after goats were introduced on the island.
**Statement II:** on the rocky sea coasts of Scotland, the larger and competitively superior barnacle Balanus dominates the intertidal area, and excludes the smaller barnacle Chathamalus from that zone.
(a) Statement I is incorrect but statement II is true.
(b*)Both Statements I and II are true
(c) Both Statements I and II are false
(d) Statement I is correct but statement II is false

**202.** Read following sentences.
**Statement I:** species facing competition might evolve mechanisms that promote co-existence rather than exclusion.
**Statement II:** If two species compete for the same resource, the competition can be avoided by resource partitioning'.
(a) Statement I is incorrect but statement II is true.
(b) Both Statements I and II are true
(c) Both Statements I and II are false
(d) Statement I is correct but statement II is false

## Parasitism

**203.** Which of the following are adaptations of parasite?
(a) Loss of unnecessary sense organ
(b) Loss of digestive system
(c) High reproductive capacity
(d) All of the above

**204.** Liver fluke belongs to class
(a) Cestoda (b) Trematoda
(c) Hirudeneria (d) Turbelleria

**205.** Liver fluke complete its cycle in how many intermediate hosts?
(a) 1 (b) 2
(c) 3 (d) 4

**206.** Human liver fluke has two intermediate hosts in its life cycle, these are
(a) Snail and Hydra
(b) Crustacean and fish
(c) Snail and fish
(d) Mosquito and Snail

**207.** Effect of parasite on host
(a) Reduce survival
(b) Reduce growth and reproduction
(c) Reduce its population density
(d) All of the above

**208.** Malaria parasites require which vector to spread to other hosts
(a) Snail (b) Fish
(c) Housefly (d) Mosquito

**209.** Following are correct example of ectoparasite
(a) Lice on humans
(b) Ticks on dogs
(c) Copepods on marine fishes
(d) All are correct

**210.** Cuscuta, a parasitic plant that is commonly found growing on hedge plants has lost its _______ and _______ in the course of evolution
(a) Root and stem
(b) leaves and chlorophyll
(c) Root and leaves
(d) Leaves and stem

**211.** Female mosquito require our blood for
(a) Respiration (b) Locomotion
(c) Digestion (d) reproduction

**212.** Which of the following is not parasite?
(a) Tapeworm
(b) Female anopheles mosquito
(c) Liver fluke
(d) Lice

**213.** Find out false statement
(a) Parasite that feeds on the external surface of the host organism are called ectoparasite.
(b) The life cycle of endoparasites are more complex because of their extreme specialization.
(c) Parasitism evolved in so many taxonomic groups from plants to higher vertebrates.
(d) Endoparasites have greatly complex morphological and anatomical feature along with high reproductive potential.

**214.** Example of brood parasitism
(a) Cuckoo (koel) and Crow
(b) Crow and Parrot
(c) Parrot and Piegon
(d) Koel and Parrot

**215.** Find out incorrect statement
(a) In brood parasitism (of Koel and Crow), the eggs of parasitic bird have evolved to resemble the host's egg in size and color to reduce the chance of the host bird detecting the foreign eggs and ejecting them from the host.
(b) Majority of parasite harming the host.
(c) Many parasites have evolved to be host specific in such a way that both host and the parasite tend to co-evolve.
(d) Monarch butterfly require chemical by feeding on a poisonous weed in its adult stage, that chemical make it high distasteful to its bird.

**216.** Adaptations found in parasites are
(A) the loss of unnecessary sense organs,
(B) presence of adhesive organs or suckers
(C) complex digestive system
(D) low reproductive capacity
(a) B and D (b) A and B
(c) A, C and D (d) B and D

**217.** A trematode parasite, liver fluke is parasite in
(A) a human
(B) a snail
(C) a fish
(a) A and B (b) A and C
(c) B and C (d) A, B and C

**218.** Endoparasites live inside the host body in
(A) liver
(B) kidney
(C) lungs
(D) red blood cells
(a) B and D (b) A and C
(c) B, C and D (d) A, B, C and D

**219.** Select set of correct statements about endoparasites:
(a) Endoparasites often have more complex life cycles compared to free-living organisms
(b) Endoparasites have evolved specific adaptations to exploit their host organisms efficiently
(c) The morphological and anatomical features of endoparasites are often simplified.
(d) Since the primary goal of an endoparasite is to reproduce and complete its life cycle within the host, there is a significant emphasis on reproductive potential.
(a) B and D (b) A and C
(c) B, C and D (d) A, B, C and D

**220.** **Assertion:** The female mosquito is considered a parasite in human
**Reason:** It needs human blood for reproduction.
(a) (A) is false but (R) is true
(b) Both (A) and (R) are true and (R) is the correct explanation of (A)

(c) Both (A) and (R) are true but (R) is not the correct explanation of (A)
(d) (A) is true but (R) is false.

**221.** Select set of incorrect statements regarding parasitism:
(A) Many marine fish are infested with endoparasitic copepods.
(B) The female mosquito is a parasite in human
(C) The life cycles of endoparasites are simple because they are residing inside the host
(D) Brood parasitism in birds is an example of parasitism
(a) B, C and D
(b) A and C
(c) A, B and C
(d) A, C and D

## Commensalism and Mutualism

**222.** Which of the following shows commensalism?
(a) Sea anemone and clown fish
(b) Lichens
(c) Lice and human
(d) Mycorrhizae

**223.** Commensalism is shown by all except
(a) Orchid on mango branch
(b) Cattle egret and grazing cattle
(c) Sea anemone and clown fish
(d) Cuckoo (Koel) and crow

**224.** Lichens are mutualistic relationship between
(a) Fungus and photosynthetic algae
(b) Fungus and cyanobacteria
(c) Fungus and roots of higher plants
(d) Both (a) and (b)

**225.** Barnacles growing on the back of a whale are example of
(a) Predation
(b) Parasitism
(c) Commensalism
(d) Mutualism

**226.** Stinging tentacles are found in
(a) Clown fish
(b) Lichens
(c) Sea anemone
(d) Egrets

**227.** Mycorrhizae are association between
(a) Fungus and photosynthetic algae
(b) Fungus and roots of higher plants
(c) Fungus and cyanobacteria
(d) Fig plant and wasp

**228.** What is function of fungus in mycorrhizae
(a) Absorption of nutrient from soil
(b) Provide energy yielding substrate to plant
(c) Provide ATP to plant
(d) All of these

**229.** Pseudo copulation helps in pollination in
(a) Fig plant
(b) Orchid
(c) Cuscuta
(d) Sunflower

**230.** Best example of co-evolution
(a) Fig trees and pollinator species of wasp
(b) Fungus and cyanobacteria
(c) Sea anemone and clown fish
(d) All of them

**231.** Fruit of fig species provide
(a) Egg laying site to female wasp for oviposition
(b) Developing seed as food for the developing wasp larvae
(c) Both (a) and (b)
(d) None of these

**232.** Select incorrect statement
(a) The Mediterranean orchid ophrys employs sexual deceit to get pollinated
(b) In mycorrhazial association fungi help the plant in the absorption of essential nutrients from the soil
(c) Pinus seeds cannot germinate and establish without the presence of mycorrhizae
(d) When resources are unlimited, the growth is usually logistic but when resources become progressively limiting, the growth pattern turns exponential

**233.** In Ophrys, one petal of female flower bears an uncanny resemblance to the female of the been in which of the following aspect
(a) Size (b) Color
(c) Markings (d) All

**234.** Plant offer following reward pollinators
(a) Pollen
(b) Nectar
(c) Juicy or nutritious fruit
(d) Any or all of these

**235.** Lichens are the associations of:
(a) Bacteria and fungus
(b) Algae and bacterium
(c) Fungus and algae
(d) Fungus and virus

**236.** Which plant is pollinated by below insect?

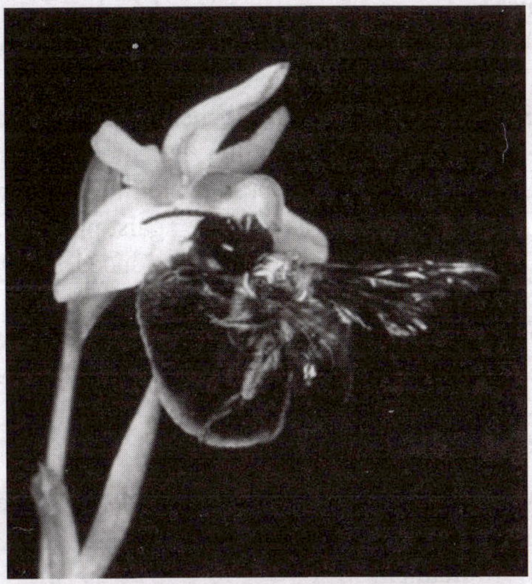

(a) Orchid flower (b) Fig flower
(c) Sunflower (d) Lotus flower

**237.** Below diagram represent which flower?

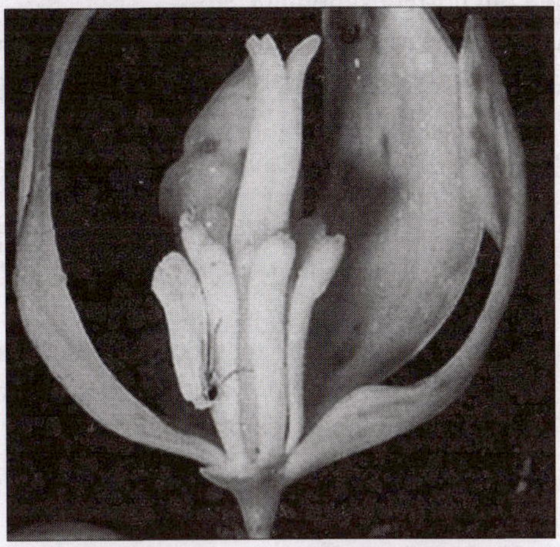

(a) Orchid flower (b) Fig flower
(c) Sunflower (d) Rose flower

**238.** Below diagram shows some insect laying eggs in fruit of figure? Find out insects from the following?

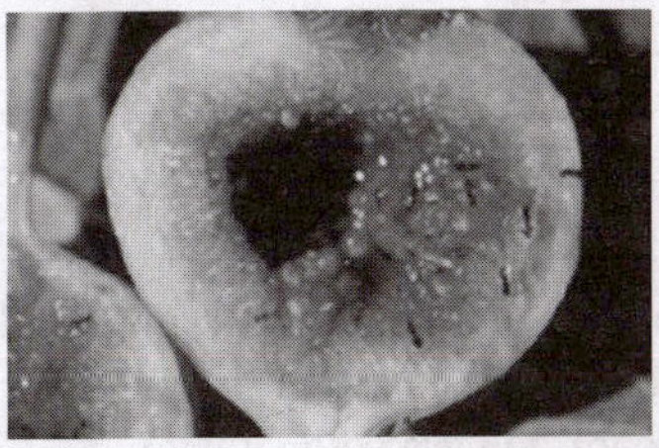

(a) Wasp (b) Female anopheles
(c) Culex (d) Honeybee

**239.** Which of the following is not example of commesalism:
(a) An orchid growing on a mango branch
(b) barnacles growing on the whale
(c) The cattle egret and grazing cattle
(d) crow and cuckoo

**240.** Select set of correct statements:
(A) Plants need the help of animals for pollination and seeds dispersal.
(B) the *mycorrhizae* are associations between fungi and the roots of higher plants.
(C) The female wasp uses the fruit for egg-laying as well as for nourishment
(D) The pollinator insects for orchids are bees and bumblebees.
(a) B and D (b) A and C
(c) B, C and D (d) A, B, C and D

## Plant interactions

**241.** Read following sentences.
**Statement I:** For any species, the minimal requirement is one more species on which it can feed.
**Statement II:** A plant species, which makes its own food can survive alone.
(a) Statement I is incorrect but statement II is true.
(b) Both Statements I and II are true
(c) Both Statements I and II are false
(d) Statement I is correct but statement II is false

**242.** Read following sentences.
**Statement I:** Interspecific interactions arise from the interaction of populations of two different species.
**Statement II:** They could be beneficial, detrimental or neutral to one of the species or both.
(a) Statement I is incorrect but statement II is true.
(b) Both Statements I and II are true
(c) Both Statements I and II are false
(d) Statement I is correct but statement II is false

**243.** Select set of correct statements:
(A) In parasitism only parasite is benefitted.
(B) In predation, the interaction is detrimental to the prey.
(C) The interaction where one species is benefitted and the other is neither benefitted nor harmed is called amensalism.
(D) In predation, parasitism and commensalism, the interacting species live closely together.
(a) A, B and D (b) A, B and C
(c) B, C and D (d) B and D only

**244.** Role of predators are:
(A) 'conduits' for energy transfer across trophic levels
(B) keep prey populations under control
(C) maintain species diversity in a community
(D) biological control of exotic, invasive and widespread species
(a) A, B and D (b) A, B and C
(c) B, C and D (d) A, B, C and D

**245.** Defence mechanisms by preys include:
(A) Camouflage
(B) distastefulness
(C) Thorns
(D) certain chemical production
(a) A, B and D (b) A, B and C
(c) B, C and D (d) A, B, C and D

**246.** Select set of correct statements:
(A) Predation is nature's way of transferring the energy fixed by plants to lower trophic levels.
(B) animals eating plants are herbivores, and can not be called as predators.
(C) predators act as 'conduits' for energy transfer across trophic Levels.
(D) Biological control methods adopted in agricultural pest control are based on the ability of the predator to regulate prey population.
(a) A, B and D (b) A, B and C
(c) B, C and D (d) C and D only

**247.** **Assertion:** predators in nature are 'prudent'.
**Reason:** overexploitation of its prey may lead to extinction of prey and followed by extinction of the predator itself.
(a) (A) is false but (R) is true
(b) Both (A) and (R) are true and (R) is the correct explanation of (A)
(c) Both (A) and (R) are true but (R) is not the correct explanation of (A)
(d) (A) is true but (R) is false.

**248.** **Assertion:** cattle or goats do not browse on Calotropis plant.
**Reason:** The plant produces highly poisonous cardiac glycosides as a defense mechanism.
(a) (A) is false but (R) is true
(b) Both (A) and (R) are true and (R) is the correct explanation of (A)
(c) Both (A) and (R) are true but (R) is not the correct explanation of (A)
(d) (A) is true but (R) is false.

**249.** Plants therefore have evolved an astonishing variety of morphological and chemical defences against herbivores. Select set of correct statements regarding this:
(A) weed Calotropis produces thorns as morphological means of defence.
(B) Many plants produce chemicals that make the herbivore sick when they are eaten.
(C) Acacia and Cactus produce highly poisonous cardiac glycosides as defence agaist predators.
(D) nicotine and caffeine are produced by plants as defences against grazers and browsers.
(a) B and D (b) A and C
(c) B, C and D (d) C and D

## Miscellaneous

**250.** In which of the following interaction only one of the species benefited
(a) Mutualism
(b) Competition
(c) Parasitism and Predation
(d) Amensalism

**251.** Find out correct statement
(a) Under particular set of selection progresses, organism evolve towards the most efficient reproductive strategy.
(b) In amensalism one species is harmed where as other is benefited.
(c) Some species of insects and frogs are cryptically colored (Camouflaged) to avoid being detected easily by the prey.
(d) 'Biological Control' methods adopted in agricultural pest control are based on the ability of the prey to regulate predator population.

**252.** Amensalism is an association between two species where:
(a) One species is harmed and other is benefitted
(b) One species is harmed and other is unaffected
(c) One species is benefitted and other is unaffected
(d) Both the species are harmed

**253.** Example of hyper parasite is
(a) *Pasteurella pestis*
(b) Rat flea
(c) Lice
(d) Plasmodium

**254.** Study the four statements (1-4) given below and select the two correct ones out of them.
(A) Ticks of dog are ectoparasite
(B) Orchid is an epiphyte
(C) Female anopheles is parasite on human
(D) Predator in nature is not prudent

(a) (B) and (C) (b) (C) and (D)
(c) (A) and (D) (d) (A) and (B)

**255.** Malaria parasites require which vector to spread to other hosts
(a) Snail (b) Fish
(c) Housefly (d) Mosquito

**256.** Which of the following is an incorrect statement?
(a) The human liver fluke depends on two intermediate hosts to complete its life cycle.
(b) The malarial parasite needs vector (mosquito to spread to other host).
(c) Parasites that feed on external surface of the host organism are called endoparasites.
(d) *Cuscuta* derives its nutrition from the host plant which it parasitizes.

**257.** Read the following statements regarding adaptation and choose the correct option.
(i) Many xerophytic plants have thick cuticle on leaf epidermis sunken stomata to prevent transpiration.
(ii) Some xerophytic plants have special photosynthetic pathway (CAM) that enables their stomata close during day.
(iii) Opuntia, have no leaves, they are reduced to spines.
(iv) All adaptation is genetically fixed in all organisms.
(v) Desert lizard has physiological ability to control its body temperature
(a) (i), (ii) and (iii) are correct.
(b) Only (iv) is correct.
(c) (iv) and (v) are correct.
(d) All are correct.

**258.** Which statement defines the Allen's rule
(a) Aquatic mammals have blubber as insulator.
(b) Mammals of colder climate have shorter ears and limbs.
(c) Mammals of humid and warmer region have more melanin in their skin.
(d) The bears undergo hibernation during winter.

**259.** Select correct statement from the following
(a) Kangaroo rat is unable to concentrate urine.
(b) Plants have mechanism to maintain their internal temperature
(c) Organisms living in extreme environment have many biochemical adaptations
(d) Nearly 75% of the insects feeds on plant sap and other parts of plant.

## Multiple Choice Questions: Level II

**260.** Consider the following four statements (1-4) about desert, certain desert animals such as kangaroo rat.
(1) They have dark colour and high rate of reproduction and excrete solid urine.
(2) They do not drink water, breathe at a slow rate to conserve water and have their body covered with thick.
(3) They feed on dry seeds and do not require drinking water.
(4) They excrete very concentrated urine and do not use water to regulate body temperature.

Which two of the above statements for such animals are true?
(a) 3 and 1 (b) 1 and 2
(c) 3 and 4 (d) 2 and 3

**261.** Geometric representation of age structure is characteristic of
(a) population (b) landscape
(c) ecosystem (d) biotic community

**262.** The population of an insect species shows an explosive increase in numbers during rainy season followed by its disappearance at the end of the season. What does this show?
(a) the food plants mature and die at the end of the rainy season.
(b) its population growth curve is of J-type.
(c) the population of its predators increases enormously.
(d) S-shaped or sigmoid growth of this insect.

**263.** A high density of elephant population in an area can result in
(a) intra specific competition
(b) inter specific competition
(c) predation on one another
(d) mutualism.

**264.** Biological organization starts with
(a) cellular level
(b) organismic level
(c) atomic level
(d) submicroscopic molecular level

**265.** Choose the incorrect statement, for predator:
(a) Acts as medium for energy transfer.
(b) Keeps prey population under control.
(c) Maintain species diversity.
(d) Predators are imprudent in nature.

**266.** Praying mantis is a good example of
(a) warning colouration (b) social insects
(c) camouflage (d) mullerian mimicry

**267.** Barophilic prokaryotes:
(a) grow and multiply in very deep marine sediments.
(b) occur in water containing high concentrations of barium hydroxide.
(c) readily grow and divide in sea water enriched in any soluble salt of barium.
(d) grow slowly in highly alkaline frozen lakes at high altitudes.

**268.** Animals have the innate ability to escape from predation. Examples for the same are given below. Select the incorrect example.
(a) Colour change in chameleon.
(b) Enlargement of body size by swallowing air in puffer fish.
(c) Poison fangs in snakes.
(d) Melanism in moths.

**269.** In which one of the following habitats does the diurnal temperature of soil surface vary most?
(a) Shrub land (b) Forest
(c) Desert (d) Grassland

**270.** The maximum growth rate occurs in
(a) Stationary phase (b) Senescent phase
(c) Lag phase (d) Exponential phase

**271.** In a population unrestricted reproductive capacity is called as
(a) biotic potential (b) fertility
(c) carrying capacity (d) birth rate

**272.** Cause of mimicry is
(a) concealment (b) attack (offence)
(c) protection (defence) (d) both (a) and (c)

**273.** An interesting modification of flower shape for insect pollination occurs in some orchids in which a male insect mistakes the pattern on the orchid flower for the female of his species and tries to copulate with it, thereby pollinating the flower. This phenomenon is called
(a) Mimicry (b) Pseudopollination
(c) Pseudocopulation (d) Pseudoparthenocarpy

**274.** What is the most important factor for the success of animal population?
(a) Natality
(b) Unlimited food
(c) Adaptability
(d) Inter-species activity

**275.** In increasing order of organizational complexity which one of the following is the correct sequence?
(a) Population, species, community, ecosystem
(b) Population, variety, species, ecosystem
(c) Population, ecosystem, species, community
(d) Species, variety, ecosystem, community

**276.** Desert plants are generally
(a) Viviparous (b) succulent
(c) herbaceous (d) heterophyllus

**277.** Which of the following does not have stomata?
(a) hydrophytes
(b) mesophytes
(c) xerophytes
(d) submerged hydrophytes

**278.** Sunken stomata is the characteristic feature of
(a) hydrophyte (b) mesophyte
(c) xerophyte (d) halophyte

**279.** Which of the following pairs is correctly matched?
(a) uricotelism – aquatic habitat
(b) parasitism – intra-specific relationship
(c) excessive perspiration – xeric adaptation
(d) stream-lined body – aquatic adaptation

**280.** People living at sea level have around 5 million RBC per cubic millimetre of their blood, whereas those living at an altitude of 5400 meters have around 8 million. This is because at high altitude
(a) atmospheric $O_2$ level is less and hence more RBCs are needed to absorb the required amount of $O_2$ to survive.
(b) there is more UV radiation which enhances RBC production.
(c) people eat more nutritive food, therefore more RBCs are formed.
(d) people get pollution-free air to breathe more oxygen is available.

**281.** Xeric environment is characterized by
(a) Precipitation
(b) Low atmospheric humidity
(c) Extremes of temperature
(d) High rate of vapourization

**282.** Animals that can tolerate a narrow range of salinity are
(a) Stenohaline (b) Euryhaline
(c) Anadromous (d) Catadromous

**283.** Largest amount of fresh water is found in
(a) Lakes and streams
(b) Underground
(c) Polar ice and glaciers
(d) Rivers

**284.** Study of inter-relationships between organisms and their environment is
(a) Ecology (b) Ecosystem
(c) Phytogeography (d) Ethology

**285.** The sum total of the populations of the same kind of organism constitute
(a) Colony (b) Genus
(c) Community (d) Species

**286.** Soil best suited for plant growth is
(a) Clay (b) Loam
(c) Sandy (d) Gravel

**287.** Association of animals when both partners are benefitted
(a) Colony
(b) Mutualism
(c) Commensalism
(d) Amensalism

**288.** A fertile agriculture soil appears deep coloured at the surface as compared to soil one metre down. The reason for colour of top soil is
(a) More moisture
(b) Rich in organic matter
(c) Rich in iron, calcium and magnesium
(d) Recent formation

**289.** Soil particle determine its
(a) Texture
(b) Field capacity
(c) Water holding capacity
(d) Soil flora

**290.** Homeostasis is
(a) Tendency of biological system to change with change in environment.
(b) Tendency of biological systems to resist change.
(c) Disturbance of self-regulatory system and natural controls.
(d) Biotic material used in homeopathic medicines.

**291.** Which one is true?
(a) Commensalism when none of the interacting population affects each other.
(b) Symbiosis when the interaction is useful to both the populations.
(c) Symbiosis when neither population affect each other.
(d) Commensalism when the interaction is useful to both the populations.

**292.** Pedology is science of
(a) Earth (b) Soil
(c) Diseases (d) Pollution

**293.** Competition for light, nutrients and space is most severe between
(a) Closely related organism growing in different niches.
(b) Closely related organisms growing in the same area/niche.
(c) Distantly related organisms growing in the same habitat.
(d) Distantly related organisms growing in different niches.

**294.** A mutually beneficial association necessary for survival of both partners is
(a) Mutualism/Symbiosis.
(b) Commensalism.
(c) Amensalism.
(d) Both A and B.

## A & R and Statement-based Questions

### Assertion and Reason questions:

***Direction for questions 295 to 299:*** *Read the* ***assertion*** *and* ***reason*** *carefully to mark the correct option out of the options given below:*

**(a)** **(A)** is **true** but **(R)** is **false**.
**(b)** **(A)** is **false** but **(R)** is **true**.
**(c)** Both **(A)** and **(R)** is **true** and **(R)** is the correct explanation of **(A)**.
**(d)** Both **(A)** and **(R)** is **true** and **(R)** is not the correct explanation of **(A)**.

**295. Assertion:** Ecology is basically concerned with four levels of biological organization, organism, populations, communities and biomes.
**Reason:** Ecology is a subject which studies the interactions among organisms and between the organism and its physical environment.

**296. Assertion:** Mammals from colder climates generally have shorter ears and limbs.
**Reason:** It is to maximize the heat loss.

**297. Assertion:** Temperature is the most ecologically relevant environmental factor.

**Reason:** Temperature affects the kinetics of enzyme.

**298. Assertion:** Photosynthesis is an essential life process of plants.

**Reason:** Small plants growing in forest are adapted to photosynthesis optimally under low light condition because they are over-shadowed by tall canopied trees.

**299. Assertion:** Any species growing exponentially can reach enormous population density in a shirt time.

**Reason:** Availability of unlimited resources makes it possible.

## Statement-based Questions:

***Direction for questions 300 to 304:** These type of questions consist of two statement each, printed as* **Statement-I** *and* **Statement-II**. *While answering such questions, a student is needed to choose any one of the following four responses.*

**(a)** **Statement I** is **correct Statement II** is **incorrect**.
**(b)** **Statement I** is **incorrect Statement II** is **correct**.
**(c)** Both **Statement I** and **Statement II** are **correct**.
**(d)** Both **Statement I** and **Statement II** are **incorrect**.

**300. Statement-I:** In both parasitism and predation interacting species live closely together.

**Statement-II:** Parasites and predators limit the population of their host species.

**301. Statement-I:** We maintain a constant body temperature to 37°C, in summer when outside temperature is more than our body temperature.

**Statement-II:** We sweat profusely in summer, which brings down the body temperature.

**302. Statement-I:** Desert lizards have physiological ability to main body temperature.

**Statement-II:** Desert lizards are warm blooded animals.

**303. Statement-I:** The size of a population for any species is not a static parameter.

**Statement-II:** It doesn't depend on food availability, predation pressure and adverse weather.

**304. Statement-I:** Immigration contributes to decrease in population.

**Statement-II:** Emigration contributes to increase in population.

## Matrix-Match Type Questions

**305.** Match the following:

| List-I (Water Body) | List-II (Salinity Parts/Thousand) |
|---|---|
| 1. Inland waters | (i) > 100 |
| 2. Sea | (ii) 5 |
| 3. Hypersaline lagoons | (iii) 30 – 35 |

**The correct matching is**

| | 1 | 2 | 3 |
|---|---|---|---|
| (a) | (ii) | (iii) | (i) |
| (b) | (iii) | (i) | (ii) |
| (c) | (i) | (iii) | (ii) |
| (d) | (ii) | (i) | (iii) |

**306.** Match the following:

| List-I | List-II |
|---|---|
| 1. Eurythermal | (i) Tolerant to wide range of salinity. |
| 2. Stenothermal | (ii) Tolerant to narrow range of salinity. |
| 3. Euryhaline | (iii) Tolerant to wide range of temperature. |
| 4. Stenohaline | (iv) Tolerant to narrow range of temperature. |

**The correct matching is**

| | 1 | 2 | 3 | 4 |
|---|---|---|---|---|
| (a) | (iii) | (iv) | (i) | (ii) |
| (b) | (i) | (iv) | (ii) | (iii) |
| (c) | (ii) | (iii) | (iv) | (i) |
| (d) | (iv) | (iii) | (i) | (ii) |

**307.** Match the following:

| List-I (Abiotic Factor) | List-II (Characteristics) |
|---|---|
| 1. Soil | (i) Salinity |
| 2. Light | (ii) Topography |
| 3. Water | (iii) Photoperiod |

**The correct matching is**

| | 1 | 2 | 3 |
|---|---|---|---|
| (a) | (ii) | (iii) | (i) |
| (b) | (ii) | (i) | (iii) |
| (c) | (i) | (iii) | (ii) |
| (d) | (iii) | (i) | (ii) |

**308.** Match the following:

| List-I (Organisms) | List-II (Responses to Unfavourable Environment) |
|---|---|
| 1. Bear | (i) Aestivation |
| 2. Snails & fish | (ii) Spores & seed formation |
| 3. Zooplankton species | (iii) Hibernation |
| 4. Plants | (iv) Diapause |

**The correct matching is**

| | 1 | 2 | 3 | 4 |
|---|---|---|---|---|
| (a) | (iii) | (i) | (iv) | (ii) |
| (b) | (iii) | (ii) | (iv) | (i) |
| (c) | (i) | (iv) | (iii) | (ii) |
| (d) | (ii) | (iv) | (i) | (iii) |

**309.** Match the following:

| I (Method) | II (Type) | III |
|---|---|---|
| 1. Regulation | (i) Physiological homeostasis | X. Temporary homeostasis (For short duration) |
| 2. Conformation | (ii) Behavioural homeostasis | Y. Lasting homeostasis (For long duration) |
| 3. Migration | | |
| 4. Suspension | | |

**The correct matching is**

(a) 1 – (i) – Y, 2 – (i) – Y, 3 – (ii) – X, 4 – (i) – X
(b) 1 – (ii) – X, 2 – (i) – X, 3 – (i) – Y, 4 – (i) – Y
(c) 1 – (i) – Y, 2 – (ii) – X, 3 – (ii) – Y, 4 – (i) – X
(d) 1 – (i) – Y, 2 – (i) – Y, 3 – (ii) – Z, 4 – (i) – X

## NCERT Exemplar Questions

**1.** Autecology is the
(a) Relation of heterogenous population to its environment
(b) Relation of an individual to its environment
(c) Relation of a community to its environment
(d) Relation of a biome to its environment

**2.** Ecotone is
(a) A polluted area
(b) The bottom of a lake
(c) A zone of transition between two communities
(d) A zone of developing community

**3.** Biosphere is
(a) A component in the ecosystem
(b) Composed of the plants present in the soil
(c) Life in the outer space
(d) Composed of all living organisms present on earth which interacts with the physical environment.

**4.** Ecological niche is
(a) The surface area of the ocean.
(b) An ecologically adapted zone.
(c) The physical position and functional role of a species within the community.
(d) Formed of all plants and animals living at the bottom of a lake.

**5.** According to Allen's Rule, the mammals from colder climates have
(a) Shorter ears and longer limbs
(b) Longer ears and shorter limbs
(c) Longer ears and longer limbs
(d) Shorter ears and shorter limbs

**6.** Salt concentration (Salinity) of the sea measured in parts per thousand is
(a) 10-15 (b) 30-70
(c) 0-5 (d) 30-35

**7.** Formation of tropical forests needs mean annual temperature and mean annual precipitation as
(a) 18-25°C and 150-400 cm
(b) 5-15°C and 50-100 cm
(c) 30-50°C and 100-150 cm
(d) 5-15°C and 100-200 cm

**8.** Which of the following forest plants controls the light conditions at the ground?
(a) Lianas and climbers
(b) Shrubs
(c) Tall trees
(d) Herbs

9. What will happen to a well growing herbaceous plant in the forest if it is transplanted outside the forest in a park?
   (a) It will grow normally.
   (b) It will grow well because it is planted in the same locality.
   (c) It may not survive because of the change in its micro climate.
   (d) It grows very well because the plant gets more sunlight.
10. If a population of 50 *Paramoecium* present in a pool increases to 150 after an hour, what would be the growth rate of population?
   (a) 50 per hour (b) 200 per hour
   (c) 5 per hour (d) 100 per hour
11. What would be the per cent growth or birth rate per individual per hour for the same population mentioned in the previous question?
   (a) 100 (b) 200
   (c) 50 (d) 150
12. A population has more young individuals compared to the older individuals. What would be the status of the population after some years?
   (a) It will decline
   (b) It will stabilize
   (c) It will increase
   (d) It will first decline and then stabilize
13. What parameters are used for the tiger census in our country's national parks and sanctuaries?
   (a) Pug marks only
   (b) Pug marks and faecal pellets
   (c) Faecal pellets only
   (d) Actual head counts
14. Which of the following would necessarily decrease the density of a population in a given habitat?
   (a) Natality > mortality
   (b) Immigration > emigration
   (c) Mortality and emigration
   (d) Natality and immigration
15. A protozoan reproduces by binary fission. What will be the number of protozoans in its population after six generations?
   (a) 128 (b) 24 (c) 64 (d) 32
16. In 2005, for each of the 14 million people present in a country, 0.028 were born and 0.008 died during the year. Using the exponential equation, the number of people present in 2015 is predicted as
   (a) 25 million (b) 17 million
   (c) 20 million (d) 18 million
17. Amensalism is an association between two species where
   (a) One species is harmed and other is benefitted.
   (b) One species is harmed and other is unaffected.
   (c) One species is benefitted and other is unaffected.
   (d) Both the species are harmed.
18. Lichens are the associations of
   (a) Bacteria and fungus
   (b) Algae and bacterium
   (c) Fungus and algae
   (d) Fungus and virus
19. Which of the following is a partial root parasite?
   (a) Sandal wood (b) Mistletoe
   (c) *Orobanche* (d) *Gonoderma*
20. Which one of the following organisms reproduces sexually only once in its life time?
   (a) Bamboo (b) Mango
   (c) Tomato (d) Eucalyptus

## Previous Years' Questions

1. Which one of the following is one of the characteristics of a biological community? [AIPMT 2010 PRE]
   (a) Stratification (b) Natality
   (c) Mortality (d) Sex-ratio
2. Which two of the following changes (1–4) usually tend to occur in the plain dwellers when they move to high altitudes (3,500 m or more)?
   (A) Increase in red blood cell size
   (B) Increase in red blood cell production
   (C) Increased breathing rate
   (D) Increase in thrombocyte count

   Changes occurring are: [AIPMT 2010 PRE]
   (a) (b) and (c) (b) (c) and (d)
   (c) (a) and (d) (d) (a) and (b)

**3.** The figure given below is a diagrammatic representation of response of organisms to abiotic factors. What do A, B and C represent, respectively?

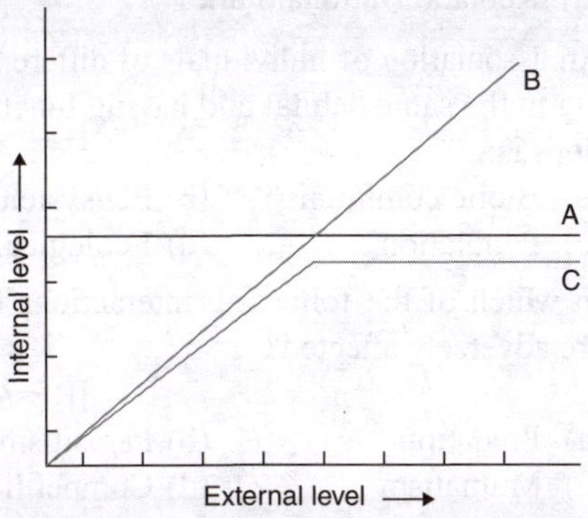


[AIPMT 2010 PRE]

(a) A: Conformer, B: Regulator, C: Partial regulator
(b) A: Regulator, B: Partial, C: Conformer regulator
(c) A: Partial, B: Regulator, C: Conformer regulator
(d) A: Regulator, B: Conformer, C: Partial regulator

**4.** Study the four statements (1–4) given below and select the two correct ones out of them.
(A) A lion eating a deer and a sparrow feeding on grain are ecologically similar in being consumers
(B) Predator starfish Pisaster helps in maintaining species diversity of some invertebrates
(C) Predators ultimately lead to the extinction of prey species
(D) Production of chemicals such as nicotine, strychnine by the plants are metabolic disorders The two correct statements are [AIPMT 2010 PRE]

(a) (B) and (c)
(b) (c) and (d)
(c) (A) and (d)
(d) (a) and (b)

**5.** Which one of the following is most appropriately defined? [AIPMT 2010 MAINS]
(a) Host is an organism which provides food to another organism
(b) Amensalism is a relationship in which one species is benefitted, whereas the other is unaffected
(c) Predator is an organism that catches and kills other organism for food
(d) Parasite is an organism which always lives inside the body of other organism and may kill it

**6.** Which one of the following is categorized as a parasite in its true sense? [AIPMT 2011 PRE]
(a) Human foetus developing inside the uterus draws nourishment from the mother
(b) Head louse living on the human scalp as well as laying eggs on human hair
(c) The cuckoo (koel) lays its eggs in crow's nest
(d) The female Anopheles bites and sucks blood from humans

**7.** What type of human population is represented by the following age pyramid?

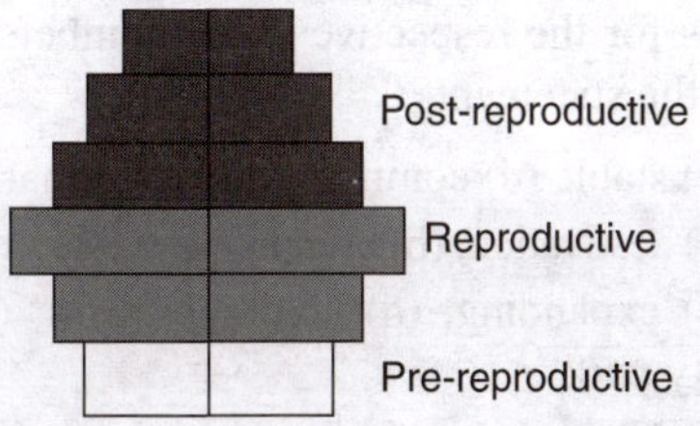


[AIPMT 2011 PRE]

(a) Stable population
(b) Declining population
(c) Expanding population
(d) Vanishing population

**8.** Consider the following four conditions (A-D) and select the correct pair out of them as adaptation to environment in desert lizards.

**The conditions:**

(A) Burrowing in soil to escape high temperature
(B) Losing heat rapidly from the body during high temperature
(C) Bask in sun when temperature is low
(D) Insulating body due to thick fatty dermis [AIPMT 2011 PRE]

(a) (a) and (c) (b) (b) and (d)
(c) (a) and (b) (d) (c) and (d)

**9.** The logistic population growth is expressed by the equation: [AIPMT 2011 MAINS]

(a) $dt/dN = Nr\left(\frac{K-N}{K}\right)$

(b) $dN/dt = rN\left(\frac{K-N}{K}\right)$

(c) $dN/dt = rN$

(d) $dN/dt = rN\left(\frac{N-K}{N}\right)$

**10.** Consider the following statements (A-D) each with one or two blanks. [AIPMT 2011 MAINS]

(A) Bears go into __(a)__ during winter to __(b)__ cold weather.

(B) A conical age pyramid with a broad base represents __(c)__ human population.

(C) A wasp pollinating a fig flower is an example of __(d)__.

(D) An area with high levels of species richness is known as __(e)__.

Which one of the following options, gives the correct fill ups for the respective blank numbers from (a) to (d) in the statements?

(a) (c) stable (d) commensalism, (e) marsh

(b) (a) aestivation, (b) escape, (c) stable, (d) mutualism

(c) (c) expanding, (d) commensalism, (e) biodiversity park

(d) (a) hibernation, (b) escape, (c) expanding (e) hot spot

**11.** People who have migrated from the planes to an area adjoining Rohtang Pass about six months back: [AIPMT 2012 PRE]

(a) Have more RBCs and their haemoglobin has a lower binding affinity to $O_2$

(b) Are not physically fit to play games like football

(c) Suffer from altitude sickness with symptoms like nausea, fatigue, etc.

(d) Have the usual RBC count but then haemoglobin has very high binding affinity to $O_2$

**12.** Cuscuta is an example of: [AIPMT 2012 MAINS]

(a) Brood parasitism (b) Predation

(c) Endoparasitism (d) Ectoparasitism

**13.** A sedentary sea anemone gets attached to the shell lining of hermit crab. The association is: [AIPMT 2013]

(a) Ectoparasitism (b) Symbiosis

(c) Commensalism (d) Amensalism

**14.** A biologist studied the population of eats in a barn. He found that the average natality was 250, average mortality 240, immigration 20 and emigration 30. The net increase in population is: [AIPMT 2013]

(a) 10 (b) 15

(c) 05 (d) Zero

**15.** Just as a person moving from Delhi to Shimla to escape the heat for the duration of hot summer, thousands of migratory birds from Siberia and other extremely cold northern regions move to: [AIPMT 2014]

(a) Western Ghat

(b) Meghalaya

(c) Corbett National Park

(d) Keolado National Park

**16.** An association of individuals of different species living in the same habitat and having functional interactions is: [RE-AIPMT 2015]

(a) Biotic community (b) Ecosystem

(c) Population (d) Ecological niche

**17.** In which of the following interactions both partners are adversely affected? [RE-AIPMT 2015]

(a) Predation (b) Parasitism

(c) Mutualism (d) Competition

**18.** The following graph depicts changes in two populations (A and B) of herbivore in a grassy field. A possible reason for these changes is that : [AIPMT 2015]

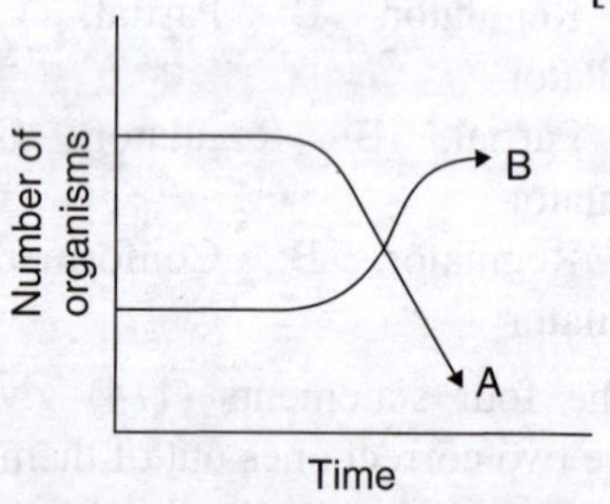


(a) Both plant populations in this habitat decreased.

(b) Population B compound more successfully for food than populations A.

(c) Population A produced more offspring than population B.

(d) Population A consumed the members of population B.

**19.** Leaves become modified into spines in [AIPMT 2015]

(a) Opuntia (b) Pea

(c) Onion (d) Skin cotton

**20.** The principle of competitive exclusion was stated by [NEET 2016 – PHASE II]

(a) G. F. Gause (b) MacArthur

(c) Verhuist and Pearl (d) C. Darwin

**21.** If '+' sign is assigned to beneficial interaction, '-' sign to detrimental and '0' sign to neutral interaction, then the population interaction represent by '+' '-' refers to [NEET 2016 – PHASE II]

(a) Amensalism (b) Commensalism

(c) Parasitism (d) Mutualism

**22.** Which of the following is correct for reselected species? [NEET 2016 – PHASE II]

(a) Large number of progeny with large size
(b) Small number of progeny with small size
(c) Small number of progeny with large size
(d) Large number of progeny with small size

**23.** It is much easier for a small animal to run uphill than for large animals, because: [NEET 2016 – PHASE I]
(a) It is easier to carry a small body weight
(b) Smaller animals have higher metabolic rate
(c) Small animals have lower $O_2$ requirement
(d) The efficiency of muscles in large animals is less than in the small animals

**24.** When does the growth rate of a population follow the logistic model equal zero? The logistic model is given as dN/dt = rN(1-N/K): [NEET 2016 – PHASE I]
(a) When N/K is exactly one
(b) When N nears the carrying capacity of the habitat
(c) When N/K equals zero
(d) When death rate is greater than birth rate

**25.** Gause's principle of competitive exclusion states that: [NEET 2016 – PHASE I]
(a) More abundant species will exclude the less abundant species through competition.
(b) Competition for the same resources excludes species having different food preferences.
(c) No two species can occupy the same niche indefinitely for the same limiting resources.
(d) Larger organisms exclude smaller ones through competition.

**26.** In a hypothetical population of 100 individual having 'r' = 0.5/female/year, what will be the population size in 6 years (with e = 2.72) showing exponential rate of growth? [NEET Regional 2017 ]
(a) 448 (b) 1218
(c) 739 (d) 2012

**27.** Asymptote in a logistic growth curve is obtained when [NEET 2017]
(a) K = N
(b) K > N
(c) K < N
(d) The value of 'r' approaches zero

**28.** Mycorrhizae are the example of: [NEET 2017]
(a) Amensalism (b) Antibiosis
(c) Mutualism (d) Fungistasis

**29.** Natality refers to [NEET 2018]
(a) Death rate
(b) Number of individuals leaving the habitat
(c) Birth rate
(d) Number of individuals entering a habitat

**30.** Which one of the following population interactions is widely used in medical science for the production of antibiotics? [NEET 2018]
(a) Commensalism (b) Parasitism
(c) Mutualism (d) Amensalism

**31.** In a growing population of a country, [NEET 2018]
(a) Pre-reproductive individuals are more than the reproductive individuals.
(b) Reproductive and pre-reproductive individuals are equal in number.
(c) Reproductive individuals are less than post-reproductive individuals.
(d) Pre-reproductive individuals are less than reproductive individuals.

**32.** Secondary metabolites such as nicotine, strychnine and caffeine are produced by plants for their: [NEET 2020]
(a) Nutritive value (b) Growth response
(c) Defence action (d) Effect on reproduction

**33.** Which of the following is **not** an attribute of a population? [NEET 2020]
(a) Sex ratio (b) Natality
(c) Mortality (d) Species interaction

**34.** In spite of interspecific competition in nature, which mechanism the competing species might have evolved for their survival? [NEET 2021]
(a) Predation (b) Resource partitioning
(c) Competitive release (d) Mutualism

**35.** Amensalism can be represented as [NEET 2021]
(a) Species A(+); Species B (0)
(b) Species A(–); Species B (0)
(c) Species A (+); Species B (+)
(d) Species A(–); Species B (–)

**36.** In the exponential growth equation, $N_t = N_0e^{rt}$, e represents: [NEET 2021]
(a) the base of geometric logarithms.
(b) the base of number logarithms.
(c) the base of exponential logarithms.
(d) the base of natural logarithms.

**37.** Match the following: [NEET 2021]

| List-I | List-II |
|---|---|
| 1. Allen's Rule | (i) Kangaroo rat |
| 2. Physiological adaptation | (ii) Desert lizard |
| 3. Behavioural adaptation | (iii) Marine fish at depth |
| 4. Biochemical adaptation | (iv) Polar seal |

**The correct matching is**

| | 1 | 2 | 3 | 4 |
|---|---|---|---|---|
| (a) | (iv) | (iii) | (ii) | (i) |
| (b) | (iv) | (ii) | (iii) | (i) |
| (c) | (iv) | (i) | (iii) | (ii) |
| (d) | (iv) | (i) | (ii) | (iii) |

**38.** **Assertion:** A person goes to high altitude and experiences 'altitude sickness' with symptoms like breathing difficulty and heart palpitations.

**Reason:** Due to low atmospheric pressure at high altitude, the body does not get sufficient oxygen. In the light of the above statements, Choose the correct answer from the options given below : [NEET 2021]

(a) (A) is false but (R) is true.
(b) Both (A) and (R) are true and (R) is the correct explanation of (A).
(c) Both (A) and (R) are true but (R) is not the correct explanation of (A).
(d) (A) is true but (R) is false.

**39.** Which one of the following statements cannot be connected to predation? [NEET 2022]

(a) It might lead to extinction of a species.
(b) Both the interacting species are negatively impacted.
(c) It is necessitated by nature to maintain the ecological balance.
(d) It helps in maintaining species diversity in a community.

**40.** While explaining interspecific interaction of population (+) sign is assigned for beneficial interaction, (–) sign is assigned for detrimental interaction and (0) for neutral interaction. Which of the following interactions can be assigned (+) for one species and (–) for another species involved in the interaction? [NEET 2022]

(a) Amensalism (b) Commensalism
(c) Competition (d) Predation

**41.** If '8' *Drosophila* in a laboratory population of '80' died during a week, the death rate in the population is_________individuals per *Drosophila* per week. [NEET 2022]

(a) 10 (b) 1.0
(c) zero (d) 0.1

**42.** Given below are two statements: [NEET 2023]

**Statement I:** Gause's 'Competitive Exclusion principle' states that two closely related species competing for the same resources cannot co-exist indefinitely inferior one will be eliminated eventually.

**Statement II:** In general, carnivores are more adversely affected by competition than herbivores.

(a) Both statement I and statement II are incorrect.
(b) Statement I is correct but statement II is incorrect.
(c) Statement I is incorrect but statement II is correct.
(d) Both statement I and statement II are correct.

**43.** Match List I with List II: [NEET 2023]

| List I (Interaction) | List II (Species A and B) |
|---|---|
| A. Mutualism | I. +(A), 0(B) |
| B. Commensalism | II. −(A), 0(B) |
| C. Amensalism | III. +(A),−(B) |
| D. Parasitism | IV. +(A), +(B) |

Choose the correct answer from the options given below:

(a) A-IV, B-I, C-II, D-III
(b) A-IV, B-III, C-I, D-II
(c) A-III, B-I, C-IV, D-II
(d) A-IV, B-II, C-I, D-III

**44.** Match List I with List II. [NEET 2023]

| List I (Interacting species) | List II (Name of Interaction) |
|---|---|
| A. A Leopard and a Lion in a forest / grassland | I. Competition |
| B. A Cuckoo laying eggs in a Crow's nest | II. Brood parasitism |
| C. Fungi and root of a higher plant in Mycorrhizae | III. Mutualism |
| D. A cattle egret and a Cattle in a field | IV. Commensalism |

Choose the correct answer from the options given below:

(a) A - I, B - II, C - IV, D - III
(b) A - III, B - IV, C - I, D - II
(c) A - II, B - III, C - I, D - IV
(d) A - I, B - II, C - III, D - IV

**45.** Match the list I with List II. [NEET 2023]

| List I | List II |
|---|---|
| A. Logistic growth | I. Unlimited resource availability condition |
| B. Exponential growth | II. Limited resource availability condition |

| | |
|---|---|
| C. Expanding age pyramid | III. The percent individuals of pre-reproductive age is largest followed by reproductive and post reproductive age groups |
| D. Stable age pyramid | IV. The percent individuals of pre-reproductive age groups are same |

Choose the correct answer from the options given below:

(a) A-II, B-III, C-I, D-IV
(b) A-II, B-IV, C-I, D-III
(c) A-II, B-IV, C-III, D-I
(d) A-II, B-I, C-III, D-IV

**46.** The equation of Verhulst-Pearl logistic growth is [NEET 2024]

$$\frac{dN}{dt} = rN\left[\frac{K-N}{K}\right]$$

From this equation, $K$ indicates:

(a) Intrinsic rate of natural increase
(b) Biotic potential
(c) Carrying capacity
(d) Population density

**47.** Given below are two statements: [NEET 2024]

**Statement I:** Gause's competitive exclusion principle states that two closely related species competing for different resources cannot exist indefinitely.

**Statement II:** According to Gause's principle during competition, the inferior will be eliminated. This may be true if resources are limiting.

In the light of the above statements, choose the correct answer from the options given below:

(a) Both statement I and statement II are true.
(b) Both statement I and statement II are false.
(c) Statement I is true but statement II is false.
(d) Statement I is false but statement II is true.

## Answer Key

### Multiple Choice Questions: Level I

| | | | | | | | | | |
|---|---|---|---|---|---|---|---|---|---|
| **1.** (c) | **2.** (b) | **3.** (b) | **4.** (d) | **5.** (c) | **6.** (c) | **7.** (b) | **8.** (d) | **9.** (d) | **10.** (d) |
| **11.** (d) | **12.** (b) | **13.** (c) | **14.** (c) | **15.** (c) | **16.** (b) | **17.** (d) | **18.** (d) | **19.** (b) | **20.** (b) |
| **21.** (b) | **22.** (d) | **23.** (b) | **24.** (d) | **25.** (b) | **26.** (b) | **27.** (a) | **28.** (a) | **29.** (b) | **30.** (b) |
| **31.** (b) | **32.** (d) | **33.** (b) | **34.** (a) | **35.** (d) | **36.** (b) | **37.** (a) | **38.** (d) | **39.** (a) | **40.** (c) |
| **41.** (d) | **42.** (b) | **43.** (c) | **44.** (a) | **45.** (a) | **46.** (b) | **47.** (d) | **48.** (b) | **49.** (c) | **50.** (b) |
| **51.** (c) | **52.** (c) | **53.** (a) | **54.** (d) | **55.** (b) | **56.** (c) | **57.** (a) | **58.** (b) | **59.** (d) | **60.** (c) |
| **61.** (b) | **62.** (d) | **63.** (b) | **64.** (d) | **65.** (c) | **66.** (c) | **67.** (b) | **68.** (c) | **69.** (a) | **70.** (d) |
| **71.** (d) | **72.** (b) | **73.** (d) | **74.** (c) | **75.** (c) | **76.** (c) | **77.** (b) | **78.** (d) | **79.** (c) | **80.** (c) |
| **81.** (a) | **82.** (c) | **83.** (b) | **84.** (a) | **85.** (b) | **86.** (a) | **87.** (c) | **88.** (a) | **89.** (c) | **90.** (d) |
| **91.** (b) | **92.** (c) | **93.** (d) | **94.** (d) | **95.** (c) | **96.** (b) | **97.** (c) | **98.** (b) | **99.** (d) | **100.** (c) |
| **101.** (b) | **102.** (b) | **103.** (a) | **104.** (b) | **105.** (b) | **106.** (a) | **107.** (d) | **108.** (d) | **109.** (b) | **110.** (c) |
| **111.** (d) | **112.** (b) | **113.** (a) | **114.** (d) | **115.** (b) | **116.** (d) | **117.** (c) | **118.** (d) | **119.** (c) | **120.** (b) |
| **121.** (c) | **122.** (a) | **123.** (d) | **124.** (d) | **125.** (b) | **126.** (c) | **127.** (d) | **128.** (c) | **129.** (c) | **130.** (c) |
| **131.** (c) | **132.** (b) | **133.** (b) | **134.** (c) | **135.** (a) | **136.** (c) | **137.** (d) | **138.** (b) | **139.** (a) | **140.** (c) |
| **141.** (b) | **142.** (c) | **143.** (b) | **144.** (d) | **145.** (d) | **146.** (d) | **147.** (d) | **148.** (a) | **149.** (c) | **150.** (c) |
| **151.** (d) | **152.** (b) | **153.** (a) | **154.** (a) | **155.** (c) | **156.** (c) | **157.** (c) | **158.** (b) | **159.** (c) | **160.** (c) |
| **161.** (b) | **162.** (b) | **163.** (c) | **164.** (b) | **165.** (b) | **166.** (b) | **167.** (b) | **168.** (b) | **169.** (c) | **170.** (d) |
| **171.** (c) | **172.** (d) | **173.** (d) | **174.** (d) | **175.** (a) | **176.** (d) | **177.** (c) | **178.** (d) | **179.** (b) | **180.** (d) |
| **181.** (c) | **182.** (d) | **183.** (a) | **184.** (a) | **185.** (c) | **186.** (b) | **187.** (c) | **188.** (b) | **189.** (c) | **190.** (a) |
| **191.** (c) | **192.** (b) | **193.** (b) | **194.** (d) | **195.** (b) | **196.** (d) | **197.** (a) | **198.** (c) | **199.** (d) | **200.** (d) |
| **201.** (b) | **202.** (b) | **203.** (d) | **204.** (b) | **205.** (b) | **206.** (c) | **207.** (d) | **208.** (d) | **209.** (d) | **210.** (b) |
| **211.** (d) | **211.** (b) | **213.** (d) | **214.** (a) | **215.** (d) | **216.** (b) | **217.** (d) | **218.** (d) | **219.** (d) | **220.** (a) |
| **221.** (c) | **222.** (a) | **223.** (d) | **224.** (d) | **225.** (c) | **226.** (c) | **227.** (b) | **228.** (a) | **229.** (b) | **230.** (a) |
| **231.** (c) | **232.** (d) | **233.** (d) | **234.** (d) | **235.** (c) | **236.** (a) | **237.** (b) | **238.** (a) | **239.** (d) | **240.** (d) |
| **241.** (d) | **242.** (b) | **243.** (a) | **244.** (d) | **245.** (d) | **246.** (d) | **247.** (b) | **248.** (b) | **249.** (a) | **250.** (c) |
| **251.** (a) | **252.** (b) | **253.** (a) | **254.** (d) | **255.** (d) | **256.** (c) | **257.** (a) | **258.** (b) | **259.** (c) | |

### Multiple Choice Questions: Level II

| | | | | | | | | | |
|---|---|---|---|---|---|---|---|---|---|
| **260.** (c) | **261.** (a) | **262.** (b) | **263.** (a) | **264.** (d) | **265.** (d) | **266.** (c) | **267.** (a) | **268.** (c) | **269.** (c) |
| **270.** (d) | **271.** (a) | **272.** (a) | **273.** (a) | **274.** (c) | **275.** (a) | **276.** (b) | **277.** (d) | **278.** (c) | **279.** (d) |
| **280.** (a) | **281.** (b) | **282.** (a) | **283.** (c) | **284.** (a) | **285.** (d) | **286.** (b) | **287.** (b) | **288.** (b) | **289.** (a) |
| **290.** (b) | **291.** (b) | **292.** (b) | **293.** (b) | **294.** (a) | | | | | |

### A & R and Statement-based Questions

| | | | | | | | | | |
|---|---|---|---|---|---|---|---|---|---|
| **295.** (d) | **296.** (a) | **297.** (c) | **298.** (d) | **299.** (c) | **300.** (a) | **301.** (c) | **302.** (d) | **303.** (a) | **304.** (d) |

### Matrix-Match Type Questions

| | | | | |
|---|---|---|---|---|
| **305.** (a) | **306.** (a) | **307.** (a) | **308.** (a) | **309.** (a) |

## NCERT Exemplar Questions

| | | | | | | | | | |
|---|---|---|---|---|---|---|---|---|---|
| **1.** (b) | **2.** (c) | **3.** (d) | **4.** (c) | **5.** (d) | **6.** (d) | **7.** (a) | **8.** (c) | **9.** (c) | **10.** (d) |
| **11.** (b) | **12.** (c) | **13.** (b) | **14.** (c) | **15.** (c) | **16.** (b) | **17.** (b) | **18.** (c) | **19.** (a) | **20.** (a) |

## Previous Years' Questions

| | | | | | | | | | |
|---|---|---|---|---|---|---|---|---|---|
| **1.** (a) | **2.** (a) | **3.** (d) | **4.** (d) | **5.** (c) | **6.** (b) | **7.** (b) | **8.** (a) | **9.** (b) | **10.** (d) |
| **11.** (a) | **12.** (d) | **13.** (b) | **14.** (d) | **15.** (d) | **16.** (a) | **17.** (d) | **18.** (b) | **19.** (a) | **20.** (a) |
| **21.** (c) | **22.** (d) | **23.** (b) | **24.** (a) | **25.** (c) | **26.** (d) | **27.** (a) | **28.** (c) | **29.** (c) | **30.** (d) |
| **31.** (a) | **32.** (c) | **33.** (d) | **34.** (b) | **35.** (b) | **36.** (d) | **37.** (d) | **38.** (b) | **39.** (b) | **40.** (d) |
| **41.** (d) | **42.** (b) | **43.** (a) | **44.** (d) | **45.** (d) | **46.** (c) | **47.** (a) | | | |

# HINTS AND EXPLANATION

## Multiple Choice Questions: Level II

**260.** (a) Characteristics of certain desert animals such as kangaroo, rat are
(b) They feed on dry seeds and do not require drinking water.
(c) They excrete very concentrated urine and do not use water to regulate body temperature.

**261.** Geometric representation of age structure is a characteristic of population.

**262.** If a population (e.g. reindeer population) is allowed to grow in a predator-free environment, the population grows beyond carrying capacity and there occurs population crash due to sudden shortage of food. Such growth curves also occur in insect populations during rainy season and in Algal blooms.

**263.** It is competition between individuals of different species. The interspecific competition may be very severe because all the members of a species have similar requirements of food, habitat mate, etc. and they also have similar adaptations to get their needs.

**264.** Biological organisms starts with submicroscopic molecular level like viruses, bacteria, etc. These organisms are unable to be seen by naked eyes without the help of microscope or even electron microscope.

**265.** Predators are prudent in nature.

**266.** Praying mantis is a good example of Camouflage. Camouflage is the natural colouring of an animal which enables it to blend with its surroundings.

A **praying** mantis, **or praying mantis,** is the common name for an insect of the order Mantodea. Often mistakenly spelled **preying mantis** (a tempting mistake, as they are notoriously predatory) they are in fact named for the typical 'prayer-like' stance. The word *mantis* derives from the Greek word mantis for prophet or fortune teller.

**267.** Barophilic bacteria grows under high pressure conditions. **Barophiles** are bacteria which live in high pressure environments, They are generally found on ocean floors, where pressure generally exceeds 380 atm (38 MPa).

**268.** Poison fangs in snakes are used by the snakes to inject poison into their prey and not for defence.

**269.** Desert shows maximum difference between day and night temperature.

**270.** In the Sigmoid growth curve, growth is slow in the lag phase. Growth rate remains stable during the stationary phase and it declines during the senescent phase. Growth increases logarithmically during the exponential phase

**271.** Carrying capacity refers to the maximum number of individuals that can be sustained by the environment. Birth rate refers to number of births per unit population.

**272.** Mimicry is resemblance of an organism to its natural surroundings, a non-living object or another organism for concealing itself from its natural predators or preys.

**273.** Mimicry is resemblance of an organ in its natural surroundings, a non-living object or another organism for concealing itself from its enemies. Flowers of *Ophrys muscifera* resemble the female wasps of Colpa aurea so that the male wasp tries to copulate with the flowers and pollinate them.

**274.**
- Natality refers to the rate at which new individuals are born.
- Adaptability refers to the capacity of the organisms to adapt themselves to their environment.

**275.** Population is an aggregation or grouping of individuals of the same species at the same time in a particular area. Species is a grouping of individuals of one or more populations resembling each other in important morphological, anatomical and biochemical characters and can potentially interbreed. Biotic community is an assemblage of interdependent. An ecosystem is a self-sufficient and self-regulating segment of nature comprising of a biotic community and its physical environment, both interacting and exchanging materials.

**276.** Succulent plants are fleshy xerophytes, which can grow in low water level area (desert). That is why they are called as desert plants.

**277.** In submerged hydrophytes, whole plant body remains under water, e.g., Ceratophyllum and Utricularia. In these plants, stomata is absent and gaseous exchange takes place through general body surface.

**278.** Sunken stomata is the characteristic feature of xerophytes which help in reducing loss of water from leaf surface. This type of stomata is found in Oleander or Pine.

**279.** The correctly matched pair: streamlined body for aquatic adaptation.

**280.** At the altitude of 5400 meters, the low atmospheric pressure of $O_2$ will be too low so the solubility of oxygen in the blood will be very less hence the oxygen carried by each RBC will be too Iow. But to fulfil the oxygen requirement of the body, blood has to carry more oxygen to the body tissue and this is done by the increased no. of RBCs.

**281.** Xeric environment is found in deserts where temperature remains high in the day and low during the night and air humidity is very low.

**282.** **Stenohaline:** Steno means narrow and haline meaning salt. A fish cannot handle a wide fluctuation in salt content in water. Many fresh water fish tend to be stenohaline and die in environment of high salinity such as the ocean. Fish living in coastal estuaries and tide pools are often euryhaline (tolerant to changes in salinity) as are many species which have lifecycle requiring tolerance to both fresh water and sea water environments such as salmon.

**283.** Polar ice and Glaciers have the largest amount of pure and fresh water without any dissolved salt or impurity.

**284.** German biologist Ernst Haeckel coined the term ecology, the inter-relationship between organisms and their environment.

**285.** A species is a group of individuals of same kind of phenotype characters and can interbreed.

**286.** Loam soil is best suited for plant growth because it possesses good aeration, nutritive salts and good water retaining capacity.

**287.** It is in case of mutualism.

**288.** High organic matter darkens the colour of soil

**289.** Soil particles size defines its texture.

**290.** **Homeostasis** is the property of an open system, especially living organisms to regulate its internal environment to maintain a stable, constant condition by means of multiple dynamic equilibrium adjustments controlled by interrelated regulation mechanisms. Homeostasis is one of the fundamental characteristics of living things.

**291.** Symbiosis when the interaction is useful to both the populations

**292.** Soil is the uppermost weathered layer or earth's crust and is composed of minerals and partly decomposed organic matter. Pedologist is a scientist who studies origin, composition and distribution of soil and the materials from which the soil is made.

**293.** Competition is most severe between the members of a population belonging to same niches.

**294.** A mutually beneficial association necessary for survival of both partners is symbiosis.

## NCERT Exemplar Questions

**1.** Autecology is the relation of an individual to its environment.

**2.** Ecotone is a zone of transition between two communities.

**3.** Biosphere is composed of all living organisms present on earth which interact with the physical environment.

**4.** Ecological niche is the physical position and functional role of a species within the community.

**5.** According to Allen's Rule, the mammals from colder climates have **shorter ears** and **shorter limbs.**

**6.** The salt concentrations is measured as salinity in parts per thousand, is less than S in inland waters, 3Q-3S in the sea and greater than 100 percent in some hypersaline lagoons.

**7.**

| Biome | MAT | MAP |
|---|---|---|
| Desert | 5°C to 20°C | 10–50 cm |
| Grassland | 0°C to 25°C | 25–100 cm |
| Tropical forest | 18°C to 25°C | 150–400 cm |
| Temperature forest | 10°C to 22°C | 60–220 cm |
| Coniferous forest | –1°C to 13°C | 50–250 cm |
| Arctic & Alpine tundra | –11°C to 1°C | 10–110 cm |

**8.** **Tall trees** control light conditions at the ground.

**9.** A well-growing herbaceous plant in the forest if it is transplanted outside the forest in a park. It may not survive because of change in its micro climate.

10. Initial population of paramecium Pi = 50

After one hour, population of paramecium Pf = 150

Growth rate after one hour = Pf – Pi

= 150 – 50 =100.

11. The per cent growth or birth rate per individual per hour = $\frac{\text{Final population} - \text{Initial population}}{\text{Initial population}} \times 100$

$= \frac{150 - 150}{50} \times 100 = 200$

12. A population has more young individuals compared to older individuals. It will increase the status of the population after some years.

13. Sometimes population size is indirectly estimated without actually counting them or seeing them. E.g. The tiger census in our National Parks and Tiger Reserves is often based on pug marks and faecal pellets.

14. **Mortality and emigration** would necessarily decrease the density of a population in a given habitat.

15. Population after $n^{th}$ generations = $2^n$

Population after $6^{th}$ generations = $2^6 = 64$.

16. $\frac{dN}{dt} = rN$

r = 0.028 – 0.008 = 0.02

dt = 2015–2005 = 10 years

$N = N_{2005}$ = 14 million

*dN* = change in population in 10 years

$\frac{dN}{dt} = 0.02 \times 14$

*dN* = 0.02 × 14 × 10

*dN* = 2.8 million

$dN = N_{2015} - N_{2005}$

$N_{2015} = dN + N_{2005}$

= 2.8 + 14

= 16.8 = 17 million.

17.

**Interspecific Population Interactions**

| Species A | Species B | Nature of interaction |
|---|---|---|
| + | + | Mutualism |
| – | – | Competition |
| + (Predator) | – (Prey) | Predator |
| + (Parasite) | – (Host) | Parasitism |
| + | 0 | Commensalism |
| – | 0 | Amensalism |

+ → Beneficial interaction

– → Detrimental interaction

0 → Neutral interaction

18. Lichens are the associations of **fungus** and **algae.**

19. Sandalwood is partial root parasite.

Mistletoe: partial stem parasite

Orobanche: total root parasite

Gonoderma : wood rotting fungi

20. Bamboo

## Previous Years' Questions

1. Stratification is the characteristic of biological community. Stratification is the vertical layering or the phenomenon of having more than one stratum formed by different plants/organisms in the same place. A forest may have 5–7 strata including large or canopy trees, medium tees, short trees, shrubs, herbs, ground flora, etc.

2. At high altitude, the body undergoes numerous changes in order to increase oxygen delivery to cells and improve the efficiency of oxygen usage. The early changes include increased breathing rate and increased red blood cell production.

3. (a) Regulator – Mammals and birds

(b) Conformer – All plants and 99% animals

(c) Partial regulators

4. Predators also help in maintaining species diversity in a community, by reducing the intensity of competition among competing prey species (e.g. Pisaster in intertidal zone of American pacific coast).

A wide variety of chemical substances (generally secondary metabolite) that we extract from plants on a commercial scale (nicotine, caffeine, quinine, strychnine, opium, etc.,) are produced by them actually as defences against grazers and browsers.

Predator control prey population but not lead to its extinction.

5. Predator is an organism which catches and kills another organism (prey) for obtaining food. The term 'host' is also used for an organism which provides food to another organism but it is not a general term. It is specific to parasitic interrelationship only.

6. Human louse (Pediculus) lives among hair and surface of human body feeding on blood. It spreads diseases like typhus.

7. An age pyramid is a graphic representation of proportion of various age groups of a population with pre-reproductive at the base, reproductive in the middle and post reproductive at the top. For human population, the age pyramids show age distribution of males and females in a combined diagram. The shape of the age pyramids reflects the growth status of the population. In a declining population, the shape of pyramid is urn-shaped.

8. Some organism show behavioural responses to cope with variations in their environment. Desert lizards bask in the sun and absorb heat when their body temperature drops below the comfort zone, but move into shade when the ambient temperature starts increasing. Some species are capable of burrowing into the soil to hide and escape from the above-ground heat.

9. A population growing in a habitat with limited resources show initially a lag phase, followed by phases of acceleration and deceleration and finally an asymptote, when the population density reaches the carrying capacity, A plot of N (population density at time r) in relation to time (t) results in sigmoid curve. This type of population grown is called Verhulst–Pearl Logistic Growth and is described by the following equation:

$$dN/dt = rN\left(\frac{K-N}{K}\right)$$

where, $N$ = Population density at time t,

$r$ = Intrinsic rate of natural increase

$K$ = Carrying capacity

Since resources for growth for most animal populations are finite and become limiting sooner or later, the logistic growth model is considered to be a more realistic one.

10. Bears go into hibernation during winter to escape cold weather.

A conical age pyramid with a broad base represents expanding human population.

A wasp pollinating a fig flower is an example of mutualism.

An area with high levels of species richness is known as hot spots.

11. Acclimatization occurrence is characterized by

(1) More number of RBCs (Polycythemia)

(2) Their haemoglobin has a lower binding affinity to $O_2$

(3) Increase in breathing rate

12. In plants four major types of parasites are present, they are ectoparasite.

(i) **Total stem parasite,** *e.g., Cuscuta*

(ii) **Total root parasite,** *e.g., Rafflesia* and *Orobanche*

(iii) **Partial stem parasite,** *e.g., Viscum* and *Loranthus*

(iv) **Partial root parasites,** *e.g., Santalum*

13. The association between sea anemone and hermit crab is symbiosis as both live together for very long duration.

14. Natality = 250, Immigration = 20

Mortality = 240, Emigration = 30

Increase in Population size

P.D. = [Natality + Immigration) – (Mortality + Emigration)]

= [(250 + 20) – (240 + 30)]

= 0.

15. Every winter the famous Keolado National Park (Bharatpur) in Rajasthan hosts thousands of migratory birds coming from Siberia and other extremely cold northern regions.

16. **Biotic community:** The assemblage of interdependent and interacting populations of different species present in an area.

17. Both the species lose in competition in their interactions with each other.

18. The numbers of organism of A is decreased and B increased with time therefore option (b) is correct.

19. Some desert plants like *Opuntia* have no leaves – they are reduced to spines to reduce the loss of water by transpiration – and the photosynthetic function is taken over by the flattened stems

20. Gause's '*Competitive Exclusion Principle*' states that two closely related species competing for the same resources cannot co-exist indefinitely and the competitively inferior one will be eliminated eventually.

This may be true if resources are limiting, but not otherwise.

**21.**

| Species A | Species B | Name of Interaction |
|---|---|---|
| + | + | *Mutualism* |
| – | – | *Competition* |
| + | – | *Predation* |
| + | – | *Parasitism* |
| + | 0 | *Commensalism* |
| – | 0 | *Amensalism* |

**22.** Selection of life history traits that are sensitive to population density is known as K-selection, or density-dependent selection.
Selection for life history traits that maximize reproductive success in uncrowded environments (low densities) is called r-selection, or density-independent selection.

**23.** It is much easier for a small animal to run uphill than for animal, because smaller animals have higher metabolic rate.

**24.** When N\K is exactly one, growth rate will be zero

**25.** Gause principle of competitive exclusion states that no species can occupy the same niche indefinitely for the same limiting resources.

**26.** $N_t = N_0\ e^{rt}$
$N_t = 100\ (2.72)^{0.5 \times 6}$
$N_t = 100 \times (2.72)^3$
$N_t = 2012$

**27.** A population growing in a habitat with limited resources show initially a lag phase, followed by phases of acceleration and deceleration and finally an asymptote, when the population density(N) reaches the carrying capacity(K).

**28.** Association between roots of higher plants and fungal hyphae is called mycorrhiza. It is of two types:
(a) **Ectotrophic or Ectophytic mycorrhiza:** In this association, fungal hyphae are on surface of roots, *e.g.,* in *Pinus*.
(b) **Endotrophic or Endophytic mycorrhiza:** Here fungal hyphae are inside the root tissue, *e.g.,* in orchids. Mycorrhiza is example of mutualism.

**29.** **Natality** (Birth rate) refers to the number of births during a given period in the population that are added to the initial density. Mortality (Death rate).

**30.** In **amensalism,** on the other hand, one species is harmed, whereas the other is unaffected. (*Penicillium notatum* and gram positive bacteria)

**31.** The shape of the pyramids reflects the growth status of the population. In a growing population of a country, pre-reproductive individuals are more than the reproductive individuals.

**32.** A wide variety of chemical substances that we extract from plants on a commercial scale (nicotine, caffeine, quinine, strychnine, opium, etc) are produced by them (plants) as defences against grazers and browsers.

**33.** The correct option is (b) because flippers of Penguins and Dolphins are an example of analogous organs. Analogous structures are a result of convergent evolution.

**34.** Inspite of interspecific competition the competing species may co-exist by doing resource partitioning.

**35.** Refer to answer 21

**36.** In the exponential growth equation $N_t = N_0 e^{rt}$,
e represents the base of natural logarithms
$N_t$ = Population density after time t
$N_0$ = Population density at time zero
r = Intrinsic rate of natural increase called biotic potential.

**37.**

| | |
|---|---|
| Allen's Rule | Polar seal generally has shorter ears and limbs (extremities) to minimise heat loss. This is with reference to Allen's rule. |
| Physiological adaptation | Kangaroo rat exhibits physiological adaptation. |
| Behavioural adaptation | Desert lizard shows behavioural adaptation. They lack the physiological ability to cope-up with extreme temperature but manage the body temperature by behavioural means. |
| Biochemical adaptation | Marine fishes at depth are adapted biochemically to survive in great depths in ocean. |

**38.** **Altitude sickness** can be experienced at high altitude where body does not get enough oxygen due to low atmospheric pressure and causes nausea, fatigue and heart palpitations.

Hence, correct option is (b) as [R] is correct explanation of [A].

39. **Important role of predators:**

- Predators help in maintaining species diversity in a community, by reducing the intensity of competition among competing prey species.
- If a predator is too efficient and overexploits its prey, then the prey might become extinct.
- One of the species in predation gains benefit on the expense of the other.

**Both species are negatively impacted in competition.**

40. In predation, one species is benefitted whereas the other is harmed. It is (+ –) type of population interaction.

| Species A | Species B | Name if Interaction |
|---|---|---|
| + | + | Mutualism |
| - | - | Competition |
| + | - | Predation |
| + | - | Parasitism |
| + | 0 | Commensalism |
| - | 0 | Amensalism |
| + | + | Protocooperation |

41. If 8 *Drosophila* in a laboratory population of 80 died during a week, the death rate in the population is $\frac{8}{10}$ 0.1 individuals per *Drosophila* per week.

42. Gause's 'Competitive Exclusion principle' states that two closely related species competing for the same resources cannot co-exist indefinitely and the competitively inferior one will be eliminated eventually

In general, herbivores and plants are more adversely affected by competition than carnivores.

43.

Mutualism: +(A), +(B) Both the species are benefitted

Commensalism: +(A), 0(B) one species is benefitted and the other is neither benefitted nor harmed

Amensalism: -(A), 0(B) one species is harmed whereas the other is unaffected

Parasitism: +(A),−(B) only
one species is benefitted and other is harmed

44.

| | |
|---|---|
| A Leopard and a Lion in a forest / grassland | Competition |
| A Cuckoo laying eggs in a Crow's nest | Brood parasitism |
| Fungi and root of a higher plant in Mycorrhizae | Mutualism |
| A cattle erget and a Cattle in a field | Commensalism |

45.

| | |
|---|---|
| Logistic growth | Limited resource availability condition |
| Exponential growth | Unlimited resource availability condition |
| Expanding age pyramid | The percent individuals of pre-reproductive age groups are same |
| Stable age pyramid | The percent individuals of pre-reproductive age is largest followed by reproductive and post reproductive age groups |

46. In the equation $\frac{dN}{dt} = rN\left[\frac{K-N}{K}\right]$, $K$ represents carrying capacity.
$N$ = Population density at time t
$r$ = Intrinsic rate of natural increase
$K$ = Carrying capacity

47. Gause's competitive exclusion principle states that two closely related species competing for the same resources cannot exist indefinitely and the competitively inferior one will be eliminated eventually. This may be true if resources are limiting.

# 6

# Ecosystem

## LEARNING OBJECTIVES

- Discuss about the ecosystem its structure, and functions
- Know more about energy flow, food chain, and energy pyramid
- Understand productivity and decomposition

## Chapter Overview

- **An ecosystem** is a structural and functional unit of nature where, the living organisms interact among themselves and also with the surrounding physical environment.
- **Categories of Ecosystem:** (i) Terrestrial: forest, grassland, desert, (ii) Aquatic: pond, lake, wetlands, river, estuary.
- **The term 'Ecosystem' was coined by Arthur Tansley.**
- The crop field and an aquarium are some examples of manmade ecosystems. Crop field is the largest manmade ecosystem and its limitation is that, it has **a least genetic variability**.
- **Structural components** of the ecosystem are comprised of species composition, **stratification**, trophic level, standing state and standing crop.
- **Stratification** is maximum in tropical rain forest and minimum in desert. In forest, the ecosystem is divided into various strata or levels namely, the top strata which comprises of trees, the middle strata which comprises of shrubs and the bottom strata which comprises of herbs and grasses.
- **Functional components** of ecosystem are **productivity, decomposition, energy flow and nutrient cycling.**
- Pond is a shallow water body which consists of basic components of ecosystem namely, fungi, bacteria and flagellates (usually abundant at the sea floor) and they acts as the decomposers.
- Energy moves unidirectional from the lower trophic level to the higher trophic level. A part of energy is also lost as heat in the environment.
- **Primary production:** It is the amount of biomass or organic matter produced per unit area over a time period by the plants during photosynthesis and it is expressed in terms of weight (g/m$^2$) or energy (kcal m$^{-2}$).
- **Primary productivity:** It is the rate of biomass production and it is expressed in terms of g/m$^2$/ yr or (kcal m$^{-2}$ yr$^{-1}$).
- **Gross primary productivity (GPP):** It is the rate of production of organic matter during photosynthesis.
- **Net primary productivity (NPP):** It is the rate at which the energy is stored as biomass by plants and makes it available for heterotrophs such as herbivores and decomposers in the ecosystem. A part of GPP is utilised by the plants during respiration (R) whereas, the remaining GPP is utilised for the next trophic level. Therefore, **NPP = GPP – R.**
- Primary productivity depends on various factors namely, plant species inhabiting that ecosystem, environmental factors, availability of nutrients and photosynthetic capacity of plants.
- In **aquatic ecosystem**, both **light and nutrients** are essential in controlling the primary productivity.
- Primary productivity varies for different types of ecosystem which can be understood by comparing the ecosystems as follows: **coral reef > estuaries > sugar-cane field > forests > grassland > ponds > lakes > oceans > deserts.**

---

Refer NCERT Ch 12: Ecosystem

- Annual net primary productivity of the whole biosphere is **170 billion tons** which is the dry weight of organic matter. Out of it, o**nly 55 billion tons** is contributed by oceans despite occupying about 70 per cent of the earth's surface.
- **Secondary productivity** is defined as the rate of formation of new organic matter by consumers.
- Some soil nutrients are held up in the biomass of decomposers and **detritivores** and they become unavailable to organisms. Such incorporation of nutrients in decomposers and detritivores is known as **nutrient immobilization.**

**Decomposition**

- It is the process where the complex organic matter is broken down into inorganic substances such as carbon dioxide, water and nutrients. Earthworm also helps in the breakdown of complex organic matter into inorganic substance which leads to loosening of soil. Hence, it is known as 'farmer's friend'.
- **Detritus:** It includes the dead remains of plants such as leaves, bark, flowers, etc. and the dead remains and faecal matters of animals.
- **Decomposition** includes three simultaneously occurring processes namely, these processes occur simultaneously.
- **Fragmentation:** It is the process in which detritus particles are broken down into smaller particles by detritivores like earthworms.
- **Leaching:** It is the movement of water-soluble inorganic nutrients into the soil horizon after which they get precipitated as unavailable salts.
- **Catabolism:** It is the process in which complex substances are broken down into small substances in which, the bacterial and fungal enzymes degrade detritus substances into simple inorganic substances.
- **Humification:** It results in accumulation of a dark colored amorphous substance called humus. Humus is highly resistant to microbial action and it undergoes decomposition at an extremely slow rate. As the humus is colloidal in nature, it serves as a reservoir of nutrients.
- **Mineralization:** Humus gets degraded by microbes and as a result, inorganic nutrients are released. This process is known as mineralization.
- Decomposition depends upon the following factors namely,
  **(a) Chemical composition of detritus:** If the detritus is rich in lignin and chitin, the decomposition rate becomes slower and if, the detritus is rich in nitrogen and water-soluble substances like sugars, the decomposition rate becomes faster.
  **(b) Climatic factors:** The rate of decomposition mainly depends upon the availability of oxygen. Anaerobic conditions which are also known as anaerobiosis decreases the decomposition and as a result of this, organic materials accumulate. Increase in temperature and soil moisture, increases the activities of soil microbes, thus, increasing the rate of decomposition. Therefore, warm and moist environment promotes decomposition.
- **Except deep sea hydrothermal ecosystem,** sun is the only source of energy for all the ecosystems on earth**.**

**Photosynthetically active radiation**

- PAR is less than 50 per cent of the total incident solar radiations.
- Plants fix only **2 to 10 per cent** of the PAR.
- The first as well as the second law of thermodynamics is applicable for energy flow in ecosystem.
- Flow of energy follows only **10 per cent of the 'Law of Lindeman'** that is, only 10 per cent of the energy present at the lower trophic level will be transferred to the higher trophic level. This is the reason, why the number of trophic levels are restricted in a food chain.
- In an aquatic ecosystem, major fraction of energy flows through GFC while, in a terrestrial ecosystem, a much larger fraction of energy flows through the DFC than through the GFC.
- DFC begins with dead organic matter which is acts upon decomposers (heterotrophic organisms mainly fungi and bacteria) and meets their energy and nutrient requirements by degrading dead organic matter or detritus.
- **Standing crop:** It refers to the total biomass (mass of living material) at a time, in a particular trophic level. It is measured in terms of mass of living organisms or their numbers per unit area.

**Ecological Pyramids**

- **Ecological Pyramids also known as 'Eltonian pyramid':** There are three types of ecological pyramids and they are described below.
  (1) **Pyramid of number:** Inverted/ Spindle-shaped in tree ecosystem.
  (2) **Pyramid of biomass:** Inverted in aquatic ecosystem.
  (3) **Pyramid of energy:** Always upright without exception.
- A sparrow which eat seeds, fruits, peas, etc., is a primary consumer and also it becomes a secondary consumer when it eats insects and worms.
- **Limitations of ecological pyramids:**
  (1) A single species cannot be given two or more trophic levels in an ecological pyramid.
  (2) An ecological pyramid does not accommodate a food web and it assumes a simple food chain that almost never exists in nature.
  (3) Saprophytes are not given any place in ecological py-ramids despite their important role in the ecosystem.
- **Standing state:** It refers to the amount of nutrients such as carbon, nitrogen, phosphorus, calcium, etc., present in the soil at any given time. It is different for different kinds of ecosystem and may vary according to the season.
- **Reservoir:** It compensates the deficit which occurs due to imbalance in the rate of influx and efflux of nutrients.

# PRACTICE EXERCISES

**Direction:** Read the question carefully and choose the correct option for each.

## Multiple Choice Questions: Level I

### Ecosystem (Type, Structure and Function)

**1.** The following are examples of terrestrial ecosystem except
(a) Forest (b) Wetland
(c) Grassland (d) Desert

**2.** Which of these are examples of aquatic ecosystem?
(a) Pond (b) River
(c) Estuary (d) All of these

**3.** Which of these are examples of man-made ecosystem?
(a) Crop field (b) Aquarium
(c) Wetland (d) Both (a) and (b)

**4.** Find out the incorrect statement.
(a) Biosphere is a global ecosystem.
(b) Transfer of energy in ecosystem explains in terms of food web and nutrient cycle.
(c) Pond, lake and wetland are aquatic ecosystems.
(d) Ecosystem is structural, not functional unit of ecosystem.

**5.** Which of the following occupy top vertical strata of forest ecosystem?
(a) Shrubs (b) Herbs and grasses
(c) Tree (d) Phytoplankton

**6.** Pond is a
(a) Shallow fresh water body
(b) Deep fresh water body
(c) Shallow marine water body
(d) Deep marine water body

**7.** The functional aspect of ecosystem can be explained in terms of
(a) Productivity
(b) Decomposition and energy flow
(c) Nutrient cycle
(d) All of these

**8.** At the bottom of ponds the decomposers found are
(a) Fungi (b) Bacteria
(c) Flagellates (d) All of these

**9.** Which of the following have only unidirectional flow?
(a) Carbon (b) Nitrogen
(c) Energy (d) Sulphur

**10.** Driving force for an ecosystem is
(a) Primary producers (b) Secondary producers
(c) Solar radiation (d) Food chain

**11.** Ecosystem shows
(a) Homeostasis (b) Mineral cycling
(c) Energy flow (d) All of these

**12.** Which of the following statements is correct?
(a) Producers produce energy
(b) Consumers consume energy
(c) Decomposers decompose energy
(d) Producers transform energy

**13.** In ecosystem, the nonliving components are
(a) Less important than the living components.
(b) Equally important as those of the living components.
(c) More important than living components.
(d) None of the above

**14.** Which of the following are the two main structural features of an ecosystem?
(A) Species composition
(B) Energy flow
(C) Decomposition
(D) Stratification
(a) A and D only
(b) B and C only
(c) A only
(d) B, C and D only

**15.** Biological equilibrium is maintained with the help of
(a) Producers and consumers
(b) Consumers and decomposers
(c) Herbivores and carnivores
(d) Photosynthesis and respiration

**16.** Select the incorrect statements
(a) An ecosystem can be visualised as a functional unit of nature
(b) Ecosystem can be a small pond as well as large forest.
(c) Forests, oceans and Crop fields are natural eco-systems.
(d) In ecosystem, transfer of energy occurs in food chain or web.

**17.** Select set of correct statements:
(A) Interaction of biotic and abiotic components result in a physical structure that is characteristic for each type of ecosystem.
(B) Identification and enumeration of plant and animal species of an ecosystem gives its species composition.
(C) Vertical distribution of different species occupying different levels is called standing crop.
(D) Productivity and decomposition are functional components of ecosystem.
(a) A, B and D (b) A, B and C
(c) B, C and D (d) B and D only

**18.** Ecosystems may exhibit variations based on
(a) nutrient availability.
(b) productivity
(c) ecological interactions.
(d) All of these.

**19.** The rate of function of the entire pond is regulated by
(A) The solar input,
(B) the cycle of temperature,
(C) day-length
(a) A and B (b) B and C
(c) A and C (d) A, B and C

**Direction of Q20–22:** Choose the most appropriate option:
(a) Statement I is incorrect but statement II is true.
(b) Both Statements I and II are true
(c) Both Statements I and II are false
(d) Statement I is correct but statement II is false

**20** Read following sentences.
**Statement I:** Interaction of biotic and abiotic components result in a physical structure that is characteristic for each type of ecosystem.
**Statement II:** Identification and enumeration of plant and animal species of an ecosystem gives its species composition.

**21.** Read following sentences.
**Statement I:** The solar input, the cycle of temperature, day-length and other climatic conditions regulate the rate of function of the entire pond.
**Statement II:** The fungi, bacteria and flagellates are the decomposers found in the pond, especially abundant on the surface of water.

**22.** Read following sentences.
**Statement I:** A unidirectional movement of energy is always towards the lower trophic levels of ecosystem.
**Statement II:** During transfer through different levels, there is dissipation and loss of energy as heat to the environment.

**23.** There is ______ movement of energy towards the ______ trophic levels and its dissipation and ______ as heat to the environment.
(a) unidirectional, lower, loss
(b) unidirectional, higher, loss
(c) bidirectional, lower, gain
(d) bidirectional, higher, gain

## Functional Aspect of Ecosystem (Productivity and Decomposition)

**24.** The amount of biomass or organic matter produced per unit area over a period of time by plants during photosynthesis is known as
(a) Primary production
(b) Secondary production
(c) Net primary productivity
(d) Net secondary production

**25.** The unit of primary production is
(a) $g/m^2$ (b) $kcal/m^2$
(c) Both (a) and (b) (d) None of these

**26.** NPP is equal to
(a) GPP + R (b) GPP – R
(c) GPP × R (d) GPP ÷ R

**27.** Secondary productivity means
(a) Rate of formation of organic matter by producer.
(b) Rate of formation of new organic matter by consumers.
(c) Rate of formation of inorganic matter by producer.
(d) Rate of formation of inorganic matter by consumers.

**28.** Primary productivity depends on which of the following factors?
(a) Environmental factor
(b) Photosynthetic capacity of plant
(c) Availability of nutrients
(d) All the above

**29.** GPP means
(a) Gross Public Partnership
(b) Gross Primary Production
(c) Gross Producer Production
(d) Gross Plant Production

**30.** The unit of productivity is
(a) $gm^{-2}yr^{-1}$ (b) $Kcal/m^2/year$
(c) Both (a) and (b) (d) None

**31.** NPP means
(a) Available biomass for the consumption to heterotrophs
(b) Biomass produced by producers
(c) Respiratory losses by consumers
(d) All of the above

**32.** The annual net primary productivity of the whole biosphere is how much billion tons (dry weight) of organic matter?
(a) 120 (b) 170
(c) 210 (d) 150

**33.** Oceans occupy ________ % of the surface of earth but productivity of ocean are ________ billion tons.
(a) 70, 45 (b) 60, 55
(c) 70, 55 (d) 60, 65

**34.** The productivity of ocean is less because
(a) It occupies 70 per cent of earth's surface.
(b) Light is a major limiting factor which decreases with increase in water depth.
(c) It contains algae as a chief producer.
(d) All the above

**35.** What is the percentage of primary productivity of oceans?
(a) 50% (b) 90%
(c) 32% (d) 70%

**36.** Earthworms help in
(a) Breakdown of complex organic matter
(b) Loosening of soil
(c) Both (a) and (b)
(d) None of these

**37.** Detritus contain
(a) Dead plant remains (leaves, bark and flower)
(b) Dead animal remains
(c) Fecal matter
(d) All the above

**38.** The important steps in the process of decomposition are
(a) Fragmentation (b) Leaching
(c) Catabolism (d) All of these

**39.** Match the columns.

| Column–I | Column–II |
|---|---|
| 1. Fragmentation | A. Break down of detritus into smaller particles |
| 2. Leaching | B. Precipitation of water soluble nutrients as unavailable salt |
| 3. Catabolism | C. Degradation of detritus by bacterial and fungal enzymes |

(a) 1–A, 2–B, 3–C
(b) 1–B, 2–C, 3–A
(c) 1–C, 2–B, 3–A
(d) 1–C, 2–A, 3–B

**40.** Which of these are true about humus?
(a) Dark coloured amorphous substance
(b) Colloidal in nature
(c) Reservoir of nutrient
(d) All of these

**41.** Humus is degraded by some microbes and release of inorganic nutrients occur by the process known as ________.
(a) Fragmentation (b) Leaching
(c) Humidification (d) Mineralization

**42.** Find out the total number of incorrect statements from the following:
(A) Decomposition is largely an anaerobic process.
(B) Fragmentation, leaching and catabolism occur simultaneously on detritus.
(C) Vertical distribution of different species occupying different level is called stratification.
(D) Pond is a deep water body.
(E) The rate of decomposition is controlled by chemical composition of detritus and climatic factors.
(a) 1 (b) 2
(c) 3 (d) 4

**43.** Decomposition is favoured by
(a) Warm and moist environment.
(b) Rich amount of nitrogen and water soluble substance like sugar in detritus.
(c) Aerobic environment
(d) All the above

**44.** The rate of decomposition process is decreased by
(a) Aerobic environment
(b) Rich amount of lignin and chitin in detritus
(c) Worm and moist environment
(d) All the above

**45.** Litter is decomposed by how many organisms among the following?
*Earthworm, Bacteria, Fungi, Mites*
(a) 1 (b) 2
(c) 3 (d) 4

**46.** In decomposition, complex organic compounds of detritus are converted to which of the following substances by decomposers?
(a) Carbon dioxide (b) Water
(c) Inorganic nutrients (d) All of these

**Direction of Q47–50:** Choose the most appropriate option:
(a) Statement I is incorrect but statement II is true.
(b) Both Statements I and II are true
(c) Both Statements I and II are false
(d) Statement I is correct but statement II is false

**47.** Read following sentences.
**Statement I:** Primary production is defined as the amount of biomass or organic matter produced per unit area over a time period by plants during photosynthesis.
**Statement II:** Gross primary productivity of an ecosystem is the rate of production of organic matter during photosynthesis.

**48.** Read following sentences.
**Statement I:** Net primary productivity is the available biomass for the consumption to heterotrophs.
**Statement II:** The rate of biomass production is called productivity.

**49.** Read following sentences.
**Statement I:** Primary production is expressed in terms of $gm^{-2}$ $yr^{-1}$.
**Statement II:** Productivity is expressed in terms of (kcal $m^{-2}$) $yr^{-1}$.

**50.** Read following sentences.
**Statement I:** Secondary productivity is defined as the rate of formation of new organic matter by consumers.
**Statement II:** Primary production can be expressed exclusively in terms of energy (kcal $m^{-2}$).

**51.** **Assertion:** the net primary productivity is Gross primary productivity minus respiration losses.
**Reason:** A considerable amount of GPP is gained by plants during respiration.
(a) (A) is false but (R) is true
(b) Both (A) and (R) are true and (R) is the correct explanation of (A)
(c) Both (A) and (R) are true but (R) is not the correct explanation of (A)
(d) (A) is true but (R) is false.

**52.** Read following sentences.
**Statement I:** The annual net primary productivity of the whole biosphere is approximately 170 billion tons (dry weight) of organic matter.
**Statement II:** the productivity on the land is 115 billion tons of organic matter.
(a) Statement I is incorrect but statement II is true.
(b) Both Statements I and II are true
(c) Both Statements I and II are false
(d) Statement I is correct but statement II is false

**53.** Read following sentences.
**Statement I:** Net primary productivity is the available biomass for the consumption to producers.
**Statement II:** Secondary productivity is defined as the rate of formation of new organic matter by consumers.
(a) Statement I is incorrect but statement II is true.
(b) Both Statements I and II are true
(c) Both Statements I and II are false
(d) Statement I is correct but statement II is false

**Direction for Q54–55:** Choose the correct option:
(a) (A) is false but (R) is true
(b) Both (A) and (R) are true and (R) is the correct explanation of (A)
(c) Both (A) and (R) are true but (R) is not the correct explanation of (A)
(d) (A) is true but (R) is false.

**54.** **Assertion:** Primary productivity varies in different types of ecosystems
**Reason:** Primary productivity depends on the plant species inhabiting a particular area, and also on a variety of environmental factors, availability of nutrients and photosynthetic capacity of plants.

**55.** **Assertion:** The productivity of the oceans are 55 billion tons.
**Reason:** Oceans occupy about 70 per cent of the surface.

**56.** Which of the following statements are true regarding secondary productivity in an ecosystem?
(a) It represents the rate at which producers convert solar energy into chemical energy.
(b) It is influenced by the efficiency of energy transfer between trophic levels.
(c) Carnivores generally have higher secondary productivity compared to herbivores.
(d) Secondary productivity is independent of the primary productivity.

**57.** Which of the following are examples of decomposers in an ecosystem?

A. Bacteria B. Fungi
C. Insects D. Plants
(a) a, b and c (b) a and b
(c) a, b and d (d) a and d

**Direction for Q58–64:** Choose the correct option:

(a) (A) is false but (R) is true
(b) Both (A) and (R) are true and (R) is the correct explanation of (A)
(c) Both (A) and (R) are true but (R) is not the correct explanation of (A)
(d) (A) is true but (R) is false.

**58. Assertion:** The earthworm being referred to as the farmer's 'friend'.
**Reason:** Earthworms help in the breakdown of complex organic matter as well as in loosening of the soil.

**59. Assertion:** The earthworm are called Detritivores.
**Reason:** Earthworms break down detritus into smaller particles.

**60. Assertion:** Humus serves as a reservoir of nutrients.
**Reason:** Humus is colloidal in nature.

**61. Assertion:** The rate of decomposition is controlled by chemical composition of detritus.
**Reason:** if detritus is rich in lignin and chitin, decomposition is quicker, and slower if detritus is rich in nitrogen and water-soluble substances.

**62. Assertion:** The rate of decomposition is controlled by climatic factors.
**Reason:** Warm and moist environment inhibit decomposition whereas low temperature and anaerobiosis favour decomposition.

**63. Assertion:** The rate of decomposition is controlled by climatic factors.
**Reason:** Warm and moist environment inhibit decomposition whereas low temperature and anaerobiosis favour decomposition.

**64. Assertion:** Anaerobiosis inhibit decomposition and result in build up of organic materials.
**Reason:** Decomposition is largely an oxygen-requiring process.

**65.** Select the correct statements regarding the decomposition of organic matter.

(A) Decomposition releases nutrients back into the environment.
(B) detritus constitutes of dead plant and animals, but not their fecal matter.
(C) Decomposition contributes to the formation of humus in the soil.
(D) Decomposition occurs more rapidly in anaerobic conditions.

(a) A and C (b) A, B and C
(c) A, B and D (d) B and D

**66.** Consider the following statements about the decomposers present in the ecosystem.

(A) Decomposers help in the recycling of nutrients.
(B) Decomposers secrete digestive enzyme extracellularly that breakdown dead material into simple organic compounds, which are absorbed by them.
(C) They are also known as saprotrophs
(D) Decomposers are not essential for the functioning of an ecosystem

How many of them are correct regarding decomposers

(a) (A) and (C) only (b) (A), (B) and (C) only
(c) (A) and (D) only (d) (B) and (D) only

**67.** Select set of correct statements about decomposition:

(A) In process of fragmentation detritus is broken down into smaller particles.
(B) In the process of leaching, water soluble inorganic nutrients go down into the soil horizon and get precipitated as unavailable salts.
(C) In catabolism bacterial and fungal enzymes degrade detritus into simpler inorganic substances.

(a) A and B (b) B and C
(c) A and C (d) A, B and C

**68.** Following statements are given regarding humus

(A) Dark coloured crystalline substance
(B) Easily degradable by microbial action
(C) Decomposition rate is extremely slow
(D) Act as reservoir of nutrients
(E) Non- colloidal in nature

How many of them are correct regarding humus

(a) (A) and (C) only (b) (A), (B) and (E) only
(c) (C) and (D) only (d) (B) and (E) only

**69.** Select the correct statements regarding the energy flow in an ecosystem.

(A) It is not exempted from the second law of thermodynamics
(B) Energy can be trapped in an organism and remain in it for ever
(C) Only producers can convert solar energy into chemical energy
(D) Only 10% of the energy transferred to each trophic level from the higher trophic levels

(a) (A) and (C) only (b) (B) and (C) only
(c) (C) and (D) only (d) (B) and (D) only

## Functional Aspect of Ecosystem (Energy Flow and Pyramids)

**70.** What is the main source of energy for all ecosystems on earth?
(a) Sun
(b) Volcano
(c) Deep sea hydro-thermal system
(d) Moon

**71.** PAR (Photosynthetically active radiation) from incident solar radiation is
(a) 50% (b) 30%
(c) 70% (d) 20%

**72.** Plant capture how much of PAR?
(a) 2–10% (b) 10–20%
(c) 50% (d) 30%

**73.** Which law is obeyed during energy flow in an ecosystem?
(a) First law of thermodynamics
(b) Second law of thermodynamics
(c) Third law of thermodynamics
(d) Both (a) and (b)

**74.** In a terrestrial ecosystem the major producers are
(A) Herbs
(B) Woody plant
(C) Algae
(a) A and B only (b) A and C only
(c) A, B and C (d) B only

**75.** Primary producers in aquatic ecosystem are
(a) Phytoplankton (b) Algae
(c) Higher plant (d) All of these

**76.** Which of these is a primary consumer?
(a) Grass (b) Goat
(c) Man (d) Tiger

**77.** Which of these is a common herbivores in aquatic ecosystem?
(a) Insect (b) Birds
(c) Mammals (d) Mollusc

**78.** Which of the following represent simple GFC (Grazing Food Chain)?
(a) Grass → Goat → Man
(b) Goat → Grass → Man
(c) Detritus → Fungi → Man
(d) Fungi → Detritus → Grass

**79.** DFC (Detritus Food Chain) begins with
(a) Dead organic matter (b) Fungi
(c) Bacteria (d) Plant

**80.** The main decomposers are
(a) Bacteria and fungus
(b) Earthworm
(c) Flagellated protozoans
(d) Flagellated diatoms

**81.** Decomposers meet their energy and nutrient requirements by degrading
(a) Phytoplanktons
(b) Zooplanktons
(c) Detritus
(d) Bacteria

**82.** GFC is a major conduit for energy flow in
(a) Terrestrial ecosystem
(b) Aquatic ecosystem
(c) Both (a) and (b)
(d) None of these

**83.** Decomposers shows
(a) Intracellular digestion
(b) Extracellular digestion
(c) Both intra and extracellular digestion
(d) No digestion at all

**84.** Find the incorrect statement.
(a) In terrestrial ecosystem larger fraction of energy flow occurs through DFC.
(b) In aquatic ecosystem a major conduit for energy flow is GFC.
(c) Detritus food chain is not at all connected with grazing food chain at any level.
(d) Natural interconnection of food chain makes it a food web.

**85.** Based on the source of their nutrient or food, organisms occupy a specific place in the food chain that is known as their ________.
(a) Hierarchy position (b) Class
(c) Order (d) Trophic level

**86.** Herbivoures are
(a) Producers (b) Primary consumers
(c) Secondary consumer (d) Tertiary consumers

**87.** Plants are
(a) Producers
(b) Primary consumers
(c) Secondary consumers
(d) Tertiary consumers

**88.** Each tropic level has a certain mass of living material at a particular time called
(a) Standing state (b) Stranding crop
(c) Ecological pyramid (d) GPP

**89.** Stranding crop is measured in terms of
(a) Biomass/unit area
(b) Number of organism/unit area
(c) Both (a) or (b)
(d) None of these

**90.** Measurement of biomass is generally done in terms of
(a) Fresh weight
(b) Dry weight
(c) Ash
(d) Numbers of organisms

**91.** What does A represent in the diagram?

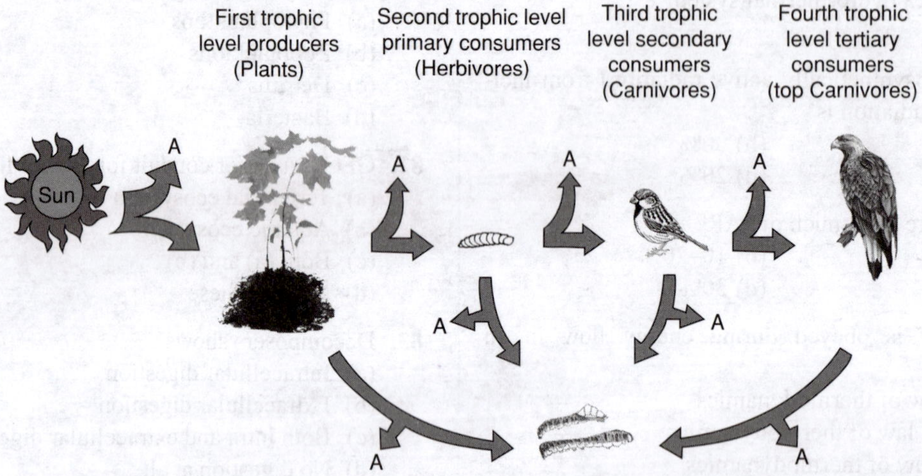


(a) Food (b) Heat (c) Water (d) $CO_2$

**92.** Transfer of energy in tropic level follows
(a) 20% law (b) 10% law
(c) 5% law (d) 15% law

**93.** A graphical representation known as ________ is required to express food or energy relationship between organisms at different trophic levels.
(a) Ecological pyramid
(b) Standing state
(c) Ecological quadrilateral
(d) Standing crop

**94.** Ecological pyramids are based on
(a) Food chain (b) Food web
(c) Nutrient cycling (d) All of these

**95.** How many ecological pyramids are usually studied?
(a) 1 (b) 2 (c) 3 (d) 4

**96.** Ecological pyramids are
(a) Pyramids of number (b) Pyramids of biomass
(c) Pyramids of energy (d) All the above

**97.** Which of the following pyramid is always upright?
(a) Energy (b) Biomass
(c) Number (d) All of these

**98.** How much energy of sunlight is converted by primary producers into NPP in the above energy pyramid?

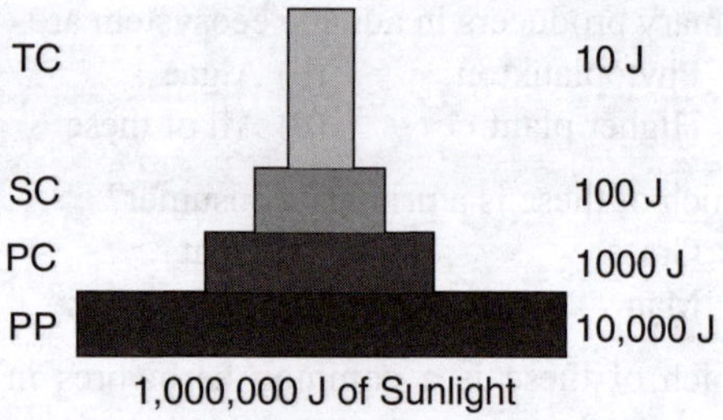


(a) 2% (b) 10% (c) 1% (d) 110%

**99.** How many top-carnivores are supported in an above grassland ecosystem based on production of nearly 6 million plants?

| Trophic level | Number of individuals |
|---|---|
| TC (Tertiary consumer) | 3 |
| SC (Secondary consumer) | 3,54,000 |
| PC (Primary consumer) | 708,000 |
| PP (Primary producer) | 5,842,000 |

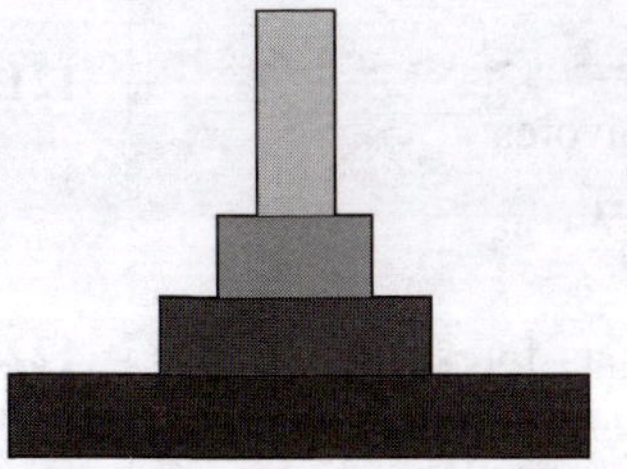

(a) 3 (b) 6 (c) 9 (d) 12

**100.** An inverted pyramid of biomass is seen in
(a) Forest ecosystem (b) Grassland ecosystem
(c) Aquatic ecosystem (d) Desert

**101.** Find out the correct statement:
(a) Trophic level represents a functional level, not a species as such.
(b) A given species never occupies more than one trophic level in the same ecosystem at the same time.
(c) In most of the ecosystems, producers are less in number and biomass than the herbivores.
(d) Pyramid of energy can never be upright.

**102.** Which of the following are limitations of ecological pyramids?
(a) It does not take into account the same species belonging to two or more trophic levels.
(b) It assumes a simple food chain that almost does not exist in nature.
(c) Saprophytes are not given at any place.
(d) All the above

**103.** Which of the following may occupy more than one trophic level in the same ecosystem at the same time?
(a) Lion (b) Sparrow
(c) Snake (d) Frog

**104.** Which of these are true about sparrows?
(a) When it eats seeds and peas, it is a primary consumer.
(b) When it eats insects and worms, it is a secondary consumer.
(c) It may occupy more than one trophic level in same ecosystem at the same time.
(d) All the above

**105.** Which of the following organisms have no space in ecological pyramid although they play vital role in the ecosystem?
(a) Birds (b) Snake
(c) Bacteria and fungi (d) Frog

**106.** The amount of nutrients such as carbon, nitrogen, phosphorus, calcium, etc., present in the soil at any given time is referred to as
(a) Standing state (b) Standing crop
(c) Hydrarch (d) Xerarch

**107.** Standing state
(a) Vary according to the type of ecosystem
(b) Vary on seasonal basis
(c) Both (a) and (b)
(d) None of these

**108.** Which of the following factors regulate the release of nutrients into the atmosphere?
(a) Soil and moisture (b) pH
(c) Temperature (d) All of these

**109.** Frog, snake and eagle belongs to
(a) Three trophic levels
(b) Two trophic levels
(c) Only one trophic level
(d) None of these

**110.** Diagrammatic representation of different trophic levels of an ecosystem presents
(a) Energy flow
(b) Mineral cycling
(c) Food chain and food web
(d) Ecological pyramids

**111.** A plant eaten by a herbivorous animal which in turn is eaten by a carnivorous animal forms a
(a) Food web (b) Food chain
(c) Food pyramid (d) Food cycle

**112.** Food chain operating on decaying cow dung or organic remains is referred to as
(a) Secondary succession
(b) Secondary food chain
(c) Food web
(d) Detritus food chain

**113.** Cycling of material in ecosystem is entirely dependent upon
(a) Producers and consumers
(b) Primary producers and herbivores
(c) Herbivores and carnivores
(d) Producers and decomposers

**114.** In a terrestrial ecosystem such as forest, maximum energy is found in which trophic level?
(a) $T_1$ (b) $T_2$
(c) $T_3$ (d) $T_4$

**115.** Trophic levels are formed by
(a) Only plants
(b) Only animals
(c) Only carnivores
(d) Organisms linked in food chains

**116.** If 20 J energy is available at producer level, then how much energy will be transferred to the lion in the food chain: producer → deer → lion?
(a) 0.2 J (b) 0.02 J
(c) 0.002 J (d) 2 J

**117.** Which one of the following has the largest population in a food chain?
(a) Producers
(b) Primary consumers
(c) Secondary consumers
(d) Decomposers

**118.** In a food chain, which trophic level is responsible for the maximum energy loss?
(a) Primary Producers
(b) Primary Consumers
(c) Secondary Consumers
(d) None of these

**Direction for Q119–125:** Choose the correct option:
(a) (A) is false but (R) is true
(b) Both (A) and (R) are true and (R) is the correct explanation of (A)
(c) Both (A) and (R) are true but (R) is not the correct explanation of (A)
(d) (A) is true but (R) is false.

**119. Assertion:** Sun is not the only source of energy for all ecosystems on Earth
**Reason:** For the deep sea ecosystem, hydro-thermal energy is the source.

**120. Assertion:** ecosystems are not exempt from the Second Law of thermodynamics.
**Reason:** ecosystems need a constant supply of energy to synthesise the molecules they require, to counteract the universal tendency toward increasing disorderliness.

**121. Assertion:** The energy trapped by the producer is either passed on to a consumer or the organism dies
**Reason:** No energy that is trapped into an organism remains in it for ever.

**122. Assertion:** animals are heterotrophs and are called consumers.
**Reason:** All animals depend on plants directly or indirectly for their food needs.

**123. Assertion:** detritus food chain is made up of decomposers which are heterotrophic organisms
**Reason:** Decomposers secrete digestive enzymes that breakdown dead and waste materials into simple, inorganic materials, which are subsequently absorbed by them.

**124. Assertion:** The natural interconnection of food chains make it a food web.
**Reason:** In a natural ecosystem, some animals are omnivores and some organisms of DFC are prey to the GFC animals.

**125. Assertion:** The number of trophic levels in the grazing food chain is restricted.
**Reason:** the transfer of energy follows 10 per cent law.

**Direction for Q126–133:** Choose the correct option:
(a) Statement I is incorrect but statement II is true.
(b) Both Statements I and II are true
(c) Both Statements I and II are false
(d) Statement I is correct but statement II is false

**126.** Read following sentences.
**Statement I:** Less than 50 per cent of the incident solar radiation is photosynthetically active radiation (PAR).
**Statement II:** Plants capture only 2-10 per cent of the PAR which is enough to sustain the entire living world.

**127.** Read following sentences.
**Statement I:** All organisms are dependent for their food on producers, either directly or indirectly.
**Statement II:** When any organism dies it is converted to detritus or dead biomass that serves as an energy source for decomposers.

**128.** Read following sentences.
**Statement I:** Common herbivores in terrestrial ecosystem are insects, birds and mammals.
**Statement II:** Common herbivores in aquatic ecosystem are molluscs.

**129.** Read following sentences.
**Statement I:** The detritus food chain (DFC) begins with dead organic matter.
**Statement II:** fungi and insects are main decomposers found in DFC.

**130.** Read following sentences.
**Statement I:** In an aquatic ecosystem, GFC is the major conduit for energy flow.
**Statement II:** in a terrestrial ecosystem, DFC is the major conduit for energy flow.

**131.** Read following sentences.
**Statement I:** Organisms occupy a place in the natural surroundings according to their feeding relationship with other organisms.
**Statement II:** Based on the source of their nutrition or food, organisms occupy a specific place in the food chain which is known as their trophic level.

**132.** Read following sentences.
**Statement I:** The biomass of a species is expressed in terms of fresh or dry weight.
**Statement II:** Measurement of biomass in terms of fresh weight is more accurate.

**133.** Read following sentences.
**Statement I:** Organisms at each trophic level depend on those at the lower trophic level for their energy demands.
**Statement II:** The standing crop is measured as the biomass of living organisms or the number in a unit area.

**134.** Choose the correct ones from the following statements regarding energy flow in an ecosystem:
(A) Energy flow is unidirectional, passing from producers to consumers and then to decomposers.
(B) Solar energy is the ultimate source of energy in most ecosystems.
(C) Only a small fraction of the energy is transferred from one trophic level to the next.
(D) Consumers obtain energy by consuming other organisms
(a) A, B and C (b) B, C and D
(c) A, B and D (d) A, B, C and D

**135.** Which of the following are consequences of the second law of thermodynamics in the context of energy flow in ecosystems?
(A) Energy is lost as heat during each energy transfer.
(B) The efficiency of energy transfer between trophic levels decreases.
(C) Energy is recycled within the ecosystem.
(D) Producers convert solar energy into chemical energy.
(a) A and B only (b) B, C and D only
(c) A, B and D only (d) A, B, C and D

**136.** Inverted pyramids of biomass are more commonly observed in
(a) forest ecosystems
(b) aquatic ecosystems
(c) grassland ecosystems
(d) desert ecosystems

**137.** Which of the following statements about ecological pyramids is/are true?
A. Pyramid of Numbers can never be inverted in a tree ecosystem.
B. Pyramid of Biomass represents the total mass of organisms at each trophic level.
C. Pyramid of Energy is always upright.
D. Inverted pyramid of biomass is common in a grassland ecosystem.
(a) a and c (b) b and c
(c) a, b and d (d) a and d

**Direction for Q138–140:** Choose the correct option:
(a) Statement I is incorrect but statement II is true.
(b) Both Statements I and II are true
(c) Both Statements I and II are false
(d) Statement I is correct but statement II is false

**138.** Read following sentences.
**Statement I:** Pyramids of ecosystem can be expressed in terms of number, biomass or energy.
**Statement II:** Organisms of different trophic levels in nature are connected to each other for food or energy relationship forming a food chain.

**139.** Read following sentences.
**Statement I:** A given organism may occupy more than one trophic level simultaneously.
**Statement II:** The trophic level represents a functional level, not a species as such.

**140.** Read following sentences.
**Statement I:** Energy at a lower trophic level is always more than at a higher level.
**Statement II:** The pyramid of biomass in sea is also generally inverted

**Direction for Q141–144:** Choose the correct option:
(a) (A) is false but (R) is true
(b) Both (A) and (R) are true and (R) is the correct explanation of (A)
(c) Both (A) and (R) are true but (R) is not the correct explanation of (A)
(d) (A) is true but (R) is false.

**141. Assertion:** Any calculations of energy content, biomass, or numbers has to include all organisms at a specific trophic level.
**Reason:** Generalisations made by considering only a few individuals at any trophic level will not be true

**142. Assertion:** A given species may occupy more than one trophic level in the same ecosystem at the same time
**Reason:** a sparrow is a primary consumer when it eats seeds, fruits, peas, and a secondary consumer when it eats insects and worms.

**143. Assertion:** The pyramid of biomass in sea is generally inverted
**Reason:** the biomass of fishes far exceeds that of phytoplankton.

**144. Assertion:** Pyramid of energy is always upright and can never be inverted,
**Reason:** energy flow from one to the next trophic level is always associated with loss as heat at each step.

**145.** Limitations of ecological pyramids are
(A) no consideration of the species belonging to two or more trophic levels.
(B) assumption of a simple food chain, which is rare in nature;
(C) no accommodation of a food web.
(D) no place for saprophytes
(a) A and B only (b) B, C and D only
(c) A, B and D only (d) A, B, C and D

## Multiple Choice Questions: Level II

**146.** Which one of the following types of organisms occupy more than one trophic level in a pond ecosystem?
(a) fish (b) zooplankton
(c) frog (d) phytoplankton

**147.** Consider the following statements concerning food chains-
(A) Removal of 80% tigers from an area resulted in greatly increased growth of vegetation
(B) Removal of most of the carnivores resulted in an increased population of deers
(C) The length of food chains is generally limited to 3–4 trophic levels due to energy loss
(D) The length of food chains may vary from 2 to 8 trophic levels.

Which two of the above statements are correct?
(a) A, D (b) A, B
(c) B, C (d) C, D

**148.** The slow rate of decomposition of fallen logs in nature is due to their-
(a) Anaerobic environment around them
(b) low cellulose content
(c) Low moisture content
(d) Poor nitrogen content

**149.** 'The table below gives the populations (in thousands) often species, (A-J) in four areas (p-s) consisting of the number of habitats given within brackets against each. Study the table and answer the question which follows

| Area and No of habitats | Species and their population (in thousands) in the areas | | | | | | | | | |
|---|---|---|---|---|---|---|---|---|---|---|
| | A | B | C | D | E | F | G | H | I | J |
| p(11) | 2.3 | 1.2 | 0.52 | 6 | – | 3.1 | 1.1 | 9 | – | 10.3 |
| q(11) | 10.2 | – | 0.62 | – | 1.5 | 3 | – | 8.2 | 1.1 | 11.2 |
| r(13) | 11.3 | 0.9 | 0.48 | 2.4 | 1.4 | 4.2 | 0.8 | 8.4 | 2.2 | 4.1 |
| s(12) | 3.2 | 10.2 | 11.1 | 4.8 | 0.4 | 3.3 | 0.8 | 7.3 | 11.3 | 2.1 |

Which area out of p–s shows maximum species diversity?
(a) q (b) r (c) s (d) p

**150.** About 70% of total global carbon is found in
(a) oceans (b) forests
(c) grasslands (d) agroecosystems

**151.** Which one of the following ecosystem types has the highest annual net primary productivity?
(a) tropical deciduous forest

(b) temperate evergreen forest
(c) temperate deciduous forest
(d) tropical rain forest

**152.** Which one of the following is not used for construction of ecological pyramids?
(a) Number of individuals
(b) Rate of energy flow
(c) Fresh weight
(d) Dry weight

**153.** Which of the following is expected to have the highest value (gm/m²/yr) in a grassland ecosystem?
(a) Secondary Production
(b) Tertiary Production
(c) Gross Primary Productivity (GPP)
(d) Net Production (NP)

**154.** Bamboo plant is growing in a fir forest then what will be the trophic level of it?
(a) First trophic level ($T_1$)
(b) Second trophic level ($T_2$)
(c) Third trophic level ($T_3$)
(d) Fourth trophic level ($T_4$)

**155.** The greatest biomass of autotrophs in the oceans is that of
(a) sea grasses and slime moulds
(b) free-floating microalgae, cyanobacteria and nanoplankton
(c) benthic brown algae, coastal red algae and daphnids
(d) benthic diatoms and marine viruses

**156.** Which part of the world has high density of organisms?
(a) Grasslands
(b) Savannahs
(c) Deciduous forests
(d) Tropical rain forests

**157.** Which of the following communities is more vulnerable to invasion by outside animals and plants?
(a) Tropical evergreen forests
(b) Oceanic island communities
(c) Mangroves
(d) Temperate forests

**158.** The rate at which light energy is converted to the chemical energy of organic molecules is the ecosystem's
(a) Net primary productivity
(b) Gross primary productivity
(c) Net secondary productivity
(d) Gross secondary productivity

**159.** Which of the following ecosystem has highest rate of gross primary production?
(a) Grasslands
(b) Mangroves
(c) Coral reefs
(d) Equatorial rain forest

**160.** In a food chain, the largest population is of
(a) decomposers
(b) producers
(c) primary consumers
(d) tertiary consumers

**161.** The transfer of energy from one trophic level to another is governed by the 2nd law of thermodynamics. The average efficiency of energy transfer from herbivores to carnivores is
(a) 5% (b) 10%
(c) 25% (d) 50%

**162.** Niche of a species in an ecosystem refers to its
(a) function at its place of occurrence
(b) place of its occurrence
(c) competitive ability
(d) centre of origin

**163.** If we completely remove the decomposers from an ecosystem, its functioning will be adversely affected, because
(a) energy flow will be blocked.
(b) herbivores will not receive solar energy.
(c) mineral movement will be blocked.
(d) rate of decomposition will be very high.

**164.** Which of the following is the most stable ecosystem?
(a) Forest (b) Desert
(c) Mountain (d) Ocean

**165.** In a biotic community, the primary consumers are
(a) carnivores
(b) omnivores
(c) detritivores
(d) herbivores

**166** The pyramid which cannot be inverted in a stable ecosystem is that of
(a) Biomass (b) Number
(c) Energy (d) All the above

**167.** In grass–deer–tiger food chain, grass biomass is one tonne. The tiger biomass shall be
(a) 100 Kg (b) 10 kg
(c) 200 kg (d) 1 kg

**168.** In a biotic community, the most important factor for survival of an animal is
(a) Day length (b) Soil moisture
(c) Green food (d) Predators

**169.** In a food chain, the largest population is that of
(a) Producers
(b) Decomposers
(c) Secondary consumers
(d) Primary consumers

**171.** Second-most important trophic level in a lake is
(a) Zooplankton
(b) Phytoplankton
(c) Benthos
(d) Neuston

**171.** Pyramid of numbers deals with number of
(a) Species in an area
(b) Individuals in a community
(c) Individuals in a tropic level
(d) Subspecies in a community

**172.** Pyramid of numbers in a pond ecosystem is
(a) Irregular
(b) Inverted
(c) Upright
(d) Spindle shaped

**173.** Food chain in which micro-organisms breakdown the food formed by primary producers is
(a) Parasitic food chain
(b) Detritus food chain
(c) Consumer food chain
(d) Predator food chain

**174.** Pick up the correct food chain
(a) Grass → Chameleon → Insect → Bird
(b) Grass → Fox → Rabbit → Bird
(c) Phytoplankton → Zooplankton → Fish
(d) Fallen leaves → Bacteria → Insect larvae

**175.** Pyramid of numbers in a grassland/true ecosystem is
(a) Always inverted
(b) Always upright
(c) Both A and B
(d) Spindle-shaped

**176.** Upper part of sea/aquatic ecosystem contains
(a) Plankton
(b) Nekton
(c) Plankton and Nekton
(d) Benthos

**177.** What is true of ecosystem?
(a) Primary consumers are least dependent upon producers.
(b) Primary consumers outnumber producers.
(c) Producers are more than primary consumers.
(d) Secondary consumers are the largest and most powerful.

**178.** In an ecosystem, which one shows one-way passage?
(a) Free energy (b) Carbon
(c) Nitrogen (d) Potassium

# A & R and Statement-based Questions

## Assertion and Reason Questions:

***Direction for questions 179 to 183:** Read the **assertion** and **reason** carefully to mark the correct option out of the options given below:*

**(a) (A)** is **true** but **(R)** is **false**.
**(b) (A)** is **false** but **(R)** is **true**.
**(c)** Both **(A)** and **(R)** is **true** and **(R)** is the correct explanation of **(A)**.
**(d)** Both **(A)** and **(R)** is **true** and **(R)** is not the correct explanation of **(A)**.

**179. Assertion:** Forest, grassland and desert are examples of terrestrial ecosystem.
**Reason:** Ecosystem is a functional unit of nature.

**180. Assertion:** Vertical distribution of different species occupying different levels is called stratification.
**Reason:** Tree occupy top vertical strata of forest.

**181. Assertion:** Secondary productivity is defined as the rate of formation of new organic matter by consumers.
**Reason:** Secondary productivity = GPP – R.

**182.** **Assertion:** Amount of nutrient present in the soil at any given time, in a given ecosystem is referred as the standing state.
**Reason:** Each trophic level has a certain mass of living material at particular time is known as the standing crop.

**183.** **Assertion:** In terrestrial ecosystem, a large amount of energy passes through detritus food chain.
**Reason:** Energy for the detritus food chain comes from the sun.

***Direction for questions 184 to 187:*** *These type of questions consist of two statement each, printed as* **Statement-I** *and* **Statement-II**. *While answering such questions, a student is needed to choose any one of the following four responses.*

**(a)** **(A)** is **correct** but **(R)** is **incorrect**.
**(b)** **(A)** is **incorrect** but **(R)** is **correct**.
**(c)** Both **(A)** and **(R)** is **true** and **(R)** is the correct explanation of **(A)**.
**(d)** Both **(A)** and **(R)** is **true** and **(R)** is the incorrect explanation of **(A)**.

**184.** **Assertion:** Biomass of a species is expressed in terms of dry weight in more accurate than fresh weight.
**Reason:** Fresh weight is affected by environment condition.

**185.** **Assertion:** Pyramid of energy is always upright.
**Reason:** Energy flow is unidirectional and some energy is always lost as heat at each step.

**186.** **Assertion:** Ecosystem is an open system.
**Reason:** Ecosystem exchange mass as well as energy from surrounding.

**187.** **Assertion:** Despite occupying about 70% of surface, the productivity of oceans is only 55 billion to us.
**Reason:** Light and minerals are limiting factor for productivity of ocean.

## Matrix-Match Type Questions

**188.** Match the following:

| List-I (Step in Decomposition) | List-II (Action) |
|---|---|
| 1. Fragmentation | (i) Release of water soluble inorganic nutrients |
| 2. Leaching | (ii) Release of inorganic substances by microbes |
| 3. Catabolism | (iii) Breakdown of detritus in smaller particles |
| 4. Humification | (iv) Enzymatic degradation of detritus into simple inorganic substance |
| 5. Mineralisation | (v) Accumulation of a dark coloured amorphous substance |

**The correct matching is**

| | 1 | 2 | 3 | 4 | 5 |
|---|---|---|---|---|---|
| (a) | (iii) | (i) | (iv) | (v) | (ii) |
| (b) | (ii) | (iii) | (iv) | (i) | (v) |
| (c) | (i) | (iv) | (iii) | (ii) | (v) |
| (d) | (ii) | (iv) | (i) | (iii) | (v) |

**189.** Match the following:

| List-I (Term) | List-II (Definition) |
|---|---|
| 1. Stratification | (i) Rate of biomass produced per unit area over a time period by plants during photosynthesis |
| 2. Primary productivity | (ii) Rate of formation of new organic matter by consumers over a time period |
| 3. Secondary productivity | (iii) Vertical distribution of different species occupying different levels |
| 4. Decomposition | (iv) Break down of complex organic matter into inorganic substances |

**The correct matching is**

| | 1 | 2 | 3 | 4 |
|---|---|---|---|---|
| (a) | (iii) | (i) | (ii) | (iv) |
| (b) | (i) | (iv) | (ii) | (iii) |
| (c) | (ii) | (iii) | (iv) | (i) |
| (d) | (iv) | (iii) | (i) | (ii) |

**190.** Match the following:

| List-I (Process) | List-II (Factors) |
|---|---|
| 1. Rate of decomposition of detritus increases | (i) Detritus rich in lignin & chitin |
| 2. Rate of decomposition of detritus decreases | (ii) Detritus rich in nitrogen & water-soluble substances |
| | (iii) Anaerobiosis |
| | (iv) Warm & moist environment |
| | (v) Aerobic environment |
| | (vi) Low temperature |

**The correct matching is**

(a) 1 – (ii), (iv), (v), 2 – (i), (iii), (vi)
(b) 1 – (i), (iii), (vi), 2 – (ii), (iv), (v)
(c) 1 – (i), (iv), (v), 2 – (ii), (iii), (vi)
(d) 1 – (ii), (iv), (vi), 2 – (i), (iii), (v)

**191.** Match the following:

| List-I | List-II |
|---|---|
| 1. Climax community | (i) Vertical distribution of different species occupying different levels |
| 2. Ecological succession | (ii) Mass of living organisms at a particular time in a trophic level |
| 3. Standing crop | (iii) Gradual & fairly predictable change in the species composition of a given area |
| 4. Stratification | (iv) Community which is in near equilibrium with environment |

**The correct matching is**

| | 1 | 2 | 3 | 4 |
|---|---|---|---|---|
| (a) | (iv) | (iii) | (ii) | (i) |
| (b) | (i) | (iv) | (ii) | (iii) |
| (c) | (ii) | (iii) | (iv) | (i) |
| (d) | (iv) | (iii) | (i) | (ii) |

## NCERT Exemplar Questions

**1.** Decomposers like fungi and bacteria are
i. Autotrophs
ii. Heterotrophs
iii. Saprotrophs
iv. Chemoautotrophs

Choose the correct answer:
(a) i and iii (b) i and iv
(c) ii and iii (d) i and ii

**2.** The process of mineralization by microorganisms helps in the release of
(a) Inorganic nutrients from humus.
(b) Both organic and inorganic nutrients from detritus.
(c) Organic nutrients from humus.
(d) Inorganic nutrients from detritus and formation of humus.

**3.** Productivity is the rate of production of biomass expressed in terms of
i. $(kcal\ m^{-3})\ yr^{-1}$
ii. $gm^{-2}\ yr^{-1}$
iii. $g^{-1}\ yr^{-1}$
iv. $(kcal\ m^{-2})\ yr^{-1}$

(a) ii (b) iii
(c) ii and iv (d) i and iii

**4.** An inverted pyramid of biomass can be found in which ecosystem?
(a) Forest (b) Marine
(c) Grassland (d) Tundra

**5.** Which of the following is not a producer?
(a) *Spirogyra* (b) *Agaricus*
(c) *Volvox* (d) *Nostoc*

**6.** Which of the following ecosystems is more productive in terms of net primary production?
(a) Deserts (b) Tropical rain forests
(c) Oceans (d) Estuaries

**7.** Pyramid of numbers is
(a) Always upright
(b) Always inverted
(c) Either upright or inverted
(d) Neither upright nor inverted

**8.** Approximately how much of the solar energy that falls on the leaves of a plant is converted to chemical energy by photosynthesis?
(a) Less than 1% (b) 2 to 10%
(c) 30% (d) 50%

**9.** Among the following, where do you think the process of decomposition would be the fastest?
(a) Tropical rain forest (b) Antarctic
(c) Dry arid region (d) Alpine region

**10.** How much of the net primary productivity of a terrestrial ecosystem is eaten and digested by herbivores?
(a) 1% (b) 10%
(c) 40% (d) 90%

**11.** The zone at the edge of a lake or ocean which is alternatively exposed to air and immersed in water is called
(a) Pelagic zone (b) Benthic zone
(c) Lentic zone (d) Littoral zone

**12.** If the carbon atoms fixed by producers already have passed through three species, then the trophic level of the last species would be
(a) Scavenger (b) Tertiary producer
(c) Tertiary consumer (d) Secondary consumer

**13.** Which of the following type of ecosystem is expected in an area where evaporation exceeds precipitation and the mean annual rainfall is below 100 mm
(a) Grassland (b) Shrubby forest
(c) Desert (d) Mangrove

## Previous Years' Questions

**1.** The biomass available for consumption by the herbivores and the decomposers is called:
[AIPMT 2010 PRE]
(a) Net primary productivity
(b) Secondary productivity
(c) Standing crop
(d) Gross primary productivity

**2.** Which of the following representations shows the pyramid of numbers in a forest ecosystem?

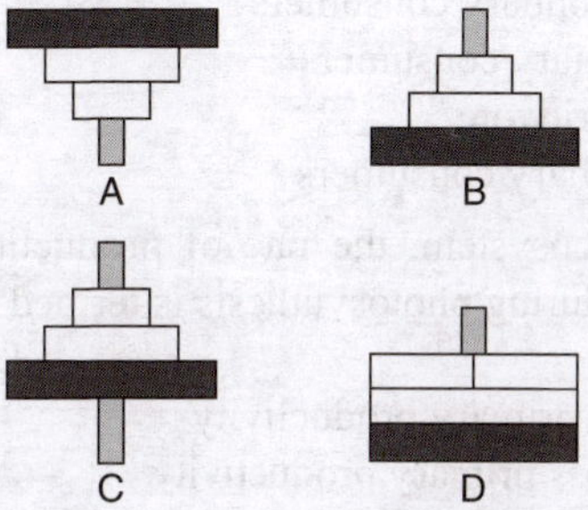


[AIPMT 2010 MAINS]
(a) D (b) A
(c) B (d) C

**3.** Of the total incident solar radiation, the proportion of PAR is: [AIPMT 2011 PRE]
(a) About 60% (b) Less than 50%
(c) More than 80% (d) About 70%

**4.** Mass of living matter at a trophic level in an area at any time is called: [AIPMT 2011 PRE]
(a) Detritus (b) Humus
(c) Standing state (d) Standing crop

**5.** Which one of the following statements for pyramid of energy is incorrect, whereas the remaining three are correct? [AIPMT 2011 PRE]
(a) It shows energy content of different trophic level organisms
(b) It is inverted in shape
(c) It is upright in shape
(d) Its base is broad

**6.** The breakdown of detritus into smaller particles by earthworm is a process called
[AIPMT 2011 MAINS]
(a) Humification (b) Fragmentation
(c) Mineralization (d) Catabolism

**7.** Which one of the following animals may occupy more than one trophic levels in the same ecosystem at the same time? [AIPMT 2011 MAINS]
(a) Sparrow (b) Lion
(c) Goat (d) Frog

**8.** The upright pyramid of number is absent in:
[AIPMT 2012 PRE]
(a) Pond (b) Forest
(c) Lake (d) Grassland

**9.** Which one of the following is not a functional unit of an ecosystem? [AIPMT 2012 PRE]
(a) Energy flow (b) Decomposition
(c) Productivity (d) Stratification

**10.** Given below is an imaginary pyramid of numbers. What could be one of the possibilities about certain organisms at some of the different levels?

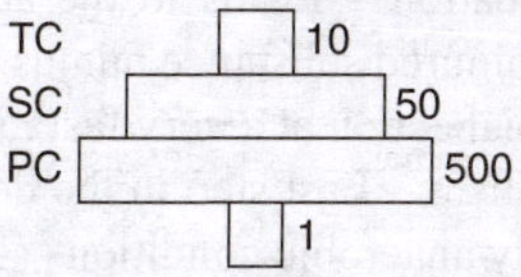


[AIPMT 2012 PRE]
(a) Level PC is 'insects' and level SC is 'small insectivorous birds'
(b) Level PP is 'phytoplanktons' in sea and 'whale' on top level TC
(c) Level one PP is 'pipal trees' and the level SC is 'sheep'
(d) Level PC is 'rats' and level SC is 'cats'

**11.** Identify the possible link 'A' in the following food chain: Plant → insert → Frog → 'A'→ Eagle [AIPMT 2012 PRE]

(a) Rabbit (b) Wolf
(c) Cobra (d) Parrot

**12.** Identify the likely organisms (a), (b), (c) and (d) in the food web shown below:

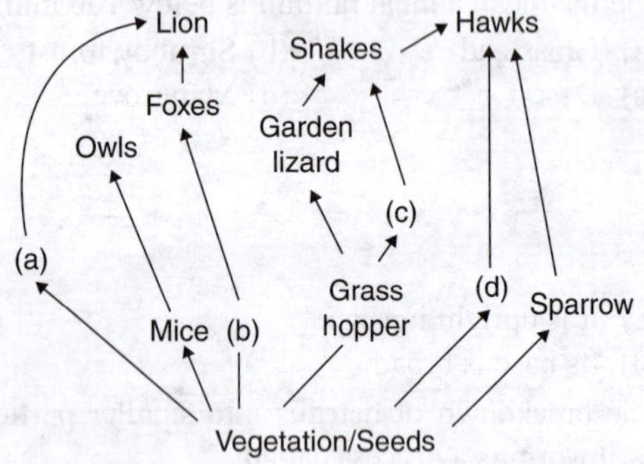


[AIPMT 2012 MAINS]

**Options:**

(a) A: Dog, B: Squirrel, C: Bat, D: Deer
(b) A: Rat, B: Dog, C: Tortoise, D: Crow
(c) A: Squirrel, B: Cat, C: Rat, D: Pigeon
(d) A: Deer, B: Rabbit, C: Frog, D: Rat

**13.** The rate of formation of new organic matter by rabbit in a grassland is called: [AIPMT 2012 MAINS]

(a) Secondary productivity
(b) Net primary productivity
(c) Gross primary productivity
(d) Net productivity

**14.** Which one of the following processes during decomposition is correctly described? [AIPMT 2013]

(a) Fragmentation – Carried out by organisms such as earthworm
(b) Humification – Leads to the accumulation of a dark-coloured substance humus which undergoes microbial action at a very fast rate
(c) Catabolism – Last step in the decomposition under fully anaerobic condition
(d) Leaching – Water-soluble inorganic nutrients rise to the top layers of soil

**15.** Secondary productivity is rate of formation of one organic matter by: [AIPMT 2013]

(a) Producer
(b) Parasite
(c) Consume
(d) Decomposer

**16.** If 20 J of energy is trapped at producer level, then how much energy will be available to peacock as food in the following chain?
Plant → Mice → Snake → Peacock [AIPMT 2014]

(a) 0.02 J (b) 0.002 J
(c) 0.2 J (d) 0.0002 J

**17.** Match the following and select the correct option. [AIPMT 2014]

| Column – I | Column – II |
|---|---|
| (A) Earthworm | (1) Pioneer species |
| (B) Succession | (2) Detritivore |
| (C) Ecosystem service | (3) Natality |
| (D) Population growth | (4) Pollination |

(a) A:1, B:2, C:3, D:4
(b) A:4, B:1, C:3, D:2
(c) A:3, B:2, C:4, D:1
(d) A:2, B:1, C:4, D:3

**18.** Most animals that live in deep oceanic waters are: [RE-AIPMT 2015]

(a) Secondary consumers
(b) Tertiary consumers
(c) Detritivore
(d) Primary consumers

**19.** In an ecosystem, the rate of production of organic matter during photosynthesis is termed as: [AIPMT 2015]

(a) Net primary productivity
(b) Gross primary productivity
(c) Secondary productivity
(d) Net productivity

**20.** The mass of living material at a trophic level at a particular time is called [AIPMT 2015]

(a) Gross primary productivity
(b) Standing state
(c) Net primary productivity
(d) Standing crop

**21.** Vertical distribution of different species occupying different levels in a biotic community is known as: [AIPMT 2015]

(a) Divergence (b) Stratification
(c) Zonation (d) Pyramid

**22.** The term ecosystem was coined by: [NEET 2016 – PHASE I]

(a) E.P.Odum (b) A.G. Tansley
(c) E. Haeckel (d) E. Warming

**23.** Which of the following is a characteristic feature of cropland ecosystem? [NEET 2016 – PHASE I]
(a) Absence of soil organisms
(b) Least genetic diversity
(c) Absence of weeds
(d) Ecological succession

**24.** The primary producers of the deep-sea hydrothermal vent ecosystem are [NEET 2016 – PHASE II]
(a) Chemosynthetic bacteria
(b) Blue–green algae
(c) Coral reefs
(d) Green algae

**25.** Which of the following statements is not true? [NEET Regional 2017]
(a) Energy pyramids of an ecosystem tend to diminish at higher trophic levels
(b) A single organism can feed at several trophic levels
(c) Detritivores feed at all trophic levels except the producer level
(d) Primary consumers are herbivores

**26.** Which ecosystem has the maximum biomass? [NEET 2017]
(a) Grassland ecosystem
(b) Pond ecosystem
(c) Lake ecosystem
(d) Forest ecosystem

**27.** Presence of plants arranged into well-defined vertical layers depending on their height can be seen best in: [NEET 2017]
(a) Tropical Rain Forest (b) Grassland
(c) Temperate Forest (d) Tropical Savannah

**28.** What type of ecological pyramid would be obtained with the following data?
Secondary consumer: 120 g
Primary consumer: 60 g
Primary producer: 10 g
[NEET 2018]
(a) Inverted pyramid of biomass
(b) Upright pyramid of numbers
(c) Pyramid of energy
(d) Upright pyramid of biomass

**29.** Which of the following ecological pyramids is generally inverted? [NEET 2019]
(a) Pyramid of energy
(b) Pyramid of biomass in a forest
(c) Pyramid of biomass in a sea
(d) Pyramid of numbers in grassland

**30.** Match the trophic levels with their correct species examples in grassland ecosystem. [NEET 2020]

| Column - I | Column - II |
|---|---|
| (A) Fourth trophic level | (i) Crow |
| (B) Second trophic level | (ii) Vulture |
| (C) First trophic level | (iii) Rabbit |
| (D) Third trophic level | (iv) Grass |

Select the correct option.

| | (A) | (B) | (C) | (D) |
|---|---|---|---|---|
| (a) | (ii) | (iii) | (iv) | (i) |
| (b) | (iii) | (ii) | (i) | (iv) |
| (c) | (iv) | (iii) | (ii) | (i) |
| (d) | (i) | (ii) | (iii) | (iv) |

**31.** In relation to Gross primary productivity and Net primary productivity of an ecosystem, which one of the following statements is correct? [NEET 2020]
(a) Gross primary productivity is always less than net primary productivity.
(b) Gross primary productivity is always more than net primary productivity.
(c) Gross primary productivity and Net primary productivity are one and same.
(d) There is no relationship between Gross primary productivity and Net primary productivity.

**32.** Which of the following statements is not correct? [NEET 2021]
(a) Pyramid of numbers in a grassland ecosystem is upright.
(b) Pyramid of biomass in sea is generally inverted.
(c) Pyramid of biomass in sea is generally upright.
(d) Pyramid of energy is always upright.

**33.** In the equation GPP – R = NPP
R represents: [NEET 2021]
(a) Respiration losses (b) Radiant energy
(c) Retardation factor (d) Environment factor

**34.** The amount of nutrients, such as carbon, nitrogen, phosphorus and calcium present in the soil at any given time, is referred as [NEET 2021]
(a) Standing crop (b) Climax
(c) Climax community (d) Standing state

**35.** Given below are two statements: [NEET 2022]
**Statement I:** Decomposition is a process in which the detritus is degraded into simpler substances by microbes.
**Statement II:** Decomposition is faster if the detritus is rich in lignin and chitin.

In the light of the above statements, choose the **correct answer** from the options given below:
(a) Both **Statement I** and **Statement II** are incorrect.
(b) **Statement I** is correct but **Statement II** is incorrect.
(c) **Statement I** is incorrect but **Statement II** is correct.
(d) Both **Statement I** and **Statement II** are correct.

**36.** Which one of the following will accelerate phosphorus cycle? [NEET 2022]
(a) Volcanic activity
(b) Weathering of rocks
(c) Rain fall and storms
(d) Burning of fossil fuels

**37.** Detritivores breakdown detritus into smaller particles. This process is called: [NEET 2022]
(a) Fragmentation (b) Humification
(c) Decomposition (d) Catabolism

**38.** Identify the correct statements: [NEET 2023]
A. Detritivores perform fragmentation.
B. The humus is further degraded by some microbes during mineralization.
C. Water soluble inorganic nutrients go down into the soil and get precipitated by a process called leaching.
D. The detritus food chain begins with living organism.
E. Earthworms break down detritus into smaller particles by a process called catabolism.

Choose the correct answer from the options given below:
(a) B,C,D only (b) C,D,E only
(c) D,E,A only (d) A,B,C only

**39.** In the equation [NEET 2023]
GPP-R= NPP
GPP is Gross Primary Productivity
NPP is Net Primary Productivity
R here is ______.
(a) Respiratory quotient
(b) Respiratory loss
(c) Reproductive allocation
(d) Photosynthetically active radiation

**40.** In an ecosystem, if the Net Primary Productivity (NPP) of first trophic level is $100x$ (kcal m$^{-2}$) yr$^{-1}$. What would be the GPP (Gross Primary Productivity) of the third trophic level of the same ecosystem? [NEET 2024]
(a) $\frac{x}{10}$ (kcal m$^{-2}$) yr$^{-1}$ (b) $x$(kcal m$^{-2}$) yr$^{-1}$
(c) $10x$ (kcal m$^{-2}$) yr$^{-1}$ (d) $\frac{100x}{3x}$ (kcal m$^{-2}$ ) yr$^{-1}$

## Answer Key

### Multiple Choice Questions: Level I

| | | | | | | | | | |
|---|---|---|---|---|---|---|---|---|---|
| **1.** (b) | **2.** (d) | **3.** (d) | **4.** (d) | **5.** (c) | **6.** (a) | **7.** (d) | **8.** (d) | **9.** (c) | **10.** (c) |
| **11.** (d) | **12.** (d) | **13.** (b) | **14.** (a) | **15.** (d) | **16.** (c) | **17.** (a) | **18.** (d) | **19.** (d) | **20.** (b) |
| **21.** (d) | **22.** (a) | **23.** (b) | **24.** (a) | **25.** (c) | **26.** (b) | **27.** (b) | **28.** (d) | **29.** (b) | **30.** (c) |
| **31.** (a) | **32.** (b) | **33.** (c) | **34.** (b) | **35.** (c) | **36.** (c) | **37.** (d) | **38.** (d) | **39.** (a) | **40.** (d) |
| **41.** (d) | **42.** (b) | **43.** (d) | **44.** (b) | **45.** (d) | **46.** (d) | **47.** (b) | **48.** (b) | **49.** (a) | **50.** (d) |
| **51.** (d) | **52.** (b) | **53.** (a) | **54.** (b) | **55.** (c) | **56.** (b) | **57.** (b) | **58.** (b) | **59.** (b) | **60.** (b) |
| **61.** (d) | **62.** (d) | **63.** (d) | **64.** (b) | **65.** (a) | **66.** (a) | **67.** (d) | **68.** (c) | **69.** (a) | **70.** (a) |
| **71.** (a) | **72.** (a) | **73.** (d) | **74.** (a) | **75.** (d) | **76.** (b) | **77.** (d) | **78.** (a) | **79.** (a) | **80.** (a) |
| **81.** (c) | **82.** (b) | **83.** (b) | **84.** (c) | **85.** (d) | **86.** (b) | **87.** (a) | **88.** (b) | **89.** (c) | **90.** (b) |
| **91.** (b) | **92.** (b) | **93.** (a) | **94.** (a) | **95.** (c) | **96.** (d) | **97.** (a) | **98.** (c) | **99.** (a) | **100.** (c) |
| **101.** (a) | **102.** (d) | **103.** (b) | **104.** (d) | **105.** (c) | **106.** (a) | **107.** (c) | **108.** (d) | **109.** (a) | **110.** (d) |
| **111.** (b) | **112.** (d) | **113.** (d) | **114.** (a) | **115.** (d) | **116.** (a) | **117.** (a) | **118.** (c) | **119.** (b) | **120.** (b) |
| **121.** (b) | **122.** (b) | **123.** (b) | **124.** (b) | **125.** (b) | **126.** (b) | **127.** (b) | **128.** (b) | **129.** (d) | **130.** (b) |
| **131.** (b) | **132.** (d) | **133.** (b) | **134.** (d) | **135.** (a) | **136.** (b) | **137.** (b) | **138.** (b) | **139.** (b) | **140.** (b) |
| **141.** (b) | **142.** (b) | **143.** (b) | **144.** (b) | **145.** (d) | | | | | |

### Multiple Choice Questions: Level II

| | | | | | | | | | |
|---|---|---|---|---|---|---|---|---|---|
| **146.** (a) | **147.** (c) | **148.** (c) | **149.** (c) | **150.** (a) | **151.** (d) | **152.** (c) | **153.** (c) | **154.** (a) | **155.** (b) |
| **156.** (d) | **157.** (b) | **158.** (b) | **159.** (c) | **160.** (b) | **161.** (b) | **162.** (a) | **163.** (c) | **164.** (d) | **165.** (d) |
| **166.** (c) | **167.** (b) | **168.** (c) | **169.** (a) | **170.** (a) | **171.** (c) | **172.** (c) | **173.** (b) | **174.** (c) | **175.** (b) |
| **176.** (a) | **177.** (c) | **178.** (a) | | | | | | | |

### A & R and Statement-based Questions

| | | | | | | | | |
|---|---|---|---|---|---|---|---|---|
| **179.** (d) | **180.** (d) | **181.** (a) | **182.** (d) | **183.** (a) | **184.** (c) | **185.** (c) | **186.** (c) | **187.** (c) |

### Matrix-Match Type Questions

| | | | |
|---|---|---|---|
| **188.** (a) | **189.** (a) | **190.** (a) | **191.** (a) |

### NCERT Exemplar Questions

| | | | | | | | | | |
|---|---|---|---|---|---|---|---|---|---|
| **1.** (c) | **2.** (a) | **3.** (c) | **4.** (b) | **5.** (b) | **6.** (b) | **7.** (c) | **8.** (b) | **9.** (a) | **10.** (b) |
| **11.** (d) | **12.** (c) | **13.** (c) | | | | | | | |

### Previous Years' Questions

| | | | | | | | | | |
|---|---|---|---|---|---|---|---|---|---|
| **1.** (a) | **2.** (c) | **3.** (b) | **4.** (d) | **5.** (b) | **6.** (b) | **7.** (a) | **8.** (b) | **9.** (d) | **10.** (a) |
| **11.** (c) | **12.** (d) | **13.** (a) | **14.** (a) | **15.** (c) | **16.** (a) | **17.** (d) | **18.** (c) | **19.** (b) | **20.** (d) |
| **21.** (b) | **22.** (b) | **23.** (b) | **24.** (a) | **25.** (c) | **26.** (d) | **27.** (a) | **28.** (a) | **29.** (c) | **30.** (a) |
| **31.** (b) | **32.** (c) | **33.** (a) | **34.** (d) | **35.** (b) | **36.** (b) | **37.** (a) | **38.** (d) | **39.** (b) | **40.** (c) |

# HINTS AND EXPLANATION

## Multiple Choice Questions: Level II

**146.** A pond ecosystem is a delicate balance of fish, plants and other animals. Fish occupy more than one tropic level in pond ecosystem. Small fishes act as secondary consumer. They feed on primary consumer. Large fishes act as tertiary consumer. They feed on smaller fish.

**147.** Removal of carnivores remove check over growth of herbivore like deer, therefore, population increases.

Trophic levels in food chain are generally limited to 3–4 level because of limitation of transfer of energy.

**148.** Following factors affect rate of decomposition of detritus (include fallen leaves):

- Oxygenic environment: Anaerobiosis decreases rate.
- Temperature: Low temperature decreases rate.
- Moisture: Decrease in moisture decreases rate.
- Composition: lignin and chitin-rich detritus shows less decomposition rate.

**149.** Area (s) and number of habitats (12) shows the maximum species diversity.

**150.** 71% of the total quantity of global carbon is found dissolved in oceans. Thus, the amount of carbon dioxide in the atmosphere is regulated by oceanic reservoirs.

**151.** They are found in the equatorial regions rainfall exceeds 140 cm The warm humid climate supports broad-leaved evergreen plants.

Productivity is very high (12000 k.cal/m$^2$/ year). The vegetation shows stratification into two or more well-defined layers.

**152.** We cannot use the fresh weight for the construction of ecological pyramids because the total fresh weight does not change into energy or we can say the fresh weight is not continuous in the tropic levels.

**153.** Gross production has highest value in grassland ecosystem.

**154.** First trophic level is occupied by producers. Second trophic level is occupied by primary consumers. Third trophic level is occupied by the secondary consumers.

**155.** The greatest biomass of autotrophs in the oceans is that of free-floating microalgae, cyanobacteria and nanoplankton.

**156.** Tropical rain forests occur in equatorial and sub-equatorial regions. The forests receive all the external inputs for optimum plant growth. Due to abundant plant growth, large number of animals live in tropical rain forests. In grasslands, fire occurs periodically which prevents tree growth. In savannah, periods of drought are common. In deciduous forests are found predominantly broad-leaved hard wood deciduous trees.

**157.** This is because oceanic islands are normally cut off from other habitats.

**158.** This is called gross primary productivity.

**159.** Productivity in aquatic ecosystems – Coral reef (even higher than tropical rain forest) > Estuary > Coastal > Open sea.

Productivity in terrestrial ecosystems – Tropical rain forest > Tropical deciduous forest > Temperate deciduous forest > Temperate coniferous forest > Savannah > Temperate grassland > Desert.

**160.** Producers are the direct and indirect source of food for all the trophic levels.

**161.** According to the Ten percent law, at each trophic level, only 10% of the energy received is transferred to the next trophic level.

**162.** Niche is a specific part of the habitat that is determined by the functioning of the population like shelter, type of food, season, etc.

**163.** The decomposers act on the dead organic matter and break them down into simpler compounds and minerals. Therefore, mineral movement will be blocked.

**164.** The oceans cover about two-third of the whole surface of our earth. Thus, it is the most stable ecosystem, because of buffering action by water.

**165.** In a biotic community, the herbivores (goat, deer) are those animals which consume the primary producers (green plants). Hence, they are primary consumers.

**166.** Energy pyramid cannot be inverted because energy always flows in one direction only.

**167.** Only 10% of the mass is flown from one tropic level to another in the form of energy.

**168.** Food is necessary for life.

**169.** In food chain, the maximum number is of producers

**170.** First tropic level in a lake is phytoplankton, second is zooplankton.

**171.** Pyramid of number represents the number of individuals on each tropic level.

**172.** Pyramid of numbers of pond ecosystem is upright. Pyramid of biomass is inverted in pond.

**173.** Food chain starts from detritus (may be of any trophic level) is called DFC.

**174.** Phytoplankton (Primary producer) → zooplankton (Primary consumer) → Fish(secondary consumer)

**175.** Pyramid of numbers in a grassland ecosystem is always upright. Pyramid of number is inverted in tree ecosystem.

**176.** Plankton → passively floating in upper water

Nekton → Actively swimming

Benthos → lead sedentary life upon the sea bottom

**177.** In an ecosystem, producers (green plants) are always more than consumers (herbivores, carnivores, etc.)

**178.** Energy flow takes place only in one direction, i.e. producers → herbivores → Carnivores. Because none of the organism use heat energy.

## NCERT Exemplar Questions

**1.** Decomposers like fungi and bacteria are heterotrophs and saprotrophs.

**2.** • The process of mineralization by microorganisms helps in the release of inorganic nutrients from humus.

• Humus is further degraded by some microbes and release of inorganic nutrients occur by the process called mineralization.

**3.** Productivity is the rate of production of biomass expressed in terms of $gm^{-2}\ yr^{-1}$ and $(kcal\ m^{-2})\ yr^{-1}$.

**4.** In terrestrial ecosystem, pyramid of biomass is generally upright. The pyramid of biomass in sea or lake is generally inverted because the biomass of fishes far exceeds that of phytoplankton.

**5.** *Spirogyra, Volvox* and *Nostoc* are producers. *Agaricus* is a fungus.

**6.** Tropical rain forests ecosystem is most productive in terms of primary production.

**7.** Pyramid of number in grassland or forest or pond ecosystem is upright.

In parasitic food chain, the pyramid of number is inverted. In an ecosystem dominated by trees, the pyramid of number is spindle-shaped/inverted.

**8.** Approximately how much of the solar energy that falls on the leaves of a plant is converted to chemical energy by photosynthesis 2–10%.

**9.** • Warm and moist environment favour decomposition. Decomposition is largely an oxygen requiring process. Low temperature and anaerobiosis inhibit decomposition resulting in build-up of organic materials.

• The process of decomposition would be the fastest is tropical rain forest.

**10.** 10% of the net primary productivity of a terrestrial ecosystem is eaten and digested by herbivores.

**11.** The zone at the edge of a lake or ocean which is alternatively exposed to air and immersed in water is called littoral zone.

**12.**

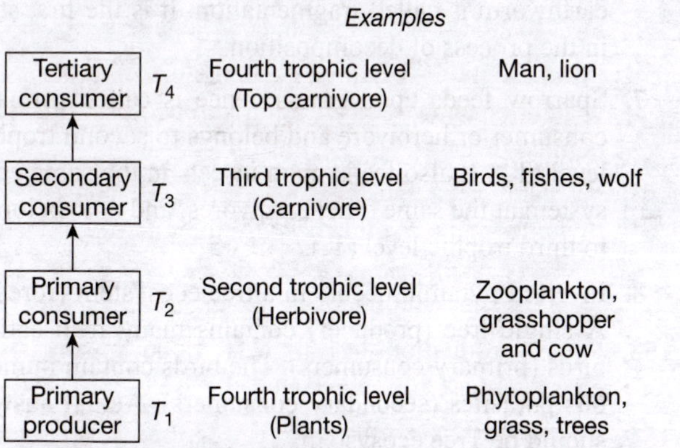


If the carbon atoms fixed by producers already have passed through three species, the trophic level of the last species would be tertiary consumer.

**13.** Desert ecosystem is expected in an area where evaporation exceeds precipitation and the mean annual rainfall is below 100 mm.

## Previous Years' Questions

1. Net primary productivity is equal to the rate of organic matter created by photosynthesis minus the rate of respiration and other losses. It is the biomass available for consumption by the herbivores and the decomposers.

2. Pyramid of number is usually upright except single tree ecosystem, parasitic food chain. So, for forest ecosystem, it is upright.

3. PAR (Photosynthetically active radiation) designates the spectral range of solar radiation from 400 to 700 nm that photosynthetic organisms are able to use in the process of photosynthesis. Of the total incident of solar radiation the proportion of PAR is less than 50%.

4. Mass of living matter at a trophic level in an area at any time is called standing crop. They are measured as the mass of living organisms in a particular area. The standing crop of each tropic level can simply be known as the biomass

5. Pyramid of energy is graphic representation of energy per unit area sequence-wise in various rising trophic levels with producers at the base and top carnivores at the apex. Pyramid of energy is upright in all the cases. It is also more accurate than other types of ecological pyramids.

6. The breakdown of detritus (dead remains of plants and animals) into smaller particle by detritivores like earthworm is called fragmentation. It is the first step in the process of decomposition.

7. Sparrow feeds upon grains hence is called primary consumer or herbivore and belongs to second trophic level ($T_2$). It also feeds upon insects in the same ecosystem at the same time, carnivores, and now belongs to third trophic level ($T_3$).

8. Inverted pyramid occurs in a tree ecosystem (forest). A single tree (producer) contains many fruit-eating birds (primary consumers). The birds contain numerous parasites (secondary consumers). Actual answer should be Tree ecosystem.

9. The components of the ecosystem are seen to function as a unit when we consider the following aspects:
   (i) Productivity
   (ii) Decomposition
   (iii) Energy flow
   (iv) Nutrient cycling.

10. It represents tree ecosystem therefore PP is tree, PC are insects, SC are small insectivorous birds and TC are large birds feeds on smaller birds.

11. Snake (cobra) is predator of frog.

12. a, b and d are herbivores and c is carnivore.

13. The productivity at consumer level is called secondary productivity and Rabbit is a consumer.

14. Humification, mineralization, catabolism, leaching and fragmentation are the steps of decomposition which operate simultaneously on the detritus. Fragmentation is breaking down detritus into smaller particles by detritivores like earthworm. By the process of leaching, water-soluble inorganic nutrients go down into soil horizon and get precipitated as unavailable salts. Humification occurs at a very slow rate.

15. Secondary productivity is the rate of formation of new organic matter by consumers. Primary productivity depends on the producers inhabiting a particular area.

16. **According to 10 percent** law of Lindeman at $4^{th}$ trophic level energy available is 0.02 J.

17. • The species that invade a bare area are called **pioneer species.**
    • Earthworm is detritivores.
    • Pollination, nutrient cycle, air purification provide habitat for wild life are some ecosystem services.

18. Most animals that live in deep oceanic waters are detritivore

19. • **Primary productivity** is the rate of capture of solar energy or biomass production of the producers. It is divided into two types: gross primary productivity (GPP) and net primary productivity (NPP). Rate of capture of solar energy or total production of organic matter is called as GPP. NPP is the remaining biomass or the energy left after utilization of producers.
    • **Secondary productivity** is the rate of assimilation of food energy by the consumers.

20. The amount of living matter present in an ecosystem in its different trophic levels is called standing crop. It is expressed in the form of number or biomass per unit area. Biomass is measured as either fresh weight. Dry weight is preferred over fresh weight as it is not viable to change with moisture content.

21. Vertical distribution of different species occupying different levels in a biotic community is known as

stratification. It refers to the vertical layering of a habitat; the arrangement of vegetation in layers. It classifies the layers of vegetation largely according to the different heights to which their plants grow. The individual layers are inhabited by different animal and plant communities.

**22.** The term ecosystem was coined by A. G. Tansley in 1935. According to Odum, an ecosystem is the basic fundamental unit of ecology which includes both the organisms and the non-living environment each influencing the properties of the other and each is necessary for the maintenance of life.

**23.** Cropland ecosystem generally used one type of high-yielding species of a crop. So, they have least genetic diversity.

**24.** Because in the deep-sea hydrothermal vent ecosystem, proper light cannot penetrate so photosynthetic organisms cannot survive, instead, chemosynthetic bacteria are primary producers.

**25.** There are certain groups of organisms which feed exclusively on the dead bodies of animals and plants. These organisms are called detritivores. Detritivores include bacteria, fungi, protozoans, insects, millipedes, centipedes, crustaceans, mussels, clams, annelid worms, nematodes, ducks, etc. They can feed at all trophic level. Rest all statements are correct.

**26.** In a forest ecosystem, comparatively more biotic components (plants, animals and microbes) are found.

**27.** Arrangement of a habitat into vertical layers known as stratification or the arrangement of vegetation in layers according to different height to which their plants grow. Stratification is clearly observed in tropical rain forests.

**28.** Inverted pyramid of biomass: small standing crop of phytoplankton supports large standing crop of zooplankton.

**29.** The pyramid of biomass in sea is generally inverted because the biomass of fishes far exceeds that of phytoplankton. Rest all other pyramids given in option are upright.

**30.** Grassland ecosystem is a terrestrial ecosystem. It includes various trophic levels

First trophic level ($T_1$) – Grass

Second trophic level ($T_2$) – Rabbit

Third trophic level ($T_3$) – Crow

Fourth trophic level ($T_4$) - Vulture

**31.** Gross primary productivity of an ecosystem is the rate of production of organic matter during photosynthesis.

Net primary productivity is GPP- Respiration. Hence, gross primary productivity is always more than NPP.

**32.** The pyramid of biomass in sea is generally inverted because the biomass of fishes far exceeds that of phytoplankton.

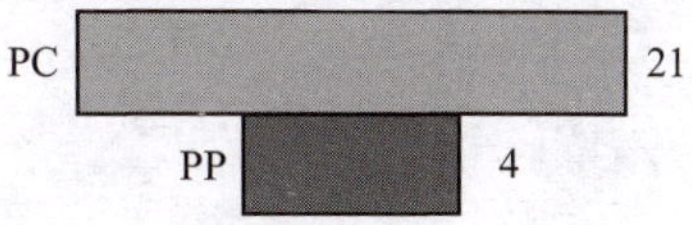


**33.** In the equation,

GPP – R = NPP

R = Respiratory loss

GPP = Gross Primary Productivity

NPP = Net Primary Productivity

**34.** The amount of nutrients, such as carbon, nitrogen, phosphorus, calcium, etc., present in the soil at any given time, is referred to as the standing state.

**35.** **The rate of decomposition is controlled** by chemical composition of detritus and climatic factors. Decomposition is slower if detritus is rich in lignin and chitin and quicker, if detritus is rich in nitrogen and water soluble substances like sugars.

**36.** Weathering of rocks accelerate phosphorus cycle. Phosphorus cycle is a sedimentary cycle. Reservoir pool of phosphorus in ecosystem is the earth's crust or lithosphere.

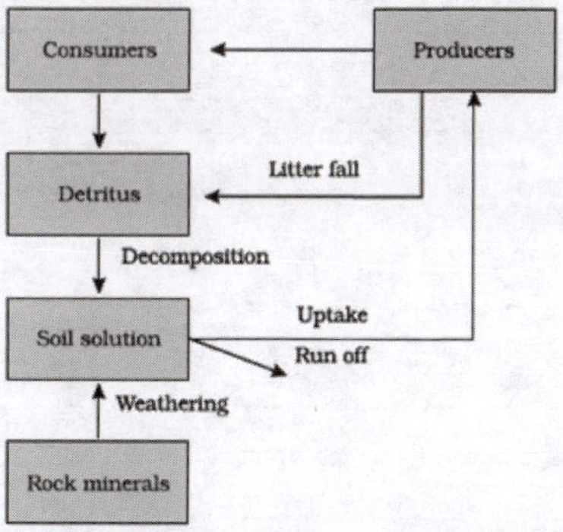


**37.** Detritivores (eg. earthworm) break down detritus into smaller particles. This process is called **fragmentation**.

**38.** The detritus food chain begins with dead organic matter. Earthworms break down detritus into smaller particles by a process called fragmentation.

**39.** GPP-R= NPP
GPP is Gross Primary Productivity.
NPP is Net Primary Productivity.
R is respiratory loss.
If we minus respiratory loss from GPP produce by plants we will get NPP which is available for the next trophic level.

**40.** NPP at first trophic level would be the GPP for second trophic level. NPP at second trophic level would be GPP for third trophic level. Therefore, $100x$ (kcal/m$^2$/yr) would be GPP at second trophic level and $100x \times 10\%$ (kcal/m$^2$/yr)
*i.e.*, $10x$ (kcal/m$^2$/yr) energy would be GPP at third trophic level.

# 7

# Biodiversity and Conservation

## LEARNING OBJECTIVES

- Understand the concepts, pattern, and importance of biodiversity
- Discuss the *In situ and ex-situ form of biodiversity* conservation
- Explain the causes and consequences of biodiversity loss

## Chapter Overview

- **The term 'Biodiversity' was popularized by Edward Wilson.** According to him, biodiversity is the combined diversity at all the levels of biological organization.
- **Biodiversity** represents the diversity in the organisms living in a particular region.
- **Niche:** It is a functional role played by the organism where it lives.
- **Species diversity:** Species diversity among amphibians is rich in the Western Ghats than in the Eastern Ghats.
- **Genetic diversity:** ***Rouwolfia vomitoria*** is a medicinal plant growing in Himalayan ranges and it produces a chemical known as reserpine which shows genetic variation in terms of potency and concentration. Genetic diversity can be nearly seen in 1000 varieties of mangoes whereas maximum genetic diversity can be seen in 50,000 varieties of rice.
- **Ecological diversity:** It is the diversity at ecosystem level.
- According to the **IUCN - International Union for Conservation of Nature (2004),** the total number of known plant and animal species so far is slightly more than **1.5 million** that is, it ranges from 1.7 to 1.8 million.
- According to **Robert May**, the global species diversity is about **7 million**. If we accept May's global estimates, only 22 per cent of the total species have been recorded so far.
- **Biodiversity of world:** Of all the total living organisms, animal species are far more than 70 per cent. Insects are forming the most species rich taxonomic group which is greater than 70 per cent of the total animals **(Fig 7.1)** and it is due to the presence of **chitinous exoskeleton.**

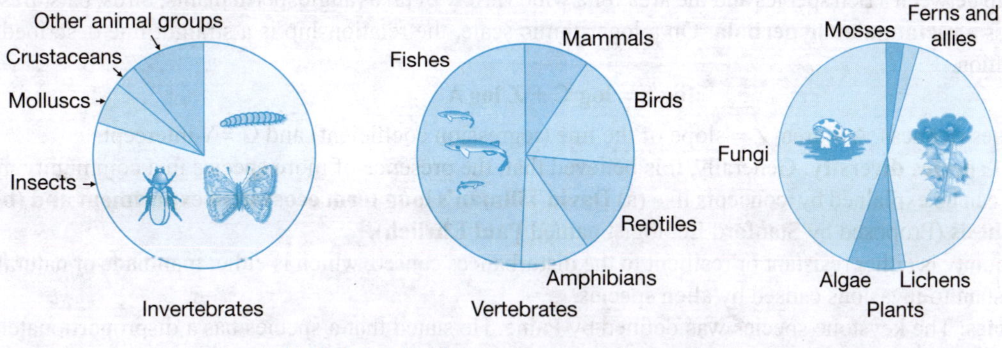


**FIGURE 7.1** Pie chart representing global biodiversity

Refer NCERT Ch 13: Biodiversity and its Conservation

- Among the vertebrates, half of the species are fishes. Plant species including algae, fungi, bryophytes, gymnosperms and angiosperms are lesser than **22 per cent** and the number of fungi species are greater than the combined number of fish species, amphibians, reptiles and mammals.
- India has only 2.4 per cent of the world's land area but the global species diversity is 8.1 per cent. India is one of the 12 mega diversity countries in the world.
- **Amazon rainforest** is a large tropical **rainforest** found in South America and it has the greatest biodiversity on earth comprising more than 40,000 species of plants, 3000 species of fishes, 1300 species of birds, 427 species of mammals, 427 species of amphibians, 378 species of reptiles and more than 1,25,000 species of invertebrates. Scientists estimate that at least 2 million insect species are yet to be discovered in rainforests.
- **Number of bird species: Colombia** (located near the equator) - nearly 1400 species > **India** (much of land area in the tropical latitudes) - nearly 1200 species > **New York** at 41° N - 105 species > **Greenland** at 71° N - only 56 species. It shows biodiversity gradient of bird species.
- **Tropical region comprises a great biodiversity and it is explained by three important hypotheses namely,**
  **(a)** Speciation is generally a function of time. Frequent glaciations have occurred in temperate regions in the past but tropical latitudes have remained relatively undisturbed for millions of years (long evolutionary time for greater species diversification).
  **(b)** There are no seasonal variations in tropical zones when compared to temperate zones. Therefore, a more constant and predictable environment is present to promote niche specialization which leads to a greater species diversity.
  **(c)** As the tropics receive more solar energy, these areas have higher productivity. This higher productivity might indirectly contribute to greater diversity.

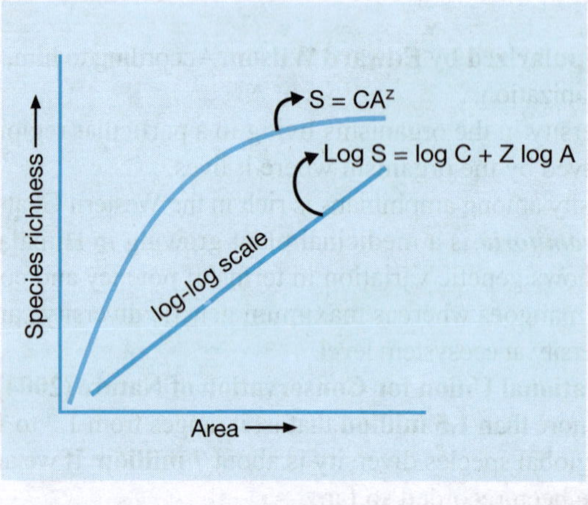


FIGURE 7.2 Showing species area relationship.

- **The Species-Area relationship was given by** the German naturalist and geographer named **Alexander von Humboldt.** The relationship between a rich species and the area for a wide variety of taxa (angiosperm plants, birds, bats, freshwater fishes) becomes a **rectangular hyperbola**. On a logarithmic scale, the relationship is a straight line described by the following equation.

$$\log S = \log C + Z \log A$$

Here, S = species richness, A = area, Z = slope of the line (regression coefficient) and C = Y-intercept.
- **Importance of species diversity:** Generally, it is believed that, the presence of more species in a community makes it more stable. It can be explained by concepts like (a) **David Tillman's long term ecosystem experiment and (b) Rivet Popper hypothesis** (Proposed by Stanford Ecologist named **Paul Ehrlich).**
- A stable community is either resistant or resilient to the disturbances caused, which is either manmade or natural. Also, it must be resistant to invasions caused by alien species.
- **Keystone species:** The keystone species was defined by Paine. He stated that a species has a disproportionately large effect on its environment relative to its abundance (in terms of biomass).
- A species facing extremely high risk in the immediate future is called **critically endangered species.**

- In the last 500 years, **IUCN Red List (2004)** highlights the extinction of 784 species (including 338 vertebrates, 359 invertebrates and 87 plants). The World Conservation Union which is formerly known as International Union for the Conservation of Nature and Natural Resources (IUCN) has recognized 8 Red List categories of species.

**TABLE 7.1** Red list category and their descriptions

| Red list category | Definition |
|---|---|
| **Extinct** | A taxon is extinct when there is no reasonable doubt that the last individual has died. *e.g:* Dodo. |
| **Extinct in the wild** | A taxon is extinct in the wild when exhaustive surveys in known and/or expected habitats have failed to record an individual. |
| **Critically endangered** | A taxon is critically endangered when it is facing an extremely high risk of extinction in the wild in the immediate future. *e.g: Sus salvanius* (Pigmy hog) and *Berberis nilghiriensus*. |
| **Endangered** | A taxon is endangered when it is not critically endangered but it is facing a very high risk of extinction in the wild in the near future. *e.g: Ailurus fulgens* (Red panda), blue whale, largest lemur Idri-Idri of Madagascar, etc. |
| **Vulnerable** | A taxon is vulnerable when it is not critically endangered or endangered, but it is facing a high risk of extinction in the wild in the impending future. *e.g: Antelope cervicapra* (Black Buck). |
| **Lower risk** | A taxon is lower risk when it has been evaluated and does not satisfy the criteria for critically endangered, endangered and vulnerable. |
| **Data deficient** | A taxon is data deficient when there is an inadequate information to make a direct or indirect assessment of its risk of extinction. |
| **Not evaluate** | A taxon is not evaluated when it has not yet been assessed. |

- Some examples of **recent extinctions** are (1) *Dodo* (Mauritius) (2) *Quagga* (Africa) (3) *Thylacine* (Australia) (4) Steller's *Sea Cow* (Russia) (5) 3 sub-species **of tiger** (Bali, Javan, Caspian) .
- Amphibians appear to be more vulnerable to extinction.
- **Extinction of species:** It refers to the large scale loss of species. Fossil records indicate that already 5 episodes of mass extinction have occurred on Earth before the evolution of human. Sixth extinction is in progress and its pace (rate of extinction of species) is estimated to be 100 to 1000 times faster than the previous 5 mass extinctions. This is because of human activities.
- Tropical rain forests, once covering more than 14 per cent of the earth's land surface are now restricted to 6 per cent. The **Amazon rainforest** (also known as the **'lungs of the planet'** because of its huge size) is the habitat for millions of species, is largely being cut and cleared for cultivation of soya beans and grasslands (for rearing beef cattle).
- **Causes of biodiversity losses (Evil quartet - 4 reasons for loss of biodiversity):**
  - **Habitat loss and fragmentation is the most important reason for biodiversity loss.**
  - **Over-exploitation (Steller's sea cow, Passenger pigeon) marine fish populations are overharvested**
  - **Alien species invasion**

    **(1) Examples:** Introduction of **Nile perch** (alien fresh water fish) into Lake Victoria in East Africa resulted in extinction of more than 200 species of **Cichlid fish** (indigenous fresh water fish).

    (2) Invasive weed species like **Carrot grass (*Parthenium hysterophorus*), Lantana** and **Water hyacinth** ***(Eicchornia crassipes*)** are potential threat to our native species.

    **(3)** Recently, illegal introduction of an **African catfish (*Clarias gariepinus*)** for aquaculture is posing a threat to the indigenous catfishes in our rivers.
  - **Co-extinction Ex. Host fish - parasite plant pollinator mutualism**

## Conservation of biodiversity

- The fast dwindling (diminishing) **Amazon forest** produces about 20 per cent of the total oxygen in the earth's atmosphere through photosynthesis.
- **Modes of conservation of biodiversity**

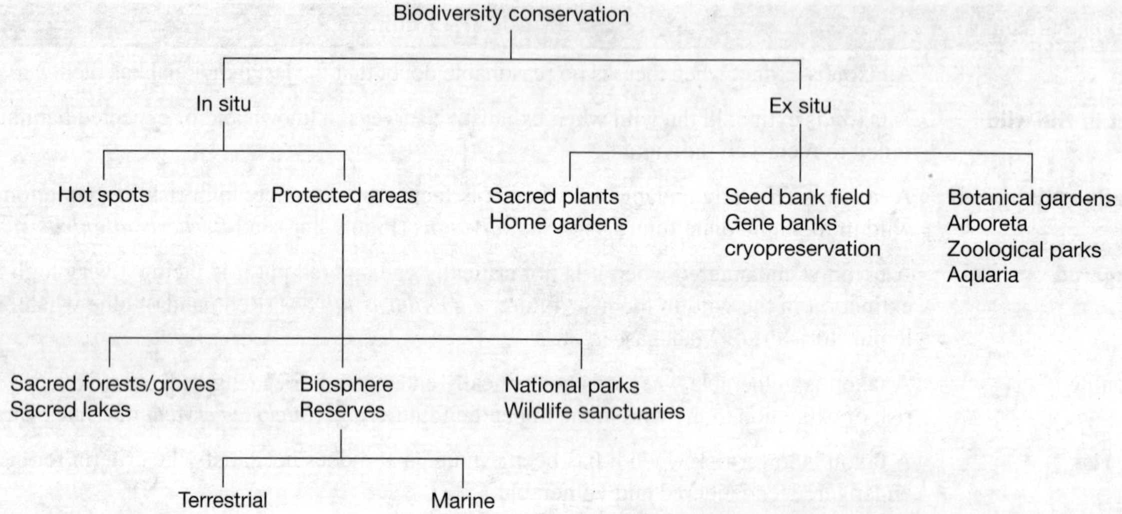


### In-situ Conservation

- **Biodiversity hotspots:** These are the regions that are characterized by a very high levels of species richness. High degree of **endemism that is species found in only a specific region and nowhere else. The** total number of biodiversity hotspots in the world is **34.** These hotspots are also the regions of accelerated habitat loss. If these hotspots are strictly protected, then it may reduce the ongoing mass extinctions by almost 30 per cent.
  **Western Ghats and Sri Lanka, Indo-Burma and the Himalaya are the three hotspots in India.** Less than 2 per cent of the earth's land area are covered by the biodiversity hotspots where, the species diversity is very high.
- In India, biodiversity rich regions are protected as biosphere reserves, national parks, sanctuaries.
- India has 14 biosphere reserves, 90 national parks and 448 wildlife sanctuaries.
- **Sacred grooves:** In India, trees and wildlife are given total protection in the name of culture. They are useful for conserving rare and threatened species. For example: Khasi and Jaintia Hills in Meghalaya (last refuges for many species of rare and threatened plants)**,** Aravalli Hills of Rajasthan**,** Western Ghats regions of Karnataka and Maharashtra, Sarguja, Chanda and Bastar areas of Madhya Pradesh.

### Ex-situ:

- Threatened plants and animals are placed in protected zones. Ex. Zoological park, botanical gardens, wildlife safari.

### Advanced:

- Gametes of species can be preserved in variables in viable and fertile conditions.
- Eggs fertilized in-vitro
- Seed bank: preservation of souls
- Plant propagation by tissue culture.

### Convention on Biological Diversity (The Earth Summit):

To take appropriate measures for conserving biodiversity and to sustainably utilise its benefits, a historic convention on biological diversity was held in Rio de Janeiro in 1992. Following this, the **World Summit on Sustainable Development was held in 2002 in Johannesburg, South Africa**. It consists of 190 member countries who pledged to achieve a significant reduction in the current rate of biodiversity loss at global, regional and local levels by 2010.

# PRACTICE EXERCISES

## Multiple Choice Questions: Level I

### Types of Biodiversity

**1.** Match Column-I (organism) with Column-II.

| Column-I | Column-II (Number of species) |
|---|---|
| 1. Ants | A. 20,000 |
| 2. Orchids | B. 25,000 |
| 3. Fishes | C. 28,000 |
| 4. Beetles | D. 3,00,000 |

(a) 1:D, 2:C, 3:B, 4:A (b) 1:B. 2:A, 3:C, 4:D
(c) 1:A, 2:B, 3:C, 4:D (d) 1:A, 2:A, 3:C, 4:D

**2.** The term 'Biodiversity' was popularized by
(a) Robert May (b) A. Von Humboldt
(c) Edward Wilson (d) Paul Ehrlich

**3.** Identify the type/level of biodiversity from the following
(a) Genetic (b) Species
(c) Ecological (d) All of these

**4.** Which of the following shows maximum genetic diversity?
(a) Rice (b) Mango
(c) *Rauwolfia vomitoria* (d) Wheat

**5.** How many different varieties of mango are found in India?
(a) 50,000 (b) 5000
(c) 2000 (d) 1000

**6.** How many genetically different strains of rice are found in India?
(a) 50,000 (b) 5000 (c) 2000 (d) 1000

**7.** Choose the incorrect statement from the following.
(A) Western Ghats have a greater amphibian species diversity than the Eastern Ghats.
(B) Diversity exists at all levels of biological organization ranging from macromolecules within cells to biomes.
(C) *Rauwolfia vomitoria* shows genetic variation in terms of potency and concentration of the reserpine produced.
(D) Norway has greater ecosystem diversity than India.
(a) A and B only (b) B and D only
(c) A, B and C only (d) D only

**8.** If the present rate of species losses continues, we will lose our biological wealth in how much time?
(a) Less than one century (b) Less than 2 centuries
(c) Less than 50 years (d) Next 20 years

**9.** Robert May places the global species diversity at about ________ million.
(a) 2 (b) 3 (c) 6 (d) 7

**10.** More than ________ % of all species recorded are animals.
(a) 60 (b) 70 (c) 90 (d) 10

**11.** Arrange the following in their decreasing order of species.

Fishes, Birds, Reptiles, Amphibian

(a) Fishes > Birds > Reptiles > Amphibian
(b) Fishes > Reptiles > Birds > Amphibian
(c) Reptiles > Fishes > Birds > Amphibian
(d) Amphibian > Fishes > Birds > Reptiles

**12.** Which of the following have more number of species?
(a) Fungi (b) Mosses
(c) Angiosperm (d) Lichens

**13.** Which order is correct with respect to the number of species?
(a) Fungi > Algae > Lichens > Angiosperm
(b) Angiosperm > Fungi > Algae > Lichen
(c) Fungi > Angiosperm > Algae > Lichen
(d) Mosses > Ferns > Algae > Lichens

**14.** What does A, B, C, D, E and F represent in this figure?

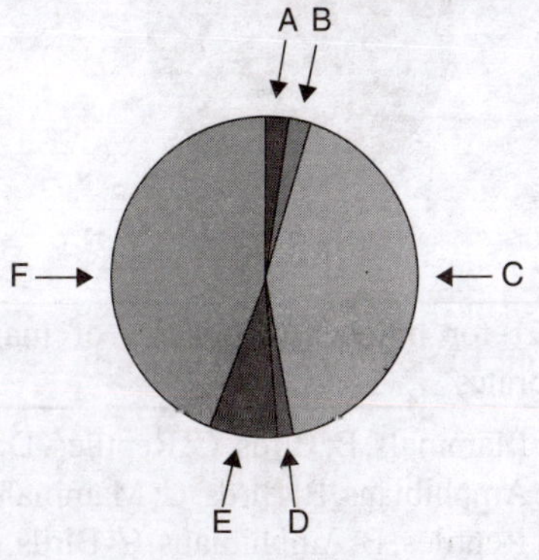


π-chart for number of species of major taxa of plants.

(a) A: Ferns and allies, B: Mosses, C: Algae, D: Fungi, E: Lichens, F: Angiosperms
(b) A: Fungi, B: Mosses, C: Lichens, D: Ferns and allies, E: Angiosperms, F: Algae
(c) A: Angiosperms, B: Ferns and allies, C: Fungi, D: Lichens, E: Algae, F: Mosses
(d) A: Mosses, B: Ferns and allies, C: Angiosperms, D: Lichens, E: Algae, F: Fungi

**15.** Find the false statement.
(a) The number of fungi species is more than the combined total of the species of fishes, amphibians, reptiles and mammals.
(b) Conventional taxonomic methods are not suitable for identifying microbial species.
(c) For many taxonomic groups, species inventories are more complete in temperate than in tropical countries.
(d) Insects forms 70 per cent part of all the species recorded.

**16.** Find the true statement.
A. If we consider biochemical or molecular criteria for microorganisms, their diversity may run into millions.
B. There are 12 mega diversity countries in the world.
C. If we accept May's global estimates, only 32 per cent of the total species have been recorded so far.
D. Western Ghats have a greater amphibian species diversity than Eastern Ghats.

(a) A and B only (b) D only
(c) A and D only (d) A, B and D only

**17.** What is A, B, C and D in this figure?

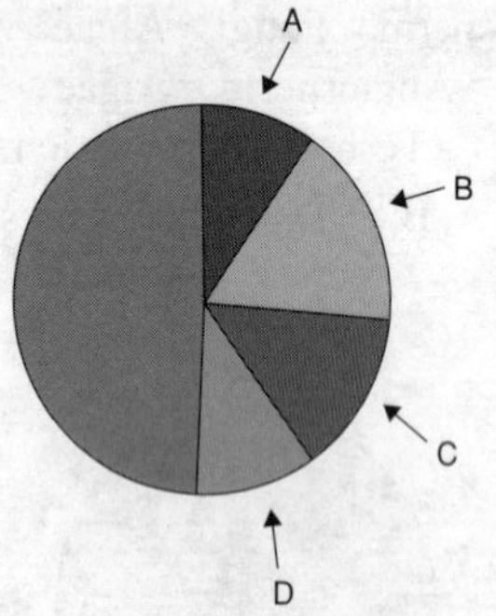


π-chart for number of species of major taxa of vertebrates

(a) A: Mammals, B: Birds, C: Reptiles, D: Amphibians
(b) A: Amphibians, B: Birds, C: Mammals, D: Reptiles
(c) A: Reptiles, B: Amphibians, C: Birds, D: mammals
(d) A: Mammals, B: Reptiles, C: Birds, D: Amphibians

**18.** Identify A, B, C and D in this figure.

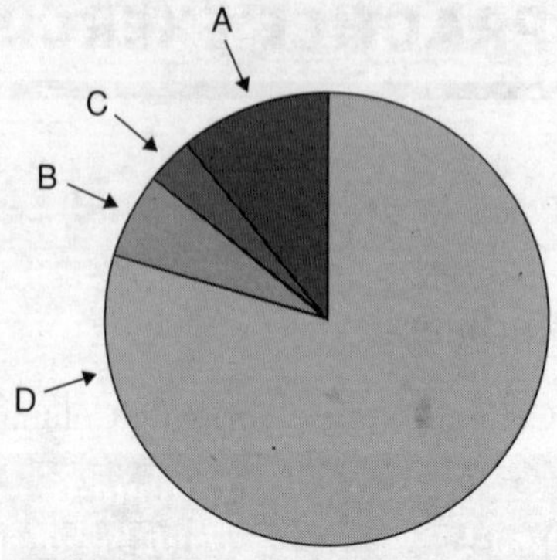


π-chart for the number of species of major taxa of Invertebrates

(a) A: Insects, B: Crustaceans, C: Molluscs, D: Other animal groups
(b) A: Other animal groups, B: Molluscs, C: Crustaceans, D: Insects
(c) A: Molluscs, B: Insects, C: Other animal groups, D: Crustaceans
(d) A: Insects, B: Molluscs, C: Crustaceans, D: Other animal groups

**19.** How do ecologists estimate the total number of species present in the world?
(a) By counting them all.
(b) By counting the number of any one species and applying this to various genus.
(c) By making statistical comparison of the temperate–tropical species richness of an exhaustively studied group of insects and extrapolating this ratio to other group of animals and plants.
(d) By calculating biomass of all the species.

**20.** Select the incorrect statements regarding biodiversity:
(A) Biodiversity and its conservation are vital environmental issues of international concern.
(B) The term Biodiversity is popularised by the sociobiologist Paul Ehrlich.
(C) Biodiversity exists only at the species level.
(D) Edward Wilson described the combined diversity at all the levels of biological organisation.

(a) A, B and D (b) A, B and C
(c) C and D only (d) B and C only

**Direction for Q21–22:** Choose the correct option:
(a) (A) is false but (R) is true
(b) Both (A) and (R) are true and (R) is the correct explanation of (A)
(c) Both (A) and (R) are true but (R) is not the correct explanation of (A)
(d) (A) is true but (R) is false.

21. **Assertion:** India has more than 50,000 genetically different strains of rice, and 1,000 varieties of mango.
**Reason:** A single species might show high diversity at the genetic level over its distributional range

22. **Assertion:** Species diversity is one of the important type of diversity of biological organisation.
**Reason:** The Eastern Ghats have a greater amphibian species diversity than the Western Ghats.

23. Rauwolfia vomitoria produces the active chemical reserpine. The genetic variation shown by it might be in terms of the
(a) potency
(b) concentration
(c) types
(d) a and b

24. Select the incorrect statements
(A) A Scandinavian country Norway has a greater ecosystem diversity than India
(B) The wealth of rich diversity in nature, can be lost in less than three centuries with the present rates of species losses.
(C) The biodiversity is critically important for survival and well- being of human on Earth.
(D) India shows a greater ecosystem diversity with its deserts, rain forests, mangroves, coral reefs, wetlands, estuaries, and alpine meadows.
(a) A, B and D
(d) A, B and C
(c) C and D only
(d) A and B only

## Biodiversity (Patterns and Importance)

25. The species diversity of plants (22%) is much less than that of animals (72%), what could be the explanation to how animals achieved greater diversification?
(a) Animal are non-motile.
(b) Their movement to diverse habitats resulted in more evolutionary changes occurring in animals.
(c) Animals use carbohydrate and lipid as a source of energy.
(d) Animal DNA is different from plant DNA in terms of type of nitrogen bases.

26. India has only ________ percent of the world's land area; its share of the global species diversity is an impressive ________ percent.
(a) 4.2, 1.8 (b) 2.4, 8.1
(c) 2.4, 13 (d) 4.2, 13

27. Match Column-I (Place) with Column-II (Number of bird species).

| Column–I | Column–II |
|---|---|
| 1. Colombia | A. 1200 |
| 2. New York | B. 1300 |
| 3. India | C. 1400 |
| 4. Amazonian rain forest | D. 105 |

(a) A:3, B:4, C:2, D:1 (b) A:2, B:1, C:4, D:3
(c) A:2, B:4, C:3, D:1 (d) A:3, B:4, C:1, D:2

28. Find the incorrect statement.
(a) India has nearly 45,000 species of plants and twice as many animals.
(b) A forest in a tropical region like equador has 10 times as many species of vascular plants as a forest of equal area in a temperate region like the mid west of the USA.
(c) Greenland 71° N has only 56 species of birds.
(d) The diversity of plant and animals is uniform throughout the world.

29. The largely tropical Amazonian rain forest in South America has the greatest biodiversity on earth. It is the home for more than ________ species of plants. ________ of fishes, ________ of birds, ________ of mammals, ________ of amphibians, ________ of reptiles and of more than ________ invertebrates.
(a) 30,000, 4000, 1200, 427, 427, 387, 1,25,000
(b) 40,000, 3000, 1200, 427, 427, 387, 1,25,000
(c) 40,000, 3000, 1300, 427, 427, 378, 1,25,000
(d) 40,000, 3000, 1200, 427, 427, 378, 1,25,000

30. What is the sum of the number of species of birds in New York 41° N and Greenland of 71° N.
(a) 112 (b) 161 (c) 170 (d) 56

31. Species richness of tropics is because of
(a) Tropics have more evolutionary time.
(b) Tropics have relatively constant environment.
(c) Tropics receive more solar energy.
(d) All/any the above

32. Species–area relationship was provided by
(a) Alexander Von Humboldt
(b) Robert May
(c) Paul Ehrlich
(d) Edward Wilson

33. The graph formed by plotting species richness against area for a wide variety of taxa (angiosperm plants, birds, bats, fresh water fishes, etc.) turns out to be a
(a) Parabola
(b) Straight line
(c) Rectangular hyperbola
(d) Any of the above

**34.** log S = log C + Z log A (Logarithmic formula for species–area relationship). True about this formula
(a) S = Species richness; A = Area
(b) Z = Regression coefficient
(c) C = Y-intercept
(d) All of these

**35.** If we analyze species–area relationship among very large area like entire continents, slope of line becomes
(a) Less steeper (b) Vertical
(c) Much steeper (d) Horizontal

**36.** Z-value in a much steeper slope ranges between
(a) 0.6 to 1.2 (b) 0.1 to 1.2
(c) 0.01 to 0.02 (d) 0.6 to 0.12

**37.** For frugivorous (fruit-eating) birds and mammals in the tropical forests of different continents, the slope of species–area relationship is found to be approximately
(a) 0.6 (b) 1.3 (c) 1.15 (d) 1

**38.** Which is the correct formula of the graph shown below? Given:

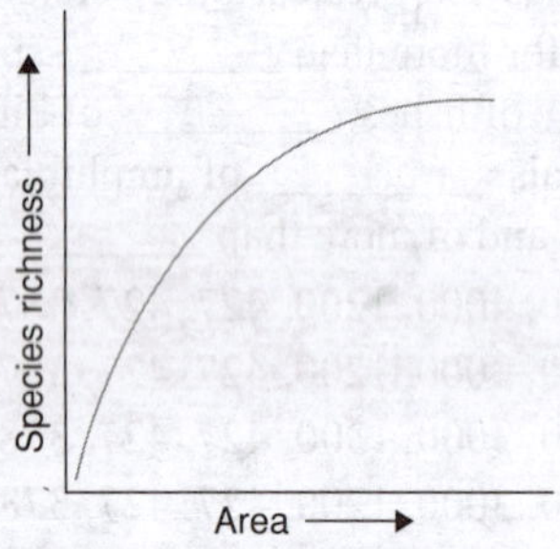


S-species richness A-Area C-Y-intercept
Z-Slope of line (regression coefficient)
(a) $S = CA^Z$ (b) $S = CZ^A$
(c) $S = ZC^A$ (d) $Z = SC^A$

**39.** 'Z' value in species–area relationship lies in the rage of 0.1 to 0.2 for
(a) Plants in Britain
(b) Birds in California
(c) Molluscs in New York State
(d) All of these

**40.** Which of the followings are the features of a stable community?
(a) Resistant or resilient to occasional disturbances (Natural or Anthropogenic).
(b) Does not show much variation in productivity.
(c) Resistant to invasion by alien species.
(d) All the above

**41.** There are two plots Plot '1' has less species and Plot '2' has more species. Which statement is true regarding the two plots?
(a) Plot '1' shows less year to year variation in total biomass.
(b) Plot '2' is less resistant to natural disturbance.
(c) Plot '1' has more productivity than plot '2'.
(d) Plot '2' has more productivity than plot '1'.

**42.** Rivet popper hypothesis was proposed by
(a) Robert May (b) A. Von Humboldt
(c) Paul Ehrlich (d) Edward Wilson

**43.** Tropical environments, unlike temperate ones, are
(a) Less seasonal
(b) Relatively more constant
(c) More predictable
(d) All of these

**44.** Find the incorrect statement.
(a) Constant environment promote niche specialization.
(b) Key species are those which derive major ecosystem functions.
(c) Increase in diversity generally increases productivity.
(d) Increased steepness in species–area relationship curve decreases species richness in a given area.

**45.** **Statement I:** The diversity of plants and animals is not uniform throughout the world but shows a rather uneven distribution.
**Statement II:** Species diversity decreases as we move away from the equator towards the poles.
(a) Statement I is incorrect but statement II is true.
(b) Both Statements I and II are true
(c) Both Statements I and II are false
(d) Statement I is correct but statement II is false

**46.** Select set of incorrect statements:
(A) Tropics harbour more species than temperate or polar areas.
(B) New York at 41° N has 56 species and Greenland at 71° N has 105 species of birds.
(C) A forest Equador has up to 10 times as many species of vascular plants as a forest Midwest of the USA.
(D) Amazonian rain forest is home to more than 1,25,000 vertebrates.
(a) B and D (b) A and C
(c) B, C and D (d) C and D

**47.** **Assertion:** Tropical latitudes have remained relatively undisturbed for millions of years and thus, had a long evolutionary time for species diversification,
**Reason:** Speciation is generally a function of time
(a) (A) is false but (R) is true
(b) Both (A) and (R) are true and (R) is the correct explanation of (A)
(c) Both (A) and (R) are true but (R) is not the correct explanation of (A)
(d) (A) is true but (R) is false.

**48.** Select set of correct statements:
(A) Tropical environments are less seasonal, relatively more constant and predictable.
(B) More solar energy in the tropics contributes to higher productivity; and thus to greater diversity.
(C) Variable environments promote niche specialisation and lead to a greater species diversity
(D) Tropical regions have been subjected to frequent glaciations in the past
(a) B and D (b) A and B
(c) B, C and D (d) C and D

**49.** Read following sentences.
**Statement I:** Within a region species richness increased with increasing explored area, but only up to a limit.
**Statement II:** The relation between species richness and area for a wide variety of taxa is represented by rectangular hyperbola
(a) Statement I is incorrect but statement II is true.
(b) Both Statements I and II are true
(c) Both Statements I and II are false
(d) Statement I is correct but statement II is false

**50.** Select set of correct statements:
(A) On a logarithmic scale, the Species-Area relationship is a straight line described by the equation $\log S = \log C + Z \log A$
(B) The value of Z, lies in the range of 0.1 to 0.2, regardless of the taxonomic group or the region
(C) Z value lies in the range of 0.6 to 1.2 for the species-area relationships among very large areas like the entire continents.
(D) Z value is found to be 1.15 for frugivorous birds and mammals in the tropical forests of different continents.
(a) A, B and D (b) A, B and C
(c) B, C and D (d) A, B, C and D

**51.** A stable community should
(a) not show too much variation in productivity from year to year
(b) be either resistant or resilient to occasional disturbances
(c) be resistant to invasions by alien species
(d) all of these

**52.** David Tilman
(a) carried out long-term ecosystem experiments using outdoor plots
(b) found that plots with more species showed less year-to-year variation in total biomass.
(c) showed that increased diversity contributed to higher productivity
(d) all of these

## Biodiversity Losses

**53.** Which extinction is presently in progress?
(a) Fifth (b) Sixth (c) Forth (d) Third

**54.** Which of the following require large territories?
(a) Birds (b) Amphibians
(c) Mammals (d) Both (a) and (c)

**55.** Presently which of the following face maximum threat of extinction?
(a) Birds (b) Amphibians
(c) Mammals (d) Gymnosperm

**56.** Loss of biodiversity in a region leads to increase in variability in certain ecosystem processes like
(a) Plant productivity
(b) Water use
(c) Pest and disease cycle
(d) All of these

**57.** The colonization of tropical Pacific Islands by humans led to the extinction of more than, ________ species of native birds
(a) 2000 (b) 50 (c) 4000 (d) 3000

**58.** IUCN Red list (2004) documents the extinction of how many species in last 500 years?
(a) 784 (b) 874 (c) 478 (d) 487

**59.** Match the Column-I (Recently extinct animals) with Column-II (Places from where they are extinct).

| Column-I | Column-II |
|---|---|
| A. Dodo | 1. Russia |
| B. Quagga | 2. Australia |
| C. Thylacine | 3. Africa |
| D. Steller's sea cow | 4. Mauritius |

(a) A:1, B:2, C:3, D:4 (b) A:4, B:3, C:2, D:1
(c) A:4, B:2, C:3, D:1 (d) A:4, B:1, C:2, D:3

**60.** Find the false statement.
(A) In the last 20 years alone there is a disappearance of 27 species.
(B) Three species (Bali, Javan and Caspian) of tiger are included in recently extinct animals.
(C) If we apply May's estimate then there are probably more than 1,00,000 plant species in India that are yet to be discovered and described.
(D) There is more solar energy available in tropics, which contribute to higher productivity; this in turn contributes directly to greater diversity.
(a) A only (b) C, D only
(c) B, D only (d) A and C only

**61.** According to the IUCN Red list (2004) how many vertebrates became extinct in the last 500 years?
(a) 359 (b) 338
(c) 487 (d) 87

**62.** According to IUCN Red list (2004) how many invertebrates became extinct in the last 500 years?
(a) 359 (b) 338
(c) 784 (d) 87

**63.** Which group is most vulnerable to extinction?
(a) Fishes (b) Amphibians
(c) Reptiles (d) Birds

**64.** Approximately how many species face the threat of extinction?
(a) 3000 (b) 1500
(c) 15,500 (d) 70,000

**65.** Presently ________ % of all bird species, ________ % of all mammals species, ________ % of all amphibian species and ________ % of all gymnosperm species in the world face the threat of extinction.
(a) 23, 32, 12, 31 (b) 12, 23, 32, 31
(c) 12, 23, 31, 32 (d) 23, 12, 32, 81

**66.** Since the origin and diversification of life on earth how many episodes of mass extinction of species have occurred till date?
(a) 2 (b) 3 (c) 4 (d) 5

**67.** The current rate of species extinction is how many times faster than the pre-human time?
(a) 10 to 50 times
(b) 100 to 1000 times
(c) 1000 to 10,000 times
(d) 10,000 to 1,00,000 times

**68.** Find the incorrect statement.
(a) 'Sixth extinction' is different from previous extinction in terms of rate of extinction.
(b) Ecologist warn that if the present trend of extinction continues, nearly 50 per cent all species on earth might be wiped out within the next 100 years.
(c) Amphibians appear to be vulnerable to extinction.
(d) Recent extinction is completely natural.

**69.** Loss of biodiversity in a region may lead to
(a) Decline in plants production.
(b) Lowered resistance to environmental perturbations such as draught.
(c) Increased variability in certain ecosystem processes such as plant productivity, water use, and pest and disease cycle.
(d) All the above

**70.** Which of the following is a major cause of loss of biodiversity?
(a) Habitat loss and fragmentation
(b) Over-exploitation
(c) Alien species invasion
(d) Co-extinction

**71.** The most dramatic examples of habitat loss comes from the
(a) Tropical rain forests (b) Temperate forests
(c) Grasslands (d) Deserts

**72.** Find the incorrect statement from the following.
(A) Tropic rain forests cover around 6 per cent of earth's land surface.
(B) Amazonian rain forest is being cut and cleared for soya bean cultivation or for conversion to grasslands for raising beef cattle.
(C) Animals with migratory habits are badly affected by habitat loss and fragmentation.
(D) Mammals and birds require small territories.
(a) A and B only
(b) A and D only
(c) D only
(d) B and C only

**73.** Steller's sea cow and Passenger pigeon became extinct due to
(a) Alien species invasion
(b) Co-extinction
(c) Habitat loss and fragmentation
(d) Over exploitation

**74.** Which of these are examples of alien species invasion?
(a) Nile perch was introduced in Lake Victoria in east Africa
(b) African catfish in Indian River
(c) Water hyacinth in India
(d) All the above

**75.** Which of these are invasive weeds?
(a) Carrot grass (*Parthenium*)
(b) Gandhari (*lantana*)
(c) Water hyacinth (*Eicchornia*)
(d) All of these

**76.** Co-extinction means
(a) Introduction of alien species leading to decline or extinction of indigenous species.
(b) Extinction due to over exploitation.
(c) Extinction due to Habitat loss.
(d) Extinction due to obligatory association of plant or animal.

**77.** Stellar's Sea cow became extinct from
(a) Mauritius (b) Africa
(c) Russia (d) Australia

**78.** Select set of correct statements:
(A) The colonisation of tropical Pacific Islands by humans have led to the extinction of more than 2,000 species of native birds.
(B) The IUCN Red List (2004) documents the extinction of 874 species in the last 500 years.
(C) Recent extinctions include the dodo, quagga, thylacine , Steller's Sea Cow and three subspecies of tiger.
(D) The last twenty years alone have witnessed the disappearance of 17 species.
(a) B and D (b) A and C
(c) B, C and D (d) C and D

**79. Assertion:** Extinctions across taxa are not random.
**Reason:** Some groups like amphibians appear to be more vulnerable to extinction.
(a) (A) is false but (R) is true
(b) Both (A) and (R) are true and (R) is the correct explanation of (A)
(c) Both (A) and (R) are true but (R) is not the correct explanation of (A)
(d) (A) is true but (R) is false.

**80.** Select the incorrect match regarding the percentage of species facing the threat of extinction
(a) Bird – 12 %
(b) Mammals – 25 %
(c) Amphibians – 32 %
(d) Gymnosperms – 31 %

**81.** Which of the following is not the cause for biodiversity loss?
(a) Habitat loss and fragmentation
(b) Over-exploitation
(c) Alien species invasions
(d) Co-existance

**82.** Select set of correct statements:
(A) Tropical rainforests present some of the most striking instances of habitat loss.
(B) At one point, tropical rainforests spanned over 14% of the Earth's land surface; however, their current extent is reduced to no more than 6%.
(C) The Amazon rainforest, which likely shelters millions of species, faces deforestation as it is being cut and cleared for soybean cultivation or transformed into grasslands for beef cattle farming.
(D) Fragmentation of large habitats, caused by human activities, adversely impacts mammals, birds needing extensive territories, and animals with migratory habits, resulting in population declines.
(a) A, B and D (b) A, B and C
(c) B, C and D (d) A, B, C and D

**Direction for Q83–84:** Choose the correct option:
(a) (A) is false but (R) is true
(b) Both (A) and (R) are true and (R) is the correct explanation of (A)
(c) Both (A) and (R) are true but (R) is not the correct explanation of (A)
(d) (A) is true but (R) is false.

**83. Assertion:** Mammals and birds requiring large territories and certain animals with migratory habits are getting badly affected, leading to population declines.
**Reason:** Large habitats are broken up into small fragments due to various human activities.

**84. Assertion:** Co-extinctions is one of the causes for biodiversity loss.
**Reason:** When a species becomes extinct, the plant and animal species associated with it in an obligatory way become extinct.

## Biodiversity Conservation

**85.** Which of these is not a narrowly utilitarian argument for conserving biodiversity?
(a) Food
(b) Medicine
(c) Construction material
(d) Pollination

**86.** All are examples of broadly utilitarian except
(a) Pollination
(b) Oxygen
(c) Aesthetic pleasure of walking through thick woods
(d) Firewood

**87.** Find the incorrect statement from the following.
(a) Introduction of Nile perch in Lake Victoria in east Africa lead to the extinction of more than 200 species of cichlid fish in the lake.
(b) Fast dwindling Amazon forest is estimated to produce, through photosynthesis, 20 per cent of the total oxygen in the earth's atmosphere.
(c) More than 25 per cent of drugs currently sold worldwide are derived from plants.
(d) Illegal introduction of American catfish Clarias gariepinus for aquaculture purpose is posing threat to indigenous cat fishes in our rivers.

**88.** 'We save the entire forest to save the tiger'. This approach of conservation is
(a) *In situ* (b) *Ex situ* (c) *In vitro* (d) *In vivo*

**89.** What percentage of the earth's land area is covered by all biodiversity hotspots put together?
(a) 6% (b) 10% (c) 2% (d) 15%

**90.** The following are examples of ex situ conservation except
(a) Zoological parks (b) Botanical garden
(c) Wildlife safari parks (d) Biosphere reserve

**91.** The following are examples of In situ conservation except?
(a) Biosphere reverse (b) National park
(c) Sacred groves (d) Gene-bank

**92.** Hotspots are characterized by
(a) Very high species richness
(b) High degree of endemism
(c) Region of accelerated habitat loss
(d) All of these

**93.** In India, ecologically unique and biodiversity rich regions are legally protected as
(a) Biosphere reserve (b) National park
(c) Sanctuaries (d) All of these

**94.** The Earth Summit (Historic Convention on Biological Diversity) was held in
(a) Johannesburg, South Africa, 2002
(b) Rio De Janeiro, 1992
(c) Kyoto, Japan
(d) Montreal, Canada

**95.** World Summit on sustainable development was held in
(a) Johannesburg, South Africa, 2002
(b) Rio De Janeiro, 1992
(c) Kyoto, Japan
(d) Montreal, Canada

**96.** Which of these are hotspots of India?
(a) Western Ghats (b) Himalaya
(c) Indo-Burma (d) All of these

**97.** Ex situ conservation includes
(a) Cryopreservation of gametes
(b) In vitro fertilization
(c) Tissue culture
(d) All of these

**98.** The reasons for biodiversity conservation are
(a) Broad utilization (b) Narrow utilization
(c) Ethical (d) All of these

**99.** The following are broadly utilitarian except
(a) Pest control (b) Flood control
(c) Climate moderation (d) Pharmaceuticals

**100.** In the World Summit on sustainable development held in 2002 in Johannesburg, South Africa, how many countries pledged their commitment to achieve a significant reduction in the current rate of biodiversity loss at global, regions and local levels, by 2010?
(a) 100 (b) 180
(c) 190 (d) 200

**101.** Sacred groves are present in
(a) Khasi and Jaintia Hills in Meghalaya
(b) Aravalli Hills of Rajasthan
(c) Western Ghat regions of Karnataka and Maharashtra
(d) All the above

**102.** Gametes of threatened species can be preserved in viable and fertile condition for long periods using
(a) PCR technique
(b) CTAB
(c) Cryopreservation technique
(d) In situ conservation

**103.** At present, how many biosphere reserves does India have?
(a) 11 (b) 14
(c) 18 (d) 20

**104.** How many biodiversity hotspots are found in the world?
(a) 25 (b) 34
(c) 9 (d) 20

**105.** Hotspot is a region of
(a) Endemism
(b) Accelerated habitat loss
(c) Low level of species richness
(d) Both (a) and (b)

**106.** The following are direct benefits from biodiversity except
(a) Firewood (b) Fibre
(c) Food (d) Pollination

**107.** The following are indirect benefits from biodiversity except
(a) Pest control
(b) Climate moderation
(c) Flood control
(d) Dyes, resins and perfumes

**108.** Which area of M.P. (Madhya Pradesh) contain sacred groves?
(a) Sarguja (b) Chanda
(c) Bastar (d) All of these

**109.** Find the incorrect match.

| | |
|---|---|
| (a) Pollinator | – Bees, Bumblebees, Bats and Birds |
| (b) Legally protected biodiversity rich region | – Biosphere reserve, National park, wildlife sanctuaries, sacred groves |
| (c) Lung of planet | – Amazonian rain forest |
| (d) Rivet popper hypothesis | – Harvard ecologist Paul Ehrlich |

**110.** Select incorrect statement of the following:
(a) The narrowly utilitarian reasons for conserving biodiversity are tannins, lubricants, dyes, resins, perfumes
(b) More than 25 per cent of the drugs currently sold in the market worldwide are derived from plants
(c) The broadly utilitarian argument says that biodiversity plays a major role in many ecosystem services that nature provides.
(d) Pollination through pollinators like bees, bumblebees, birds and bats is narrowly utilitarian reason.

**111.** Select set of correct statements:
(A) When the whole ecosystem conserved and protected, its biodiversity at all levels is protected. This approach is called in situ conservation.
(B) When an animal or plant is endangered or threatened and needs urgent measures to save it from extinction, in situ conservation is the desirable approach.
(C) 'Bio prospecting' means exploring molecular, genetic and species-level diversity for products of economic importance
(D) Endemism means species is critically endangered or threatened
(a) B and D only (b) A and C only
(c) B, C and D only (d) C and D only

**112.** Select set of correct statements:
(A) Biodiversity hotspots regions with very high levels of species richness and high degree of endemism
(B) Biodiversity hotspots are regions of accelerated habitat loss
(C) The total number of biodiversity hotspots in the world are 25.
(D) All the biodiversity hotspots put together cover around 5 percent of the earth's land area.
(E) Strict protection of biodiversity hotspots could reduce the ongoing mass extinctions by almost 30 per cent.
(a) A, B and E only (b) A, B and C only
(c) B, C and E only (d) C and D only

**113.** Select set of correct statements:
(A) In India, ecologically unique and biodiversity-rich regions are legally protected as biosphere reserves, national parks and sanctuaries.
(B) India now has 14 biosphere reserves, 90 national parks and 448 wildlife sanctuaries.
(C) Sacred groves in India are found in Khasi and Jaintia Hills in Meghalaya, Aravalli Hills of Rajasthan, Western Ghat regions of Karnataka and Maharashtra
(D) In Meghalaya, the sacred groves are the last refuges for a large number of rare and threatened plants.
(a) A, B and D only (b) A, B and C only
(c) B, C and D only (d) A, B, C and D

**114.** Select set of correct statements:
(A) In Ex situ Conservation, threatened animals and plants are taken out from their natural habitat and placed in special setting where they can be protected and given special care.
(B) Zoological parks, botanical gardens and wildlife safari parks are examples of Ex situ Conservation.
(C) cryopreservation techniques, in vitro fertilizartion, and tissue culture methods are advanced Ex situ Conservation methods
(D) Seeds of different genetic strains of commercially important plants can be kept for long periods in seed banks.
(a) A, B and D only (b) A, B and C only
(c) B, C and D only (d) A, B, C and D

**115.** Ex situ conservation methods include protective maintenance of threatened species by
(A) zoological parks and botanical gardens
(B) in vitro fertilisation
(C) tissue culture propagation
(D) cryopreservation of gametes.
(E) sacred groves
(a) A, B and E only (b) A, B and C only
(c) B, C and E only (d) A, B, C and D

**116.** Long form of IUCN is
(a) Indian Union for Conservation of Nature and Natural resources
(b) International Union for Conservation of Nature and Natural resources
(c) International Union for Conservation of Nature
(d) International United for Conservation of Nature and Natural resources

**117. Assertion:** Biologists make a statistical comparison of the temperate-tropical species richness of an exhaustively studied group of insects and extrapolate this ratio to other groups of animals and plants to come up with a gross estimate of the total number of species on earth.

**Reason:** It is considered that an overwhelmingly large proportion of the species waiting to be discovered are in the tropics.
(a) (A) is false but (R) is true
(b) Both (A) and (R) are true and (R) is the correct explanation of (A)

(c) Both (A) and (R) are true but (R) is not the correct explanation of (A)
(d) (A) is true but (R) is false.

**118.** Select set of correct statements:
(A) Long form of IUCN is International Union for Conservation of Nature and Natural resources
(B) According to the IUCN (2004), the total number of plant and animal species described so far is slightly more than 1.5 million
(C) For many taxonomic groups, species inventories are more complete in temperate than in tropical countries.
(D) Estimate by Robert May places the global species diversity at about 7 million.
(a) A, B and D only (b) A, B and C only
(c) B, C and D only (d) A, B, C and D

**119.** Select set of correct statements:
(A) More than 70 per cent of all the species on earth's biodiversity recorded are animals.
(B) Plants comprise more than 22 per cent of the total biodiversity.
(C) The number of fungi species in the world is more than the combined total of the species of fishes, amphibians, reptiles and mammals.
(D) Embracing biochemical or molecular criteria for defining species within the prokaryotic group could result in a diversity that might encompass millions of species.
(a) A, B and D (b) A, B and C
(c) A, C and D (d) B and D only

**Direction for Q120–123:** Choose the correct option:
(a) (A) is false but (R) is true
(b) Both (A) and (R) are true and (R) is the correct explanation of (A)
(c) Both (A) and (R) are true but (R) is not the correct explanation of (A)
(d) (A) is true but (R) is false.

**120. Assertion:** Among animals, insects are the most species-rich taxonomic group.
**Reason:** Insects make up more than 80 per cent of the total animals.

**121. Assertion:** Biologists are unable to give estimates for prokaryotic species on the Earth.
**Reason:** Traditional taxonomic approaches may be unsuitable for microbial species identification due to the fact that many species cannot be cultured using standard laboratory methods.

**122. Assertion:** The share of India in the global species diversity is an impressive 8.1 per cent.
**Reason:** India has only 2.4 per cent of the world's land area.

**123. Assertion:** India is one of the 12 mega diversity countries of the world.
**Reason:** The share of India in the global species diversity is an impressive 8.1 per cent.

**124.** Select set of correct statements:
(A) Nearly 45,000 species of plants and twice as many of animals have been recorded from India.
(B) According to May's global estimates, only 22 per cent of the total species have been recorded so far.
(C) A large fraction of these species faces the threat of becoming extinct even before their discovery
(D) The diversity of plants and animals is not uniform throughout the world but shows a rather uneven distribution.
(a) A, B and D only (b) A, B and C only
(c) B, C and D only (d) A, B, C and D

## Multiple Choice Questions: Level II

**125.** Which one of the following has maximum genetic diversity in India?
(a) Mango (b) Wheat
(c) Tea (d) Teak

**126.** Which one of the following is not observed in biodiversity hotspots?
(a) Lesser inter-specific competition
(b) Species richness
(c) Endemism
(d) Accelerated species loss

**127.** Which one of the following pairs of organisms are exotic species introduced in India?
(a) *Lantana camara*, water hyacinth
(b) Qater hyacinth, *Prosopis cinereria*
(c) Nile perch, *Licus religiosa*
(d) *Ficus religiosa*, *Lantana camara*

**128.** Which one of the following is not included under in-situ conservation?
(a) Botanical garden (b) Biosphere reserve
(c) National park (d) Sanctuary

**129.** Which of the following is considered to be a hot-spot of biodiversity in India?
(a) Indo-Gangetic Plain (b) Eastern Ghats
(c) Aravalli Hills (d) Western Ghats

**130.** One of the most important functions of botanical gardens is that
(a) they provide a beautiful area for recreation
(b) one can observe tropical plants there
(c) they allow ex-situ conservation of germ plasm
(d) they provide natural habitats for wildlife

**131.** In your opinion, which is the most effective way to conserve plant diversity of an area?
(a) By tissue culture method
(b) By creating biosphere reserve
(c) By creating botanical garden
(d) By developing seed bank

**132.** Which group of vertebrates comprises the highest number of endangered species?
(a) Birds (b) Mammals
(c) Fishes (d) Reptiles

**133.** Reason of diversity in living beings is due
(a) Mutation
(b) Long-term evolutionary change
(c) Gradual change
(d) Short-term evolutionary change

**134.** An institution where valuable plant material likely to become irretrievably lost in the wild or in cultivation is preserved in a viable condition is known as
(a) Genome (b) Herbarium
(c) Gene library (d) Gene bank

**135.** At present, the most significant cause extinction of biodiversity is probably
(a) the deterioration of ozone layer
(b) the destruction of habitat
(c) biological magnification of DDT
(d) global warming

**136.** A high density of a protected animal in a National Park can result into
(a) Mutualism (b) Intraspecific competition
(c) Emigration (d) Predation

**137.** A number of natural reserves have been created to conserve specific wild life species. Identify the correct combination from the following
(a) Gir Forest - Tiger
(b) Kaziranga - Elephants
(c) Rann of Kutch - Wild Ass
(d) Manas wild life Sanctuary - Musk deer

**138.** Which of the following is the main factor of desertification?
(a) Tourism (b) Irrigated agriculture
(c) Over-grazing (d) All of these

**139.** Species diversity increases as one proceeds from
(a) High altitude to low altitude and high latitude to low latitude
(b) Low altitude to high altitude and high latitude to low latitude
(c) Low altitude to high altitude and low latitude to high latitude
(d) High altitude to low altitude and low latitude to high latitude

**140.** Which animal has become extinct from India?
(a) Snow Leopard (b) Hippopotamus
(c) Wolf (d) Cheetah

**141.** Wildlife is destroyed most when
(a) There is lack of proper care
(b) Mass scale hunting for foreign trade
(c) Its natural habitat is destroyed
(d) Natural calamity

## A & R and Statement-based Questions

### Assertion and Reason Questions:

***Direction for questions 142 to 146:** Read the **assertion** and **reason** carefully to mark the correct option out of the options given below:*

**(a)** **(A)** is **true** but **(R)** is **false**.
**(b)** **(A)** is **false** but **(R)** is **true**.
**(c)** Both **(A)** and **(R)** is **true** and **(R)** is the correct explanation of **(A)**.
**(d)** Both **(A)** and **(R)** is **true** and **(R)** is not the correct explanation of **(A)**.

**142. Assertion:** Sixth extinction presently in progress which is different from the previous episode.
**Reason:** Current species extinction rates are estimated to be 100 to 1000 times faster than in the pre-human times.

**143. Assertion:** Bioremediation is the use of living organisms, usually prokaryotes, fungi plants, to detoxify polluted ecosystems.
**Reason:** Biological augmentation uses organisms to add essential materials to a degraded ecosystem.

**144. Assertion:** Amazon rain forest is called lung of our planet.

**Reason:** Amazon rain forest produces 20% of total oxygen in Earth's atmosphere through the process of photosynthesis.

**145. Assertion:** There are 30 biodiversity hotspots in the world.

**Reason:** High level of species richness is a criterion for selection of a biodiversity hotspot.

**146. Assertion:** If we take entire continent the slope of the line of logarithmic graph of species area relationship to be less steep.

**Reason:** The species area relationship is generally a rectangle hyperbolic function.

## Statement-based Questions:

***Direction for questions 147 to 151:*** *These type of questions consist of two statement each, printed as* **Statement-I** *and* **Statement-II.** *While answering such questions, a student is needed to choose any one of the following four responses.*

**(a) Statement I** is **correct Statement II** is **incorrect**.
**(b) Statement I** is **incorrect Statement II** is **correct**.
**(c)** Both **Statement I** and **Statement II** are **correct**.
**(d)** Both **Statement I** and **Statement II** are **incorrect**.

**147. Statement-I:** Biodiversity hotspots are example of in-situ conservation.

**Statement-II:** It is a conservation of biological wealth on site.

**148. Statement-I:** Ex-situ conservation is carried out in biosphere reserves, national parks and sanctuaries.

**Statement-II:** NGOs are only involved in the maintenance of these protected areas.

**149. Statement-I:** Habitat loss and fragmentation is the most important cause driving animals and plants to extinction.

**Statement-II:** Habitat loss and fragmentation causes alien species invasion.

**150. Statement-I:** Temperate regions have greater biological diversity.

**Statement-II:** More solar energy in tropics, contributes to higher productivity, which in turn may contribute indirectly to greater biodiversity.

**151. Statement-I:** Endemism is high in biodiversity hotspot.

**Statement-II:** Pollination is broadly utilitarian argument of conservation of biodiversity.

# Matrix-Match Type Questions

**152.** Match the following:

| List-I (Scientist) | List-II (Work) |
|---|---|
| 1. Alexander Von Humboldt | (i) Popularised term 'Biodiversity' |
| 2. Edward Wilson | (ii) Rivet popper hypothesis |
| 3. Paul Ehrlich | (iii) Hyperbolic relation between species richness & area |

The correct matching is

| | 1 | 2 | 3 |
|---|---|---|---|
| (a) | (iii) | (i) | (ii) |
| (b) | (i) | (iii) | (ii) |
| (c) | (ii) | (i) | (iii) |
| (d) | (iii) | (ii) | (i) |

**153.** Match the following:

| List-I (Place) | List-II (Extinct Species) |
|---|---|
| 1. Mauritius | (i) Quagga |
| 2. Africa | (ii) Stellar's Sea Cow |
| 3. Australia | (iii) Dodo |
| 4. Russia | (iv) Tiger (3 subspecies) |
| 5. Bali | (v) Thylacine |

The correct matching is

| | 1 | 2 | 3 | 4 | 5 |
|---|---|---|---|---|---|
| (a) | (iii) | (i) | (v) | (ii) | (iv) |
| (b) | (ii) | (iii) | (iv) | (i) | (v) |
| (c) | (i) | (iv) | (iii) | (ii) | (v) |
| (d) | (ii) | (iv) | (i) | (iii) | (v) |

**154.** Match the following:

| List-I (Species) | List-II (% Facing Threat of Extinction) |
|---|---|
| 1. Bird | (i) 23 |
| 2. Mammal | (ii) 32 |
| 3. Amphibia | (iii) 12 |
| 4. Gymnosperms | (iv) 31 |

The correct matching is

| | 1 | 2 | 3 | 4 |
|---|---|---|---|---|
| (a) | (iii) | (i) | (ii) | (iv) |
| (b) | (iv) | (iii) | (ii) | (i) |
| (c) | (ii) | (i) | (iii) | (iv) |
| (d) | (ii) | (ii) | (i) | (iv) |

**155.** Match the following:

| List-I (Causes of Biodiversity) | List-II (Reasons) |
|---|---|
| 1. Habitat loss & fragmentation | (i) Introduction of foreign species which cause extinction of indigenous species |
| 2. Over exploitation | (ii) Extinction of species which are in close association with extinct species |
| 3. Alien species invasions | (iii) Over use of resources |
| 4. Co-extinctions | (iv) Breaking up of large habitats into small fragments due to human activities |

The correct matching is

| | 1 | 2 | 3 | 4 |
|---|---|---|---|---|
| (a) | (iv) | (iii) | (ii) | (i) |
| (b) | (i) | (iv) | (ii) | (iii) |
| (c) | (ii) | (iii) | (iv) | (i) |
| (d) | (iv) | (iii) | (i) | (ii) |

**156.** Match the following:

| List-I (In India) | List-II (Numbers) |
|---|---|
| 1. Biosphere reserves | (i) greater than 448 |
| 2. National parks | (ii) 148 |
| 3. Wildlife sanctuaries | (iii) 90 |

The correct matching is

| | 1 | 2 | 3 |
|---|---|---|---|
| (a) | (ii) | (i) | (iii) |
| (b) | (i) | (iii) | (ii) |
| (c) | (ii) | (iii) | (i) |
| (d) | (iii) | (ii) | (i) |

## NCERT Exemplar Questions

**1.** Which of the following countries has the highest biodiversity?
(a) South America (b) South Africa
(c) Russia (d) India

**2.** Which of the following is not a cause for the loss of biodiversity?
(a) Destruction of habitat
(b) Invasion by alien species
(c) Keeping animals in zoological parks
(d) Over-exploitation of natural resources

**3.** Which of the following is not an invasive alien species in the Indian context?
(a) *Lantana* (b) *Cynodon*
(c) *Parthenium* (d) *Eichhornia*

**4.** Where among the following will you find the pitcher plant?
(a) Rain forest of North-East India
(b) Sunderbans
(c) Thar Desert
(d) Western Ghats

**5.** Which one of the following is not a characteristic feature of biodiversity hotspots?
(a) Large number of species
(b) Abundance of endemic species
(c) Mostly located in the tropics
(d) Mostly located in the Polar Regions

**6.** Match the animals given in column A with their location in column B.

| List-I | List-II |
|---|---|
| (i) Dodo | (A) Africa |
| (ii) Quagga | (B) Russia |
| (iii) Thylacine | (C) Mauritius |
| (iv) Steller's sea cow | (D) Australia |

Choose the correct match from the following:
(a) i-A, ii-C, iii-B, iv-D
(b) i-D, ii-C, iii-A, iv-B
(c) i-C, ii-A, iii-B, iv-D
(d) i-C, ii-A, iii-D, iv-B

7. What is common to the following plants: *Nepenthes, Psilotum, Rauwolfia* and *Aconitum*?
(a) All are ornamental plants
(b) All are phylogenic link species
(c) All are prone to over exploitation
(d) All are exclusively present in the Eastern Himalayas.

8. The one-horned rhinoceros is specific to which of the following sanctuary
(a) Bhitar Kanika (b) Bandipur
(c) Kaziranga (d) Corbett park

9. Amongst the animal groups given below, which one appears to be more vulnerable to extinction?
(a) Insects (b) Mammals
(c) Amphibians (d) Reptiles

10. Which one of the following is an endangered plant species of India?
(a) *Rauvolfia serpentina*
(b) *Santalum album* (Sandal wood)
(c) *Cycas beddonei*
(d) All of the above

11. What is common to *Lantana*, *Eichhornia* and African catfish?
(a) All are endangered species of India.
(b) All are keystone species.
(c) All are mammals found in India.
(d) All the species are neither threatened nor indigenous species of India.

12. The extinction of passenger pigeon was due to
(a) Increased number of predatory birds
(b) Over exploitation by humans
(c) Non-availability of the food
(d) Bird flu virus infection

13. Which of the following statements is correct?
(a) *Parthenium* is an endemic species of our country.
(b) African catfish is not a threat to indigenous catfishes.
(c) Steller's sea cow is an extinct animal.
(d) *Lantana* is popularly known as carrot grass.

14. Among the ecosystem mentioned below, where can one find maximum biodiversity?
(a) Mangroves (b) Desert
(c) Coral reefs (d) Alpine meadows

15. Which of the following forests is known as the '**lungs of the planet Earth**'?
(a) Tiaga forest
(b) Tundra forest
(c) Amazon rain forest
(d) Rain forests of North-East India

16. The active chemical drug reserpine is obtained from
(a) *Datura* (b) *Rauwolfia*
(c) *Atropa* (d) *Papaver*

17. Which of the following group exhibit more species diversity?
(a) Gymnosperms (b) Algae
(c) Bryophytes (d) Fungi

18. Which of the below mentioned regions exhibit less seasonal variations?
(a) Tropics (b) Temperates
(c) Alpines (d) Both (a) and (b)

19. The historic convention on Biological Diversity held in Rio de Janeiro in 1992 is known as
(a) CITES Convention (b) The Earth Summit
(c) G-16 Summit (d) MAB Programme

20. What is common to the techniques (i) *in vitro* fertilization, (ii) Cryo preservation and (iii) tissue culture?
(a) All are *in situ* conservation methods.
(b) All are *ex situ* conservation methods.
(c) All require ultra-modern equipment and large space.
(d) All are methods of conservation of extinct organisms.

## Previous Years' Questions

1. Which one of the following is an example of ex-situ conservation? [AIPMT 2010 PRE]
(a) Wildlife sanctuary (b) Seed bank
(c) Sacred groves (d) National park

2. A renewable exhaustible natural resource is [AIPMT 2010 PRE]
(a) Coal (b) Petroleum
(c) Minerals (d) Forest

**3.** Which one of the following shows maximum genetic diversity in India? [AIPMT 2011 PRE]
(a) Rice (b) Maize
(c) Mango (d) Groundnut

**4.** Large woody vines are more commonly found in [AIPMT 2011 PRE]
(a) Mangroves (b) Tropical rainforests
(c) Alpine forests (d) Temperate forests

**5.** Which one of the following has the highest number of species in nature? [AIPMT 2011 PRE]
(a) Insects (b) Birds
(c) Angiosperms (d) Fungi

**6.** Biodiversity of a geographical region represents [AIPMT 2011 MAINS]
(a) Endangered species found in the region
(b) The diversity in the organism living in the region
(c) Genetic diversity in the dominant species of the region
(d) Species endemic to the region

**7.** The highest number of species in the world is represented by: [AIPMT 2012 PRE]
(a) Fungi (b) Mosses
(c) Algae (d) Lichens

**8.** Which one of the following areas in India is a hotspot of biodiversity? [AIPMT 2012 PRE]
(a) Eastern Ghats (b) Gangetic Plain
(c) Sunderbans (d) Western Ghats

**9.** Sacred groves are especially useful in: [AIPMT 2012 MAINS]
(a) Preventing soil erosion
(b) Year-round flow of water in rivers
(c) Conserving rare and threatened species
(d) Generating environmental awareness

**10.** Select the correct statement about biodiversity [AIPMT 2012 MAINS]
(a) Large-scale planting of Bt cotton has no adverse effect on biodiversity
(b) Western Ghats have a very high degree of species richness and endemism
(c) Conservation of biodiversity is just a fad pursued by developed countries
(d) The desert areas of Rajasthan and Gujarat have very high level of desert animal species as well as numerous rare animals

**11.** Which of the following represent maximum number of species among global biodiversity? [AIPMT 2013]
(a) Algae (b) Lichens
(c) Fungi (d) Mosses and Ferns

**12.** Which of the following is not used for ex-situ plant conservation? [AIPMT 2013]
(a) Field gene banks (b) Seed banks
(c) Shifting cultivation (d) Botanical Gardens

**13.** Given below is the representation of the extent of global diversity of invertebrates. What groups the four portions (A–D) represent, respectively? [AIPMT 2014]

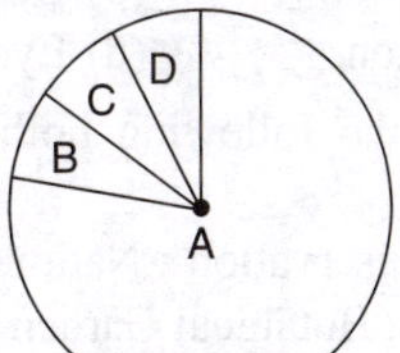


(a) A: Insects, B: Crustaceans, C: Other animal groups, D: Molluscs
(b) A: Crustaceans, B: Insects, C: Molluscs, D: Other animal groups
(c) A: Molluscs, B: Other animal groups, C: Crustaceans, D: Insects
(d) A: Insects, B: Molluscs, C: Crustaceans, D: Other animal groups

**14.** The organization which publishes the red list of species is: [AIPMT 2014]
(a) ICFRE (b) IUCN
(c) UNEP (d) WWF

**15.** A species facing extremely high risk of extinction in the immediate future is called: [AIPMT 2014]
(a) Vulnerable
(b) Endemic
(c) Critically Endangered
(d) Extinct

**16.** An example of ex-situ conservation is: [AIPMT 2014]
(a) National Park (b) Seed Bank
(c) Wildlife Sanctuary (d) Sacred Grove

**17.** The species confined to a particular region and not found elsewhere is termed as: [RE-AIPMT 2015]
(a) Alien (b) Endemic
(c) Rare (d) Keystone

**18.** Cryopreservation of gametes of threatened species in viable and fertile condition can be referred to as [AIPMT 2015]
(a) In-situ conservation of biodiversity
(b) Advanced ex-situ conservation of biodiversity
(c) In-situ conservation by sacred groves
(d) In-situ cryoconservation of biodiversity

**19.** Most animals are tree dwellers in a [AIPMT 2015]
(a) Coniferous forest
(b) Thorn woodland
(c) Temperature deciduous forest
(d) Tropical rain forest

**20.** Which of the following characteristics is mainly responsible for diversification of insects of land? [AIPMT 2015]
(a) Segmentation (b) Bilateral symmetry
(c) Exoskeleton (d) Eyes

**21.** In which of the following both pairs have correct combination? [AIPMT 2015]
(a) In-situ conservation : National park Ex-situ conservation : Botanical Garden
(b) In-situ conservation : Cryopreservation Ex-situ conservation : Wildlife Sanctuary
(c) In-situ conservation : Seed Bank Ex-situ conservation : National park
(d) In-situ conservation : Tissue culture Ex-situ conservation : Sacred groves

**22.** Which of the following National Parks is home to the famous musk deer or hangul? [NEET 2016 – PHASE II]
(a) Bandhavgarh National Park, Madhya Pradesh
(b) Eaglenest Wildlife Sanctuary, Arunanchal Pradesh
(c) Dachigam National Park, Jammu and Kashmir
(d) Keibul Lamjao National Park, Manipur

**23.** Red list contains date or information on [NEET 2016 – PHASE II]
(a) Plants whose products are in international trade
(b) Threatened species
(c) Marine vertebrate only
(d) All economically important plants

**24.** How many hot spots biodiversity in the world have been identified till date by Norman Myers? [NEET 2016 – PHASE II]
(a) 25 (b) 34 (c) 43 (d) 17

**25.** Which of the following is the most important causes of animals and plants being driven to extinction? [NEET 2016 – PHASE I]
(a) Over-exploitation
(b) Alien species invasion
(c) Habitat loss and fragmentation
(d) Co-extinctions

**26.** Which of the following is the National Aquatic Animal of India? [NEET 2016 – PHASE I]
(a) Gangetic shark (b) River dolphin
(c) Blue whale (d) Sea horse

**27.** Which of the following is correctly matched? [NEET 2016 – PHASE II]
(a) Age pyramid–Biome
(b) Parthenium hysterophorus–threat to biodiversity
(c) Stratification–Population
(d) Aerenchyma–Opuntia

**28.** Which scientist proposed 'Rivet popper hypothesis' related to biodiversity and ecosystems? [NEET Regional 2017]
(a) Tansley
(b) Alexander von Humboldt
(c) Paul Ehrlich
(d) David Tilman

**29.** Alexander Von Humbolt described for the first time [NEET 2017]
(a) Laws of limiting factor
(b) Species area relationships
(c) Population Growth equation
(d) Ecological Biodiversity

**30.** The region Biosphere Reserve which is legally protected and where no human activity is allowed is known as: [NEET 2017]
(a) Buffer zone (b) Transition zone
(c) Restoration zone (d) Core zone

**31.** Which one of the following is related to ex-situ conservation of threatened animals and plants? [NEET 2017]
(a) Biodiversity hot spots
(b) Amazon rainforest
(c) Himalayan region
(d) Wildlife Safari parks

**32.** All of the following are included in '*Ex-situ* conservation' except [NEET 2018]
(a) Wildlife safari parks (b) Botanical gardens
(c) Sacred groves (d) Seed banks

**33.** Niche is [NEET 2018]
(a) All the biological factors in the organism's environment
(b) The range of temperature that the organism needs to live
(c) The physical space where an organism lives
(d) The functional role played by the organism where it lives

**34.** Which one of the following is **not** a method of *in-situ* conservation of biodiversity? [NEET 2019]
(a) Wildlife Sanctuary (b) Botanical Garden
(c) Sacred Grove (d) Biosphere reserve

**35.** The Earth Summit held in Rio de Janeiro in 1992 was called: [NEET 2019]

(a) For conservation of biodiversity and sustainable utilization of its benefits
(b) To assess threat posed to native species by invasive weed species
(c) For immediate steps to discontinue use of CFCs that were damaging the ozone layer
(d) To reduce $CO_2$ emissions and global warming

**36.** Which of the following is the most important causes for animals and plants being driven to extinction? [NEET 2019]
(a) Drought and floods
(b) Economic exploitation
(c) Alien species invasion
(d) Habitat loss and fragmentation

**37.** According to Robert May, the global species diversity is about: [NEET 2020]
(a) 1.5 million (b) 20 million
(c) 50 million (d) 7 million

**38.** Which of the following regions of the globe exhibits highest species diversity? [NEET 2020]
(a) Western Ghats of India
(b) Madagascar
(c) Himalayas
(d) Amazon forests

**39.** Habitat loss and fragmentation, over exploitation, alien species invasion and co-extinction are causes for: [NEET 2022]
(a) Competition
(b) Biodiversity loss
(c) Natality
(d) Population explosion

**40.** Which of the following is not a method of *ex situ* conservation? [NEET 2022]
(a) National Parks
(b) Micropropagation
(c) Cryopreservation
(d) *In-vitro* fertilization

**41.** *In-situ* conservation refers to: [NEET 2022]
(a) Conserve only high risk species.
(b) Conserve only endangered species.
(c) Conserve only extinct species.
(d) Protect and conserve the whole ecosystem.

**42.** Among 'The Evil Quartet' which one is considered the most important cause driving extinction of species? [NEET 2023]
(a) Over-exploitation for economic gain
(b) Alien species invasions
(c) Co-extinctions
(d) Habitat loss and fragmentation

**43.** The historic convention on Biological Diversity, 'The Earth Summit' was held in Rio de Janeiro in the year: [NEET 2023]
(a) 1992 (b) 1986
(c) 2002 (d) 1985

**44.** Tropical regions show greatest level of species richness because [NEET 2024]
A tropical latitudes have remained relatively undisturbed for millions of years, hence more time was available for species diversification.
B tropical environments are more seasonal.
C more solar energy is available in tropics.
D constant environments promote niche specialization.
E tropical environments are constant and predictable.

Choose the correct answer from the options given below:
(a) A, C, D and E only
(b) A and B only
(c) A, B and E only
(d) A, B and D only

**45.** These are regarded as major causes of biodiversity loss: [NEET 2024]
A Over exploitation
B Co-extinction
C Mutation
D Habitat loss and fragmentation
E Migration

Choose the correct option:
(a) A, C and D only
(b) A, B, C and D only
(c) A, B and E only
(d) A, B and D only

**46.** List of endangered species was released by: [NEET 2024]
(a) GEAC (b) FOAM
(c) WWF (d) IUCN

**47.** The type of conservation in which the threatened species are taken out from their natural habital and placed in special setting where they can be protected and given special care is called: [NEET 2024]
(a) *in-situ* conservation
(b) Biodiversity conservation
(c) Semi-conservative method
(d) Sustainable development

**48.** Match List-I with List-II. [NEET 2024]

| List-I | List-II |
|---|---|
| (A) Robert May | (i) Species-Area relationship |
| (B) Alexander von Humboldt | (ii) Long-term ecosystem experiment using out door plots |
| (C) Paul Ehrlich | (iii) Global species diversity at about 7 million |
| (D) David Tilman | (iv) Rivet popper hypothesis |

Choose the correct answer from the options given below:

(a) (A)-(ii), (B)-(iii), (C)-(i), (D)-(iv)
(b) (A)-(iii), (B)-(i), (C)-(iv), (D)-(ii)
(c) (A)-(i), (B)-(iii), (C)-(ii), (D)-(iv)
(d) (A)-(iii), (B)-(iv), (C)-(ii), (D)-(i)

## Answer Key

### Multiple Choice Questions: Level I

| | | | | | | | | | |
|---|---|---|---|---|---|---|---|---|---|
| **1.** (d) | **2.** (c) | **3.** (d) | **4.** (a) | **5.** (d) | **6.** (a) | **7.** (d) | **8.** (b) | **9.** (d) | **10.** (b) |
| **11.** (a) | **12.** (a) | **13.** (c) | **14.** (d) | **15.** (d) | **16.** (d) | **17.** (a) | **18.** (b) | **19.** (c) | **20.** (d) |
| **21.** (b) | **22.** (d) | **23.** (d) | **24.** (d) | **25.** (b) | **26.** (b) | **27.** (d) | **28.** (d) | **29.** (c) | **30.** (b) |
| **31.** (d) | **32.** (a) | **33.** (c) | **34.** (d) | **35.** (c) | **36.** (a) | **37.** (c) | **38.** (a) | **39.** (d) | **40.** (d) |
| **41.** (d) | **42.** (c) | **43.** (d) | **44.** (d) | **45.** (b) | **46.** (a) | **47.** (b) | **48.** (b) | **49.** (b) | **50.** (d) |
| **51.** (d) | **52.** (d) | **53.** (b) | **54.** (d) | **55.** (b) | **56.** (d) | **57.** (a) | **58.** (a) | **59.** (b) | **60.** (c) |
| **61.** (b) | **62.** (a) | **63.** (b) | **64.** (c) | **65.** (b) | **66.** (d) | **67.** (b) | **68.** (d) | **69.** (d) | **70.** (a) |
| **71.** (a) | **72.** (c) | **73.** (d) | **74.** (d) | **75.** (d) | **76.** (d) | **77.** (c) | **78.** (b) | **79.** (b) | **80.** (b) |
| **81.** (d) | **82.** (d) | **83.** (b) | **84.** (b) | **85.** (d) | **86.** (d) | **87.** (d) | **88.** (a) | **89.** (c) | **90.** (d) |
| **91.** (d) | **92.** (d) | **93.** (d) | **94.** (b) | **95.** (a) | **96.** (d) | **97.** (d) | **98.** (d) | **99.** (d) | **100.** (c) |
| **101.** (d) | **102.** (c) | **103.** (c) | **104.** (b) | **105.** (d) | **106.** (d) | **107.** (d) | **108.** (d) | **109.** (d) | **110.** (d) |
| **111.** (b) | **112.** (a) | **113.** (d) | **114.** (d) | **115.** (d) | **116.** (b) | **117.** (b) | **118.** (d) | **119.** (c) | **120.** (d) |
| **121.** (b) | **122.** (c) | **123.** (b) | **124.** (d) | | | | | | |

### Multiple Choice Questions: Level II

| | | | | | | | | | |
|---|---|---|---|---|---|---|---|---|---|
| **125.** (a) | **126.** (a) | **127.** (a) | **128.** (a) | **129.** (d) | **130.** (c) | **131.** (b) | **132.** (b) | **133.** (b) | **134.** (d) |
| **135.** (b) | **136.** (b) | **137.** (c) | **138.** (c) | **139.** (a) | **140.** (d) | **141.** (c) | | | |

### A & R and Statement-based Questions

| | | | | | | | | | |
|---|---|---|---|---|---|---|---|---|---|
| **142.** (c) | **143.** (d) | **144.** (c) | **145.** (b) | **146.** (b) | **147.** (c) | **148.** (d) | **149.** (a) | **150.** (b) | **151.** (c) |

### Matrix-Match Type Questions

| | | | | |
|---|---|---|---|---|
| **152.** (a) | **153.** (a) | **154.** (a) | **155.** (d) | **156.** (c) |

### NCERT Exemplar Questions

| | | | | | | | | | |
|---|---|---|---|---|---|---|---|---|---|
| **1.** (a) | **2.** (c) | **3.** (b) | **4.** (a) | **5.** (d) | **6.** (d) | **7.** (c) | **8.** (c) | **9.** (c) | **10.** (d) |
| **11.** (d) | **12.** (b) | **13.** (c) | **14.** (c) | **15.** (c) | **16.** (b) | **17.** (d) | **18.** (a) | **19.** (b) | **20.** (b) |

### Previous Years' Questions

| | | | | | | | | | |
|---|---|---|---|---|---|---|---|---|---|
| **1.** (b) | **2.** (d) | **3.** (a) | **4.** (b) | **5.** (a) | **6.** (b) | **7.** (a) | **8.** (d) | **9.** (c) | **10.** (b) |
| **11.** (c) | **12.** (c) | **13.** (d) | **14.** (b) | **15.** (c) | **16.** (b) | **17.** (b) | **18.** (b) | **19.** (d) | **20.** (c) |
| **21.** (a) | **22.** (c) | **23.** (b) | **24.** (b) | **25.** (c) | **26.** (b) | **27.** (b) | **28.** (c) | **29.** (b) | **30.** (d) |
| **31.** (d) | **32.** (c) | **33.** (d) | **34.** (b) | **35.** (a) | **36.** (d) | **37.** (d) | **38.** (d) | **39.** (b) | **40.** (a) |
| **41.** (d) | **42.** (d) | **43.** (a) | **44.** (a) | **45.** (d) | **46.** (d) | **47.** (b) | **48.** (b) | | |

# HINTS AND EXPLANATION

## Multiple Choice Questions: Level II

**125.** Among the following mango has maximum biodiversity in India.

**126.** Biodiversity hot spot is characterized by species richness, endemism and accelerated habitat and species loss.

**127.** Exotic Species has been introduced from another geographic region to an area outside its natural range. Examples are water hyacinth, Lantana camara.

**128.** Botanical garden, zoological park are example of ex-situ conservation.

**129.** Three hotspots – Western Ghats and Sri Lanka, Indo-Burma and Himalaya – cover our country's exceptionally high biodiversity regions.

**130.** Ex-situ conservation means off-site conservation. It is the process of protecting an endangered species of plant of animal by removing it from an unsafe or threatened habitat and placing it or part of it under the care of man. Botanical garden is one of the methods of ex-situ conservation.

**131.** Creating biosphere reserve conserves both flora and fauna. Research and scientific management are carried out. Botanical gardens can conserve only a few specific varieties of plants.

**132.** Mammals. Almost one in four mammals are at risk of extinct.

**133.** Diversity is due to the long-term evolutionary changes. Adaptability to continuous changes in environmental conditions is important for natural selection of variants and variations generation after generation leading to emergence of diverse descendants.

**134.** An institution where valuable plant material likely to become irretrievably lost in the wild or in cultivation is preserved in a viable condition is known as Gene Bank.

**135.** Habitat destruction affects the survival of populations and reduces biodiversity.

**136.** Competition between organisms of the same species is called intraspecific competition. Mutualism is obligatory and mutually beneficial relationship occurring between two interacting organisms. Predation is the act of capturing, killing and eating. It is a negative interaction between two organisms. Migration is a permanent outward movement of individuals from a population for settling into a new area.

**137.** Refer to solution 93.

**138.** Desertification is the process leading to formation of desert. The main factor of desertification of land is over-grazing by herbivorous animals.

**139.** At low altitude and latitude more habitats is found, i.e., more species and individuals occur at lower latitude and altitude places.

**140.** The 'Cheetah' has become extinct from India.

**141.** If natural habitat is destroyed, wild life is affected badly.

## NCERT Exemplar Questions

**1.** **Brazil** has the highest biodiversity because it is located near the equator.

**2.** Destruction of habitat, invasion by alien species, and over-exploitation of natural resources are cause for loss of biodiversity.

**3.** Carrot grass *(Parthenium), Lantana* and water hyacinth *(Eichhornia crassipe)* are invasive weeds that cause environment damage.

**4.** Pitcher plants are found at rain forest of North-East India.

**5.** Characteristic feature of biodiversity hot spots are large number of species, abundance of endemic species and mostly located in the tropics.

**6.**

| Column A | Column B |
|---|---|
| (i) Dodo | (C) Mauritius |
| (ii) Quagga | (A) Africa |
| (iii) Thylacine | (D) Australia |
| (iv) Stellar's sea cow | (B) Russia |

**7.** *Nepenthes, Psilotum, Rauwolfia* and *Aconitum* all are prone to overexploitation.

**8.**

| Name | Site | For protecting |
|---|---|---|
| Jim Corbett National Park | Uttarakhand | Project Tiger |
| Rajaji National Park | Uttarakhand | Project Tiger |
| Dudhwa National Park | UP. | Project Tiger |
| Kanha National Park | M.P. | Project Tiger |
| Sunderbans National Park | West Bengal | Project Tiger |
| Bandipur National Park | Mysore (Karnataka) | Project Tiger, Elephant |

**9.** Presently, 12% all the birds species, 23% all mammals species, 31 % all gymnosperms species and 32% all amphibian species in world face threat of extinctions.

**10. Endangered (ER):** It is facing a high risk of extinction in the wild in the near future if conservation measures are not promptly taken.

E.g.: Red panda *(Ailurus fulgens)*

- Giant panda
- Largest lemur *ldri idri* of Madagascar
- Asiatic Wild Ass *(Asinus hernionus khur* now restricted to Rann of Kutch)
- Lion Tailed Macaque
- Bald Eagle
- Asiatic lion
- *Drosera indica*
- *Nepenthes*
- Hornbill
- Indian Aconite
- *Bentinckia nicobarica*
- Snow leopard
- *Rauwolfia serpentina*
- *Santalurn album* (Sandal wood)
- *Cycas beddonei*

**11.** *Lantana, Eichhornia* and African catfish all the species are neither threatened nor indigenous species of India.

**12.** Humans have always depended on nature for food and shelter but when 'need' turns to 'greed' it leads to over-exploitation of natural resources. In the last 500 years, many species' extinctions (Steller's sea cow, passenger's pigeon) were due to over-exploitation by human.

**13.** Steller's sea cow is an extinct animal.

**14.** Coral reefs have maximum biodiversity among above options.

**15.** Amazon rain forest is known as the 'lungs of the planet Earth'.

**16.** The genetic variation shown by the medicinal plant *Rauwolfia vomitoria* growing in different Himalayan ranges might be in terms of potency and concentration of the active chemical (Reserpine) obtained from roots of plants.

**17.** Fungi plants exhibit more species diversity.

**18.** Tropical regions exhibit less seasonal variations.

**19. The Earth Summit:** This historical convention on biological diversity held in Rio-de-Janeiro, Brazil in 1992. Attending nations take appropriate measure for conservation of biodiversity and sustainable utilization of its benefits.

**20.**

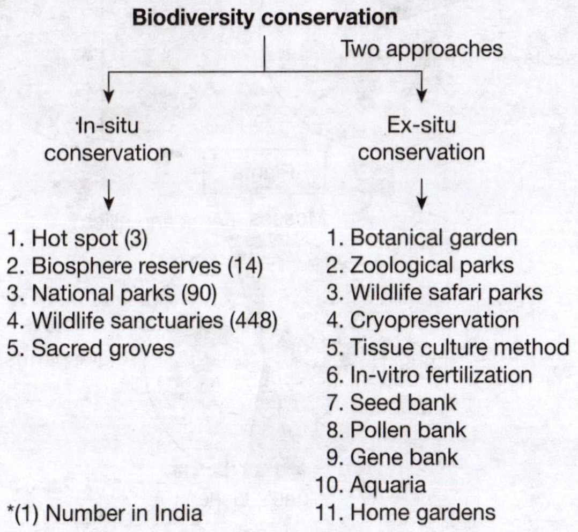

## Previous Years' Questions

1. Seeds of different genetic strains of commercially important plants can be kept for long periods in seed banks.
2. Mineral is not a renewable exhaustible natural resource.
3. India has more than 50,000 genetically different strains of rice and 1,000 varieties of mango.
4. Lianas (vascular plants) or Large woody vines are rooted in soil and they only get support of trees for climbing to top) and epiphytes (air plants) are common in this biome due to excess of moisture.
5. More than 70 percent of all the species recorded are animals. Among animals, insects are the richest in the taxonomic group; making more than 70 per cent of the total. It means out of every 10 animals on this planet, 7 are insects.
6. Biodiversity is the term popularized by the socio-biologist Edward Wilson to describe the combined diversity at all levels of biological organization. The most important of them are genetic diversity, species diversity and ecological diversity.
7. 

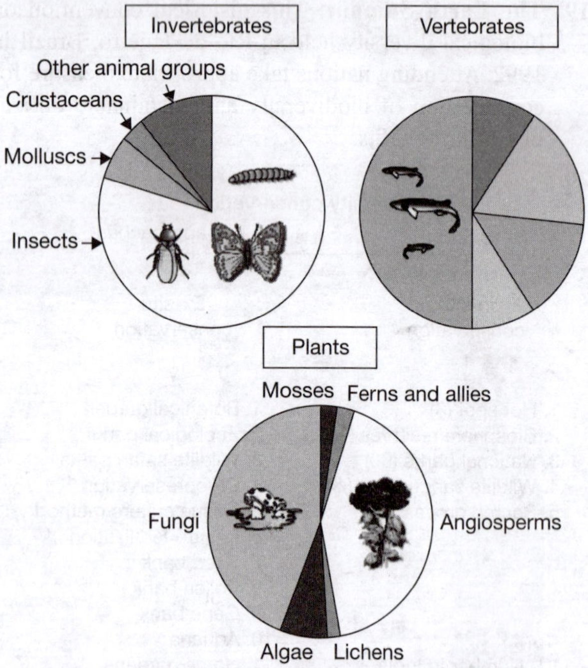


Representing global biodiversity: proportionate number of species of major taxa of plants, invertebrates and vertebrates.

8. Hot spots are the areas with high density of diversity or megadiversity which are also the most threatened ones. Today, the number of hot spots identified by ecologists are 25 out of which two hotspots are present in India.
9. Sacred groves are important to conserve rare and threatened species as it is a part of in-situ conservation.
10. Western Ghat is a biodiversity-rich zone along with high degree of endemism, it is one of the biodiversity hotspots in India.
11. Fungi have highest species diversity among all plant groups. Fungi also possess chitinous cell wall.
12. Shifting cultivation or Jhum cultivation is a kind of deforestation not conservation.
13. Bonus According AIPMT answer key 2014.

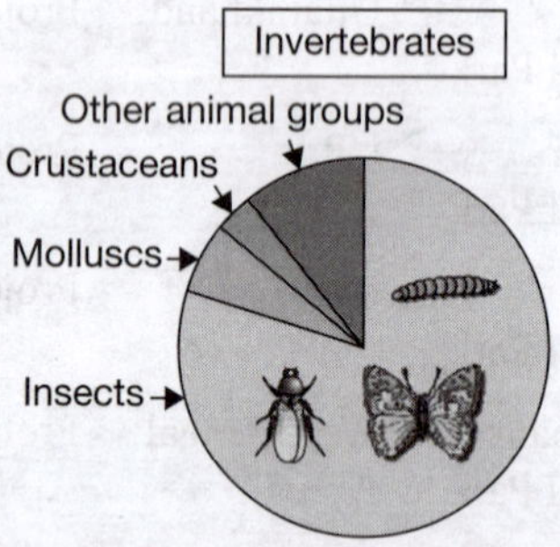


14. The IUCN Red List (2004) documents the extinction of 784 species (including 338 vertebrates, 359 invertebrates and 87 plants) in the last 500 years.
15. The extremely highest risk category assigned by the ICUN Red List for wild species is critically endangered species. These are those species that are facing a very high risk of extinction in the wild. There are currently 2129 animals and1821 plants which have been recorded in this category.
16. Seeds of different genetic strains of commercially important plants can be kept for long periods in seed banks.
17. **Endemism**: Species confined to that region and not found anywhere else.
18. Preservation at –196°C in liquid nitrogen is an advanced method for ex-situ conservation of gametes, tissue culture, embryos, etc., for indefinite periods. To prevent extinction of threatened species, cryopreservation is done.

    In-situ conservation occurs at ecosystem level of threatened or endangered species.

**19.** Tree dwelling or arboreal animals are particularly well adapted to spending most or all of their time in trees. They are found in tropical rain forest.

**20.** Chitinous (Monomer-N-acetyl glucosamine) exoskeleton is a characteristic feature responsible for diversification of insect.

**21.** In-situ conservation means the conservation of ecosystems and natural habitats and the maintenance and recovery of viable populations of species in their natural surroundings. *Ex-situ* conservation is the conservation and maintenance of samples of living organisms outside their natural habitat in the form of whole plants, seed, pollen, vegetative propagules, tissue or cell cultures.

**22.** The Kashmir stag (cervus Canadensis hangul) also called hangul is a subspecies of elk. In Kashmir, it is found in the Dachigam National Park where it is protected.

**23.** The IUCN Red List (2004) documents the extinction of 784 species (including 338 vertebrates, 359 invertebrates and 87 plants) in the last 500 years. Some examples of recent extinctions include the Dodo (Mauritius), Quagga (Africa), Thylacine (Australia), Steller's Sea Cow (Russia) and three subspecies (Bali, Javan, Caspian) of tiger.

Red list (IUCN 2004) or Red data book is a catalogue facing risk of extinction. Threatened species.

**Red list has eight categories**

| Red list category | Definition |
|---|---|
| Extinct | A taxon is extinct when there is no reasonable doubt that the last individual has died. *e.g.* Dodo. |
| Extinct in the wild | A taxon is extinct in the wild when exhaustive surveys in known and/or expected habitats have failed to record an individual. |
| Critically endangered | A taxon is critically endangered when it is facing an extremely high risk of extinction in the wild in the immediate future. *e.g. Sus salvanius* (Pigmy hog) *Berberis nilghiriensus*. |
| Endangered | A taxon is endangered when it is not critically endangered but is facing a very high risk of extinction in the wild in the near future. *e.g. Ailurus fulgens* (Red panda), Blue whale, Largest Lemur Idri-Idri of Madagascar, etc. |
| Vulnerable | A taxon is vulnerable when it is not critically endangered or endangered, but is facing high risk of extinction in the wild in the medium-term future. *e.g. Antelope cervicapra* (Black Buck). |
| Lower risk | A taxon is lower risk when it has been evaluated and does not satisfy the criteria for critically endangered, endangered or vulnerable. |
| Data deficient | A taxon is data-deficient when there is inadequate information to make a direct or indirect assessment of its risk of extinction. |
| Not evaluate | A taxon is not evaluated when it has not yet been assessed. |

**24.** Hot spots are the richest and the most threatened reservoirs of plant and animal life on earth. Ecologically hot spots are determined by four factors.

(i) Number of species/species diversity
(ii) Degree of endemism
(iii) Degree of threat to habitat due to its degradation and fragmentation
(iv) Degree of exploitation

Total number of biodiversity hotspots in the world is **34**. Three of these hotspots – Western Ghats and Sri Lanka, Indo-Burma and Himalaya – cover our country's exceptionally high biodiversity regions.

**25.** The accelerated rates of species extinctions that the world is facing now are largely due to human activities. There are four major causes (The Evil Quartet) out of this four habitat loss and fragmentation is the most important cause.

**26.** River dolphin (*Platanista gangetica*) is National Aquatic Animal of India.

**27.**
- Stratification found in ecosystem.
- Aerenchyma found in aquatic plants.
- Age pyramid is for population.

**28.** The 'rivet popper hypothesis' used by Stanford ecologist Paul Ehrlich to explain biodiversity is necessary for ecosystem to be stable and sustainable. He explained analogy of airplane with the ecosystem.

**29.** The German naturalist and geographer Alexander von Humboldt observed that within a region species richness increased with increasing explored area, but only up to a limit. i.e., Species area relationship.

**30.** Each biosphere reserve has three zones

(1) **Core or natural zone:** No human activity is allowed. The area is undisturbed and legally protected ecosystem.

(2) **Buffer zone:** It surrounds the core area. Limited human activity is allowed like resource use strategies, research and education.

(3) **Transition zone:** It is outermost or peripheral part of biosphere reserve where an active cooperation is present between reserve management and local people for activities like cropping, forestry.

**31.** (i) **In-situ conservation:** It is protection and management of important components of biological diversity through a network of protected areas.

**Example:**

(a) Protected areas: Wild life sanctuary and national park

(b) Biosphere reserves

(c) Sacred forests and scared lakes

(d) Hot spots of biodiversity rest Wild life safari park is example of ex-situ conservation

**32. Sacred groves** are found in Khasi and Jaintia Hills in Meghalaya, Aravalli Hills of Rajasthan, Western Ghat regions of Karnataka and Maharashtra and the Sarguja, Chanda and Bastar areas of Madhya Pradesh. ***(In-situ conservation: National park , wildlife sanctuary, biosphere reserve, biodiversity hotspot and sacred groves)***

**33.** Each organism has an invariably defined range of conditions that it can tolerate, diversity in the resources it utilizes and a distinct functional role in the ecological system, all these together comprise its niche.

**34.** *Ex situ* Conservation: In this approach, threatened animals and plants are taken out from their natural habitat and placed in special setting where they can be protected and given special care. Zoological parks, botanical gardens and wildlife safari parks serve this purpose. In-situ conservation of biodiversity includes wildlife sanctuary, sacred grove, biosphere reserve, national park and biodiversity hotspots.

**35.** The historic Convention on Biological Diversity ('The Earth Summit') held in Rio de Janeiro in 1992, called upon all nations to take appropriate measures for conservation of biodiversity and sustainable utilization of its benefits.

- **Kyoto protocol** – To reduce greenhouse gas (i.e., $CO_2$, Methane) emissions and global warming
- **Montreal Protocol** – For immediate steps to discontinue use of CFCs that were damaging the ozone layer

**36.** Habitat loss and fragmentation is the most important cause driving animals and plants to extinction.

**37.** • Robert May estimated global species diversity at about 7 million.

• Although some extreme estimates range from 20 to 50 million.

**39.** The largely tropical Amazonian rain forest in South America has the greatest biodiversity on earth.

**39. Causes for biodiversity loss:**

**Four major causes-'The Evil Quartet'.**

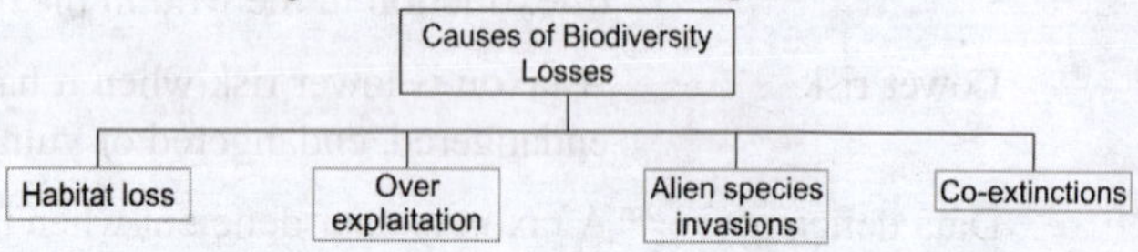


**40.** There are two basic strategies of biodiversity conservation

1. In Situ Conservation
2. Ex Situ Conservation

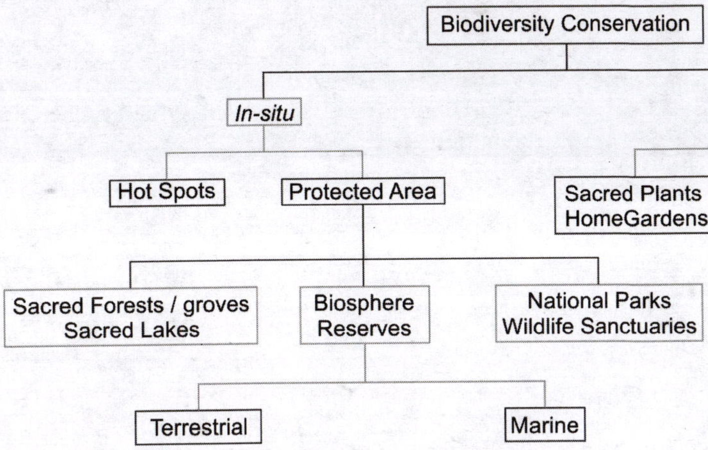


Here,
-Micropropagation,
-In vitro fertilization is also part of Ex-situ Conservation.

**41.** The approach of conserving and protecting the whole ecosystem, to protect its biodiversity at all the levels, is called in-situ conservation.

**42.** According to 'The Evil Quartet' Habitat loss and fragmentation is the most important cause driving extinction of species.

**43.** The historic convention on Biological Diversity, 'The Earth Summit' was held in Rio de Janerio in the year 1992 to take appropriate measures for conservation of biodiversity and sustainable utilisation of its benefits.

**44.** Only statement B is incorrect because tropical environments unlike temperate ones, are less seasonal, relatively more constant and predictable.
Thus statements A, C, D and E are correct.

**45.** Major causes of biodiversity losses are:
(1) habitat loss and fragmentation
(2) over-exploitation
(3) alien species invasions
(4) co-extinctions
Hence correct option is A, B and D only.

**46.** List of endangered species was released by IUCN.

**47.** The type of conservation in which threatened species are taken out from their natural habitat and placed in special setting where they can be protected and given special care is called *ex-situ* conservation which is a type of biodiversity conservation. Whereas *in-situ* conservation is onsite conservation.

**48.** Robert May places the global species diversity at about 7 million.
Alexander von Humboldt gave species-area relationship.
Paul Ehrlich used an analogy "Rivet popper hypothesis" to explain the role of species in the ecosystem.
David Tilman performed long term ecosystem experiments using out door plots.

# ZOOLOGY

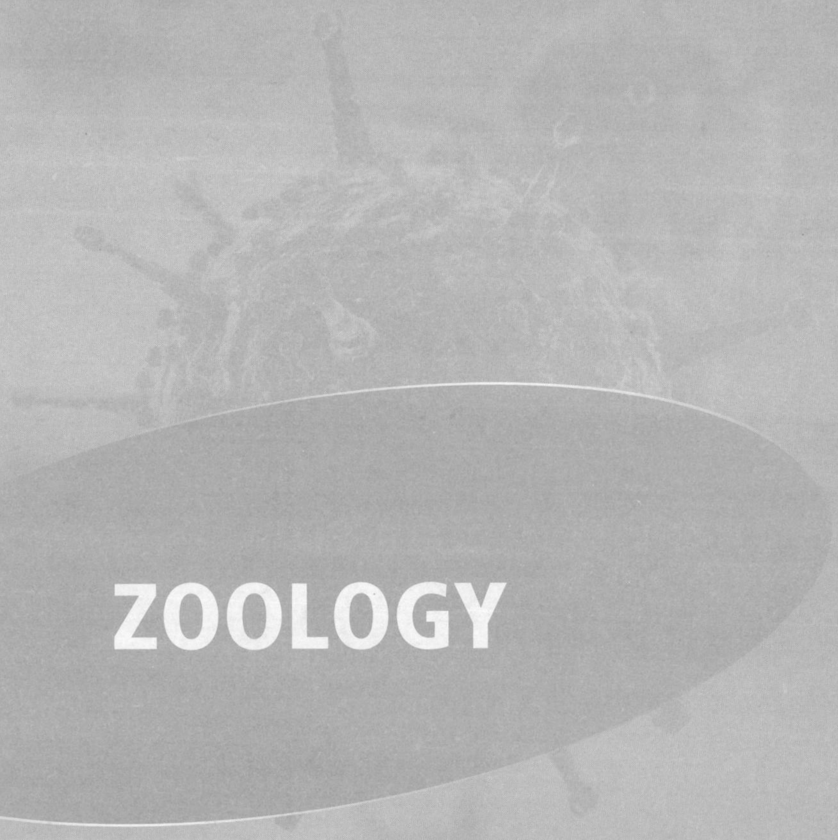

8

# Human Reproduction

## LEARNING OBJECTIVES

- Learn the process of double fertilization and post-fertilization process
- Understand the various male and female reproductive parts with their important functions
- To know more about the complete process of gametogenesis including the spermatogenesis and oogenesis
- Understand the different stages in humans from production of gametes to development of embryo
- Understand the elementary idea of lactation
- Discuss menstrual cycle
- Explain fertilization and implantation
- Understand parturition

## Chapter Overview

### Introduction

- Humans reproduce sexually only and are **viviparous** (i.e., give birth to the young ones). They are **unisexual** i.e., male and female sexes are separate.
- All reproductive events in human occur after puberty.
- In human beings the major reproductive events include:
  - **Gametogenesis:** Formation of gametes i.e., sperms in males and ovum in females.
  - **Insemination:** Transfer of sperms into the female genital tract.
  - **Fertilization:** Fusion of male and female gametes, leading to the formation of zygote.
  - **Implantation:** Formation and development of blastocyst and its attachment to the uterine wall.
  - **Gestation:** Embryo development or the time from conception to birth.
  - **Parturition:** Delivery of the baby or the process of birth.
- When the reproductive organs start functioning, the reproductive events in the males and females differ remarkably.
- Example:
  - the mammary glands are well developed in the females and rudimentary in males; the females do not develop beard and moustache but males do;
  - the voice in females is pitched higher than in males;
  - in men formation of sperms continues even in old age, but in women the formation of ovum ceases at around the age of fifty years.

Refer NCERT Ch 2: Human Reproduction

## Male Reproductive System

- Male reproductive system is located in pelvic region.

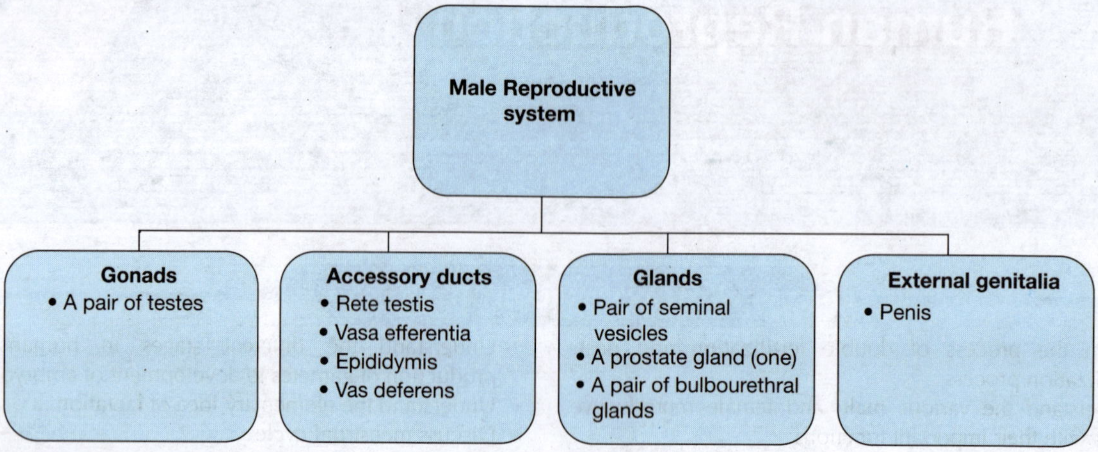


- **Gonads (or Testes):** It is located outside the abdominal cavity within a skin pouch called scrotum. Scrotum helps to maintain temperature of testis 2–2.5°C lower than that of body for optimum spermatogenesis. The length of testis is 4 to 5 cm and width is 2 to 3 cm **(Fig. 8.1)**. It is oval in shape. The testis is surrounded by three dense coverings called **tunicae.** These are:
  - **Tunica vaginalis** is the outer covering of the testis
  - **Tunica albuginea** is a fibrous covering surrounding the testis situated under the tunica vaginalis.
  - **Tunica vasculosa** consists of a network of capillaries supported by delicate connective tissue which lines the tunica albuginea.

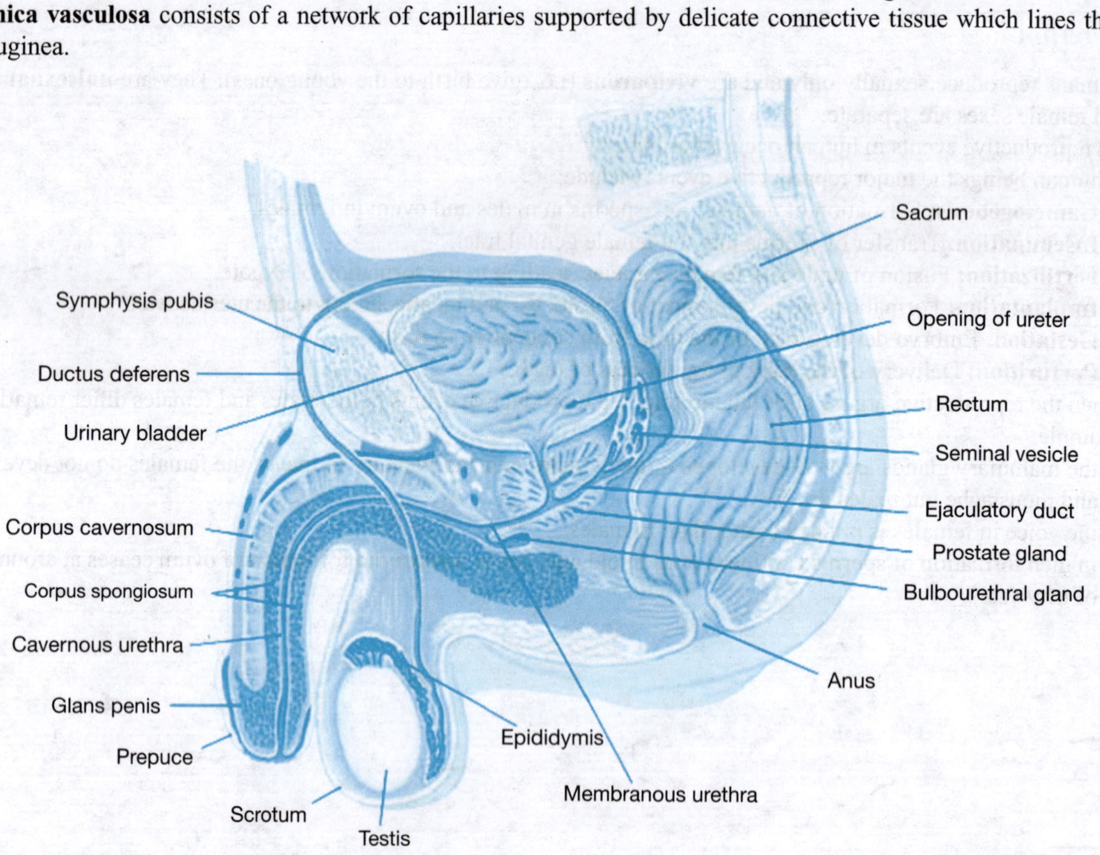


**FIGURE 8.1** Diagrammatic sectional view of male pelvis showing reproductive system

- **Testicular lobules**: Each testis has about 250 compartments called **testicular lobules (Fig 8.2).** Each lobule have one to three highly coiled structures:
  **Seminiferous tubules,** in which spermatogenesis occur. Lining of each seminiferous tubule is having two types of cells:
  **(1) Male germ cells** (or **Spermatogonia**): These cells undergo meiosis and result in sperm formation.
  **(2) Sertoli cells:** These cells provide nourishment to the germ cells and developing sperms.

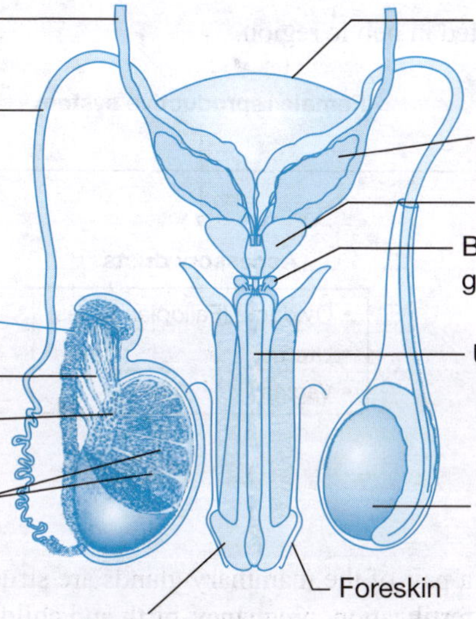


**FIGURE 8.2** Diagrammatic view of male reproductive system (part of testis is open to show inner details)

- In the testicular lobules but outside the seminiferous tubules, interstitial spaces are present which possess **interstitial cells** (or **Leydig cells**) and small blood vessels. These **Leydig** cells manufacture and secrete testicular hormone called androgens.
- Other immunologically competent cells are also present in the interstitial spaces. Testis performs two functions such as production of sperms and secretion of male sex hormones.
- **Accessory ducts:** Sperms formed in seminiferous tubules pass thorough following path which include **accessory ducts.** Functions of accessory ducts are storage and transport of the sperms from the testis upto the urethra. The epididymis stores the sperms and also secretes fluid which is considered to nourish the sperms.

**Path of sperms in male reproductive tract**

**Seminiferous tubules** → **Rete testis** → **Vasa efferentia** → **Epididymis** (located along the posterior surface of each testis) → **Vas deferens** (It ascends to the abdomen, loops around the urinary bladder and receives a duct from seminal vesicle) → **Ejaculatory duct** (duct formed by fusion of Vas deferens and duct from seminal vesicle) → **Urethra** → **Urethral Meatus**

- **External genitalia (or Penis):** Urethra starts at the urinary bladder, passes through the penis and open outside by **urethral meatus**. Penis is also the copulatory organ of male and is made up of special tissue that helps in its erection to facilitate insemination. Under the skin, penis contains three columns of erectile tissue—two dorsal **corpora cavernosa** and one ventral **corpus spongiosum. Glans penis** is the enlarged end of the penis and is covered by **foreskin or prepuce** (a loose skin fold).
- **Male accessory glands:** The secretion of the seminal vesicle contains spermatozoa activating substances such as **fructose, citrate, inositol, prostaglandins** and **several proteins**. Fructose is a source of energy for the sperm.

  These glands together secrete **seminal plasma (Rich in fructose, calcium and certain enzymes).** Secretion from **Bulbourethral glands** helps in the **lubrication of penis** also. Secretions of epididymis, vas deferens, seminal vesicle and prostate play very important role in maturation and motility of sperms. **Semen** is the mixture of spermatozoa and seminal plasma (the secretions of the seminal vesicles, prostate gland and Cowper's glands). It is ejected from the penis during ejaculation. A single ejaculate may contain 200 to 300 million spermatozoa (sperms). **Semen** is slightly alkaline (pH 7.35 to 7.50).

## Female Reproductive System

- Female reproductive system located in pelvic region.

**Female reproductive system**

- **Gonads**
  - A pair ovaries
- **Accessory ducts**
  - Oviducts (Fallopian tubes)
  - Uterus
  - Vagina
- **External genitalia (Vulva, pudendum)**
  - Mons pubis
  - Labia majora
  - Labia minora
  - Hymen
  - Clitoris

- Female reproductive system and a pair of the mammary glands are structurally and functionally integrated to promote various processes like ovulation, fertilization, pregnancy, birth and child care.
- The oviduct, uterus, vagina, clitoris, the accessory genital glands and mammary glands constitute the secondary sexual organs of human female **(Fig. 8.3)**.

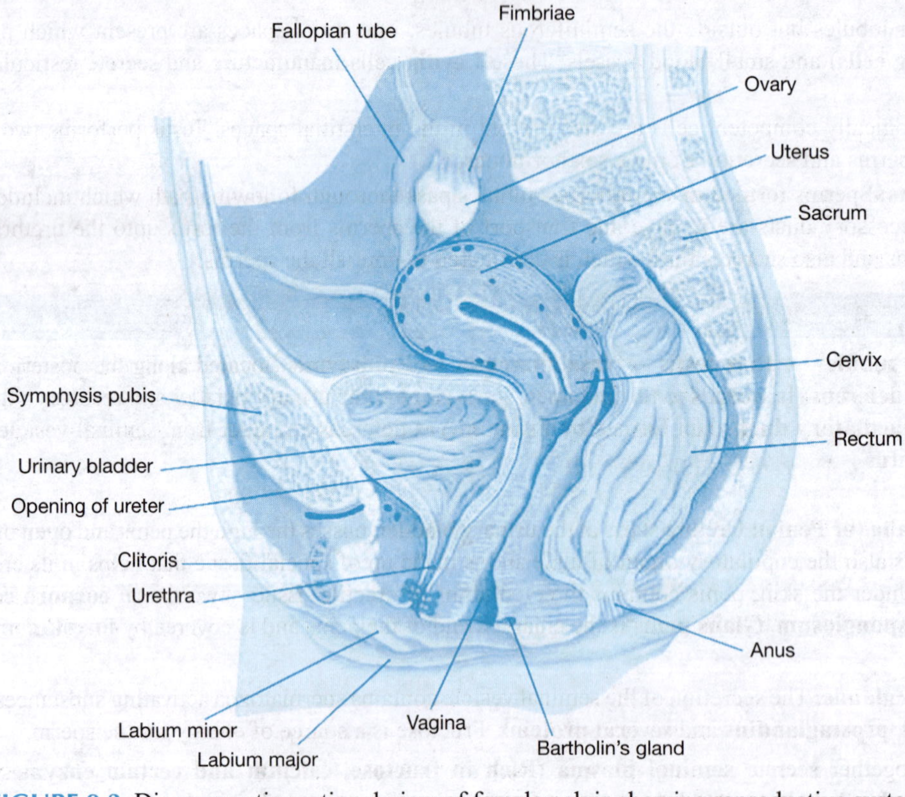


**FIGURE 8.3** Diagrammatic sectional view of female pelvis showing reproductive system

- **Gonads (or Ovaries)**: These are primary female sex organs as gametogenesis (oogenesis) occur in it. Ovary is located one on each side of the lower abdomen, connected to the pelvic wall and uterus by ligaments. Length of ovary is 2 to 4 cm. Ovary perform oogenesis and secrete ovarian hormones (steroid hormones). Each ovary is covered by a thin layer of cubical epithelium called **germinal epithelium.** A layer of connective tissue lies beneath the epithelium called **tunica albuginea.** It encloses the **ovarian stroma.** The ovarian stroma consists of a dense outer layer called **cortex** and a less dense inner portion called **medulla.** During the embryonic development stage millions of gamete mother cells (oogonia) are formed within each fetal ovary. No more oogonia are formed and added after birth.

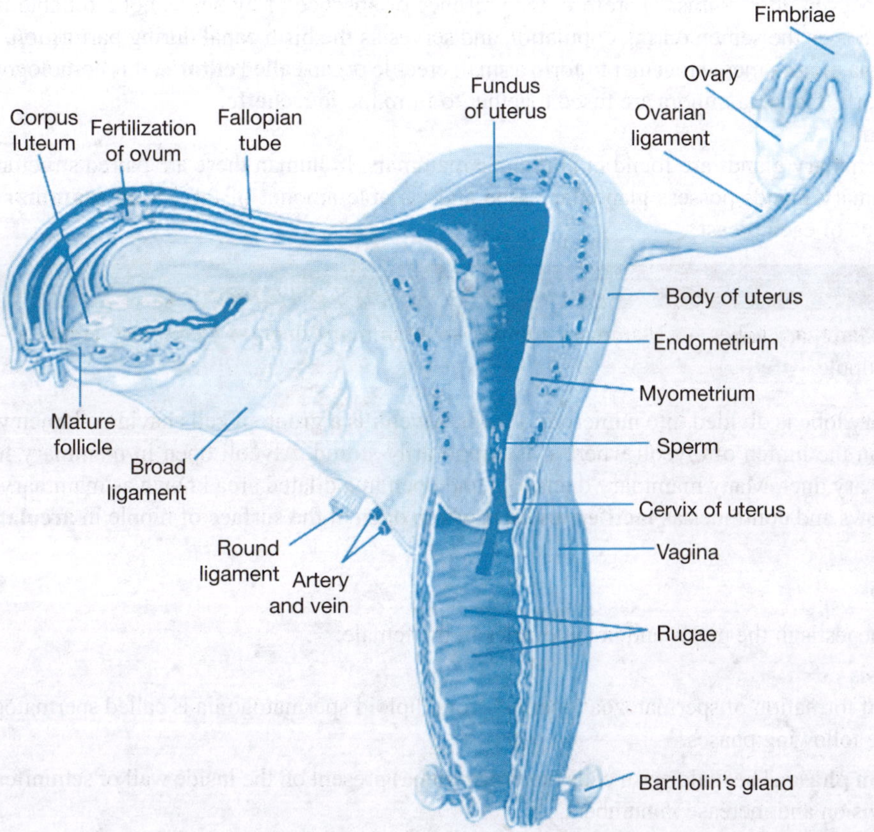


**FIGURE 8.4** Diagrammatic sectional view of the female reproductive system

- **Accessory ducts**

The fallopian tubes (oviducts), uterus and vagina constitute the female accessory ducts **(Fig 8.4)**.

1. **Fallopian tubes:** Each fallopian tube is about 10–12 cm long and extends from the periphery of each ovary to the uterus. The fallopian tube closer to ovary has a funnel like opening called **infundibulum.** The margin of infundibulum possesses finger like projections called **fimbriae** which help in collection of the ovum after ovulation. The infundibulum leads to a wider part of the fallopian tube called **ampulla.** The last part of the fallopian tube that joins the uterus is narrow and is called **isthmus.** The fallopian tubes convey the ovum from the ovary to the uterus. It is achieved by peristalsis. Fertilization of ovum generally takes place in the ampulla portion of the fallopian tube.
2. **Uterus (womb)**: The uterus is a hollow muscular and inverted pear-shaped structure. It lies in the pelvic cavity between the urinary bladder and the rectum, and is attached by ligaments to the pelvic wall. The uterus consists of a body called **corpus** which is a narrow uterine cavity called **internal Os** and the lower cylindrical structure called **cervix.** The wall of the uterus has three layers of tissue. The outer thin covering is called **perimetrium.** The middle thick layer of smooth muscle is **myometrium.** It shows strong contraction during delivery of the baby. The inner glandular layer that lines the uterine cavity is called **endometrium.** The endometrium undergoes cyclical changes during menstrual cycle.
3. **Vagina**: The cervix projects slightly into an elastic muscular tube called vagina. The vagina is about 10 cm long and opens to the exterior by an aperture called **vaginal orifice. Cervical canal along with vagina forms the birth canal.**

- **Female external genitalia:** The female external genitalia include mons pubis, labia majora, labia minora, hymen and clitoris.
  1. **Mons pubis** is a cushion of fatty tissue covered by skin and pubic hair.
  2. The **labia majora** are fleshy folds of tissue which extend down from the mons pubis and surround the vaginal opening.
  3. The **labia minora** are smaller folds which lie under the labia majora.
  4. The opening of the vagina remains partially covered by a thin ring of a membrane called **hymen.** It is often torn during the first coitus (intercourse). However, it can also be ruptured due to vigorous physical activities. In some women the hymen persists even after coitus. Therefore, the presence or absence of hymen is not a reliable indicator of virginity. The vagina receives the semen during copulation and serves as the birth canal during parturition.
  5. Anteriorly, labia minora merge together to form a small erectile organ called **clitoris.** It is homologous to the male's glans penis. Posteriorly, the labia minora are fused together to form the **fourchette.**
- **Mammary Gland**
  - Functional mammary glands are found in all female mammals. In human these are paired structures and are termed as breasts. Mammary glands possess glandular tissue and variable amount of fat. **15–20 mammary** lobes are found in glandular tissue of each breast.

| Path of milk secretion |
|---|
| Alveoli in Mammary lobes → Mammary tubules → Mammary duct → Mammary ampulla → Lactiferous duct opening at nipple |

  - Each mammary lobe is divided into numerous alveoli. Alveoli is a group of cells having a lumen within. Alveolar cells secrete milk in the lumen of alveoli where it is temporarily stored. Alveoli open in mammary tubules which join to form a mammary duct. Many mammary ducts join and open in a dilated area known as mammary ampulla. Mammary ampulla narrows and continues as **lactiferous duct** which open at the surface of nipple in **areolar part.**

## Gametogenesis

- It occurs in the testis in the males and in the ovaries in the female.

**1. Spermatogenesis**

- The process of formation of spermatozoa (sperms) from diploid spermatogonia is called spermatogenesis **(Fig. 8.5)**.
- It includes the following phases:

**(a) Multiplication phase:** The male germ cells (spermatogonia) present on the inside wall of seminiferous tubules multiply by mitotic division and increase in numbers.

**(b) Growth phase:** Spermatogonia grow and increase in size and forms primary spermatocytes. Each spermatogonia is diploid and contains 46 chromosomes.

**(c) Maturation phase or formation of spermatids:** Some of the spermatogonia called primary spermatocytes periodically undergo meiosis. A primary spermatocyte completes the first meiotic division (reduction division) leading to formation of two equal haploid cells called secondary spermatocytes, which have only 23 chromosomes each. The secondary spermatocytes undergo the second meiotic division to produce four equal haploid spermatids.

**(d) Differentiation phase:** The spermatids are transformed into spermatozoa (sperms) by the process of **spermiogenesis.** The sperm's head gets attached to Sertoli cells to draw nourishment and are finally released from the seminiferous tubules by the process called spermiation.

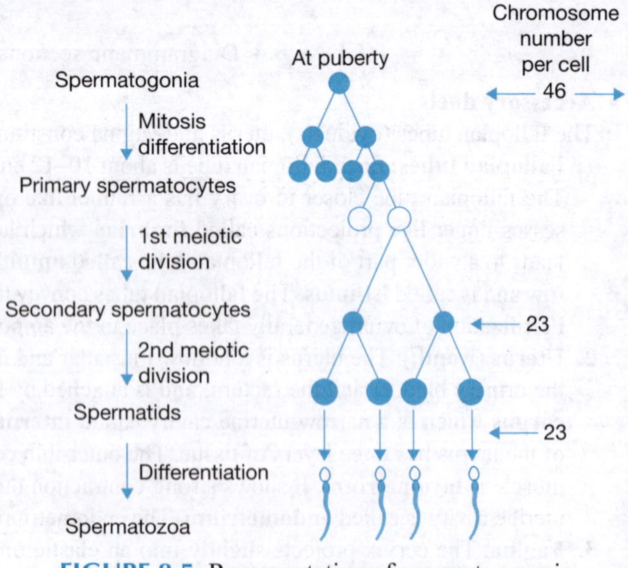


**FIGURE 8.5** Representation of spermatogenesis

- The sperm's head gets attached to Sertoli cells to draw nourishment and are finally released from the seminiferous tubules by the process called spermiation **(Fig. 8.6)**.

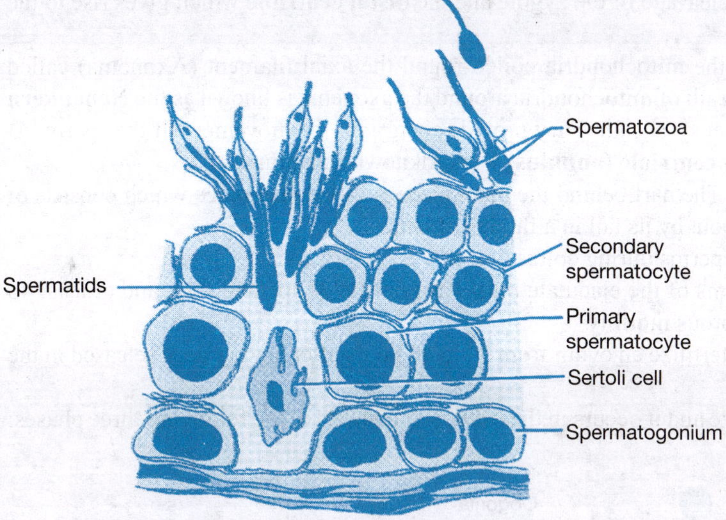


**FIGURE 8.6** Diagrammatic sectional view of a seminiferous tubule (enlarged)

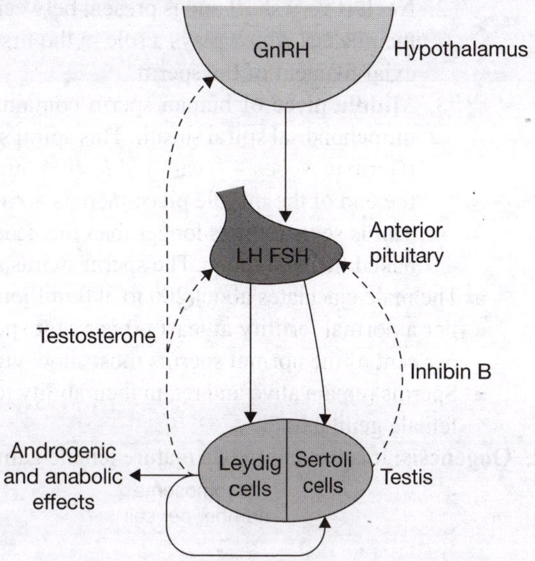


**FIGURE 8.7** Hormonal control of spermatogenesis

- **Hormonal Control of Spermatogenesis:** Spermatogenesis begins at the age of puberty due to significant increase in the secretion of gonadotropin releasing hormone (GnRH) from hypothalamus **Fig. 8.7**.
  - The increased level of GnRH stimulates the anterior lobe of pituitary gland to secrete two gonadotropin—luteinizing hormone (LH) and follicle stimulating hormone (FSH).
  - LH stimulates Leydig cells (interstitial cells) in the testes to synthesize and secrete androgens. Testosterone is the principal androgen and the testosterone is essential for sperm formation.
  - FSH stimulates sertoli cells to secrete two factors—**androgen binding protein** (ABP) that concentrates testosterone in the seminiferous tubules and a protein hormone **inhibin** which suppresses FSH synthesis.
  - FSH acts directly on spermatogonia to stimulate sperm production. The level of testosterone is under negative feed-back control.
  - A rising level of testosterone suppresses the release of GnRH from the hypothalamus.
- **Structure of spermatozoa:** The sperms are microscopic and motile cell. Each sperm is composed of four parts such as a head, neck, a middle piece and a tail. A plasma membrane covers the whole body of sperm **(Fig. 8.8)**.

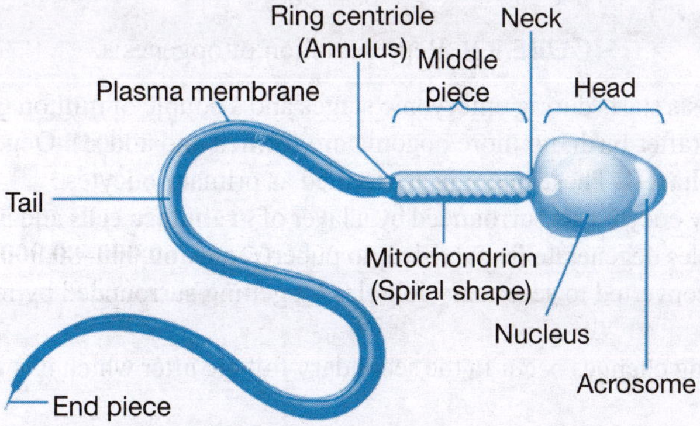


**FIGURE 8.8** Structure of a sperm

1. **Head** is the enlarged end of the sperm and containing an elongated haploid nucleus. The anterior of the nucleus is covered by a cap like structure called **acrosome.**

The acrosome is containing hydrolytic enzymes known as **sperm lysins** which are used to contact and penetrate the ovum at the time of fertilization.

2. **Neck** is very short and is present between the head and middle piece. It contains the **proximal centriole** towards the nucleus which plays a role in the first cleavage of the zygote and the **distal centriole** which gives rise to the axial filament of the sperm.
3. **Middle piece** of human sperm contains the mitochondria coiled round the axial filament (Axonema) called mitochondrial spiral sheath. This spiral sheath of mitochondria around the axonema is known as the **Nebenkern** (German *Neben* – 'near' and *Kern* – 'nucleus') sheath. They provide energy for the movement of the sperm. At the end of the middle piece there is a **ring centriole (annulus)** with unknown function.
4. **Tail** is several times longer than the head. The part behind the main piece is called **end piece** which consists of naked filament alone. The sperm swims about by its tail in a fluid medium.

- The male ejaculates about 200 to 300 million sperms during coitus.
- For a normal fertility at least 60 per cent sperms of the ejaculate must have normal shape and size, and at least 40 per cent of the normal sperms must show vigorous motility.
- Sperms remain alive and retain their ability to fertilize an ovum from 24 to 48 hours after having been released in the female genital tract.

2. **Oogenesis:** It is formation of a mature female gamete and it occurs in the ovaries. It consists of the following three phases:

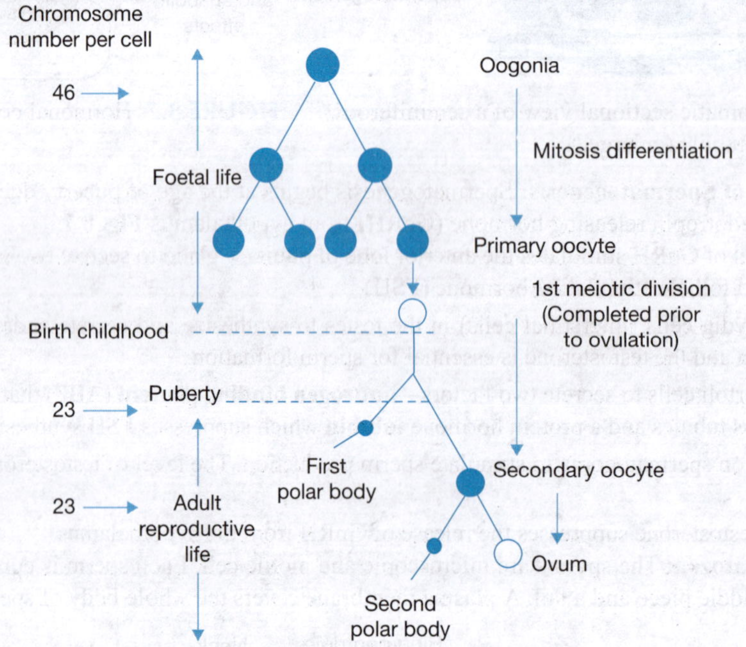


**FIGURE 8.9** Representation of oogenesis.

- **Multiplication phase:** Genesis starts during embryonic stages and a couple of million gamete mother cells (oogonia) are formed in each foetal ovary (after birth, no more oogonia are formed and added). Oogonia enters the **Meiosis-I** and get temporarily arrested at **Prophase-I.** These oogonia are termed as primary oocytes.
- **Growth phase:** Each primary oocyte gets surrounded by a layer of **granulosa cells** and is now termed as **primary follicle.** As most of the primary follicles degenerate from birth upto puberty, only **60,000–80,000 primary follicles** are left in each ovary. Primary follicles are converted to secondary follicles by getting surrounded by few more layers of granulosa cells and a new theca.
- **Maturation phase:** Following changes occur in the secondary follicle after which it is immediately converted to tertiary follicle:

1. Development of a fluid filled cavity called **Antrum.**
2. Differentiation of Theca layer into—**Theca interna** (inner) and **Theca externa** (outer).
3. Primary oocyte grows in size, completes Meiosis-I (unequal division) resulting in the formation of a large haploid **Secondary oocyte** and a small **First polar body.**

- Tertiary follicle changes into the **Mature follicle** (or **Graafian follicle). (Fig. 8.9).**
- Secondary oocyte develops a new membrane around it—Zona pellucida.
- **Ovulation:** The Graafian follicle now ruptures to release the Secondary oocyte (or ovum) from the ovary.
- When sperm comes in contact of **Secondary oocyte**, it completes Meiosis-II and results in the formation of **Ovum (n)** alongwith release of **Second polar body (n).**

**TABLE 8.1** Difference between Spermatogenesis and Oogenesis

| Spermatogenesis | Oogenesis |
|---|---|
| **1.** It occurs in the testis. | **1.** It occurs in the ovaries. |
| **2.** Spermatogonia change to primary spermatocytes. | **2.** Oogonia change to primary oocytes. |
| **3.** A primary spermatocyte divides to form two secondary spermatocytes. | **3.** A primary oocyte divides to form one secondary oocyte and one polar body. |
| **4.** The secondary spermatocyte divides to form two spermatids. | **4.** A secondary oocyte divides to form one ootid and one polar body. |
| **5.** A spermatogonium forms four spermatozoa. | **5.** An oogonium forms on ovum. |
| **6.** It is completed in the testis. | **6.** It begins in the ovary and is completed in the female reproductive tract. |

## Menstrual Cycle

- Menstrual cycle is the reproductive cycle in the female primates and it is shown in **Fig. 8.10** (monkeys, apes and human beings).

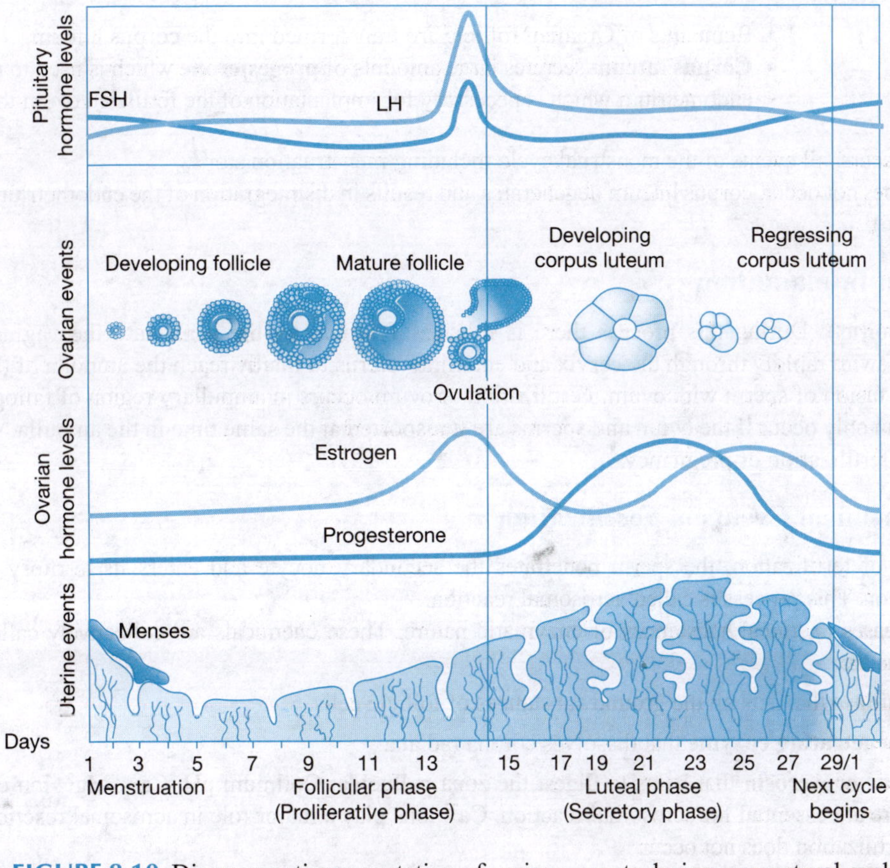


**FIGURE 8.10** Diagrammatic presentation of various events during a menstrual cycle

- **Menarche:** It is the first menstruation that begins at puberty.
- **Menopause:** Menstrual cycle ceases at about **50 years** of age.
- **Reproductive phase:** It extends between menarche and menopause.
- Duration of menstrual cycle in human females is **about 28–29 days.**

TABLE 8.2 Events during a menstrual cycle

| Phase | Description |
|---|---|
| **Menstrual Phase (Duration: 3– 5 days)** | • First phase of menstrual cycle.<br>• Breakdown of endometrial lining of the uterus and its blood vessels occur that comes out of the vagina as menstrual fluid.<br>• Absence of menstruation may be indicative of pregnancy (sometimes due to poor health, stress, etc.) as menstruation does not occur if the egg is fertilized. |
| **I. Ovary-Follicular phase Uterus-Proliferative phase** | • Important events: Primary follicles grow to become Graafian follicle. Endometrium of uterus regenerate by proliferation regeneration.<br>• **Hormonal changes:** Gradual increase in release of gonadotropins (LH and FSH) → Stimulates 1. Follicular development. 2. Oestrogen release (by the growing follicles).<br>• In the middle of menstrual cycle (about 14th day), both LH and FSH attains their peak level. |
| **II. Ovary-Ovulatory phase Uterus-Luteal phase (14th day)** | • LH surge (peak concentration of LH) during the mid-cycle. Rupture of Graafian follicle and release of an ovum (ovulation). |
| **III. Luteal phase** | • Remnants of Graafian follicle are transformed into the corpus luteum.<br>• **Corpus luteum** secretes large amounts of **progesterone** which is used to maintain the endometrium which is necessary for implantation of the fertilized ovum that is pregnancy. |

- If pregnancy occurs, all events of the menstrual cycle including menstruation stops.
- If pregnancy does not occur, corpus luteum degenerates and results in disintegration of the endometrium (starting of next menstrual cycle).

## Fertilization and Implantation

- **Copulation (coitus)**: During this process there is release of semen by the penis into the vagina (insemination). Motile sperms swim rapidly through the cervix and enter into uterus to finally reach the ampulla of the fallopian tube. Fertilization is fusion of sperm with ovum. Fertilization of ovum occurs in ampullary region of fallopian tube.
- Fertilization can only occur if the ovum and sperms are transported at the same time in the ampulla, so all copulations cannot lead to fertilization or pregnancy.

## Physical and Chemical Events of Fertilization

- In the process of fertilization, the sperm penetrates the secondary oocyte and enters its territory through intricate chemical reaction. This process is called acrosomal reaction.
- The sperm releases chemical substances of enzymatic nature. These chemicals are collectively called **sperm lysins.** Important lysins are:

  (i) **Hyaluronidase** that acts on the ground substances of follicle cells.

  (ii) **Corona penetrating enzyme** that dissolves corona radiata.

  (iii) **Zona lysine** or **Acrosin** that helps to digest the zona pellucida. Optimum pH, $Ca^{2+}$, $Mg^{2+}$ ion concentration and temperature are essential for acrosomal reaction. $Ca^{2+}$ ions play a major role in acrosomal reaction and in absence of $Ca^{2+}$ fertilization does not occur.

- Due to acrosomal reaction, plasma membrane of the sperm fuses with the plasma membrane of the secondary oocyte, so that the sperm contents enter the oocyte. Binding of the sperm to the secondary oocyte induces depolarization of the oocyte plasma membrane.
- Depolarization ensures **monospermy** (entry of one sperm into the oocyte) and prevents **polyspermy** (entry of more than one sperm into the oocyte). When the sperm fuses with the plasma membrane of the oocyte, the secondary oocyte shows a **cortical reaction.**
- The cortical granules present below the plasma membrane of the oocyte fuse with the latter and release their enzymatic content between the plasma membrane and the zona pellucida.
- The enzymes harden the zona pellucida which helps in prevention of the entry of additional sperms (polyspermy) into the secondary oocyte. At the point of contact with the sperm, the secondary oocyte forms a projection called **cone of reception** or **fertilization cone** which receives the sperm. The distal centriole of the sperm divides and forms two centrioles to generate the mitotic spindle formation for cell division.
- The mammalian secondary oocyte (ovum) does not have centrioles of its own. The entry of sperm stimulates the secondary oocyte to complete the suspended second meiotic division. This produces a haploid mature ovum and a second polar body.
- The head of the sperm containing the nucleus which is separates from the middle piece and tail, and becomes the **male pronucleus.** The second polar body and the tail of the sperm degenerate. The nucleus of the ovum is now called **female pronucleus.**
- The male and female nuclei move towards each other and get fused. It is called **karyogamy or amphimixis.** The fertilized ovum is now called **zygote.** The zygote is a diploid cell that has 46 chromosomes.
- **Sex determination:** Female produces only one type of ovum while male produces two types of sperms. This clearly indicates that scientifically the sex of the foetus is determined by the father and not by the mother.

## Cleavage and Blastocyst Formation

- About thirty hours after fertilization, the zygote (fertilized ovum), undergoes a series of mitotic divisions and forms (2, 4, 8, 16 daughter cells called **blastomeres).**
- The embryo with 8 to 16 blastomeres looks like a mulberry and is called **morula.** During cleavage the young embryo slowly moves down the fallopian tube towards the uterus. The morula continues to divide and transforms into a sphere of cells with a cavity in the centre. This cavity is called **blastocoel** and the embryo is termed the **blastocyst.**
- The blastocyst consists of an outer envelope of cells, the **trophoblast** or **trophoectoderm** and **inner cell mass** (= embryoblast). The side of the blastocyst to which the inner cell mass is attached is called the **embryonic** or **animal pole,** while the opposite side is the **anembryonic pole.**
- The inner cell mass of the blastocyst is the precursor of the embryo, i.e., it gives rise to embryo. The cells of trophoblast help to provide nutrition to the embryo.
- They later form the extra embryonic membranes namely **chorion** and **amnion** and part of the placenta.
- **Implantation** → The attachment of the blastocyst to the uterine wall is called implantation. It occurs after seven days of fertilization.

## Pregnancy and Embryonic Development

- **Placenta:** In humans placenta develops from chorion. Because the chorion takes part in the formation of placenta, the human placenta is called the **chorionic placenta.** It consists of fetal part, the chorion and a maternal part the decidua basalis. The foetal part of placenta grows to invade the uterine mucosa with its chorionic villi. The degree of intimacy is so strong that the blood vessels of the chorionic villi are bathed in the mother's blood. This is due to erosion of the uterine mucosa, including its epithelium, connective tissue and the endothelial lining. This type of placenta which is based on the intimacy between foetal and maternal parts of the placenta which is termed as **hae-mochorial placenta.**
- **Chorionic villi** (finger—like projections) develop on the trophoblast which are surrounded by the uterine tissue and maternal blood. Interdigitations between the chorionic villi and uterine tissue forms placenta (a structural and functional unit between developing embryo and maternal body).

- **Functions of placenta:** It provides oxygen and nutrients to the embryo. It removes carbon dioxide and excretory waste, produced by the embryo. It also acts as an **endocrine tissue** and produces following hormones:
  - **Human chorionic gonadotropin (hCG).**
  - **Human placental Lactogen (hPL).**
  - **Estrogen**
  - **Progestogens.**
- Hormones produced in women only during pregnancy: **hCG, hPL** and **relaxin.**
- The placenta is connected to the embryo through **umbilical cord.**
- Ovary produces **relaxin** hormone in the later phase of pregnancy.
- Hormones that are increased in concentration (by several folds) in maternal blood during pregnancy: **Estrogens, progesterons, cortisol, prolactin, thyroxine,** etc.
- **Formation of three germ layers:** Immediately after implantation inner cell mass differentiates into an outer layer **(Ectoderm)** and an inner layer **(Endoderm)** appearance of mesoderm between the ectoderm and the endoderm. These three germ layers give rise to all tissues (organs) of body. **Stem cells** are those cells of inner cell mass that have the potency to give rise to all the tissues and organs **(totipotent).**

## Embryonic Development at Various Stages

| | | |
|---|---|---|
| **1.** End of first month | — | **Heart** is formed (listening of heart sound by stethoscope is the first sign of growing foetus). |
| **2.** End of second month | — | **limbs** and **digits** are formed. |
| **3.** End of first trimester | — | Formation of major organ systems, e.g., **limbs** and **external genitalia.** |
| **4.** Fifth month | — | First movements and appearance of hair on head. |
| **5.** End of second trimester | — | Body is covered with fine hairs. **Eyelids separate** and **eyelashes** are developed. |

## Parturition and Lactation

- Gestation period (duration of pregnancy) in human: **Approximately 9 months.**
- **Parturition**
  (1) It refers to the vigorous contraction of the uterus at the end of pregnancy that causes expulsion/delivery of foetus through the birth canal.
  (2) It is induced by a complex neuroendocrine mechanism.
- **Mechanism of neuroendocrine reflex**
  (1) **Fully developed foetus** and the **placenta** gives signals for parturition.
  (2) Initiation of mild uterine contractions called **foetal ejection reflex.**
  (3) Release of oxytocin from the maternal pituitary.
  (4) Oxytocin causes stronger uterine contractions which further stimulates secretion of oxytocin.
  (5) Stimulatory reflex between the uterine contraction and oxytocin secretion continues making the uterine contractions stronger and stronger, finally leading to parturition.
  (6) Placenta is also expelled out of the uterus soon after parturition.
  (7) Oxytocin is injected by doctors to induce delivery.
- Recently a hormone called **corticotrophin releasing hormone** (CRH), which in non-pregnant women is secreted only by neurosecretory cells of hypothalamus, which is produced by the placenta in pregnant women.

- CRH is now thought to be a part of the 'clock' that establishes the timing of birth. Secretion of CRH by placenta increases enormously towards the end of pregnancy.
- Women who have higher levels of CRH earlier in pregnancy are more likely to deliver prematurely, whereas those have low levels and are more likely to deliver after their due date.
- Differentiation of mammary glands of the female occurs during pregnancy.
- **Lactation**: Milk production at the end of pregnancy. Lactation helps the mother to feed the new-born. Breast-feeding is essential for the proper growth and development of infant.
- **Colostrum:** Colostrum is milk produced during the initial few days of lactation. It possesses antibodies (**Mainly IgA-passive immunity**) which are essential for the development of resistance against antigen/pathogen in the new-born.

# PRACTICE EXERCISES

**Direction:** Read the question carefully and choose the correct option for each.

## Multiple Choice Questions: Level I

### Reproduction in Human (Introduction)

**1.** Humans are _________ and ___________ organisms.
(a) Sexually reproducing, oviparous
(b) Asexually reproducing, ovoviviparous
(c) Asexually reproducing, viviparous
(d) Sexually reproducing, viviparous

**2.** The formation of gametes is termed as
(a) Gametogamy (b) Syngamy
(c) Gametogenesis (d) Gestation

**3.** The transfer of sperms into the female genital tract is called
(a) Insemination (b) Gametogenesis
(c) Fertilization (d) Gestation

**4.** The fusion of male and female gametes is known as
(a) Insemination (b) Fertilization
(c) Implantation (d) Parturition

**5.** Match the following correctly.

| Column-I | Column-II |
|---|---|
| 1. Gestation | A. Fusion of male and female gametes |
| 2. Parturition | B. Formation of gametes |
| 3. Gametogenesis | C. Attachment to the uterine wall |
| 4. Implantation | D. Delivery of the baby |
| | E. Embryonic development |

(a) 1:A, 2:C, 3:B, 4:D (b) 1:E, 2:D, 3:A, 4:C
(c) 1:E, 2:D, 3:B, 4:C (d) 1:C, 2:D, 3:A, 4:C

**6.** The correct chronological order of the following events is
(a) Gametogenesis → Fertilization → Insemination → Gestation → Implantation → Parturition
(b) Gametogenesis → Insemination → Fertilization → Impanation → Parturition → Gestation
(c) Gametogenesis → Insemination → Fertilization → Implantation → Gestation → Parturition
(d) None of these

**7.** The following statements are true except
(a) In an individual, reproductive changes occur after puberty.
(b) Sperm formation occurs even in old men.
(c) Formation of ovum continues in women after fifty years.
(d) Humans are sexually producing and viviparous.

### Male Reproductive System

**8.** The testes are situated __________ the abdominal cavity within a pouch called __________.
(a) inside, testicular lobules
(b) outside, scrotum
(c) outside, vas deferens
(d) inside, scrotum

**9.** The scrotum helps in maintaining a temperature ________ lower than the internal body temperature.
(a) 1 to 1.5°C (b) 2 to 2.5°C
(c) 3 to 3.5°C (d) 4 to 4.5°C

**10.** An adult testes is oval in shape. Its width is about ____ and length is about ____ respectively.
(a) 4 to 5 cm, 2 to 3 cm (b) 2 to 5 cm, 1 to 3 cm
(c) 2 to 3 cm, 4 to 5 cm (d) 2 to 5 cm, 4 to 7 cm

**11.** Label a, b, c, d, and e in the diagram below:

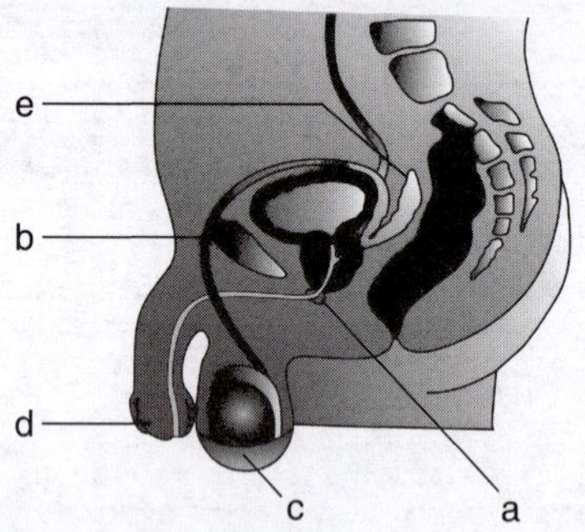


(a) a: Ureter, b: vas deferens c: Scrotum d: glans penis e: Seminal vesicle
(b) a: Bulbourethral gland, b: vas deferens c: Scrotum d: glans penis e: Seminal vesicle
(c) a: Bulbourethral gland, b: vas deferens c: Testis d: glans penis e: vasa efferentia
(d) a: Epididy, b: vas deferens c: Scrotum d: glans penis e: Seminal vesicle

**12.** An adult testes bears ____ compartments called testicular lobules.
(a) 150 (b) 250
(c) 350 (d) 500

**13.** Each testicular lobule contains ____ seminiferous tubule.
(a) Only three
(b) Only one
(c) One to three
(d) More than three

**14.** Male germ cells are known as
(a) Sperms (b) Spermatogonia
(c) Spermatid (d) Sertoli cells

**15.** Seminiferous tubules contain ____ cells for providing nutrition to sperm cells.
(a) Leydig cells
(b) Interstitial cell
(c) Sertoli cells
(d) Germ cells

**16.** The cells which secrete androgens are
(a) Spermatozoa
(b) Interstitial cells
(c) Sertoli cells
(d) Germ cells

**17.** Select the correct anatomical sequence.
(a) Seminiferous tubules → Rete testis → Vasa efferentia → Vasa deferens → Epididymis
(b) Seminiferous tubules → Rete testis → Vasa efferentia → Epididymis → Vasa deferens
(c) Seminiferous tubules → Vasa efferentia → Rete testis → Vasa deferens → Epididymis
(d) None of these

**18.** The enlarged end of penis is known as
(a) Glans
(b) Foreskin
(c) Urethra
(d) Prostate

**19.** If A stands for seminal vesicles, B stands for bulbourethral glands, C stands for prostate gland, then which of the following is true?
(a) A and C occurs in pair
(b) A and B occur in pair
(c) B and C occur in pair
(d) None of these

**20.** Seminal plasma is rich in which sugar?
(a) Sucrose (b) Glucose
(c) Fructose (d) Maltose

**21.** Label a, b, c, d and e in the given figure:

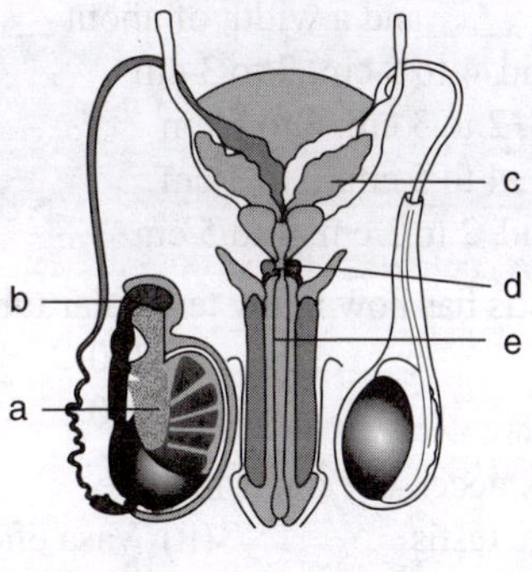


(a) a: Rete testis, b: Epididymis c: Seminal vesicle, d: Prostate, e: Urethra
(b) a: Rete testis, b: Epididymis c: Seminal vesicle, d: Bulbourethral gland, e: Urethra
(c) a: Vasa efferentia, b: Epididymis c: Seminal vesicle, d: Bulbourethral gland, e: Ureter
(d) a: Rete testis, b: Epididymis c: Seminal vesicle, d: Urinary bladder e: Urethra

**22.** The secretion of which gland helps in the lubrication of penis?
(a) Seminal vesicle (b) Prostate
(c) Bulbourethral (d) Epididymis

**23.** Label a b c and d in the given figure:

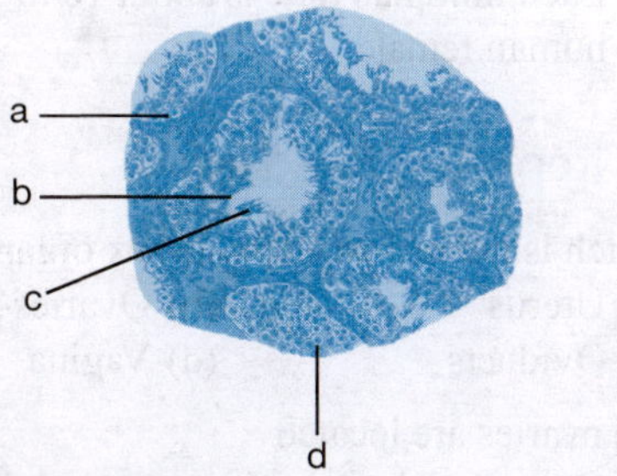


(a) a: Interstitial cells, b: Spermatogonia, c: Spermatozoa, d: Sertoli cells
(b) a: Sertoli cells, b: Spermatogonia, c: Spermatozoa, d: Interstitial cells
(c) a: Interstitial cells, b: Sertoli cells, c: Spermatozoa, d: Spermatogonia
(d) a: Spermatogonia, b: Sperm, c: Spermatozoa, d: Sertoli cells

**24.** Which one of the following is not an accessory male duct in context of male reproductive system?
(a) Rete testis (b) Testes
(c) Epididymis (d) Vas deferens

**25.** Which one of the following is not a male sex accessory gland?
(a) Seminal vesicle (b) Epididymis
(c) Prostate (d) bulbourethral

**26.** In an adult, each testis is ____ in shape, with a length of about ____ and a width of about ____.
(a) round, 4 to 5 cm, 2 to 3 cm
(b) oval, 2 to 3 cm, 4 to 5 cm
(c) oval, 4 to 5 cm, 2 to 3 cm
(d) round, 2 to 3 cm, 4 to 5 cm

**27.** Each testis has how many testicular tubules?
(a) 200 (b) 250
(c) 300 (d) 150

**28.** Male sex accessory ducts include
(i) Rete testis (ii) Vasa efferentia
(iii) Epididymis (iv) Vas deferens
(a) i, ii (b) ii, iii
(c) i, ii, iii (d) i, ii, iii, iv

**29.** Which of the following duct stores sperm?
(a) Vasa efferentia (b) Rete testis
(c) Epididymis (d) All of these

**30.** Find the false statement.
(a) A pair of seminal vesicles is present in human males.
(b) A pair of prostates is present in human males.
(c) Glans penis is covered by a loose fold of skin called foreskin.
(d) Each fallopian tube is about 10 to 12 cm long in a human female.

## Female Reproductive System

**31.** Which is the primary female sex organ?
(a) Uterus (b) Ovaries
(c) Oviducts (d) Vagina

**32.** The ovaries are located
(a) One on each side of the upper abdomen
(b) Two on each side of the lower abdomen
(c) Two on each side of the upper abdomen
(d) One on each side of the lower abdomen

**33.** Which of the following statements about ovary is not true?
(a) Ovaries are responsible for the production of several steroid hormones.
(b) Each ovary is about 4 to 6 cm in length.
(c) Ovary is connected to the pelvic wall.
(d) Ovary produces female gamete (Ovum).

**34.** Ovarian stroma is enclosed by ____.
(a) Endothelium
(b) Epithelium
(c) Mesothelium
(d) Ciliated epithelium

**35.** The ovarian stroma is divided into zones
(a) Peripheral medulla and inner cortex
(b) Peripheral epithelia and inner endothelia
(c) Peripheral cortex and inner medulla
(d) Peripheral endothelia and inner epithelia

**36.** The tubes which conducts ovum to the uterus are known as
(a) Fallopian tube (b) Oviduct
(c) Cervical opening (d) Both (a) and (b)

**37.** Which one of the following is not a female accessory duct?
(a) Vagina (b) Uterus
(c) Oviduct (d) Ovary

**38.** Each oviduct is about ____ long.
(a) 5 to 6 mm (b) 10 to 12 cm
(c) 10 to 12 mm (d) 5 to 6 cm

**39.** The funnel shaped part of fallopian tube which traps ovum is known as
(a) Isthmus (b) Ampulla
(c) Infundibulum (d) Cervix

**40.** Isthmus a part of oviduct, is a narrow lumen and joins ____.
(a) Uterus (b) Ampulla
(c) Infundibulum (d) Both (a) and (b)

**41.** The anatomical structure which succeeds infundibulum is
(a) Isthmus (b) Ampulla
(c) Uterus (d) Ovary

**42.** Finger-like projection of infundibulum are known as
(a) Cilia (b) Flagella
(c) Fimbriae (d) None

**43.** Uterus is commonly known as
(a) Birth canal
(b) Womb
(c) Primary female sex organ
(d) Female external genitalia

**44.** The uterus opens into vagina through ____.
(a) Ampulla (b) Isthmus
(c) Cervix (d) Labia minora

**45.** Birth canal is formed by
(a) Cervical canal + Uterus
(b) Cervical canal + Vagina
(c) Cervical canal + Isthmus
(d) Cervical canal + Fallopian tube

**46.** The wall of uterus is made up of ____ layers of tissue.
(a) 2 (b) 3
(c) 1 (d) 4

**47.** External thin membranous layer of uterus is known as
(a) Pleura (b) Pericardium
(c) Perimetrium (d) Periosteum

**48.** Thick muscular layer of ____ muscle constitutes middle layer of uterus.
(a) Smooth (b) Striated
(c) Intercalated (d) Voluntary

**49.** Which layer of uterus undergoes cyclic changes during menstrual cycle?
(a) Mesoderm (b) Myometrium
(c) Endothelium (d) Endometrium

**50.** The layer of uterine tissues responsible for strong contractions during childbirth is
(a) Perimetrium (b) Mesometrium
(c) Mesoderm (d) Myocardium

**51.** Of the following statements, which one is true for Mons Pubis?
(a) It is the region of pubic hair growth found in females as well as males.
(b) It is a cushion of proteins covered by skin and pubic hair.
(c) It is a cushion of fats covered by skin and pubic hair.
(d) It is a part of female internal genitalia.

**52.** Clitoris lies at the junction of
(a) Labia majora (b) Labia minora
(c) Mons pubis (d) Pubis symphysis

**53.** The clitoris is a tiny ____ shaped structure which lies above the urethral opening
(a) Flagellated (b) Finger like
(c) Bean shaped (d) Pear

**54.** The only statement correct about hymen is
(a) It is an opening of cervix.
(b) It is a reliable indicator of virginity.
(c) It is always torn after first coitus.
(d) It can be broken by a sudden fall or jolt, insertion of vaginal tampon, cycling, etc.

**55.** Cluster of cells in mammary lobes is known as
(a) Mammary duct (b) Alveoli
(c) Ampulla (d) Lactiferous duct

**56.** The terminal structure of the mammary glands through which milk is sucked out is known as
(a) Lumen of alveoli (b) Mammary duct
(c) Lactiferous duct (d) Mammary lobe

**57.** Several mammary ducts join to form
(a) Mammary lobe (b) Alveoli
(c) Mammary ampulla (d) Lactiferous duct

**58.** Label a, b, c, d and e in the diagram below:

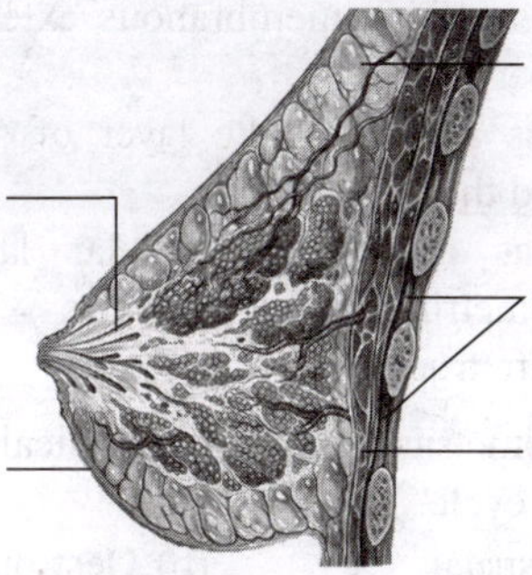


(a) a: Fat, b: Ampulla, c: Areola, d: Muscle b/w ribs, e: Pectoralis major muscle
(b) a: Protein, b: Ampulla, c: Areola, d: Muscle b/w ribs, e: Pectoralis major muscle
(c) a: Fat, b: Areola, c: ampulla, d: Muscle b/w ribs, e: Pectoralis minor muscle
(d) a: Proteins, b: Ampulla, c: Areola, d: Muscle b/w ribs, e: Pectoralis minor muscle

**59.** The female reproductive system along with a pair of mammary glands is integrated structurally and functionally to support the process of
(a) Ovulation and fertilization
(b) Pregnancy and birth
(c) Child care
(d) All the above

**60.** Find out the incorrect statement about ovaries.
(a) Each ovary is connected to the pelvic wall and uterus by ligaments.
(b) The ovarian stroma is divided into two zones, i.e., a peripheral cortex and an inner medulla.
(c) Each ovary is covered by thick epithelium which encloses the ovarian stroma.
(d) Ovaries are the primary female sex organs.

**61.** The fallopian tube is about ____ long.
(a) 10 to 12 cm (b) 8 to 10 cm
(c) 12 to 14 cm (d) 14 to 16 cm

**62.** The part of the fallopian tube closer to the ovary is
(a) Infundibulum (b) Ampulla
(c) Isthmus (d) Womb

**63.** Which facts about the uterus (in human females) is true?
(a) Single (b) Also called womb
(c) Inverted pear shape (d) All of these

**64.** Birth canal is formed by
(i) Uterus (ii) Cervix
(iii) Vagina
(a) i and ii (b) i and iii
(c) ii and iii (d) iii only

**65.** Which statement is true about the walls of the uterus?
(a) It has a thick membranous external wall called the perimetrium.
(b) It has a thin middle layer of smooth muscles called the myometrium.
(c) It has an inner glandular layer called the endometrium.
(d) All are true

**66.** The endometrium undergoes cyclical changes during the ____ cycle.
(a) Menstrual (b) Oestrous
(c) Thermal (d) None of these

**67.** The opening of vagina is often covered partially by
(a) Mons pubis (b) Labia majora
(c) Labia minora (d) Hymen

**68.** Which of the facts is true about clitoris?
(i) It is a tiny finger-like structure.
(ii) It lies at the upper junction of two labia minora.
(iii) It lies at the upper junction of two labia majora.
(iv) It lies above the utheral opening.
(v) It lies below the urethral opening.
(a) i, ii and iii (b) i, ii and v
(c) i, ii and iv (d) iii and v

**69.** Hymen can be torn or broken by
(i) First coitus
(ii) Sudden fall or jolt
(iii) Horse riding
(iv) Cycling
(v) Insertion of a vaginal tampon
(a) i, ii and iv only (b) iii, iv and v only
(c) i, iv and v only (d) All of these

**70.** Select the true statement.
(a) Presence of hymen is a reliable indicator of virginity.
(b) Absence of hymen is a reliable indicator of sexual experience.
(c) Presence of hymen is a reliable indicator of sexual experience.
(d) Presence or absence of hymen is not a reliable indicator of virginity.

**71.** Which is the correct path for the secretion and transport of milk in mammary gland?
(a) Alveoli → Cavity of alveoli → Mammary tubule → Mammary duct → Mammary ampulla → Lactiferous duct
(b) Mammary duct → Mammary tubule → Alveoli → Lactiferous duct → Mammary ampulla → Cavity of alveoli
(c) Mammary duct → Cavity of alveoli → Lactiferous duct → Mammary ampulla → Mammary tubule → Alveoli
(d) Alveoli → Mammary tubule → Mammary ampulla → Cavity of alveoli → Mammary duct → Lactiferous duct

**72.** Which fact about the mammary glands in humans is false?
(a) A non-functional mammary gland is the characteristic of all male mammals.
(b) Mammary glands are paired structures.
(c) It is a glandular tissue containing fixed amount of fat.
(d) Glandular tissue of each breast is divided into 15 to 20 mammary lobes containing clusters of cells called alveoli.

**73.** Label b, d, e, f, h and j in the figure given below:

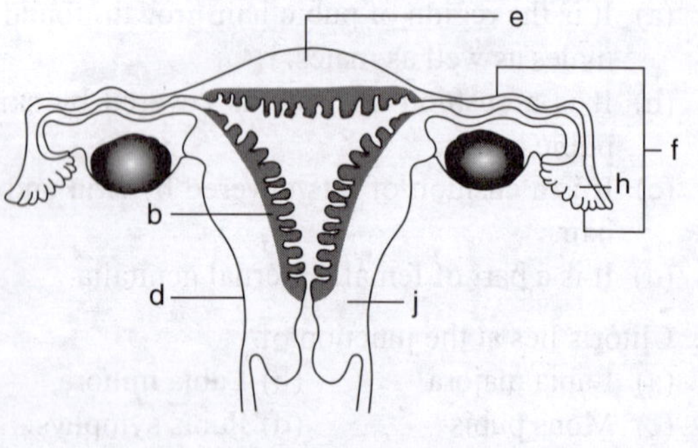


(a) b: Endometrium d: Perimetrium e: Uterine fundus f: Fallopian tube h: Infundibulum j: Cervix
(b) b: Endometrium d: Perimetrium e: Isthmus f: Fallopian tube h: Infundibulum j: Uterus
(c) b: Endometrium d: Uterine fundus e: Perimetrium f: Fallopian tube h: Infundibulum j: Cervix
(d) b: Endometrium d: Perimetrium e: Uterine fundus f: Ovary h: Infundibulum j: Uterus

**74.** Label b, c, d, f and k in the below diagram:

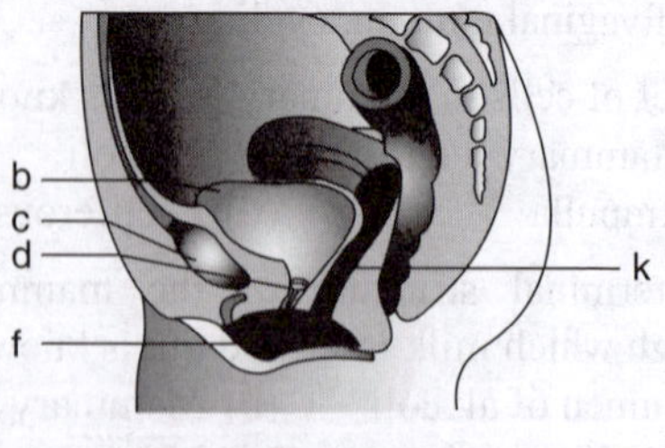


(a) b: Urinary bladder, c: Pubic symphysis, d: Urethra, f: Labia minora, k: Vagina
(b) b: Urinary bladder, c: Pubic symphysis, d: Ureter, f: Labia majora, k: Clitoris

(c) b: Urinary bladder, c: Pubic symphysis, d: Urethra, f: Labia minora, k: Clitoris
(d) b: Urinary bladder, c: Pubic symphysis, d: Ureter, f: Labia minora, k: Vagina

## Gametogenesis

**75.** Immature male germ cells are known as
(a) Spermatid (b) Spermatozoa
(c) Spermatogonia (d) Sperm

**76.** Spermatogonium undergoes ____.
(a) Reduction division (b) Meiotic division
(c) Mitotic division (d) None of these

**77.** Label a, c, e and f in the below figure:

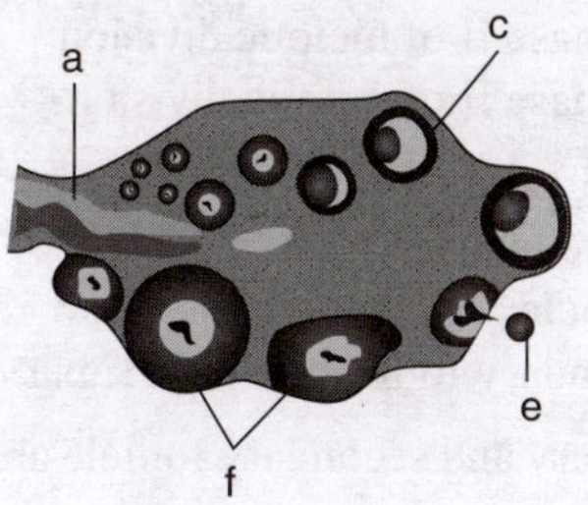


(a) a: Blood vessels, c: Tertiary follicle, e: Ovum, f: Corpus luteum
(b) a: Blood vessels, c: primary follicle, e: Nerve fibres, f: Antrum
(c) a: Blood vessels, c: Corpus luteum, e: Ovum, f: Tertiary follicle
(d) a: Blood vessels, c: Secondary follicle, e: Ovum, f: Corpus luteum

**78.** Each spermatogonium is ____ and has ____ number of chromosomes.
(a) n, 45 (b) 2n, 23
(c) 2n, 46 (d) n, 46

**79.** The spermatogonia which undergo meiosis are known as
(a) Sperm
(b) Spermatid
(c) Secondary spermatocyte
(d) Primary spermatocyte

**80.** The difference between primary and secondary spermatocyte lies in ____.
(a) Presence/absence of a tail
(b) Number of chromosomes
(c) Being hormone producing/non-hormone producing
(d) Primary gamete/secondary gamete in males

**81.** Secondary spermatocytes give rise to
(a) Diploid spermatids (b) Haploid sperm
(c) Diploid sperm (d) Haploid spermatid

**82.** Sperms are synonymous with
(a) Spermatid
(b) Spermatogonia
(c) Primary spermatocyte
(d) Spermatozoa

**83.** Spermiogenesis is
(a) Transformation of sperm into spermatids.
(b) Transformation of spermatogonia into primary spermatocyte.
(c) Transformation of secondary spermatocyte into spermatids.
(d) Transformation of spermatid into spermatozoa.

**84.** After spermiogenesis, the sperm head is embedded in the ____ cells.
(a) Sertoli (b) Leydig
(c) Interstitial (d) Both (a) and (b)

**85.** The release of sperms from seminiferous tubules is known as ____
(a) Ejaculation (b) Copulation
(c) Spermiation (d) None of these

**86.** Spermatogenesis starts at puberty due to the secretion of
(a) Luteinizing hormone
(b) Gonadotropin releasing hormone
(c) Follicle stimulating Hormone
(d) Testosterone

**87.** Luteinizing hormone (LH) acts on ____ cells and stimulates synthesis and secretion of ____.
(a) Leydig cells, FSH
(b) Interstitial cells, androgens
(c) Leydig cells, GnRH
(d) None of these

**88.** Androgens stimulate ____.
(a) Spermiation (b) Insemination
(c) Spermatogenesis (d) Oogenesis

**89.** The function of FSH in male is
(a) Act on leydig cells and stimulates secretion of factors responsible for spermiation.
(b) Act on sertoli cells and stimulates secretion of factors responsible for spermatogenesis.
(c) Act on interstitial cells and stimulates secretion of factors responsible for spermiogenesis.
(d) Act on sertoli cells and stimulates secretion of factors responsible for spermiogenesis.

**90.** The microscopic structure of sperm consists of
(a) Head, Neck, Tail
(b) Head, Neck, Middle piece, Tail
(c) Head, Middle piece, Tail
(d) Neck, Middle piece, Tail

**91.** Label a, b, c and d in the below figure:

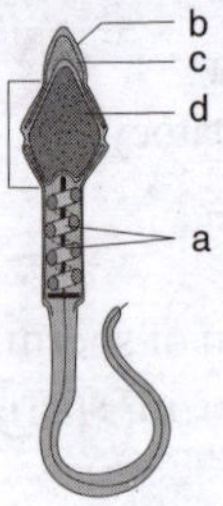


(a) a: Mitochondria, b: Plasma membrane, c: Acrosome, d: Nucleus
(b) a: Neck, b: Plasma membrane, c: Acrosome, d: Tail
(c) a: Plasma membrane, b: Mitochondria, c: Acrosome, d: Nucleus
(d) a: Tail, b: Plasma membrane, c: Aseosome, d: Nucleus

**92.** The sperm head contains:
(a) Antherosome (b) Acrosome
(c) Arthosome (d) Ascosome

**93.** The function of acrosome is
(a) Stimulates synthesis of ovum
(b) Stimulates release of ovum
(c) Stimulates fertilization of ovum
(d) Stimulates degradation of ovum

**94.** The middle piece of sperm contains cell organelles like
(a) Filaments (b) Mitochondria
(c) Nucleus (d) Ribosomes

**95.** How many sperm cells are there in an average human ejaculation?
(a) 200 to 300 billion (b) 200 to 300 million
(c) 200 to 300 trillion (d) 200 to 300 lacs

**96.** For a normal male fertility, which of the following statements is correct?
(a) 60 per cent sperm must have normal motility and 40 per cent must have normal shape.
(b) 60 per cent sperm must have normal shape and 40 per cent must have acrosome.
(c) 60 per cent sperm must have normal shape and 40 per cent must have vigorous motility.
(d) None of these

**97.** Semen consists of
(a) Seminal plasma + Spermatid
(b) Seminal plasma + Spermatozoa
(c) Seminal plasma + Spermatogonia
(d) None of these

**98.** The process of formation of mature female gamete is known as
(a) Gametogenesis (b) Spermatogenis
(c) Oogenesis (d) Morphogenesis

**99.** Oogenesis initiates after/at
(a) Fertilization
(b) Puberty
(c) Embryonic development
(d) Time of birth

**100.** Each female ovary consists of
(a) Millions of ova
(b) Millions of primary oocytes
(c) Millions of oogonia
(d) Millions of secondary oocytes

**101.** The primary oocytes are in which stage of cell division?
(a) Prophase I of mitotic division
(b) Prophase I of meiotic division
(c) Prophase II of meiotic division
(d) Prophase II of mitotic division

**102.** From the period of birth till puberty, which cells degenerate in ovary?
(a) Oogonia (b) Ova
(c) Secondary follicle (d) Primary follicle

**103.** The primary and secondary follicle are surrounded by cells known as
(a) Granulosa (b) Mucosa
(c) Serosa (d) Granuloma

**104.** The tertiary follicle in ovary is characterized by the presence of
(a) Fundus (b) Antrum
(c) Vacuole (d) Cavity

**105.** The mature tertiary follicle is also known as
(a) Ovum (b) Oogonia
(c) Graafian follicle (d) Polar body

**106.** The membrane around Graafian follicle is known as
(a) Zona fasciculata (b) Zona reticularis
(c) Zona externa (d) Zona pellucida

**107.** Spermatogonia is
(a) Immature male germ cells
(b) Mature male germ cells
(c) Immature male gamete
(d) Mature male gamete

**108.** The spermatids are transformed into spermatozoa (sperm) by the process called
(a) Spermatogenesis (b) Spermiogenesis
(c) Spermiation (d) Capacitation

**109.** Select the correct sequence:
(a) GnRH → LH → Leydig cells → Androgens → Spermatogenesis
(b) GnRH → FSH → Sertoli cells → Some factors → Spermiogenesis

(c) Both are correct
(d) Both are incorrect

**110.** Acrosome is a modified
(a) Golgi body (b) ER
(c) Vacuole (d) Ribosome

**111.** Antrum is present in
(a) Primary follicle (b) Secondary follicle
(c) Tertiary follicle (d) All of these

**112.** Primary oocyte grows in size and completes its first meiotic division inside the
(a) Primary follicle
(b) Secondary follicle
(c) Tertiary follicle
(d) All of these

**113.** Which of the following undergoes unequal division?
(a) Primary oocyte
(b) Pollen grain of angiosperm
(c) Yeast cell during bud formation
(d) All the above

**114.** Secondary oocyte develops zona pellucida around it in the ____.
(a) Primary follicle (b) Secondary follicle
(c) Tertiary follicle (d) Graafian follicle

**115.** Theca layer is organized into theca interna and externa in which follicle?
(a) 1° (b) 2°
(c) 3° (d) Mature follicle

**116.** The ploidy of spermatogonia, primary spermatocyte, secondary spermatocyte and spermatid is
(a) 2n, 2n, 2n, n (b) n, 2n, 2n, n
(c) n, 2n, n, n (d) 2n, 2n, n, n

## Menstrual Cycle

**117.** The first menstruation which begins at puberty is called
(a) Menstrual cycle (b) Menarche
(c) Oogenesis (d) Ovulation

**118.** An average interval of menstrual cycle in females is about ____ days.
(a) 15/16 (b) 30/31
(c) 28/29 (d) 25/26

**119.** One ovum is released during the ____ of each menstrual cycle.
(a) Initial (b) Middle
(c) Terminal (d) Alternative

**120.** The menstrual flow in menstrual cycle lasts for about
(a) 6 to 7 days (b) Almost 7 days
(c) 3 to 5 days (d) 1 to 2 days

**121.** Lack of menstruation may be indicative of
(a) Pregnancy (b) Routine work stress
(c) Poor health (d) All of these

**122.** In females, gonadotropins attain a peak level at about ____ day of the menstrual cycle.
(a) 15th (b) 14th (c) 28th (d) 29th

**123.** LH surge causes
(a) Rupture of graafian follicle
(b) Release of ovum
(c) Endometrial shedding
(d) Both (a) and (b)

**124.** The ovulation phase is followed by ____ phase.
(a) Gestation (b) Luteal
(c) Menstrual (d) Oogenesis

**125.** After ovulation, Graafian follicle transforms into
(a) Corpus cavernosa (b) Corpus pellucida
(c) Corpus luteum (d) Corpus metrium

**126.** Large amounts of progesterone is secreted by
(a) Corpus germinativum
(b) Corpus luteum
(c) Corpus cavernosa
(d) Corpus pellucida

**127.** If fertilization does not occur corpus luteum ____.
(a) Proliferates (b) Degenerates
(c) Regenerates (d) Divides

**128.** The stage in human female when menstrual cycle ceases at the age of 50 is known as
(a) Ovopause (b) Menarche
(c) Menopause (d) Menstruation

**129.** Label a, b, c and d in the below figure:

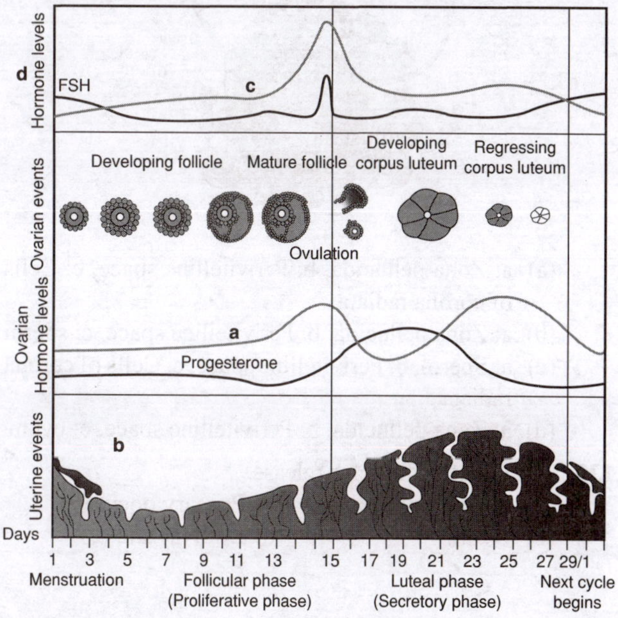

(a) a: Oestrogen, b: Menses, c: Progesterone, d: Pitutary
(b) a: FSH, b: Menses, c: LH, d: Pitutary,
(c) a: Oestrogen, b: Menses, c: LH, d: Pitutary
(d) a: Oestrogen, b: Menses, c: LH, d: Ovaries

**130.** How many ovum(s) is/are released in one menstruation?
(a) 1 (b) 2
(c) 3 (d) 4

**131.** Which of the facts is true about menstruation?
(a) It occurs only when the released ovum is not fertilized.
(b) It occurs due to the breakdown of endometrial lining.
(c) Menstrual flow lasts for 3 to 5 days.
(d) All the above

**132.** Menopausal age in human being is
(a) 45 years (b) 55 years
(c) 50 years (d) 60 years

**133.** The time required to convert primary follicle into mature follicle is
(a) 4 days (b) 9 to 11 days
(c) 18 to 20 days (d) 2 days

## Fertilization and Implantation

**134.** Label a, b and c in the below figure:

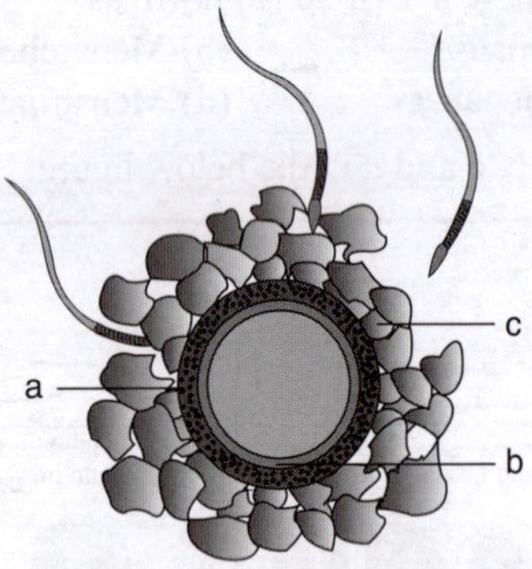


(a) a: Zona pellucida, b: Perivitelline space, c: Cells of corona radiata
(b) a: Zona pellucida, b: Perivitelline space, c: sperm
(c) a: Sperm, b: Perivitelline space, c: Cells of corona radiata
(d) a: Zona pellucida, b: Perivitelline space, c: ovum

**135.** The Graafian follicles release
(a) Secondary oocyte (b) Primary oocyte
(c) Ovum (d) Both (a) and (c)

**136.** The release of ovum from ovary is known as
(a) Ovulation (b) Oogenesis
(c) Parturition (d) Gametogenesis

**137.** Total number of polar bodies formed in oogenesis?
(a) 2 (b) 1
(c) 3 (d) 0

**138.** What does ‘a’ represent in this figure?

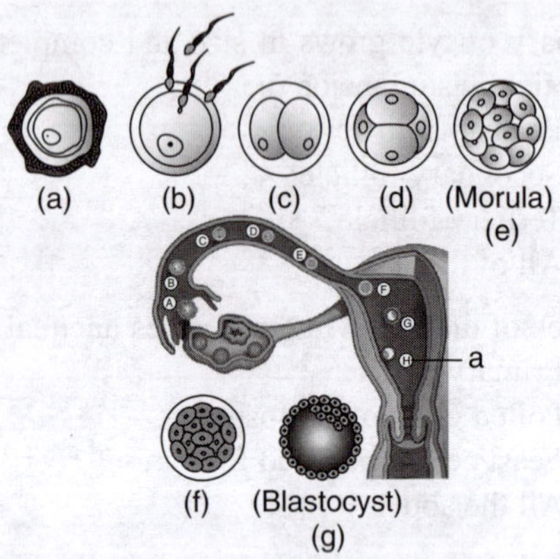


(a) Blastocyst
(b) Blastocyst implantation
(c) Morula
(d) Cells

**139.** Once the sperm is injected into the female genital tract, which junction is primarily concerned with meeting of sperm with ovum?
(a) Utero-ampullary junction
(b) Ampullary-region
(c) Isthmic-infundibullary junction
(d) Uterine-cervical junction

**140.** All copulations do not lead to pregnancy. The most appropriate reason to support this statement is
(a) The ovum and sperm should be transported randomly to ampullary-isthmic region.
(b) The ovum and sperm should be continuously transported to ampullary-isthmic region.
(c) The ovum and sperm should be simultaneously transported to ampullary- isthmic region.
(d) None of these

**141.** The sperm comes into contact with the ____ layer of ovum to cause fertilization.
(a) Corona radiata
(b) Perivitelline layer
(c) Zona pellucida
(d) Zona fasciculata

**142.** Once a sperm fuses with an ovum, the remaining sperms cannot fertilize ovum. What changes are responsible for such phenomenon?
(a) Selective permeation through ovum.
(b) Specific spatial arrangement of corona radiata cells.
(c) Change in the membrane zona pellucida.
(d) Ovum releases toxic substances thereby killing other sperms.

**143.** After entry of sperm into cytoplasm of ovum which of the following event takes place?
(a) Mitotic division of secondary oocyte
(b) Meiotic division of primary oocyte
(c) Mitotic division of secondary oocyte
(d) Meiotic division of secondary oocyte

**144.** The human female has which of the following sex chromosome pattern?
(a) XX (b) YY (c) XY (d) XYX

**145.** The human male has which of the following sex chromosome pattern?
(a) XYX (b) XY (c) XX (d) YY

**146.** Female produces only
(a) One type of gamete Y
(b) One type of gamete X
(c) Either X or Y type of gamete
(d) All of these

**147.** Scientifically, sex of the baby is determined by
(a) Only mother (b) Only father
(c) Either mother or father (d) Gestational phase

**148.** After formation of zygote, it cleaves into 2, 4, 8, 16 daughter cells called
(a) Blastocyst (b) Morula
(c) Trophoblast (d) Blastomere

**149.** The embryo with $2^3$ or $4^2$ blastomeres is known as
(a) Blastocyst (b) Morula
(c) Trophoblast (d) Zygote

**150.** Morula divides and transforms into
(a) Inner cell mass (b) Blastocyst
(c) Trophoblast (d) Blastomere

**151.** The outer layer of blastocyst is known as
(a) Zona pellucida (b) Trophoblast
(c) Blastomere (d) Corona radiata

**152.** Which layer of blastocyst gets attached to the endometrium during implantation?
(a) Trophoblast (b) Blastomere
(c) Inner cell mass (d) Morula

**153.** The inner cell mass of blastocyst develops into
(a) Morula (b) Trophoblast
(c) Embryo (d) Zygote

**154.** Label a b, c, and d in the given figure:

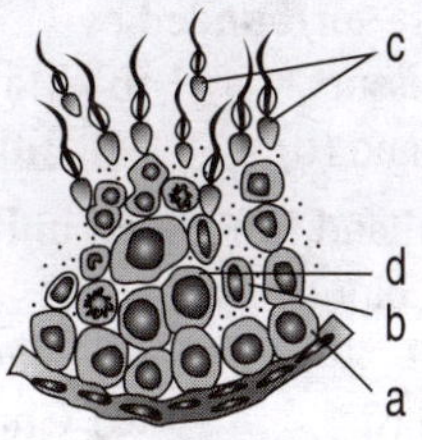


(a) a: spermatogonium, b: Sertoli cells, c: spermatozoa, d: Primary spermatocytes
(b) a: spermatogonium, b: Sertoli cells, c: spermatozoa, d: Spermatocytes
(c) a: Spermatid, b: spermatozoa, c: Sertoli cell, d: Primary spermatocytes
(d) a: Spermatid, b: Sertoli cells, c: spermatozoa, d: Primary spermatocytes

**155.** Secretion of which part of sperm require for entry of sperm into the cytoplasm of the ovum through zona pellucida and the plasma membrane
(a) Mitochondria (b) Nucleus
(c) Acrosome (d) Centriole

**156.** Stem cells which have the potential to produce all types of cells, tissues and organs are present in
(a) Ectoderm (b) Inner cell mass
(c) Trophoblast (d) Endoderm

## Pregnancy, Embryonic Development, Parturition and Lactation

**157.** Label a, b, c and d in the figure below:

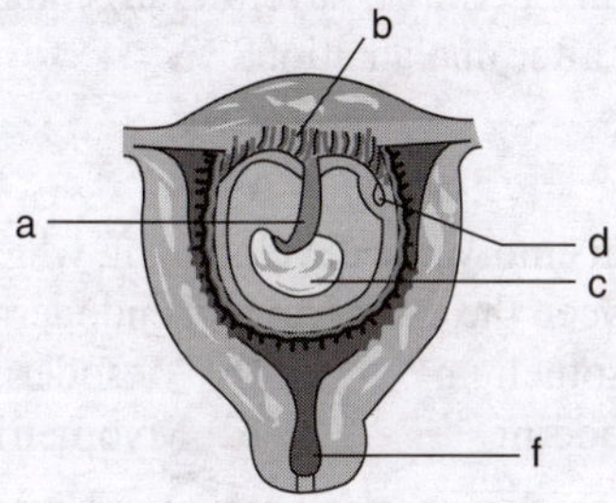


(a) a: Umbilical cord, b: Placental villi, c: Cavity of uterus, d: Yolk sac
(b) a: Umbilical cord, b: Placental villi, c: Embryo, d: Yolk sac
(c) a: Embryo, b: Placental villi, c: cavity of uterus, d: Yolk sac
(d) a: Umbilical cord, b: Placental villi, c: Embryo, d: cavity of uterus

**158.** After implantation the finger-like projection which appears on the trophoblast are known as
(a) Intestinal villi (b) Ampullary villi
(c) Chorionic villi (d) Amniotic villi

**159.** After implantation the finger-like projections on the trophoblast are surrounded by
(a) Uterine tissue (b) Maternal blood
(c) Both (a) and (b) (d) Either (a) and (b)

**160.** The structural and functional unit between the foetus and maternal blood is known as
(a) Inner cell (b) Placenta
(c) Trophoblast (d) Chorionic villi

**161.** Placenta does not perform which of the following function?
(a) Supply of $O_2$
(b) Supply of excretory materials
(c) Supply of nutrients
(d) Removal of $CO_2$

**162.** The placenta is connected to embryo through ____ cord.
(a) Chorionic (b) Umbilical
(c) Amniocentic (d) Uterine

**163.** Placenta also acts as a/an ____ tissue.
(a) Endocrine (b) Exocrine
(c) Paracrine (d) Mepacrine

**164.** Which of the following hormone is released by placenta?
(a) FSH (b) HCG
(c) Relaxin (d) LH

**165.** Relaxin is secreted by
(a) Ovary (b) Uterus
(c) Cervix (d) Oviduct

**166.** How many germinal layers does embryo consist of initially, after implantation?
(a) 3 (b) 2
(c) 4 (d) 5

**167.** In human embryonic development, which layer develops between the ectoderm and endoderm?
(a) Mesothelium (b) Mesoderm
(c) Myoderm (d) Myometrium

**168.** In humans, the inner cell mass (embryo) contains certain cells called ____ cells which have the potential to give rise to all the tissues and organs.
(a) Root (b) Leaf
(c) Stem (d) Seed

**169.** The average time span of human gestation is
(a) 8 months (b) 9 months
(c) 10 months (d) 1 year

**170.** The pregnancy phase in humans is divided into how many trimesters?
(a) 2 (b) 4 (c) 3 (d) 5

**171.** After one month of pregnancy which vital organ is formed in the foetus?
(a) Brain (b) Heart
(c) Lungs (d) Liver

**172.** In a developing foetus, most of the major organ systems are developed by the end of ____ weeks.
(a) 14 (b) 12
(c) 10 (d) 16

**173.** Foetal limbs and digits are formed in the ____ month of embryonic development.
(a) 4th (b) 2nd
(c) 3rd (d) 7th

**174.** The second trimester of human pregnancy is characterized by
(a) Appearance of heart and aorta
(b) Appearance of external genital organs
(c) Appearance of fine hair, eye-lashes on the eye-lids
(d) Appearance of limbs and digits

**175.** The scientific name of childbirth is
(a) Gestation (b) Parturition
(c) Implantation (d) Foetal development

**176.** During parturition, the mild uterine contractions which lead to expulsion of the foetus is known as
(a) Foetal ejection release
(b) Foetal ejection reflex
(c) Foetal uterine reflex
(d) Foetal placental reflex

**177.** Which hormone is responsible for severe uterine contractions during parturition?
(a) Oestrogen (b) Oxytocin
(c) Progesterone (d) Relaxin

**178.** After the delivery of the foetus which of the following structure is also expelled out?
(a) Uterus (b) Corpus luteum
(c) Placenta (d) Ovary

**179.** The production of milk in mammary gland occurs
(a) During parturition
(b) After parturition
(c) Before embryogenesis
(d) At the end of pregnancy

**180.** The milk produced during the initial days of lactation is called
(a) Menstrum (b) Colostrum
(c) Gynostrum (d) None of these

**181.** The first foetal movement is observed during the ____ month of embryonic development.
(a) $4^{th}$ (b) $5^{th}$
(c) $3^{rd}$ (d) $7^{th}$

**182.** Fertilization takes place at
(a) Isthmus
(b) Ampulla
(c) Infundibulum
(d) Ampullary-isthmic junction

**183.** Which part of the sperm helps in penetration into the ovum?
(a) Mitochondria (b) Acrosome
(c) Tail (d) All of these

**184.** Second meiotic division in secondary oocyte is
(a) Unequal
(b) Complete after sperm penetration
(c) Both (a) and (b)
(d) Equal

**185.** The embryo with 8 to 16 blastomeres is called
(a) Blastula (b) Gastrula
(c) Morula (d) None of these

**186.** Implantation leads to
(a) Formation of trophoblast in blastocyst
(b) Formation of inner cell mass in blastocyst
(c) Pregnancy
(d) All the above

**187.** Which of these hormones is/are produced in women during pregnancy?
(a) HCG (b) HPL
(c) Relaxin (d) All of these

**188.** Which of these statements is incorrect about embryo development?
(a) After one month of pregnancy the heart is formed.
(b) By the end of first trimester most of the major organ systems are formed.
(c) First movement of foetus is observed in the seventh month.
(d) At the end of second trimester, the body is covered with fine hair, eyelids separate and eye lashes are formed.

**189.** The process of delivery of foetus is called
(a) Parturition (b) Gestation
(c) Ejaculation (d) Capacitation

## Multiple Choice Questions: Level II

**190.** Which one of the following is the most likely root cause why menstruation is not taking place in regularly cycling human female?
(a) maintenance of the hypertrophical endometrial lining
(b) maintenance of high concentration of sex hormones in the blood stream
(c) retention of well-developed corpus luteum
(d) fertilization of the ovum

**191.** The correct sequence of spermatogenetic stages leading to the formation of sperms in a mature human testes is
(a) spermatogonia – spermatocyte – spermatid – sperms
(b) spermatid – spermatocyte – spermatogonia – sperms
(c) spermatogonia – spermatid – spermatocyte – sperms
(d) spermatocyte – spermatogonia – spermatid – sperms

**192.** Which one of the following is correct matching of process occurring during menstrual cycle?
(a) Proliferative phase: Rapid regeneration of myo- and maturation of Graafian follicle.
(b) Secretory phase: Development of corpus luteum, and increased secretion of progesterone.
(c) Menstruation: breakdown of myometrium and ovum not fertilized.
(d) Ovulation: LH and FSH attain peak level and sharp fall in the secretion of progesterone.

**193.** Seminal plasma in humans is rich in
(a) Fructose and calcium but has no enzymes
(b) Glucose and certain enzymes but has no calcium
(c) Fructose and certain enzymes but poor in calcium
(d) Fructose, calcium and certain enzymes

**194.** Given below is a diagrammatic sketch of a portion of human male reproductive system. Select the correct set of names of the parts labelled A, B, C, D.

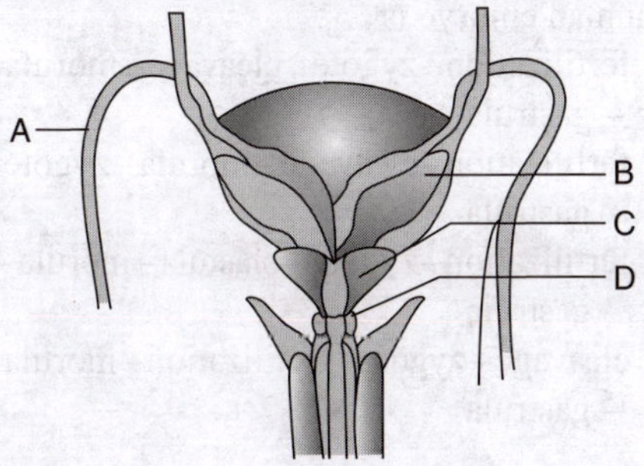

(a) A: Vas deferens, B: Seminal vesicle, C: Prostate, D: Bulbourethral gland
(b) A: Vas deferens, B: Seminal vesicle, C: Bulbo-urethral gland, D: Prostate
(c) A: Ureter, B: Seminal vesicle, C: Prostate, D: Bulbourethral gland
(d) A: Ureter, B: Prostate, C: Seminal vesicle, D: Bulbourethral gland

**195.** Which one of the following statements is incorrect about menstruation?
(a) At menopause in female, there is especially abrupt increase in gonadotropic hormones.
(b) The beginning of the cycle of menstruation is called menarche.
(c) During normal menstruation, about 40 ml blood is lost.
(d) The menstrual fluid can easily clot.

**196.** Which extra embryonic membrane in humans prevents desiccation of the embryo inside the uterus?
(a) yolk sac (b) amnion
(c) chorion (d) allantosis

**197.** In human adult females oxytocin
(a) stimulates pituitary to secrete vasopressin
(b) causes strong uterine contractions during parturition
(c) is secreted by anterior pituitary
(d) stimulates growth of mammary glands

**198.** In humans, at the end of the first meiotic division, the male germ cells differentiate into the
(a) Spermatids
(b) Spermatozonia
(c) Primary spermatocytes
(d) Secondary spermatocytes

**199.** Withdrawal of which of the following hormones is the immediate cause of menstruation?
(a) FSH (b) FSH-RH
(c) Progesterone (d) Estrogen

**200.** The correct sequence in the process of development of human embryo is
(a) fertilization–zygote–cleavage–morula–blastula – gastrula
(b) fertilization–cleavage–morula–zygote–blastula – gastrula
(c) fertilization–zygote–blastula–morula–cleavage – gastrula
(d) cleavage–zygote–fertilization–morula–blastula – gastrula

**201.** If mammalian ovum fails to get fertilized, which one of the following is unlikely?
(a) Corpus luteum will disintegrate
(b) Progesterone secretion rapidly declines
(c) Estrogen secretion further decreases
(d) Primary follicle starts developing

**202.** Ovulation in the human female normally takes place during the menstrual cycle
(a) at the mid secretory phase
(b) just before the end of the secretory phase
(c) at the beginning of the proliferative phase
(d) at the end of the proliferative phase

**203.** Bartholin's glands are situated
(a) on either side of vas deferens in humans
(b) on the sides of the head of some amphibians
(c) at the reduced tail end of birds
(d) on either side of vagina in humans

**204.** What is true for cleavage?
(a) size of embryo increases
(b) size of cells decrease
(c) size of cells increase
(d) size of embryo decreases

**205.** The growth of corpus luteum is initiated by
(a) Human chorionic gonadotropin
(b) Follicle stimulating hormone
(c) Luteinizing hormone
(d) Prolactin

**206.** Which of the following processes is associated with a change in the cellular DNA amount?
(a) Spore germination (b) Cytokinesis
(c) Fertilization (d) Blastulation

**207.** After ovulation the collapsed ovarian follicle shrinks and becomes filled with cell to form
(a) corpus luteum (b) corpus albicans
(c) corpus atresia (d) corpus adiposum

**208.** The correct sequence in the process of development of human embryo is
(a) fertilization – zygote – cleavage – morula – blasula – gastrula
(b) fertilization – cleavage – morula – zygote – blatula – gastrula
(c) fertilization – zygote – blastula – morula – cleavage – gastrula
(d) cleavage – zygote – fertilization – morula – blastula – gastrula

**209.** The mammalian corpus luteum produces
(a) estrogen (b) progesteron
(c) luteotropic hormone (d) luteinizing hormone

**210.** In 28-day human ovarian cycle, ovulation occurs on
(a) Day 1 (b) Day 5
(c) Day 14 (d) Day 28

**211.** At the end of first meiotic division, male sperm differentiates into
(a) Secondary spermatocyte
(b) Primary spermatocyte
(c) Spermatogonium
(d) Spermatid

**212.** What is true about cleavage in fertilized egg of humans?
(a) Meroblastic
(b) Starts when egg reaches uterus
(c) Starts in fallopian tube
(d) It is identical to normal mitosis

**213.** Extra-embryonic membranes of the mammalian embryo are derived from
(a) Inner cell mass (b) Trophoblast
(c) Formative cells (d) Follicle cells

**214.** Acrosome reaction in sperm is triggered by
(a) Capacitation (b) Release of lysin
(c) Influx of $Na^+$ (d) Release of fertilizin

**215.** Extrusion of second polar body from egg nucleus occurs
(a) After entry of sperm before completion of fertilization
(b) After completion of fertilization
(c) Before entry of sperm
(d) Without any relation of sperm entry

**216.** Middle piece of mammalian sperm possesses
(a) Mitochondria and centriole
(b) Mitochondria only
(c) Centricle only
(d) Nucleus and mitochondria

**217.** Location and secretion of Leydig's cells are
(a) Liver – cholesterol
(b) Ovary – estrogen
(c) Testes – testosterone
(d) Pancreas – glucagon

**218.** Freshly released human egg has
(a) One Y-chromosome
(b) One X-chromosome
(c) Two X-chromosomes
(d) One X-chromosome and one Y-chromosome

**219.** During cleavage, what is true about cells?
(a) Nucleocytoplasmic ratio remains unchanged
(b) Size does not increase
(c) There is less consumption of oxygen
(d) The division is like meiosis

**220.** Fertilizins are emitted by
(a) Immature eggs (b) Mature eggs
(c) Sperms (d) Polar bodies

**221.** How many sperms are formed from a secondary spermatocyte?
(a) 4 (b) 8
(c) 2 (d) 1

**222.** Gonads develop from embryonic
(a) Ectoderm
(b) Endoderm
(c) Mesoderm
(d) Both mesoderm and endoderm

**223.** Sperm and egg nuclei fuse due to
(a) Base pairing of their DNA and RNA
(b) Formation of hydrogen bonds
(c) Mutual attraction due to differences in electrical charges
(d) Attraction of their protoplasts

**224.** Egg is liberated from ovary in
(a) Secondary oocyte stage
(b) Primary oocyte stage
(c) Oogonial stage
(d) Mature ovum stage

**225.** Human eggs are
(a) Alecithal (b) Microlecithal
(c) Mesolecithal (d) Macrolecithal

**226.** Cells become variable in morphology and function in different regions of the embryo. The process is
(a) Differentiation
(b) Metamorphosis
(c) Organization
(d) Rearrangement

## A & R and Statement-based Questions

### Assertion and Reason Questions:

***Direction for questions 227 to 231:** Read the **assertion** and **reason** carefully to mark the correct option out of the options given below:*

(a) **(A)** is **true** but **(R)** is **false**.
(b) **(A)** is **false** but **(R)** is **true**.
(c) Both **(A)** and **(R)** is **true** and **(R)** is the correct explanation of **(A)**.
(d) Both **(A)** and **(R)** is **true** and **(R)** is not the correct explanation of **(A)**.

**227. Assertion:** Testis are situated outside the abdominal cavity with in a pouch called scrotum.

**Reason:** Scrotum helps in maintaining the low temperature of the testes which is necessary for spermatogenesis.

**228. Assertion:** Ampulla helps in collection of ovum just after ovulation.

**Reason:** Infundibulum is part of fallopian tube.

**229. Assertion:** Milk is sucked out from lactiferous duct in lactating women.

**Reason:** Lactiferous duct are distil part of lactating tree in mammary gland.

**230. Assertion:** Spermatogonia are diploid cells.

**Reason:** Spermatogonia multiply by binary fission.

**231. Assertion:** There is increased production of hormones like progesterone, oestrogen, cortisol and thyroxine during pregnancy.

**Reason:** These hormones help in supporting foetal growth, metabolic changes in mother and maintenance of pregnancy.

### Statement-based Questions:

***Direction for questions 232 to 236:** These type of questions consist of two statement each, printed as **Statement-I** and **Statement-II**. While answering such questions, a student is needed to choose any one of the following four responses.*

(a) **Statement I** is **correct Statement II** is **incorrect**.
(b) **Statement I** is **incorrect Statement II** is **correct**.
(c) Both **Statement I** and **Statement II** are **correct**.
(d) Both **Statement I** and **Statement II** are **incorrect**.

**232. Statement-I:** Oogenesis is different from spermatogenesis.

**Statement-II:** Oogenesis is initiated during embryonic stages.

**233. Statement-I:** Secretions of epididymis, vas deference, seminal vesical and prostate are essential for maturation and motility of sperm.

**Statement-II:** Primary follicle contain antrum.

**234. Statement-I:** Corpus luteum secretes small amount of progesterone required for maintenance of endometrium.

**Statement-II:** Menstrual cycle is an indicator of normal reproductive phase.

**235. Statement-I:** Acrosome help in penetration of sperm through zona pellucida of ovum.

**Statement-II:** Implantation of blastocyst in the wall of uterus leads to pregnancy.

**236. Statement-I:** First foetal movement observed during fifth month.

**Statement-II:** Colostrum contain antibodies.

## Matrix-Match Type Questions

**237.** Which is the correct order of reproductive events in human?

(a) Gametogenesis → Insemination → Fertilisation → Implantation → Gestation → Parturition.
(b) Gametogenesis → Fertilisation → Insemination → Implantation → Gestation → Parturition.
(c) Gametogenesis → Gestation → Implantation → Insemination → Fertilisation → Parturition.
(d) Parturition → Gestation → Implantation → Insemination → Fertilisation → Gametogenesis

**238.** Match the following:

| List-I | List-II |
|---|---|
| 1. Spermatogonia | (i) Nutrition of germ cells |
| 2. Sertoli cells | (ii) Secrete testicular hormones |
| 3. Leydig cells | (iii) Store sperms |
| 4. Epididymis | (iv) Male germ cells |

**The correct matching is**

| | 1 | 2 | 3 | 4 |
|---|---|---|---|---|
| (a) | (iv) | (i) | (ii) | (iii) |
| (b) | (i) | (iv) | (ii) | (iii) |
| (c) | (iii) | (ii) | (i) | (iv) |
| (d) | (ii) | (i) | (iv) | (iii) |

**239.** Match the following:

| List-I | List-II |
|---|---|
| 1. Gametogenesis | (i) Attachment to uterine wall |
| 2. Implantation | (ii) Delivery of baby |
| 3. Gestation | (iii) Embryonic development |
| 4. Parturition | (iv) Formation of gametes |

**The correct matching is**

| | 1 | 2 | 3 | 4 |
|---|---|---|---|---|
| (a) | (iv) | (i) | (iii) | (ii) |
| (b) | (iv) | (i) | (ii) | (iii) |
| (c) | (i) | (ii) | (iv) | (iii) |
| (d) | (ii) | (i) | (iv) | (iii) |

**240.** Match the following:

| List-I (Type of Waste) | List-II (Effect on Water) |
|---|---|
| 1. Head | (i) Enzyme for fertilization of ovum |
| 2. Acrosome | (ii) Mitochondria for energy |
| 3. Middle piece | (iii) Movement for motility |
| 4. Tail | (iv) Haploid nucleus |

**The correct matching is**

| | 1 | 2 | 3 | 4 |
|---|---|---|---|---|
| (a) | (iv) | (i) | (ii) | (iii) |
| (b) | (ii) | (i) | (iii) | (iv) |
| (c) | (iv) | (ii) | (i) | (iii) |
| (d) | (ii) | (iii) | (i) | (iv) |

**241.** Match the following:

| List-I | List-II |
|---|---|
| 1. Corpus luteum | (i) Collection of the ovum for ovulation |
| 2. Acrosome | (ii) Motility |
| 3. Fimbriae | (iii) Contributes in menstrual cycle |
| 4. Endometrium | (iv) Enzymes for fertilisation of ovum |
| 5. Sperm tail | (v) Secretion of progestrone |

**The correct matching is**

| | 1 | 2 | 3 | 4 | 5 |
|---|---|---|---|---|---|
| (a) | (v) | (iv) | (i) | (iii) | (ii) |
| (b) | (ii) | (i) | (iii) | (iv) | (v) |
| (c) | (v) | (iii) | (i) | (iv) | (ii) |
| (d) | (ii) | (i) | (iv) | (iii) | (v) |

## NCERT Exemplar Questions

**1.** Choose the incorrect statement from the following:
(a) In birds and mammals internal fertilization takes place.
(b) Colostrum contains antibodies and nutrients.
(c) Polyspermy in mammals is prevented by the chemical changes in the egg surface.
(d) In humans, female implantation occurs almost seven days after fertilization.

**2.** Identify the correct statement from the following:
(a) High levels of oestrogen triggers the ovulatory surge.
(b) Oogonial cells start to proliferate and give rise to functional ova in regular cycles from puberty onwards.
(c) Sperms released from seminiferous tubules are highly motile.
(d) Progesterone level is high during the post ovulatory phase of menstrual cycle.

**3.** Spot the odd one out from the following structures with reference to the male reproductive system.
(a) Rete testis (b) Epididymis
(c) Vasa efferentia (d) Isthmus

**4.** Seminal plasma, the fluid part of semen, is contributed by
i. Seminal vesicle
ii. Prostate gland
iii. Urethra
iv. Bulbourethral gland
(a) i and ii (b) i, ii and iv
(c) ii, iii and iv (d) i and iv

**5.** Spermiation is the process of the release of sperms from
(a) Seminiferous tubules
(b) Vas deferens
(c) Epididymis
(d) Prostate gland

6. Mature Graafian follicle is generally present in the ovary of a healthy human female around
(a) 5 – 8 day of menstrual cycle
(b) 11 – 17 day of menstrual cycle
(c) 18 – 23 day of menstrual cycle
(d) 24 – 28 day of menstrual cycle

7. Acrosomal reaction of the sperm occurs due to
(a) Its contact with zona pellucida of the ova.
(b) Reactions within the uterine environment of the female.
(c) Reactions within the epididymal environment of the male.
(d) Androgens produced in the uterus.

8. Which one of the following is not a male accessory gland?
(a) Seminal vesicle
(b) Ampulla
(c) Prostate
(d) Bulbourethral gland

9. The spermatogonia undergo division to produce sperms by the process of spermatogenesis. Choose the correct option with reference to the above.
(a) Spermatogonia have 46 chromosomes and always undergo meiotic cell division.
(b) Primary spermatocytes divide by mitotic cell division.
(c) Secondary spermatocytes have 23 chromosomes and undergo second meiotic division.
(d) Spermatozoa are transformed into spermatids.

10. Match between the following representing parts of the sperm and their functions and choose the correct option.

| Column A | | Column B |
|---|---|---|
| A. | Head | i. Enzymes |
| B. | Middle piece | ii. Sperm motility |
| C. | Acrosome | iii. Energy |
| D. | Tail | iv. Genetic material |

(a) A-ii, B-iv, C-i, D-iii
(b) A-iv, B-iii, C-i, D-ii
(c) A-iv, B-i, C-ii, D-iii
(d) A-ii, B-i, C-iii, D-iv

11. Which among the following has 23 chromosomes?
(a) Spermatogonia (b) Zygote
(c) Secondary oocyte (d) Oogonia

12. Match the following and choose the correct options:

| Column A | | Column B |
|---|---|---|
| A. | Trophoblast | i. Embedding of blastocyst in the endometrium |
| B. | Cleavage | ii. Group of cells that would differentiate as embryo |
| C. | Inner cell mass | iii. Outer layer of blastocyst attached to the endometrium |
| D. | Implantation | iv. Mitotic division of zygote |

**Options:**
(a) A-ii, B-i, C-iii, D-iv
(b) A-iii, B-iv, C-ii, D-i
(c) A-iii, B-i, C-ii, D-iv
(d) A-ii, B-iv, C-iii, D-i

13. Which of the following hormones is not secreted by human placenta?
(a) hCG (b) Oestrogens
(c) Progesterone (d) LH

14. The vas deferens receives duct from the seminal vesicle and opens into urethra as
(a) Epididymis (b) Ejaculatory duct
(c) Efferent ductule (d) Ureter

15. Urethral meatus refers to the
(a) Urinogenital duct
(b) Opening of vas deferens into urethra
(c) External opening of the urinogenital duct
(d) Muscles surrounding the urinogenital duct

16. Morula is a developmental stage
(a) Between the zygote and blastocyst
(b) Between the blastocyst and gastrula
(c) After the implantation
(d) Between implantation and parturition

17. The membranous cover of the ovum at ovulation is
(a) Corona radiata (b) Zona radiata
(c) Zona pellucida (d) Chorion

18. Identify the odd one from the following:
(a) Labia minora (b) Fimbriae
(c) Infundibulum (d) Isthmus

## Previous Years' Questions

**1.** Secretions from which one of the following are rich in fructose, calcium and some enzymes? [AIPMT MAINS 2010]

(a) male accessory glands (b) liver
(c) pancreas (d) salivary glands

**2.** In human female, the blastocyst [AIPMT MAINS 2010]

(a) forms placenta even before implantation.
(b) gets implanted into uterus 3 days after ovulation.
(c) gets nutrition from uterine endometrial secretion only after implantation.
(d) gets implanted in endometrium by the trophoblast cells.

**3.** Signals from fully developed foetus, and placenta ultimately lead to a parturition which requires the release of [AIPMT MAINS 2010]

(a) estrogen from placenta
(b) oxytocin from maternal pituitary
(c) oxytocin from foetal pituitary
(d) relaxin from placenta

**4.** The first movements of the foetus and appearance of hair on its head are usually observed during which month of pregancy? [AIPMT PRE 2010]

(a) Fourth month (b) Fifth month
(c) Sixth month (d) Third month

**5.** The signals for parturition originate from [AIPMT PRE 2010]

(a) placenta only
(b) placenta as well as fully developed foetus
(c) oxytocin released from maternal pituitary
(d) fully developed foetus only

**6.** The part of fallopian tube closest to the ovary is [AIPMT PRE 2010]

(a) isthmus (b) infundibulum
(c) cervix (d) ampulla

**7.** Which one of the following statements about human sperm is correct? [AIPMT PRE 2010]

(a) Acrosome has a conical pointed structure used for piercing and penetrating the egg, resulting in fertilization
(b) Sperm lysins in the acrosome dissolve the egg envelope facilitating fertilization
(c) Acrosome serves as a sensory structure leading the sperm towards the ovum
(d) Acrosome serves no particular function

**8.** The second maturation division of the mammalian ovum occurs [AIPMT PRE 2010]

(a) shortly after ovulation before the ovum makes entry into the fallopian tube.
(b) until after the ovum has been penetrated by a sperm.
(c) until the nucleus of the sperm has fused with that of the ovum.
(d) in the Graafian follicle following the first maturation division.

**9.** Seminal plasma in human males is rich in [AIPMT PRE 2010]

(a) fructose and calcium
(b) glucose and calcium
(c) DNA and testosterone
(d) ribose and potassium

**10.** Vasa efferentia are the ductules leading from [AIPMT MAINS 2010]

(a) testicular lobules to rete testis
(b) rete testis to vas deferens
(c) vas deferens to epididymis
(d) epididymis to urethra

**11.** Sertoli cells are found in [AIPMT MAINS 2010]

(a) ovaries and they secrete progesterone.
(b) adrenal cortex and they secrete adrenalin.
(c) seminiferous tubules and provide nutrition to germ cells.
(d) pancreas and they secrete cholecystokinin.

**12.** What happens during fertilization in humans after many sperms reach close to the ovum? [AIPMT MAINS 2011]

(a) secretions of acrosome helps one sperm enter cytoplasm of ovum through zona pellucid.
(b) all sperms except the one nearest to the ovum lose their tails.
(c) cells of corona radiata trap all the sperms except one.
(d) only two sperms nearest to the ovum penetrate zona pellucid.

**13.** About which day in a normal human menstrual cycle does rapid secretion of LH (popularly called LH surge) normally occurs? [AIPMT MAINS 2011]

(a) 14th day (b) 20th day
(c) 5th day (d) 11th day

**14.** If for some reason, the vasa efferentia in the human reproductive system get blocked, the gametes will not be transported from [AIPMT PRE 2011]

(a) Epididymis to vas deferens
(b) Ovary to uterus
(c) Vagina to uterus
(d) Testes to epididymis

**15.** The testes in humans are situated outside the abdominal cavity inside a pouch called scrotum. The purpose served is for [AIPMT PRE 2011]

(a) escaping any possible compression by the visceral organs.
(b) providing more space for the growth of epididymis.
(c) providing a secondary sexual feature for exhibiting the male sex.
(d) maintaining the scrotal temperature lower than the internal body temperature.

**16.** The figure given below depicts a diagrammatic sectional view of the female reproductive system of humans. Which one set of three parts out of A–F have been correctly identified? [AIPMT PRE 2011]

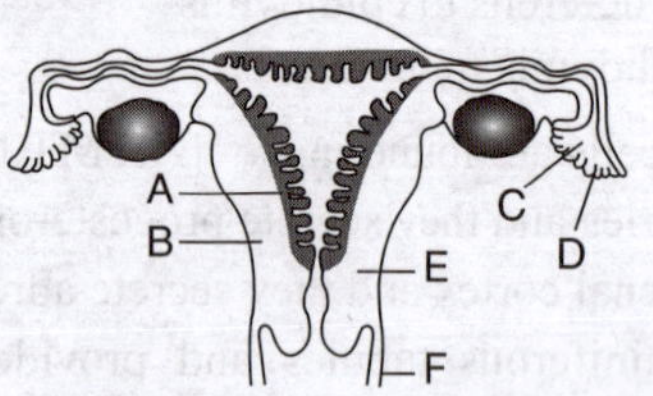


(a) C – Infundibulum, D – Fimbriae, E – Cervix
(b) D – Oviducal funnel, E – Uterus, F – Cervix
(c) A – Perimetrium, B – Myometrium, C – Fallopian tube
(d) B – Endometrium, C – Infundibulum, D – Fimbriae

**17.** The secretory phase in the human menstrual cycle is also called: [AIPMT MAINS 2012]

(a) Follicular phase lasting for about 6 days
(b) Luteal phase that lasts for about 13 days
(c) Follicular phase that lasts for about 13 days
(d) Luteal phase that lasts for about 6 days

**18.** Identify the human development stage shown below as well as the right place of its occurrence in a normal pregnant women and select the right option for the two together: [AIPMT MAINS 2012]

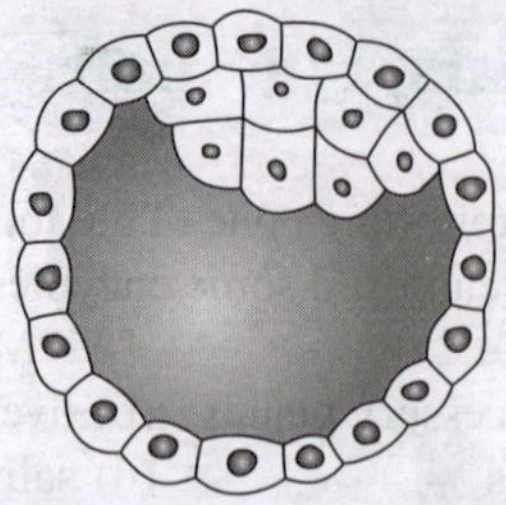

| Developmental stage | Site of occurrence |
|---|---|
| (a) Blastula | End part of Fallopian tube |
| (b) Blastocyst | Uterine wall |
| (c) 8-celled morula | Starting point of Fallopian tube |
| (d) Late morula | Middle part of Fallopian tube |

**19.** The Leydig cells as found in the human body are the secretory source of : [AIPMT PRE 2012]

(a) progesterone (b) intestinal mucus
(c) glucagon (d) androgens

**20.** In normal pregnant woman, the amount of total gonadotropin activity was assessed. The result expected was [AIPMT PRE 2012]

(a) High levels of FSH and LH in uterus to stimulate endometrial thickening.
(b) High levels of circulating HCG to stimulate estrogen and progesterone synthesis.
(c) High level of circulating FSH and LH in the uterus to stimulate implantation of the embryo.
(d) High level of circulating HCG to stimulate endometrial thickening.

**21.** Which one of the following statements is false in respect of viability of mammalian sperm? [AIPMT PRE 2012]

(a) Sperm is viable for only up to 24 hours
(b) Survival of sperm depends on the pH of the medium and is more active in alkaline medium
(c) Viability of sperm is determined by its motility
(d) Sperms must be concentrated in a thick suspension

**22.** Signals for parturition originate from: [AIPMT PRE 2012]

(a) Both placenta as well as fully developed foetus
(b) Oxytocin released from maternal pituitary
(c) Placenta only
(d) Fully developed foetus only

**23.** Which one of the following is not the function of placenta? It : [AIPMT 2013]
(a) facilitates supply of oxygen and nutrients to embryo.
(b) secretes estrogen.
(c) facilitates removal of carbon dioxide and waste material from embryo.
(d) secretes oxytocin during parturition.

**24.** Menstruel flow occurs due to lack of [AIPMT 2013]
(a) Progesterone (b) FSH
(c) Oxytocin (d) Vasopressin

**25.** What is the correct sequence of sperm formation? [AIPMT 2013]
(a) Spermatid, spermatocyte, spermatogonia, spermatozoa
(b) Spermatogonia, spermatocyte, spermato-zoa, spermatid
(c) Spermatogonia, spermatozoa, spemato-cyte, spermatid
(d) Spermatogonia, spermatocyte, spermatid, spermatozoa

**26.** Select the correct option describing gonadotropin activity in a normal pregnant female : [AIPMT 2014]
(a) High level of FSH and LH stimulates the thickening of endometrium.
(b) High level of FSH and LH facilitate implantation of the embryo.
(c) High level of hCG stimulates the synthesis of estrogen and progesterone.
(d) High level of hCG stimulates the thickening of endometrium.

**27.** The main function of mammalian corpus luteum is to produce: [AIPMT 2014]
(a) Estrogen only
(b) Progesterone
(c) Human chorionic gonadotropin
(d) Relaxin only

**28.** Which of these is not an important component of initiation of parturition in humans? [AIPMT 2015]
(a) Increase in estrogen and progesterone ratio
(b) Synthesis of prostaglandins
(c) Release of oxytocin
(d) Release of prolactin

**29.** Which of the following cells during gametogenesis is normally diploid? [AIPMT 2015]
(a) Primary polar body
(b) Spermatid
(c) Spermatogonia
(d) Secondary polar body

**30.** Capacitation refers to changes in the [AIPMT 2015]
(a) Sperm before fertilization
(b) Ovum before fertilization
(c) Ovum after fertilization
(d) Sperm after fertilization

**31.** Which of the following events is not associated with ovulation in human female? [RE–AIPMT 2015]
(a) Full development of Graafian follicle
(b) Release of secondary oocyte
(c) LH surage
(d) Decrease in estradiol

**32.** In human female, meiosis-II is not completed until? [RE–AIPMT 2015]
(a) Fertilization
(b) Uterine implantation
(c) Birth
(d) Puberty

**33.** Which of the following layers in an antral follicle is acellular? [RE–AIPMT 2015]
(a) Theca interna (b) Stroma
(c) Zona pellucida (d) Granulosa

**34.** Ectopic pregnancies are referred to as [RE–AIPMT 2015]
(a) Implantation of embryo at side other than uterus
(b) Implantation of defective embryo in the uterus
(c) Pregnancies terminated due to hormonal imbalance
(d) Pregnancies with genetic abnormality

**35.** Fertilization in humans is practically feasible only if– [NEET 2016 PHASE – I]
(a) The sperms are transported into vagina just after the release of ovum in fallopian tube.
(b) The ovum and sperms are transported simultaneously to ampullary–isthmic junction of the fallopian tube.
(c) The ovum and sperms are transported simultaneously to ampullary–isthmic junction of the cervix.
(d) The sperms are transported into cervix within 48 hrs of release of ovum in uterus.

**36.** Select the incorrect statement: [NEET 2016 PHASE – I]
(a) FSH stimulates sertoli cells which help in spermiogenesis
(b) LH triggers ovulation in ovary.
(c) LH and FSH decrease gradually during the follicular phase.
(d) LH triggers secretion of androgens from the Leydig cells.

**37.** Several hormones like hCG, hPL, estrogen, progesterone are produced by [NEET 2016 PHASE – II]

(a) Placenta (b) Fallopian tube
(c) Pituitary (d) Ovary

**38.** Match the column – I With Column – II and select the correct option using the codes given below:

| Column – I | Column – II |
|---|---|
| (A) Mono pubis | (1) Embryo formation |
| (B) Antrum | (2) Sperm |
| (C) Trophectoderm | (3) Female external genitalia |
| (D) Nebenkern | (4) Graffian follicle |

[NEET 2016 – PHASE II]

(a) A:3, B:4, C:1, D:2 (b) A:2, B:1, C:4, D:2
(c) A:1, B:4, C:3, D:2 (d) A:3, B:4, C:2, D:1

**39.** Which of the following depicts the correct pathway of transport of sperms? [NEET 2016 – PHASE II]

(a) Rete testis → Epididymis → Efferent ductules → Vas deferens
(b) Rete testis → Vas deferens → Efferent ductules → Epididymis
(c) Efferent ductules → Rete testis → Vas deferens → Epididymis
(d) Rete Testis → Efferent ductules → Epididymis → Vas deferens

**40.** Capacitation occurs in: [NEET 2017]

(a) Epididymis
(b) Vas deferens
(c) Female Reproductive tract
(d) Rate testis

**41.** Trace the correct path of sperm from seminiferous tubules: [NEET Regional 2017]

(a) Rete testis → vasa efferentia → epididymis → vas deferens
(b) Rete testis → epididymis → vasa efferentia → vas deferens
(c) Vasa efferentia → rete testis → vas deferens → epididymis
(d) Epididymis → vasa efferentia → rete testis → vas deferens

**42.** Signals for the onset of parturition originate from: [NEET Regional 2017]

(a) Mothers hypothalamus
(b) Foetus and placenta
(c) Mothers uterus
(d) Mothers pituitary

**43.** Hormones secreted by the placenta to maintain pregnancy are [NEET 2018]

(a) hCG, hPL, progestogens, prolactin
(b) hCG, hPL, progestogens, estrogens
(c) hCG, hPL, estrogens, relaxin, oxytocin
(d) hCG, progestogens, estrogens, glucocorticoids

**44.** The amnion of mammalian embryo is derived from [NEET 2018]

(a) Ectoderm and mesoderm
(b) Mesoderm and trophoblast
(c) Endoderm and mesoderm
(d) Ectoderm and endoderm

**45.** The difference between spermiogenesis and spermiation is [NEET 2018]

(a) In spermiogenesis spermatids are formed, while in spermiation spermatozoa are formed.
(b) In spermiogenesis spermatozoa from sertoli cells are released into the cavity of seminferous tubules, while in spermiation spermatozoa are formed.
(c) In spermiogenesis spermatozoa are formed, while in spermiation spermatids are formed.
(d) In spermiogenesis spermatozoa are formed, while in spermiation spermatozoa are released from sertoli cells into the cavity of seminiferous tubules.

**46.** Match the items given in Column-I with those in Column-II and select the correct option given below: [NEET 2018]

| Column-I | Column-II |
|---|---|
| a. Proliferative phase | i. Breakdown of endometrial lining |
| b. Secretory phase | ii. Follicular phase |
| c. Menstruation | iii. Luteal phase |

| | a | b | c |
|---|---|---|---|
| (a) | iii | ii | i |
| (b) | ii | iii | i |
| (c) | i | iii | ii |
| (d) | iii | i | ii |

**47.** Select the correct sequence for transport of sperm cells in the male reproductive system. [NEET 2019]

(a) Seminiferous tubules → Rete testis → Vasa efferentia → Epididymis → Vas deferens → Ejaculatory duct → Urethra → Urethral meatus
(b) Seminiferous tubules → Vasa efferentia → Epididymis → Inguinal canal → Urethra
(c) Testis → Epididymis → Vasa efferentia → vas deferens → Ejaculatory duct → Inguinal canal → Urethra → Urethral meatus
(d) Testis → Epididymis → Vasa efferentia → Rete testis → Inguinal canal → Urethra

**48.** Extrusion of second polar body from egg nucleus occurs: [NEET 2019]
(1) After fertilization
(2) Before entry of sperm into ovum
(3) Simultaneously with first cleavage
(4) After entry of sperm but before fertilization

**49.** Meiotic division of the secondary oocyte is completed: [NEET 2020]
(a) Prior to ovulation
(b) At the time of copulation
(c) After zygote formation
(d) At the time of fusion of a sperm with an ovum

**50.** Which of the following hormone levels will cause release of ovum (ovulation) from the graffian follicle? [NEET 2020]
(a) High concentration of Estrogen
(b) High concentration of Progesterone
(c) Low concentration of LH
(d) Low concentration of FSH

**51.** Match the following columns and select the correct option. [NEET 2020]

| Column – I | Column – II |
|---|---|
| (A) Placenta | (i) Androgens |
| (B) Zona pellucid | (ii) Human Chorionic Gonadotropin (HCG) |
| (C) Bulbo urethral glands | (iii) Layer of the ovum |
| (D) Leydig cells | (iv) Lubrication of the Penis |

| | (A) | (B) | (C) | (D) |
|---|---|---|---|---|
| (a) | (iv) | (iii) | (i) | (ii) |
| (b) | (i) | (iv) | (ii) | (iii) |
| (c) | (iii) | (ii) | (iv) | (i) |
| (d) | (ii) | (iii) | (iv) | (i) |

**52.** Receptors for sperm binding in mammals are present on: [NEET 2021]
(a) Zona pellucida
(b) Corona radiata
(c) Vitelline membrane
(d) Perivitelline space

**53.** Which of these is not an important component of initiation of parturition in humans? [NEET 2021]
(a) Release of Prolactin
(b) Increase in estrogen and progesterone ratio
(c) Synthesis of prostaglandins
(d) Release of Oxytocin

**54.** Which of the following secretes the hormone, relaxin, during the later phase of pregnancy? [NEET 2021]
(a) Uterus
(b) Graafian follicle
(c) Corpus luteum
(d) Foetus

**55.** Given below are two statements: [NEET 2022]

**Statement I:** The release of sperms into the seminiferous tubules is called Spermiation.

**Statement II:** Spermiogenesis is the process of formation of sperms from spermatogonia.

In the light of the above statements, choose the **most appropriate** answer from the options given below:
(a) Both **Statement I** and **Statement II** are incorrect.
(b) **Statement I** is correct but **Statement II** is incorrect.
(c) **Statement I** is incorrect but **Statement II** is correct.
(d) Both **Statement I** and **Statement II** are correct.

**56.** Which of the following statements are true for spermatogenesis but **do not** hold true for Oogenesis? [NEET 2022]
(A) It results in the formation of haploid gametes.
(B) Differentiation of gamete occurs after the completion of meiosis.
(C) Meiosis occurs continuously in a mitotically dividing stem cell population.
(D) It is controlled by the Luteinising hormone (LH) and Follicle Stimulating Hormone (FSH) secreted by the anterior pituitary.
(E) It is initiated at puberty.

Choose the **most appropriate** answer from the options given below:
(a) (B) and (C) only
(b) (B), (D) and (E) only
(c) (B), (C) and (E) only
(d) (C) and (E) only

**57.** At which stage of life the oogenesis process is initiated? [NEET 2022]
(a) Embryonic development stage
(b) Birth
(c) Adult
(d) Puberty

**58.** Which of the following statement are correct regarding female reproductive cycle? [NEET 2023]
A. In non-primate mammals cyclical changes during reproduction are called oestrus cycle.

B. First menstrual cycle begins at puberty and is called menopause.
C. Lack of menstruation may be indicative of pregnancy.
D. Cyclic menstruation extends between menarche and menopause.
(a) A and B only (b) A, B and C only
(c) A, C and D only (d) A and D only

**59.** Given below statements: one is labelled as Assertion A and the other is labelled as Reason R. [NEET 2023]
**Assertion A:** Endometrium is necessary for implantation of blastocyst.
**Reason R:** In the absence of fertilization, the corpus luteum degenerates that causes disintegration of endometrium.
(a) Both A and R are true but R is NOT the correct explanation of A.
(b) A is true but R is false.
(c) A is false but R is true.
(d) Both A and R are true and R is the correct explanation of A.

**60.** Which of the following is not a cloning vector? [NEET 2023]
(a) YAC (b) pBR322
(c) Probe (d) BAC

**61.** Given below are two statements: [NEET 2023]
**Statement I:** Vas deferens receives a duct from seminal vesicle and opens into urethra as the ejaculatory duct.
**Statement II:** The cavity of the cervix is called cervical canal which along with vagina forms birth canal.
In the light of the above statements, choose the correct answer from the options given below:
(a) Both Statement I and Statement II are false.
(b) Statement I is correct but Statement II is false.
(c) Statement I is incorrect but Statement II is true
(d) Both Statement I and Statement II are true.

**62.** Which of the following is not a component of Fallopian tube? [NEET 2024]
(a) Uterine fundus (b) Isthmus
(c) Infundibulum (d) Ampulla

**63.** Given below are two statements: [NEET 2024]
**Statement I:** The presence or absence of hymen is not a reliable indicator of virginity.
**Statement II:** The hymen is torn during the first coitus only.
In the light of the above statements, choose the correct answer from the options given below:
(a) Both Statement I and Statement are true.
(b) Both Statement I and Statement II are false.
(c) Statement I is true but Statement II is false.
(d) Statement I is false but Statement II is true.

**64.** Give below are two statements: One is labelled as Assertion A and the other is labelled as Reason R: [NEET 2024]
**Assertion A:** FSH acts upon ovarian follicles in female and Leydig cells in male.
**Reason R.** Growing ovarian follicles secrete estrogen in female while interstitial cells secrete androgen in male human being.
In the light of the above statements, choose the correct answer from the options given below:
(a) Both A and R are true and R is the correct explanation of A.
(b) Both A and R are true but R is NOT the correct explanation of A.
(c) A is true but R is false.
(d) A is false but R is true.

**65.** Given below ate two statement: one is labelled as Assertion A and the other is labelled as Reason R: [NEET 2024]
**Assertion A:** Breast feeding during initial period of infant growth is recommended by doctors for bringing a healthy baby.
**Reason R:** Colostrum contains several antibodies absolutely essential to develop resistance for the new born baby.
In the light of the above statement, choose the most appropriate answer from the options given below:
(a) Both A and R are correct and R is the correct explanation of A.
(b) Both A and R are correct but R is NOT the correct explanation of A.
(c) A is correct but R is not correct.
(d) A is not correct out R is correct.

**66.** Identify the correct option (A), (B), (C), (D) with respect to spermatogenesis. [NEET 2024]

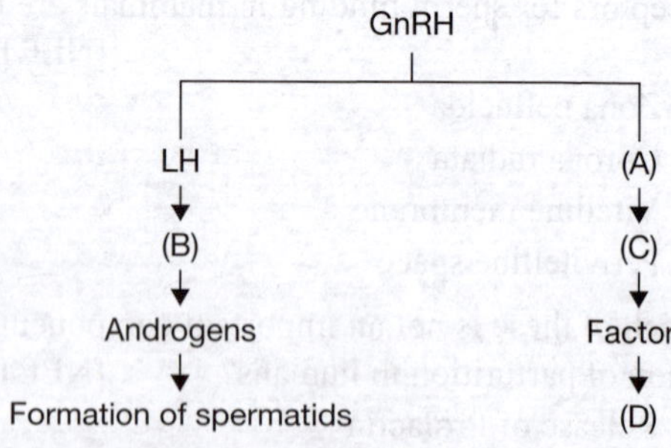


(a) FSH, Leydig cells, Sertoli cells, Spermiogenesis
(b) ICSH, Interstitial cells, Leydig cells, Spermiogenesis
(c) FSH, Sertoli cells, Leydig cells, spermatogenesis.
(d) ICSH, Leydig cells, Sertoli cells, spermatogenesis.

## Answer Key

### Multiple Choice Questions: Level I

| | | | | | | | | | |
|---|---|---|---|---|---|---|---|---|---|
| **1.** (d) | **2.** (c) | **3.** (a) | **4.** (b) | **5.** (c) | **6.** (c) | **7.** (c) | **8.** (b) | **9.** (b) | **10.** (c) |
| **11.** (b) | **12.** (b) | **13.** (c) | **14.** (b) | **15.** (c) | **16.** (b) | **17.** (b) | **18.** (a) | **19.** (b) | **20.** (c) |
| **21.** (b) | **22.** (c) | **23.** (a) | **24.** (b) | **25.** (b) | **26.** (c) | **27.** (b) | **28.** (d) | **29.** (d) | **30.** (b) |
| **31.** (b) | **32.** (d) | **33.** (b) | **34.** (b) | **35.** (c) | **36.** (d) | **37.** (d) | **38.** (b) | **39.** (c) | **40.** (d) |
| **41.** (b) | **42.** (c) | **43.** (b) | **44.** (c) | **45.** (b) | **46.** (b) | **47.** (c) | **48.** (a) | **49.** (d) | **50.** (b) |
| **51.** (c) | **52.** (b) | **53.** (b) | **54.** (d) | **55.** (b) | **56.** (c) | **57.** (c) | **58.** (a) | **59.** (d) | **60.** (c) |
| **61.** (a) | **62.** (a) | **63.** (d) | **64.** (c) | **65.** (c) | **66.** (a) | **67.** (d) | **68.** (c) | **69.** (d) | **70.** (d) |
| **71.** (a) | **72.** (c) | **73.** (a) | **74.** (a) | **75.** (c) | **76.** (c) | **77.** (a) | **78.** (c) | **79.** (d) | **80.** (b) |
| **81.** (d) | **82.** (d) | **83.** (d) | **84.** (a) | **85.** (c) | **86.** (b) | **87.** (b) | **88.** (c) | **89.** (d) | **90.** (b) |
| **91.** (a) | **92.** (b) | **93.** (c) | **94.** (b) | **95.** (b) | **96.** (c) | **97.** (b) | **98.** (c) | **99.** (c) | **100.** (c) |
| **101.** (b) | **102.** (d) | **103.** (a) | **104.** (b) | **105.** (c) | **106.** (d) | **107.** (a) | **108.** (b) | **109.** (c) | **110.** (a) |
| **111.** (c) | **112.** (c) | **113.** (d) | **114.** (d) | **115.** (c) | **116.** (d) | **117.** (b) | **118.** (c) | **119.** (b) | **120.** (c) |
| **121.** (d) | **122.** (b) | **123.** (d) | **124.** (b) | **125.** (c) | **126.** (b) | **127.** (b) | **128.** (c) | **129.** (c) | **130.** (a) |
| **131.** (d) | **132.** (c) | **133.** (b) | **134.** (a) | **135.** (d) | **136.** (a) | **137.** (a) | **138.** (b) | **139.** (b) | **140.** (c) |
| **141.** (c) | **142.** (c) | **143.** (d) | **144.** (a) | **145.** (b) | **146.** (b) | **147.** (b) | **148.** (d) | **149.** (b) | **150.** (b) |
| **151.** (b) | **152.** (a) | **153.** (c) | **154.** (a) | **155.** (a) | **156.** (b) | **157.** (b) | **158.** (c) | **159.** (c) | **160.** (b) |
| **161.** (b) | **162.** (b) | **163.** (a) | **164.** (b) | **165.** (a) | **166.** (b) | **167.** (b) | **168.** (c) | **169.** (b) | **170.** (c) |
| **171.** (b) | **172.** (b) | **173.** (b) | **174.** (c) | **175.** (b) | **176.** (b) | **177.** (b) | **178.** (c) | **179.** (d) | **180.** (b) |
| **181.** (b) | **182.** (b) | **183.** (b) | **184.** (c) | **185.** (c) | **186.** (c) | **187.** (d) | **188.** (c) | **189.** (a) | |

### Multiple Choice Questions: Level II

| | | | | | | | | | |
|---|---|---|---|---|---|---|---|---|---|
| **190.** (d) | **191.** (a) | **192.** (b) | **193.** (d) | **194.** (a) | **195.** (d) | **196.** (b) | **197.** (b) | **198.** (d) | **199.** (c) |
| **200.** (a) | **201.** (d) | **202.** (d) | **203.** (d) | **204.** (b) | **205.** (c) | **206.** (c) | **207.** (a) | **208.** (a) | **209.** (b) |
| **210.** (c) | **211.** (a) | **212.** (c) | **213.** (b) | **214.** (d) | **215.** (a) | **216.** (a) | **217.** (c) | **218.** (b) | **219.** (b) |
| **220.** (b) | **221.** (c) | **222.** (c) | **223.** (d) | **224.** (a) | **225.** (a) | **226.** (a) | | | |

### A & R and Statement-based Questions

| | | | | | | | | | |
|---|---|---|---|---|---|---|---|---|---|
| **227.** (c) | **228.** (b) | **229.** (c) | **230.** (a) | **231.** (c) | **232.** (c) | **233.** (a) | **234.** (b) | **235.** (c) | **236.** (c) |

### Matrix-Match Type Questions

| | | | | |
|---|---|---|---|---|
| **237.** (a) | **238.** (a) | **239.** (a) | **240.** (a) | **241.** (a) |

### NCERT Exemplar Questions

| | | | | | | | | | |
|---|---|---|---|---|---|---|---|---|---|
| **1.** (c) | **2.** (d) | **3.** (d) | **4.** (b) | **5.** (a) | **6.** (b) | **7.** (a) | **8.** (b) | **9.** (c) | **10.** (b) |
| **11.** (c) | **12.** (b) | **13.** (d) | **14.** (b) | **15.** (c) | **16.** (a) | **17.** (a) | **18.** (a) | | |

### Previous Years' Questions

| | | | | | | | | | |
|---|---|---|---|---|---|---|---|---|---|
| **1.** (a) | **2.** (d) | **3.** (b) | **4.** (b) | **5.** (b) | **6.** (b) | **7.** (b) | **8.** (b) | **9.** (a) | **10.** (b) |
| **11.** (c) | **12.** (a) | **13.** (a) | **14.** (d) | **15.** (d) | **16.** (a) | **17.** (b) | **18.** (b) | **19.** (d) | **20.** (b) |
| **21.** (a) | **22.** (a) | **23.** (d) | **24.** (a) | **25.** (d) | **26.** (c) | **27.** (b) | **28.** (d) | **29.** (c) | **30.** (a) |
| **31.** (d) | **32.** (a) | **33.** (c) | **34.** (a) | **35.** (b) | **36.** (c) | **37.** (a) | **38.** (a) | **39.** (d) | **40.** (c) |
| **41.** (a) | **42.** (b) | **43.** (b) | **44.** (a) | **45.** (d) | **46.** (b) | **47.** (a) | **48.** (d) | **49.** (d) | **50.** (a) |
| **51.** (d) | **52.** (a) | **53.** (a) | **54.** (c) | **55.** (b) | **56.** (c) | **57.** (a) | **58.** (c) | **59.** (a) | **60.** (c) |
| **61.** (d) | **62.** (d) | **63.** (a) | **64.** (d) | **65.** (c) | **66.** (b) | | | | |

# HINTS AND EXPLANATION

## Multiple Choice Questions: Level II

**190.** Fertilization of ovum is the most likely root cause for menstruation not taking place in regular cycles inhuman female. In order for fertilization to occur, one of these sperm must attach itself to the ovum and penetrate its outer surface. The fertilized ovum will then continue travelling down the fallopian tube, taking several days until it reaches the uterus. When it arrives, it attaches itself to the lining of the uterus and continues to grow. If the ovum is not fertilized, it will die and the progesterone and oestrogen hormone levels will drop. Without these hormones, the prepared uterus lining breaks up and is released through the vagina. This is known as a 'period'.

**191.** In testis, the immature male germ cells or spermatogonia (2n) multiply by mitotic division and increase in number. Some spermatogonia (2n) known as primary spermatocytes divide by meiotic division to form secondary spermatocytes (n). The secondary spermatocytes undergo second meiotic division to produce spermatid which are transformed into spermatozoa (sperms) by the process called spermiogenesis.

**192.** **Proliferative phase:**

- It is also known as follicular phase or post-menstrual phase or pre-ovulatory phase (first oestrogen than FSH).
- It continues for 10–20 days.

**193.** Seminal plasma in human males is rich in fructose, calcium and certain enzymes. They provide a medium for transport of sperms, nourishes and activates sperms.

**194.** The human male reproductive system consists of a number of sex organs that are part of the human reproductive process. In diagrammatic representation of male reproductive system of human, points indicated by A, B, C, D are vas deferens, seminal vesicle, prostate and bulbourethral gland.

**195.** In human female, the periodic discharge of blood, mucus and cellular debris from uterine wall from non-pregnant women of sexual maturity is known as menstrual cycle. Few hours before the start of mensuration, the spiral arterioles constrict one by one resulting into the blanch mucosa. The mucosa shrinks and the death of the blood deprived tissues takes place. Blood clotting doesn't occur due to presence of fibrinolysin.

**196.** Amnion is an extra-embryonic membrane in human which prevents desiccation of the embryo inside the uterus. Amnion is a membrane that encloses the embryo of reptiles, birds and mammals within the amniotic cavity. This cavity is filled with amniotic fluid, in which the embryo is protected from desiccation and external pressure.

**197.** It causes strong uterine contraction during childbirth.

**198.** In human, at the end of the first meiotic division, the male germ cells differentiate into the secondary spermatocytes.

**199.** Progesterone hormone which is secreted by the corpus luteum in the ovaries is responsible to stop ovulation (during, pregnancy) and fixes the foetus to uterine wall, facilitates placenta formation and controls the foetus development in uterus. If this hormone is withdrawn, then fixation of foetus to uterine wall will also take place, formation of placenta will also not take place, ovulation starts from ovaries and hence in human female menstruation starts.

**200.** Fusion of male and female gamete produces a zygote. Repeated division of the zygote is called cleavage forming a solid morula. After further division and rearrangement, a fluid filled cavity surrounded by blastomeres, blastula, is formed. The appearance of germ layers marks the gastrula.

**201.** Since corpus luteum degenerates, progesterone also decreases rapidly (progesterone is essential for maintenance of pregnancy). Also estrogen continues to curve growth of the endometrium which ultimately becomes thick enough to break down and cause menstruation. Hence, choice (c) is incorrect, as estrogen secretion does not decrease further. Primary follicles start developing.

**202.** **It occurs at the end of proliferative phase.**

**Stage of ovulation:**

- As the concentration of LH increases (LH surge), it results in release of secondary oocyte (ovulation).
- It usually occurs on $14^{th}$ day of menstrual cycle.

**203.** Bartholin's glands secrete a slimy liquid at the time of excitement and copulation. This slimy liquid acts as lubricant for vaginal treat and facilitates copulation.

**204.** Cleavage involves repeated division without increase in size.

**205.** Luteinizing hormone causes ovulation. The remaining cells of ovarian follicle are stimulated by LH to develop corpus luteum.

**206.** Cytokinesis involves division of cytoplasm of the parent cell into its daughter cells. Fertilization involves fusion of two haploid gametes. Blastulation refers to the process of cleavage in the zygote to form a blastula.

**207.** After ovulation, ovarian follicles undergo several stages of degeneration: corpus Iuteum, corpus albicans and finally corpus atresia or the atretic follicle.

**208.** Fusion of male and female gamete produces a zygote. Repeated division of the zygote is called cleavage forming a solid morula. After further division and rearrangement, a fluid-filled cavity surrounded by blastomeres, or blastula, is formed. The appearance of germ layers marks gastrula.

**209.** Mammalian corpus luteum produces progesterone. It is essential for continuation of pregnancy and it also stimulates acini glands.

**210.** It occurs in mid of cycle or 14th day before onset of menstruation.

**211.** After first meiotic division, primary spermatocyte (diploid) gives rise to two secondary spermatocytes (haploid).

**212.** After ovulation, egg comes in fallopian tube where it is fertilized by the sperm and cleavage starts here only.

**213.** Four extra-embryonic membranes are present in mammals which originally arise from trophoblast viz. amnion, chorion, allantois and yolk sac. The trophoblast is the outermost layer of cells in morula.

**214.** Egg secretes fertilizin due to which acrosome of sperm secretes antifertilizine and due to their reaction sperm adheres to egg. The acrosome reaction occurs in the acrosome of the sperm as it approaches the zona pellucida. ln mammals, the acrosome reaction releases hyaluronidase and acrosin; their role in fertilization is not yet clear. It also alters a patch of pre-existing sperm plasma membrane so that it can fuse with the egg plasma membrane.

**215.** The entry of sperm stimulates the secondary oocyte to resume and complete the suspended meiosis II. This produces a haploid mature ovum and a second polar body. The second polar body and sperm tail immediately degenerate.

**216.** Sperm has:

(i) head in which acrosome and nucleus are present.

(ii) middle piece in which it contains many mitochondria.

(iii) A long and highly motile tail.

(A short neck is also present between middle piece and head which has centric and may sometimes regarded as a part of middle piece)

**217.** Interstitial cells = Leydig's cells are present in testes and secrete male hormone testosterone.

**218.** Human female has XX chromosomes. When eggs formed each egg carries 22 autosomes and one X chromosome. In human male, each sperm carries 22 autosomes either X or Y chromosomes.

**219.** During cleavage, size of cells do not increase (in fact the resultant blastomeres are smallest in size, because size of embryo doesn't increase and mitosis occurs repeatedly).

**220.** A glycoprotein fertilizin (composed of monosaccharides and amino acids) is secreted by a mature egg. Penetrating sperm also has some proteinaceous substance on its surface called antifertilizin. Due to the interaction between fertilizin and antifertilizin, the sperm adheres to the egg.

**221.** Primary spermatocyte (46) divides through meiosis to give two secondary spermatocytes (23). Each secondary spermatocyte divides through mitosis giving rise to two spermatids (23) which on spermeogenesis mature as sperms.

**222.** Ectoderm produces: Liver, Epidermis, glands, hair, nervous system, etc.

Endoderm produces: Pancreas, lining of urinary bladder, etc.

Mesoderm produces: Dermis, most muscles, Kidneys, Gonads, etc.

**223.** Sperm or male gamete fuses with egg or female gamete because of the attraction of their protoplast. Some chemicals are secreted by ovule or egg wall to attract the male gamete or sperm.

**224.** Egg is liberated from the ovary (ovulation) at secondary oocyte stage when the meiosis II is arrested in secondary oocyte. It will be induced by the sperm.

**225.** Eggs are of 4 types based on the amount of yolk present in them:

(i) Alecithal egg: Almost free of yolk, e.g. Most mammals like man.

(ii) Microlecithal egg: Very small amount of yolk, E.g. Branchiostoma.

(iii) Mesolecithal egg: Moderate amount of yolk e.g. Frog's egg

(iv) Macrolecithal egg: Large amount of yolk, e.g. Reptiles, birds and egg-laying mammals

**226.** Cells become variable in shape, size and getting their specialization for the formation of particular tissue or organ in future foetus. They place themselves at some specific regions in embryo for further organogeny.

## NCERT Exemplar Questions

**1.** During fertilization, a sperm comes in contact with zona pellucida layer of the ovum and induces changes in the membrane that block the entry of additional sperms. Thus, it ensures that only one sperm can fertilise an ovum.

**2.**
- Rapid secretion of LH leading to its maximum level during the mid-cycle called LH surge.
- Oogenesis is initiated during the embryonic development stage when a couple of million gamete mother cells (oogonia) are formed within each fetal ovary (about third month of foetal ovary), no more oogonia are formed and added after birth.
- In the head of epididymis sperms undergo physiological maturation, acquiring increased motility and fertilizing capacity.

**3.**
- Male reproductive system contains rete testis, vasa efferentia, epididymis and vas deferens, etc.
- Female reproductive system contains isthmus, ampulla, infundibulum and uterus, etc.

**4.** Secretion of seminal vesicle (paired), prostate gland (unpaired) and bulbourethral glands or Cowper's glands (paired) constitute the seminal plasma which is rich in fructose, calcium and certain other enzymes.

**5.**

| | |
|---|---|
| Spermiation | Process of release of sperms from seminiferous tubules |
| Gametogenesis | Formation of gametes |
| Insemination | Transfer of sperms into female genital tract |
| Fertilization | Fusion of male and female gametes |
| Implantation | Attachment of blastocyst to the uterine wall |
| Gestation | Embryonic development |
| Parturition | Delivery of baby |

**6.** Mature Graafian follicle is generally present in ovary of a healthy human female around 11–17 days of menstrual cycle.

**7.** Acrosome reaction in sperm is triggered by release of fertilizing. The secretion of acrosome helps the sperm to enter into cytoplasm of the ovum through zona pellucida and the plasma membrane.

**8.**
- Male accessory gland is seminal vesicle, prostate gland and bulbourethral gland.
- Ampulla is a part of female reproductive system.

**9.**
- Secondary spermatocytes have 23 chromosomes and undergo second meiotic division.
- Spermatogonia have 46 chromosomes and always undergo mitotic cell division.
- Primary spermatocytes divide by meiotic cell division.
- Spermatids are transformed into spermatozoa.

**10.**

| | |
|---|---|
| A. Head | iv. Genetic material |
| B. Middle piece | iii. Energy |
| C. Acrosome | i. Enzymes |
| D. Tail | ii. Sperm motility |

**11.** Secondary oocyte (D = 23)

**12.** A. Trophoblast iii. Outer layer of blastocyst attached to the endometrium

B. Cleavage iv. Mitotic division of zygote

C. Inner cell mass ii: Group of cells that would differentiate as embryo

D. Implantation i. Embedding of blastocyst in the endometrium

**13.**
- Placenta acts as an endocrine tissue and produces several hormones like human chorionic gonadotropin (hCG), human placental lactogen (hPL), estrogens, progestogens, etc.
- LH is secreted by pituitary gland.

**14.** Vas deferens receives duct from seminal vesicle and opens into urethra as ejaculatory duct.

**15.** Urethra originates from the urinary bladder and extends through the penis to its external opening called urethral meatus (external opening of the urino-genital duct).

**16.** The embryo with 8–16 blastomeres is called morula. Morula is the solid mass of cells and is mulberry like. Morula is a developmental stage between the zygote and blastocyst.

**17.** The membranous cover of ovum at ovulation is corona radiata.

**18.** Fimbriae, infundibulum, isthmus and ampulla are part of fallopian duct, while labia minora is female external genitalia.

## Previous Years' Questions

**1.** Male accessory glands include seminal vesicles, prostate gland and bulbourethral glands (Cowper's glands).

**2.** (a) gets implanted into uterus 7–8 days after ovulation.

(b) starts getting nutrition from uterine endometrial secretion just after entering the uterus.

(c) forms placenta after implantation.

**3.** Parturition is induced by a complex neuroendocrine mechanism. The signals for parturition originate from the fully developed foetus and the placenta which induce mild uterine contractions called foetal ejection reflex. This triggers release of oxytocin from the maternal pituitary. Oxytocin acts on the uterine muscles and causes stronger uterine contractions, which in turn stimulates further secretion of oxytocin. The stimulatory reflex between the uterine contraction and oxytocin secretion continues resulting in stronger and stronger contractions. This leads to expulsion of the baby out of the uterus through the birth canal, i.e., parturition.

**4.** Following changes occur during the 4th month (week 13–16):

- The foetus reaches a length of about 15 cm (6 inches).
- A fine hair called lanugo develops on the head.
- The foetus makes active movement.
- Meconium is made in the intestinal tract.
- The liver and pancreas produce fluid seretions.
- From week 13, sex prediction by obstetric ultrasonography can be done.
- At week 15, main development of external genitalia is finished.

**5.** The process of delivery of the foetus (childbirth) is called parturition which is induced by a complex neuroendocrine mechanism. The signals for parturition originate from the fully developed foetus and the placenta which induce mild uterine contractions called foetal ejection reflex. This triggers release of oxytocin from maternal pituitary. Oxytocin causes stronger uterine contractions which in turn stimulate further secretion of oxytocin.

**6.** The part of fallopian tube closest to the ovary is infundibulum. Infundibulum possess finger-like projections called fimbriae that help in collection of ovum after ovulation. It leads to wider part of oviduct called ampulla.

**7.** Acrosome a small pointed structure at the tip of nucleus. It breaks down just before fertilization, releasing hydrolytic enzymes that assist penetration between follicle cells that surrounds the ovum, thus facilitating fertilization.

**8.** In Oogenesis, the second maturation division occurs until after the ovum has been penetrated by a sperm. Oogenesis involves formation of haploid female gametes, ova, from this diploid egg mother cells, oogonia of ovary of female organism.

**9.** Seminal plasma in human males are rich in fructose, calcium and certain enzymes. They provide a medium for transport of sperms, nourishes and activates sperms.

**10.** Vasa efferentia are ductules leading from rete testis to vas deferens. The rete testis is an anastomosing network of tubules located in the hilum of the testicles that carries sperm from the seminiferous tubules to the vasa efferentia.

**11.** Sertoli cells are found in the walls of seminiferous tubules of the testes. They anchor and provide nutrition to the developing germ cells especially the seprmatids.

**12.** During fertilization in humans, many sperms reach close to the ovum. As sperm comcs in contact with the zona pellucid layer of the ovum, it induces changes in the membrane that blocks the entry of additional sperm. The secretions of acrosome helps one sperm enter cytoplasm of ovum through zona pellucida.

**13.** Rapid secretion of LH leading to its maximum level during the mid-cycle, i.e about the 14th day of menstrual cycle, popularly called LH surge induces rupture of Graafian follicle and thereby the release of ovum (ovulation).

**14.** If the vasa efferentia in the human reproductive system get blocked, the gametes will not be transformed from testes to epididymis.

**15.** Humans are warm-blooded and the body temperature is fixed (37°C). Optimum temperature required for spermatogenesis is 2–2.5°C lower than that of body temperature. That is the reason why the testis are extra-abdominal in location.

**16.** C: marked portion is Infundibulum

D: marked portion is Fimbriae

E: marked portion is Cervix

**17. Menstrual cycle :**

- It is also known as weeping of uterus for lost ovum or funeral of unfertilized ovum.
- 28 days cycle.
- Menarche is the first menstruation (onset of puberty) while menopause is the last menstruation (45 to 50 yrs of age)

**Menstrual Phase :**

- It continues for 3–5 days.
- Menstrual fluid possess – endometrium, blood (50–100 ml), mucous and secondary oocyte.
- This phase starts due to decrease in progesterone levels.
- 1st day of menses is considered as 1st day of menstrual cycle.

**Proliferative Phase :**

- It is also known as follicular phase or post-menstrual phase or pre-ovulatory phase (first oestrogen than FSH).
- It continues for 10–20 days.

**Stage of ovulation :**

- As the concentration of LH increases (LH surge), it results in release of secondary oocyte (ovulation).
- It usually occurs on 14th day of menstrual cycle.

**Luteal Phase/Secretory Phase :**

- The empty Graffian follicle is convented to corpus luteum which starts secreting progesterone hormone for the next 14 days (if pregnancy do not occur). Progesterone hormone maintains endometrium.
- It continues for 14 days.
- Endometrium further thicken to 5 mm and becomes secretory.
- Meant for receiving of fertilized ovum and its implantation.

**18.** The cavity seen in the diagram is blastocoels, so the stage is blastocyst.

**19. Interstitial cells of Leydig**

- These are located in between the seminiferous tubules in the lobule.
- These cells secrete androgens :
  (1) Testosterone hormone
  (2) Androstenedione
  (3) Dehydro epi androstenedione (DHEA)
- These cells are stimulated by ICSH (LH)

**20.** β-hCG (Beta human chorionic gonadotropin) – it is a placental hormone that ensures the secretion of oestrogen and progesterone to maintain pregnancy, especially during first two months. Thereafter, it is not required as it itself starts producing progesterone hormone. This hormone is also excreted in the urine. Its presence indicates pregnancy (pregnancy test).

**21.**

| Fertilizability Period | |
|---|---|
| Sperm (viability) | 24–48 Hrs (after ejaculation at temperature equivalent to body temperature) |
| Ovum (viability) | 24–48 Hrs |

**22.** The process of delivery of the foetus (childbirth) is called parturition which is induced by a complex neuroendocrine mechanism. The signals for parturition originate from the fully developed foetus and the placenta which induce mild uterine contractions called foetal ejection reflex. This triggers release of oxytocin from maternal pituitary. Oxytocin causes stronger uterine contractions which in turn stimulate further secretion of oxytocin.

**23.** Oxytocin is secreted by posterior pituitary.

**24.** Progesterone supports pregnancy. FSH stimulates gonadal activity called as gonadotrophins. Oxytocin stimulates contraction in uterus during childbirth

**25.** In testis, the immature male germ cells or spermatogonia (2n) multiply by mitotic division and increase in number. Some spermatogonia (2n) known as primary spermatocytes divide by meiotic division to form secondary spermatocytes (n). The secondary spermatocytes undergo second meiotic division to produce spermatid which are transformed into spermatozoa (sperms) by the process called spermiogensis.

**26.** hCG (human Chorionic Gonadotrophin) secretion occurs about 48–72 hours after implantation. Its level increases and excess of hCG leaks into urine which is indication of pregnancy.

**27.** Corpus luteum secretes large amounts of progesterone which is essential for maintenance of endometrium.

**28.** Parturition is the birth process; triggered by oxytocin which initiates uterine contractions.

Prostaglandins are produced in response to oxytocin and CRH production. They are effective at causing uterine contractions at times. Oestrogen, progesterone levels mark the beginning of parturition.

Prolactin hormone is responsible for milk secretion at the end of pregnancy. It is not significant during the birthing or initiation of parturition process.

**29.** The **spermatogonia** (sing. spermatogonium) present on the inside wall of Seminiferous tubules multiply by mitotic division and increase in numbers. Each spermatogonium is diploid and contains 46 chromosomes.

**30.** Capacitation of sperms (5–6 Hrs.) : It is development of capacity of fertilization in sperms while passing through the female genital tract. It involves:

**(1)** Neutralization of inhibitory factors of semen.

**(2)** Dissociaton of cholesterol → weaking of membrane of acrosome head.

**(3)** $Ca^{2+}$ enters → Undulating movement of sperms become whiplash movement.

**31.** At ovulation, LH surge occurs due to hypersecretion of estrogen, which gives positive feedback to anterior pituitary for secretion of LH.

**32.** Sperm enters in ovum induces completion of the meiotic division of secondary oocyte. The second meiotic division is also unequal and results in formation of a **second polar body** and haploid ovum (ootid).

**33.** Zona pellucida is secreted by secondary oocyte around itself and it is acellular.

**34.** **An ectopic pregnancy** occurs when an embryo implants somewhere other than the uterus, such as in one of the fallopian tubes.

**35.** Fertilization human is possible when ovum and sperms are transported simultaneously to ampullary–isthmic junction of the fallopian tube.

**36.** LH and FSH decrease gradually during the follicular phase of menstrual cycle.

**37.** **Placenta** also acts as an endocrine tissue and produces following hormones:

- Human chorionic gonadotropin (hCG)
- Human placental lactogen (hPL)
- Estrogens
- Progestogens

**38.** • **Mons pubis (part of Female external genitalia):** It is the fatty tissue cushion which is covered by skin and pubic hair.

• Tertiary Graffian follicle contain a fluid-filled cavity called **antrum.**

**39.** The correct path of sperm from seminiferous tubules: Seminiferous tubules → Rete Testis → Efferent ductules (vasa efferentia) → Epididymis → Vas deferens

**40.** Capacitation is a process, where the spermatozoa acquires the capacity to fertilize eggs. It occurs in female reproductive tract.

**41.** The correct path of sperm from seminiferous tubules:

Seminiferous tubules → Rete Testis → Efferent ductules (vasa efferentia) → Epididymis → Vas deferens

**42.** **Fully developed foetus** and **the placenta** gives signals for parturition. Initiation of mild uterine contractions called **foetal ejection reflex.** Release of oxytocin from the maternal pituitary. Oxytocin causes stronger uterine contractions which further stimulates secretion of oxytocin. Stimulatory reflex between the uterine contraction and oxytocin secretion continues making the uterine contractions more stronger, finally leading to parturition.

**43.** Placenta also acts as an endocrine tissue and produces several hormones like **human chorionic gonadotropin** (hCG), **human placental lactogen** (hPL), **estrogens, progestogens,** etc.

**44.** Amnion (embryonic membrane) is formed around the embryo. It is formed by outer somatic mesoderm and inner ectoderm. It encloses a cavity called amniotic cavity in which embryo is present. Amniotic cavity is filled with amniotic fluid.

**45.** Spermatids are transformed into **spermatozoa (sperms)** by a process called **spermiogenesis**. After spermiogenesis, sperm heads become embedded in the **Sertoli cells** and are finally released from the seminiferous tubules by a process called **spermiation**.

**46.** During proliferative phase, the follicles start developing, hence, called follicular phase. Secretory phase is also called as luteal phasc mainly controlled by progesterone secreted by corpus luteum. Estrogen further thickens the endometrium maintained by progesterone. Menstruation occurs due to decline in progesterone level and involves breakdown of overgrown endometrial lining.

**47.** The seminiferous tubules of the testis open into the vasa efferentia through rete testis. The vasa efferentia leave the testis and open into epididymis located along the posterior surface of each testis. The epididymis leads to vas deferens that ascends to the abdomen and loops over the urinary bladder. It receives a duct from seminal vesicle and opens into urethra as the ejaculatory duct. These ducts store and transport tsperms from the testis to the outside through urethra. The urethra originates from the urinary bladder and extends through the penis to its external opening called **urethral meatus.**

**48.** Secretions of acrosome helps the sperm enter into the cytoplasm of the ovum through zona pellucida and plasma membrane. This induces completion of the meiotic division of secondary oocyte. The second meiotic division is also unequal and results in e formation of a second polar body and a haploid ovum (ootid).

**49.** Meiotic division of secondary oocyte is completed after the entry of sperm in secondary oocyte which lead to the formation of a large ovum and a tiny II[nd] polar body.

**50.**
- High level of estrogen will send positive feedback to anterior pituitary for release of LH.
- FSH, LH and estrogen are at peak level during mid of menstrual cycle (28 day cycle).
- LH surge leads to ovulation.

**51.** The correct option is (d) becuase
(A) placenta secretes human chorionic gonadotropin (hCG)
(B) zona pellucida is a primary egg membrane secreted by the secondary oocyte
(C) the secretions of bulbourethral glands help in lubrication of the penis
(D) Leydig cells synthesise and secrete testicular hormones called androgens

**52.** **Zona pellucida** has receptors for sperm binding in mammals.

**53.** **Prolactin** is a lactation hormone that has no role in initiation of parturition.

**54.** The hormone **relaxin** is produced in the later phase of pregnancy. It is produced by the ovary.
**Relaxin is produced by the corpus luteum present in the ovary.** Ruptured Graafian follicle is called corpus luteum, which has endocrine function.

**55.** The, option (b) is the correct answer because Statement II is incorrect as the transformation of spermatids into spermatozoa (sperms) are called spermiogenesis. After this, sperm head becomes embedded in the sertoli cells and are finally released from the seminiferous tubules by the process called spermiation. Hence, Statement I is a correct statement.
Spermatogenesis is the process of formation of sperms from spermatogonia.

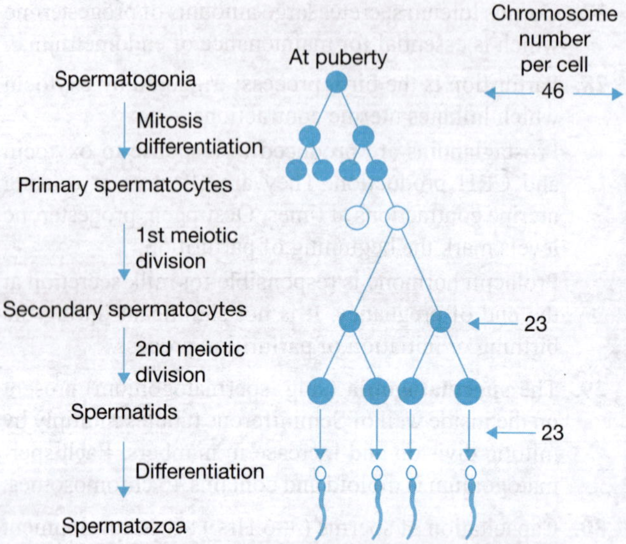


**56.** (a) Both spermatogenesis & oogenesis produce haploid gametes through the process of meiosis.
(b) Differentiation of gamete ocurs after the completion of mitosis in case of oogenesis.
(c) In oogenesis, cells start division & enter into prophase-I of meiotic division & gets temporarily arrested at that stage (primary oocytes).
(d) In both oogenesis & spermatogenesis, the process is controlled by LH & FSH.
(e) Oogenesis is initiated during the embryonic development stage.

Spermatogenesis starts at age of puberty.
LH acts on leydig cells.
FSH acts on sertoli cells.

**57.** Oogenesis process initials during embryonic development stage when a couple of million gamete mother cell (oogonia) are formed within each foetal ovary. No more oogonia are formed & added after birth.
Process of spermatogenesis initiates at puberty age.

**58.** First menstrual cycle begins at puberty and is called Menarche.

**59.** Both Assertion and Reason are true but Reason is NOT the correct explanation of Assertion.

**60.** Commonly used vectors are:
BAC (bacterial artificial chromosomes)
YAC (yeast artificial chromosomes)
pBR322 (*E. coli* cloning vector)

**61.** Both the statements are true.

**62.** The correct answer is option (a) as uterine fundus is the upper, dome-shaped part of the uterus, above the opening of Fallopian tubes.

- Option (b) is incorrect as isthmus is the last and narrow part of the oviduct that links to the uterus.
- Option (c) is incorrect as infundibulum is the part of oviduct which is closer to the ovary.
- Option (d) is incorrect as ampulla is the wider part of the oviduct.

**63.** The correct answer is option no. (c) because the presence or absence of hymen is not a reliable indicator of virginity because hymen can also be broken by a sudden jolt, insertion of a vaginal tampon, active participation in some sports and in some women the hymen persists even after coitus.

**64.** The correct answer is option (d) as **FSH** is a gonadotropin **affecting ovarian follicles in** females and causing their growth but in males **LH affects Leydig cells** leading to secretion of androgens.
Growing ovarian follicles secrete estrogen in females while interstitial cells secrete androgen in male human being.
Hence, Assertion is false and Reason is true.

**65.** Correct answer is option (a).
Breast-feeding during initial period of infant growth is highly recommended by doctors for bringing a healthy baby as colostrum contains several antibodies absolutely necessary to develop resistance for the new born baby.

**66.** The correct answer is option no. (a).

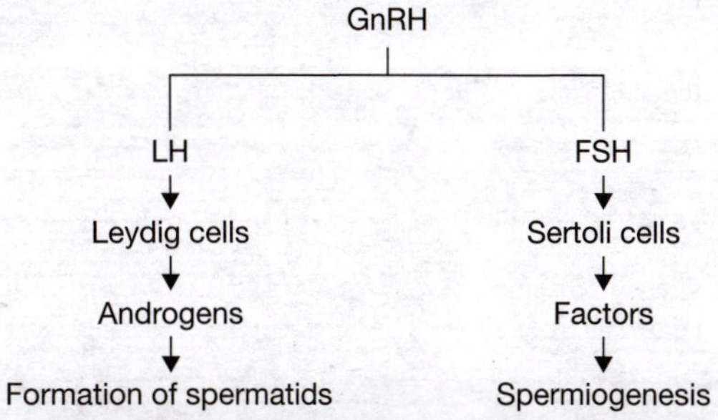


(A) FSH (follicle stimulating hormone) is secreted by anterior pituitary
(B) Leydig cells (interstitial cells) which are found in the interstitial space outside of the seminiferous tubules in testis.
(C) Sertoli cells or sustentacular cells are found inside the seminiferous tubules secrete some factors which help in process of spermiogenesis
(D) Spermiogenesis is a process that helps in transformation of spermatids into spermatozoa.

# 9

# Reproductive Health

**LEARNING OBJECTIVES**

- Discuss the major problems associated with the reproductive health.
- Understand the importance of Family planning and sex education
- Know more about the sources, causes, prevention: Sexually transmitted diseases and Infections (STIs)
- Learn about the child immunization programme
- Learn more about the various contraceptive methods

## Chapter Overview

### Introduction

- According to the **World Health Organization (WHO):** Reproductive health means a total well-being in all aspects of reproduction, i.e., physical, emotional, behavioural and social. Thus, the persons having physically and functionally normal reproductive organs, and normal emotional and behavioral interactions among them in all sex related aspects may be called reproductively healthy.

### Reproductive Health—Problems and Strategies

- In India, **'Family planning programmes'** were initiated in **1951**. Later, improved program like **Reproductive and Child Health Care (RCH)** was launched with following objectives: The major objectives of these programmes are to create awareness among people about various aspects related to reproduction and to provide facilities and support for building up a reproductively healthy society.

  **Strategies**:
  - **Awareness about reproduction**
  - **Sex education**
  - **Adolescence related changes and STDs**
  - **Birth control and care of mother and child**
  - **Sex abuse and sex related crimes**
  - **Infrastructural facilities and material support**
- Statutory **ban on amniocentesis** (a foetal sex determination test) proves to be an important legal check on increasing female foeticides. In **amniocentesis** some of the amniotic fluid of the developing foetus is taken to analyse the foetal cells and dissolved substances. This procedure is used to test for the presence of certain **genetic disorders such as down's syndrome, haemophilia, sickle-cell anaemia**, etc., determine the survivability of the foetus.

### Population Stabilization and Birth Control

- **Population Stabilization and Birth Control**
  - **World population:** 2 billion (2000 million) in 1900 which increased to about 6 billion in 2000 and 7.2 billion in 2011.

---

Refer NCERT Ch 3: Reproductive Health

- **Population of India:** 350 million in 1947 which crossed 1 billion in 2000 and crossed 1.2 billion in May 2011. According to the 2011 census report, the population growth rate was less than two percent, i.e., 20/1000/year, a rate at which our population could increase rapidly.
- A rapid decline in death rate, maternal mortality rate (MMR) and infant mortality rate (IMR) and an increase in number of people in reproducible age have contributed to the increasing population.
- Government has taken various measures to check the increasing population:
  (a) To motivate smaller families to use various contraceptive methods (most important method).
  (b) Many urban couples have adopted 'one child norm'.
  (c) Marriageable age of the female is increased to 18 years and that of males is increased to 21 years.
  (d) Incentives are given to the couples with small families.
  (e) Advertisement of **Slogan: Hum Do Hamare Do** (we two, our two).

## Contraception

- An ideal contraceptive should be user-friendly, effective easily available, reversible with no or least side-effects and should not interfere with the sexual drive or act.
- **Birth Control Methods:**
  - The contraceptive methods are divided into following categories:
    (i) Natural/traditional methods
    (ii) Barrier methods
    (iii) Intra uterine devices (IUDs)
    (iv) Oral contraceptives
    (v) Injectable and implants
    (vi) Surgical methods
- **Natural methods**
  - These are natural methods that work on the principle of avoiding the meeting of ovum and sperm.
    **(a) Periodic abstinence** is a method in which a couple avoids or abstains from coitus from day 10–17 of the menstrual cycle, when ovulation is expected to occur.
    **(b) Coitus interruptus** or withdrawal is a method in which male partner withdraws his penis from the vagina just before ejaculation to avoid insemination.
    **(c) Lactational amenorrhea** is based on the principle that during the period of lactation after parturition, ovulation does not occur.
- **Barrier methods**
  - These methods prevent the contact of sperm and ovum with the help of barriers. Such methods are available for both males and females.
    **(a) Condoms** are barriers made of thin rubber/latex sheath used to cover the penis in the male or vagina and cervix in females **(Fig. 9.1)**. It prevents the deposition of ejaculated semen into the vagina of the female.**'Nirodh':** Popular brand of condom for the male. **Additional benefit: Protection from STDs and AIDS.**
    **(b) Diaphragms, cervical caps and vaults (Fig. 9.2)** are the barriers made of rubber that are inserted into the female reproductive tract to cover the cervix during coitus. They prevent the entry of sperms through cervix.
    **(c) Spermicidal creams, jellies and foams** are used along with these barriers to increase their contraceptive efficiency.

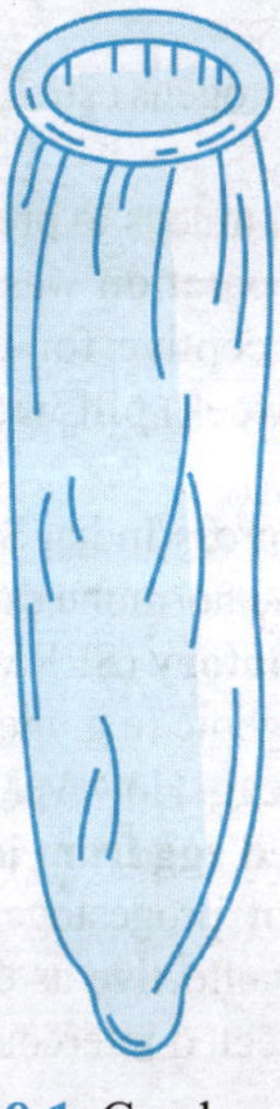

FIGURE 9.1 Condom for male

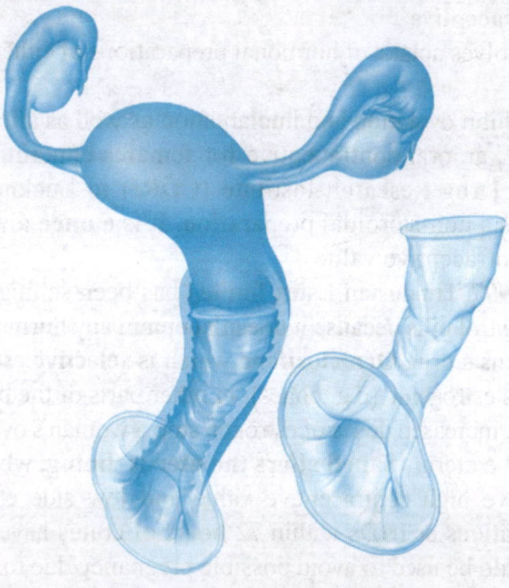

FIGURE 9.2 Condom for female

- **Intra uterine devices (IUDs)**
  - These devices are inserted by doctors in the uterus through vagina. In India, it is one of most widely accepted methods of contraception **(Fig. 9.3)**.
  - There are three types of IUDs available:
    **(a) Non-medicated IUDs:** These increase phagocytosis of sperms within the uterus, e.g., Lippes loop.
    **(b) Copper releasing IUDs:** Along with phagocytosis of sperms, the copper ions released suppress sperm motility and fertilizing capacity of sperms, e.g., **CuT, Cu 7 and Multiload 375.**
    **(c) Hormone releasing IUDs:** These make the uterus unsuitable for implantation and the cervix hostile to sperms, e.g., **Progestasert, LNG-20.**

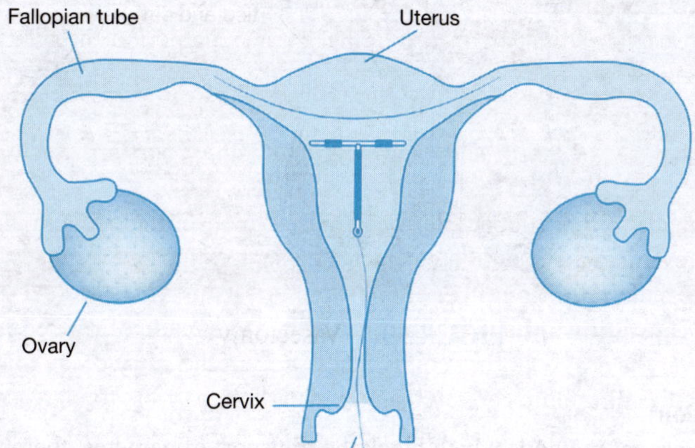


FIGURE 9.3 Intra-Uterine Devices

- **Oral contraceptive**
  - This involves uptake of hormonal preparations of either progestogens or progestogens estrogen combinations in the form of pills.
  - They inhibit ovulation and implantation as well as after the quality of cervical mucus to prevent entry of sperms.
  - 'Saheli', an oral contraceptive for females containing a non-steroidal preparation was developed by scientists at Central Drug Research Institute (CDRI) in Lucknow. A new oral contraceptive for the female named **'Saheli'** contains a non-steroidal preparation. It is a **once a week** (taken once in a week) pill with very few side effects and high contraceptive value.
  - Since 1997, Hindustan Latex limited has been selling Saheli to women all across India. Saheli is different from other birth control pills because it doesn't contain any hormones. Instead of using the hormone estrogen to prevent pregnancy, it contains a drug **Ormeloxifene** which is **selective estrogen receptor modulatory** (SERM). In some parts of body its action is estrogenic (e.g. bones), in other parts of the body its action antiestrogenic (e.g. uterus, breasts).
  - Usually, increased doses of estrogen stop a woman's ovaries from releasing an egg. However, by blocking estrogen receptors in the uterus, **Saheli alters the uterus' lining, which prevents a fertilized egg from implanting.**
  - Pills have high contraceptive value and few side effects. Administration of progestogens or progestogen estrogen combinations or IUDs within 72 hours of coitus have been found to be very effective as emergency contraceptives as they could be used to avoid possible pregnancy due to a rape or casual unprotected intercourse.
- **Injections and implants**
  - Progestogens or progestogen-estrogen combination can also be used by females as injections or implants under the skin.
  - Their mode of action is similar to that of pills but their effective periods are longer.

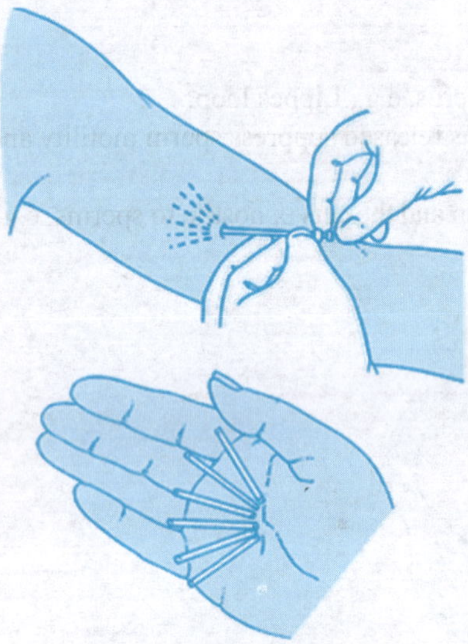

FIGURE 9.4 Implants

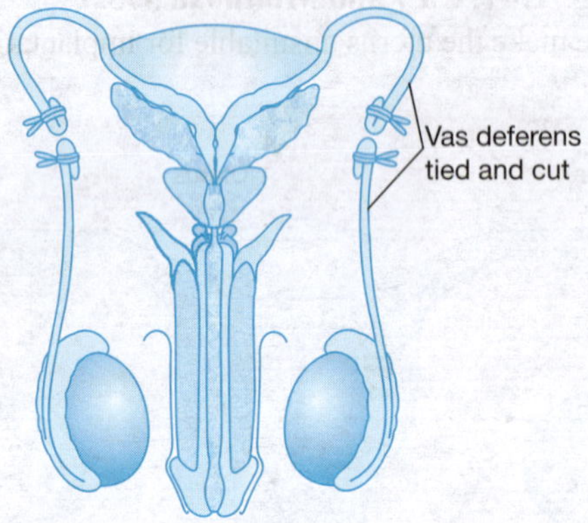


FIGURE 9.5 Vasectomy

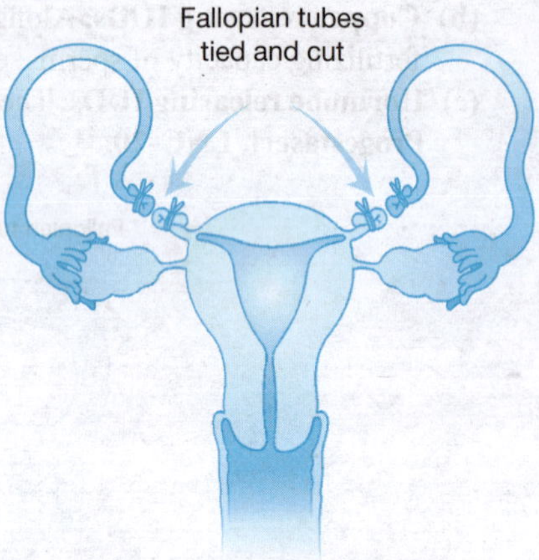


FIGURE 9.6 Tubectomy

- **Surgical methods (Sterilization)**
  - These are terminal and permanent methods which block the transport of gametes, thereby preventing conception.
  - In males, a small part of the vas deferens is removed and tied up through a small incision on the scrotum. This is called **vasectomy (Fig. 9.5)**.

    In females, a small part of the fallopian tube is removed and tied up through a small incision in the abdomen or vagina. This is called **tubectomy (Fig. 9.6).**
- **Side-effects of contraceptive methods:** Although not significant and involves nausea, breakthrough bleeding, abdominal pain, irregular menstrual bleeding, breast cancer, etc.

- **Emergency contraception:** Emergency contraception is used to avoid possible pregnancy due to a rape or casual unprotected intercourse. It can be done by using either of the following within 72 hours of coitus.
  (1) Administration of **progestogens** or **progestogen-estrogen** combinations.
  (2) **IUDs**

## Medical Termination of Pregnancy (MTP)

- **MTP** (or **induced abortion**) is intentional or voluntary termination of pregnancy before full term.
- About 45 to 50 million MTPs are done in a year all over the world (l/5th of the total conceived pregnancies in a year).
- Government of India has legalised MTP in 1971 with some strict conditions.
- The Medical Termination of Pregnancy (Amendment) Act, 2017 was enacted by the government of India with the intension of reducing the incidence of illegal abortion and consequent maternal mortality and morbidity. According to this Act, a pregnancy may be terminated on certain considered grounds within the first 12 weeks of pregnancy on the opinion of one registered medical practitioner. If the pregnancy has lasted more than 12 weeks, but fewer than 24 weeks, two registered medical practitioners must be of the opinion, formed in good faith, that the required ground exist. The grounds for such termination of pregnancies are: (i) The continuation of the pregnancy would involve a risk to the life of the pregnant woman or of grave injury physical or mental health: or (ii) There is a substantial risk that of the child were born, it would suffer from such physical or mental abnormalities as to be seriously handicapped.

## Sexually Transmitted Infections (STIs)

- Infections or diseases which are transmitted through sexual intercourse are collectively called **sexually transmitted infections (STIs) or venereal diseases (VD) or reproductive tract infections (RTI).**
- **Examples are: Gonorrhoea, Syphilis, Genital herpes, Chlamydiasis, Genital warts, Trichomoniasis, Hepatitis-B** and **AIDS.**
- AIDS is most dangerous STI. STIs are completely curable if detected early and treated properly. **Hepatitis-B, Genital herpes** and **AIDS** are **incurable.**
- STIs are very common among persons of age group— 15 to 24 years.
- **General symptoms of STIs: Early symptoms:** Itching, fluid discharge, slight pain, swellings, etc., in the genital region. Often the infected females may remain asymptomatic. Later complications include **pelvic inflammatory diseases (PID)**, abortions, still births, infertility, ectopic pregnancies, cancer of the reproductive tract, etc.
- In addition to sexual transmission, **AIDS** and **Hepatitis–B** can also be transmitted by:
  - Sharing needles and surgical instruments.
  - Transfusion of blood.
  - Infected mother to the foetus.
- STIs can be prevented by the following principles:
  - Avoid sex/intercourse with unknown partners/multiple partners.
  - Always use condoms during coitus.
  - Any doubtful situation, should be consulted with a qualified doctor so that early detection and complete treatment taken care of.

## Infertility

- There are many couples who are infertile or are unable to produce children in spite of unprotected sexual activities. Thus, 'the inability to conceive or produce children even after 2 years of unprotected sexual cohabitation is called infertility'.
- There are many reasons for infertility. These reasons may be physical, congenital, diseases, drugs, immunological or even psychological. Presently, there are specialized health care units (infertility clinics, etc.) in our country, which could help in diagnosis and corrective treatment of some of the infertility related disorders, and enable the childless couples to have children.

- The childless couples are assisted to have children through certain special techniques commonly called **Assisted Reproductive Technologies (ART).** Some important ARTs are described below.

**1. In Vitro Fertilization (IVF)**

- It involves fertilization of ovum outside the body (in almost similar conditions as that in the body) followed by **Embryo Transfer (ET).** This technique is popularly known as 'test-tube baby' programme. In this technique, ova from the wife/donor female and sperms from the husband/donor male are collected and are induced to get fuse to form zygote under simulated conditions in the laboratory.
- The zygote can divide (undergo cleavage). The zygote or early embryos (with upto 8 blastomeres) is then transferred into the fallopian tube. It is called **Zygote Intra Fallopian Transfer (ZIFT).**
- If the embryo is with more than 8 blastomeres, it is transferred into the uterus. It is called **Intra Uterine Transfer (IUT).** The transferred embryos complete their further developed within the uterus.
- It is to be noted that in test tube baby programme, the baby is not reared in the test tube. The success rate of this technique of producing test tube babies is less than 20%.
- The embryo formed by **in vivo fertilization** i.e., fusion of gametes within the female can be used for such transfer to assist such **females who cannot conceive** due to one reason or the other.
- The world's first test tube baby was **Louise Joy Brown**, was born on July 25, 1978 in Oldham, Lancashire, England. The Indian's first test tube baby was **Kum Harsha**. She was born on August 6, 1986 at K.E.M. Hospital, Mumbai with the help of **Dr. Idra Hinduja**.

**2. Gamete Intra Fallopian Transfer (GIFT)**

- In this technique, ovum is collected from a donor female and is transferred into the fallopian tube of another female who cannot produce the ovum, but can provide suitable environment for fertilization and further development of embryo.
- Such transfer of the ovum is called **'Gamete Intra Fallopian Transfer' or (GIFT)**.

**3. Intra-Cytoplasmic Sperm Injection (ICSI)**

- In this technique a sperm is directly injected into the ovum under appropriate conditions in the laboratory.

**4. Artificial Insemination (AI)**

- It is a technique by which the infertility cases of male partner either due to inability to inseminate the female or due to very low sperm counts in the ejaculates could be corrected. In artificial insemination, the semen collected either from the husband or a healthy donor is artificially introduced either into the vagina or into the uterus of the female.
- The introduction of the semen directly into the uterus is termed as **Intra-Uterine Insemination (IUI).**
- Presently, many options are available to deal with the problems of infertility, but all these techniques require expensive instrumentation and handling by specialized professionals having high precision.
- Therefore, there are only few such centres in the country and hence their benefits are affordable to only a limited number of people.
- The adoption of these methods is also interfered by emotional, religious and social factors. The ultimate aim of these procedures is to have children. In country like ours, there are so many orphaned and destitute children.
- Adoption of such children, which is also permitted by our country's law, could be one of the best methods for couples looking for parenthood.

# PRACTICE EXERCISES

**Direction:** Read the question carefully and choose the correct option for each.

## Multiple Choice Questions: Level I

### Reproductive Health

1. What is the full form of WHO?
(a) Ware House Organization
(b) War and Health Organization
(c) World Health Office
(d) World Health Organization

2. What are the various aspects of reproduction covered by WHO?
(a) Physical, Emotional, Behavioural
(b) Physical, Emotional, Behavioural, Social
(c) Physical, Emotional, Gestational, Social
(d) Physical, Emotional, Social

3. Which was the first country in the world to initiate a nationwide programme for reproductive health?
(a) China (b) USA (c) India (d) Russia

4. The figure indicates which contraceptive device?

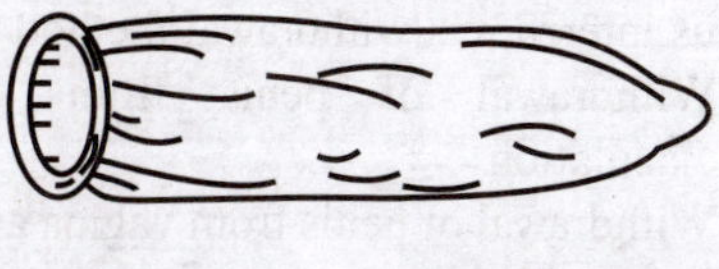

(a) Condom for female (b) Condom for male
(c) Diaphragm (d) Cervical cap

5. The programme of '*Family Planning*' was initiated in the year ________.
(a) 1950 (b) 1947 (c) 1949 (d) 1951

6. The reproductive program RCH stands for
(a) Reproductive and Community Health Care
(b) Restorative and Communal Health Care
(c) Reproductive and Child Health Care
(d) Reproductive and Congenital Health Care

7. In context of reproductive health, STD stands for
(a) Sexually Terminal Disease
(b) Sexually Transmitted Disease
(c) Sexually Transformed Disease
(d) Sexually Transducted Disease

8. The fluid which envelops the developing foetus is called
(a) Chorionic fluid (b) Placental fluid
(c) Amniotic fluid (d) Uterine fluid

9. Statutory ban has been laid on ________ to check female foeticide.
(a) Choriocentesis (b) Amniocentesis
(c) Uterocentesis (d) Embryocentesis

10. The amniocentesis test is based on ________ to determine the sex of developing foetus.
(a) External genitalia
(b) Secondary sexual characters
(c) Chromosomal pattern
(d) Embryonic enzymes

11. WHO refers reproductive health as
(a) Physically healthy reproductive organ
(b) Functionally healthy reproductive organ
(c) Normal emotional and behavioural interaction among people in all sex related aspects.
(d) All the above

12. In 2011 the world population and Indian population was:
(a) 7.2 billion and 1 billion respectively
(b) 6 billion and 1.2 billion respectively
(c) 7.2 billion and 1.2 billion respectively
(d) 6 billion and 1 billion respectively

13. Every ________ person in the world is an Indian.
(a) 4th (b) 6th (c) 8th (d) 10th

### Birth Control Method

14. What is shown in the figure?

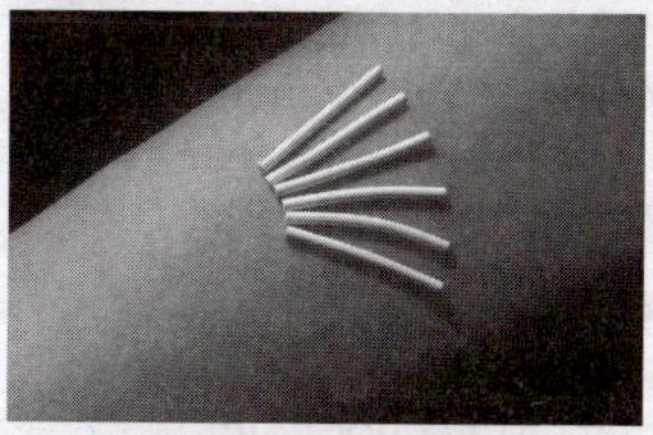

(a) Copper T (b) Implants
(c) Stents (d) Vault

15. 'Saheli', oral contraceptive for the females was developed by which institute?
(a) CDRI, Lucknow (b) NBG, Lucknow
(c) Kazari, Jodhpur (d) NIV, Pune

**16.** The following are indicative signs which indicate improved reproductive health of society. Choose the correct combination.
 (i) Better awareness about sex related problem
 (ii) Better detection and cure of STDs
 (iii) Better postnatal care
 (iv) Increased number of couples with large families
 (a) i and iv only (b) ii, iii and iv only
 (c) i and ii only (d) i, ii and iii only

**17.** CDRI, Lucknow developed which new female contraceptive?
 (a) 'Sakhi' (b) 'Saheli'
 (c) 'Saloni' (d) 'Smiti'

**18.** CDRI stands for
 (a) Contraceptive Drug Research Institute
 (b) Central District Research Institute
 (c) Central Drug Research Institute
 (d) Central Dermatologic Research Institute

**19.** The world population was 2000 million in the year
 (a) 1980 (b) 1970 (c) 1960 (d) 1900

**20.** Which IUD is shown in the given figure?

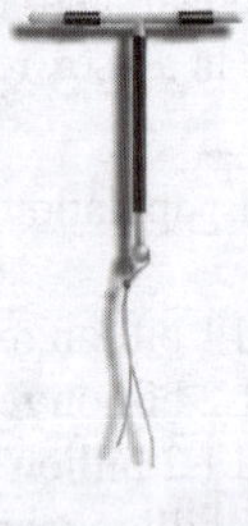

 (a) Lippes loop (b) Progestasert
 (c) Copper T (d) Multiload-375

**21.** By the year 2000, the world population rocketed to
 (a) 6 million (b) 6 billion
 (c) 6 trillion (d) 600 million

**22.** MMR stands for
 (a) Magnetic Maxima Resonance
 (b) Mortality Memorandum Rate
 (c) Mortality Maternal Rate
 (d) Maternal Mortality Rate

**23.** IMR stands for
 (a) Indigenous Mortality Rate
 (b) Infant Migratory Rate
 (c) Infant Mortality Rate
 (d) Infant Mitigation Rate

**24.** According to 2011 census report, our population growth rate was less than
 (a) 1% (b) 2% (c) 0.5% (d) 0.2%

**25.** Smaller families can be encouraged by using various
 (a) Educational methods (b) Contraceptive methods
 (c) Abortive methods (d) Rhythm method

**26.** A wise way to encourage small families is by raising the marriageable age of female to ________ years and that of male to ________ years respectively.
 (a) 16, 18 (b) 18, 20
 (c) 18, 21 (d) 17, 22

**27.** Many couples in the urban working areas have adopted the ________ norm.
 (a) Two child (b) One child
 (c) No child (d) Three child

**28.** Identity the characteristic which an ideal contraceptive should not have.
 (a) User friendly (b) Easily available
 (c) Non reversible (d) Least side effect

**29.** A natural method of contraception, periodic abstinence is
 (a) Abstaining from coitus from day 1 to 5 of the menstrual cycle.
 (b) Abstaining from coitus from day 17 to 22 of the menstrual cycle.
 (c) Abstaining from coitus from day 10 to 17 of the menstrual cycle.
 (d) Abstaining from coitus from day 5 to 10 of the menstrual cycle.

**30.** Coitus interruptus/withdrawal method concerns with
 (a) Withdrawal of penis from vagina before ejaculation
 (b) Withdrawal of penis from vagina after ejaculation
 (c) Prevention of coitus
 (d) Alternate prevention of coitus

**31.** After parturition, which natural contraception way can be utilized?
 (a) Lactational menorrhea
 (b) Lactational amenorrhea
 (c) Lactational deficiency
 (d) Lactational prevention

**32.** The figure indicates which contraceptive device?

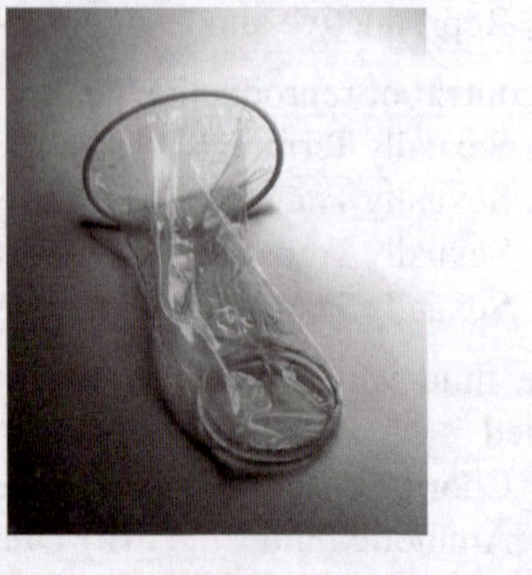

(a) Condom for female
(b) Condom for male
(c) Diaphragm
(d) Cervical cap

**33.** In lactational amenorrhea, which event does not occur in menstrual cycle?
(a) Follicular phase (b) Ovulation
(c) Luteal phase (d) All of these

**34.** Lactational amenorrhea is effective only up to a maximum of ________ months.
(a) Two (b) Four
(c) Six (d) Eight

**35.** In the ________ method of contraception ovum and sperms are prevented from physically meeting by the use of a membranous sheath.
(a) Barrier (b) Sterilization
(c) Natural (d) Pills

**36.** ________ is a popular brand of condom for males.
(a) 'Nishodh' (b) 'Nirodh'
(c) 'Nidosh' (d) 'Nirdosh'

**37.** Which of the following is not applicable to females for contraception?
(a) Diaphragms (b) Vasectomy
(c) Condoms (d) Cervical caps

**38.** Multiload 375 is a
(a) Disease resistant crop
(b) New viral vector
(c) Intrauterine Device
(d) Biological warfare device

**39.** IUD stands for
(a) Intra Ureter Device
(b) Intrinsic Uterine Device
(c) Intrauterine Device
(d) Intra Urinogenital Device

**40.** Lippes loop is a
(a) Structure associated with nephron
(b) Structure associated with male reproductive system
(c) Structure associated with ligamentous tissue
(d) A non-medicated IUD

**41.** Which of the following is a copper releasing IUD?
(a) CUT (b) Multiload 375
(c) Cu 7 (d) All of these

**42.** Progestasert is a
(a) Oral contraceptive (b) Natural contraceptive
(c) Hormonal IUD (d) Implant contraceptive

**43.** LNG-20 is a
(a) Fuel (b) Modified crop
(c) Hormonal IUD (d) Cu releasing IUD

**44.** Which of the following is a most widely used contraceptive in India?
(a) IUD (b) Pills
(c) Barrier method (d) Natural method

**45.** The pills used by females to prevent conception contain
(a) Only oestrogen
(b) Only progestogen
(c) Combination of oestrogen progestogen
(d) Both (b) and (c)

**46.** The 'Pills' have to be taken for contraception continuously for a period ________ days.
(a) 22 (b) 21 (c) 24 (d) 25

**47.** Oral pills work by
(a) Inhibiting ovulation
(b) Inhibiting implantation
(c) Altering the quality of mucus
(d) All of these

**48.** Which procedure is carried out in the below figure and which portion of male reproductive organ is cut and ligated.

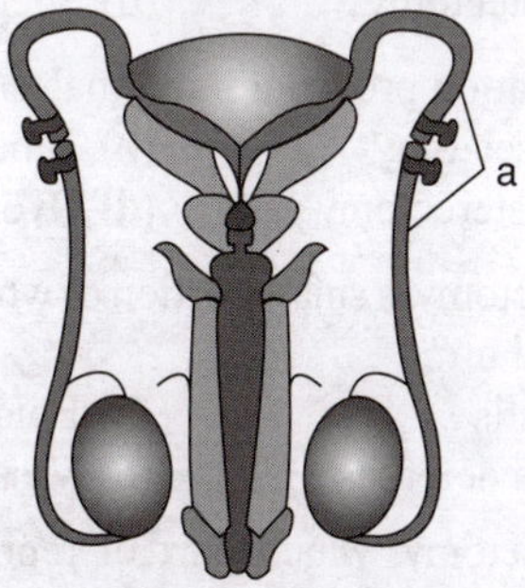


(a) Vasectomy, Vas deferens
(b) Tubectomy, Urethra
(c) Vasectomy, Rete testis
(d) vasectomy, Vasa efferentia

**49.** 'Saheli', the new oral contraceptive for females, contains a ________ preparation.
(a) Steroidal (b) Peptide
(c) Non steroidal (d) Inorganic

**50.** 'Saheli' is a/an ________ contraceptive pill.
(a) Emergency (b) Once a week
(c) 72 hour (d) Once a month

**51.** Apart from pills of progestogen alone or in combination with oestrogen, which other means can be used for contraception?
(a) Implants (b) Injections
(c) Syrups (d) Both (a) and (b)

**52.** Emergency contraceptive should be under which of the following conditions

(a) Casual unprotected intercourse
(b) In conjunction with pills
(c) Rape
(d) Both (a) and (c)

**56.** Emergency contraceptive should be used within ________ hours of unprotected intercourse.
(a) 48 (b) 72 (c) 36 (d) 86

**54.** To prevent further pregnancies, a surgical method called ________ is advised for male/female partner as a means of contraception.
(a) Radiation (b) Sterilization
(c) Abortion (d) Neutralization

**55.** Surgical method for terminal contraception work on which of the following grounds?
(a) Block gamete transport
(b) Block gamete generation
(c) Alter biochemical nature of gamete
(d) Destroys gamete permanently

**56.** Sterilization procedure in males is known as
(a) Tubectomy (b) Vasectomy
(c) Testectomy (d) Spermectomy

**57.** Sterilization procedure in females is known as
(a) Vasectomy (b) Tubectomy
(c) Hysterectomy (d) Ovotomy

**58.** In vasectomy, a small portion of which duct is removed and tied up?
(a) Testis (b) Epididymis
(c) Vas deferens (d) Vasa efferentia

**59.** In tubectomy, which part of reproductive system is removed and/or tied up?
(a) Cervix (b) Oviduct
(c) Uterus (d) Ovary

**60.** Which of the following is/are the ill-effect/effects of using contraceptives?
(a) Abdominal pain
(b) Breast cancer
(c) Irregular menstrual bleeding
(d) All of these

**61.** Which procedure is carried out in the below figure and which portion of female reproductive organ is cut and ligated.

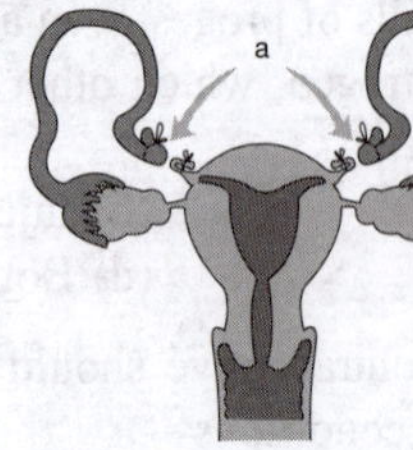


(a) Tubectomy, Fallopian tube
(b) Tubectomy, uterus
(c) Vasectomy, Fallopian tube
(d) vasectomy, Vasa efferentia

**62.** Full form of RCH is
(a) Reproduction and Contraception Hazard
(b) Reproductive and Child Health Care
(c) Research and Care Development
(d) Reproductive Community Health Centre

**63.** India's population grew from 350 million to a billion in 2000 mainly due to
(i) Rapid decline in death rate (MMR and IMR).
(ii) Increase in number of people in reproducecible age group.
(iii) Increase in number of people in post-reproductive age group.
(a) (iii) only
(b) (i) and (iii) only
(c) (i) and (ii) only
(d) (i) only

**64.** Motivation for smaller families in India can be provided by
(a) Slogans like 'Hum Do Hamare Do'.
(b) Raising marriageable age (female–18 years and male–21 years).
(c) Giving incentive to couples with small families.
(d) All the above

**65.** An ideal contraceptive should be
(A) User-friendly
(B) Easily available
(C) Effective and reversible
(D) With nor or least side-effects
(a) A, B and C only (b) A and D only
(c) B and C only (d) All

## MTP, STD and Infertility

**66.** Intentional or voluntary termination of pregnancy before full term is called ________.
(a) Medical transformation of pregnancy
(b) Median terminal pregnancy
(c) Medical Termination of Pregnancy
(d) None of these

**67.** Nearly ________ MTPs are preformed in a year all over the world.
(a) 45 to 50 billion
(b) 45 to 50 million
(c) 45 to 50 thousands
(d) 45 to 50 lacs

**68.** Government of India legalized MTP in the year ________.

(a) 1970 (b) 1971 (c) 1972 (d) 1973

**69.** MTPs are considered relatively safe during ________ trimester of pregnancy.

(a) 1st (b) 2nd
(c) 3rd (d) None of these

**70.** MTPs are harmful to mother and foetus during ________ trimester of pregnancy.

(a) 1st (b) 2nd
(c) 3rd (d) None of these

**71.** Misuse of amniocentesis has led to the misuse of ________.

(a) MTP (b) STD
(c) RTI (d) HIV

**72.** Sexually transmitted diseases are also known as

(a) Venereal disease
(b) Vulnerable diseases
(c) Reproductive tract infections
(d) Both (a) and (c)

**73.** Which infections can be transmitted by sharing of injection needles, surgical instruments, etc., with infected persons; through transfusion of blood, or from an infected mother to the foetus?

(a) AIDS (b) Hepatitis B
(c) Genital herpes (d) Both (a) and (b)

**74.** Which of the following STD is not completely curable?

(a) Gonorrhoea (b) Genital warts
(c) Genital herpes (d) Chlamydiasis

**75.** Which of these options is correct with regards to statements X and Y?

**Statement X:** Some STDs do not show symptoms in females.

**Statement Y:** Some STDs in females may remain undetected for long time.

(a) Statement 'X' and 'Y' are correct and 'X' is the correct explanation for 'Y'.
(b) Only statement 'X' is correct.
(c) Only statement 'Y' is correct.
(d) Statement 'X' and 'Y' are correct.

**76.** Severe complications of STDs lead to further complications like

(a) Abortion (b) Still birth
(c) Ectopic pregnancy (d) All of these

**77.** The age group of ________ years is quite vulnerable to STDs.

(a) 10 to 19 (b) 15 to 22
(c) 17 to 27 (d) 15 to 24

**78.** In order to prevent STDs, one of the following is not correct?

(a) Avoid sex with unknown partners/multiple partners.
(b) Go to an unqualified doctor at earliest instance of STD.
(c) Always use condoms during coitus.
(d) Participate in sex education sessions.

**79.** The reasons for infertility can be

(a) Physical (b) Diseases
(c) Psychological (d) All of these

**80.** In India, which gender is generally wrongly blamed for being infertile?

(a) Woman
(b) Man
(c) Either man or woman
(d) Genetic factors

**81.** In India, most of the infertility cases are because of the

(a) Male (b) Female
(c) Either (a) and (b) (d) Hereditary disorders

**82.** In order to combat infertility, special techniques are used like ________.

(a) Stimulated reproductive technologies
(b) Assisted reproductive technologies
(c) Fertile reproductive technologies
(d) In vitro fertilization

**83.** Fertilization outside the body in almost similar conditions as that in the body is termed as

(a) In vitro fertilization (b) Ex vivo fertilization
(c) In vivo fertilization (d) Ex vitro fertilization

**84.** Which of the following defines 'Test Tube Baby' correctly?

(a) Ova and sperms are collected and mixed in test tube to form zygote.
(b) Ova and sperms are centrifuged in test tube to form zygote.
(c) Ova and sperms are induced to form zygote under controlled condition.
(d) Embryogenesis is allowed to continue in test tube under controlled conditions.

**85.** Under ZIFT procedure, zygote or embryos, with up to 8 blastomeres can be transferred into the

(a) Uterus (b) Placenta
(c) Fallopian tube (d) Cervix

**86.** Transfer of an ovum from a donor to another female who can provide a suitable environment for fertilization is called

(a) ZIFT (b) GIFT
(c) ICSI (d) IUT

**87.** Intracytoplasmic sperm injection is a specialized procedure in which the sperm is directly injected into the ________.
(a) Ovary (b) Fallopian tube
(c) Ovum (d) Uterus

**88.** In artificial insemination, the semen from husband/ healthy donor is artificially introduced into the ________.
(a) Vagina (b) Oviduct
(c) Uterus (d) Both (a) and (c)

## Multiple Choice Questions: Level II

**89.** Given below are four methods (A–D) and their row action (i–iv) in achieving contraception. Select their co matching from the four options that follow.

| Method | Mode of Action |
|---|---|
| (A) The pill | (i) Prevents sperms reaching cervix |
| (B) Condom | (ii) Prevents implantation |
| (C) Vasectomy | (iii) Prevents ovulation |
| (D) Copper T | (iv) Semen contains no sperms |

(a) A – (iii), B – (iv), C (i), D – (ii)
(b) A – (ii), B – (iii), C – (i), D – (iv)
(c) A – (iii), B – (i), C – (iv), D – (ii)
(d) A – (iv), B – (i), C – (ii), D – (iii)

**90.** Consider the statements given below regarding contraception and answer as directed thereafter:
(A) Medical termination of pregnancy (MTP) during first trimester is generally safe.
(B) Generally, chances of conception are nil until mother breastfeeds the infant up to two years.
(C) Intrauterine devices like copper-T are effective contraceptives.
(D) Contraception pills may be taken up to one week after coitus to prevent conception.

Which two of the above statements are correct?
(a) A, C (b) A, B
(c) B, C (d) C, D

**91.** In the human female, menstruation can be deferred by the administration of
(a) combination of FSH and LH
(b) combination of estrogen and progesterone
(c) FSH only
(d) LH only

**92.** Certain characteristic demographic features of developing countries are
(a) high fertility, low or rapidly falling mortality rate, rapid population growth and very young age distribution.
(b) high fertility, high density, rapidly rising mortality rate and very young age distribution.
(c) high infant mortality, low fertility, uneven population growth and very young age distribution
(d) high mortality, high density, uneven population growth and very old age distribution

**93.** Copper-T is a device that prevents
(a) implantation of blastocyst
(b) ovulation
(c) fertilization
(d) egg maturation

**94.** Correctly match sexually transmitted disease with its pathogen
(a) Syphilis– *Treponema pallidum*
(b) AIDS– *Bacillus anthracis*
(c) Urethritis– *Entamoeba gingivalis*
(d) Gonorrhoea–*Leishmania donovani*

**95.** Amniocentesis is a technique
(a) by which the essential amino acids in the body can be estimated
(b) by which any chromosomal anomalies in the foetus can be detected
(c) in which the sex of' the foetus can be reversed
(d) that can be used for correcting genetic disorders of the foetus

**96.** The population of the world in year 1999 was about
(a) 500 million (b) 100 billion
(c) 6 billion (d) 15 billion

**97.** Test-tube baby is one who
(a) is born out of artificial insemination
(b) has undergone development in a test tube
(c) is born out of *in vitro* fertilization
(d) has been developed without fertilization

**98.** Human population growth in India
(a) tends to follow a sigmoid curve as in case of many other animal species.
(b) tends to reach zero growth as in case of some animal species.
(c) can be reduced by permitting natural calamities and enforcing birth control measures.
(d) can be regulated by following national programme of family planning.

**99.** In India, human population is heavily weighted towards the younger age groups as a result of
(a) short life span of many individuals and low birth rate.
(b) long life span of many individuals and low birth rate.
(c) short life span of many individuals and high birth rate.
(d) long life span of many individuals and high birth rate.

## A & R and Statement-based Questions

### Assertion and Reason Questions:

***Direction for questions 100 to 104:*** *Read the* ***assertion*** *and* ***reason*** *carefully to mark the correct option out of the options given below:*

**(a)** **(A)** is **true** but **(R)** is **false**.
**(b)** **(A)** is **false** but **(R)** is **true**.
**(c)** Both **(A)** and **(R)** is **true** and **(R)** is the correct explanation of **(A)**.
**(d)** Both **(A)** and **(R)** is **true** and **(R)** is not the correct explanation of **(A)**.

**100.** **Assertion:** There is statuary ban on amniocentesis for sex determination.
**Reason:** There is increase is female foeticides.

**101.** **Assertion:** There is decrease in maternal & infant mortality ratio now a days.
**Reason:** Better awareness about sex related matter, increased number of medical assisted deliveries and better post-natal care leading to it.

**102.** **Assertion:** We can prevent STIs by use of diaphragms during coitus.
**Reason:** Diaphragms are type of barrier contraceptives.

**103.** **Assertion:** IUDs can be used as emergency contraceptives.
**Reason:** IUDs are most accepted method of contraception in India.

**104.** **Assertion:** Amniocentesis is use to detect genetic disorder like haemophilia in foetus.
**Reason:** Amniocentesis is ART.

### Statement-based Questions:

***Direction for questions 105 to 109:*** *These type of questions consist of two statement each, printed as* **Statement-I** *and* **Statement-II**. *While answering such questions, a student is needed to choose any one of the following four responses.*

**(a)** **Statement I** is **correct Statement II** is **incorrect**.
**(b)** **Statement I** is **incorrect Statement II** is **correct**.
**(c)** Both **Statement I** and **Statement II** are **correct**.
**(d)** Both **Statement I** and **Statement II** are **incorrect**.

**105.** **Statement-I:** IUI is used as contraceptives.
**Statement-II:** IUI releases copper ion.

**106.** **Statement-I:** Trichomoniasis can be completely curable, if detected early and treated properly.
**Statement-II:** Trichomoniasis is fungal disease.

**107.** **Statement-I:** GIFT is gamete Intra Fallopian Transfer, done in those female which cannot produce ovum.
**Statement-II:** Reason for infertility may be physical, psychological and immunological.

**108.** **Statement-I:** In AI, semen can be taken from either husband or healthy donor.
**Statement-II:** IVF embryo is transfer from uterus to fallopian tube (more than 8 blastomere) for further development.

**109.** **Statement-I:** Inability to conceive or produce children even after years of unprotected sexual cohabitation is called infertility.
**Statement-II:** Lactational amenorrhea is natural method of contraception.

## Matrix-Match Type Questions

**110.** Match the following:

| List-I | List-II |
|---|---|
| 1. Periodic abstinence | (i) Avoid insemination in female |
| 2. Coitus interrupts | (ii) Avoid coitus during fertile period |
| 3. Lactational amenorrhea | (iii) Absence of menstruation during lactation |

**The correct matching is**

| | 1 | 2 | 3 |
|---|---|---|---|
| (a) | (ii) | (i) | (iii) |
| (b) | (iii) | (ii) | (i) |
| (c) | (i) | (iii) | (ii) |
| (d) | (iii) | (i) | (ii) |

**111.** Match the following:

| List-I | List-II |
|---|---|
| 1. Barrier | (i) Pills |
| 2. IUD | (ii) Diaphragms / Condoms / Vaults |
| 3. Injectables | (iii) Vasectomy / Tubectomy |
| 4. Oral | (iv) CuT / Cu7 / Multilod 375 |
| 5. Surgical | (v) Progesteron – estrogen combo |

**The correct matching is**

| | 1 | 2 | 3 | 4 | 5 |
|---|---|---|---|---|---|
| (a) | (ii) | (iv) | (v) | (i) | (iii) |
| (b) | (ii) | (iii) | (iv) | (iv) | (iii) |
| (c) | (i) | (iii) | (ii) | (v) | (iv) |
| (d) | (ii) | (iv) | (v) | (iii) | (i) |

**112.** Match the following:

| List-I (Method) | List-I (Mode of Action) |
|---|---|
| 1. Natural | (i) Suppression of sperm fertility & motility |
| 2. Barrier | (ii) Blocking of gamete transport |
| 3. IUD | (iii) Inhibition of ovulation & Implantation |
| 4. Implants | (iv) Avoid fertile period |
| 5. Surgical | (v) Prevent physical meeting of sperm & ovum |

**The correct matching is**

| | 1 | 2 | 3 | 4 | 5 |
|---|---|---|---|---|---|
| (a) | (iv) | (v) | (i) | (iii) | (ii) |
| (b) | (iii) | (ii) | (i) | (iv) | (v) |
| (c) | (ii) | (iii) | (i) | (v) | (iv) |
| (d) | (ii) | (i) | (iii) | (iv) | (v) |

**113.** Match the following:

| List-I | List-II |
|---|---|
| 1. Non-medicated IUD | (i) Suppress sperm motility and fertility |
| 2. Copper releasing IUD | (ii) Make uterus unsuitable for implantation |
| 3. Hormone releasing IUD | (iii) Phagocytosis of sperms in uterus |

**The correct matching is**

| | 1 | 2 | 3 |
|---|---|---|---|
| (a) | (iii) | (i) | (ii) |
| (b) | (ii) | (i) | (iii) |
| (c) | (i) | (iii) | (ii) |
| (d) | (iii) | (ii) | (i) |

**114.** Match the following:

| List-I | List-II | List-III |
|---|---|---|
| 1. Tubectomy | (i) Female | X. Vas deference |
| 2. Vasectomy | (ii) Male | Y. fallopian tube |

**The correct matching is**

(a) 1 – (i) – Y, 2 – (ii) – X
(b) 1 – (ii) – X, 2 – (i) – Y
(c) 1 – (i) – X, 2 – (ii) – Y
(d) 1 – (ii) – Y, 2 – (i) – X

## NCERT Exemplar Questions

**1.** The method of directly injecting a sperm into ovum in Assisted Reproductive Technology is called
(a) GIFT (b) ZIFT
(c) ICSI (d) ET

**2.** Increased IMR and decreased MMR in a population will
(a) Cause rapid increase in growth rate
(b) Result in the decline in growth rate
(c) Not cause significant change in growth rate
(d) Result in an explosive population

**3.** Intensely lactating mothers do not generally conceive due to the
(a) Suppression of gonadotropins
(b) Hyper secretion of gonadotropins
(c) Suppression of gametic transport
(d) Suppression of fertilization

**4.** Sterilization techniques are generally fool proof methods of contraception with least side effects. Yet, this is the last option for the couples because
i. It is almost irreversible
ii. Of the misconception that it will reduce sexual urge
iii. It is a surgical procedure
iv. Of lack of sufficient facilities in many parts of the country

Choose the correct option:
(a) i and iii (b) ii and iii
(c) ii and iv (d) i, ii, iii and iv

**5.** A national level approach to build up a reproductively healthy society was taken up in our country in
(a) 1950s (b) 1960s (c) 1980s (d) 1990s

**6.** Emergency contraceptives are effective if used within
(a) 72 hours of coitus
(b) 72 hours of ovulation
(c) 72 hours of menstruation
(d) 72 hours of implantation

**7.** Choose the right one among the statements given below:
(a) IUDs are generally inserted by the user herself.
(b) IUDs increase phagocytosis reaction in the uterus.
(c) IUDs suppress gametogenesis.
(d) IUDs once inserted need not be replaced.

**8.** The following statements are given regarding MTP. Choose the correct options given below:
i. MTPs are generally advised during the first trimester.
ii. MTPs are used as a contraceptive method.
iii. MTPs are always surgical.
iv. MTPs require the assistance of qualified medical personnel.
(a) i and iii (b) ii and iii
(c) i and iv (d) and ii

**9.** From the sexually transmitted diseases mentioned below, identify the one which does not specifically affect the sex organs.
(a) Syphilis (b) AIDS
(c) Gonorrhoea (d) Genital warts

**10.** Condoms are one of the most popular contraceptives because of the following reasons:
(a) These are-effective barriers for insemination
(b) They do not interfere with coital act
(c) These help in reducing the risk of STDs
(d) All of the above

**11.** Choose the correct statement regarding the ZIFT procedure:
(a) Ova collected from a female donor are transferred to the fallopian tube to facilitate zygote formation.
(b) Zygote is collected from a female donor and transferred to the fallopian tube.
(c) Zygote is collected from a female donor and transferred to the uterus.
(d) Ova collected from a female donor and transferred to the uterus.

**12.** The correct surgical procedure as a contraceptive method is
(a) Ovariectomy (b) Hysterectomy
(c) Vasectomy (d) Castration

**13.** Diaphragms are contraceptive devices used by the females. Choose the correct option from the statements given below:
i. They are introduced into the uterus.
ii. They are placed to cover the cervical region.
iii. They act as physical barriers for sperm entry.
iv. They act as spermicidal agents.
(a) i and ii (b) i and iii
(c) ii and iii (d) iii and iv

## Previous Years' Questions

**1.** Cu ions released from copper-releasing Intra Uterine Devices (IUDs): [AIPMT PRE 2010]
(a) Make uterus unsuitable for implantation
(b) Increase phagocytosis of sperms
(c) Suppress sperm motility
(d) Prevent ovulation

**2.** The permissible use of technique amniocentesis is for: [AIPMT PRE 2010]
(a) Detecting sex of the unborn foetus
(b) Artificial insemination
(c) Transfer of embryo into the uterus of a surrogate mother
(d) Detecting any genetic abnormality

**3.** In vitro fertilization is a technique that involves transfer of which one of the following into the fallopian tube? [AIPMT PRE 2010]
(a) Embryo only, up to 8 cell stage
(b) Either zygote or early embryo up to 8 cell stage
(c) Embryo of 32 cell stage
(d) Zygote only

**4.** The technique called Gamete Intra Fallopian Transfer (GIFT) is recommended for those females [AIPMT MAINS 2011]
(a) who cannot produce an ovum
(b) who cannot retain foetus inside uterus
(c) whose cervical canal is too narrow to allow passage for sperms
(d) who cannot provide suitable environment for fertilization

**5.** Which one of the following is the most widely accepted method of contraception in India, at present? [AIPMT PRE 2011]
(a) Tubectomy
(b) Diaphragms
(c) IUDs (Intra Uterine Devices)
(d) Cervical caps

**6.** If for some reason, the vasa efferentia in the human reproductive system get blocked, the gametes will not be transported from [AIPMT PRE 2011]
(a) Epididymis to vas deferens
(b) Ovary to uterus
(c) Vagina to uterus
(d) Testes to epididymis

**7.** Medical Termination of Pregnancy (MTP) is considered safe up to how many weeks of pregnancy? [AIPMT PRE 2011]
(a) Twelve weeks (b) Eighteen weeks
(c) Six weeks (d) Eight weeks

**8.** What is the figure given below showing in particular? [AIPMT PRE 2012]

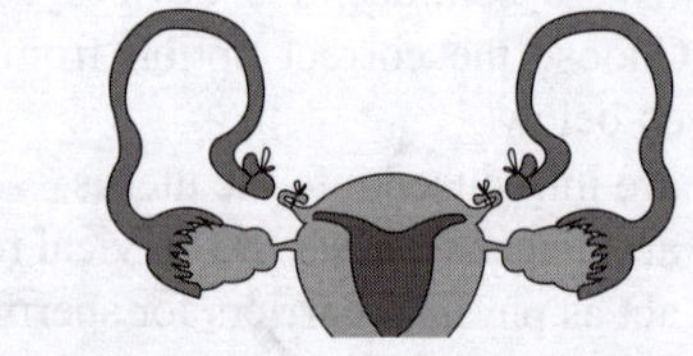

(a) Ovarian cancer (b) Uterine cancer
(c) Tubectomy (d) Vasectomy

**9.** The test-tube baby programme employs which one of the following techniques [AIPMT PRE 2012]
(a) Gamete intra fallopian transfer (GIFT)
(b) Zygote intra fallopian transfer (ZIFT)
(c) Intra cytoplasmic sperm injection (ICSI)
(d) Intra uterine insemination (IUI)

**10.** Artificial insemination means: [AIPMT 2013]
(a) Transfer of sperms of a healthy donor to a test tube containing ova
(b) Transfer of sperms of donor to a test tube containing ova
(c) Artificial introduction of sperms of a healthy donor into the vagina
(d) Introduction of sperms of a healthy donor directly into the ovary

**11.** Which of the following cannot be detected in a developing foetus by amniocentesis? [AIPMT 2013]
(a) Klinefelter syndrome (b) Sex of the foetus
(c) Down syndrome (d) Jaundice

**12.** One of the legal methods of birth control is: [AIPMT 2013]
(a) Abortion by taking an appropriate medicine
(b) By abstaining from coitus from day 10 to 17 of the menstrual cycle
(c) By having coitus at the time of day break
(d) By a premature ejaculation during coitus

**13.** Assisted reproductive technology, IVF involves transfer of: [AIPMT 2014]
(a) Ovum into the fallopian tube
(b) Zygote into the fallopian tube
(c) Zygote into the uterus
(d) Embryo with 16 blastomeres into the fallopian tube

**14.** Which of the following is a hormone releasing Intra Uterine Device (IUD)? [AIPMT 2014]
(a) Multiload 375 (b) LNG – 20
(c) Cervical cap (d) Vault

**15.** Tubectomy is a method of sterilization in which: [AIPMT 2014]
(a) Small part of the fallopian tube is removed or tied up
(b) Ovaries are removed surgically
(c) Small part of vas deferens is removed or tied up
(d) Uterus is removed surgically

**16.** A childless couple can be assisted to have a child through a technique called GIFT. The full form of GIFT is: [RE-AIPMT 2015]
(a) Gamete intra fallopian transfer
(b) Gamete internal fertilization and transfer
(c) Germ cell internal fallopian transfer
(d) Gamete inseminated fallopian transfer

**17.** Which of the following is not a sexually transmitted disease? [AIPMT 2015]
(a) Syphilis
(b) Acquired Immuno Deficiency Syndrome disease (AIDS)
(c) Trichomoniasis
(d) Encephalitis

**18.** Which of the following viruses is not transferred through semen of an infected male? [AIPMT 2015]
(a) Hepatitis B virus
(b) Human immunodeficiency virus
(c) Chikunguniya virus
(d) Ebola virus

**19.** Hysterectomy is surgical removal of [RE-AIPMT 2015]
(a) Uterus (b) Prostate gland
(c) Vas-deference (d) Mammary glands

**20.** Embryo with more than 16 blastomeres formed due to *in vitro* fertilization is transferred into [NEET 2016 – PHASE II]

(a) Fallopian tube (b) Fimbriae
(c) Cervix (d) Uterus

**21.** Which of the following is incorrect regarding vasectomy? [NEET 2016 – PHASE II]

(a) No sperm occurs in epididymis
(b) Vasa deferentia is cut and tied
(c) Irreversible sterility
(d) No sperm occurs in seminal fluid

**22.** Which of the following is hormone releasing IUD? [NEET 2016 – PHASE II]

(a) Multiload 375 (b) Lippes loop
(c) Cu7 (d) LNG-20

**23.** Which of the following approaches does not give the defined action of contraceptive? [NEET 2016 – PHASE I]

| | |
|---|---|
| (a) Barrier methods | Prevent fertilization |
| (b) Intra uterine devices | Increase phagocytosis of sperms suppresses sperm motility and fertilizing capacity of sperms. |
| (c) Hormonal contraceptives | Prevent retard entry of sperms, prevent ovulation and fertilization |
| (d) Vasectomy | Prevents spermatogenesis |

**24.** In context of amniocentesis, which of the following statements is incorrect? [NEET 2016 – PHASE I]

(a) It is usually done when a woman is between 14–16 weeks pregnant.
(b) It is used for prenatal sex determination.
(c) It can be used for detection of Down's syndrome.
(d) It can be used for detection of Cleft palate.

**25.** Match the following sexually transmitted diseases (Column-I) with their causative agent (Column-II) and select the correct option. [NEET 2017]

| Column – I | Column – II |
|---|---|
| (a) Gonorrhoea | (i) HIV |
| (b) Syphilis | (ii) Neisseria |
| (c) Genital Warts | (iii) Treponema |
| (d) AIDS | (iv) Human Papilloma – Virus |

**Options:**

| | (a) | (b) | (c) | (d) |
|---|---|---|---|---|
| (a) | (iii) | (iv) | (i) | (ii) |
| (b) | (iv) | (ii) | (iii) | (i) |
| (c) | (iv) | (iii) | (ii) | (i) |
| (d) | (ii) | (iii) | (iv) | (i) |

**26.** The function of copper ions in copper releasing IUDs is: [NEET 2017]

(a) They inhibit gametogenesis
(b) They make uterus unsuitable for implantation
(c) They inhibit ovulation
(d) They suppress sperm motility and fertilizing capacity of sperms

**27.** In case of a couple, where the male is having very low sperm count, which of the following techniques will be suitable for fertilization? [NEET 2017]

(a) Gamete instracytoplasmic fallopian transfer
(b) Artificial insemination
(c) Intracytoplasmic sperm injection
(d) Intrauterine transfer

**28.** Which one of following is not an IUD? [NEET Regional 2017]

(a) Vaults (b) Cu T
(c) Multiload 375 (d) Progestasert

**29.** Select the correct option: [NEET Regional 2017]

(a) IUI can help a woman with premature menopause to bear a child.
(b) GIFT involves IVF to help women who cannot produce ovum to bear a child.
(c) ZIFT involves IVF to help women who cannot produce ovum to bear a child.
(d) ZIFT involves IVF to help women who have damaged fallopian tubes to bear a child.

**30.** In lactational amenorrhoea, ovulation does not occur during the period of intense lactation because of : [NEET Regional 2017]

(a) High level of FSH and LH
(b) Surge of Estrogen
(c) Stimulation of GnRH
(d) High level of Prolactin

**31.** The contraceptive SAHELI [NEET 2018]

(a) blocks estrogen receptors in the uterus, preventing eggs from getting implanted.
(b) is an IUD
(c) increases the concentration of estrogen and prevents ovulation in females.
(d) is a post-coital contraceptive.

**32.** Which of the following contraceptive methods play the role of a hormone? [NEET 2019]
(a) Barrier method, Lactational amenorrhea, Pills
(b) CuT, Pills, Emergency contraceptives
(c) Pills, Emergency Contraceptives, Barrier methods
(d) Lactional amenorrhea, Pills, Emergency contraceptives

**33.** Select the hormone-releasing Intra-Uterine Devices. [NEET 2019]
(a) Multiload 375, Progestasert
(b) Progestasert, LNG – 20
(c) Lippes Loop, Multiload 375
(d) Vaults, LNG – 20

**34.** Which of the following sexually transmitted disease is not completely curable? [NEET 2019]
(a) Genital warts (b) Genital herpes
(c) Chlamydiasis (d) Gonorrhoea

**35.** In which of the following techniques, the embryos are transferred to assist those females who cannot conceive? [NEET 2020]
(a) ZIFT and IUT (b) GIFT and ZIFT
(c) ICSI and ZIFT (d) GIFT and ICSI

**36.** Select theoption including all sexually transmitted diseases. [NEET 2020]
(a) Gonorrhoea, Syphilis, Genital herpes
(b) Gonorrhoea, Malaria, Genital herpes
(c) AIDS, Malaria, Filaria
(d) Cancer, AIDS, Syphilis

**37.** Veneral diseases can spread through:
(A) Using sterile needles
(B) Transfusion of blood from infected person
(C) Infected mother to foetus
(D) Kissing
(E) Inheritance
Choose the correct answer from the options given below. [NEET 2021]
(a) (A) and (C) only
(b) (A), (B) and (C) only
(c) (B), (C) and (D) only
(d) (B) and (C) only

**38.** Match the following: [NEET 2021]

| Column – I | Column – II |
|---|---|
| 1. Vaults | (i) Entry of sperm through cervix is blocked |
| 2. IUDs | (ii) Removal of Vas deferens |
| 3. Vasectomy | (iii) Phagocytosis of sperms within the uterus |
| 4. Tubectomy | (iv) Removal of fallopian tube |

**The correct matching is**

| | 1 | 2 | 3 | 4 |
|---|---|---|---|---|
| (a) | (iii) | (i) | (iv) | (ii) |
| (b) | (iv) | (ii) | (i) | (iii) |
| (c) | (i) | (iii) | (ii) | (iv) |
| (d) | (ii) | (iv) | (iii) | (i) |

**39.** Which one of the following is an example of Hormone releasing IUD? [NEET 2021]
(a) Multiload 375 (b) CuT
(c) LNG 20 (d) Cu7

**40.** Lippes loop is a type of contraceptive used as: [NEET 2022]
(a) Vault barrier
(b) Non-Medicated IUD
(c) Copper releasing IUD
(d) Cervical barrier

**41.** Match **List-I** with **List-II** with respect to methods of Contraception and their respective actions. [NEET 2022]

| List-I | | List-II | |
|---|---|---|---|
| (A) | Diaphragms | (i) | Inhibit ovulation and implantation |
| (B) | Contraceptive Pills | (ii) | Increase phagocytosis of sperm within uterus |
| (C) | Intra Uterine Devices | (iii) | Absence of menstrual cycle and ovulation following parturition |
| (D) | Lactational Amenorrhea | (iv) | They cover the cervix blocking the entry of sperms. |

Choose the **correct answer** from the options given below:
(a) (A)-(iv), (B)-(i), (C)-(ii), (D)-(iii)
(b) (A)-(ii), (B)-(iv), (C)-(i), (D)-(iii)
(c) (A)-(iii), (B)-(ii), (C)-(i), (D)-(iv)
(d) (A)-(iv), (B)-(i), (C)-(iii), (D)-(ii)

**42.** Which one of the following common sexually transmitted diseases is completely curable when detected early and treated properly? [NEET 2023]
(a) Gonorrhoea (b) Hepatitis - B
(c) HIV Infection (d) Genital herpes

**43.** Given below are two statements: one is labelled as Assertion A and the other labelled as Reason R. [NEET 2023]

**Assertion A:** Amniocentesis for sex determination in one of the strategic of reproductive and child health care programme.

**Reason R:** Ban on amniocentesis checks increasing menace of female foeticide.

In the light of the above statements, choose the correct answer from the options given below:

(a) Both A and R are true but R is NOT the correct explanation of A.
(b) A is true but R is false.
(c) A is false but R is true.
(d) Both A and R are true and R is the correct explanation of A.

**44.** Match List I with List II. [NEET 2023]

| List I | List II |
|---|---|
| A. Vasectomy | I. Oral method |
| B. Coitus interruptus | II. Barrier method |
| C. Cervical caps | III. Surgical method |
| D. Saheli | IV. Natural method |

Choose the correct answer from the options given below:

(a) A - III, B - IV, C - II, D - I
(b) A - II, B - III, C - I, D - IV
(c) A - IV, B - II, C - I, D - III
(d) A - III, B - I, C - IV, D - II

**45.** Match List-I with List-II [NEET 2024]

| List-I | List-II |
|---|---|
| (A) Non-medicated IUD | (i) Multiload 375 |
| (B) Copper releasing IUD | (ii) Progestogens |
| (C) Hormone releasing IUD | (iii) Lippes loop |
| (D) Implants | (iv) LNG-20 |

Choose the correct answer from the options given below:

(a) (A)-(iii), (B)-(i), (C)-(ii), (D)-(iv)
(b) (A)-(i), (B)-(iii), (C)-(iv), (D)-(ii)
(c) (A)-(iv), (B)-(i), (C)-(ii), (D)-(iii)
(d) (A)-(iii), (B)-(i), (C)-(iv), (D)-(ii)

**46.** Which of the following is not a natural/traditional contraceptive method? [NEET 2024]

(a) Coitus interruptus
(b) Periodic abstinence
(c) Lactational amenorrhea
(d) Vaults

## Answer Key

### Multiple Choice Questions: Level I

| | | | | | | | | | |
|---|---|---|---|---|---|---|---|---|---|
| **1.** (d) | **2.** (b) | **3.** (c) | **4.** (b) | **5.** (d) | **6.** (c) | **7.** (b) | **8.** (c) | **9.** (b) | **10.** (c) |
| **11.** (d) | **12.** (c) | **13.** (b) | **14.** (b) | **15.** (a) | **16.** (d) | **17.** (b) | **18.** (c) | **19.** (d) | **20.** (c) |
| **21.** (b) | **22.** (d) | **23.** (c) | **24.** (b) | **25.** (b) | **26.** (c) | **27.** (b) | **28.** (c) | **29.** (c) | **30.** (a) |
| **31.** (b) | **32.** (a) | **33.** (d) | **34.** (c) | **35.** (a) | **36.** (b) | **37.** (b) | **38.** (c) | **39.** (c) | **40.** (d) |
| **41.** (d) | **42.** (c) | **43.** (c) | **44.** (a) | **45.** (d) | **46.** (b) | **47.** (d) | **48.** (a) | **49.** (c) | **50.** (b) |
| **51.** (d) | **52.** (d) | **53.** (b) | **54.** (b) | **55.** (a) | **56.** (b) | **57.** (b) | **58.** (c) | **59.** (b) | **60.** (d) |
| **61.** (a) | **62.** (b) | **63.** (c) | **64.** (d) | **65.** (d) | **66.** (c) | **67.** (b) | **68.** (b) | **69.** (a) | **70.** (b) |
| **71.** (a) | **72.** (d) | **73.** (d) | **74.** (c) | **75.** (a) | **76.** (d) | **77.** (d) | **78.** (b) | **79.** (d) | **80.** (a) |
| **81.** (a) | **82.** (b) | **83.** (a) | **84.** (c) | **85.** (c) | **86.** (b) | **87.** (c) | **88.** (d) | | |

### Multiple Choice Questions: Level II

| | | | | | | | | | |
|---|---|---|---|---|---|---|---|---|---|
| **89.** (c) | **90.** (a) | **91.** (b) | **92.** (a) | **93.** (c) | **94.** (a) | **95.** (b) | **96.** (c) | **97.** (c) | **98.** (d) |
| **99.** (c) | | | | | | | | | |

### A & R and Statement-based Questions

| | | | | | | | | | |
|---|---|---|---|---|---|---|---|---|---|
| **100.** (c) | **101.** (c) | **102.** (b) | **103.** (d) | **104.** (a) | **105.** (d) | **106.** (a) | **107.** (c) | **108.** (a) | **109.** (c) |

### Matrix-Match Type Questions

| | | | | |
|---|---|---|---|---|
| **110.** (a) | **111.** (a) | **112.** (a) | **113.** (a) | **114.** (a) |

### NCERT Exemplar Questions

| | | | | | | | | | |
|---|---|---|---|---|---|---|---|---|---|
| **1.** (c) | **2.** (c) | **3.** (a) | **4.** (d) | **5.** (a) | **6.** (a) | **7.** (b) | **8.** (c) | **9.** (b) | **10.** (d) |
| **11.** (b) | **12.** (c) | **13.** (c) | | | | | | | |

### Previous Years' Questions

| | | | | | | | | | |
|---|---|---|---|---|---|---|---|---|---|
| **1.** (c) | **2.** (d) | **3.** (b) | **4.** (a) | **5.** (c) | **6.** (d) | **7.** (a) | **8.** (c) | **9.** (b) | **10.** (c) |
| **11.** (d) | **12.** (a) | **13.** (b) | **14.** (b) | **15.** (a) | **16.** (a) | **17.** (d) | **18.** (c) | **19.** (a) | **20.** (d) |
| **21.** (a) | **22.** (d) | **23.** (d) | **24.** (d) | **25.** (d) | **26.** (d) | **27.** (b) | **28.** (a) | **29.** (c) | **30.** (d) |
| **31.** (a) | **32.** (d) | **33.** (b) | **34.** (b) | **35.** (a) | **36.** (a) | **37.** (d) | **38.** (c) | **39.** (c) | **40.** (b) |
| **41.** (a) | **42.** (a) | **43.** (c) | **44.** (a) | **45.** (c) | **46.** (d) | | | | |

# HINTS AND EXPLANATION

## Multiple Choice Questions: Level II

**89.** A. The pill – Prevents ovulation
B. Condom - Prevents sperms reaching cervix
C. Vasectomy – Semen contains no sperms
D. Copper-T – Prevents implantation

**90.** Statements A and C are correct.
- Medical Termination of Pregnancy (MTP) during first trimester is generally safe.
- Intrauterine devices like copper-T are effective contraceptive

**91.** The progesterone and estradiol continue hypertrophy of endometrial lining of the uterus and fallopian tubes and maintain it throughout pregnancy; progesterone is also necessary for proper implantation of foetus in the uterine wall by stimulating the endometrial glands – secrete a nutrient fluid for the foetus, hence the term secretory phase. Progesterone inhibits the release of FSH so that it may not develop additional follicles and eggs.

**92.** Demography is the study of population in all aspects. Fertility refers to the number of children per couple. Mortality rate is the average number of natural deaths per unit population per unit time. Age distribution refers to the proportionate occurrence of individuals of three age groups. Developing countries usually have high rate of population growth, because of increasing fertility and declining mortality.

**93.** Copper T is a device and its shape is T. It is inserted such that egg and sperm will not undergo fertilization process. The insertion process is also simple, non-surgical. Only known side effect till now is excessive bleeding and for some, there are chances of getting other symptoms too, but it's very rare.

**94.** AIDS is caused by HIV, and Gonorrhoea is caused by *Neisseria gonorrhoea.*

**95.** It is use to detect chromosomal defects in foetus.

**96.** Human population in world is estimated to have crossed 6 billion in the year 1999.

**97.** In test-tube baby, fertilization of sperm and ova is carried out in lab conditions (in vitro) and when the embryos have reached the 32-celled stage, it is implanted back into the uterus of the surrogate mother.

**98.** Human population growth in India can be regulated by following the national programme of family planning.

**99.** In India, there is short life span of individuals and high birth rate as compared to other countries. Thus, the human population is heavily weighted towards younger age groups.

## NCERT Exemplar Questions

**1.** Intracytoplasmic sperm injection (IESI) is a method in which embryo is formed in the laboratory by directly injecting sperm into the ovum.

**2.** Increased IMR and decreased MMR in a population will **not cause significance change in growth rate.**

**3.** There is suppression of gonadotropins which inhibits ovulation and thus women miss their menstrual cycle during this period. Thus, coitus during this time will not lead to conception.

**4.** Sterilization techniques are generally foo-proof methods of contraception with least side effects. Yet, this is the last option for couples because of (i), (ii), (iii) and (iv).

**5.** A national level approach to build up a reproductively healthy society was taken up in our country in **1950s.**

**6.** Combination or IUDs within 72 hours of coitus have been found to be very effective as emergency contraceptives as they could be used to avoid possible pregnancy due to rape or casual unprotected intercourse.

**7.**
- Hormone-releasing IUDs: Progestasert, LNG-20
- IUDs increases phagocytes of sperm within the uterus

**8.**
- MTPs are considered relatively safe during the first trimester (up to 12 weeks of pregnancy).
- 2nd trimester abortions are highly risky
- MTPs require assistance of qualified medical personnel.

**9.** Diseases or infections which are transmitted through sexual intercourse are called sexually transmitted diseases (STD) or VD (Venereal diseases) or RTI (Reproductive tract infections).

**Examples of STDs:**

(i) HIV (AIDS)
(ii) Hepatitis-B
(iii) Genital herpes
(iv) Chlamydiasis
(v) Gonorrhoea
(vi) Genital warts
(vii) Syphilis
(viii) Trichomoniasis

**10.** Condoms are barriers made of thin rubber/latex sheath. Condoms are used to cover the penis in male or vagina and cervix in the female, just before coitus so that the ejaculated semen would not enter into the female reproductive tract. This can prevent conception. Use of condoms has increased in recent years due to its additional benefit of protecting the user from contracting STDs and AIDS. Both male and female condoms are disposable and give privacy to the user. Nirodh is a popular brand of condom for the male. Condom is the most widely used contraceptive by males in India as it is cheap and easily available. It is simple and effective and has no side effects.

**11.** *ZIFT (Zygote Intra Fallopian Transfer)*

**12.** Vasectomy and tubectomy are surgical procedure as a contraceptive method.

**13.** **Diaphragms, Cervical caps and Vaults:** These are also barriers made of rubber that are inserted into the female reproductive tract to cover the cervix during coitus. They prevent conception by blocking entry of sperms through the cervix. They are reusable. Spermicidal creams, jellies and foams are usually used along with these barriers to increase their contraceptive efficiency.

## Previous Years' Questions

**1.** Copper releasing IUDs (CuT, Cu7, Multiload 375) increase phagocytosis of sperms within the uterus and the Cu ions released suppress sperm motility and the fertilizing capacity of sperms.

**2.** Amniocentesis is a technique for diagnosis of congenital abnormalities before birth. By karyotypic studies of somatic cells, abnormalities due to changes in chromosome number like Down's syndrome, Turner's syndrome, Klinefelter's syndrome, etc., can be determined. It can be used as a pre-natal diagnostic technique. These days, amniocentesis is being misused also. Mothers even get their normal foetus aborted if it is a female.

**3.** Refer to solution 20

**4.** Refer to solution 16

**5.** At present, the most widely accepted method of contraception in India is IUDs (Intra Uterine Devices). These devices are effective and popular. These devices are inserted by doctors and expert nurses in the uterus through the vagina.

**6.** Vasa efferentia (Ductuli efferences) are 10–20 fine tubules which connect rete testis with an epididymis (Ductus epididymis). The latter is a pair of ducts from each testis which is formed by union of its vasa efferentia. If the vasa efferentia gets blocked, sperms will not be transported from testis to epididymis.

**7.** Intentional or voluntary termination of pregnancy before full term is called medical termination of pregnancy (MTP) or induced abortion. MTPs are considered relatively safe during the first trimester, i.e., up to 12 weeks of pregnancy. Second trimester abortions are much more riskier.

**8.** **Tubectomy :**

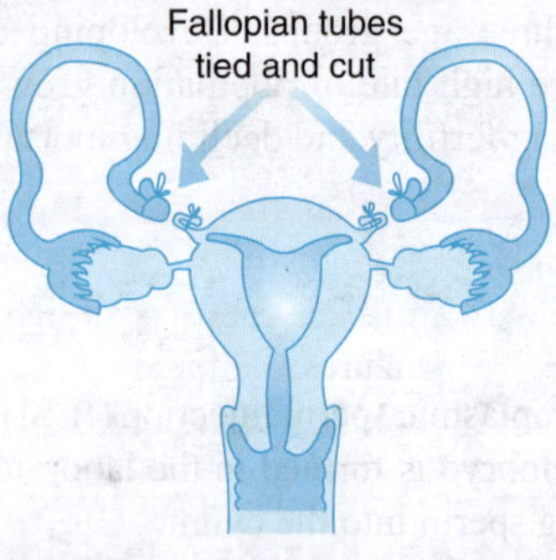


Surgical methods, also called sterilization, are generally advised for male/female partner as a terminal method to prevent any more pregnancies. Surgical intervention blocks gamete transport and thereby prevents conception. Sterilization procedure in the male is called 'vasectomy' and that of the female is 'tubectomy'. In tubectomy, a small part of the fallopian tube is removed (Figure) or tied up through a small incision in the abdomen or through vagina. These techniques are highly effective but their reversibility is very poor.

**9.** Refer to solution 20

**10.** During artificial insemination, semen is collected from a donor and artificially introduced into the vagina.

**11.** Amniocentesis is a foetal sex determination test based on the chromosomal pattern in the amniotic fluid surrounding the developing embryo. Jaundice is a condition not based on chromosomal pattern. It is a disease related to dysfunctions.

**12.** MTP can be performed non-surgically on prescription of mifepristone + Prostaglandins by registered medical practitioner under his supervision.
This is legal method of termination of pregnancy.
Duration of menstrual cycle in all female is not fixed hence ovulation can occur anytime between 8 to 19th day hence this method of abstinence is not practically possible for birth control.

**13.** *In vitro* fertilization (IVF–fertilization outside the body in almost similar conditions as that in the body) followed by embryo transfer (ET) is one of such methods.

**14.** Hormone releasing IUDs (Progestasert, LNG-20)

**15.** Tubectomy is a surgical strategy for cleansing in which a lady's fallopian tubes are clasped and blocked or separated and fixed, both of which keeps eggs from achieving the uterus for implantation. Tubal ligation is viewed as a lasting technique for disinfection and conception prevention.

**16.** Transfer of an ovum collected from a donor into the fallopian tube (GIFT – **gamete intra fallopian transfer**) of another female who cannot produce one but can provide suitable environment for fertilization and further development is another method attempted.

**17.** Encephalitis is inflammation of the brain. Severity is variable. Symptoms may include headache, fever, confusion, a stiff neck, and vomiting. Complications may include seizures, hallucinations, trouble speaking, memory problems, and problems with hearing.

**18.** Chikungunya is an infection caused by the chikungunya virus (CHIKV). Symptoms include fever and joint pain. These typically occur two to twelve days after exposure. Other symptoms may include headache, muscle pain, joint swelling, and a rash.
Chikunguniya virus transfers through Aedes mosquito.

**19.**

| Term | Surgical removal of |
|---|---|
| Prostate gland | Prostatectomy |
| Vas deferens | Vasectomy |
| Mammary glands / Breast | Mastectomy |
| Gall bladder | Cholecystectomy |
| Stomach | Gastrectomy |
| Intestine | Ileectomy |
| Pituitary | Hypophysectomy |

**20.** ***In vitro* fertilization** (IVF fertilization outside the body in almost similar conditions to that of inside the body) followed by **embryo transfer** (ET) is one of such methods. In this method, popularly known as **test-tube baby** programme, ova from the wife/donor (female) and sperms from the husband/donor (male) are collected and are induced to form zygote under simulated conditions in the laboratory. The zygote or early embryos (with up to 8 blastomeres) could then be transferred into the fallopian tube (ZIFT–**zygote intra fallopian transfer**) and embryos with more than 8 blastomeres, into the uterus (IUT – **intra uterine transfer**), to complete its further development. Embryos formed by **in-vivo fertilization** (fusion of gametes within the female) also could be used for such transfer to assist those females who cannot conceive.

**21.** Vasectomy is a surgical procedure for male sterilization or permanent contraception. During the procedure, the male vas deferens are severed and then tied or sealed in a manner so as to prevent sperm from entering into the ejaculate and thereby prevent fertilization.

**22.** Refer to solution 28

**23.** (a) In barrier methods, ovum and sperms are prevented from physically meeting with the help of barriers.
(b) IUDs increase phagocytosis of sperms within the uterus and the Cu ions released suppress sperm motility and the fertilizing capacity of sperms. The hormone-releasing IUDs, in addition, make the uterus unsuitable for implantation and the cervix hostile to the sperms.
(c) Hormonal contraceptives inhibit ovulation and implantation as well as alter the quality of cervical mucus to prevent/retard entry of sperms.
(d) Surgical methods, also called sterilization, are generally advised for e male/female partner as a terminal method to prevent any more pregnancies. In male, it is vasectomy and in female, it is tubectomy.

**24.** Amniocentesis (amniotic fluid test or AFT) procedure used in prenatal diagnosis of chromosomal abnormalities (like Down syndrome) and fetal infections and also used for sex determination. It is usually done when women is between 14 and 16 weeks pregnant.

**25.** Some STDs

| Disease | Causative organism |
|---|---|
| **AIDS (Acquired Immuno deficiency Syndrome)** | Retrovirus – HIV |
| **Genital Herpes** | Herpes Simplex Virus |
| **Genital warts** | Human papilloma virus (HPVs) |
| **Gonorrhoea** | *Neisseria gonorrhoea* |
| **Chlamydiasis** | *Chlamydia trachomatis* |
| **Syphilis** | *Treponema pallidum* |
| **Trichomoniasis** | *Trichomonas vaginalis* |
| **Chancroid** | *Haemophilus ducreyi* |
| **Lymphogranuloma venerum** | *Lymphogranuloma psittacosis bacteria* |

**26.** Refer to solution 23

**27.** **Artificial insemination (AI) technique :** If the male partner is unable to inseminate due to very low sperm counts, then the semen is collected (from husband or healthy donor) and artificially introduced either into the vagina or into the uterus **(IUI– Intra-uterine Insemination)** of the female.

**28.** **Types of IUDs:**

(1) Non-–medicated IUDs–**Lippes loop.**

(2) Copper-releasing IUDs–**CuT, Cu7, Multiload 375.**

(3) Hormone-releasing IUDs–**Progestasert, LNG-20.**

**29.** ZIFT involves IVF to help women who cannot produce ovum to bear a child.

**30.** Nursing stimulates prolactin secretion and evidence suggests that pro-lactin inhibits GnRH secretion, inhibits the action of GnRH on the pituitary and antagonizes the action of gonadotropins on the ovaries. Ovulation is inhibited and the ovaries are inactive, so estrogen and progesterone output falls to low levels.

**31.** **SAHELI** contain Ormeloxifene, also known as centchroman, is one of the selective estrogen-receptors modulators, or SERMs, a class of medication which acts on estrogen receptor. It is best known as a non-steroidal oral contraceptive which is taken once per week.

**32.** In barrier methods, ovum and sperms are prevented from physically meeting with the help of barriers. CuT is a copper-releasing IUD. Lactional amenorrhea, Pills, Emergency contraceptives all play the role of hormones.

- In lactational amenorrhoea, due to high prolactin level, gonadotropin level decreases.
- Oral pills are either progestogens or progestogen–estrogen combination used by the females.
- Emergency contraceptives include the administration of progestogens or progestogen–estrogen combination or IUDs within 72 hours of coitus.

**33.** Hormone-releasing IUDs (Progestasert, LNG-20)

**34.** Gonorrhoea, syphilis, genital herpes, chlamydiasis, genital warts, trichomoniasis, hepatitis-B and of course, the most discussed infection in the recent years, HIV leading to AIDS are some of the common STDs. Except for hepatitis-B, genital herpes and HIV infections, other diseases are completely curable if detected early and treated properly.

**35.** Option (a) is the answer because ART in which embryos are transferred, include ZIFT and IUT i.e. Zygote Intrafallopian Transfer and Intra Uterine Transfer respectively, both are embryo transfer (ET) methods.

Option (b), (c) and (d) are incorrect because in GIFT (Gamete Intrafallopian Transfer), gamete is transferred into the fallopian tube of female who cannot produce ova. ICSI is Intra cytoplasmic sperm injection in which sperm is directly injected into the ovum.

**36.** Gonorrhoea, Syphilis, Genital herpes are sexually transmitted diseases.

Gonorrhoea is caused by a bacterium *Neisseria gonorrhoeae.*

Syphilis is caused by a bacterium *Treponema pallidum.*

Genital herpes is caused by a virus Type- II Herpes simplex virus.

**37.**
- Venereal diseases or sexually transmitted diseases or infections are transmitted by sharing of infected needles, surgical instruments with infected person, transfusion of blood from an infected mother to foetus.
- Venereal diseases are not transmitted through kissing or inheritance.

**38.**

| | |
|---|---|
| Vaults | Diaphragms, cervical caps and vaults are barrier methods of contraception for female which works by blocking the entry of sperms through the cervix. |
| IUDs | IUDs increase phagocytosis of sperms within the uterus. |
| Vasectomy | Vasectomy is a surgical method of contraception in males in which a small part of the vas deferens is removed or tied up through a small incision on the scrotum. |
| Tubectomy | Tubectomy is a surgical method of contraception in females where a small part of the fallopian tube is removed or tied up through a small incision in the abdomen or through vagina. |

**39.** **Hormone releasing IUDs**- Progestasert, LNG-20

These IUDs make the uterus unsuitable for implantation and the cervix hostile to sperms.

**40.** Vaults are barriers made of rubber that are inserted into the female reproductive tract to cover the cervix during coitus

Vaults are cervical barriers.

**Copper releasing IUDs -** CuT, Cu7, Multiload 375.

**Non – medicated IUD -** Lippes loop.

Diaphragms, cervical caps & vaults are cervical barriers.

**41.**

| | List-I | | List-II |
|---|---|---|---|
| (a) | Diaphragms | (i) | They cover the cervix blocking the entry of sperms |
| (b) | Contraceptive Pills | (ii) | Inhibit ovulation and Implantation |
| (c) | Intra Uterine Devices | (iii) | Increase phagocytosis of sperm within Uterus |
| (d) | Lactational Amenorrhea | (iv) | Absence of Menstrual cycle and ovulation following parturition |

**42.** Gonorrhoea, syphilis, genital herpes, chlamydiasis, genital warts, trichomoniasis, hepatitis-B and AIDS are some of the common STIs.. Except for hepatitis-B, genital herpes and HIV infections, other diseases are completely curable if detected early and treated properly.

**43.** Statutory ban on amniocentesis (a foetal sex determination test based on the chromosomal pattern in the amniotic fluid surrounding the developing embryo) for sex-determination to legally check increasing female foeticides, In amniocentesis some of the amniotic fluid of the developing foetus is taken to analyse the fetal cells and dissolved substances. This procedure is used to test for the presence of certain genetic disorders such as, down syndrome, haemophilia, sickle-cell anemia, etc., determine the survivability of the foetus.

**44.**

| | |
|---|---|
| Vasectomy | Surgical method |
| Coitus interruptus | Natural method |
| Cervical caps | Barrier method |
| Saheli | Oral method |

**45.** Correct answer is option (d) because
- Lippes loop is a non-medicated IUD.
- Multiload 375, Cu T and Cu 7 is a copper releasing IUD.
- LNG -20, Progestasert is a hormone releasing IUD.
- Progestogens are used as implants.

**46.** The correct answer is option (d) as
Vault is a barrier method of contraception which is made of rubber that is inserted into the female reproductive tract to cover the cervix during the coitus.
- Option (a) is incorrect as coitus interruptus is a natural method of contraception in which male partner withdraws his penis from the vagina just before ejaculation so as to avoid insemination.
- Option (b) is incorrect as periodic abstinence is also a natural method of contraception in which couples avoid coitus during the fertile period.
- Option (c) is incorrect as lactational amenorrhea is also a natural method of contraception which is based on the fact that ovulation and therefore the cycle do not occur during the period of intense lactational following parturition.
- Therefore first three are natural or traditional contraceptive methods.

# 10

# Evolution

## LEARNING OBJECTIVES

- Understand the major evidences of evolution
- Discuss origin of life
- Know more about the Lamarckism and Darwinism theory of evolution
- Discuss major theory of evolution
- Explain adaptive radiation
- Discuss the modern views on evolution and also the organic view of evolution
- Understand the importance of Hardy-Weinberg principle
- Discuss how peppered Moth is considered an example to understand the phenomenon of natural selection
- Explain origin and evolution of man

## Chapter Overview

- **Evolutionary Biology:** It is the study of history of life forms on earth.

### Origin of Life

- **Origin of universe:** Almost 20 billion years old based on Big Bang theory.

| | |
|---|---|
| Origin of universe | – 20 billion years ago |
| Origin of earth | – 4.5 billion years ago |
| First life | – 4 billion years ago |
| Origin of first non-cellular forms of life (RNA, protein) | – 3 billion years ago |
| Origin of first cellular form of life (probably single-cells) | – 2 billion years ago |

- Our galaxy: Milky Way galaxy.
- Clouds of gas and dust and stars forms galaxy.
- There was no atmosphere on early earth.
- Hydrogen and helium formed after big bang explosion.
- Formation of atmosphere.
  (1) Molten mass released some gases: Water vapour, methane, carbon dioxide and ammonia. These gases covered the surface of earth.
  (2) Water $\xrightarrow{\text{(UV radiation from Sun)}}$ Hydrogen + Oxygen.
  (3) Hydrogen was lighter so it escaped out.
  (4) Oxygen reacted with Ammonia and Methane to form water, $CO_2$ and other gases.
  (5) Formation of ozone layer.
- As the earth further cooled, the water vapour reached the earth as rain. Finally oceans were formed.

Refer NCERT Ch 6: Evolution

## Theories Regarding the Origin of Life

- **Theory of Panspermia or Cosmozoic Theory or Spore Theory**: It was proposed by Richter. According to this theory protoplasm come from some other planets in the form of spores (units of life).
- **Theory of Spontaneous Generation** (Abiogenesis or Autogenesis): Life Originated from nonliving things spontaneously. Life came out of decaying and rotting matter like straw, mud, etc.

  **Evidences against Theory of Spontaneous Generation by Louis Pasteur's experiments, Redi's experiment and Spallanzani's experiment.**

  (1) Louis Pasteur proved that life comes only from pre-existing life.
  Killed yeast if placed in pre-sterilized flasks → No life originated.
  Killed yeast if placed in another flask open to air → New living organisms formed.

  (2) Although spontaneous generation theory was totally discarded, but this did not explain that how the **first life** on earth came.
- **Theory of Chemical Evolution (by Oparin of Russia and Haldane of England)**

  (1) They proposed that first life come from organic molecule and organic molecule arises from inorganic molecule by process of chemical evolution.

  (2) Conditions on earth at that time were: High temperature and Volcanic storms, reducing atmosphere containing $CH_4$, $NH_3$, water and hydrogen, etc.
- Experimental proof of theory of chemical evolution was given by S.L. Miller (American scientist) in 1953 **(Fig. 10.1)**.

  (1) He develops similar atmospheric conditions in laboratory - Electric discharge in a closed flask containing $CH_4$, $H_2$, $NH_3$ and water vapour at 800°C.

  (2) Few Amino acids were obtained in flask.

  (3) Later on, similar experiments were done and formation of sugars, nitrogen bases, pigments and fats were observed.

  (4) Analysis of meteorite also revealed similar compounds which indicate that such processes are also occurring elsewhere in space.

  (5) With this limited evidence there was acceptance of theory of chemical evolution.

  (6) All life forms were originated in water only.

  (7) The first life forms have originated slowly through evolutionary forces from non-living molecules but once the living molecules have formed they have given rise to complex biodiversity of today.

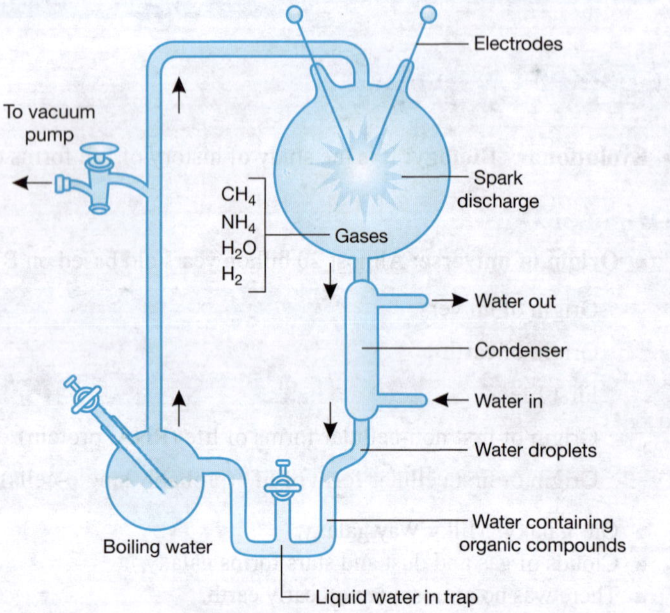


**FIGURE 10.1** Diagrammatic representation of Miller's experiment

## Evolution of Life Forms–A theory

### Theory of Special Creation

A. All living organisms that we observe today were created as such.
B. Diversity was same since creation and will remain same in future.
C. The earth is 4000 years old.

### Theory of Natural Selection (by Charles Darwin)

- Charles Darwin has done a sea voyage in a sail ship called H.M.S. Beagle around the world.
- Charles Darwin concluded that existing living forms share similarities up to varying degrees

- Characteristics of any population show built-in variations (based on climate, food, physical factors, etc.) which help them to survive better in natural conditions and outbreed others.
- According to Darwin, 'fitness' refers to reproductive fitness, i.e., more fit individuals will survive more and leave more offsprings than others.
- Better fit individuals are said to be selected by nature. Darwin gave the **term natural selection** to this and implied it as a mechanism of evolution.
- Around the same time, same conclusion was drawn by **Alfred Wallace**, a naturalist who worked in Malay Archipelago.
- All the existing life forms share similarities and common ancestors. Their ancestors were present at different periods in the history of earth smaller time scale to larger i.e. epochs, periods and eras.
- The geological history of earth runs parallel with the biological history of earth.

## Evidences for Evolution

1. Paleontological evidences (Evidence from fossils)
2. Evidences from comparative Anatomy and Morphology
3. Embryological evidences
4. Biogeographical evidences
5. Evidences from biochemistry and comparative physiology: Similarities in proteins and genes among diverse organisms also indicates about the common ancestry
6. Cytological evidence
7. Evidences from taxonomy
8. Evidences from genetics
9. Evidences from Plant and animal breeding

- **Fossils:** These are remains of hard parts of life-forms and usually found in sedimentary rocks. Fossils are direct evidence of evolution and age of fossils are calculated by radioactive dating method.
- **Evidences by embryological studies: Ernst Haeckel** observed that some features appear during embryonic development common to all vertebrates (for example, row of vestigial gill slits) and proposed embryological evidences. This proposal was disapproved by Karl Ernst von Baer. He noted that embryo never pass via the adult stages of other animals.
- Evidences based on Comparative anatomy and morphology:

| Type of Organs | Features/Description | Examples |
|---|---|---|
| **1.** Homologous organs | • Those organs which share common origin (or ancestors) but have different function.<br>• Such organs show divergent evolution. | **Example 1:** Pattern of bones of forelimbs in whales, bats, Cheetah and human (all mammals) share similarities in anatomical structure (all have humerus, radius, ulna, carpals, metacarpals and phalanges in their forelimbs) but perform different function.<br>**Example 2:** Vertebrate hearts<br>**Example 3:** Vertebrate brains.<br>**Example 4:** Thorn of Bougainvillea and tendrils of Cucurbita.<br>**Example 5:** Heart of frog and heart of human.<br>**Example 6:** Penis / Glans penis of male Rabbit and Clitoris of female Rabbit.<br>**Example 7:** Horns* of cattle and claws of cat.<br>**Example 8**: Wings of birds and wings of bat.<br>**Example 9:** Endostyle of Amphioxus and thyroid of Rabbit. |

| Type of Organs | Features/Description | Examples |
|---|---|---|
| **2.** Analogous organs | • Those organs which have different origin but have similar functions.<br>• Such organs show convergent evolution. | **Example 1:** Wings of butterfly and birds.<br>**Example 2:** Eyes of the octopus and mammals.<br>**Example 3:** Flippers of penguins and Dolphins.<br>**Example 4:** Sweet potato (root modification) and potato (stem modification).<br>**Example 5:** Trunk of an elephant and arm of a monkey.<br>**Example 6:** Fins of fishes and flippers of whale.<br>**Example 7:** Food vacuole of *paramecium* and alimentary canal of rabbit.<br>**Example 8:** Wings of *Draco* and wings of bat.<br>**Example 9**: Eyes of *Octopus* and eyes of monkey. |

- In a common habitat, similar adaptive features have developed in different groups of organisms but towards the same function.
- Homology indicates common ancestry **(Fig. 10.2).**

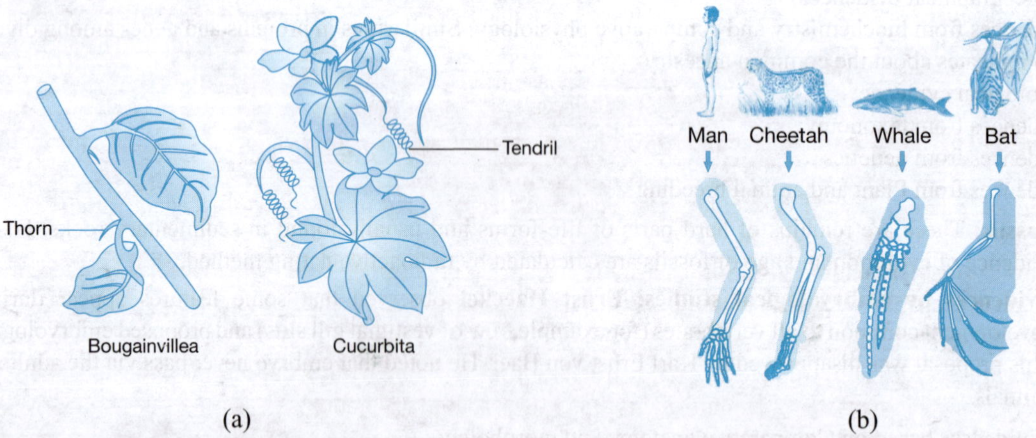


FIGURE 10.2 Examples of homologous organs in (a) Plants and (b) Animals

- Evidences from plant and animal breeding: Within hundreds of years, man has created breeds by intensive breeding programme that differ from other breeds (e.g., dogs) but still are of the same group. Nature will take over millions of years to perform the same work.

- **Evolution by natural selection:**
  - Evolution is not a directed process in the sense of determinism. It is a stochastic process which is based on chance events in nature and mutation in the organisms. Industrial melanism: **Examples of Evolution by anthropogenic action**
  - Industrial melanism is an observation made in England that supports 'evolution by natural selection'.
  - ***Biston betularia*** is commonly called peppered moth because of the presence of black dots on creamy-white body. These moths during 1850 were mostly gray *(Biston betularia typicas)* and during day time used to rest on tree-trunks which had lichens grown on them. They resembled with the background and could not be detected by their predators, mainly birds.
  - During industrial revolution in England, the coal was burnt and the soot got deposited on the tree-trunk. Moreover, sulphur-dioxide killed lichens. In such polluted areas all the moths of gray color now could be spotted by birds **(Fig. 10.3)**.
  - A few black individuals which had mutant gene were selected by nature. Such individuals got more chances of reproduction and the gray were reduced in number.

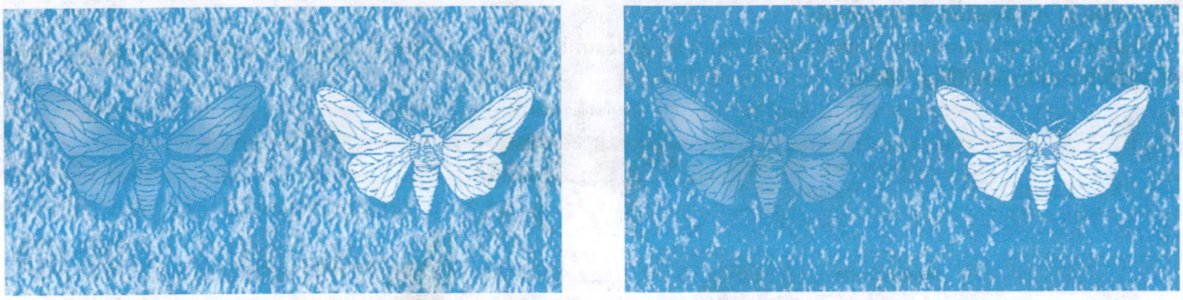

FIGURE 10.3 Figure showing white – winged moth and dark – winged moth (melanised) on a tree trunk (a) In unpolluted area (b) In polluted area

- After about 100 years (by 1950), more than 90 per cent of the individuals had become black, known as 'Melanic form' *(Biston betularia carbonaria)*. Here biologists could see the evolution occurring before their eyes. This evolution from gray to black (Melanic) forms was not due to mutation but due to *selection of pre-existing mutant allele* by nature (Natural selection).
- Now, when electricity is being used in industries, the numbers of gray moths are again increasing. This also indicates that industrial pollution has not eliminated the genes responsible for light colour of the moth. The above hypothesis was also tested by **Dr. H. B. D. Kettlewell** after releasing equal number of dark and light moths.
- **Examples of Evolution by Anthropogenic Action**

  **Example 1:** The count of melanic moths was low in rural areas. Also, this is a fact that no variant is completely wiped out.

  **Example 2:** Excess use of herbicides, pesticides, etc., has resulted in selection of resistant varieties in a much lesser time.

  **Example 3:** Use of antibiotics or drugs against eukaryotic organisms / cells / microbes has resulted in appearance of resistant organisms / cells / microbes in a time scale of months or years and not centuries.

- **Adaptive Radiation (Divergent Evolution)**
  - Development of different functional group structure from a common ancestral form is called adaptive radiation. This concept was given by Osborn. Homologous organ shows adaptive radiation.
  - The process of evolution of different species in given geographical area starting from a point and radiating to other areas of geography (habitats) is called adaptive radiation.

    **Example 1: Darwin's Finches (one of the classic examples of Adaptive Radiation)**
  - He observed that there were many varieties of small black birds (later on called Darwin's Finches) in the same island and also, they have evolved on the island itself. The original birds were seed-eating from which many forms with altered beaks arose making those in to insectivorous and vegetarian finches **(Fig. 10.4)**.

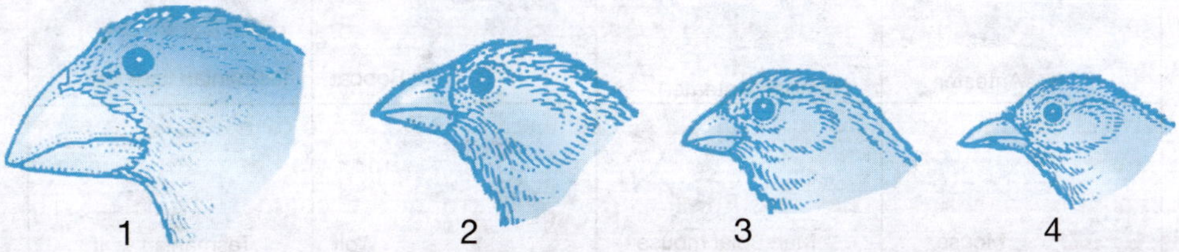


FIGURE 10.4 Variety of beaks of finches that Darwin found in Galapagos Island

**Example 2: Australian Marsupials**

- Evolution of many numbers of marsupials from an ancestral stock within the Australian island continent is an example of adaptive radiation **(Fig. 10.5).**

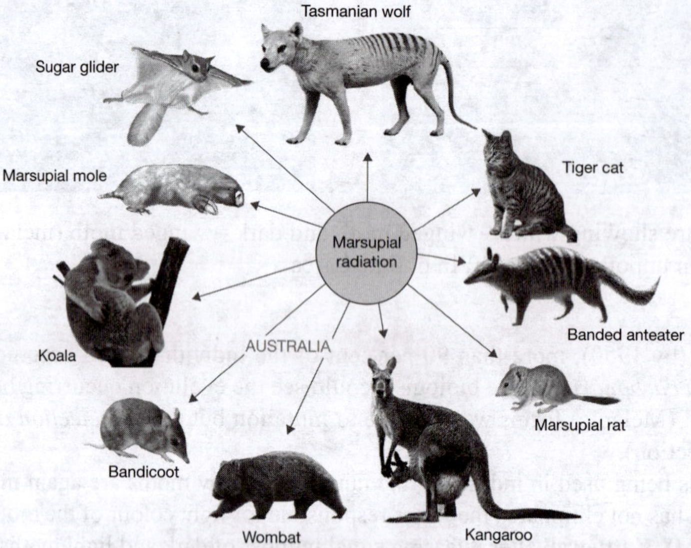


**FIGURE 10.5** Adaptive radiation of marsupials of Australia

**Example 3: Placental Mammals in Australia**

- Evolution of many types of Placental Mammals from an ancestral stock within the Australian island continent is another example of adaptive radiation.

- **Convergent Evolution (Adaptive Convergence):**
  - Development of similar adaptive functional structures in unrelated group of organism is called convergent evolution.
  - If more than one adaptive radiation occurs in the same geographical area (adaptive radiation in marsupials and placental mammals in the same Australian continent) representing different habitats, similar functional structure develops among the organisms of same habitat.

  **Example 1.** Australian Marsupials and Australian Placental Mammals **(Fig. 10.6).**
  **Example 2.** Wings of insect, bird and bats.

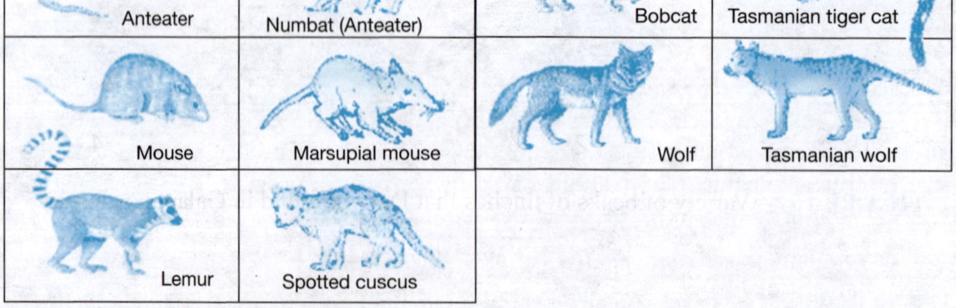


**FIGURE 10.6** Picture showing convergent evolution of Australian Marsupials and placental mammals

**TABLE 10.1** Convergent evolution of Australian Marsupials and Australian Placental Mammals

| Placental Mammals | Australian Marsupials |
|---|---|
| Mole | Marsupial mole |
| Anteater | Numbat (anteater) |
| Mouse | Marsupial mouse |
| Lemur | Spotted cuscus |
| Flying squirrel | Flying phalanger |
| Bobcat | Tasmanian tiger cat |
| Wolf | Tasmanian wolf |

## Biological Evolution

- Evolution by natural selection would have started since the cellular forms of life have originated on earth with different metabolic abilities.
- Rate of appearance of new forms is linked to the life cycle or the life span, i.e., longer the life span and slower the rate of appearance of new forms. Microbes have smaller life span evolved faster.
  **Example:** Fishes and fowl may take millions of years for speciation in a natural way while the microbes may do the same in within few days.
- Nature selects for fitness. Fitness is the end result of the ability to adapt and get selected by nature. In an organism, the so-called fitness depends upon the inherited characteristics, so there must be a genetic basis for getting selected and to evolve. Adaptive ability is inherited and has a genetic basis.
- Theories of evolution: Four theories have been put forward to explain process of evolution.
  1. Lamarckism (**Theory of inheritance of acquired characters)**
  2. Darwinism (Theory of natural selection)
  3. Hugo de Vries' mutation theory
  4. Modern theory of evolution
- Lamarck (a French naturalist) has given his view that the evolution is driven by **use and disuse of organs**.
  **Example 1:** Giraffes attempted to forage leaves on tall trees which has resulted in elongation of their necks. This acquired character of elongated necks was passed on to the succeeding generations. Nobody believes this concept anymore.
  **Example 2: Disappearance of limbs in snake**
  **Example 3: Webbed toes of Aquatic birds**
- **Mendel's law of inheritance and Weismann theory of Continuity of Germplasm** discarded Lamarck concept
- Two key concepts of Darwinian Theory of Evolution:
  (1) Branching descent
  (2) Natural selection
- Darwin was influenced by the work of Thomas Malthus on populations.
- Natural selection is based on certain observations which are factual.
  1. Rapid multiplication 2. Stability of populations 3. Limited food and space: all these leads to struggle for existence.
  2. Struggle for existence and variation (most are inherited) will lead to natural selection. Only those individuals will survive which are fittest to nature (survival of fittest = by Herbert Spencer).
  3. Natural selection and inheritance of useful variation over many generation leads to speciation.
- Darwin was unable to explain cause of variation and mode of transmission of the variation to next generation.
- **Modern concept of evolution includes** – Genetic variation in population (causes: mutation, gene recombination, gene flow, non-random mating and hybridization), Isolation, Natural selection and Speciation.

## Modern Synthetic Theory

The synthetic theory of evolution, often referred to as the modern synthesis or neo-Darwinism, is indeed the most widely accepted theory of evolution in the field of biology. It represents the integration of several key concepts and ideas from different fields of biology into a comprehensive framework for understanding how evolution works.

The theory is based on:

(i) Genetic variation in population
(ii) Isolation
(iii) Heredity
(iv) Natural selection
(v) Speciation

### *Genetic Variation in Population*

Genetic variation within populations is a crucial aspect of evolutionary biology. It provides the raw material upon which natural selection and other evolutionary processes act.

- The key mechanisms that contribute to genetic variation in populations:
  - **Mutation**: Mutations are spontaneous changes in an organism's DNA sequence. They can introduce new genetic variation by creating new alleles (gene variants). Mutations can be caused by various factors, including environmental factors, errors during DNA replication, and radiation.
  - **Recombination**: Recombination occurs during the formation of gametes (sperm and eggs) through processes like crossing over during meiosis. It shuffles existing genetic variation by mixing genetic material from two parents, resulting in offspring with combinations of alleles different from their parents.
  - **Gene Flow (Gene Migration)**: Gene flow refers to the movement of genes from one population to another. It occurs when individuals or their gametes migrate and interbreed with members of other populations. Gene flow can introduce new alleles into a population and reduce genetic differences between populations.
  - **Genetic Drift (Sewall Wright Effect)** : Genetic drift is a random change in frequency of alleles in a population. Thus, it changes the gene frequency of remaining population which causes variation. It is named after the American geneticist Sewall Wright who realised its evolutionary significance. Although genetic drift occurs in all populations, its effects are most marked in very small isolated population. Two important example of genetic drift are **founder effect** and **bottleneck effects:**

    **(a) Founder Effect** and **Founder Principle.** It is an important example of genetic drift in human population. It is noted when a small group of persons called **founders,** leave their homes to find a new settlement, the population in a new settlement may have different genotype frequencies from that of the parent population. Formation of a different genotype in new settlement is called the **founder effect.** Sometimes they form a new species.

    **(b) Bottleneck Effect.** The term was introduced by **Stebbibns** for annual and binual cycle phenomenon of decrease and increase of a size of a population. It is a form of genetic drift in which fluctuations in gene frequencies occur when a population is reduced in size (population crash) and later expands in number (population flush). The enlarged population that result may have gene frequencies distinctly different than before the bottleneck. It often prevents the species from extinction.

**Significance of genetic drift:** Genetic drift is an evolutionary force. Most interbreeding animal population are small. Genetic drift helps the populations to become different because of the probability that each population fixes different genotypes by chance.

- **Non-Random Mating**: Non-random mating occurs when individuals preferentially choose mates with specific traits or genetic characteristics. This can lead to an increase in the frequency of certain alleles within a population. Examples include assortative mating (mates with similar traits) and disassortative mating (mates with dissimilar traits).
- **Hybridization**: Hybridization occurs when individuals from different species or populations interbreed, producing hybrid offspring. Hybrids may have unique combinations of alleles from each parent population, contributing to genetic diversity. In some cases, hybridization can lead to the formation of new species.

These mechanisms collectively contribute to the genetic variation observed within and between populations. Genetic variation is the substrate upon which natural selection acts, allowing populations to adapt to changing environments and driving the evolutionary processes that lead to the diversity of life on Earth.

## Isolation Top of Form

- Isolation mechanisms play a crucial role in the process of speciation by preventing or reducing gene flow between populations. These mechanisms can be categorized into prezygotic and postzygotic isolation, depending on when they occur in the reproductive process. Here's an overview of prezygotic and postzygotic isolation, including subtypes:

  **(i) Prezygotic Isolation:**

  - Prezygotic isolation mechanisms prevent the formation of a viable zygote (fertilized egg) between individuals from different populations or species. They act before mating or during the mating process.

  **Example:** Geographic Isolation (Ecological Isolation), Temporal Isolation, Behavioural Isolation, Mechanical Isolation, Gametic Isolation.

  **(ii) Postzygotic Isolation:**

  - Postzygotic isolation mechanisms occur after mating and fertilization have taken place, but they reduce the fitness of hybrid offspring.

  **Example:** Hybrid Inviability (Hybrid Mortality, Hybrid Sterility, Hybrid Breakdown.

These isolation mechanisms collectively contribute to the formation of distinct species by reducing or eliminating gene flow between populations. Over time, the accumulation of genetic differences between isolated populations can lead to the evolution of new species.

- **Mechanism of Evolution:** What is the cause of variation in population and how these variations lead to evolution?
- **Mutation:** Sudden large change in genetic material

  1. **Hugo de Vries** did his work on **Evening primrose** (*Oenothera lamarckiana*). He is one of the rediscoverer of Mendelism and also he coined the term mutation.
  2. He put forward idea of **Mutation** (sudden large variations in a population).
  3. Mutations were random and directionless.
  4. According to Hugo deVries, speciation is caused by mutation so called it – **saltation** (single step large mutation).

- **Darwinian variations:**

  1. Based on his theory of Natural selection. He proposes that new species are formed by continuous minor heritable variations.
  2. Darwinian variations were minor variations.
  3. Darwin variations were small and directional.
  4. Evolution for Darwin was gradual.

- **Hardy-Weinberg's Principle (Evolution is departing from this principle)**

  - According to Hardy-Weinberg's Principle - In a given population, allele frequencies of a gene (or a locus) are stable and constant from generation to generation.
  - The gene pool (total genes and their alleles in a population) remains a constant. This is called genetic equilibrium.
  - Hardy-Weinberg principle stated it using algebraic equations.

    Frequency of dominant allele (A) = p

    Frequency of recessive allele (a) = q

    Sum total of all the allelic frequencies is 1, i.e., $p + q = 1$

    Frequency of AA (homozygous dominant) individuals in population = $p \times p = p^2$

    Frequency of aa (homozygous recessive) individuals in population = $q \times q = q^2$

    Frequency of Aa (heterozygous) individuals in population = $2pq$

Binomial expression is $(p + q)^2 = p^2 + 2pq + q^2 = 1$

- Disturbance in genetic equilibrium (or Hardy-Weinberg equilibrium) → Change of allele frequency → leads to evolution.
- **Five factors are known to affect Hardy-Weinberg equilibrium:**

**(1) Gene migration or gene flow:** When a section of a population migrates to another place and set up new population, then gene frequencies of original as well as the new population changes. New genes / alleles are added to the new population while some genes / alleles are lost from the old population.

If the above-mentioned gene migration happens multiple times, it leads to gene flow.

**(2) Genetic drift**: If the change in gene frequency occurs by chance, it is called genetic drift. It is non- directional and it will always operate in small population. Sometimes, the genetic drift so prominent in the new sample of population that newly formed population may become a different species. In this case original drifted population is termed as founders and the effect is called **founder effect**. **(Sewell Wright effect)**

**(3) Mutation:** Experiments on microbes show that pre-existing advantageous mutations help the organisms to get selected and the result is observed in new phenotypes. This may lead to speciation over few generations. It is a source of variation. Mutation is sudden change in genetic material.

**(4) Genetic re-combination:** These occur during gametogenesis and it is also a source of variation

**(5) Natural selection:** In this process, heritable variations help the organism for better survival and enable it to reproduce and leave more number of progeny.

- In a population, natural selection can be of three types

**(1) Stabilizing selection (Balancing selection):** More individuals acquire mean character value. For example when human baby delivered the overweight and underweight generally not survived.

**(2) Directional selection (Progressive selection):** More individuals acquire value other than the mean character value. In directional selection it is always the 'extreme' which is favored. Example: (i) Evolution of DDT resistant mosquitoes, (ii) Evolution of giraffe and (iii) Industrial melanism in peppered moth.

**(3) Disruptive selection (Diversifying selection):** More individuals acquire peripheral character value at both ends of the distribution curve. Such types of selections are rare in nature. Example: Sickle cell anemia **(Fig. 10.7)**.

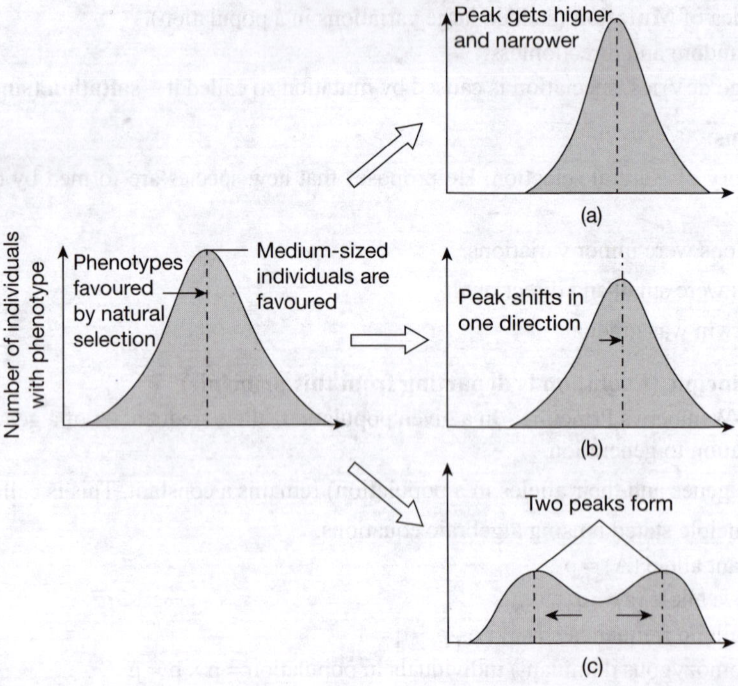


**FIGURE 10.7** Diagrammatic representation of the operation of natural selection on different traits (a) Stabilizing (b) Directional and (c) Disruptive

**TABLE 10.2** Brief account of evolution

| Geological time | Important Events |
|---|---|
| About 2000 mya | • Appearance of first cellular forms of life on earth (mechanism not known).<br>• Some cell had the ability of release $O_2$ (by a reaction similar to light reaction of photosynthesis).<br>• Gradual conversion of single-celled organisms into multi-cellular organisms. |
| 500 mya | • Origin of Invertebrates. |
| 350 mya | • Origin of Jawless fishes.<br>• Fishes that have stout and strong fins could move on land and again go back to the water.<br>• In 1938, a Coelacanth fish (lobe finned fish) was caught in South Africa which was thought to be extinct. These lobefins have evolved into the first amphibians (capable of living on both land and in water). These were ancestors of modern day frogs and salamanders.<br>• Later on amphibians evolved into reptiles which lay thick-shelled eggs which were resistant to xeric condition.<br>• Giant ferns (pteridophytes) were initially present but later on these all slowly fell to form coal deposits. |
| 320 mya | • Origin of Sea weeds and few other plants. |
| 200 mya | • Some land reptiles went back into water and evolved into fish like reptiles (e.g., *Ichthyosarus*).<br>• Tyrannosaurus rex was one of the huge land reptiles (Height is about 20 feet, with huge fearsome dagger like teeth). |
| 65 mya | • Sudden disappearance of dinosaurs from the earth.<br>• Probable reasons: Climatic changes / Evolution of most of them into birds, etc.<br>• Small sized reptiles of that era still exist today. |

A family of dinosaurs and their existing counterparts are depicted in **Fig. 10.8.**

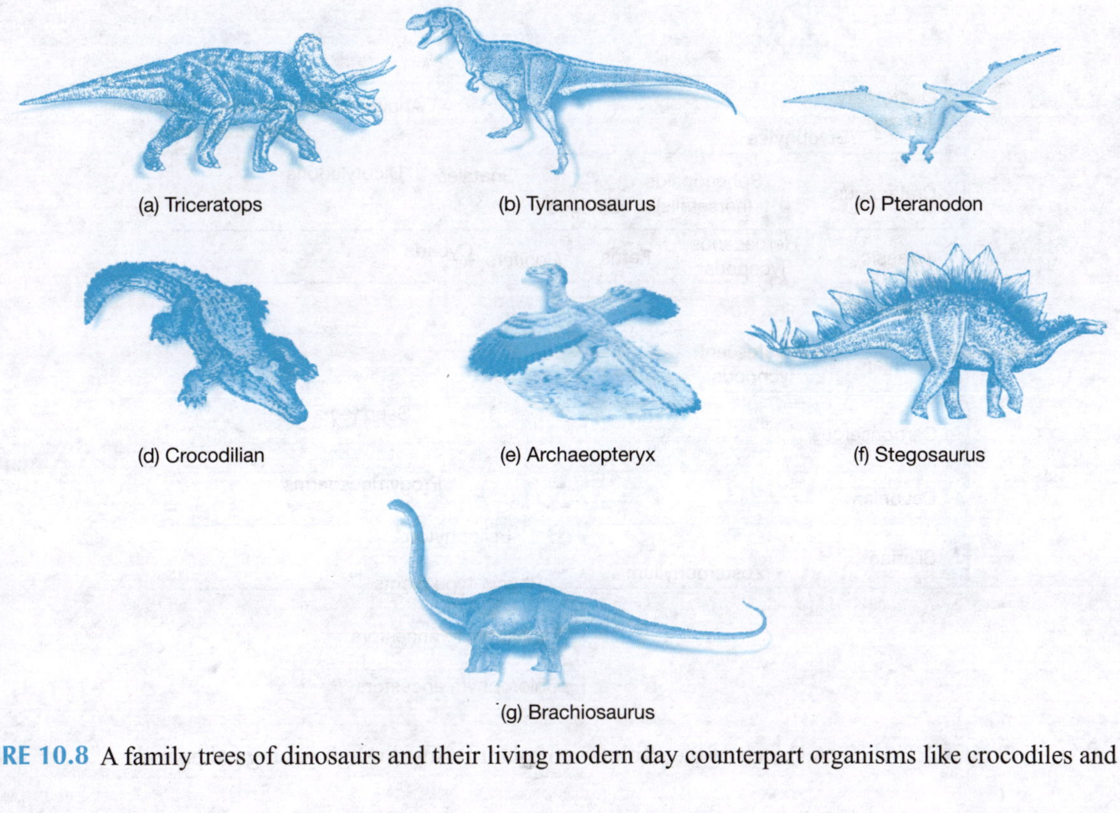


**FIGURE 10.8** A family trees of dinosaurs and their living modern day counterpart organisms like crocodiles and birds

**Note:**

- It is of common opinion that the first organisms that invaded land were plants.
- The first evolved mammals were shrew like (small size).
- After reptiles, earth was dominated by mammals.
- In comparison to other animals, mammals are more intelligent in sensing and avoiding danger at least.
- Due to continental drift:
  1. When South America joined North America, mammals of South America (resembling horse, hippopotamus, bear, rabbit, etc.) were overridden by North American fauna.
  2. Pouched mammals of Australia (marsupials) survived because of absence of any other mammal as there is lack of competition.
- Example of aquatic mammals: whales, dolphins, seals, sea cows, etc.
- Evolution can also be seen specifically during evolution of horse, elephant, dog, etc.
- Evolution of man is the most successful story in which language skills and self-consciousness has also developed.
- **Devonian period: Age of Fishes**
- **Carboniferous period: Age of Amphibians**
- **Jurassic period: Age of Reptiles**
- **Paleozoic** Era divided in four periods namely: Silurian, Devonian, Carboniferous ,Permian
- **Mesozoic** Era divided in three period namely: Triassic, Jurassic, Cretaceous
- **Cenozoic** Era divided in two period namely: Tertiary and Quaternary
- **Therapsids** (reptiles) are direct ancestors of mammals

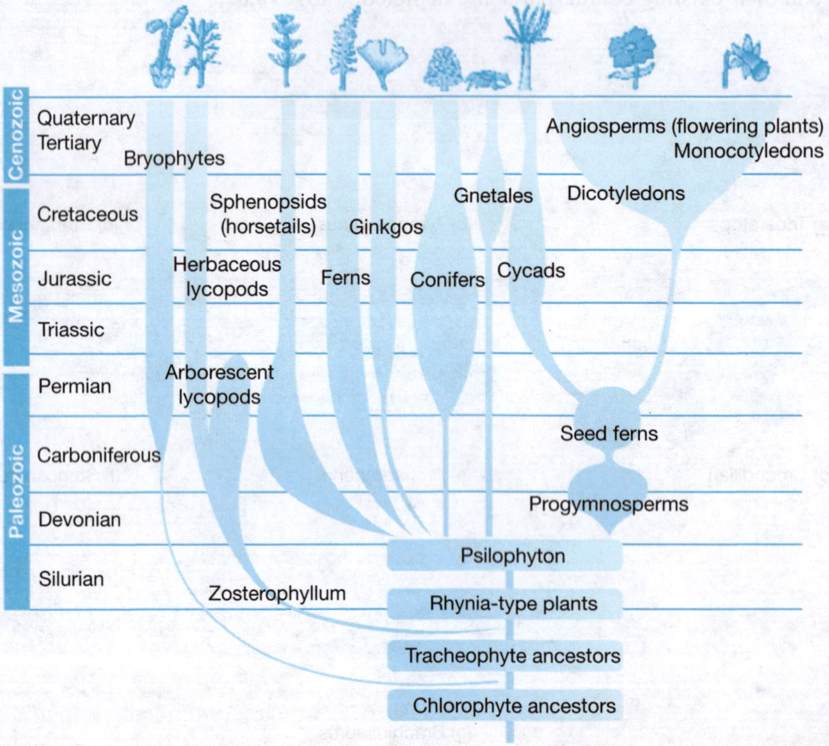


**FIGURE 10.9** A sketch of the evolution of plant forms through geological periods

**Fig. 10.10** illustrates the representative evolutionary history of vertebrates across geological periods.

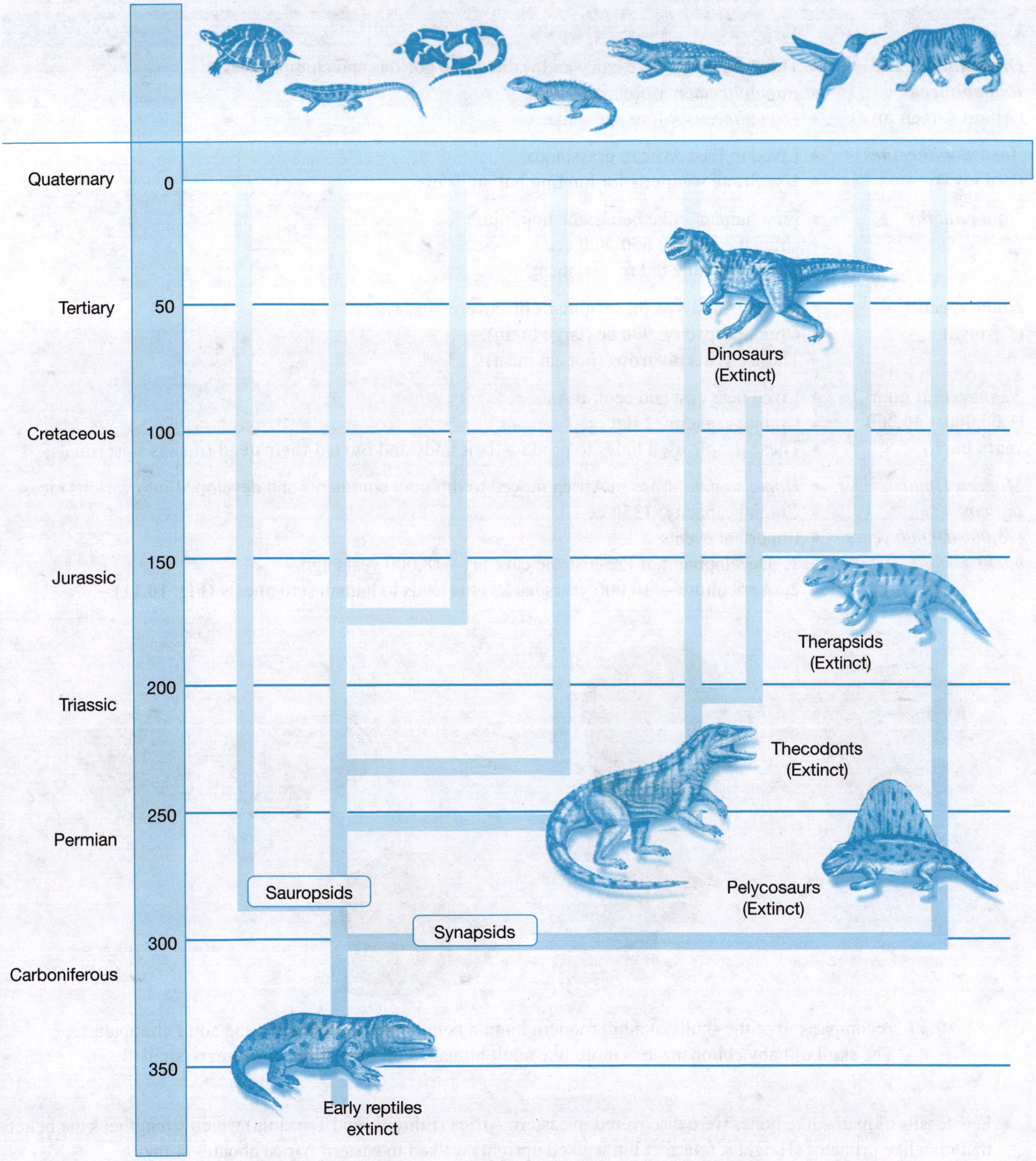


**FIGURE 10.10** Representative evolutionary history of vertebrates through geological periods

## Origin and Evolution of Man

**TABLE 10.3** Events in human evolution

| Human Evolution | Description |
|---|---|
| ***Dryopithecus* and *Ramapithecus* (About fifteen mya)** | • These primates were hairy and walked like gorillas and chimpanzees.<br>• *Ramapithecus*: More man – like.<br>• *Dryopithecus*: More ape – like. |
| ***Australopithecines* (two mya)** | • Lived in East African grasslands.<br>• **Use Stone weapons** for hunting but ate fruits. |
| ***Homo habilis*** | • First human – like being: the hominid.<br>• Cranial capacity: **650–800 cc.**<br>• These probably did not eat meat. |
| ***Homo erectus* (1.5 mya)** | • In 1891 fossils of these humans discovered in Java<br>• Cranial capacity: **900 cc** (large brain).<br>• These are **herbivorous** (not eat meat) |
| ***Neanderthal* man (1,00,000 – 40,000 years back)** | • Lived near east and central Asia.<br>• Cranial capacity: **1400 cc.**<br>• These people used hides to product their body and **buried their dead** (means start rituals) |
| ***Modern Homo sapiens (75,000-10,000 years back)*** | • *Homo sapiens* arose in Africa moved to different continents and developed into various races.<br>• Cranial capacity: **1350 cc**<br>• Important events:<br>**1.** Development of Pre-historic cave art—18,000 years ago.<br>**2.** Agriculture— 10,000 years back. This leads to human settlements **(Fig. 10.11)**. |

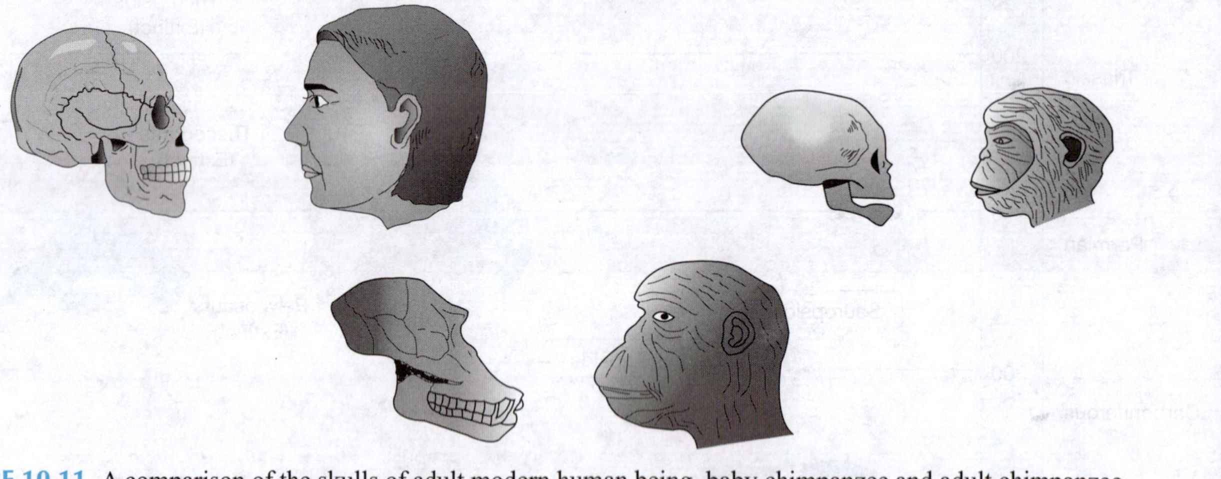

**FIGURE 10.11** A comparison of the skulls of adult modern human being, baby chimpanzee and adult chimpanzee. The skull of baby chimpanzee is more like adult human skull than adult chimpanzee skull

- Few fossils of man – like bones were discovered in eastern Africa (Ethiopia and Tanzania) which strengthens the belief that man like primates (Height < four feet but walked upright) walked in eastern Africa about 3–4 mya.
- Pre-historic human's cave painting can be seen at Bhimbetka rocks in Raisen district of Madhya Pradesh.

# PRACTICE EXERCISES

**Direction:** Read the question carefully and choose the correct option for each.

## Multiple Choice Questions: Level I

### Origin of Life and Theories for Origin of Life

1. Evolutionary biology is related to the
   (a) Origin of universe
   (b) Origin of earth
   (c) Study of history of life forms on earth
   (d) Origin of stars
2. Stellar distances are measured in
   (a) km (b) m
   (c) Light year (d) pm
3. How old is the universe?
   (a) 10 billion years (b) 20 billion years
   (c) 5 billion years (d) 15 billion years
4. Galaxies contain
   (a) Stars (b) Clouds of gas and dust
   (c) Both (d) None of these
5. Select the false statement from the following.
   (a) Big bang theory is used to explain the origin of the universe.
   (b) Expansion of the universe after the explosion lead to a decrease in temperature.
   (c) Hydrogen and helium had formed before the explosion.
   (d) Gases condensed under gravitation and formed galaxies.
6. Earth was formed ________ billion years back.
   (a) 4.5 (b) 5.5 (c) 3.5 (d) 1.5
7. Molten mass on early earth produced
   (a) Water vapour and $CH_4$
   (b) $CO_2$
   (c) $NH_3$
   (d) All of these
8. Which part of solar radiation can break $H_2O$?
   (a) Visible radiation (b) Ultraviolet radiation
   (c) Infrared (d) None of these
9. Life appeared ________ years after the formation of earth.
   (a) 1000 million (b) 100 million
   (c) 10 million (d) 500 million
10. Which of the following is related to the origin of life on earth?
   (a) Panspermia
   (b) Theory of spontaneous generation
   (c) Chemical evolution
   (d) All of these
11. Who proposed the theory of chemical evolution for the first time?
   (a) Oparin and Haldane (b) Miller
   (c) Louis Pasteur (d) Darwin
12. Identify the parts A, B, C and D in the figure.

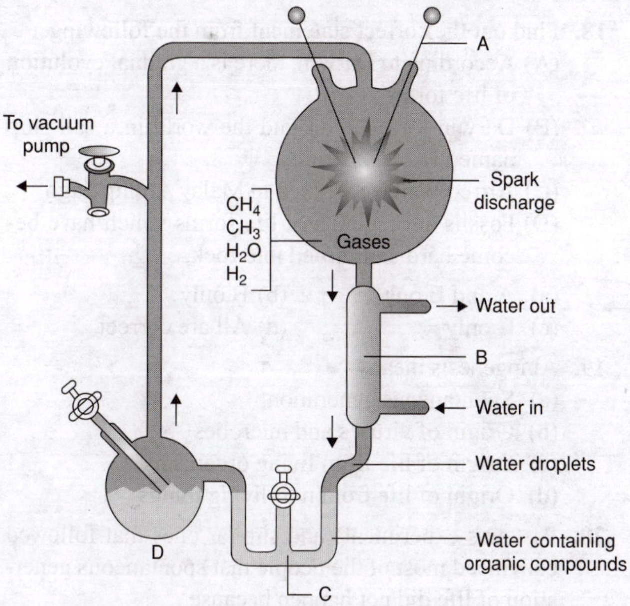


   (a) A: Liquid water in trap, B: Electrode, C: Boiling water, D: Condenser
   (b) A: Boiling water, B: Condenser, C: Electrode, D: Liquid water in trap
   (c) A: Electrode, B: Condenser, C: Liquid water in trap, D: Boiling water
   (d) A: Condenser, B: Liquid water in trap, C: Boiling water, D: Electrode
13. Miller simulated early Earth conditions in a laboratory by passing electric discharge through a closed flask raising its temperature to 800°C and containing
   (a) $CH_4$ and $H_2$ (b) $NH_3$
   (c) Water vapour (d) All of these

**14.** The first non-cellular form of life could have originated ________ billion years back.
(a) 1 (b) 2
(c) 3 (d) 4

**15.** Which of the given statement is wrong as per the 'Theory of Special Creation'?
(a) All living organism created as such
(b) Diversity change as time changes
(c) Earth is about 4000 years old
(d) All are correct

**16.** The fitness referred to in Darwin's theory is
(a) Physical fitness (b) Mental fitness
(c) Reproductive fitness (d) All of these

**17.** Evidence of evolution from fossils is known as
(a) Paleontological evidence
(b) Embryological evidence
(c) Physiological evidence
(d) Biochemical evidence

**18.** Find out the correct statement from the following.
(A) According to Darwin, there is a gradual evolution of life forms.
(B) Darwin travelled around the world in a sail ship named H.M.S. Beagle.
(C) Alfred Wallace worked in Malay Archipelago.
(D) Fossils are remains of life forms which have become hard and turned into rock.
(a) A and B only (b) B only
(c) C only (d) All are correct

**19.** Abiogenesis means
(a) Spontaneous generation
(b) Origin of viruses and microbes
(c) Origin of life from living organisms
(d) Origin of life from non-living things

**20.** Pasteur's experiments and similar ones that followed convinced most of the people that spontaneous generation of life did not happen because
(a) Pasteur was extremely meticulous.
(b) Pasteur did not boil his flask for a long time.
(c) Pasteur used very fine mesh screens to cover his flask.
(d) Pasteur's swan-necked flasks ruled out the objection that spoiled air could have contaminated his experiments.

**21.** The early belief of the spontaneous origin of life was disproved by
(a) Lederberg (b) Robert Koch
(c) Louis Pasteur (d) Charles Darwin

**22.** Who said that organisms develop from pre-existing organisms?
(a) Aristotle
(b) Louis Pasteur
(c) Alexander Oparin
(d) Thomas Hunt Morgan

**23.** The idea that life originates from pre-existing life is referred to as
(a) Biogenesis theory
(b) Abiogenesis theory
(c) Extraterrestrial theory
(d) Special creation theory

**24.** Life was created by some supernatural power. This theory is
(a) Abiogenesis
(b) Spore theory
(c) Special creation theory
(d) Spontaneous generation

**25.** Life came from outer space, this theory is called
(a) Spore theory
(b) Naturalistic theory
(c) Special creation theory
(d) Spontaneous generation

**26.** About how long ago was the Earth formed?
(a) 3.0 billion years ago (b) 10 billion years ago
(c) 4.6 billion years ago (d) 20 billion years ago

**27.** '*Modern theory of origin of life*' was propounded by
(a) Oparin (b) Miller
(c) Darwin (c) Khorana

**28.** A. I. Oparin was a
(a) Polish biologist (b) Russian biochemist
(c) Belgian nutritionist (d) Swedish cosmologist

**29.** Oparin's theory of 'Origin of life' is based on
(a) Chemical evolution (b) Cosmic evolution
(c) Artificial synthesis (d) Organic evolution

**30.** According to Oparin, which one of the following was not present in the primitive atmosphere of the Earth?
(a) Oxygen (b) Methane
(c) Hydrogen (d) Water vapour

**31.** The basic components of atmosphere of primitive Earth were
(a) Ammonia, methane and water
(b) Methane, ozone, nitrogen and water
(c) Hydrogen, nitrogen, methane and water
(d) Ammonia, methane, hydrogen and water

**32.** Which of the following is a true statement?
(a) The primitive atmosphere had 20 per cent oxygen, just like it is today.
(b) The reducing primitive atmosphere contributed to the origin of life and the oxidizing one today would hinder it.

(c) The primitive atmosphere was an oxidizing one and today's is a reducing one, making photosynthesis possible.
(d) It took so long for prokaryote evolution because the primitive atmosphere screened out the ultraviolet radiation from the sun.

**33.** Life originated in
(a) Air (b) Water
(c) Land (d) All of these

**34.** Stanley Miller proposed the origin of life by
(a) Biogenesis (b) Abiogenesis
(c) Chemical synthesis (d) None of these

**35.** The first experiment on chemical evolution and origin of life was carried out by
(a) Watson and Crick (b) Miller and Urey
(c) Beadle and Tatum (d) Darwin and Wallace

**36.** The spark-discharge apparatus to test chemical evolution of life was designed by
(a) Urey and Miller (b) Dixon and Jolly
(c) Jacob and Monod (d) Oparin and Haldane

**37.** The diagram represents Miller's experiment. Choose the correct combination of labelling:

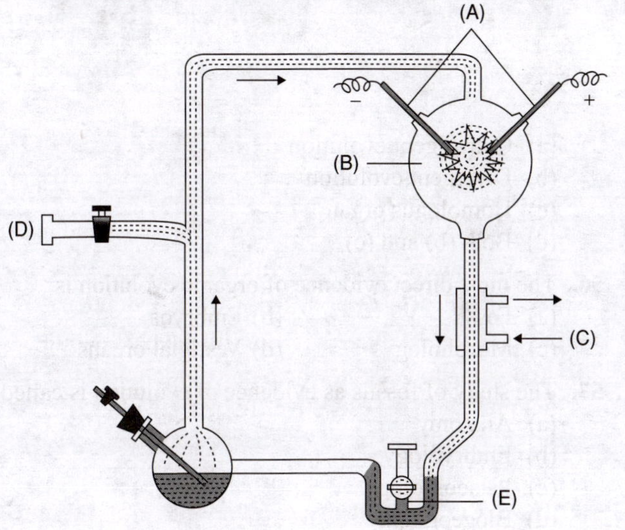


(a) A: Electrodes, B: $NH_3 + H_2 + H_2O + CH_4$, C: Hot water, D: Vacuum, E: U trap
(b) A: Electrodes, B: $NH_3 + H_2O$, C: Hot water, D: Tap, E: U trap
(c) A: Electrodes, B: $NH_3 + H_2 + H_2O$, $CH_4$, C: Cold water, D: Vacuum, E: U trap
(d) A: Electrodes, B: $NH_3 + H_2 + H_2O + CH_4$, C: Steam, D: Vacuum, E: U Trap
(e) A: Electrodes, B: $NH_3 + CH_4$, C: Cold water, D: Sink, E: U trap

**38.** The findings of Miller's experiment on origin of life have provided evidence for
(a) Theory of biogenesis
(b) Oparin-Haldane theory
(c) Theory of special creation
(d) Theory of organic evolution

**39.** The category of molecules produced by the Miller–Urey experiment was
(a) Organic polymers (b) Inorganic polymers
(c) Organic monomers (d) Inorganic monomers

**40.** Stanley Miller who is famous for 'simulation experiments' belonged to
(a) USA (b) UK (c) USSR (d) Canada

**41.** Stanley Miller conducted his experiments and produced amino acids by electric discharge passed through $NH_3$, $H_2O$, $CH_4$ and ______.
(a) Oxygen (b) Hydrogen
(c) Nitrogen (d) Carbon dioxide

**42.** The energy used in the Miller–Urey experiment was
(a) Photo energy (b) Electric spark
(c) Atomic radiation (d) Mechanical energy

**43.** Earliest life forms on the earth were
(a) Autotrophs
(b) Cyanobacteria
(c) Photoautotrophs
(d) Chemoheterotrophs

**44.** The concept of chemical evolution is based on
(a) Crystallization of chemicals.
(b) Effect of solar radiation on chemicals.
(c) Interaction of water, air and clay under intense heat.
(d) Possible origin of life by combination of chemicals under suitable environmental conditions.

**45.** Which one of the following is incorrect about the characteristic of protobionts (coacervates and microspheres) as envisaged in abiogenic origin of life?
(a) They were able to reproduce.
(b) They could maintain an internal environment.
(c) They were partially isolated from the surroundings.
(d) They could separate the combination of molecule from the surroundings.

**46.** Biologists define evolution as
(a) Heritable change in a line of descent over generations
(b) Inheritance of characteristics acquired by the individual
(c) The origin of species
(d) None of the above

47. Basic idea of evolution is
(a) Cosmic evolution
(b) Special creation
(c) Spontaneous generation
(d) Descent with modification

48. The process of evolution is
(a) Continuous
(b) Discontinuous
(c) Continuous in the past but discontinuous presently
(d) Discontinuous in the past but continuous presently

49. The concept of evolution is an excellent working hypothesis to approach the problem of
(a) Matter, energy and life
(b) Environmental conditions
(c) Prodigality in reproduction
(d) Diversity of organisms upon earth

## Evidences of Evolution

50. Homologous organ represents
(a) Convergent evolution
(b) Divergent evolution
(c) Anthropogenic evolution
(d) Genetic drift

51. Analogous organs represent
(a) Convergent evolution
(b) Divergent evolution
(c) Anthropogenic evolution
(d) Genetic drift

52. Which of the following shows analogy?
(a) Eye of octopus and mammals
(b) Vertebrate hearts
(c) Thorn of Bougainvillea and tendril of Cucurbita
(d) Vertebrate brains

53. What does this diagram show?

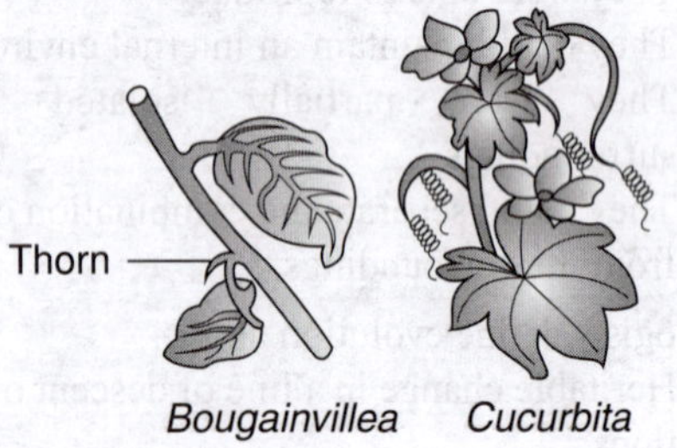


(a) Convergent evolution
(b) Divergent evolution
(c) Homologous organ
(d) Both (b) and (c)

54. What does this diagram show?

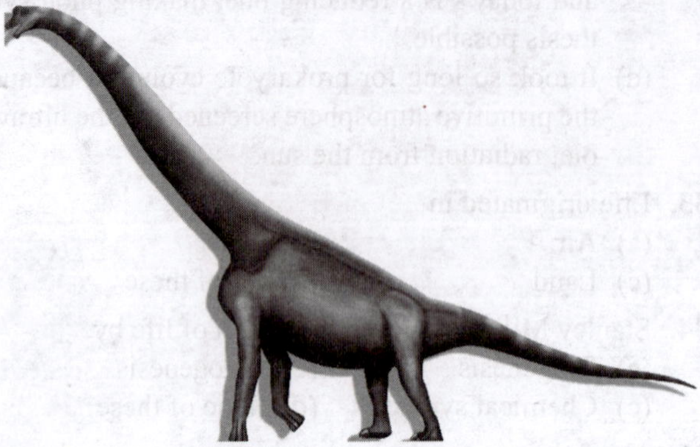

(a) Brachiosaurus (b) Stegosaurus
(c) Triceratops (d) Tyrannosaurus

55. This diagram shows

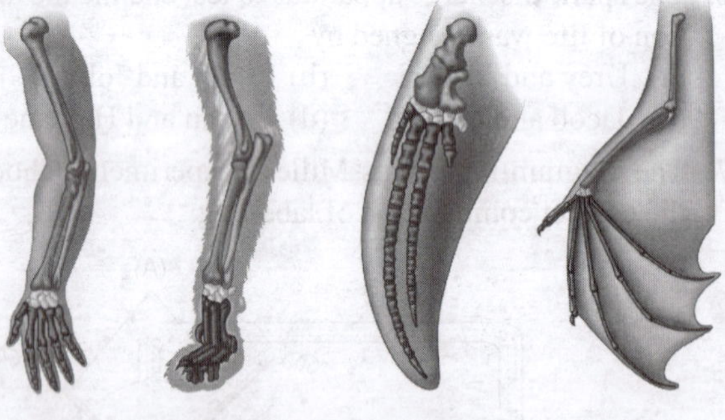

(a) Convergent evolution
(b) Divergent evolution
(c) Homologus organ
(d) Both (b) and (c)

56. The most direct evidence of organic evolution is
(a) Fossils (b) Embryos
(c) Morphology (d) Vestigial organs

57. The study of fossils as evidence of evolution is called
(a) Anatomy
(b) Embryology
(c) Palaeontology
(d) Biogeography

58. The fossils are preserved in
(a) Sedimentary rocks (b) Igneous rocks
(c) Metamorphic rocks (d) None of these

59. Fossil X is older than fossil Y because
(a) Fossil Y was found in deeper sedimentation.
(b) Fossil X was found in deeper sedimentation.
(c) Fossil Y has some vestigial organs functional in X.
(d) Fossil Y has homologous and analogous organs of X.

**60.** Our best estimate for the age of Earth, which is 4.5 billion years is supported by
(a) Gradualism
(b) Big bang theory
(c) Assumption of uniformitarianism
(d) Radioactive dating of the oldest rocks found

**61.** Darwin's finches are found in
(a) Tahiti (b) Tundra
(c) Galapagos Island (d) None of these

## Adaptive Radiation and Biological Evolution (Theories)

**62.** Which of the following shows convergent evolution?
(a) Mouse and Marsupial mouse
(b) Bobcat and Spotted cuscus
(c) Anteater and Marsupial mole
(d) Lemur and Tasmanian wolf

**63.** Which of the following is an example of anthropogenic evolution?
(a) Selection of resistant varieties due to herbicides.
(b) Selection of resistant varieties due to pesticides.
(c) Industrial melanism
(d) All the above

**64.** This diagram shows:

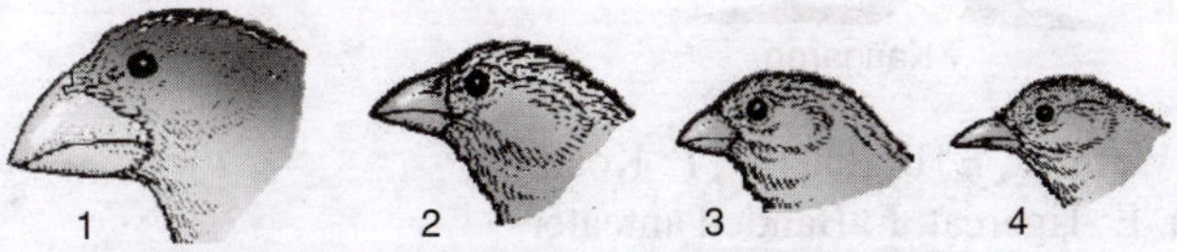


(a) Adaptive radiation (b) Genetic drift
(c) Founder effect (d) Mutation

**65.** Which of the following diagrams is not a correct representation of convergent evolution?

(a) 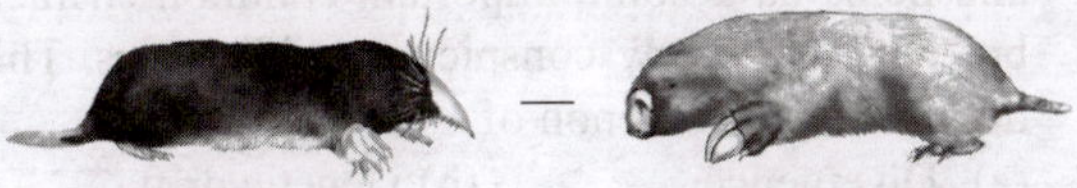

(b) 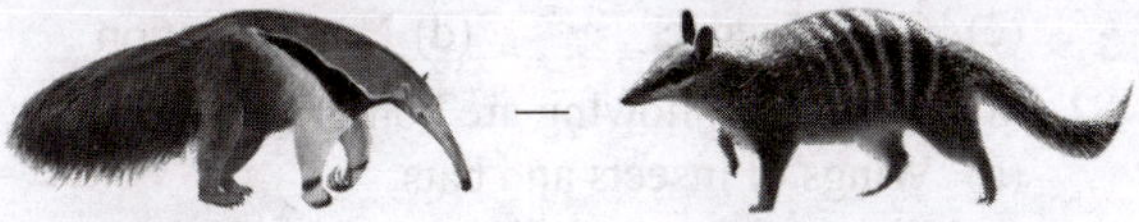

(c) 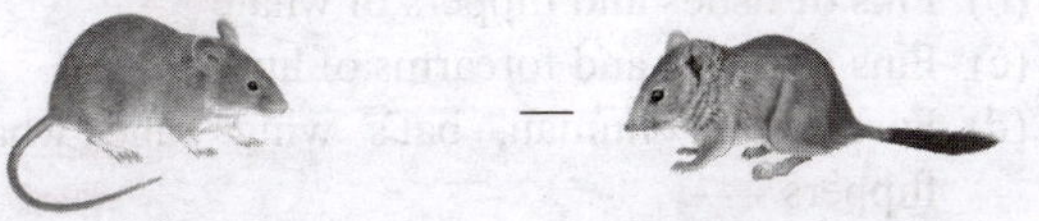

(d) 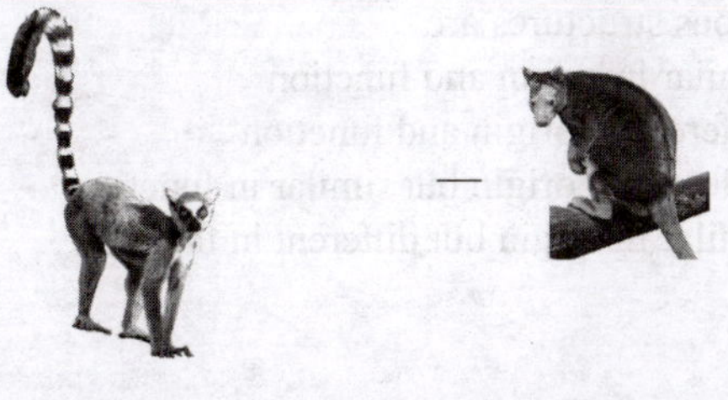

**66.** Which of the following diagram does not correctly represent the convergent evolution?

(a) 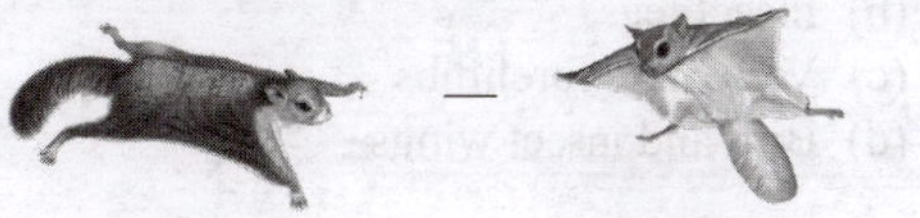

(b) 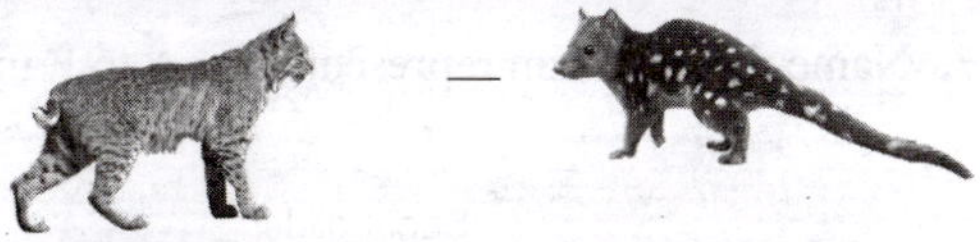

(c) 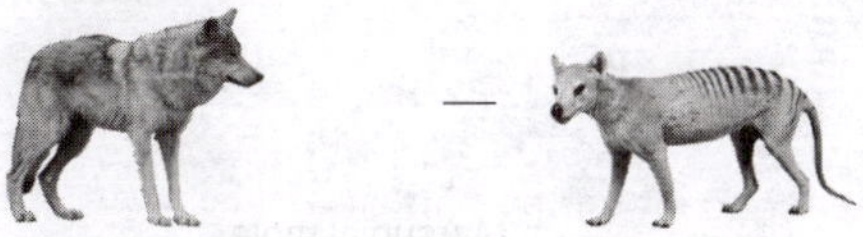

(d) None of these

**67.** Darwin's finches provide excellent evidence in favour of evolution. This evidence comes from the field of
(a) Anatomy (b) Biogeography
(c) Embryology (d) Palaeontology

**68.** The evolution of numerous species, such as Darwin's finches from a single ancestor is called
(a) Gradualism (b) Adaptive radiation
(c) Sympatric speciation (d) Geographical isolation

**69.** Darwin's finches discovered from the Galapagos Islands serve as a good example of
(a) Mimicry
(b) Camouflage
(c) Seasonal migration
(d) Biogeographical evidence of evolution

**70.** The classical example of adaptive radiation in development of new species is
(a) Darwin's finches (b) Marsupials of Australia
(c) Both (a) and (b) (d) None of these

**71.** The organs of different species that are related to each other through common descent though becomes functionally different are called
(a) Vestigial (b) Analogous
(c) Homologous (d) None of these

**72.** Organs which have the same fundamental structure but different in functions are called
(a) Vestigial organs (b) Analogous organs
(c) Homoplastic organs (d) Homologous organs

**73.** Homology does not refer to
(a) Divergent evolution (b) Common descent
(c) Convergent evolution (d) Adaptive radiation

**74.** The homologous organs are wings of
(a) Pigeon and bat
(b) Butterfly and bat
(c) Sparrow and honeybee
(d) Parrot and limbs of man

**75.** Which of the following are not homologous?
(a) Insect mouthparts
(b) Insect legs
(c) Vertebrate forelimbs
(d) Bird and insect wings

**76.** Which of the following is a set of homologous organs?
(a) Wings of grasshopper, flippers of whale
(b) Wings of birds, front feet of horse
(c) Wings of housefly, wings of birds
(d) None of these

**77.** Name the organism represented by A to F in the illustration.

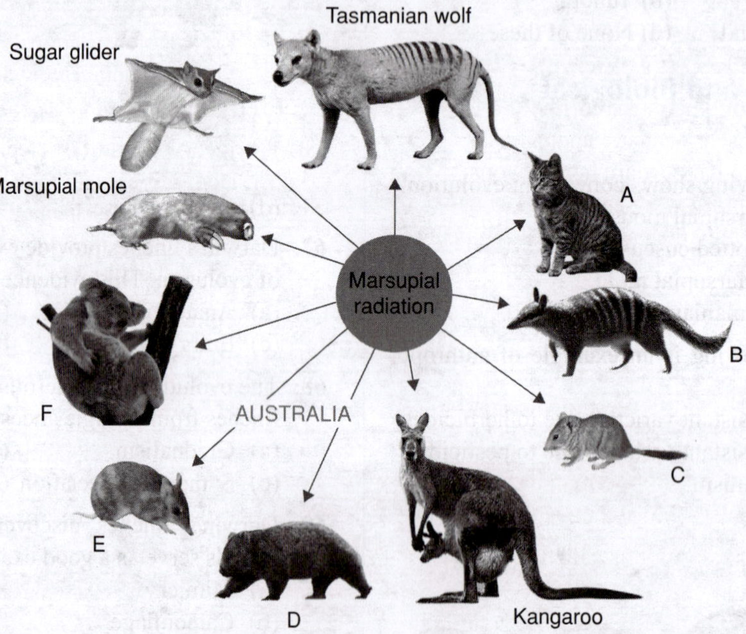


(a) A: Tigercat, B: Banded anteater, C: Marsupial rat, D: Wombat, E: Bandicoot, F: Koala
(b) A: Bandicoot, B: Wombat, C: Marsupial rat, D: Koala, E: Tigercat, F: Banded anteater
(c) A: Koala, B: Banded anteater, C: Tigercat, D: Bandicoot, E: Marsupial rat, E: Wombat
(d) A: Wombat, B: Tigercat, C: Koala, D: Bandicoot, E: Banded anteater, F: Marsupial rat

**78.** Which group includes homologous organs?
(a) Wings of butterfly, flying fish and bird
(b) Tentacles of hydra and arms of starfish
(c) Fins of seal, wings of birds and forelimbs of man
(d) Horns of cattle, tail of horse and teeth of mammals

**79.** Which of the following are homologous organs?
(a) Hand of man, wings of bat
(b) Eyes of man, eyes of squid
(c) Gills of fish, lungs of man
(d) Leaf of moss, frond of fern

**80.** Thorn of bougainvillea and tendril of cucurbita are examples of
(a) Vestigial organs
(b) Analogous organs
(c) Homologous organs
(d) Retrogressive evolution

**81.** Although all mammals whale, dolphin, bat, monkey and horse have some important common characters, but they also show conspicuous differences. This is due to the phenomenon of
(a) Divergence
(b) Genetic drift
(c) Convergence
(d) Normalization

**82.** Which of the following are homologous organs?
(a) Wings of insects and bats
(b) Fins of fishes and flippers of whale
(c) Fins of fishes and forearms of human
(d) Forearm of human, bat's wings and whale's flippers

**83.** Analogous structures are
(a) Similar in origin and function
(b) Different in origin and function
(c) Different in origin but similar in function
(d) Similar in origin but different in function

**84.** Analogy is found between
(a) Wings of birds and bats
(b) Wings of bat and butterfly
(c) Hands of man and flippers of whale
(d) Hands of man and forelimbs of horse

**85.** Which pair of organs are analogous in nature?
(a) Gills of fish and gills of prawn
(b) Ear of frog and ear of rabbit
(c) Arm of man and limbs of horse
(d) Wings of bat and flippers of seal

**86.** Which of the following pairs are correct?
(a) Bat wing and insect wing are analogous.
(b) Seal flippers and bat paw are homologous.
(c) Insect wing and bird wing are homologous.
(d) Thorn of bougainvillea and tendril of pea are analogous.

**87.** Which type of evolution is shown by the wings of bats, mosquitoes and pigeons?
(a) Divergent (b) Atavism
(c) Convergent (d) Vestigial organs

**88.** Lamarck was a
(a) French naturalist (b) German biologist
(c) British evolutionist (d) American biochemist

**89.** Lamarck's theory of evolution is called
(a) Inheritance of acquired characters
(b) Theory of special creation
(c) Survival of the fittest
(d) None of these

**90.** The theory of use and disuse of organs was given by
(a) Lamarck (b) Darwin
(c) Weissmann (d) Hugo de Vries

**91.** The most important theory of evolution was proposed by
(a) Beadle and Tatum (b) Watson and Crick
(c) Darwin and Wallace (d) Mendel and Morgan

**92.** Darwin's finches are an excellent example of
(a) Connecting links (b) Brood parasitism
(c) Adaptive radiation (d) Seasonal migration

**93.** Sweet potato and potato are examples of
(a) Homologous structures
(b) Analogous structures
(c) Both (a) and (b)
(d) None of these

**94.** The concepts of natural selection in evolution were proposed by
(a) Hugo de Vries
(b) Charles Darwin
(c) August Weismann
(d) Jean Baptiste de Lamarck

**95.** Darwin travelled in which ship?
(a) H.N.S. Eagle (b) Titanic
(c) H.M.S. Beagle (d) D. Matrica

**96.** The main point of Darwin's theory is
(a) Variation (b) Mutation
(c) Enormous fertility (d) Natural selection

**97.** Survival of the fittest is possible due to
(a) Overproduction
(b) Favourable variations
(c) Environmental changes
(d) Inheritance of acquired characters

**98.** The theory of natural selection of Darwin
(a) Does not explain fossils
(b) Is completely changed
(c) Has the first theory of organic evolution
(d) Has failed in explaining the origin of variations

**99.** Darwin was influenced by reading the essays of
(a) Wallace (b) Spencer
(c) Mendel (d) Malthus

**100.** Which one provides the correct sequence of events in origin of species according to Darwinism?
(A) Natural selection
(B) Variations and their inheritance
(C) Survival of the fittest
(D) Struggle for existence
(a) A, B, C, D (b) B, D, C, A
(c) D, B, C, A (d) B, C, A, D

**101.** Which of the following is not under Darwin's theory of natural selection?
(a) Over production (b) Survival of the fittest
(c) Causes of variation (d) Struggle for existence

**102.** Which one of the following phenomena supports Darwin's concept of natural selection in organic evolution?
(a) Development of transgenic animals.
(b) Prevalence of pesticide resistant insects.
(c) Production of 'Dolly' the sheep by cloning.
(d) Development of organs from 'stem cells' for organ transplantation.

**103.** The breeding of plants and animals by humans is termed as
(a) Natural selection (b) Founder effect
(c) Neutral variation (d) Artificial selection

**104.** Improved race of pigeons have been developed by
(a) Natural selection
(b) Artificial selection
(c) Protective selection
(d) Environmental selection

**105.** Most modern breeds of domestic dog have been evolved through
(a) Isolation (b) Sexual selection
(c) Artificial selection (d) Natural selection

**106.** In which condition does the gene ratio remain constant for any species?
(a) Mutation (b) Gene flow
(c) Sexual selection (d) Random mating

**107.** The phenomenon of 'Industrial melanism' demonstrates
(a) Natural selection
(b) Induced mutation
(c) Reproductive isolation
(d) Geographical isolation

**108.** The change of the lighter coloured variety of peppered moth, Biston betularia, to its darker variety (carbonaria) is due to
(a) Deletion of a segment of genes due to industrial pollution.
(b) Mutation of single Mendelian gene for survival in smoke laden industrial environment.
(c) Industrial carbon deposited on the wings of the moth resulting in darker variety.
(d) Translocation of a block of genes in chromosomes in response to heavy carbons.

**109.** The classical example of adaptive radiation in the development of new species is
(a) Darwin finches (b) Marsupials of Australia
(c) Giant turtles (d) All of these

**110.** In the developmental history of mammalian heart, it is observed that it passes through a two chambered fishlike heart, three chambered frog-like heart and finally four chambered stage. To which hypothesis can this above cited statement be approximated?
(a) Biogenetic law (b) Lamarck's principle
(c) Hardy-Weinberg law (d) Mendelian principles

## Mechanism of Evolution

**111.** The first attempt to solve the problem of mechanism of organic evolution was made by
(a) Oparin (b) Darwin
(c) Wallace (d) Lamarck

**112.** Mutation theory explaining organic evolution was proposed by
(a) E. Darwin (b) W. Harvey
(c) Hugo de Vries (d) Louis Pasteur

**113.** The material in which Hugo de Vries experimented to explain the mechanism of evolution thus pioneering the theory of mutations was
(a) Fruitfly (b) China rose
(c) Garden pea (d) Evening primrose

**114.** Hugo de Vries gave his mutation theory on organic evolution while working on
(a) *Althea rosea*
(b) *Pisum sativum*
(c) *Oenothera lamarckiana*
(d) *Drosophila melanogaster*

**115.** For natural selection the important factor is
(a) Disuse (b) Variation
(c) Catastrophe (d) Special creation

**116.** Initiating the force of evolution is
(a) Variation (b) Adaptation
(c) Competition (d) Natural selection

**117.** The raw material for organic evolution is
(a) Asexual reproduction
(b) Mutation
(c) Nutritive substances
(d) Effect of hormones

**118.** Lederberg replica experiment explains
(a) Mutation theory (b) Darwin's theory
(c) Lamarck's theory (d) None of these

**119.** Some bacteria are able to grow in streptomycin containing medium due to
(a) Genetic drift
(b) Natural selection
(c) Induced mutation
(d) Reproductive isolation

**120.** The processes of ________ and ________ generate variation and ________ produces adaptation to the environment.
(a) Sexual selection, natural selection, mutation
(b) Mutation, sexual recombination, genetic drift
(c) Genetic drift, mutation, sexual recombination
(d) Mutation, sexual recombination, natural selection

**121.** Industrial melanism was highlighted by
(a) Polar bear (b) Rock python
(c) *Mimosa pudica* (d) *Biston betularia*

**122.** Speciation usually occurs
(a) Suddenly
(b) By genetic drift
(c) When populations are geographically isolated
(d) When populations are not geographically isolated

**123.** Which is the basis for evolution?
(a) Cell (b) Species
(c) Individual (d) Population

**124.** Hugo de Vries, based on his work on ________, brought forth the idea of mutations.
(a) *Pisum sativum* (b) *Lathyrus odoratus*
(c) Evening primrose (d) *Lathyrus sativus*

**125.** Mutations are
(a) Directionless and random
(b) Random and directional
(c) Small variations and directional
(d) Not responsible for evolution

**126.** Select the false statement from the following.
(a) Darwinian variations are small and directional.
(b) Saltation is a single large step mutation.
(c) Branching descent and natural selection are the two key concepts of Darwinian theory of evolution.
(d) Mutation is random and progressive in nature.

## Hardy-Weinberg Concept

**127.** When a given population is in genetic equilibrium, then
(a) Gene pool remains constant.
(b) Allele frequencies in population is constant from generation to generation.
(c) Sum total of all allelic frequencies is 1.
(d) All the above

**128.** How many factors affect the Hardy–Weinberg equilibrium?
(a) 1 (b) 3
(c) 4 (d) 5

**129.** The factors affecting genetic equilibrium are the following except
(a) Gene flow (b) Mutation
(c) Somatic variation (d) Genetic recombination

**130.** The five factors affecting genetic equilibrium are
(a) Gene flow, genetic drift
(b) Mutation, genetic recombination
(c) Natural selection
(d) All of these

**131.** Natural selection is which of the following types?
(a) Stabilizing (b) Disruptive
(c) Directional (d) Any of these

**132.** Variation may be due to
(a) Mutation
(b) Genetic recombinant during gametogenesis
(c) Gene flow or genetic drift
(d) All the above

**133.** Sum of all the genes in a population is called
(a) Genome (b) Gene pool
(c) Germplasm (d) Gene bank

**134.** At a particular locus, frequency of 'A' allele is 0.6 and that of 'a' is 0.4. What would be the frequency of heterozygotes in a random mating population at equilibrium?
(a) 0.36 (b) 0.48
(c) 0.16 (d) 0.24

**135.** Genetic drift operates in
(a) Large isolated population
(b) Small isolated population
(c) Fast reproductive population
(d) Slow reproductive population

**136.** Match the following concepts of evolution in List-I with List-II and select the correct answer using the codes given below the lists:

| List-I | List-II |
|---|---|
| (A) Mutation | (1) Changes in population's allele frequencies due to chance alone. |
| (B) Gene flow | (2) Differences in survival and reproduction among variant individuals. |
| (C) Natural selection | (3) Immigration, emigration change allele frequencies. |
| (D) Genetic drift | (4) Source of new alleles |

(a) A:1, B:2, C:3, D:4 (b) A:4, B:2, C:3, D:1
(c) A:3, B:1, C:4, D:2 (d) A:4, B:3, C:2, D:1

**137.** Which of the following concepts is known as the Sewall Wright effect?
(a) Genetic drift (b) Isolation
(c) Gene pool (d) Gene flow

**138.** Which of the following would stop evolution by barring the occurrence of the natural selection?
(a) If humans became extinct because of a disease or epidemic.
(b) If ozone depletion led to increased ultraviolet radiation which caused many new mutations.
(c) If a thermonuclear war killed most of the living organisms and changed the environment drastically.
(d) If genetic recombination, sexual reproduction and mutation stopped so that all offspring of all organisms were exact copies of their parents.

**139.** Directional selection ________.
(a) Works against adaptive traits
(b) Favours intermediate forms of a trait
(c) Eliminates uncommon forms of alleles
(d) Shifts allele frequencies in a steady, consistent direction

**140.** Disruptive selection ________.
(a) Eliminates uncommon forms of alleles
(b) Does not favour intermediate forms of a trait
(c) Shifts allele frequencies in a steady, consistent direction
(d) All the above

**141.** The spread of genes from one breeding population to another by migration which may result in change in gene frequency is
(a) Gene flow
(b) Genetic drift
(c) Gene frequency
(d) None of these

**142.** The presence of recessive trait is 16 per cent. The frequency of dominant allele in population is
(a) 0.6 (b) 0.32
(c) 0.84 (d) 0.92

**143.** The frequency of an autosomal lethal gene is 0.4. The frequency of carrier in a population of 200 individual is
(a) 72 (b) 96
(c) 104 (d) 36

**144.** The principle that gives the geneticists a tool to determine when evolution is occurring is
(a) Hardy–Weinberg principle
(b) Chemiosmotic theory
(c) Malthusian principle
(d) Cloning theory

**145.** Which of the following defines Hardy–Weinberg's law?
(a) $p^2 + 2pq + q^2 = 0$
(b) $q^2 + p^2 + 2pq = 0$
(c) $p^2 + 2pq + q^2 = 1$
(d) $p^2 + 3pq + q^2 = 1$

**146.** Hardy–Weinberg equilibrium is known to be affected by gene flow, genetic drift, mutation, genetic recombination and ________.
(a) Saltation (b) Evolution
(c) Limiting factors (d) Natural selection

**147.** In this figure, which kind of selection does A, B and C represent respectively?

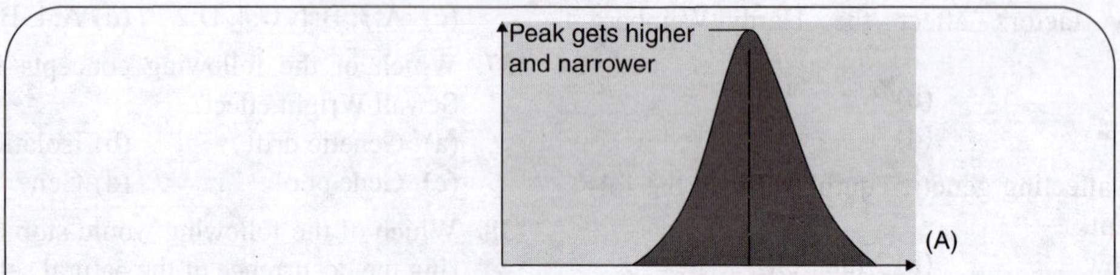


(a) A: Stabilizing, B: Disruptive, C: Directional
(b) A: Stabilizing, B: Directional, C: Disruptive
(c) A: Disruptive, B: Stabilizing, C: Directional
(d) A: Directional, B: Disruptive, C: Stabilizing

## Evolution in Brief

**148.** The first cellular form of life appeared _______ mya.
(a) 1000 (b) 2000
(c) 3000 (d) 4000

**149.** Match the columns.

| | |
|---|---|
| (A) Invertebrates | (1) 500 mya |
| (B) Jawless fish | (2) 320 mya |
| (C) Seaweeds | (3) 350 mya |
| (D) Dryopithecus and Ramapithecus | (4) 15 mya |

(a) A:2, B:1, C:4, D:3
(b) A:1, B:3, C:2, D:4
(c) A:1, B:4, C:2, D:3
(d) A:4, B:3, C:1, D:2

**150.** The first organisms that invaded land were
(a) Animals (b) Plants
(c) Amphibians (d) Reptiles

**151.** Which of the following is a lobe finned fish?
(a) Coelacanth (b) Hippocampus
(c) Catla (d) Pteropus

**152.** Amphibians evolved from
(a) Synapsids (b) Sauropside
(c) Lobed fin fishes (d) Cycads

**153.** Which of these is a direct ancestor of turtles?
(a) Sauropsids (b) Synapsids
(c) Pelycosaurs (d) Thecodonts

**154.** Find out the total number of correct statements from the following.
(A) Pteridophytes forms coal deposits.
(B) Fishlike reptiles (Ichthyosaurs) evolved 200 million years ago.
(C) About 65 million years ago dinosaurs suddenly disappeared from earth.
(D) Tyrannosaurus rex was the biggest dinosaurs which is about 20 feet in height.
(E) Because of continental drift, pouched mammals of Australia survived as there was a lack of competition from any other mammals.
(a) 2 (b) 3
(c) 4 (d) 5

**155.** Which of these is/are aquatic mammals?
(a) Whale
(b) Dolphin
(c) Seals and Sea cows
(d) All of these

**156.** Find the total number of organisms evolved from Psilophyton in the following.
*Bryophytes, Herbaceous lycopods, Sphenopsids, Ferns, Ginkgos, Conifers, Gnetales, Arborescent lycopods*
(a) 2 (b) 3 (c) 5 (d) 6

**157.** All these are animals except
(a) Synapsids (b) Therapsids
(c) Sphenopsids (d) Sauropsids

**158.** Seed fern evolved into
(a) Cycads (b) Dicot
(c) Monocot (d) All of these

**159.** Which of the following were extinct in the Permian period?
(a) Ferns
(b) Cycads
(c) Arborescent lycopodus
(d) Bryophytes

**160.** Bryophytes evolved in which of these periods?
(a) Carboniferous (b) Permian
(c) Triassic (d) Cretaceous

**161.** How many of these periods belong to the paleozoic era?
*Cretaceous, Jurrasic, Triassic, Permian, Carboniferous, Devonian, Silurin*
(a) 1 (b) 2 (c) 3 (d) 4

**162.** Synapsids existed
(a) 300 mya (b) 150 mya
(c) 350 mya (d) 50 mya

**163.** Zosterophyllum belonged to which period?
(a) Silurian (b) Devonian
(c) Carboniferous (d) Permian

**164.** Which of the following was/were the most abundant in cenozoic era?
(a) Angiosperm (b) Cycads
(c) Conifers (d) Ginkgos

**165.** Which of these features belong/s to mammals?
(a) Viviparous, avoid danger
(b) More intelligent in sensing
(c) Both (a) and (b)
(d) None of these

**166.** Conifers were most abundant in
(a) Paleozoic era (b) Mesozoic era
(c) Cenozoic era (d) All eras

**167.** Seed ferns evolved from
(a) Cycads (b) Gnetales
(c) Conifers (d) Progymnosperm

**168.** Arrange the ascending order of extinction (reptiles):
(a) Pelycosaurs, Thecodonts, Therapsids, Dinosaurs
(b) Thecodonts, Dinosaurs, Pelycosaurs, Therapsids
(c) Dinosaurs, Therapsids, Thecodonts, Pelycosaurs
(d) Therapsids, Thecodonts, Pelycosaurs, Dinosaurs

**169.** Correct order is
(a) Palaeozoic → Mesozoic → Cenozoic
(b) Mesozoic → Archaeozoic → Proterozoic
(c) Palaeozoic → Archaeozoic → Cenozoic
(d) Archaeozoic → Palaeozoic → Proterozoic

**170.** The largest subdivision in geological time scale is
(a) Era (b) Period
(c) Epoch (d) Century

**171.** Which of the following is called 'age of fish'?
(a) Silurian (b) Permian
(c) Devonian (d) Cretaceous

**172.** Carboniferous period of coal deposition was
(a) 50 million years ago
(b) 300 million years ago
(c) 500 million years ago
(d) 2000 million years ago

**173.** What is A, B, C and D in the diagram?

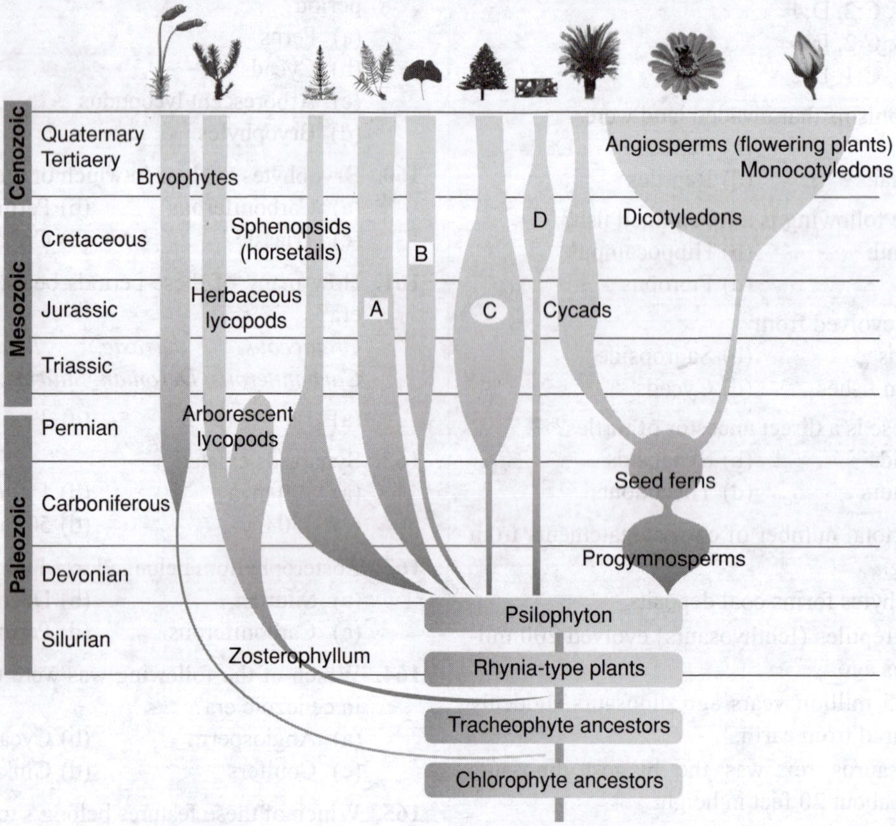


(a) A: Conifers, B: Ginkgos, C: Ferns, D: Gnetales
(b) A: Ferns, B: Ginkgos, C: Conifers, D: Gnetales
(c) A: Gnetales, B: Conifers, C: Ginkgos, D: Ferns
(d) A: Ginkgos, B: Gnetales, C: Ferns, D: Conifers

**174.** Mesozoic era is the age of
(a) Birds (b) Fishes
(c) Reptiles (d) Mammals

**175.** Dinosaurs were the
(a) First mammals (b) Extinct reptiles
(c) Giant mammals (d) First amphibians

**176.** If you want to see a dinosaur, it would be the best to set the controls of your time machine for the
(a) Mesozoic era (b) Precambrian era
(c) Palaeozoic era (d) Pleistocene period

**177.** Dinosaurs became extinct during
(a) Jurassic (b) Triassic
(c) Permian (d) Cretaceous

**178.** Which era was dominated by reptiles?
(a) Mesozoic era (b) Cenozoic era
(c) Palaeozoic era (d) Archaeozoic era

**179.** The golden age of reptile was
(a) Mesozoic era (b) Cenozoic era
(c) Palaeozoic era (d) Proterozoic era

**180.** The Jurassic period belongs to the era
(a) Cenozoic (b) Mesozoic
(c) Palaeozoic (d) Archaeozoic

**181.** Evolution of unique groups of mammals in South America, Africa and Australia is an evidence supporting
(a) Continental drift
(b) Glaciation
(c) Crustal movement
(d) Geographical juxtaposition

**182.** Occurrence of endemic species in South America and Australia is due to
(a) Progressive evolution
(b) Continental separation
(c) Absence of terrestrial route to these places
(d) Extinction of these species in other regions

**183.** What is A, B, C and D in this figure?

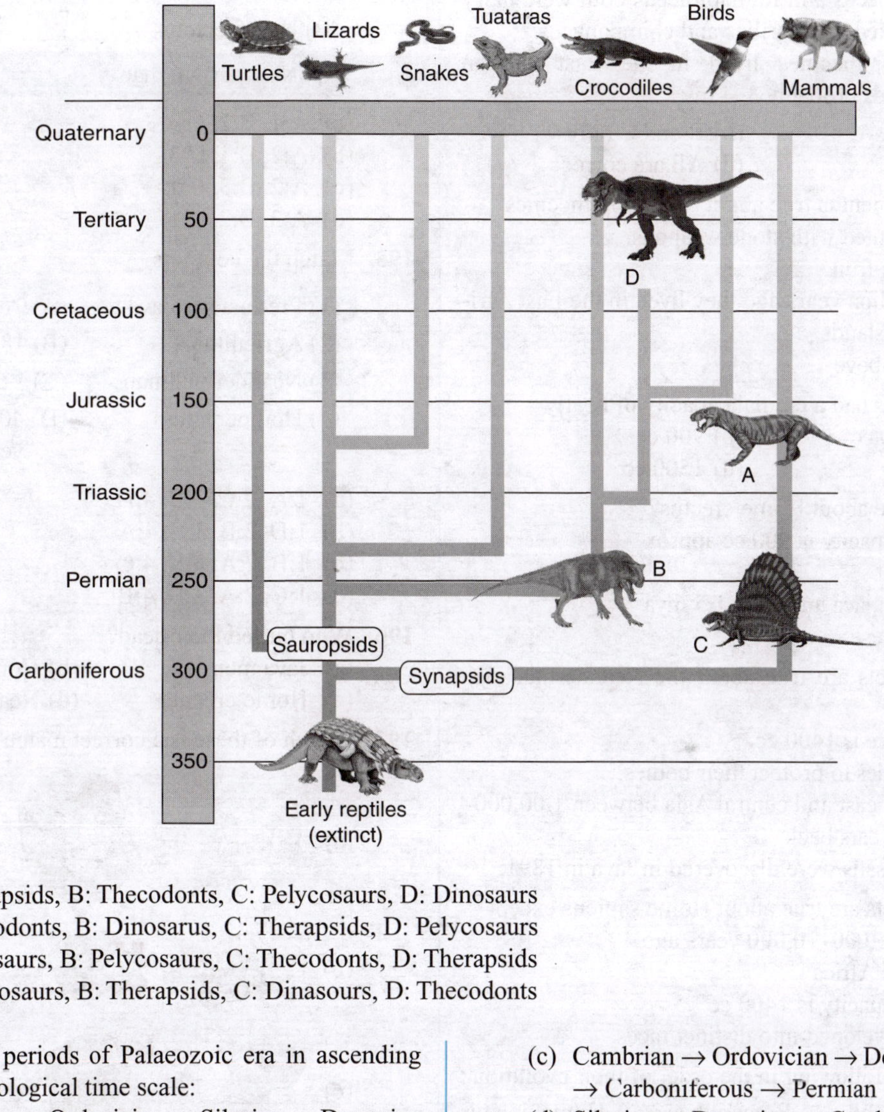


(a) A: Therapsids, B: Thecodonts, C: Pelycosaurs, D: Dinosaurs
(b) A: Thecodonts, B: Dinosarus, C: Therapsids, D: Pelycosaurs
(c) A: Dinosaurs, B: Pelycosaurs, C: Thecodonts, D: Therapsids
(d) A: Pelycosaurs, B: Therapsids, C: Dinasours, D: Thecodonts

**184.** Arrange the periods of Palaeozoic era in ascending order in a geological time scale:
(a) Cambrian → Ordovician → Silurian → Devonian → Carboniferous → Permian
(b) Cambrian → Devonian → Ordovician → Silurian → Carboniferous → Permian
(c) Cambrian → Ordovician → Devonian → Silurian → Carboniferous → Permian
(d) Silurian → Devonian → Cambrian → Ordovician → Permian → Carboniferous

## Origin and Evolution of Man

**185.** What can be said to be the success story of man in evolution?
(a) Language skills
(b) Self-consciousness
(c) Increased cranial capacity
(d) All of these

**186.** Dryopithecus and Ramapithecus existed ______ mya.
(a) 5 (b) 10 (c) 15 (d) 25

**187.** Select the false statements.
(A) Dryopithecus was more Ape-like.
(B) Ramapithecus was more Man-like.
(C) Dryopithecus and Ramapithecus both were hairy and walked like gorillas and chimpanzees.
(D) Australopithecines lived in the East African grasslands probably 3–4 mya.
(a) B only (b) B and C only
(c) D only (d) All are correct

**188.** Which statement is true about Australopithecines?
(a) They hunted with stone weapons.
(b) They ate fruit.
(c) Two million years ago they lived in the East African grasslands.
(d) All the above

**189.** Homo habilis had a cranial capacity of nearly
(a) 650–800 cc (b) 900 cc
(c) 1400 cc (d) 1500 cc

**190.** Which is true about Homo erectus?
(a) Brain capacity is 900 cc approx
(b) Ate meat
(c) Found in java and exist 1.5 mya
(d) All of these

**191.** All these facts are true about the Neanderthal man except
(a) Brain size is 1400 cc.
(b) Used hides to protect their bodies.
(c) Lived in east and central Asia between 1,00,000–40,000 years back.
(d) Their fossils were discovered in Java in 1891.

**192.** All these facts are true about Homo sapiens except
(a) Arose 75,000–10,000 years ago
(b) Arose in Africa
(c) Brain capacity is 1400 cc
(d) They developed into distinct races

**193.** Arrange the following in the order of their evolution.
(a) Homo habilis → Ramapithecus → Homo erectus → Dryopithecus → Homo sapiens → Australopithecines → Neanderthal man
(b) Dryopithecus → Ramapithecus → Australopithecus → Homo habilis → Homo erectus → Neanderthal man → Homo sapiens
(c) Australopithecines →Homo sapiens → Ramapithecus → Dryopithecus → Homo habilis → Homo erectus → Neanderthal man
(d) Neanderthal man → Australopithecines → Homo sapiens → Homo erectus →Homo habilis → Ramapithecus → Dryopithecus

**194.** Match the columns.

| Column-I | Column-II |
|---|---|
| (A) Homo habilis | (1) 650–800 cc |
| (B) Homo erectus | (2) 900 cc |
| (C) Neanderthal man | (3) 1400 cc |

(a) A:1, B:2, C:3
(b) A:2, B:1, C:3
(c) A:2, B:3, C:1
(d) A:3, B:2, C:1

**195.** Match the columns.

| | |
|---|---|
| (1) Pre-historic cave art | (A) 10,000 years back |
| (2) Agriculture | (B) 18,000 years back |
| (3) Neanderthal man | (C) 1.5 million years ago |
| (4) Homoerectus | (D) 40,000 – 1,00,000 years back |

(a) 1:A, 2:C, 3:B, 4:D
(b) 1:D, 2:B, 3:C, 4:A
(c) 1:B, 2:A, 3:D, 4:C
(d) 1:C, 2:A, 3:D, 4:B

**196.** Who buried their dead?
(a) Java men (b) Homo habilis
(c) Homo erectus (d) Neanderthal man

**197.** Which of these is a correct match?

(a) 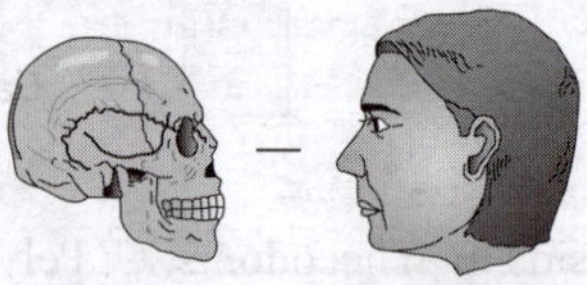

(b) 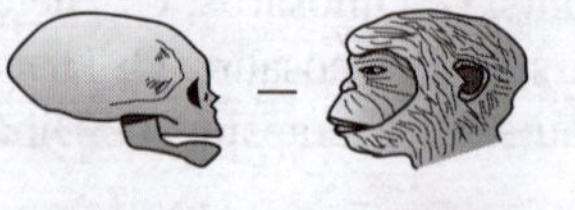

(c) 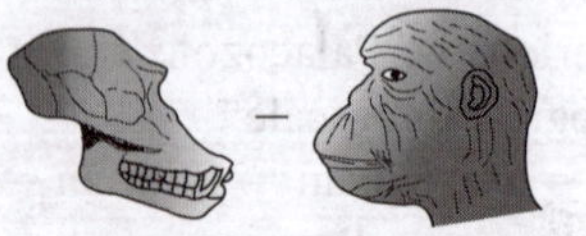

(d) All the above

## Multiple Choice Questions: Level II

**198.** In the case of peppered moth (*Biston betularia*), the black-coloured form became dominant over the light-coloured form in England during industrial revolution. This is an example of
(a) appearance of the darker coloured individuals due to very poor sunlight
(b) protective mimicry
(c) inheritance of darker colour character acquired due to the darker environment
(d) natural selection whereby the darker forms were selected

**199.** What is true about the isolated small tribal populations?
(a) Wrestlers who develop strong body muscles in time pass this character on to their progeny
(b) There is no change in population size as the large gene pool
(c) There is a decline in population as boys marry from their own tribe
(d) Hereditary diseases like colour blindness don in the isolated population

**200.** Thorn of Bougainvillea and tendril of Cucurbita are examples of
(a) Vestigial organs
(b) Retrogressive evolution
(c) Analogous organs
(d) Homologous organs

**201.** Darwin's finches are excellent examples of
(a) Brood parasitism
(b) Connecting links
(c) Adaptive radiation
(d) Seasonal migration

**202.** The most likely reason for development of resistance against pesticides in insects damaging a crop is
(a) random mutations
(b) genetic recombination
(c) directed mutations
(d) acquired heritable changes

**203.** Which one of the following pairs of items correctly belongs to the category of organs mentioned against it?
(a) Nephridia of earthworm and Malpighian tubules of cockroach – excretory organs
(b) Wings of honey bee and wings of crow – homologous organs
(c) Thorn of Bougainvillea and tendrils of Cucurbita – analogous organs
(d) Nictitating membrane and blind spot in human eye – vestigial organs

**204.** Which one of the following in birds indicates their reptilian ancestry?
(a) Two special chambers crop and gizzard in their digestive tract
(b) Eggs with a calcareous shell
(c) Scales on their hind limbs
(d) four-chambered heart

**205.** Which one of the following scientists name is correctly matched with the theory put forth by him?
(a) De Vries – Natural selection
(b) Mendel – Theory of Pangenesis
(c) Weismann – Theory of continuity of germ plasm
(d) Pasteur – Inheritance of acquired characters

**206.** Industrial melanism as observed in peppered moth proves that
(a) melanic form of the moth has no selective advantage over lighter form in industrial area
(b) lighter-form moth has no selective advantage either in polluted industrial area or non-polluted area
(c) melanism is pollution-generated feature
(d) true black melanic forms arise by a recurring random mutation

**207.** Two plants can be conclusively said to belong to the same species if they
(a) have more than 90 per cent similar genes
(b) look similar and possess identical secondary metabolites
(c) have same number of chromosomes
(d) can reproduce freely with each other and form seed

**208.** Adaptive radiation refers to
(a) evolution of different species from a common ancestor
(b) migration of members of a species to different geographical area
(c) power of adaptation in an individual to a variety of environments
(d) adaptations due to geographical isolation

**209.** One of the important consequences of geographical isolation is
(a) preventing speciation
(b) speciation through reproductive isolation
(c) random creation of new species
(d) no change in the isolated fauna

**210.** Select the correct statement from the following?
(a) Fitness is the result of the ability to adapt and gets selected by nature
(b) All mammals except whales and camels have seven cervical vertebrae
(c) Mutations are random and directional
(d) Darwinian variations are small and directionless

**211.** At a locus, frequency of 'A' allele is 0.6 and that of 'a' is 0.4. What would be the frequency of heterozygotes in a random mating population at equilibrium?
(a) 0.36 (b) 0.16
(c) 0.24 (d) 0.48

**212.** Which of the following is not true for a species?
(a) Members of a species can interbreed.
(b) Gene flow does not occur between the populations of a species.
(c) Each species is reproductively isolated from every other species.
(d) Variations occur among members of a species.

**213.** According to Oparin, which one of the following was not present in the primitive atmosphere of the earth?
(a) Methane (b) Oxygen
(c) Hydrogen (d) Water vapour

**214.** Diversification in plant life appeared
(a) Due to long periods of evolutionary changes
(b) due to abrupt mutations
(c) suddenly on earth
(d) by seed dispersal

**215.** Angiosperms have dominated the land flora primarily because of their
(a) power of adaptability in diverse habitat
(b) property of producing large number of seeds
(c) nature of self-pollination
(d) domestication by man

**216.** Which of the following is most important for speciation?
(a) seasonal isolation
(b) reproductive isolation
(c) behavioural isolation
(d) tropical isolation

**217.** Forthcoming generation are less adaptive than their parental generation due to
(a) Natural selection (b) Mutation
(c) Genetic drift (d) Adaptation

**218.** Frequency of an allele in an isolated population may change due to
(a) Genetic drift (b) Gene flow
(c) Mutation (d) Natural selection

**219.** First life on earth was
(a) Cyanobacteria
(b) Chemoheterotrophs
(c) Autotrophs
(d) Photoautotrophs

**220.** Darwin's finches provide an excellent evidence in favour of evolution. This evidence comes from the field of
(a) Biogeopraphy (b) Anatomy
(c) Embryology (d) Paleontology

**221.** Phenomenon of 'Industrial melanism' demonstrates
(a) natural selection
(b) induced mutation
(c) geographical
(d) reproductive isolation

**222.** Species occurring in different geographical areas are called as
(a) Sibling (b) Sympatric
(c) Allopatric (d) Neopatric

**223.** Diversity in the type of beaks of finches adapted to different feeding habits on the Galapagos Islands, as observed by Darwin, provides evidence for
(a) Intraspecific variations
(b) Intraspecific competition
(c) Interspecific competition
(d) Origin of species by natural selection

**224.** The change of the light-coloured variety of peppered moth (*Biston betularia*) to its darker variety (*Biston carbonaria*) is due to
(a) mutation
(b) regeneration
(c) genetic isolatio
(d) temporal isolation

**225.** Study of fossils is
(a) Palaeontology (b) Herpetology
(c) Saurology (d) Organic evolution

**226.** Phenomenon of organisms resembling others for escaping from enemies is
(a) Adaptation (b) Mimicry
(c) Homology (d) Analogy

# A & R and Statement-based Questions

## Assertion and Reason Questions:

***Directions for questions 227 to 231:** Read the **assertion** and **reason** carefully to mark the correct option out of the options given below:*

**(a)** **(A)** is **true** but **(R)** is **false**.
**(b)** **(A)** is **false** but **(R)** is **true**.
**(c)** Both **(A)** and **(R)** is **true** and **(R)** is the correct explanation of **(A).**
**(d)** Both **(A)** and **(R)** is **true** and **(R)** is not the correct explanation of **(A).**

**227. Assertion:** Homo erectus has brain capacity of 900 cc
**Reason:** Homo erectus probably eat meat.

**228. Assertion:** Antibiotic resistance is an example of anthropogenic evolution.
**Reason:** Antibiotic resistant cells appearing in months or years because of excess use of antibiotics.

**229. Assertion:** Pouched mammals survived in Australia.
**Reason:** Due to continental drift they lack competition from other mammals.

**230. Assertion:** Sweet potato and potato is an example of analogous organ.
**Reason:** Both are modification of stem meant for storage of food.

**231. Assertion:** Big Bang theory attempts to explain the origin of life.
**Reason:** Universe is almost 20 billion year old.

## Statement-based Questions:

***Direction for questions 232 to 236:** These type of questions consist of two statement each, printed as **Statement-I** and **Statement-II**. While answering such questions, a student is needed to choose any one of the following four responses.*

**(a)** **Statement I** is **correct Statement II** is **incorrect**.
**(b)** **Statement I** is **incorrect Statement II** is **correct**.
**(c)** Both **Statement I** and **Statement II** are **correct**.
**(d)** Both **Statement I** and **Statement II** are **incorrect**.

**232. Statement-I:** Homology shows common ancestry.
**Statement-II:** Analogous structures are result of convergent evolution.

**233. Statement-I:** Darwin finches are example of adaptive radiation.
**Statement-II:** Fitness is the end result of the ability to adapt and get selected by nature.

**234. Statement-I:** Only two factors affect Hardy-Weinberg equilibrium.
**Statement-II:** Hugo deVries gave idea of mutation by working on evening primrose.

**235. Statement-I:** Devonian period belongs to Palaeozoic era.
**Statement-II:** Seed ferns are evolved from progymnosperms.

**236. Statement-I:** Bryophytes are evolved from Psilophyton.
**Statement-II:** Therapsids are direct ancestors of mammals.

# Matrix-Match Type Questions

**237.** Match the following:

| I (Type of Evolution) | II (Based On) | III |
|---|---|---|
| 1. Divergent evolution | (i) Analogy | X. Anatomically similar |
| 2. Convergent evolution | (ii) Homology | Y. Functionally similar |

**The correct matching is**

(a) 1 – (ii) – X, 2 – (i) – Y
(b) 1 – (i) – X, 2 – (ii) – Y
(c) 1 – (i) – Y, 2 – (ii) – X
(d) 1 – (ii) – Y, 2 – (i) – X

**238.** Match the following:

| List-I (Type of Evolution) | List-II (Examples) |
|---|---|
| 1. Divergent evolution | (i) Eye of octopus & mammals |
| 2. Convergent evolution | (ii) Bones of forelimb in whale & human |
| | (iii) Thorn & tendrils of Bougainvillea & Cucurbita |
| | (iv) Potato & Sweet potato |
| | (v) Flippers of Penguins and Dolphins |

**The correct matching is**

(a) 1 – (ii) & (iii), 2 – (i), (iv) & (v)
(b) 1 – (i) & (iii), 2 – (iv), (ii) & (v)
(c) 1 – (iii) & (v), 2 – (i), (iv) & (ii)
(d) 1 – (v) & (ii), 2 – (i), (iv) & (iii)

**239.** Match the following:

| List-I (Scientist) | List-II (Work) |
|---|---|
| 1. Louis Pasteur | (i) Proposed that first form of life was non-living organic molecules (RNA, protein) |
| 2. Oparin & Haldane | (ii) Proposed natural selection as mechanism of evolution |
| 3. Miller | (iii) Proposed that life come from pre-existing life only & killed spontaneous generation theory |
| 4. Darwin | (iv) Experimented the formation of amino acid in a laboratory scale by creating similar conditions present in earlier time on earth |

**The correct matching is**

| | 1 | 2 | 3 | 4 |
|---|---|---|---|---|
| (a) | (iii) | (i) | (iv) | (ii) |
| (b) | (iii) | (ii) | (iv) | (i) |
| (c) | (ii) | (iv) | (iii) | (i) |
| (d) | (i) | (iii) | (iv) | (ii) |

**240.** Match the following:

| List-I (Scientist) | List-II (Proposed Theories ) |
|---|---|
| 1. Charles Darwin | (i) Based on heritable variations |
| 2. Hugo de Vries | (ii) Based on mutations |
| | (iii) Evolution is directionless |
| | (iv) Evolution is directional |
| | (v) Evolution is gradual |
| | (vi) Evolution is saltation (single step large mutation) |

**The correct matching is**

(a) 1 – (i), (iv), (v) 2 – (ii), (iii), (vi)
(b) 1 – (i), (iii), (vi) 2 – (ii), (iv), (v)
(c) 1 – (i), (iv), (vi) 2 – (ii), (iii), (vi)
(d) 1 – (ii), (iv), (v) 2 – (i), (iii), (vi)

**241.** Match the following:

| List-I (Organism) | List-II (Existence on Earth) |
|---|---|
| 1. Single-celled organism | (i) 500 |
| 2. Jawless fish | (ii) 320 |
| 3. Sea weeds | (iii) 350 |
| 4. Invertebrates | (iv) 2000 |

**The correct matching is**

| | 1 | 2 | 3 | 4 |
|---|---|---|---|---|
| (a) | (iv) | (iii) | (ii) | (i) |
| (b) | (ii) | (iii) | (iv) | (i) |
| (c) | (i) | (iv) | (iii) | (ii) |
| (d) | (iii) | (i) | (iv) | (ii) |

## NCERT Exemplar Questions

**1.** Which of the following is used as an atmospheric pollution indicator?
(a) Lepidoptera (b) Lichens
(c) *Lycopersicum* (d) *Lycopodium*

**2.** The theory of spontaneous generation stated that
(a) Life arose from living forms only.
(b) Life can arise from both living and non-living.
(c) Life can arise from non-living things only.
(d) Life arises spontaneously, neither from living nor from the non-living.

**3.** Animal husbandry and plant breeding programmes are the examples of
(a) Reverse evolution (b) Artificial selection
(c) Mutation (d) Natural selection

**4.** Paleontological evidences for evolution refers to the
(a) Development of embryo
(b) Homologous organs
(c) Fossils
(d) Analogous organs

**5.** The bones of forelimbs of whale, bat, cheetah and man are similar in structure, because
(a) One organism has given rise to another
(b) They share a common ancestor
(c) They perform the same function
(d) They have biochemical similarities

**6.** Analogous organs arise due to
(a) Divergent evolution (b) Artificial selection
(c) Genetic drift (d) Convergent evolution

7. $(p + q)^2 = p^2 + 2pq + q^2 = 1$ represents an equation used in
(a) Population genetics (b) Mendelian genetics
(c) Biometrics (d) Molecular genetics

8. Appearance of antibiotic-resistant bacteria is an example of
(a) Adaptive radiation
(b) Transduction
(c) Pre-existing variation in the population
(d) Divergent evolution

9. Evolution of life shows that life forms had a trend of moving from
(a) Land to water
(b) Dry land to wet land
(c) Fresh water to sea water
(d) Water to land

10. Viviparity is considered to be more evolved because
(a) The young ones are left on their own.
(b) The young ones are protected by a thick shell.
(c) The young ones are protected inside the mother's body and are looked after they are born leading to more chances of survival.
(d) The embryo takes a long time to develop.

11. Fossils are generally found in
(a) Sedimentary rocks
(b) Igneous rocks
(c) Metamorphic rocks
(d) Any type of rock

12. For the MN-blood group system, the frequencies of M and N alleles are 0.7 and 0.3, respectively. The expected frequency of MN-blood group bearing organisms is likely to be
(a) 42 per cent (b) 49 per cent
(c) 9 per cent (d) 58 per cent

13. Which type of selection explains industrial melanism observed in moth, *Biston bitularia*?
(a) Stabilizing (b) Directional
(c) Disruptive (d) Artificial

14. The most accepted line of descent in human evolution is
(a) Australopithecus → Ramapithecus → *Homo* sapiens → *Homo* habilis
(b) *Homo* erectus → *Homo* habilis → *Homo* sapiens
(c) Ramapithecus → *Homo* habilis → *Homo* erectus → *Homo* sapiens
(d) Australopithecus → Ramapithecus → *Homo* erectus → *Homo* habilis → *Homo* sapiens

15. Which of the following is an example for link species?
(a) Lobe fish (b) Dodo bird
(c) Sea weed (d) Chimpanzee

16. Match the scientists listed under column 'A' with 'ideas listed in column 'B'.

| Column A | Column B |
|---|---|
| i. Darwin | M. Abiogenesis |
| ii. Oparin | N. Use and disuse of organs |
| iii. Lamarck | O. Continental drift theory |
| iv. Wagner | P. Evolution by natural selection |

(a) i - M; ii - P; iii - N; iv - O
(b) i - P ; ii - M; iii - N; iv - O
(c) i - N; ii - P; iii - O; iv - M
(d) i - P; ii - O; iii - N; iv - M

17. In 1953, S. L. Miller created the primitive earth conditions in the laboratory and gave experimental evidence for the origin of first form of life from pre-existing non-living organic molecules. The primitive earth conditions created include
(a) Low temperature, volcanic storms, atmosphere rich in oxygen.
(b) Low temperature, volcanic storms, reducing atmosphere.
(c) High temperature, volcanic storms, non-reducing atmosphere.
(d) High temperature, volcanic storms, reducing atmosphere containing $CH_4$, $NH_3$, etc.

18. Variations during mutations of meiotic recombination are
(a) Random and directionless
(b) Random and directional
(c) Random and small
(d) Random, small and directional

## Previous Years' Questions

1. Darwin's finches are a good example of [AIPMT 2010 PRE]
   (a) Industrial melanism
   (b) Connecting link
   (c) Adaptive radiation
   (d) Convergent evolution

2. Given below are four statements (A–D) each with one or two blanks. Select the option which correctly fills up the blanks in two statements.

   **Statements:**

   (A) Wings of butterfly and birds look alike and are the results of ____ evolution.
   (B) Miller showed that $CH_3$, $H_2$, $NH_3$ and ____ when exposed to electric discharge in a flask resulted in formation of ____.
   (C) Vermiform appendix is a ____ organ and are ____ evidence of evolution.
   (D) According to Darwin, evolution took place due to ____ and ____ of the fittest.

   [AIPMT 2010 MAINS]

   (a) (D) – (i) small variations, (ii) survival, (A) – (i) convergent
   (b) (A) – (i) convergent, (B) – (i) oxygen, (ii) nucleosides
   (c) (B) – (i) water vapour, (ii) amino acids (C) – rudimentary, (ii) anatomical
   (d) (C) – (i) vestigial, (ii) anatomical (D) – (i) mutations, (ii) multiplication

3. The most apparent change during the evolutionary history of Homo sapiens can be traced in [AIPMT 2010 MAINS]
   (a) Loss of body hair
   (b) Walking upright
   (c) Shortening of the jaws
   (d) Remarkable increase in the brain size

4. Sweet potato is homologous to [AIPMT 2011 MAINS]
   (a) Potato (b) Colocasia
   (c) Ginger (d) Turnip

5. Mutations can be induced with: [AIPMT 2011 PRE]
   (a) IAA
   (b) Ethylene
   (c) Gamma radiations
   (d) Infra-red radiations

6. What was the most significant trend in the evolution of modern man (Homo sapiens) from his ancestors? [AIPMT 2011 PRE]
   (a) Shortening of jaws
   (b) Binocular vision
   (c) Increasing brain capacity
   (d) Upright posture

7. The extinct human who lived 1,00,000 to 40,000 years ago, in Europe, Asia and parts of Africa, with short stature, heavy eye brows, retreating foreheads, large jaws with heavy teeth, stocky bodies, a lumbering gait and stooped posture was: [AIPMT 2012 PRE]
   (a) Homo hibilis
   (b) Neanderthal human
   (c) Cro-magnan human
   (d) Ramapithecus

8. What was the most significant trend in the evolution of modern man (Homo sapiens) from his ancestors? [AIPMT 2012 PRE]
   (a) Shortening of jaws
   (b) Binocular vision
   (c) Increasing cranial capacity
   (d) Upright posture

9. Which one of the following options gives one correct example each of convergent evolution and divergent evolution? [AIPMT 2012 PRE]

| Convergent evolution | | Divergent evolution |
|---|---|---|
| (a) Eyes of octopus and mammals | - | Bones of forelimbs of vertebrates |
| (b) Thorns of bougainvillea cucurbita | - | Wings of butterflies and birds |
| (c) Bones of forelimbs if vertebrates | - | Wings of butterfly and birds |
| (d) Thorns of bougainvillea and tendrils of cucurbita | - | Eyes of octopus and mammals |

10. Evolution of different species in a given area starting from a point and spreading to other geographical areas is known as: [AIPMT 2012 PRE]
    (a) Adaptive radiation (b) Natural selection
    (c) Migration (d) Divergent evolution

**11.** Which one of the following sets of items in options 1–4 are correctly categorized with one exception in it? [AIPMT 2012 MAINS]

| Items | Category | Exception |
|---|---|---|
| (a) Kangaroo, Koala, Wombat | Australian marsupials | Wombat |
| (b) Plasmodium, Cuscuta, Trypanosoma | Protozoan parasites | Cuscuta |
| (c) Typhoid, Pneumonia, Diphtheria | Bacterial diseases | Diphtheria |
| (d) UAA, UAG, UGA | Stop codons | UAG |

**12.** The idea of mutations was brought forth by: [AIPMT 2012 MAINS]
(a) Gregor Mendel, who worked on pisum sativum
(b) Hardy Weinberg, who worked on allele frequencies in a population
(c) Charles Darwin, who observed a wide variety of organisms during his sea voyage
(d) Hugo de Vries, who worked on evening primrose

**13.** According to Darwin, the organic evolution is due to: [AIPMT 2013]
(a) Intraspecific competition
(b) Interspecific competition
(c) Competition within closely related species
(d) Reduced feeding efficiency in one species due to the presence of interfering species

**14.** The eye of octopus and eye of cat show different patterns of structure, yet they perform similar function. This is an example of: [AIPMT 2013]
(a) Homologous organs that have evolved due to convergent evolution
(b) Homologous organs that have evolved due to divergent evolution
(c) Analogous organs that have evolved due to convergent evolution
(d) Analogous organs that have evolved due to divergent evolution

**15.** The tendency of population to remain in genetic equilibrium may be disturbed by: [AIPMT 2013]
(a) Random mating
(b) Lack of migration
(c) Lack of mutations
(d) Lack of random mating

**16.** The process by which organisms with different evolutionary history evolve similar phenotypic adaptations in response to a common environmental challenge is called [AIPMT 2013]
(a) Natural selection
(b) Convergent evolution
(c) Non-random evolution
(d) Adaptive radiation

**17.** Variation in gene frequencies within populations can occur by chance rather than by natural selection. This is referred to as: [AIPMT 2013]
(a) Genetic flow
(b) Genetic drift
(c) Random mating
(d) Genetic load

**18.** Which one of the following are analogous structures? [AIPMT 2014]
(a) Wings of bat and wings of pigeon
(b) Gills of prawn and lungs of man
(c) Thorns of bougainvillea and tendrils of cucurbita
(d) Flippers of dolphin and legs of horse

**19.** Forelimbs of cat, lizard used in walking; forelimbs of whale used in swimming and forelimb of bats used in flying are an example of: [AIPMT 2014]
(a) Analogous organs
(b) Adaptive radiation
(c) Homologous organs
(d) Convergent evolution

**20.** In a population of 1000 individuals, 360 belong to genotype AA, 480 to Aa and the remaining 160 to aa. Based on this data, the frequency of allele A in the population is: [AIPMT 2014]
(a) 0.4 (b) 0.5
(c) 0.6 (d) 0.7

**21.** Industrial melanism is an example of: [RE-AIPMT 2015]
(a) Natural selection
(b) Mutation
(c) Leo Lamarckism
(d) Neo-Darwinism

**22.** A population will not exist in Hardy–Weinberg equilibrium if: [AIPMT 2015]
(a) Individuals mate selectively
(b) There are no mutations
(c) There is no migration
(d) The population is large

**23.** Which of the following had the smallest brain capacity? [AIPMT 2015]
(a) *Homo erectus*
(b) *Homo sapiens*
(c) *Homo neanderthalensis*
(d) *Homo habilis*

**24.** Which is the most common mechanism of genetic variation in the population of the sexually reproducing organisms? [AIPMT 2015]
(a) Transduction
(b) Chromosomal aberrations
(c) Genetic drift
(d) Recombination

**25.** Which of the following is the correct sequence of events in the origin of life?

**I.** Formation of protobionts
**II.** Synthesis of organic monomers
**III.** Synthesis of organic polymers
**IV.** Formation of DNA-based genetic systems
[NEET 2016 – PHASE II]

(a) I, III, II, IV
(b) II, III, I, IV
(c) II, III, IV, I
(d) I, II, III, IV

**26.** The chronological order of human evolution from early to the recent is [NEET 2016 – PHASE II]
(a) Ramapithecus → Australopithecus → Homo habilis → Homo erectus
(b) Ramapithecus → Homo habilis → Australopithecus → Homo erectus
(c) Australopithecus → Homo habilis → Ramapithecus → Homo erectus
(d) Australopithecus → Ramapithecus → Homo habilis → Homo erectus

**27.** In Hardy–Weinberg equation, the frequency of heterozygous individual is represented by [NEET 2016 – PHASE II]
(a) 2pq
(b) pq
(c) $q^2$
(d) $p^2$

**28.** Genetic drift operates in [NEET 2016 – PHASE II]
(a) Large isolated population
(b) Non-reproductive population
(c) Slow reproductive population
(d) Small isolated population

**29.** Analogous structures are a result of: [NEET 2016 – PHASE I]
(a) Divergent evolution
(b) Convergent evolution
(c) Shared ancestry
(d) Stabilizing selection

**30.** Following are the two statements regarding the origin of life: [NEET 2016 – PHASE I]
(1) The earliest organisms that appeared on the earth were non-green and presumably anaerobes.
(2) The first autotrophic organisms were the chemoautotrophs that never released oxygen of the above statements.

Which one of the following options is correct?
(a) (1) is correct but (2) is false
(b) (2) is correct but (1) is false
(c) Both (1) and (2) are correct
(d) Both (1) and (2) are false

**31.** Which of the following structures is homologous to the wing of birds? [NEET 2016 – PHASE I]
(a) Dorsal fin of a Shark
(b) Wing of a Moth
(c) Hind limb of Rabbit
(d) Flipper of Whale

**32.** The wings of a bird and the wings of an insect are: [RE-AIPMT 2015]
(a) Analogous structures and represent convergent evolution.
(b) Phylogenetic structures and represent divergent evolution.
(c) Homologous structures and represent convergent evolution.
(d) Homologous structures and represent divergent evolution.

**33.** Artificial selection to obtain cows yielding higher milk output represents: [NEET 2017]
(a) directional as it pushes the mean of the character in one direction.
(b) disruptive as it splits the population into two, one yielding higher output and the other lower output.
(c) stabilizing followed by disruptive as it stabilizes the population to produce higher yielding cows.
(d) stabilizing selection as it stabilizes this character in the population.

**34.** Flippers of Penguins and Dolphins are the example of: [NEET Regional 2017]
(a) Radiation
(b) Homologous structure
(c) Analogous structure
(d) Divergent evolution

**35.** Continental drift led to disappearance of a number of South American mammals, because: [NEET Regional 2017]
(a) alteration of vegetation was not conducive to their survival.
(b) there was an outbreak of numerous infectious diseases.
(c) sudden change in the climatic conditions.
(d) they were outcompeted by more highly evolved animals reaching here from North America.

**36.** Among the following sets of examples for divergent evolution, select the incorrect option: [NEET 2018]
(a) Forelimbs of man, bat and cheetah
(b) Brain of bat, man and cheetah
(c) Heart of bat, man and cheetah
(d) Eye of octopus, bat and man

**37.** The similarity of bone structure in the forelimbs of many vertebrates is an example of [NEET 2018]
(a) Homology (b) Convergent evolution
(c) Analogy (d) Adaptive radiation

**38.** According to Hugo de Vries, the mechanism of evolution is [NEET 2018]
(a) Multiple step mutations
(b) Phenotypic variations
(c) Saltation
(d) Minor mutations

**39.** A gene locus has two alleles A, a. If the frequency of dominant allele A is 0.4, then what will be the frequency of homozygous dominant, heterozygous and homozygous recessive individuals in the population? [NEET 2019]
(a) 0.16 (AA); 0.24 (Aa); 0.36 (aa)
(b) 0.16 (AA); 0.48 (Aa); 0.36 (aa)
(c) 0.16 (AA); 0.36 (Aa); 0.48 (aa)
(d) 0.36 (AA); 0.48 (Aa); 0.16 (aa)

**40.** Match the hominids with their **correct** brain size:

| | |
|---|---|
| (A) *Homo habilis* | (i) 900 cc |
| (B) *Homo neanderthalensis* | (ii) 1350 cc |
| (C) *Homo erectus* | (iii) 650–800 cc |
| (D) *Homo sapiens* | (iv) 1400 cc |

[NEET 2019]

Select the **correct** option.

| | (A) | (B) | (C) | (D) |
|---|---|---|---|---|
| (a) | (iii) | (ii) | (i) | (iv) |
| (b) | (iii) | (iv) | (i) | (ii) |
| (c) | (iv) | (iii) | (i) | (ii) |
| (d) | (iii) | (i) | (iv) | (ii) |

**41.** Variations caused by mutation, as proposed by Hugo de Vries, are: [NEET 2019]
(a) Random and directionless
(b) Small and directional
(c) Small and directionless
(d) Random and directional

**42.** In a species, the weight of new-born ranges from 2 to 5 kg. 97% of the new-born with an average weight between 3 to 3.3 kg survive, whereas 99% of the infants born with weights from 2 to 2.5 kg or 4.5 to 5 kg die. Which type of selection process is taking place? [NEET 2019]
(a) Stabilizing Selection
(b) Disruptive Selection
(c) Cyclical Selection
(d) Directional Selection

**43.** Which of the following refer to **correct** example(s) of organisms which have evolved due to changes in environment brought about by anthropogenic action? [NEET 2020]
(A) Darwin's Finches of Galapagos islands.
(B) Herbicide resistant weeds.
(C) Drug resistant eukaryotes
(D) Man-created breeds of domesticated animals like dogs.
(a) Only (A) (b) (A) and (C)
(c) (B), (C) and (D) (d) Only (D)

**44.** Embryological support for evolution was disapproved by: [NEET 2020]
(a) Karl Ernst von Baer (b) Alfred Wallace
(c) Charles Darwin (d) Oparin

**45.** From his experiments, S. L. Miller produced amino acids by mixing the following in a closed flask: [NEET 2020]
(a) $CH_4$, $H_2$, $NH_3$ and water vapour at 800°C
(b) $CH_3$, $H_2$, $NH_4$ and water vapour at 800°C
(c) $CH_4$, $H_2$, $NH_3$ and water vapour at 600°C
(d) $CH_3$, $H_2$, $NH_4$ and water vapour at 600°C

**46.** Flippers of Penguins and Dolphins are examples of: [NEET 2020]
(a) Adaptive radiation (b) Convergent evolution
(c) Industrial melanism (d) Natural selection

**47.** The factor that leads to founder effect in a population is: [NEET 2021]
(a) Genetic drift
(b) Natural selection
(c) Genetic recombination
(d) Mutation

**48.** Match the following: [NEET 2021]

| List-I | List-II |
|---|---|
| 1. Adaptive radiation | (i) Selection of resistant varieties due to excessive use of herbicides and pesticides |
| 2. Convergent evolution | (ii) Bones of forelimbs in Man and Whale |
| 3. Divergent evolution | (iii) Wings of Butterfly and Bird |
| 4. Evolution by anthropogenic action | (iv) Darwin Finches |

**The correct matching is**

| | 1 | 2 | 3 | 4 |
|---|---|---|---|---|
| (a) | (i) | (iv) | (iii) | (ii) |
| (b) | (iv) | (iii) | (ii) | (i) |
| (c) | (iii) | (ii) | (i) | (iv) |
| (d) | (ii) | (i) | (iv) | (iii) |

**49.** Natural selection where more individuals acquire specific character value other than the mean character value, leads to: [NEET 2022]

(a) Directional change
(b) Disruptive change
(c) Random change
(d) Stabilising change

**50.** Which of the following statements is **not** true? [NEET 2022]

(a) Sweet potato and potato is an example of analogy.
(b) Homology indicates common ancestry.
(c) Flippers of penguins and dolphins are a pair of homologous organs.
(d) Analogous structures are a result of convergent evolution.

**51.** Select the correct group/set of Australian Marsupials exhibiting adaptive radiation. [NEET 2023]

(a) Numbat, Spotted cuscus, Flying phalanger
(b) Mole, Flying squirrel, Tasmanian tiger cat
(c) Lemur, Anteater, Wolf
(d) Tasmanian wolf, bobcat, Marsupial mole

**52.** The flippers of the Penguins and Dolphins are the example of the [NEET 2024]

(a) Adaptive radiation
(b) Natural selection
(c) Convergent evolution
(d) Divergent evolution

**53.** Which one of the following factors will not affect the Hardy-Weinberg equilibrium? [NEET 2024]

(a) Genetic recombination
(b) Genetic drift
(c) Gene migration
(d) Constant gene pool

**54.** Given below are some stages of human evolution. Arrange them in correct sequence. (Past to Recent). [NEET 2024]

A. *Homo habilis*
B. *Homo sapiens*
C. *Homo neanderthalensis*
D. *Homo erectus*

Choose the correct sequence of human evolution from the options given below:

(a) D-A-C-B (b) B-A-D-C
(c) C-B-D-A (d) A-D-C-B

**55.** Match List-I with List-II: [NEET 2024]

| List-I | List-II |
|---|---|
| (A) Mesozoic Era | (i) Lower invertebrates |
| (B) Proterozoic Era | (ii) Fish and Amphibia |
| (C) Cenozoic Era | (iii) Birds and Reptiles |
| (D) Paleozoic Era | (iv) Mammals |

Choose the correct answer from the options given below:

(a) (A)-(ii), (B)-(i), (C)-(iii), (D)-(iv)
(b) (A)-(iii), (B)-(i), (C)-(ii), (D)-(iv)
(c) (A)-(i), (B)-(ii), (C)-(iv), (D)-(iii)
(d) (A)-(iii), (B)-(i), (C)-(iv), (D)-(ii)

## Answer Key

### Multiple Choice Questions: Level I

| | | | | | | | | | |
|---|---|---|---|---|---|---|---|---|---|
| **1.** (c) | **2.** (c) | **3.** (b) | **4.** (c) | **5.** (c) | **6.** (a) | **7.** (d) | **8.** (b) | **9.** (d) | **10.** (d) |
| **11.** (a) | **12.** (c) | **13.** (d) | **14.** (c) | **15.** (b) | **16.** (c) | **17.** (a) | **18.** (d) | **19.** (a) | **20.** (d) |
| **21.** (c) | **22.** (b) | **23.** (a) | **24.** (c) | **25.** (a) | **26.** (c) | **27.** (a) | **28.** (b) | **29.** (a) | **30.** (a) |
| **31.** (d) | **32.** (b) | **33.** (b) | **34.** (c) | **35.** (b) | **36.** (a) | **37.** (c) | **38.** (b) | **39.** (c) | **40.** (a) |
| **41.** (b) | **42.** (b) | **43.** (d) | **44.** (d) | **45.** (a) | **46.** (a) | **47.** (d) | **48.** (a) | **49.** (d) | **50.** (b) |
| **51.** (a) | **52.** (a) | **53.** (d) | **54.** (a) | **55.** (d) | **56.** (a) | **57.** (c) | **58.** (a) | **59.** (b) | **60.** (d) |
| **61.** (c) | **62.** (a) | **63.** (d) | **64.** (a) | **65.** (c) | **66.** (d) | **67.** (b) | **68.** (b) | **69.** (d) | **70.** (c) |
| **71.** (c) | **72.** (d) | **73.** (c) | **74.** (d) | **75.** (d) | **76.** (b) | **77.** (a) | **78.** (c) | **79.** (a) | **80.** (c) |
| **81.** (a) | **82.** (d) | **83.** (c) | **84.** (b) | **85.** (a) | **86.** (a) | **87.** (c) | **88.** (a) | **89.** (a) | **90.** (a) |
| **91.** (c) | **92.** (c) | **93.** (b) | **94.** (b) | **95.** (c) | **96.** (d) | **97.** (b) | **98.** (d) | **99.** (d) | **100.** (c) |
| **101.** (c) | **102.** (b) | **103.** (d) | **104.** (b) | **105.** (c) | **106.** (d) | **107.** (a) | **108.** (b) | **109.** (a) | **110.** (a) |
| **111.** (d) | **112.** (c) | **113.** (d) | **114.** (c) | **115.** (b) | **116.** (a) | **117.** (b) | **118.** (b) | **119.** (b) | **120.** (d) |
| **121.** (d) | **122.** (c) | **123.** (b) | **124.** (c) | **125.** (a) | **126.** (d) | **127.** (d) | **128.** (d) | **129.** (c) | **130.** (d) |
| **131.** (d) | **132.** (d) | **133.** (b) | **134.** (b) | **135.** (b) | **136.** (d) | **137.** (a) | **138.** (d) | **139.** (d) | **140.** (b) |
| **141.** (a) | **142.** (a) | **143.** (b) | **144.** (a) | **145.** (c) | **146.** (d) | **147.** (b) | **148.** (b) | **149.** (b) | **150.** (b) |
| **151.** (a) | **152.** (c) | **153.** (a) | **154.** (d) | **155.** (d) | **156.** (c) | **157.** (c) | **158.** (d) | **159.** (c) | **160.** (a) |
| **161.** (d) | **162.** (a) | **163.** (a) | **164.** (a) | **165.** (c) | **166.** (b) | **167.** (d) | **168.** (a) | **169.** (a) | **170.** (a) |
| **171.** (c) | **172.** (b) | **173.** (b) | **174.** (c) | **175.** (b) | **176.** (a) | **177.** (d) | **178.** (a) | **179.** (a) | **180.** (b) |
| **181.** (a) | **182.** (b) | **183.** (a) | **184.** (a) | **185.** (d) | **186.** (c) | **187.** (c) | **188.** (d) | **189.** (a) | **190.** (d) |
| **191.** (d) | **192.** (c) | **193.** (b) | **194.** (a) | **195.** (c) | **196.** (d) | **197.** (d) | | | |

### Multiple Choice Questions: Level II

| | | | | | | | | | |
|---|---|---|---|---|---|---|---|---|---|
| **198.** (d) | **199.** (c) | **200.** (d) | **201.** (c) | **202.** (a) | **203.** (a) | **204.** (b, c) | **205.** (c) | **206.** (d) | **207.** (d) |
| **208.** (a) | **209.** (b) | **210.** (a) | **211.** (d) | **212.** (b) | **213.** (b) | **214.** (a) | **215.** (a) | **216.** (b) | **217.** (b) |
| **218.** (a) | **219.** (b) | **220.** (a) | **221.** (a) | **222.** (c) | **223.** (d) | **224.** (a) | **225.** (a) | **226.** (b) | |

### A & R and Statement-based Questions

| | | | | | | | | | |
|---|---|---|---|---|---|---|---|---|---|
| **227.** (d) | **228.** (c) | **229.** (c) | **230.** (b) | **231.** (a) | **232.** (c) | **233.** (c) | **234.** (b). | **235.** (c) | **236.** (b) |

### Matrix-Match Type Questions

| | | | | |
|---|---|---|---|---|
| **237.** (a) | **238.** (a) | **239.** (a) | **240.** (a) | **241.** (a) |

### NCERT Exemplar Questions

| | | | | | | | | | |
|---|---|---|---|---|---|---|---|---|---|
| **1.** (b) | **2.** (c) | **3.** (b) | **4.** (c) | **5.** (b) | **6.** (d) | **7.** (a) | **8.** (c) | **9.** (d) | **10.** (c) |
| **11.** (a) | **12.** (a) | **13.** (b) | **14.** (c) | **15.** (d) | **16.** (b) | **17.** (d) | **18.** (a) | | |

### Previous Years' Questions

| | | | | | | | | | |
|---|---|---|---|---|---|---|---|---|---|
| **1.** (c) | **2.** (a) | **3.** (d) | **4.** (d) | **5.** (c) | **6.** (c) | **7.** (b) | **8.** (c) | **9.** (a) | **10.** (a) |
| **11.** (b) | **12.** (d) | **13.** (b) | **14.** (c) | **15.** (d) | **16.** (b) | **17.** (b) | **18.** (b) | **19.** (c) | **20.** (c) |
| **21.** (a) | **22.** (a) | **23.** (d) | **24.** (d) | **25.** (b) | **26.** (a) | **27.** (a) | **28.** (d) | **29.** (b) | **30.** (c) |
| **31.** (d) | **32.** (a) | **33.** (a) | **34.** (c) | **35.** (d) | **36.** (d) | **37.** (a) | **38.** (c) | **39.** (b) | **40.** (b) |
| **41.** (a) | **42.** (a) | **43.** (c) | **44.** (a) | **45.** (a) | **46.** (b) | **47.** (a) | **48.** (b) | **49.** (a) | **50.** (c) |
| **51.** (a) | **52.** (d) | **53.** (b) | **54.** (a) | **55.** (a) | | | | | |

# HINTS AND EXPLANATION

## Multiple Choice Questions: Level II

**198.** In the case of peppered moth (*Biston betularia*), the black-coloured form became dominant over the light-coloured form in England during industrial revolution. This is an example of natural selection. This group is about species that gain protection from predators due to selection caused by nature.

**199.** It is because there is in-breeding depression.

**200.**

| Homologous organs | Analogous organs |
|---|---|
| 1. These organs are similar in origin but different in function. | 1. These organs are different in origin but similar in function. |
| 2. They indicate divergent evolution and adaptive radiation. | 2. They indicate divergent evolution. |
| 3. They differ phenotypically. | 3. They show superficial resemblance. |
| 4. Homologous organs have similar internal structure. | 4. Internal structure is quite different. |
| 5. They arise from similar position over the body. | 5. They often arise from different positions over the body. |
| **Examples:** a. Forelimbs of vertebrates – pectoral fins of fish, flippers of whales, wings of bats and birds, hand of human and legs of horse. | **Examples:** a. Wings of insects, birds and bat. |
| b. Legs of insects are meant for various activities like digging, jumping, collecting pollens, swimming, prey grassing, etc. | b. Trachea of insects and lungs of vertebrates. |
| c. Mouthparts of insects. | c. Eyes of cephalopod and mammal. |
| d. Thorns in Bougainvillea and tendrils in Passiflora and Cucurbita. | d. Leaf of plant, cladode of Ruscus and Asparagus. |
| e. Phylloclade in Opuntia and cladode of Ruscus. | e. Sweet potato and potato tuber. |

**201.** It is classical example of adaptive radiation.

**202.** According to Darwin, resistance to pesticides has a genetic basis due to presence of certain alleles. In the presence of pesticides, insects devoid of allele for resistance die while the ones having them survive. They are selected by nature.

**203.** Nephridia of earthworm and malphigian tubules of cockroach belong to excretory organs. Earthworm has a well-developed excretory system which is composed of large number of minute, coiled and glandular segmentally arranged excretory tubules called the hephridia. Malphigian tubules of cockroach are extremely fine yellowish unbranched thread-like structure present at the function of the midgut and hindgut.

**204.** Cleidoic eggs and scales on their hind limbs.

**205.** The theory of continuity of germplasm published by August Weismann (1834–1914) in 1886. It proposes that the contents of the reproductive cells (sperms and ova) are passed on unchanged from one generation to the next, unaffected by any changes undergone by the rest of the body. It thus rules out any possibility of the inheritance of acquired characteristics and has become fundamental to neo-Darwinian theory.

**206.** During the period when the number of coal-burning factories in England was increasing (during the so- called Industrial Revolution) it was noticed that the number of melanic individuals of the species of Peppered Moth (*Biston betularia*) was becoming more common. *Originally* rare in the population of normally light-coloured moths, the frequency of the melanic form increased in polluted areas until it was over 90%. This change in colour has come to be known as 'industrial melanism'

**207.** When the members of a species are interfertile and produce fertile offsprings.

**208.** It refers to evolution of different species from the common ancestor.

**209.** Speciation takes places via reproductive isolation which is the most important consequence of geographical isolation.

**210.** To survive in an environment, an organism needs to adapt in that environment. If the organism becomes success in adapting then that organism is selected by nature.

**211.** According to Hardy–Weinberg principle
Frequency of heterozygous individuals = 2pq
$= 2 \times 0.6 \times 0.4 = 0.48$

**212.** Species is the basic unit of classification. The term was coined by John Ray. Most taxonomists define species as morphologically distinct and reproductively *isolated natural population* or groups of populations where individuals resemble one another more closely than the members of other species, interbreed freely and form a genetically closed system. Gene transfer occurs between populations of a species by gene flow, *i.e.* emigration and immigration.

**213.** According to Oparin, primitive atmosphere was reducing. Hence, there was no oxygen. It had $H_2$, $CH_4$, $NH_3$ and water vapour.

**214.** According to Darwin, gradual accumulation of small variations gives rise to new species. Abrupt mutations do not give rise to new species. Plants arose by gradual adaptation to diverse habitats and not suddenly on earth. Seeded plants are just one group in the plant kingdom.

**215.** Angiosperms have adapted themselves to all kinds of habitat: terrestrial, aquatic, tropical, deciduous and alpine. Self-pollination is seen in very few angiosperms. Production of large number of seeds ensures that at least some will germinate. Not all plants have been domesticated by man.

**216.** Seasonal isolation refers to differences in season of breeding that can isolate two varieties. Behavioural or ethological isolation refers to differences in behaviour like courtship rituals, etc. to prevent mating. Mechanical isolation refers to differences in the position, size and structure of animal genitalia which prevent reproductive contact and thus bring about isolation.

**217.** Natural selection operates through differential reproduction. Genetic drift is random change in the allele number and frequency in a gene pool.

**218.** Mutations are sudden inheritable variations which develop in the genetic system. Natural selection operates through differential reproduction. Frequency of an allele in isolated population may change due to genetic drift (selection by chance).

**219.** The earliest cells were chemoheterotrophs, later they become chemoautotroph and then came photoautotroph.

**220.** Biogeography is the study of geographical distribution of organisms.
Paleontology is the study of past life based on fossils and fossil impressions.
Anatomy is the study of internal structure. Embryology is the study of development of embryo from zygote to offspring.

**221.** During industrial evolution in England, the frequency of melanic forms of species of Peppered Moth *(Biston betularia)* increased in prohibited areas. Generally, the moths are light-coloured. This change in colour is known as 'Industrial Melanism'. The change was presumed to be a result of natural selection since the melanic moths better matched the blacked trunks where they rest during day.

**222.** Two or more species which are reproductively isolated from each other but are morphologically quite similar are known as sibling species. Sympatric species are developed due to reproductive isolation and occur in overlapping or same area of geographical distribution. Parapatric species are developed in adjacent geographical areas meeting in very narrow regions of overlap.

**223.** Nature selects those set of characters that are best adapted to the environment. This has resulted in great diversity seen in the population of finches.

**224.** The change in the colour of peppered moth is due to mutation of single Mendelian gene for the survival in the smoke-laden industrial environment. It is called industrial melanism.

**225.** The study of fossils or remains of past organisms present in the rocks of different ages is called palaeontology or palaeobiology. It has two branches:

(i) Study of fossil plants – Palaeobotany

(ii) Study of fossil animals – Palaeozoology

- Herpetology is the study of reptiles, but specific study of lizards is saurology.
- Organic evolution deals with study of origin of life and origin of new species.

**226.** Mimicry is an example of long-term adaptation, in which there is close resemblance of an organism to the surrounding in order to avoid detection, e.g. Leaf insect phyllium. The term mimicry was introduced by Bates (1862).

## NCERT Exemplar Questions

**1.** Lichens are sensitive to $SO_2$ pollution. Lichens are very good pollution indicators; they do not grow in polluted areas.

**2.**
- For a long time, it was also believed that life came out of decaying and rotting matter like straw, mud, etc.
- According to theory of abiogenesis, life originated from non-living.

**3.** Animal husbandry and plant breeding programmes are examples of artificial selection.

**4.** Paleontological evidences for evolution refer to the fossils. Fossils provide direct and solid evidence in favour of organic evolution through ages. Fossils are studied for knowing about extinct organisms. Birbal Sahni Institute of Palaeobotany is situated at Lucknow. Birbal Sahni is called 'Father of Indian Palaeobotany'. Age of fossils is determined by Uranium-Lead method ($U^{238}$) or Potassium-Argon method or Radioactive Carbon dating ($C^{14}$). ESR (electron-spin-resonance method) is the most accurate method of dating of fossils.

**5.** Organs having same origin but different functions are called homologous organs. For example, whales, bats, cheetah and human (all mammals) share similarities in the pattern of bones of forelimbs. Homology indicates common ancestry.

**6.** Organs having different origin but similar function are called analogous.

**7.** $(p + q)^2 = p^2 + 2pq + l = \text{I}$ represents an equation used in population genetics.

Above equation is known as Hardy–Weinberg principle in which

$p^2$ – Dominant homozygous

$2pq$ – Heterozygous

$q^2$ – Recessive homozygous

**8.** Appearance of antibiotic-resistant bacteria is an example of **pre-existing variation** in the population.

**9.** Evolution of life shows that life forms have a trend of moving from water to land.

**10.** Viviparity is considered to be more evolved because the young ones are protected inside the mother's body and are looked after they are born leading to more chances of survival.

**11.** Fossils are generally found in **sedimentary rocks.**

**12.** By the equation $(p + q)^2 = p^2 + 2pq + q^2 = \text{I}$

$MN = 2pq = 2 \times 0.7 \times 0.3$

Expected frequency of MN group

$$= \frac{2 \times 0.7 \times 0.3}{1} \times 100 = 42\%$$

**13. Directional** type of selection is industrial melanism observed in moth, *Biston bitularia.*

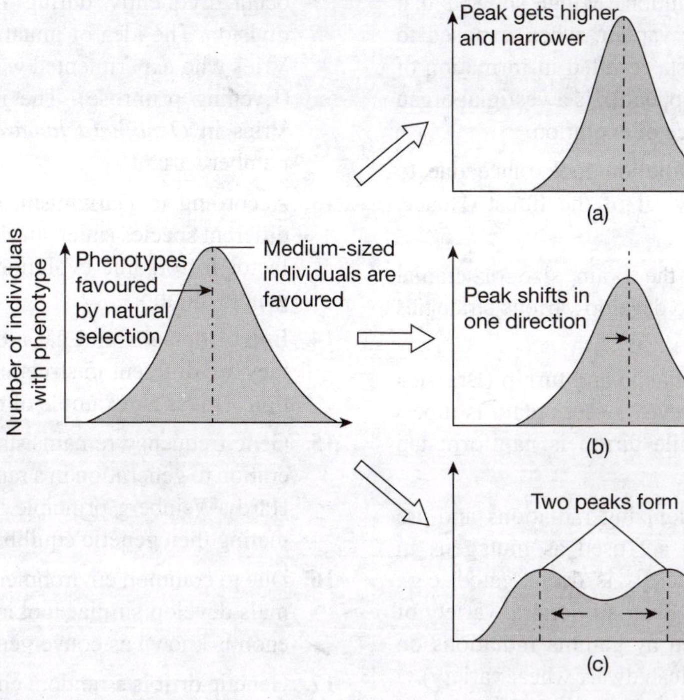


Operation of naturals selection on different traits (a) Stabilising (b) Directional and (c) Disruptive

**14.** *Ramapithecus* → *Homo habilis* → *Homo erectus* → *Homo sapiens*

**15. Chimpanzee** is an example for link species.

**16.** (i) Darwin P. Evolution by natural selection
(ii) Oparin M. Abiogenesis'
(iii) Lamarck N. Use and disuse of organs
(iv) Wagner O. Continental drift theory

**17.** In 1953 S. L. Miller created primitive earth conditions in the laboratory and gave experimental evidence for origin of first form of life from pre-existing non-living organic molecules. The primitive earth conditions created include high temperature, volcanic storms, reducing atmosphere containing $CH_4$, $NH_3$ etc.

**18.** Variations during mutations of meiotic recombination are **random** and **directionless**.

## Previous Years' Questions

**1. Adaptive radiation:**

- It is the evolution of ecological and phenotypic diversity within a rapidly multiplying lineage.
- Starting with a recent single ancestor, this process results in formation of a group of species (speciation), having different morphological and physiological traits with which they can exploit and survive in different environments.
- Adaptive radiation is a characteristic example of cladogenesis that can be indicated as a bush of coexisting species (on the tree of life).

**Four features can be used to identify an adaptive radiation:**

**(1)** A common recent ancestry
**(2)** Rapid speciation
**(3)** A significant association between environment and the morphological and physiological traits used to exploit those environments (phenotype–environment correlation)
**(4)** The performance of trait values in their corresponding environments (trait utility).

2. Wings of butterfly and birds look alike and are the result of convergent evolution. Miller showed that $CH_4$, $H_2$, $NH_3$ and water vapour, when exposed to electric discharge in a flask, resulted in formation of amino acids. Vermiform appendix is a vestigial organ and an anatomical evidence of evolution.

   According to Darwin, evolution took place due to small variations and survival of the fittest. Hence, option (a) is correct.

3. Remarkable increase in the brain size or cranial capacity enabled human to develop various strategies for his survival.

4. Sweet potato (Ipomoea batatas) and turnip (Brassica rapa) both are roots. However, sweet potato is tuberous adventitious root while turnip is napiform tap root.

5. **Gamma radiations** are ionizing radiations and are physical mutagens. They are used as mutagens in such materials, where nucleus is deep seated, e.g., seeds, stem cuttings, etc. 'Sharbati Sonora' variety of wheat has been developed by gamma radiations on 'Sonora-64' variety (Mexican dwarf wheat variety).

6. The most significant trend in the evolution of modern man is the increased brain capacity from the ancestors.

7. (b) **Neanderthal man (1,00,000–40,000 years back)** Lived near east and central Asia.
   Cranial capacity: 1400cc.These people used hides to protect their body and buried their dead
   (a) Homo hibilis – lived 2 million years ago
   (c) Cro-magnan human – originated 2 lakh years ago
   (d) Ramapithecus – lived 2 million years ago

8. Remarkable increase in the brain size or cranial capacity enabled human to develop various strategies for his survival.

9. Convergent evolution involves independent development of similar structures in organisms that are not directly related. It is represented by analogous organs, e.g., eyes of octopus and mammals, wings of insects and birds.

10. Process of evolution of different species in a given area starting from a point and radiating to other area of geographical areas is called adaptive radiations. Example: Darwin's finches, Australian marsupials.

11. Cuscuta is plant.

12. Mutations are alterations of genetic material. They occur frequently during DNA duplication in cell division. The idea of mutations was brought forth by Vries who experimented was *Oenothera lamarckiana* (Evening primrose). The mutation observed by de Vries in *Oenothera lamarckiana* was chromosomal number variant.

13. According to Darwinism, competition between two different species (inter specific competition) is the key factor for organic evolution since it results in divergent evolution.

14. Eye of octopus and cat are analogous organs, since they are different in structure but perform same function. This is an example of divergent evolution.

15. Gene frequency remains stable or constant from generation to generation in a random mating population is Hardy Weinberg principle if population lack random mating then genetic equilibrium will be disturbed.

16. Due to common environmental changes, different animals develop similar looking features. This phenomenon is known as convergent evolution.

17. Genetic drift is a random change in allele frequencies over the generations. It is brought by chance alone. Gene flow or gene migration is the physical movement of alleles into and out of a population.

18. Analogous structures are a result of convergent evolution. Eyes of the octopus and mammals, Flippers of penguins and Dolphins, Sweet potato (root modification) and potato (stem modification).

19. Organs which have a common fundamental anatomical plan and similar embryonic origin whatever varied functions they may perform are regarded as homologous organs. For examples, the flippers of a whale, a bat's wing, forelimb of a horse, a bird's wing and forelimbs of human are structurally as well as functionally different.

20. According to Hardy–Weinberg Principle.
    AA is 360 out of 1000 means $0.36 = p^2$.
    Therefore, $p = 0.6$ (frequency of 'A' allele in population)

21. Interesting observation supporting evolution by natural selection comes from England. In a collection of moths made in 1850s, i.e., before industrialization set in, it was observed that there were more white-winged moths on trees than dark-winged or melanized moths. However, in the collection carried out from the same area, but after industrialization, i.e., in 1920, there were more dark-winged moths in the same area, i.e., the proportion was reversed.

**22.** The theory of Hardy–Weinberg equilibrium states that in the absence of disturbance on the level of genetic structure, a population's existence will not continue. Thus, mating should be in a random way.

**23.** This creature was called the first human-like being the hominid and was called *Homo habilis*. The brain capacities were between 650 and 800cc.

**24.** Critical analysis makes us believe that variation due to mutation or variation due to recombination during gametogenesis or due to gene flow or genetic drift results in changed frequency of genes and alleles in future generation.

**25.** The correct sequence of event is:

Synthesis of organic monomers → Synthesis of organic polymers → Formation of protobionts → Formation of DNA-based genetic systems.

**26.** Chronological order of human evolution is Ramapithecus / *Dryopithecus* → Australopithecus → Homo habilis → Homo erectus → *Neanderthal* man→ homo sapiens

**27.** Hardy–Weinberg principle stated it using algebraic equations.

Frequency of dominant allele (A) = p
Frequency of recessive allele (a) = q
Sum total of all the allelic frequencies is 1, i.e., $p + q = 1$
Frequency of AA individuals(homozygous dominant) $= p \times p = p^2$
Frequency of aa individuals(homozygous recessive) $= q \times q = q^2$
Frequency of Aa individuals(heterozygous) = 2pq
$(p + q)^2 = p^2 + 2pq + q^2 = 1$

**28.** Genetic drift (Allelic drift or Sewall wright effect) is a change in the frequency of gene variant in a population due to random sampling of organism or occurrence by chance. It operates in small isolated population.

**29.** Analogous structures are a result of convergent evolution. When organisms with completely different organization, living in the same habitat come to possess superficial resemblance, this is known as convergent evolution.

**30.** Both statements are correct because primitive atmosphere was reducing and chlorophyll appeared later on. Chemoautotrophs were the first autotrophic organism unable to perform photolysis of water and never released oxygen.

**31.** Wings of birds and Flipper of Whale are example of homologues organ because their origin is same but functions are different. Both are modification of forelimb.

**32.** Analogous organs which have different origin but have similar functions, such organs show convergent evolution, e.g. Wings of butterfly and birds, Eyes of the octopus and mammals.

**33.** Here we are selecting breed which will produce higher milk output, we are selecting one of the breed which means its directional selection and it pushes mean character in one direction.

**34.** Analogous organs: Those organs which have different origin but have similar functions, such organs show convergent evolution, e.g. Wings of butterfly and birds, eyes of the octopus and mammals, flippers of penguins and dolphins, sweet potato (root modification) and potato (stem modification).

**35.** Due to continental drift:

**(1)** When South America joined North America, mammals of South America (resembling horse, hippopotamus, bear, rabbit, etc.) were overridden by North American fauna.

**(2)** Pouched mammals of Australia (marsupials) survived because of absence of any other mammal.

**36.** **Convergent evolution** - Different structures evolving for the same function and hence having similarity. Examples of analogy are the eye of the octopus and of mammals or the flippers of Penguins and Dolphins. Rest of the options are examples of divergent evolution.

**37.** The similarity of bone structure in the forelimbs of many vertebrates is an example of homology. Because their basic plan is same but functions may be different.

**38.** Hugo de Vries based on his work on evening primrose brought forth the idea of mutations – large difference arising suddenly in a population. He believed that it is mutation which causes evolution and not the minor variations (heritable) that Darwin talked about. Mutations are random and directionless while Darwinian variations are small and directional. Evolution for Darwin was gradual while de Vries believed mutation caused speciation and hence called its **saltation (single large step mutation).**

**39.** P(dominant allele) = 0.4 (By using Hardy–Weinberg Principle $p + q = 1$)
q(Recessive allele) $= 1 - 0.4 = 0.6$
Frequency of homozygous dominant AA($P^2$) $= (0.4)^2 = 0.16$
Frequency of heterozygous Aa(2 pq) $= 2 \times 0.4 \times 0.6 = 0.48$
Frequency of homozygous recessive aa($q^2$) $= (0.6)^2 = 0.36$

**40.** *Homo habilis* – The brain capacities were between 650 and 800cc. *Homo erectus* had a large brain around 900cc. Neanderthal man had a brain size of 1400cc and homo sapiens is 1350 cc.

**41.** In the first decade of the twentieth century, Hugo de Vries based on his work on evening primrose brought forth the idea of mutations – large difference arising suddenly in a population. He believed that it is mutation which causes evolution and not the minor variations (heritable) that Darwin talked about. Mutations are **random and directionless** while Darwinian variations are small and directional.

**42.** The given data shows stabilizing selection as most of the new-born having average weight between 3 and 3.3 kg survive and babies with less and more weight have low survival rates.

**43.** The correct answer is option (c) because

- Herbicide resistant weeds, drug resistant eukaryotes and man-created breeds of domesticated animals like dogs are examples of evolution by anthropogenic action.
- Darwin's Finches of Galapagos islands are example of natural selection, adaptive radiation and founder's effect.

**44.** Embryological support for evolution was disapproved by Karl Ernst von Baer, he noted that embryos never pass through the adult stages of other animals during embryonic development.

**45.** In 1953, S.L. Miller, an American scientist created electric discharge in a closed flask containing $CH_4$, $H_2$, $NH_3$ and water vapor at 800°C.

**46.** The correct option is (b) because flippers of Penguins and Dolphins are an example of analogous organs. Analogous structures are a result of convergent evolution.

**47.** Change in gene frequency in a small population by chance is known as genetic drift. Genetic drift has two ramifications, one is bottle neck effect and another is founder's effect.

**48.**

| | |
|---|---|
| Adaptive radiation | Adaptive radiation is the process of evolution of different species in a given geographical area starting from a point and literally radiating to other areas of geography, for example : Darwin's finches. |
| Convergent evolution | Analogous organs which are not anatomically similar structures though they perform similar functions, are a result of convergent evolution, for example: Wings of butterfly and birds. |
| Divergent evolution | Homologous organs which are anatomically similar structures but perform different functions according to their needs, are a result of divergent evolution, for example : Bones of forelimbs in man and whale |
| Evolution by anthropogenic action | Evolution by anthropogenic action means evolution due to human interference, for example: antibiotic resistant microbes, herbicides resistant varieties and pesticide resistant varieties. |

**49.** Natural selection leads to stabilising change where more individuals acquire mean character value.

It leads to directional change where more individuals acquire specific character value other than means character value.

It leads to disruptive change when more individuals acquire peripheral character value of both ends of distribution curve.

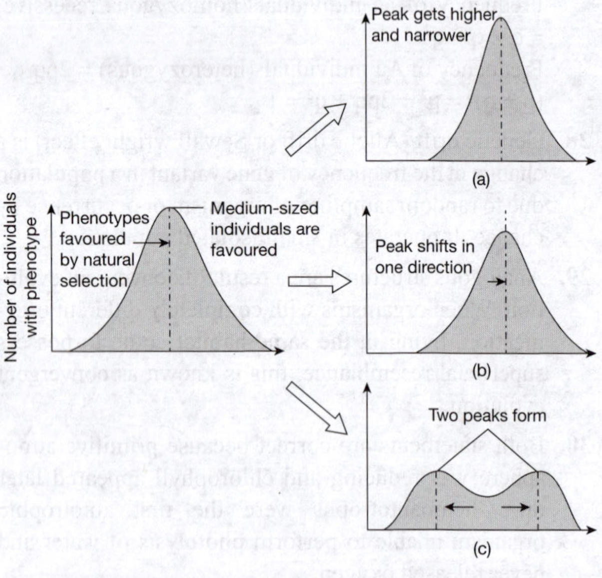


*Figure: Diagrammatic representation of the operation of natural selection on different traits (a) Stabilizing (b) Directional and (c) Disruptive*

**50.** Sweet potato is a root modification for food storage whereas potato is an underground stem modification for storage. Hence, they are analogous.

Analogous structures developed as a result of convergent evolution.

Homologous organs have the same structure but have different functions according to the needs of the organisms. Hence, homology indicates common ancestry.

Option (c) is the correct answer because flippers of penguins and dolphins are analogous organs as they help in swimming but do not have the same structure.

**51.** Placental mammals: Mole, anteater, mouse, Lemur, Flying squirrel, Bobcat, Wolf

Australian marsupials: marsupial mole, Numbat, Marsupial mouse, Spotted cuscus, Flying Phalanger, Tasmanian tiger cat, Tasmanian wolf

**52.** The correct answer is option (c), because the flippers of the Penguins and Dolphins perform similar function but they are not anatomically similar structures. This is example of analogous structures.

- Option (a) is incorrect as adaptive radiation is the process of evolution of different species in a given geographical area starting from a point and literally radiating to the other areas of geography.
- Option (b) is incorrect as natural selection is a key mechanism of evolution.
- Option (d) is incorrect as divergent evolution results in the formation of homologous structures.

**53.** The correct answer is option (d) as a constant gene pool will not disturb the Hardy-Weinberg equilibrium. Option (a), (b) and (c) will affect the equilibrium leading to evolution.

**54.** Correct answer is option (d) because the correct sequence of stages of human evolution from past to recent is

*Homo habilis* → *Homo erectus* → *Homo neanderthalensis* → *Homo sapiens*

**55.** The correct answer is option no. (d).

| | |
|---|---|
| (A) Mesozoic Era | (iii) Birds and Reptiles |
| (B) Proterozoic Era | (i) Lower invertebrates |
| (C) Cenozoic Era | (iv) Mammals |
| (D) Paleozoic Era | (ii) Fish & Amphibia |

# 11

# Human Health and Disease

## LEARNING OBJECTIVES

- Understand the importance and awareness of healthy well-being
- Discuss different types of diseases, their causative agents, and also their preventive measures
- Learn about the importance of immunization, their types and also essential immunization recommendation
- Understand about the aids and cancer its causative agent, and treatment
- Discuss drugs and alcohol abuse

## Chapter Overview

### Introduction

- **Health:** It is defined as a state of complete physical, mental and social well-being.
- **Blood circulation** was discovered by William Harvey.
- Health is affected by genetic disorders like, infections, lifestyle (food/water/rest/exercise), drugs and alcohol abuse.
- Personal hygiene, balanced diet and regular exercise are important for good health.
- **Disease:** It is characterized by various sign and symptoms manifested by abnormal functioning of one or more organ and organ system of our body. Disease is broadly divided into two types.
  - **(i) Infectious diseases:** It is easily transmitted from one person to another. It very common type of disease. Example: common cold, some fatal infectious disease is **AIDS.**
  - **(ii) Non-infectious diseases:** Not transmitted from one person to another. Example: diabetes, cancer and obesity. Among these **cancer** is major cause of death.

### Common Human Diseases

- **Pathogens**: These are disease-causing organisms. **Examples:** Bacteria, Viruses, Fungi, Protozoans, Helminthes, etc. Most of parasites are also pathogens. They harm host by living inside or on the body of host organism. Pathogens adapt within the environment of the host accordingly. Gut pathogens survive in the stomach at low pH and resist the action of various digestive enzymes.
- **Infection:** Invagination and multiplication of micro-organism inside the body those are not normally present in our body. Example: virus, bacteria and fungus, etc.
- **Infestation:** Invagination and multiplication of macro-organism in host organism.
- Life cycle pathogen:
  - (i) Entry of pathogen in our body by various means
  - (ii) Multiplication
  - (iii) Interference with normal vital activities
  - (iv) Morphological and functional damage (Disease).

Refer NCERT Ch 7: Human Health and Disease

- Brief of some common diseases in human

**(1) Bacterial Disease: Typhoid, Pneumonia, Dysentery, Plague and Diphtheria, etc.**

**A. Typhoid fever:**

- **Causative organism**: ***Salmonella typhi***
- **Mode of infection**: Faeco-oral route, by contaminated water and food. Inside body it migrates via blood.
- **Sign and symptoms:** Sustained high fever (39°C to 40°C) i.e., ladder step fever, constipation, headache, weakness, stomach pain and loss of appetite. In severe case **intestinal perforation** and death may occur.
- **Diagnostic Test: Widal test**

**B. Pneumonia :**

- **Causative organism***:* Streptococcus pneumonia and Haemophilus influenza.
- **Mode of infection:** By inhaling the droplets / aerosols released by an infected person and by sharing glasses and utensils with an infected person. Pathogen enters in respiratory tract and infect of alveoli.
- **Sign and symptoms:** Alveoli filled with fluid and severe problem in respiration, fever, chills, cough and headache. Lips and finger nails may turn gray to bluish in severe cases.

**(2) Viral diseases:** These are caused by viruses e.g., influenza, small pox, chicken pox, mumps, rabies, polio, AIDS, yellow fever, common cold, etc.

**A. Common cold:** Most common infectious viral disease.

- **Causative organism:** Rhino viruses.
- **Mode of infection:** Inhalation of droplets from cough or sneezes of an infected person either directly or transmitted through contaminated object and utensils. It will affect nose and respiratory passes (URT) and not the lungs.
- **Sign and symptoms:** Nasal congestion and discharge, sore throat, hoarseness, cough, headache, tiredness, etc.

**B. Dengue fever**

- **Pathogen:** Dengue fever is cause by mosquito borne flavi-ribo virus.
- **Mode of Transmission:** The virus of dengue fever is transmitted by the bite of Aedes aegypti (tiger mosquito). Aedes mosquito breeds in clean water and bites only during day times. Dengue is found in many parts of India.
- **Incubation Period:** 3 to 8 days.
- **Types of Dengue fever:** Two types of dengue fever are common: classical dengue fever and dengue haemorrhagic.
- **Symptoms of Classical Dengue Fever:**
  (i) Sudden onset of high fever.
  (ii) Severe frontal headache.
  (iii) Pain behind the eyes which worsens with eye movement.
  (iv) Muscles and joint pains.
  (v) Loss of appetite.
  (vi) Rashes on the body.
  (vii) Nausea and vomiting.
- **Symptoms of dengue Haemorrhagic Fever:**
  (i) Symptoms similar to classical dengue fever except the following:
  (ii) Bleeding from the nose, mouth, gums and skin bruising.
  (iii) Severe and continuous stomach pains.
  (iv) Frequent vomiting with or without blood.
  (v) Pale cold or clammy skin.
  (vi) Excessive thirst (dry mouth).
  (vii) Rapid weak pulse.
  (viii) Difficulty in breathing.
  (ix) Restlessness and constant crying.
- **Prevention:** Mosquitoes and their eggs should be eliminated. Wear clothes that cover the body. No vaccine for Dengue fever is available. Dengue test is available.
- **Treatment:** No specific therapy is available.
  Symptomatic care including bed rest, adequate fluid intake and analgesic medicine is recommended. Do not take aspirin and dispirin because they are harmful in this disease. Use Paracetamol (tablet, syrup) for fever.

**C. Chikungunya**

- **Pathogen:** It is caused by Chikungunya virus. This virus was first isolated form human patients and Aedes aegypti mosquitoes from Tanzania in 152. The name 'Chikungunya' is derived from the native word for the disease in which patient lies "Doubled up" due to severe joint pains. Epidemics of chikungunya have occurred in many African countries.
- **Mode of Transmission:** By the bite of Aedes aegypti mosquito. No vaccine is available.
- **Symptoms:** Its symptoms include sudden onset of fever, crippling joint pains, lymphadenopathy and **conjunctivitis**. Some show haemorrhagic manifestations.
  The fever is typically biphasic. Chikungunya is also found in many parts of India.
- **Incubation Period:** Usually 3-6 days.
- **Prevention:** Preventive measures include elimination of mosquitoes and their eggs.

**D. AIDS: (Acquired Immuno Deficiency Syndrome)**

It is an acquired condition (not congenital) of deficiency of immune system by an individual during his lifetime which leads to a syndrome (group of symptoms). AIDS was first reported in 1981.

- **Causative organism:** HIV (Human immuno deficiency Virus)—A member of retrovirus **(Fig. 11.1)** group. It is enveloped virus with RNA genome. There are **two ss RNA and two restriction endonuclease** in AIDS virus.

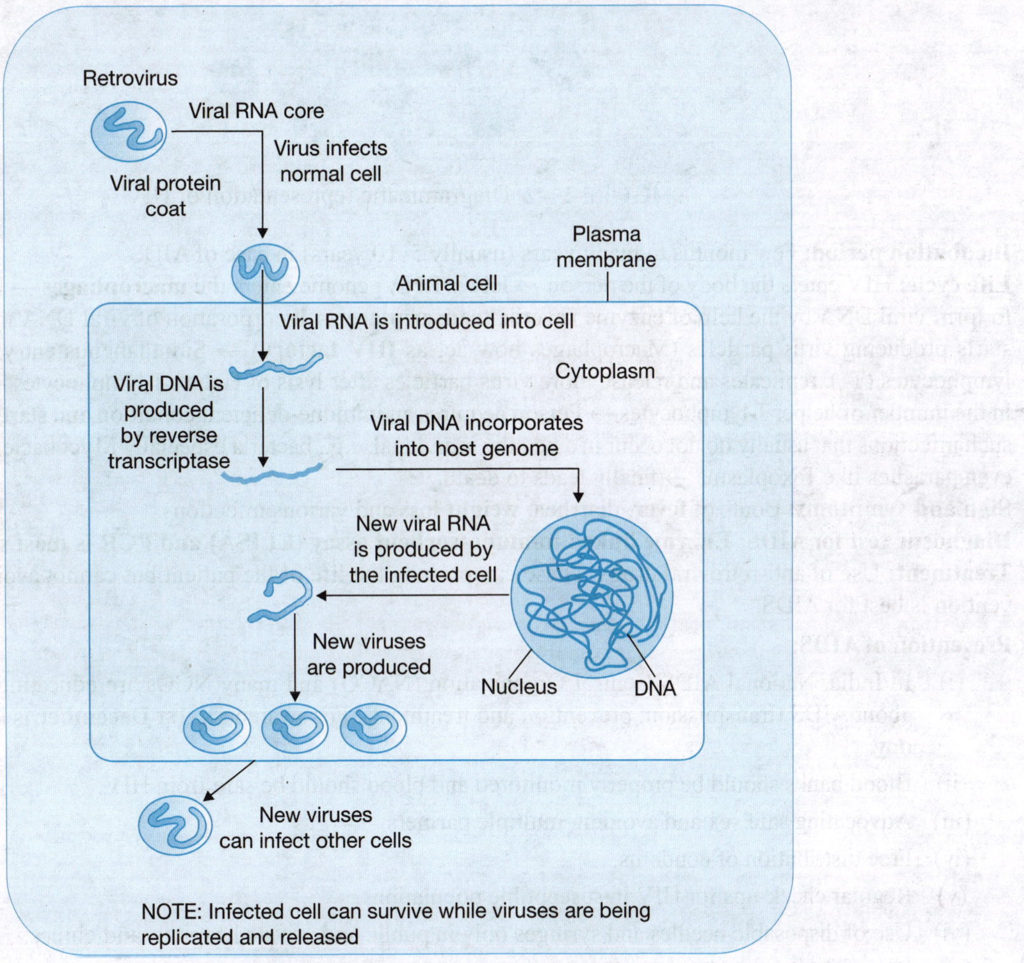


**FIGURE 11.1** Replication of retrovirus

- **Means of Transmission of HIV-infection:** Sexual contact with infected person, transfusion of infected blood and blood products, sharing infected needles (in case of intravenous drug abusers) and Infected mother to the foetus through placenta (vertical transmission). HIV **(Fig. 11.2)** spreads only through the body fluids, not by touch or physical contact.

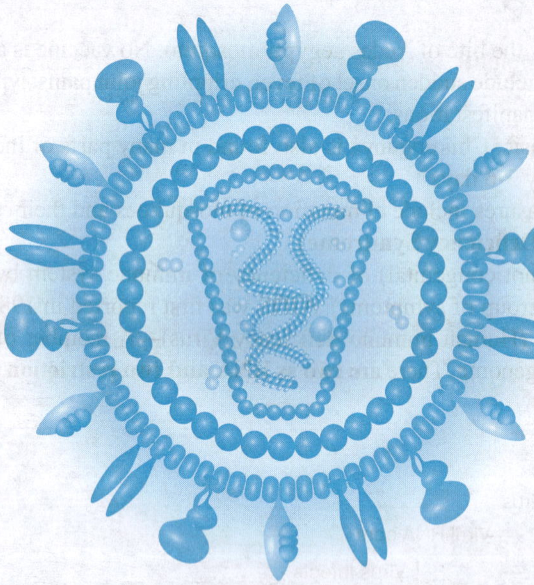

FIGURE 11.2 Diagrammatic representation of HIV

- **Incubation period:** Few months to many years (usually 5–10 years) in case of AIDS.
- **Life cycle:** HIV enters the body of the person → HIV's RNA genome enters the **macrophages** → RNA genome replicates to form viral DNA by the help of enzyme **reverse transcriptase** → Incorporation of viral DNA into host cell's DNA and starts producing virus particles (Macrophages now act as **HIV factory**) → Simultaneous entry of HIV into Helper T-lymphocytes ($T_H$), replicates and release more virus particles after lysis of Helper T-lymphocytes → Progressive decrease in the number of helper T-lymphocytes → Person acquires an immune-deficient condition and starts suffering from various such infections that usually do not occur in a healthy individual, e.g., bacteria especially Mycobacterium, viruses, fungi and even parasites like Toxoplasma → finally leads to death.
- **Sign and symptoms:** Bouts of **fever**, diarrhea, **weight loss** and various infections.
- **Diagnostic test for AIDS: Enzyme linked immuno-sorbent assay (ELISA) and PCR is most sensitive test.**
- **Treatment:** Use of anti-retroviral drugs. These can prolong the life of the patient but cannot avoid death (no cure). Prevention is best for AIDS.
- **Prevention of AIDS:**
  - (i) In India, National AIDS Control Organization (NACO) and many NGOs are educating the people everything about AIDS (transmission, prevention and treatment). For awareness, **1st December** is known as **worlds AIDS day.**
  - (ii) Blood banks should be properly monitored and blood should be safe from HIV.
  - (iii) Advocating safe sex and avoiding multiple partners.
  - (iv) Free distribution of condoms.
  - (v) Regular check-ups for HIV in susceptible populations.
  - (vi) Use of disposable needles and syringes only in public and private hospitals and clinics.
  - (vii) Drug abuse should be controlled.
  - (viii) Having AIDS should not be hidden as it may spread to other people.
  - (ix) AIDS patients should be given proper counseling, sympathy and treatment.

**(3) Protozoan diseases:** These are caused by protists e.g., malaria, amoebic dysentery, kala-azar, oriental sore, sleeping sickness, etc.

**A. Malaria:**

- **Causative organism**: ***P. vivax, P. malaria, P. falciparum*** (causes **malignant malaria** which is very serious and may be fatal) ***and P. Ovale***. Its vector is female anopheles mosquito. **Infectious form of Plasmodium: Sporozoites. Mode of infection**: Bite of **female Anopheles mosquito.**
- **Life cycle:** Plasmodium requires two hosts to complete its life cycle- **Human (host)** and **female Anopheles mosquito (vector).**
  Female Anopheles mosquito bites the human and releases **sporozoites** in the blood. Then there is multiplication of parasites in the liver cells. Entry of parasite into RBCs → Rupture of RBCs → Release of a toxic substance -**Haemozoin** → Haemozoin causes chills and high fever repeating in every 3 to 4 days. Female Anopheles mosquito bites an infected person → Parasites enter the mosquito's body (gut) and undergo further development. Multiplication of parasites within body of mosquito to form **sporozoites** → Sporozoties are stored in the salivary glands **(Fig. 11.3)**.
- **Sign and symptoms:** chill and high fever recurring in every 3 to 4 days.

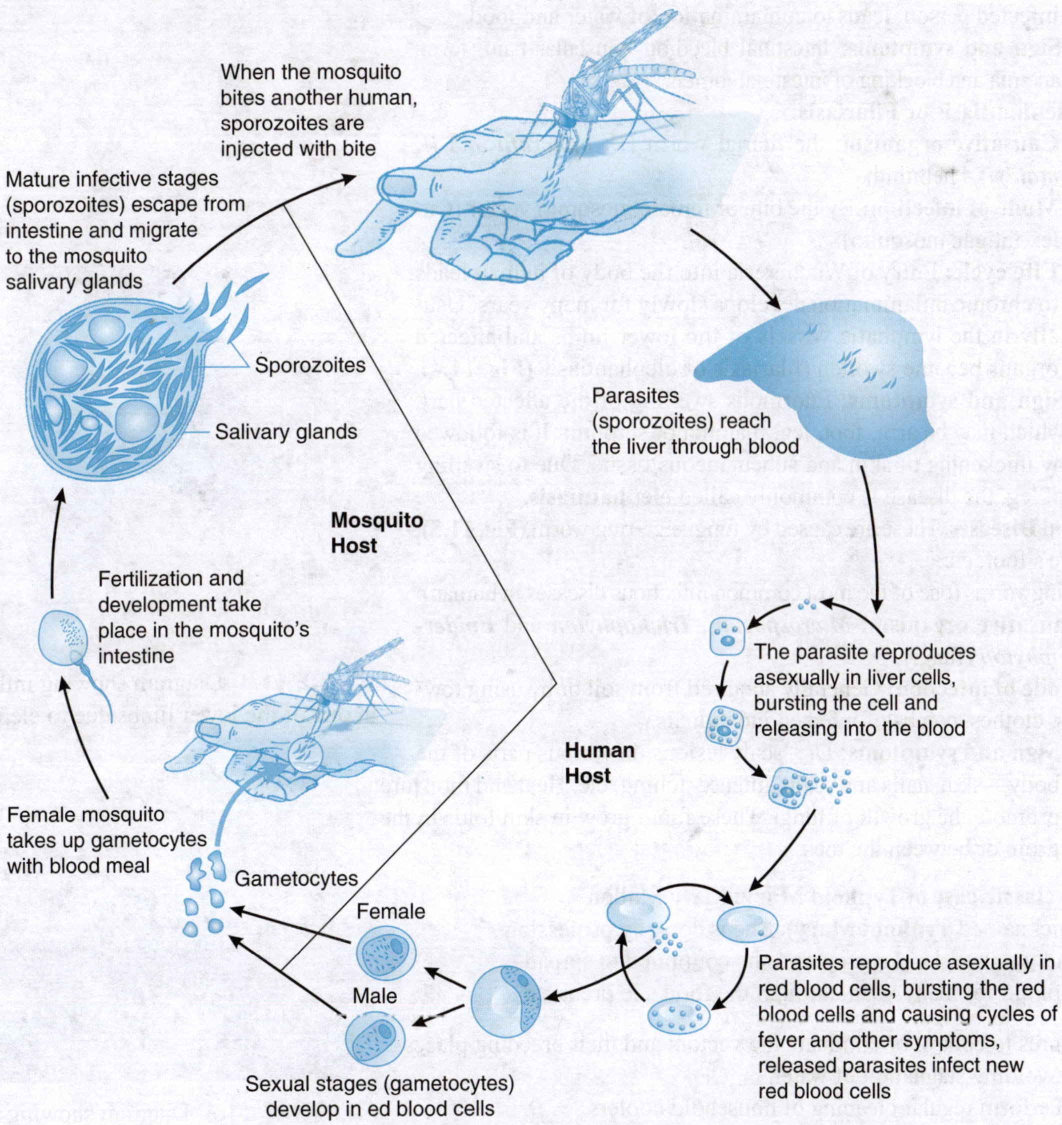


**FIGURE 11.3** Stages in the life cycle of plasmodium

**B. Amoebiasis: (Amoebic dysentery)**

- **Causative organism:** ***Entamoeba histolytica***
- **Mode of infection:** Contamination of food and water by Houseflies (carrying the parasite mechanically from the faeces of infected person to food). It is parasite of large intestine.
- **Sign and symptoms:** Abdominal pain and cramps, constipation, stools with excess mucous and blood clots. It injures intestinal lining and feeds on erythrocytes and cell debris. Periodically, it forms rounded cysts which escape with host's faeces. Entamoeba secretes a proteolytic enzyme, **cytolysin** that erodes the mucous membrane of the intestine. This may form bleeding ulcers that produce dysentery.

**(4) Helminth Diseases:** These are caused by helminths (flatworms and roundworms) taeniasis schistosomiasis (liver rot) are caused by flatworms and ascariasis, Filariasis (elephantiasis), enterobiasis, trichinosis, hook worm disease and guinea worm disease are caused by round worms.

**A. Ascariasis:**

- **Causative organism: Ascaris** the common round-worm (an intestinal parasite)
- **Mode of infection:** Faeco-oral route, by contaminated water and food. Release of parasite eggs along with the faeces of infected person, leads to contamination of water and food.
- **Sign and symptoms:** Intestinal bleeding, muscular pain, fever, anemia and blocking of intestinal lumen.

**B. Elephantiasis or Filariasis:**

- **Causative organism:** the filarial worm ***(W. bancrofti*** and ***W. malayi*)** a helminth.
- **Mode of infection:** By the bite of female mosquito vector (Culex fatigan mosquito).
- **Life cycle:** Entry of Wuchereria into the body of human leads to chronic inflammation develops slowly for many years. Usually in the lymphatic vessels of the lower limbs and affected organs become swollen (filariasis or elephantiasis **(Fig. 11.4)**.
- **Sign and symptoms:** Enormous swelling of the affected part, which may be arm, foot, leg, mamma or scrotum. It is followed by thickening of skin and subcutaneous tissue. Due to swelling of leg, the disease is commonly called **elephantiasis.**

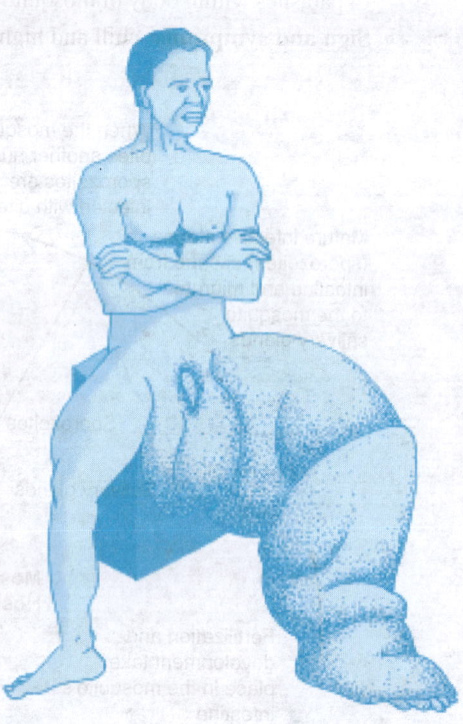

**FIGURE 11.4** Diagram showing inflammation in one of the lower limbs due to elephantiasis

**(5) Fungal Diseases.** These are caused by fungi e.g., ring worm **(Fig. 11.5)**, athlete's foot, etc.

**A.** Ringworms (one of the most common infectious diseases in human).
**Causative organism:** ***Microsporum***, ***Trichophyton*** and ***Epidermophyton*** (fungi)
**Mode of infection:** Generally acquired from soil or by using towels, clothes, combs of infected individuals.

- **Sign and symptoms:** Dry, scaly lesions on various parts of the body—skin, nails and scalp, intense itching, etc. Heat and moisture promote the growth of fungi. These fungi grow in skin folds in the groin or between the toes.

**FIGURE 11.5** Diagram showing ringworm affected area of the skin

> **A classic case of Typhoid Mary:** Mary Mallon (nicknamed **Typhoid Mary).** She is cook by profession and was a typhoid carrier and she continued to spread typhoid for many years through the food she prepared.

- Measures to control or eliminate the vectors and their breeding places :
  (i) Avoiding stagnation of water.
  (ii) Perform regular cleaning of household coolers.
  (iii) Spraying of insecticides in ditches, drainage areas and swamps, etc.

**TABLE 11.1** Types of innate immunity

| Innate immunity consist of four types of barriers | |
|---|---|
| **1. Physical barriers** | **Skin:** It is the main barrier that prevents entry of the pathogens.<br>**Mucus:** It covers the epithelium lining of respiratory, gastrointestinal and urogenital tracts, therefore, the microbes may not enter our body. |
| **2. Physiological barriers** | These prevent microbial growth and include:<br>**1.** Acid in the stomach.<br>**2.** Saliva in the mouth and tears. |
| **3. Cellular barriers** | Phagocytosis and destruction of microbes by certain types of WBCs and body cells:<br>**1.** Neutrophils (Polymorpho-nuclear leucocytes or PMNL).<br>**2.** Monocytes.<br>**3.** Natural killer (a type of lymphocytes)<br>**4.** Tissue macrophages. |
| **4. Cytokine barriers** | **Interferons:** It is a protein secreted by the virus-infected cells to protect the spread of infection to healthy or non-infected cells. |

(iv) Introducing fishes like **Gambusia** (feed on mosquito larvae) in ponds.
(v) Use of mosquito nets.
(iv) Doors and windows should be provided with wire mesh to restrict the entry of mosquitoes.

- Such precautions have become more important especially in case of the vector-borne **(Aedes mosquitoes)** diseases like **Dengue** and **Chikungunya and yellow fever (all are viral diseases)** in many parts of India.
- Use of vaccines has resulted in eradication of **smallpox** and control on infectious diseases like **polio, diphtheria, pneumonia** and **tetanus**.

## Immunity

- It refers to the overall ability of the host to fight the disease-causing organisms, conferred by the immune system.
- Types of Immunity:
  **(1) Innate immunity** (non-specific type of defense present since birth).
  **(2) Acquired immunity** (pathogen specific, not presence since birth): It is characterized by memory.
  - **Primary response:** It is a low intensity response given by the body when it encounters a pathogen for the first time.
  - **Secondary or anamnestic response:** It is a highly intensified response which is evoked by the subsequent encounter with the same pathogen. This somehow indicates that perhaps our body has memory of the first encounter.

  Two special types of lymphocytes in our blood mediate the primary and secondary immune responses:
  (i) **T. lymphocytes:** These help the B-cells to produce antibodies.
  (ii) **B. lymphocytes:** Involved in the synthesis of proteins called antibodies.
- **Structure of antibody**
  - Each antibody molecule **(Fig. 11.6)** is made up of four peptide chains-two light chains (small) and two heavy chains (longer). This is the reason why an antibody is represented as $H_2L_2$.
  - Various types of antibodies are produced in our body-IgA, IgM, IgE, IgG, etc.

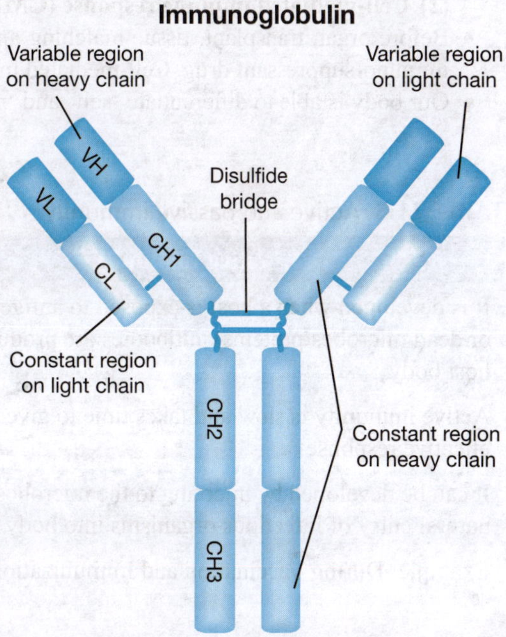


**FIGURE 11.6** Structure of an antibody molecule

**TABLE 11.2** Different classes of immunoglobulins and their functions

| Immunoglobulin Class | Presence | Functions |
|---|---|---|
| 1. IgA | (i) Second most abundant class, constituting about ten per cent of serum immunoglobulins.<br>(ii) Present in colostrums, saliva and tears.<br>(iii) Also in gastro-intestinal tract and respiratory tract. | (i) Protects from inhaled and ingested pathogens.<br>(ii) Protects eyes. |
| 2. IgD | Present on the surface of B lymphocytes which are destined to differentiate into antibody producing plasma cells. | Activates B cells to secrete antibody. |
| 3. IgE | Remain free and heat labile (inactivated at 56°C in one hour). | Acts as mediator in allergic response and also mediates type I hypersensitivity (anaphylaxis). |
| 4. IgG | (i) Most abundant class constituting about seventy five per cent of the total immunoglobulins.<br>(ii) Only antibody that can cross placenta.<br>(iii) Present in milk. | (i) Stimulates phagocytes and complement system.<br>(ii) Provide natural passive immunity in the fetus and new born.<br>(iii) Protects the body fluids. |
| 5. IgM | (i) Largest immunoglobulin (at least five times larger than IgG).<br>(ii) Earliest Ig to be synthesized by the fetus. | (i) Activates B cells.<br>(ii) Protects the blood serum. |

- As these antibodies are found in blood and the response provoked is also called humoral immune response.
- There are two types of acquired immune responses in our body:
  **(1) Antibody mediated immune response (AMI) or B cell mediated immunity or Humoral immunity.**
  **(2) Cell-mediated immune response (CMI) or T cell mediated immunity.**
- Before organ transplant, tissue matching and blood group matching are essential. After transplant patient has to take immuno-suppressant drug. Cell-mediated immune response is responsible for the graft rejection.
- Our body is able to differentiate 'self' and 'non-self'.

**TABLE 11.3** Active and passive immunity

| Active Immunity | Passive Immunity |
|---|---|
| It is developed when a host is exposed to antigens (living or dead microbes/proteins) antibodies are produced in the host body. | Prior exposure to antigens is not required. |
| Active immunity is slow and takes time to give its full effective response. | Passive immunity is fast and gives full effective response in short period of time. |
| It can be developed by injecting to the microbes or by the natural entry of infectious organisms into body. | It can be developed by injecting ready-made antibodies to combat against foreign agents. |
| Example: During Vaccination and Immunization. | Example: Tetanus antitoxin, Anti-venom. |

- The yellowish fluid **colostrum** (first milk) secreted by mother during the initial days of lactation has abundant antibodies (IgA) to protect the infant. This is the reason, that mother's milk is considered very essential for the new born infants. The fetus also receives some antibodies from mother through placenta during pregnancy. Such passive immunity is called **natural passive immunity**.
- **Vaccination and Immunization**
  - Immunization or vaccination is based on the property of 'memory' of the immune system.
  - **Mechanism:** Vaccine (antigenic proteins of pathogen / inactivated or weakened pathogen) is injected into the body → Body produces antibodies against the antigens to neutralize them → Generation of memory-B and T-cells which recognize the pathogen quickly on next exposure of antigens by massive production of antibodies.

**TABLE 11.4** Different types of vaccine preparations

| Types of vaccine | Preparation | Examples | Duration of immunity |
|---|---|---|---|
| 1. Live Vaccines Attenuated Vaccines . | Prepared from live (generally attenuated - the pathogen made weakened to make it non-virulent organism. | OPV (Oral Polio Vaccine), BCG (Bacillus Calamite Guerin), small pox, yellow fever vaccine, Influenza vaccine. | Provide life ling immunity. |
| 2. Killed Vaccines or Inactivated Vaccines | Prepared by killing the pathogenic organism by heat/ultraviolet rays/ alcohol/formalin/ phenol. | Typhoid vaccine, Sulk Polio vaccine, Typhus vaccine, Rabies vaccine, Plague vaccine, TAB vaccine (Typhoid, Para typhoid A and Paratyphoid B vaccine). | Immunity for a definite period. |
| 3. Toxoids | Prepared from toxins produced by pathogen after detoxification. | Diphtheria toxoid and tetanus toxoid. | Provide passive immunity for short period. |
| 4. Cellular Fractions | Prepared from extracted cellular fraction. | Meningococcal vaccine from the polysaccharide antigen of the cell wall and the pneumococcal vaccine from the polysaccharide contained in the capsule of the bacterium and hepatitis B polypeptide vaccine. | Duration of experience with these vaccine is limited, their efficiency and safety appear to be high. |
| 5. Combinations (Mixed or combined Vaccines) | By mixing more than one kind of immunizing agent. | DPT (diphtheria + pertussis + tetanus), DT (Diphtheria + tetanus), DP (Diphtheria + pertussis). Tetanus + Influenza vaccine, MMR (Measles + mumps + rubella) Measles + rubella | |

- Vaccines are also classified as follows:

**1. First Generation Vaccines**

These are vaccines which are produced by conventional technique using the whole microorganism. Such vaccines may produce side effects as they are not of uniform quality.

**2. Second Generation Vaccines**

These vaccines are prepared by recombinant **DNA technology/Genetic Engineering,** e.g., Hepatitis B virus vaccine (from transgenic yeast by recombinant DNA technology), Herpes virus vaccine and Pneumonia vaccine.

**3. Third Generation Vaccine (Synthetic Vaccines)**

These are chemically synthesised multivalent vaccines, which maintain high purity e.g., Leukemia virus vaccine, vaccine against diphtheria toxin developed by **Audibert** et. al. 1981.

- **Tetanus Antitoxin**
  - If a person is exposed to some deadly microbes (as tetanus causing microbe), treatment requires quick immune response in tetanus. So preformed antibodies are directly injected in the form of tetanus antitoxin (a preparation containing antibodies to the toxin).
- **Anti-venom**
  - Venom is injected into the body by snakebite and **anti-venom (preformed antibodies)** is immediately given to the patient for treatment. Anti-venom provides passive immunity.
- **Allergies**
  - **Allergy:** It refers to the exaggerated response of the immune system to certain antigens present in the environment. Common allergens (substance evoking immune response) are **pollens, mites in dust, animal dander,** etc. Lowering of immunity and more sensitivity to allergens has occurred due to present day life style and because of which, children in metro cities of India suffer from allergies and asthma due to sensitivity to the environment. This could be because of the protected environment provided early in life.
  - Antibodies produced during allergy is **IgE type.**
  - **Symptoms of allergy:** Sneezing, running nose, difficulty in breathing and watery eyes.
  - Allergic response is mediated by the release of chemicals like histamine and serotonin from the mast cells. To determination the cause of allergy very small doses of possible allergens are injected into the patient and the reactions are studied. Drugs used in allergy are **Anti-histamine, adrenaline and steroids.**
- **Auto Immunity**
  - Our memory-based acquired immunity (also in other higher vertebrates) can differentiate foreign molecules as well as foreign organisms (non-self) from our cells (self).
  - Sometimes our immunity fails to do so and attacks the self-cells. This may be due to some genetic and other unknown reasons. Such damage results in conditions known as auto-immune disease.
  - **Rheumatoid arthritis, Insulin dependent diabetes, chronic anemia, chronic hepatitis** and **Hashimoto's disease** are some other examples of auto immune diseases.

## Immune System in the Body

- Human immune system consists of:
  1. Lymphoid organs and tissues.
  2. Lymphocytes and other cells.
  3. Antibodies (soluble molecules).
- **Lymphoid organs**
  **(i)** In these organs origin and/or maturation and proliferation of lymphocytes occur.
  **(ii) Types of Lymphoid organs:**

| | | |
|---|---|---|
| 1. Primary lymphoid organs | Bone marrow and Thymus | Immature lymphocytes differentiate here into antigen sensitive lymphocytes. |
| 2. Secondary lymphoid organs | Spleen, Lymph nodes, Tonsils, Peyer's patches of small intestine and Appendix. | After maturation in primary lymphoid organs, lymphocytes migrate to the secondary lymphoid organs, which provide the sites for interaction of lymphocytes with the antigen and then proliferate to become effector cells. |

- **Bone marrow:** It is the main lymphoid organ in which all the blood cells (including lymphocytes) are produced.
- **Thymus:** It is a lobed organ near the heart, beneath the breastbone. Thymus is of large size at the time of puberty but it continuously reduces in size with age. Thymus along with the bone-marrow provide micro-environments for development and maturation of T-lymphocytes by the secretion of Thymosin hormone.

- **Spleen:** Large sized. Bean-shaped and purple coloured. It mainly possesses lymphocytes and phagocytes. It also acts as a large reservoir of RBCs. (it can store 8per cent of RBCs, hence known as blood bank of the body). It traps the blood-borne micro-organisms and acts as a filter of the blood. It help to destroy dead RBCs so referred as graveyard if RBCs.
- **Lymph Nodes:** They are small sized solid structures which are located at different points in the lymphatic system **(Fig. 11.7)**. They use to trap the micro-organisms or antigens from the lymph and tissue fluid activation of lymphocytes present Immune response.
- **Mucus-associated lymphoid tissue (MALT):** MALT is lymphoid tissue located within the lining of the major tracts (respiratory, digestive and urinogenital tracts). i.e., Payer's patches in duodenum and Brunner's gland in ileum. It forms about **50 per cent** of the lymphoid tissue in our body.

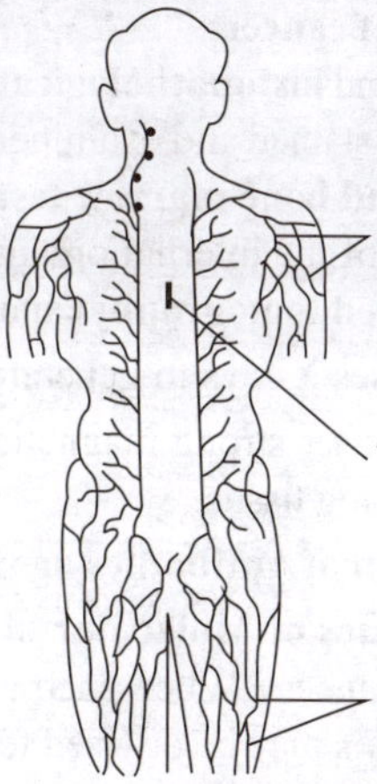


**FIGURE 11.7** Diagrammatic representation of Lymph nodes

## Cancer

- It is a major cause of death all over the world.
- **Tumour:** Cancerous cell divide and form masses of cells called tumour.
- **Contact inhibition:** This is a property of normal cells because of which have contact with other cells to keep a check on their uncontrolled growth. In cancerous cell this property is absent.
- **Types of Tumours:**

  **(A) Benign tumours:** Such tumours remain confined to their original position. These tumours cause little damage and metastasis absent.

  **(B) Malignant tumours:** Such tumours are a mass of proliferating cells called neoplastic or tumour cells. These tumours invade and extensively damaging the surrounding normal tissues. These cells grow very rapidly. Active division of these cells starve the normal cells for vital nutrients. **Metastasis** (cells sloughed from tumours reach the distant sites through blood and get lodged in the body to form a new tumour there).
- **Types of cancers on the basis of pathology**

  Pathologically, cancers are classified on the basis of the original tissue from where they arose. As such cancers are of four types:

  1. **Carcinomas**: Cancers of this type arise from epithelial and glandular tissues. They include cervical cancer of cervix), breast cancer, skin cancer, brain cancer, lung cancer, stomach cancer etc. About eighty five per cent of all tumours are carcinomas.
  2. **Melanomas**: These are cancerous growth of melanocytes (a type of skin cells).
  3. **Sarcomas**: These are the cancers of tissues of mesodermal origin (e.g., connective and muscular tissues). Thus, they include the cancers of bones (osteoma) such as, cartilages, tendons, adipose tissue (lipomas), lymphoid tissue and muscles. They are rare in human, as only about one per cent of all tumours are sarcomas.
  4. **Leukemias and Lymphomas**: These are the tumours of haematopoietic cells. Leukemias result from excessive formation of WBCs in the bone marrow and lymphatic nodes. Leukemias are commonly called **blood cancers.** Cancers of lymphatic tissue are called **lymphomas** e.g., Hodgkin's disease characterised by chronic enhancement of the production of lymphocytes by lymph nodes and spleen. In India most common cancers are mouth-throat cancer in men and uterine-cervical cancer in women.
- **Causes of Cancer**

  Cancer may be induced by physical, chemical or biological agents. These are collectively termed as **carcinogens.**

  1. Lonizing radiations (like **X-rays** and **gamma rays)** and non-ionizing radiations (like UV **rays)** cause DNA damage resulting in cancerous/neoplastic changes.
  2. Chemical carcinogens (like tobacco smoke) act as a major cause of lung cancer.
  3. Virus can also cause cancer. Such viruses are termed as oncogenic viruses and these have **viral oncogenes** (cancer causing genes).Even normal cells possess several genes called **cellular oncogenes** (c-one) or **proto-oncogenes,** which when activated under certain conditions, may lead to oncogenic transformation of the cells.

- **Diagnosis of cancer**
  - **Biopsy** and **histopathological studies** of the tissue. **In** biopsy, a piece of the suspected tissue is taken out, cut into thin sections, stained and examined under microscope (histopathological studies) by a pathologist for a proper suggestion.
  - **Blood and bone marrow tests:** These analyze the increased cell counts in case of **leukemias.**
  - Cancers of the internal organs are mainly detected by the use of techniques like **radiography (use of X-rays), CT (computed tomography)** and **MRI (magnetic resonance imaging).**

    **CT:** It uses X-rays to generate a three-dimensional image of the internals of an object.

    **MRI:** It uses strong magnetic fields and non-ionizing radiations to detect the pathological / physiological changes in the living tissue.
  - **Detection of Antibodies against cancer-specific antigens.**
  - **Techniques of Molecular biology (most sensitive)** to detect genes in individuals with inherited susceptibility to certain cancers. When such genes are identified, which predispose an individual to certain cancers and then these individuals may be advised to avoid exposure to particular carcinogens to which they are susceptible (e.g., tobacco smoke in case of lung cancer).
- **Treatment of Cancer**
  - **Surgery:** Surgical removal of benign tumours.
  - **Radiation therapy:** Tumour cells are exposed to lethal dose of radiations and taking proper care of the normal tissues surrounding the tumour mass.
  - **Chemotherapy:** Many chemotherapeutic drugs are used to kill cancerous cells. Few of them are specific for particular tumours. Common side effects of majority of drugs are hair loss, anemia, etc.
  - **Immunotherapy:** Biological response modifiers such as alpha-interferon are given to the patients which activates their immune system and destroy the tumours.
  - Most cancers are treated by combination of surgery, radiotherapy and chemotherapy.

## Drugs and Alcohol Abuse

- **Drug abuse:** When the drugs are taken for a purpose other than medicinal use or in amounts / frequency that impairs one's physical, physiological or psychological functions.
- Commonly abused drugs are obtained mainly from flowering plants and some from fungi.
- When drugs and alcohol for taken for purposes other than medicinal or taken in amounts or frequencies that impairs physical, physiological or psychological functions, it is called **drug abuse** and **alcohol abuse**, respectively.
- Drugs belong to different categories which are as follows:

(i) **Opioids**

- Heroin is a depressant and slows down body functions.
- **Source:** Morphine is extracted from the latex of poppy plant Papaver somaniferum. Heroin or smack is obtained by acetylation of morphine as a white, odorless, bitter and crystalline compound **(Fig. 11.8)**.
- **Mode of intake:** By snorting and injection.
- **Mode of action:** They bind to specific opioid receptors in the central nervous system (CNS) and gastrointestinal tract.
- Effects: Heroin is a depressant and slows down body functions. Morphine is an effective sedative and painkiller **(Fig. 11.9)**.

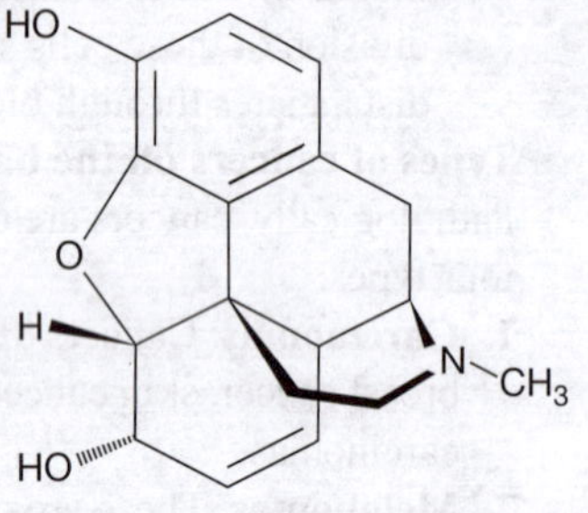

FIGURE 11.8 Chemical structure of Morphine

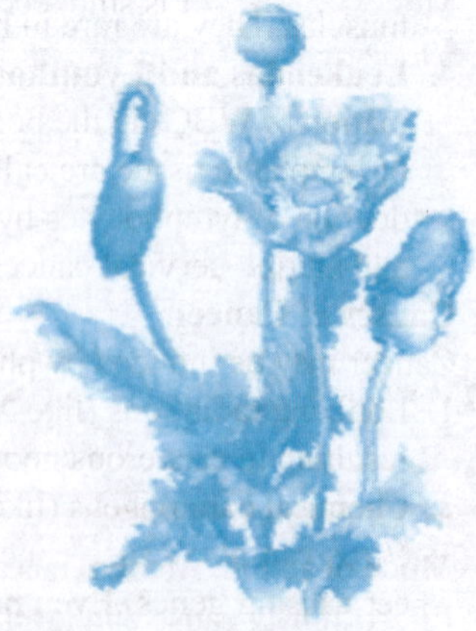
FIGURE 11.9 Opium poppy

(ii) **Cannabinoids**

- **Source:** Obtained from inflorescence of the plant Cannabis sativa **(Fig. 11.10 and 11.11)**. Flower tops, leaves and resins of C. Sativa in various combinations produce hashish, charas, marijuana and ganja.

- **Mode of intake:** By inhalation and oral ingestion.

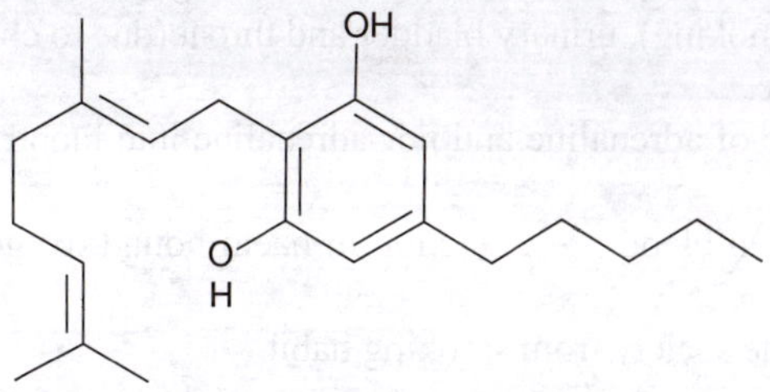


FIGURE 11.10 Skeletal structure of cannabinoid molecule

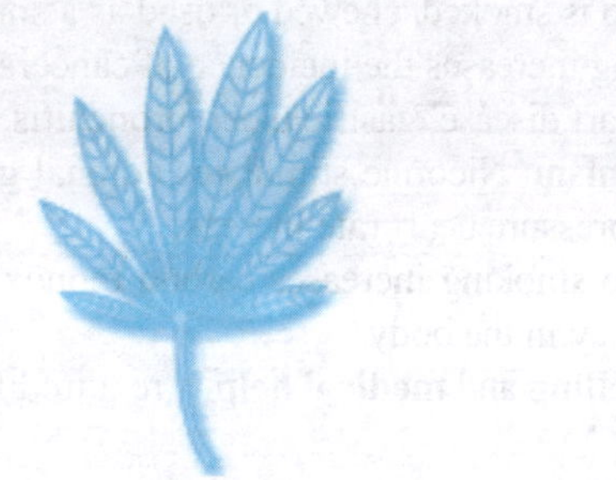

FIGURE 11.11 Leaves of *Cannabis sativa*

- **Mode of action:** They interact with the cannabinoid receptors present in the brain.
- **Effects:** Effect the cardiovascular system of the body.

(iii) **Coca alkaloid or cocaine**

- **Source:** Derived from the leaves and young branches of South American Plant called Erythroxylum coca.
- Characteristics of withdrawal symptoms: (1) Anxiety (2) Shakiness (3) Nausea (4) Sweating (5) Vomiting (6) Diarrhoea (7) Insomnia (8) Muscular and abdominal cramps (9) Restlessness
- Mode of intake: By sniffing and snorting.
- Mode of action: It has a potent stimulating action on central nervous system and interferes with the transport of the neurotransmitter dopamine.
- Effect: It is a strong stimulant and when taken in overdose causes headache, convulsions, hallucinations and death due to cardiovascular or respiratory failure.

(iv) **Hallucinogens**

- Source: Obtained from plants like *Atropa belladonna* and Datura sp. **(Fig. 11.12)** Lysergic acid diethyl amide (LSD) is derived from the fungus *Claviceps purpurea*.
- Mode of action: These drugs are called psychedelic drugs because of their effect on the cerebrum and sense organs.
- Effect: These drugs affect thoughts, feelings and perceptions of an individual. Medically these are given to patients to cope with mental illnesses like depression and insomnia.

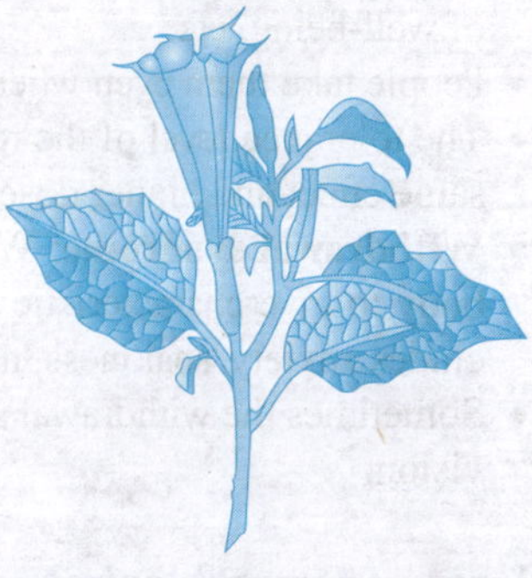

FIGURE 11.12 Flowering branch of Datura

(v) **Tobacco**

- Source: Tobacco plant.
- Mode of intake: It is smoked, chewed or used as a snuff.
- Mode of action: It has nicotine which stimulates the adrenal gland to release adrenaline and noradrenaline which in turn increases the blood pressure and heart rate.
- Effects:
  (a) It increases the chances of lung cancer, bronchitis, emphysema, coronary heart disease, cancer of throat, gastric ulcer, cancer of urinary bladder, etc.
  (b) Smoking leads to increase in carbon monoxide content of blood and reduces concentration of haem-bound oxygen, as a result of which oxygen deficiency in the body is created.
  (c) Chewing of tobacco causes oral cancer which becomes fatal in extreme conditions.

(vi) **Alcohol**

- Mode of intake: Oral intake.
- Mode of action: Alcohol has an anaesthetic effect on nervous system affecting cerebrum, cerebellum and the other parts.
- Effect: It may cause euphoria, peptic ulcer, gastric carcinoma, hepatitis, liver failure and liver cell carcinoma.

## Smoking

- Tobacco is smoked, chewed or used as a snuff. Large number of chemical substances including **nicotine (an alkaloid).**
- Smoking increases the incidence of cancers [lung (due to smoking), urinary bladder and throat (due to chewing)], coronary heart disease, gastric ulcer, bronchitis, emphysema, etc.
- **Mechanism**: Nicotine stimulates adrenal gland → Release of adrenaline and nor-adrenaline into blood circulation → Blood pressure heart rate increase.
- Tobacco smoking increases carbon monoxide (CO) levels in blood → Reduction in haem bound oxygen → Oxygen deficiency in the body.
- **Counselling** and **medical help** is required for preventing the society from smoking habit.

## Adolescence

- It is the bridge period (and process) between the childhood and adulthood during which a child becomes mature in terms of his / her attitudes and beliefs for effective participation in society.
- **Adolescence period:** between 12–18 years.
- As this period involves various biological and behavioral changes, individual undergoes a very vulnerable phase of mental and psychological development. Because of various factors, youngsters may move towards drug and alcohol abuse:

## Addiction and Dependence

- Addiction due to drugs and alcohol is a psychological attachment to their certain effects like euphoria, temporary feeling of well-being, etc.
- People take them even when these are not needed or even when their use becomes highly hazardous.
- The tolerance level of the receptors in our body also increases with repeated use of drugs because of which to produce same effect and higher doses of drugs or alcohol is required, leading to addiction.
- **Withdrawal syndrome**: Whenever a regular dose of drugs/alcohol is abruptly discontinued, there is tendency of the body to give characteristic and unpleasant .symptoms and that are collectively termed as withdrawal syndrome. It includes anxiety, shakiness, nausea and sweating. These are relieved when the drug or alcohol use is again continued.
- Sometimes the withdrawal symptoms may be severe / life threatening, therefore, the addict may need the medical supervision.

## Effects of Drug/Alcohol Abuse

- **The immediate adverse effects:** Reckless behaviour, vandalism and violence.
- Excessive doses of drugs → Respiratory failure / Heart failure / Cerebral hemorrhage → Coma and death.
- Combination of drugs / Drugs + alcohol → Overdosing and deaths.
- Most common warning signs of drug and alcohol abuse among youth:
  (1) Decreasing academic performance.
  (2) Unexplained absence from school/college.
  (3) Loss of interest in relationships with family and friends.
  (4) Loss of interest in hobbies.
  (5) Withdrawal, depression, fatigue, aggressive, isolation and rebellious behavior.
  (6) Lack of interest in personal hygiene.
  (7) Sleeping patterns and eating habits change.
  (8) Fluctuations in weight, appetite, etc.
- If an abuser is short of money to buy drugs or alcohol, he/she may start stealing.
- Family and friends of a drug/alcohol abuser may also undergo mental and financial distress because of him.
- Sharing of infected and syringes among the drug abusers increases the change of acquiring serious infection like AIDS and Hepatitis B.
- Long term or chronic use of drugs and alcohol damages CNS and causes liver cirrhosis.

- Drugs and alcohol also induces adverse effects on the foetus during pregnancy.
- Sportspersons can also misuse certain drugs (like narcotic analgesics, anabolic steroids, diuretics, hormones, etc.) for enhancing their performance by increasing their muscle strength and bulk and to promote aggressiveness.

- **Prevention and Control**
  - **Avoid undue peer pressure:** A child should not be forced to perform beyond his/her threshold limits either in studies, sports or any other activities. Education and counseling of child, seeking professional and medical help from highly qualified psychologists, psychiatrists, de-addiction and rehabilitation programmes for the individuals who have unfortunately addicted to the drugs/alcohol abuse.

# PRACTICE EXERCISES

**Direction:** Read the question carefully and choose the correct option for each.

## Multiple Choice Questions: Level I

### Diseases in Humans

**1.** Disease causing organism are known as
(a) Mutagens (b) Pathogens
(c) Carcinogens (d) Allergens

**2.** Disease which are easily transmitted from one person to another are called
(a) Cancer
(b) Infectious disease
(c) Non-infectious disease
(d) Cardiac disease

**3.** Greeks like Hippocrates and Indian Ayurveda system considered health as ________.
(a) Imbalance of certain 'humors'
(b) Absence of certain 'humors'
(c) Balance of certain 'humors'
(d) Presence of certain 'humors'

**4.** Who discovered blood circulation?
(a) William Harvey (b) Landsteiner
(c) J. F. Watson (d) Edison

**5.** Which device was used by William Harvey to disprove 'good humor' hypothesis of health?
(a) Cardiograph
(b) Sphygmomanometer
(c) Thermometer
(d) Barometer

**6.** Which system of the human body is actually responsible for maintaining health?
(a) Neuronal system (b) Circulatory system
(c) Endocrine system (d) Immune system

**7.** Health is affected by
(a) Genetic disorders (b) Infections
(c) Life style (d) All of these

**8.** A state of complete physical, mental and social well-being is termed as
(a) Disease (b) Comfort
(c) Health (d) Hygiene

**9.** Good health can be maintained by
(a) Balanced diet (b) Personal hygiene
(c) Regular exercise (d) All of these

**10.** Which disease is shown in the figure?

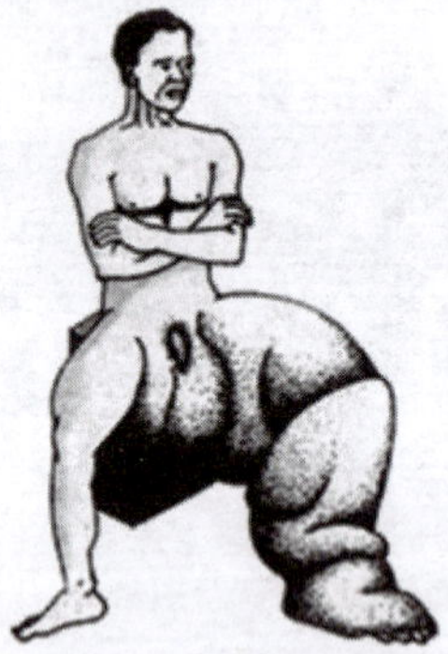

(a) Malaria (b) Kala azar
(c) Filariasis (d) Ascariasis

**11.** Diseases which are transmitted from person to person are called
(a) Non-infectious (b) Genetic
(c) Infectious (d) Deadly

**12.** An infectious disease which is fatal is
(a) Cold
(b) Conjunctivitis
(c) AIDS
(d) Cholera

**13.** Disease causing organisms are known as
(a) Vectors (b) Pathogens
(c) Carriers (d) Parasites

**14.** Typhoid fever in humans is caused by
(a) Rotavirus
(b) *Salmonella typhi*
(c) *Escherichia coli*
(d) Amoeba

**15.** *Salmonella typhi* generally enters which part of the alimentary canal?
(a) Stomach (b) Large intestine
(c) Small intestine (d) Mouth

**16.** S. *typhi* spreads through
(a) Air
(b) Sexual contact
(c) Contaminated food and water
(d) Physical touch

**17.** Sustained high fever (39° to 40° C) and intestinal perforation in severe cases is a symptom of which disease?
(a) Malaria (b) Typhoid
(c) Cholera (d) Common cold

**18.** Which test is performed to confirm typhoid fever?
(a) ELISA test (b) Widal test
(c) Biopsy (d) Schick test

**19.** I was a cook by profession and spread typhoid through the food I used to cook.
(a) Madam Curie (b) Mary Mallon
(c) Rosalind Franklin (d) G. J Mendel

**20.** Pneumonia is caused by
(a) *Streptococcus pneumoniae*
(b) *Pneumococcal pneumonia*
(c) *Haemophilus influenzae*
(d) All of these

**21.** Which part of the lungs is infected in pneumonia?
(a) Alveoli (b) Trachea
(c) Bronchus (d) Terminal bronchioles

**22.** In which disease, lips and fingernails turn grey and in severe cases bluish?
(a) Jaundice (b) Pneumonia
(c) Typhoid (d) Malaria

**23.** Which of the following is not a bacterial disease?
(a) Dysentery (b) Plague
(c) Polio (d) Diphtheria

**24.** Pneumonia is spread by
(a) Inhaling droplets/aerosols
(b) Mosquito
(c) Reusing syringes
(d) Genetic disease

**25.** Common cold is caused by
(a) Tobacco mosaic virus
(b) Rhino virus
(c) Rota virus
(d) Adeno virus

**26.** How is dengue fever transmitted?
(a) Bite of an infected mosquito.
(b) Bite of an infected male Aedes mosquito.
(c) Bite of an infected female Anopheles mosquito.
(d) Bite of an infected female Aedes mosquito.

**27.** Incubation Period refers to
(a) Time between exposure and onset of symptoms.
(b) Time between appearance of symptoms and recovery phase.
(c) Time between exposure and course of illness.
(d) Time between febrile phase and critical phase.

**28.** The following are signs and symptoms manifested by a patient in the Classical phase of Dengue Fever, except:
(a) High fever (b) Rash
(c) Frontal headache (d) Bleeding

**29.** Which mosquito species are primarily responsible for Dengue fever?
(a) Aedes albopictus
(b) Anopheles gambiae
(c) Aedes aegypti mosquito
(d) Culiseta annulated

**30.** Which of the following is a symptom of Dengue?
(a) Fever
(b) Rash
(c) Sever muscle and joint pains
(d) All of the above

**31.** Which of the following are important for dengue prevention?
(a) Using mosquito repellents
(b) Going outside in the evening
(c) Keeping the doors and windows open
(d) All of the above

**32.** Dengue fever is caused by a/an
(a) Bacteria (b) Plasmodium
(c) Virus (d) Fungi

**33.** The vector of 'break bone fever' is
(a) Culex
(b) Aedes
(c) Anopheles
(d) None of the above

**34.** Aedes aegypti is a vector for
(a) Chikungunya
(b) Dengue fever
(c) Japanese encephalitis
(d) Both A and B.

**35.** Which one of the following is not a viral disease?
(a) Dengue (b) AIDS
(c) Typhoid (d) Influenza

**36.** When dengue infection was suspected, which of the following statements regarding the dengue virus is incorrect?
(a) Spreads via ticks
(b) Is prevalent in tropical and subtropical regions of the world
(c) The virus exhibits many antigenic types
(d) Is a member of the Flavivirus family

**37.** The disease chikungunya is transmitted by
(a) House flies (b) Aedes mosquitoes
(c) Cockroach (d) Female Anopheles

**38.** The symptoms of chikun gunya are
(a) Sudden onset of fever
(b) Crippling joint pains
(c) Lymphadenopathy
(d) All of these

**39.** The incubation period for chikungunya is
(a) 1-2 days
(b) 2-4 days
(c) 3-6 days
(d) 6-8 days

**40.** The disease chikungunya is caused by
(a) Bacteria
(b) Protozoan
(c) Virus
(d) None of these

**41.** The most common symptoms in chikungunya are:
(a) Fever with cough
(b) Fever and severe joint pains
(c) Fever with severe stomach ache
(d) Fever with severe diarrhoea and vomiting

**42.** Besides Chikungunya, the Aedes mosquito also spreads:
(a) Dengue
(b) Malaria
(c) Both of the above
(d) None of the above

**43.** In common cold, which part of respiratory system is not infected?
(a) Nose (b) Respiratory passage
(c) Lungs (d) All of these

**44.** What is the one thing that is common between common cold and pneumonia?
(a) Both are caused by same pathogen.
(b) Both are caused by same vector.
(c) Both are caused by droplet infection.
(d) Both are incurable.

**45.** Malaria is caused by which species of plasmodium?
(a) *P. vivax* (b) *P. malaria*
(c) *P. falciparum* (d) All of these

**46.** *Plasmodium* is a
(a) Bacterium (b) Virus
(c) Protozoan (d) Fungi

**47.** The most serious form of malaria, malignant malaria is caused by
(a) *P. falciparum* (b) *P. vivax*
(c) *P. malariae* (d) All of these

**48.** *Plasmodium* enters the human body as ________.
(a) Merozoite (b) Trophozoite
(c) Hypnozoite (d) Sporozoite

**49.** The vector of plasmodium is
(a) Male anopheles mosquito
(b) Female anopheles mosquito
(c) *Aedes aegypti*
(d) Sandworm

**50.** In malaria, fever and chills occur every 3 to 4 days due to rupture of RBCs and release of which toxic substance?
(a) Haemophilia
(b) Hematocrit
(c) Hemozoin
(d) Haemoglobin

**51.** Sporozoites in mosquitoes are stored in
(a) Intestine (b) Mouth
(c) Salivary glands (d) Proboscis

**52** Malarial parasites require two hosts. They are
(a) Humans, female anopheles mosquito
(b) Humans, *Aedes Egypti*
(c) Cattle, female *anopheles* mosquito
(d) Cattle, *Aedes Egypti*

**53.** After the injection of sporozoites in the blood of humans, which organ do they travel initially?
(a) Lymph nodes (b) Brain
(c) Lungs (d) Liver

**54.** The plasmodium parasite reproduces in liver by ________ and in blood by ________.
(a) Sexual reproduction, asexual reproduction
(b) Asexual reproduction, sexual reproduction
(c) Spore formation, sexual reproduction
(d) Sexual reproduction, spore formation

**55.** *Entamoeba histolytica* causes ________ in humans.
(a) Histolysis (b) Amoebiasis
(c) Catharsis (d) Sporogenesis

**56.** Stool with excess of mucous and blood clots is known as
(a) Diarrhoea
(b) Dysentery
(c) Both (a) and (b)
(d) None of these

**57.** Carrier for amoebiasis is
(a) *Entamoeba histolytica*
(b) Mosquito
(c) House flies
(d) *Plasmodium vivax*

**58.** Ascaris is also known as
(a) Common roundworm
(b) Common whipworm
(c) Common threadworm
(d) Common pinworm

**59.** In humans, ascaris causes
(a) Filariasis (b) Ascites
(c) Ascariasis (d) Malaria

**60.** Symptoms like internal bleeding, muscular pain, fever, anaemia and blockage of intestinal passage occur in which disease?
(a) Typhoid (b) Ascariasis
(c) Malaria (d) Pneumonia

**61.** Contaminated water, vegetables and fruits with eggs of round worm causes
(a) Filariasis (b) Ascariasis
(c) Malaria (d) Pneumonia

**62.** Filariasis is also known as
(a) Ascariasis
(b) Elephantiasis
(c) Ringworm
(d) Amoebiasis

**63.** *Wuchereria* causes which disease in humans?
(a) Amoebiasis (b) Filariasis
(c) Ascariasis (d) Ringworm

**64.** *W. bancrofti* infects which part of the human body?
(a) Blood vessels of upper limbs
(b) Lymph vessels of lower limb
(c) Blood vessels of lower limb
(d) Lymph vessels of upper limb

**65.** Wuchereria causes
(a) Acute inflammation
(b) Chronic inflammation
(c) Bacterial inflammation
(d) Viral inflammation

**66.** Elephantiasis is caused by the bite of
(a) W. malayi (b) Elephants
(c) Female mosquito (d) Male mosquito

**67.** Ringworm is caused by
(a) Round worm (b) Bacteria
(c) Fungi (d) Virus

**68.** Which fungal genera are not responsible for causing ringworm?
(a) Megasporum
(b) Trichophyton
(c) Epidermophyton
(d) None of these

**69.** Which are the main symptoms of ringworm?
(a) Appearance of worms on skin
(b) Appearance of dry scaly lesions
(c) Inflammation of limbs
(d) Fever and chills

**70.** Which factors are necessary for the growth of fungi?
(a) Moisture and sebum
(b) Heat and hair
(c) Body odour
(d) Heat and moisture

**71.** In ringworm which parts of the body are usually affected?
(a) Skin, hair and scalp
(b) Skin, nails and hands
(c) Skin, hair and lips
(d) Skin, nails and scalp

**72.** Combs of individuals infected with ________ can transmit the disease.
(a) Sebborhiasis
(b) Dermatitis
(c) Ringworm
(d) Dandruff

**73.** Ringworms are generally acquired from
(a) Water (b) Air
(c) Soil (d) Food

**74.** The mosquito larvae are fed upon by
(a) Ambrosia (b) Gambusia
(c) Mosquito repellent (d) Turtles

**75.** Dengue is caused by which vector?
(a) *Anopheles* mosquito
(b) *Aedes* mosquito
(c) *Apollo* mosquito
(d) *Plasmodium*

**76.** A deadly disease, small pox has been eradicated through
(a) Antiserum
(b) Vaccination
(c) Cauterisation
(d) Antidote

**77.** Chikungunya is spread by the vector
(a) Fungal spores (b) Housefly
(c) Mosquito (d) Reptiles

**78.** Label a, b, c, and d in the below Figure:

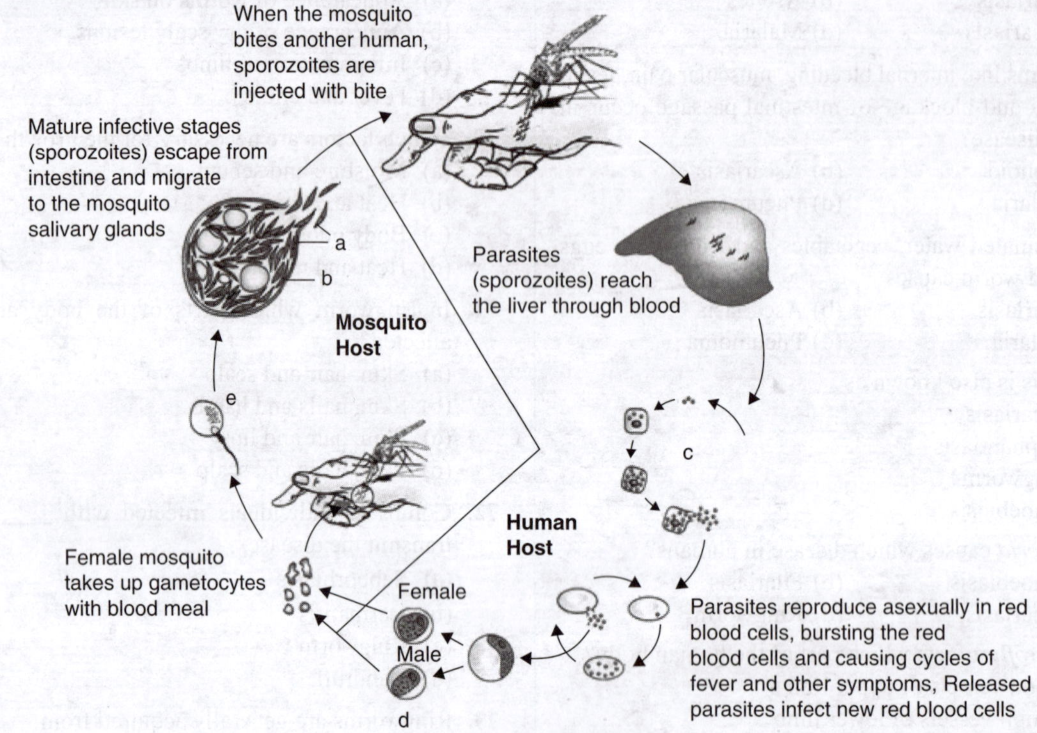


(a) a: Sporozoites, b: salivary gland c: Hepatocytes d: WBC
(b) a: Sporozoites, b: salivary gland c: Hepatocytes d: RBC
(c) a: Hypnozoites, b: salivary gland c: Hepatocytes d: RBC
(d) a: Merozoites, b: salivary gland c: Hepatocytes d: WBC

**79.** Which disease is indicated in the figure ?

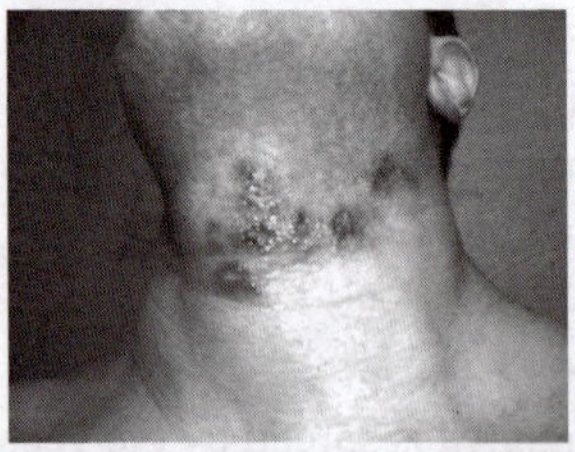

(a) Facial palsy (b) Dermatitis
(c) Ringworm (d) Round worm

**80.** Select the set of correct statements
(A) The discovery of blood circulation was done by William Harvey.
(B) Diseases which are easily transmitted from one person to another, are called infectious diseases.
(C) Drug and alcohol abuse affect the health adversely.
(D) Among non-infectious diseases, AIDS is the major cause of death.
(a) A, B and D (b) A, B and C
(c) B, C and D (d) B and D

**81.** Select set of correct statements:
(A) Disease causing organisms are called pathogens.
(B) Most parasites are pathogens.
(C) Pathogens have to adapt to life within the environment of the host.
(D) The pathogens that enter the gut must know a way of surviving in the stomach at low pH and resisting the various digestive enzymes.
(a) A, B and D (b) A, B and C
(c) B, C and D (d) A, B, C and D

**82.** Select set of correct statements about typhoid:
(A) Salmonella typhi is a pathogenic bacterium which causes typhoid fever in human beings.
(B) These pathogens generally enter the small intestine through contaminated air
(C) Sustained high fever (39° to 40°C), weakness, stomach pain, constipation, headache and loss of appetite are common symptoms of this disease.
(D) Intestinal perforation and death Are symptoms occuring in severe cases.

(a) A, B and D (b) A, B and C
(c) A, C and D (d) B and D only

**83.** Select set of correct statements about pneumomia:
(A) Haemophilus influenza are responsible for the disease pneumonia
(B) These pathogen infects the Bronchi and trachea of the lungs.
(C) The symptoms of pneumonia include fever, chills, cough and headache.
(D) In severe cases, the lips and finger nails may turn gray to bluish in colour.
(a) A, B and D (b) A, B and C
(c) A, C and D (d) B and D only

**84.** Select set of correct statements about viral diseases:
(A) Rhino viruses cause the most infectious human ailments – the common cold.
(B) They infect the nose and respiratory passage as well as the lungs.
(C) The common cold is characterised by nasal congestion and discharge, sore throat, hoarseness, cough, headache, tiredness, etc.
(D) Droplets resulting from an infected person are either inhaled directly or transmitted through contaminated objects and cause infection in a healthy person.
(a) A, C and D (b) A, B and C
(c) B, C and D (d) B and D only

**85.** Select set of incorrect statements about malaria:
(A) Plasmodium enters the human body as infectious form called sporozoin
(B) The parasites initially multiply within the RBCs and then attack the liver cells, resulting in their rupture.
(C) The bite of infected male Anopheles mosquito causes entry of pathogen in human
(D) Haemozoin is responsible for the chill and high fever recurring every three to four days.
(a) A, B and D (b) A, B and C
(c) B, C and D (d) B and D only

**86.** Read following sentences.
Statement I: The malarial parasites multiply within mosquitoes to form sporozoites that are stored in their intestine.
Statement II: In malaria, the female Anopheles mosquito acts as the vector as well as transmitting agent.
(a) Statement I is incorrect but statement II is true.
(b) Both Statements I and II are true
(c) Both Statements I and II are false
(d) Statement I is correct but statement II is false

**87.** Select set of correct statements about malaria:
(A) When infected mosquito bite a human, sporozoites are injected with bite.
(B) The parasite reproduces sexually in liver cells and result in its bursting.
(C) Sexual stages .i.e., gametocytes develop in red blood cells in human.
(D) Fertilization and development take place in gut of mosquito.
(a) A, B and D
(b) A, B and C
(c) A, C and D
(d) B and D only

**88.** Select set of correct statements about amoebiasis:
(A) Entamoeba histolytica is a bacterial parasite in the large intestine of human
(B) Symptoms of this disease include constipation, abdominal pain and cramps, stools with excess mucous and blood clots.
(C) Mosquitoes act as mechanical carriers for the disease.
(D) Drinking water and food contaminated by the faecal matter are the main source of infection.
(a) B and D (b) A and C
(c) B, C and D (d) C and D

**89.** **Assertion:** Houseflies act as mechanical carriers in amoebiasis.
**Reason:** Houseflies transmit the parasite from faeces of infected person to food.
(a) (A) is false but (R) is true
(b) Both (A) and (R) are true and (R) is the correct explanation of (A)
(c) Both (A) and (R) are true but (R) is not the correct explanation of (A)
(d) (A) is true but (R) is false.

**90.** Read following sentences.
**Statement I:** Ascaris, the filarial worm and Wuchereria, the common round worm, are pathogenic to man.
**Statement II:** In both ascariasis and filariasis, the pathogens are transmitted to a healthy person through the bite by the female mosquito vectors.
(a) Statement I is incorrect but statement II is true.
(b) Both Statements I and II are true
(c) Both Statements I and II are false
(d) Statement I is correct but statement II is false

**91.** Select set of correct statements about ringworm:
(A) Genera Microsporum, Trichophyton and Epidermophyton are responsible for ringworms.
(B) Appearance of dry, scaly lesions on skin, nails and scalp is observed

(C) Ringworms are generally acquired from soil or by using towels, clothes, comb of infected individuals.
(D) Cold and dryness help these fungi to grow.
(a) A, B and D (b) A, B and C
(c) B, C and D (d) B and D only

**92.** Read following sentences.
**Statement I:** Typhoid, amoebiasis and ascariasis are food and water borne diseases.
**Statement II:** pneumoniA and Common cold are air-borne diseases.
(a) Statement I is incorrect but statement II is true.
(b) Both Statements I and II are true
(c) Both Statements I and II are false
(d) Statement I is correct but statement II is false

**93.** The diseases in which mosquitoes act as vector are
(A) Malaria (B) elephantiasis
(C) dengue (D) chikungunya
(a) A, B and D (b) A, B and C
(c) B, C and D (d) A, B, C and D

**94.** Which of the following are bacterial diseases?
(A) pneumonia (B) Dysentery
(C) plague (D) diphtheria
(E) common cold (F) malaria
(a) A, B, D and F (b) A, B, C and D
(c) B, C, E and F (d) A, C, D and E

## Immunity

**95.** Label a, b and c in the given figure:

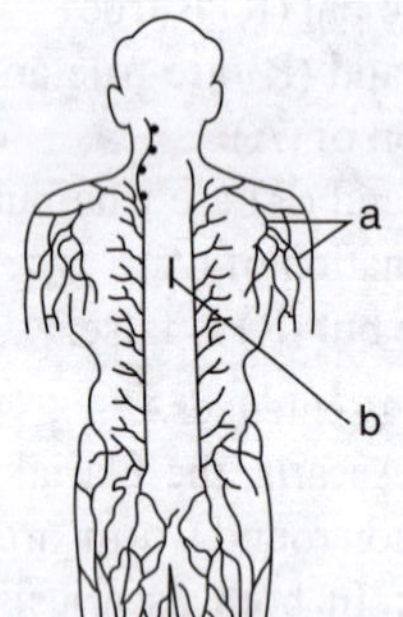


(a) a: Lymph node b: Thymus c: Lymph vessels
(b) a: Lymph node b: Lymph vessels c: Thymus
(c) a: Lymph vessels b: Thymus c: Lymph node
(d) a: Thymus b: Lymph node c: Lymph vessels

**96.** Every day our body is exposed to a large number of infectious agents. But all are not capable of causing disease. This is due to
(a) Decreased virulence of pathogen
(b) Immunity of an individual
(c) Genotype of an individual
(d) Lifestyle of an individual

**97.** Innate immunity is a _______ type of defense mechanism.
(a) Specific (b) Non-specific
(c) Congenital (d) Both (b) and (c)

**98.** Skin and mucus is which type of barrier under innate immunity?
(a) Physiological (b) Morphological
(c) Physical (d) Cellular

**99.** Saliva in mouth and tears from eye protects from microbial infection. This type of barrier is known as
(a) Cellular (b) Physical
(c) Physiological (d) Cytokine

**100.** Which of the following is not a cellular barrier of innate immunity?
(a) PMNL-Neutrophils (b) Monocytes
(c) Lymphocytes (d) Thrombocytes

**101.** Virus infected cells secrete a protein called _______ to protect other non-infected cells.
(a) Cytokine (b) Immunoglobulin
(c) Interferon (d) Clotting factors

**102.** Acquired immunity is
(a) Pathogen specific (b) Pathogen non-specific
(c) Congenital (d) Non-effective

**103.** Acquired immunity has which of the following features?
(a) Non-specific (b) Memory
(c) Anti-cancer (d) Congenital

**104.** When a pathogen comes in contact with body for the first time, it causes a _______ response of low intensity.
(a) Anamnestic (b) Anaphylactic
(c) Primary (d) Secondary

**105.** Given below is a diagrammatic sketch an Antibody, select the correct names of a, b, and c.

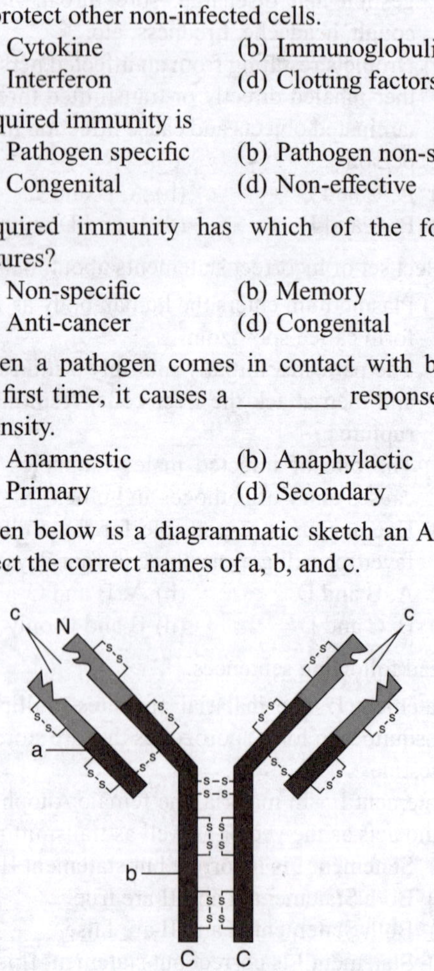

(a) a: Heavy Chain b: Light chain c: Antigen binding site
(b) a: Light Chain b: heavy chain c: Antigen binding site
(c) a: Light Chain b: heavy chain c: Antibody binding site
(d) a: Heavy Chain b: heavy chain c: Antibody binding site

**106.** If a pathogen gains access to the body the second time then a highly intensified response called ______ may occur.
(a) Analgesia (b) Anamnestic
(c) Anthropologic (d) Arthus reaction

**107.** The army of proteins produced by B-lymphocytes is called
(a) Antigen (b) Interferons
(c) Cytokines (d) Antibodies

**108.** The two types of lymphocytes responsible for immune response are
(a) A-type (b) B-type
(c) T-type (d) Both (b) and (c)

**109.** The immunity conferred by B-lymphocytes is also known as
(a) Immediate (b) Histological
(c) Humoral (d) Cell-mediate

**110.** Which lymphocytes help B-cells to secrete antibodies?
(a) Nature killer (b) Macrophages
(c) T-cells (d) Monocytes

**111.** An antibody has ______ heavy chains and ______ light chains respectively.
(a) 2, 4 (b) 4, 2 (c) 2, 2 (d) 1, 2

**112.** An antibody is represented as
(a) $H_1L_2$ (b) $H_2L_2$ (c) $H_4L_1$ (d) $H_4L_4$

**113.** Select the correct option
(a) Ig A, Ig G, Ig E, Ig D, Ig I
(b) Ig G, Ig A, Ig G, Ig H, Ig J
(c) Ig A, Ig G, Ig E, Ig D, Ig M
(d) Ig M, Ig A, Ig E, Ig I, Ig G

**114.** The chains of antibodies are held together by
(a) Dihydrogen (b) Covalent
(c) Disulfide (d) Ionic

**115.** The immunity conferred by T-lymphocyte is known as
(a) Humoral mediated (b) Tissue mediated
(c) Cell mediated (d) Neurally mediated

**116.** After any graft/transplant which medications does a patient have to take all his/her life?
(a) Immunomodulators
(b) Immunosuppressants
(c) Immuno Competors
(d) Immuno depressants

**117.** Before any graft/organ transplant, which procedure should be performed?
(a) Tissue matching (b) Pedigree analysis
(c) CT scan (d) X-ray

**118.** Which immune response makes graft rejection obvious?
(a) Humoral mediated (b) Innate immunity
(c) Cell mediated (d) Acquired immunity

**119.** Which immunity is slow and takes time for full effective response?
(a) Active (b) Passive
(c) Acquired (d) Innate

**120.** When a host is exposed to antigens, antibodies are produced in the host body. This type of immunity is known as ______.
(a) Passive (b) Active
(c) Innate (d) Cell mediated

**121.** Active immunity is induced by
(a) Injecting prepared antibodies
(b) Injecting live infectious microbes
(c) Injecting medicine
(d) Injecting vaccine

**122.** When readymade antibodies are given to protect the body against foreign agents, it is called ______ immunity.
(a) Passive (b) Active
(c) Innate (d) Humoral

**123.** In initial days of lactation, the mother's milk 'Colostrum' is rich in which antibody?
(a) Ig A (b) Ig E (c) Ig M (d) Ig G

**124.** Foetus receives ______ from mother through the placenta during pregnancy.
(a) Antigens (b) Antibodies
(c) T-cells (d) B-cells

**125.** Principle of ______ is based on the property of 'memory' of the immune system.
(a) Passive immunity (b) Antigen antibody
(c) Immunization (d) Agglutination

**126.** Immunization is also known as
(a) Passive immunity (b) Innate immunity
(c) Vaccination (d) Resistance

**127.** A vaccine is
(a) Prepared antigenic proteins
(b) Inactivated/weakened pathogen
(c) Live pathogens
(d) Both (a) and (b)

**128.** When a quick immune response is required, we can
(a) Directly inject weakened pathogen at times of emergency.
(b) Directly inject preformed antigens.
(c) Directly inject preformed antibodies.
(d) Directly inject immunosuppressants.

**129.** In Tetanus case we inject
(a) Antigenic proteins (b) Antibodies
(c) Weakened pathogen (d) Saline

**130.** When a person is bitten by snake, we inject antitoxin in the patient. This type of immunity is known as
(a) Active immunization
(b) Passive immunization
(c) Innate immunization
(d) Humoral immunity

**131.** Antigenic polypeptides of pathogen has been produced on a large scale. This is due to ________ technology.
(a) Polymerase chain reaction
(b) DNA fingerprinting
(c) Recombinant DNA technology
(d) In vitro fertilization

**132.** By using recombinant DNA technology, hepatitis B vaccine is produced from ________.
(a) Bacteria (b) Yeast
(c) Fungi (d) Lichen

**133.** A sudden episode of sneezing-wheezing when you travel to a new place is due to ________ response.
(a) Inflammation
(b) Allergic
(c) Autoimmune
(d) Cell mediated immunity

**134.** Substances which cause allergy are known as
(a) Mutagens (b) Irritants
(c) Allergens (d) Agglutinogens

**135.** The antibodies primarily participating in allergic response are
(a) IgA (b) IgE (c) IgG (d) IgM

**136.** Which of the following is an allergen?
(a) Dust (b) Pollen
(c) Animal dander (d) All the above

**137.** Which of the following is not an allergic reaction symptom?
(a) Sneezing
(b) Watery eyes
(c) Difficulty in breathing
(d) Hiccups

**138.** Which cells actively participate in allergic reaction?
(a) Mast cell (b) Monocytes
(c) Lymphocytes (d) macrophages

**139.** In an allergic reaction, which chemicals are released by the mast cells?
(a) Histamine and serotonin
(b) Histamine and secretin
(c) Serotonin and adrenalin
(d) Serotonin and Noradrenaline

**140.** In case of allergy, which drugs reduce the symptoms?
(a) Antihistamine (b) Adrenaline
(c) Steroids (d) All the above

**141.** In autoimmune disorders, the cells
(a) Produce more antibodies
(b) Produce less antibodies
(c) Start attacking other body cells
(d) Have exaggerated immune response

**142.** An example of autoimmune disease is
(a) Tetanus (b) Allergy
(c) Rheumatoid arthritis (d) Asthma

**143.** Which of the following is a primary lymphoid organ?
(a) Thymus (b) Spleen
(c) Tonsils (d) Lymph nodes

**144.** Immature lymphocytes differentiate in
(a) Liver and Spleen
(b) Bone morrow and Thyroid
(c) Thymus and Bone marrow
(d) Spleen and Thymus

**145.** Which of the following is a secondary lymphoid organ?
(a) Brunner glands (b) Peyer's patches
(c) Crypts of lieberkuhn (d) Glisson's capsule

**146.** Which structure of the lymph system keeps degenerating from birth to puberty?
(a) Spleen (b) Tonsils
(c) Peyer's patches (d) Thymus

**147.** The spleen is
(a) Butterfly shaped (b) Bean shaped
(c) Button shaped (d) Wedge shaped

**148.** Thymus is responsible for maturation of which cells?
(a) Tendons (b) B-cells
(c) T-cells (d) Mast cells

**149.** Which organ act as filter of the blood by trapping blood borne microorganisms?
(a) Spleen (b) Liver
(c) Tonsils (d) Bone marrow

**150.** Respiratory, digestive and urogenital tract has a lining of mucus along with lymph. This lining is known as
(a) Mucosa associated tissue
(b) Mucosa assisted lymphoid tissue
(c) Mucosa associated lymphoid tissue
(d) Mucosa assisted tissue

**151.** In the context of lymphoid tissue, MALT constitutes about ________ of all the lymphoid tissue in human body.
(a) 25% (b) 60% (c) 50% (d) 90%

**152.** Select set of incorrect statements:
(A) Innate immunity is specific type of defence
(B) Mucus coating of the epithelium lining the gastrointestinal tracts is a Physiological barriers
(C) Virus-infected cells secrete proteins called immunoglobulins
(D) interferons protect non-infected cells from further bacterial infection.
(a) A, B and D (b) A, B and C
(c) B, C And D (d) A, B, C and D

**Direction for Q153–154:** Choose the correct option:
(a) Statement I is incorrect but statement II is true.
(b) Both Statements I and II are true
(c) Both Statements I and II are false
(d) Statement I is correct but statement II is false

**153.** Read following sentences.
**Statement I:** Skin on human body is the main Physical barrier of immunity.
**Statement II:** Mucus coating of the epithelium lining the respiratory tract is Physiological barrier of immunity

**154.** Read following sentences.
**Statement I:** Acid in the stomach, saliva in the mouth, tears from eyes prevent microbial growth.
**Statement II:** Virus-infected cells secrete proteins called interferons which protect non-infected cells from further viral infection.

**Direction for Q155–157:** Choose the correct option:
(a) (A) is false but (R) is true
(b) Both (A) and (R) are true and (R) is the correct explanation of (A)
(c) Both (A) and (R) are true but (R) is not the correct explanation of (A)
(d) (A) is true but (R) is false.

**155. Assertion:** the immune response by antibodies is called as humoral immune response.
**Reason:** antibodies are found in the blood.

**156. Assertion:** Subsequent encounter with the same pathogen elicits a highly intensified secondary or anamnestic response in human body.
**Reason:** Human body appears to have memory of the first encounter.

**157. Assertion:** Tissue matching is essential before any transplant and patient has to take immuno–suppresants all its life.
**Reason:** The body is able to differentiate 'self ' and 'nonself' and the cell-mediated immune response is responsible for the graft rejection.

**Direction for Q158–159:** Choose the correct option:
(a) Statement I is incorrect but statement II is true.
(b) Both Statements I and II are true
(c) Both Statements I and II are false
(d) Statement I is correct but statement II is false

**158.** Read following sentences.
**Statement I:** Immunization confers passive immunity.
**Statement II:** Immunization stimulates the body's immune system to produce memory cells.

**159.** Read following sentences.
**Statement I:** Autoimmune diseases occur when the immune system fails to recognize self-antigens.
**Statement II:** Rheumatoid arthritis is an example of an autoimmune disease.

**Direction for Q160–161:** Choose the correct option:
(a) (A) is false but (R) is true
(b) Both (A) and (R) are true and (R) is the correct explanation of (A)
(c) Both (A) and (R) are true but (R) is not the correct explanation of (A)
(d) (A) is true but (R) is false.

**160. Assertion (A):** Immunization provides long-term protection against specific pathogens.
**Reason (R):** Immunization stimulates the production of memory cells by the immune system.

**161. Assertion:** mother's milk is considered very essential for the newborn infant.
**Reason:** The yellowish fluid colostrum secreted by mother during the initial days of lactation has abundant IgG antibodies to protect the infant.

**162.** Consider the following statements regarding the immune system:
(A) The immune system consists of innate and adaptive immunity.
(B) Innate immunity is non-specific and provides immediate defense against pathogens.

(C) Adaptive immunity involves the production of antibodies by B cells.
(D) T cells are involved in both innate and adaptive immunity.

Select set of correct statements:

(a) A, B and D (b) A, B and C
(c) B, C and D (d) B and D only

**163.** Select the correct statements regarding antibodies:
(A) Antibodies are proteins produced by T cells in response to antigen stimulation.
(B) Antibodies neutralize pathogens by binding to them and preventing their interaction with host cells.
(C) Each antibody molecule has two small light chains and four longer heavy chains.
(D) Antibodies are specific to a particular antigen and provide long-term immunity.
(a) A, B and D (b) A, B and C
(c) B, C and D (d) B and D only

**164.** Consider the following statements about vaccinations:
(A) Vaccinations involve the administration of weakened or killed pathogens to induce immunity.
(B) Vaccinations stimulate the production of memory cells for long-term immunity.
(C) The injection containing preformed antibodies is categorised under passive immunisation.
(D) Vaccinations are effective only against bacterial infections.

Select set of correct statements:

(a) A, B and D (b) A, B and C
(c) B, C and D (d) A, B, C and D

**165.** Select the correct statements
(A) The exaggerated response of the immune system to certain antigens present in the environment is called allergy.
(B) The antibodies produced in allergies are of IgA type.
(C) Allergy is due to the release of chemicals like histamine and serotonin from the mast cells.
(D) The use of drugs like adrenalin and steroids quickly reduce the symptoms of allergy.
(a) B and D only (b) A and C only
(c) A, C and D only (d) C and D only

**166.** Consider the following statements regarding lymphoid organs and tissues:
(A) Bone marrow and thymus are primary lymphoid organs involved in the differentiation and maturation of lymphocytes.
(B) Lymph nodes serve to trap microorganisms or antigens from the lymph and tissue fluid.
(C) Mucosa-associated lymphoid tissue (MALT) constitutes about 50% of the lymphoid tissue in the human body and is located within the lining of major tracts.
(D) The spleen acts as a filter of the blood by trapping blood-borne microorganisms and contains a large reservoir of leukocytes.

Select set of correct statements:

(a) A, B and D (b) A, B and C
(c) B, C and D (d) A, B, C and D

**167.** Which of the following statements about lymphoid organs and tissues are incorrect?
(A) The thymus is a lobed organ located near the liver.
(B) Lymph nodes are large bean-shaped organs mainly containing erythrocytes.
(C) Spleen acts as a reservoir of phagocytes.
(D) Bone marrow is the main lymphoid organ involved in the production of all blood cells, including lymphocytes.
(a) A, B and D (b) A, B and C
(c) B, C and D (d) A, B, C and D

**168.** Consider the following statements regarding lymphoid organs and tissues:
(A) Secondary lymphoid organs provide sites for the interaction of lymphocytes with antigens, leading to their proliferation into effector cells.
(B) The thymus keeps reducing in size after birth and eventually disappears by the time puberty is attained.
(C) Lymph nodes are solid structures located at various points along the circulatory system and primarily contain erythrocytes.
(D) Mucosa-associated lymphoid tissue (MALT) is found within the lining of major tracts like the respiratory, digestive, and urogenital tracts.

Select set of incorrect statements:

(a) B and D (b) A and C
(c) B, C and D (d) b and c

**169.** Select the correct statements regarding lymphoid organs and tissues:
(A) Bone marrow is responsible for the production of erythrocytes but not lymphocytes.
(B) spleen, lymph nodes, tonsils, Peyer's patches of small intestine and appendix are secondary lymphoid organs
(C) Lymphoid organs are the organs where origin, maturation and proliferation of lymphocytes occur.

(D) MALT is located within the lining of the respiratory, digestive and urogenital tracts and constitutes 20% of the lymphoid tissue in the human body.
(a) B and D (b) A and C
(c) B, C and D (d) b and c

## AIDS

**170.** Label a, b and c in the given figure:

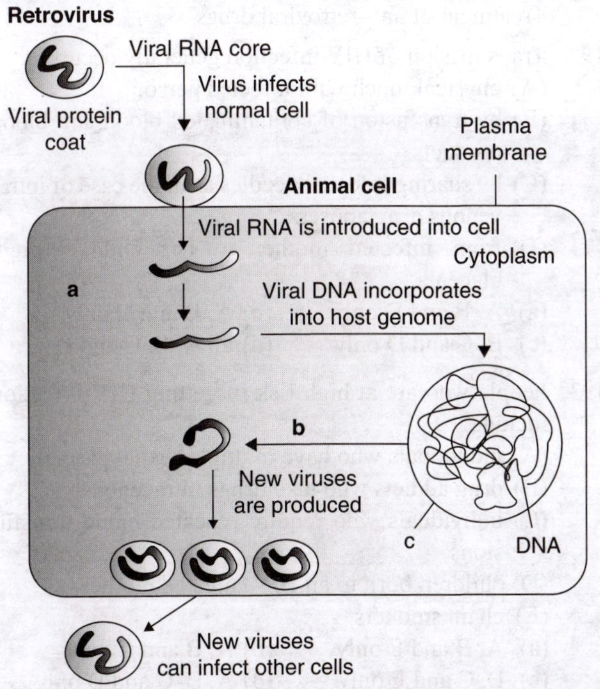


(a) a: Viral DNA produced by Reverse transcriptase., b: New Viral RNA , c: Nucleus
(b) a: Viral RNA produced by Reverse transcriptase., b: New Viral DNA , c: infected cell survives
(c) a: Viral DNA produced by Reverse transcriptase., b: New Viral DNA , c: infected cell survives
(d) a: Viral RNA produced by Reverse transcriptase., b: New Viral RNA , c: infected cell survives

**171.** A group of symptoms is known as
(a) Infection (b) Syndrome
(c) Disease (d) Collection

**172.** AIDS was first reported in the year ________.
(a) 1971 (b) 1981
(c) 1991 (d) 1960

**173.** The death toll due to AIDS has crossed ________ globally.
(a) 2.5 billion (b) 2500 million
(c) 25 million (d) 250 million

**174.** AIDS is caused due to
(a) HIV (b) DNA virus
(c) TMV (d) Bacteriophage

**175.** HIV belongs to a group of viruses known as
(a) Inverto virus (b) Retro virus
(c) Metro virus (d) Flavo virus

**176.** Retro virus causing AIDS has which kind of genome?
(a) DNA (b) RNA
(c) mRNA (d) Proteins

**177.** Which of the following is not a means of transmission of AIDS?
(a) Sexual contact with uninfected person
(b) Transfusion of contaminated blood
(c) Sharing infected needles
(d) Child born to an HIV infected mother

**178.** Time lag between infection and appearance of AIDS symptoms can be few months to ________ years.
(a) 2 to 3 (b) 5 to 10
(c) >15 (d) 1 to 2

**179.** Retro virus contains an enzyme to carry out biochemical activities in host. Name the enzyme.
(a) Polymerase
(b) Exonuclease
(c) Reverse transcriptase
(d) Ligase

**180.** The virus responsible for causing AIDS primarily infects?
(a) Monocytes (b) Mast cells
(c) Macrophages (d) Mucosal cells

**181.** HIV enters which T-cells?
(a) Helper ($T_H$) (b) Promoter ($T_P$)
(c) Suppressor ($T_S$) (d) Cytotoxic ($T_C$)

**182.** Death in AIDS is due to
(a) Aggravated immune response
(b) Due to opportunistic infections
(c) Due to inflammation of genitilia
(d) Due to diarrhoea and fever

**183.** AIDS can be detected by which diagnostic test?
(a) Widal (b) ELISA
(c) SGPT (d) Blood cell count

**184.** The organization in India which is spreading awareness and educating people regarding AIDS is
(a) Gramin Yojna
(b) Health Ministry
(c) National AIDS Control Organization
(d) None of these

**185.** NGO stands for
(a) Non Governing Organization
(b) Non Governmental Organization
(c) Non Guaranteed Object
(d) Non Granted Organization

**Direction for Q186–189:** Choose the correct option:

(a) (A) is false but (R) is true
(b) Both (A) and (R) are true and (R) is the correct explanation of (A)
(c) Both (A) and (R) are true but (R) is not the correct explanation of (A)
(d) (A) is true but (R) is false.

**186. Assertion:** HIV enters macrophages and helper T-lymphocytes, leading to a decrease in the number of helper T-lymphocytes in the body.
**Reason:** The virus replicates inside macrophages and helper T-lymphocytes, producing progeny viruses that attack other helper T-lymphocytes, ultimately leading to immunodeficiency in the infected person.

**187. Assertion:** The decrease in the number of helper T-lymphocytes in AIDS patients leads to immunodeficiency.
**Reason:** HIV infects helper T-lymphocytes and replicates inside them, leading to the destruction of these immune cells and compromising the body's ability to defend against infections.

**188. Assertion:** AIDS stands for Aggregated Immuno Deficiency Syndrome.
**Reason:** In AIDS, deficiency of immune system is gained during the lifetime of an individual and it is a group of symptoms.

**189. Assertion:** the HIV infected person starts suffering from infections that could have been otherwise overcome such as those due to bacteria especially Mycobacterium, viruses, fungi and even parasites like Toxoplasma.
**Reason:** After getting into the body of the person, the virus enters into macrophages where RNA genome of the virus replicates to form viral DNA.

**Direction for Q190–191:** Choose the correct option:

(a) Statement I is incorrect but statement II is true.
(b) Both Statements I and II are true
(c) Both Statements I and II are false
(d) Statement I is correct but statement II is false

**190.** Read following sentences.
**Statement I:** AIDS is caused by non-enveloped retrovirus enclosing the RNA genome.
**Statement II:** There is always a time-lag between the infection and appearance of AIDS symptoms.

**191.** Read following sentences.
**Statement I:** A widely used diagnostic test for AIDS is PCR.
**Statement II:** AIDS can be completely cured by Treatment of anti-retroviral drugs .

**192.** Transmission of HIV-infection generally occurs by
(A) physical touch with infected person,
(B) by transfusion of contaminated blood and blood products,
(C) by sharing infected needles as in the case of intravenous drug abusers
(D) from infected mother to her child through placenta
(a) A, B and D only (b) A, B and C only
(c) B, C and D only (d) all A, B, C and D

**193.** People who are at high risk of getting HIV infection include
(A) individuals who have multiple sexual partners,
(B) drug addicts who take drugs intravenously,
(C) individuals who require repeated blood transfusions
(D) children born to an HIV infected mother
(E) chain smokers
(a) A, B and E only (b) A, B and C only
(c) B, C and E only (d) A, B, C and D only

## Cancer

**194.** Normal cells in our body inhibit the uncontrolled growth of cells which they are in contact with. This is known as
(a) Cell-cell contact (b) Cell cycle regulation
(c) Contact inhibition (d) Contact response

**195.** Tumour is an abnormal mass of
(a) Muscles
(b) Cells
(c) Inorganic salts
(d) Cartilagenous membrane

**196.** The tumour which does not spread to other parts of body is known as ________.
(a) Benign (b) Malignant
(c) Neoplastic (d) Lymphoma

**197.** The cancerous cells which have the ability to proliferate and cause cancer in new locations of the body are known as
(a) Benign (b) Lymphoma
(c) Leukemia (d) Malignant

**198.** Cancer cells actively divide and grows due to
(a) Competition for vital nutrients with normal cells.
(b) Competition for space with normal cells.
(c) Competition for only support.
(d) Excess food materials stored in body.

**199.** Metastasis is
(a) Normal equilibrium condition of body.
(b) Morphological changes from larva to adult.
(c) Generation of new tumour in different sites of body.
(d) Abnormal growth of the body muscles.

**200.** The agents which can cause neoplastic cell generation are
(a) Gamma rays (b) X-rays
(c) UV rays (d) All of these

**201.** Which radiations can cause cancer?
(a) Visible light (b) UV rays
(c) Infra red light (d) Microwaves

**202.** Cancer causing viruses are known as
(a) Retro virus (b) Oncogenic virus
(c) Flavo virus (d) Adeno virus

**203.** The genes present in normal cells of the body which can cause cancer are known as
(a) Oncogenes (b) Carcinogenes
(c) Neogenes (d) Tumerogenes

**204.** Proto-oncogenes are also abbreviated as
(a) p-onc (b) c-onc
(c) p-con (d) c-con

**205.** Blood and bone marrow tests are usually performed to detect
(a) Anaemia (b) Leukaemia
(c) Thrombocytopenia (d) Filariasis

**206.** In case of ________, a piece of suspected tissue is cut into thin sections, stained and examined under microscope.
(a) Post mortem
(b) Biopsy
(c) DNA fingerprinting
(d) Pedigree analysis

**207.** Cancers of internal organs can be detected by
(a) Radiography (b) CT
(c) MRI (d) All of these

**208.** In which technique 3-D the image of the internals of an objected are generated?
(a) Electron microscopy
(b) Radiography
(c) Computed tomography
(d) Magnetic Resonance Imaging

**209.** MRI uses strong magnetic field and ________ radiations to detect pathological and physiological changes.
(a) Ionizing (b) Non-ionizing
(c) LASER (d) X-ray

**210.** Tobacco smoke primarily causes
(a) Mouth cancer (b) Lung cancer
(c) Breast cancer (d) Bladder cancer

**211.** The common approaches for treatment of cancer are
(a) Surgery (b) Radiation therapy
(c) Immuno therapy (d) All of these

**212.** Anti-cancer drugs have the following side effects
(a) Hair loss (b) Anaemia
(c) Vomiting (d) All of these

**213.** For the treatment of cancer, biological response modifiers such as ________ are given.
(a) β-interferons (b) γ-interferons
(c) α-interferons (d) δ-interferons

**214.** Select set of correct statements:
(A) Carcinogens can be physical, chemical or biological agents.
(B) Ionising radiations like X-rays and gamma rays and non-ionizing radiations like UV cause DNA damage.
(C) The chemical carcinogens present in tobacco smoke have been identified as a major cause of lung cancer.
(D) Cancer causing viruses called oncogenic viruses have genes called viral oncogenes.
(E) Several proto oncogenes in normal cells get activated under certain conditions leading to oncogenic transformation of the cells.
(a) A, B and E (b) A, B, D and E
(c) B, C and D (d) all are correct

**215.** Select set of correct statements:
(A) In biopsy, a piece of the suspected tissue cut into thin sections is stained and examined for histopathological studies by a pathologist.
(B) Techniques like radiography CT and MRI are very useful to detect cancers of the external organs.
(C) Computed tomography uses UV-rays to generate a three-dimensional image of the internals of an object.

(D) MRI uses strong magnetic fields and non-ionising radiations to accurately detect changes in the living tissue.
(a) A, B and D only (b) A, B and C only
(c) B, C and D only (d) A and D only

**216.** The common approaches for treatment of cancer are
(A) surgery
(B) physiotherapy
(C) radiation therapy
(D) immunotherapy
Select set of correct measures:
(a) A, B and D only (b) A, B and C only
(c) A, C and D only (d) C and D only

**217.** Read following sentences.
**Statement I:** Cancer detection is based on biopsy and histopathological studies of the tissue and blood and bone marrow tests.
**Statement II:** The cancer patients are given biological response modifiers such as $\alpha$-interferon which activates their immune system and helps in destroying the tumor.
(a) Statement I is incorrect but statement II is true.
(b) Both Statements I and II are true
(c) Both Statements I and II are false
(d) Statement I is correct but statement II is false

**218. Assertion:** Cancerous cells just continue to divide giving rise to masses of cells called tumors.
**Reason:** Cancer cells appears to have lost the property of contact inhibition.
(a) (A) is false but (R) is true
(b) Both (A) and (R) are true and (R) is the correct explanation of (A)
(c) Both (A) and (R) are true but (R) is not the correct explanation of (A)
(d) (A) is true but (R) is false.

**219. Assertion:** Techniques of molecular biology can be applied to detect genes in individuals with inherited susceptibility to certain cancers.
**Reason:** Identification of such genes, which predispose an individual to certain cancers, may be very helpful in prevention of cancers.
(a) (A) is false but (R) is true
(b) Both (A) and (R) are true and (R) is the correct explanation of (A)
(c) Both (A) and (R) are true but (R) is not the correct explanation of (A)
(d) (A) is true but (R) is false.

**220.** Read following sentences.
Statement I: Normal cells show a property called contact inhibition.
Statement II: By virtue of this property, contact with other cells inhibits their controlled growth.
(a) Statement I is incorrect but statement II is true.
(b) Both Statements I and II are true
(c) Both Statements I and II are false
(d) Statement I is correct but statement II is false

**221. Assertion:** The property called metastasis is the most feared property of malignant tumors.
**Reason:** Cells sloughed from malignant tumors reach distant sites through blood, and wherever they get lodged in the body, they start a new tumor.
(a) (A) is false but (R) is true
(b) Both (A) and (R) are true and (R) is the correct explanation of (A)
(c) Both (A) and (R) are true but (R) is not the correct explanation of (A)
(d) (A) is true but (R) is false.

**222. Assertion:** Benign tumors generally cause little damage.
**Reason:** Benign tumors normally remain confined to their original location and do not spread to other parts of the body.
(a) (A) is false but (R) is true
(b) Both (A) and (R) are true and (R) is the correct explanation of (A)
(c) Both (A) and (R) are true but (R) is not the correct explanation of (A)
(d) (A) is true but (R) is false.

## Drugs and Alcohol Abuse

**223.** What is shown in the figure?

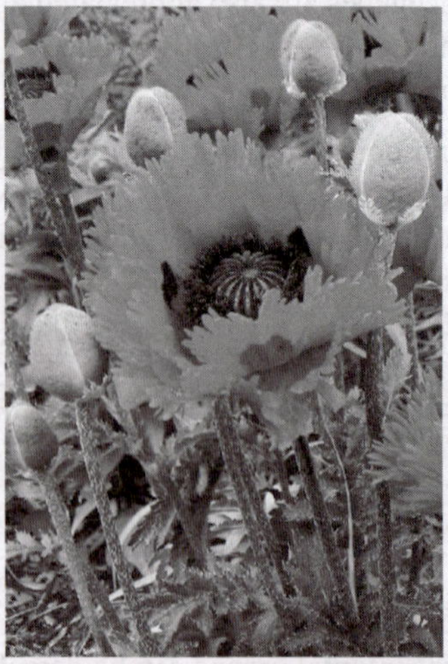

(a) Sunflower plant (b) Poppy plant
(c) Datura plant (d) Tobacco plant

**224.** What is shown in the figure?

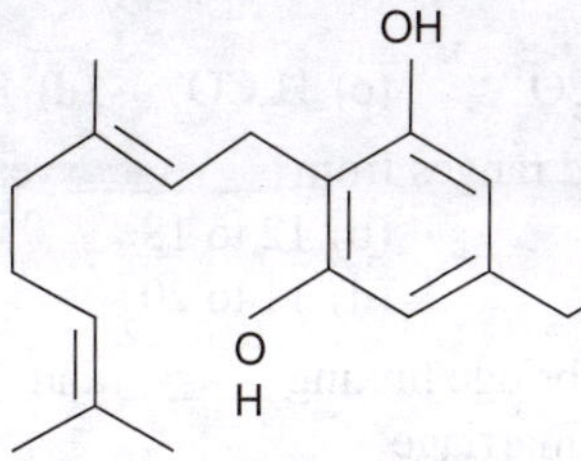


(a) Cannabinoid molecule (b) Morphine
(c) Nicotine (d) Lobeline

**225.** What is shown in the figure?

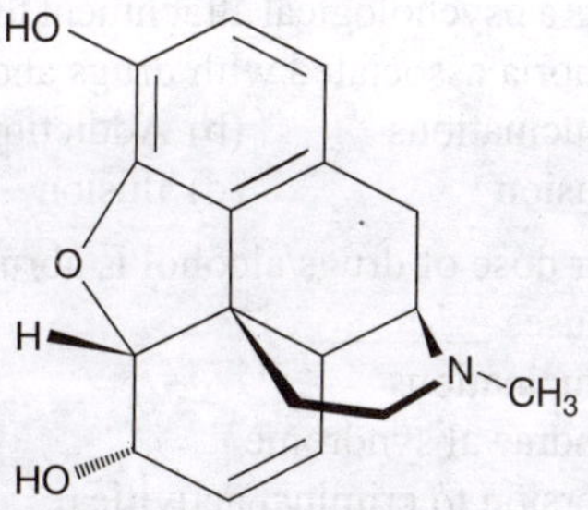


(a) Cannabinoid molecule
(b) Morphine
(c) Nicotine
(d) Lobeline

**226.** Heroine is locally known as ________.
(a) Smack (b) Angel dust
(c) Coke (d) Marijuana

**227.** Smack is chemically
(a) Dicetylmorphine
(b) Diacetylmorphine
(c) Dimethyl morphine
(d) Dihydromorphine

**228.** Morphine is obtained from
(a) Erythroxylum coca
(b) Atropa belladonna
(c) Cannabis sativa
(d) Papaver somniferum

**229.** Heroin is a ______ drug.
(a) Excitatory (b) Depressant
(c) Hallucinogenic (d) Euphoric

**230.** Morphine is extracted from ________ of poppy plant.
(a) Leaf (b) Latex (c) Stem (d) Flower

**231.** Cannabinoids are obtained from ________, ________ and ________ of cannabis sativa.
(a) leaves, flowers, fruits
(b) leaves, flower tops, resin
(c) leaves, flowers, latex
(d) flower, seed, tannins

**232.** What is shown in the figure?

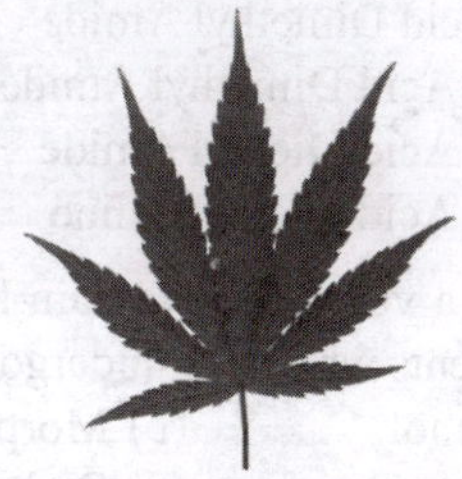

(a) Opium (b) Datura
(c) Cannabis (d) Tobacco

**233.** Cannabinoids are mainly known to affect?
(a) Cardio vascular system
(b) Nervous system
(c) Sensory system
(d) Excretory system

**234.** Charas, ganja, hashish and marijuana are all
(a) Opioids (b) Cannabinoids
(c) Coca alkaloids (d) Barbiturates

**235.** Cocaine is obtained from
(a) *Erythroxylum coca*
(b) *Paper somniferum*
(c) *Atropa belladonna*
(d) *Connalris sativa*

**236.** Coca plant is a native to
(a) North America (b) South America
(c) South Africa (d) Australia

**237.** Cocaine is commonly known as
(a) Smack (b) Coke
(c) Crack (d) Both (b) and (c)

**238.** Cocaine produces a sense of ________.
(a) Euphoria (b) Dysphoria
(c) Depression (d) Androgenic effects

**239.** Excessive dosage of cocaine causes ________.
(a) Cardiovascular collapse
(b) Hallucinations
(c) Nerve damage
(d) Vomiting

**240.** *Atropa belladonna* is
(a) Ornamental plant
(b) Hallucinogenic plant
(c) Immunomodulator plant
(d) Depressant plant

**241.** Generally, cannabinoids are taken
(a) Intravenously
(b) Intramuscularly
(c) Through oral route
(d) Through implants

**242.** LSD is
(a) Lauric Acid Dimethyl Amide
(b) Lysergic Acid Dimethyl Amide
(c) Lysergic Acid Diethyl Amide
(d) Lysergic Acid Diethyl amine

**243.** ________ is a very effective pain-killer and sedative used for patients who have undergone surgery.
(a) Paracetamol (b) Morphine
(c) LSD (d) Barbiturate

**244.** Datura is a ________ plant.
(a) Sedative (b) Hallucinogenic
(c) Excitatory (d) Health tonic

**245.** AIDS do not spread by
(a) Sexual contact
(b) Body fluids
(c) Physical touch
(d) Blood transfusion

**246.** Treatment of AIDS with anti-retro viral drugs is
(a) Not at all effective
(b) Fully effective
(c) Partially effective
(d) Leads to secondary infections

**247.** When plants having hallucinogenic properties are administered in more than required amount/frequency, it causes
(a) Addiction (b) Drug abuse
(c) Cancer (d) Both (a) and (b)

**248.** Barbiturates and Benzodiazepines are used in clinical conditions like
(a) Cancer and its prevention
(b) Euphoria and sense of well-being
(c) Depression and insomnia
(d) Increasing body strength and vigour

**249.** Tobacco has been used by human beings for more than ________ years.
(a) 400 millions (b) 40 millions
(c) 4000 millions (d) 400

**250.** Tobacco contains an alkaloid known as ________.
(a) Morphine (b) Piperine
(c) Nicotine (d) Anabasine

**251.** Nicotine stimulates which gland primarily?
(a) Salivary (b) Pancreas
(c) Spleen (d) Adrenal

**252.** What is the effect of nicotine?
(a) Relieves stress and anxiety
(b) It gives a sense of well-being and happiness
(c) It raises blood pressure and heart rate
(d) It causes excess of acidity

**253.** Smoking increases the content of which compound in blood?
(a) $CO_2$ (b) CO (c) $H_2CO_3$ (d) $H_2O_2$

**254.** Adolescent period ranges from ________ years.
(a) 10 to 16 (b) 12 to 18
(c) 13 to 19 (d) 11 to 20

**255.** Adolescence is a bridge linking ________ and ________.
(a) Teenage and marriage
(b) Childhood and adulthood
(c) Teenage and adulthood
(d) Birth and adulthood

**256.** ________ is a psychological attachment to certain effects like euphoria associated with drugs and alcohol?
(a) Hallucinations (b) Addiction
(c) Delusion (d) Ilusion

**257.** If regular dose of drugs/alcohol is abruptly discontinued it causes ________.
(a) Hallucinations
(b) Withdrawal syndrome
(c) Diversion to criminal activities
(d) Severe depression

**258.** Death in case of overdose of drugs occurs due to
(a) Respiratory failure (b) Heart failure
(c) Cerebral hemorrhage (d) All of these

**259.** Drug abusers can suffer from infections like
(a) Hepatitis (b) Depression
(c) Euphoria (d) Cirrhosis

**260.** Chronic alcoholism damages which vital organ of the body?
(a) Heart (b) Kidney
(c) Liver (d) Brain

**261.** Generally sportsmen abuse which categories of drugs?
(a) Immuno modulators
(b) Anabolic steroids
(c) Cannabinoids
(d) Potent pain killers

**262.** Which categories of drugs are used by sportsmen?
(a) Certain hormones (b) Anabolic steroids
(c) Diuretics (d) All of these

**263.** Liver damage is termed as
(a) Leeching (b) Cirrhosis
(c) Aplasia (d) Haemorrhage

**264.** If females are administered anabolic steroids, which of the following symptoms are observed?
(a) Abnormal menstruation
(b) Excessive hair growth
(c) Enlargement of clitoris
(d) All of these

**265.** The commonly abused drugs are opioids, cannabinoids and coca alkaloids. Most of these are obtained from

(A) algae
(B) fungi
(C) animals
(D) flowering plants

(a) A, B and D (b) A, B and C
(c) B, C and D (d) B and D only

**266.** Read following sentences.
**Statement I:** Heroin commonly called smack is chemically dimethylmorphine
**Statement II:** opioid receptors are present in human central nervous system and blood circulatory tract.

(a) Statement I is incorrect but statement II is true.
(b) Both Statements I and II are true
(c) Both Statements I and II are false
(d) Statement I is correct but statement II is false

**267.** Select set of correct characteristics about morphine:

(A) colourless
(B) odourless
(C) bitter in taste
(D) amorphous compound
(E) obtained by dehydration of morphine
(F) extracted from the latex of poppy plant.

(a) A, C and D (b) A, D and E
(c) B, C and F (d) C and D only

**268.** Select set of correct characteristics about Cannabinoids:

(A) obtained from the fruits of the plant
(B) receptors present in the brain
(C) used to produce marijuana, hashish, charas and ganja
(D) taken intravenously

(a) A, C and D (b) A, B and D
(c) B, C and D (d) B and C only

**269.** Select set of incorrect characteristics about cocaine:

(A) obtained from coffee plant Erythroxylum coca
(B) interferes with the transport of dopamine
(C) commonly called croke
(D) lead to hallucination

(a) A, C and D (b) A, B and C
(c) B, C and D (d) A and C only

**270.** The drugs leading to halluciations are

(A) morphine
(B) cocaine
(C) drug from Datura
(D) drug from Atropa
(E) heroin
(F) barbiturates
(G) amphetamines

Select set of correct ones:

(a) A, B and F (b) A, E and G
(c) B, C and D (d) D and G only

**Direction for Q271–273:** Choose the correct option:

(a) Statement I is incorrect but statement II is true.
(b) Both Statements I and II are true
(c) Both Statements I and II are false
(d) Statement I is correct but statement II is false

**271.** Read following sentences.
**Statement I:** Smoking is associated with increased incidence of cancer, bronchitis, emphysema, coronary heart disease, gastric ulcer.
**Statement II:** Smoking increases carbon dioxide content in blood and reduces the concentration of haembound oxygen.

**272.** Read following sentences.
**Statement I:** The chronic use of drugs and alcohol damages nervous system and liver (cirrhosis).
**Statement II:** In males, the side-effects of the use of anabolic steroids includes acne, increased aggressiveness, mood swings, depression, potential for kidney and liver dysfunction, premature baldness.

**273.** Read following sentences.
**Statement I:** cannabinoid receptors are present in gastrointestinal tract.
**Statement II:** opioid receptors are present in respiratory tract.

**Direction for Q274–275:** Choose the correct option:

(a) (A) is false but (R) is true
(b) Both (A) and (R) are true and (R) is the correct explanation of (A)
(c) Both (A) and (R) are true but (R) is not the correct explanation of (A)
(d) (A) is true but (R) is false.

**274. Assertion:** Continuous cigarette smoking leads to raised blood pressure and increased heart rate.
**Reason:** Nicotine stimulates adrenal gland to release adrenaline and nor-adrenaline into blood circulation.

**275. Assertion:** The people taking drugs intravenously are much more likely to acquire serious infections like AIDS and Hepatitis B.
**Reason:** The viruses, which are responsible for AIDS and Hepatitis B are transferred from one person to another by sharing of infected needles and syringes.

## Multiple Choice Questions: Level II

**276.** A person likely to develop tetanus is immunized by administering
(a) preformed antibodies
(b) wide spectrum antibiotics
(c) weakened germs
(d) dead germs

**277.** The letter T in T-lymphocyte refers to
(a) thalamus
(b) tonsil
(c) thymus
(d) thyroid

**278.** Which of the following is a pair of viral diseases?
(a) common cold, AIDS
(b) dysentery, common cold
(c) typhoid, tuberculosis
(d) ringworm, AIDS

**279.** Which one of the following statements is correct?
(a) benign tumours show the property of metastasis
(b) heroin accelerates body functions
(c) malignant tumours may exhibit metastasis
(d) patients who have undergone surgery are given cannabinoids to relieve pain

**280.** Use of anti-histamines and steroids give a quick relief from
(a) nausea (b) cough
(c) headache (d) allergy

**281.** Cornea transplant in humans is almost never rejected. This is because
(a) it is composed of enucleated cells
(b) it is a non-living layer
(c) its cells are least penetrable by bacteria
(d) it has no blood supply

**282.** Match the disease in column-I with the appropriate i (pathogen/prevention/treatment) in column-II

| Column I | Column II |
|---|---|
| A. Amoebiasis | i. *Treponema pallidum* |
| B. Diphtheria | ii. Use only sterilized food and water |
| C. Cholera | iii. DPT vaccine |
| D. Syphilis | iv. Use oral rehydration therapy |

(a) A - (i), B - (ii), C - (iii), D - (iv)
(b) A - (ii), B - (iii), C - (iv), D - (i)
(c) A - (i), B - (ii), C - (iii), D - (iv)
(d) A - (ii), B - (iv), C - (i), D - (iii)

**283.** To which type of barriers under innate immunity do the saliva in the mouth and the tears from the eyes belong?
(a) Physiological barriers
(b) Physical barriers
(c) Cytokine barriers
(d) Cellular barriers

**284.** Which one of the following is the correct statement regarding psychotropic drug specified?
(a) Morphine leads to delusions and disturbed emotions
(b) Barbiturates cause relaxation and temporary euphoria
(c) Hashish causes after-thought perceptions and hallucinations
(d) Opium stimulates nervous system and causes hallucinations

**285.** If you suspect major deficiency of antibodies in a person to which of the following would you look for confirmatory evidence?
(a) serum globulins (b) fibrinogen in the plasma
(c) haemocytes (d) serum albumins

**286.** Increased asthmatics attacks in certain seasons are related to
(a) eating fruits preserved in tin containers
(b) inhalation of seasonal pollen
(c) low temperature
(d) hot and humid environment

**287.** AIDS is caused by HIV that principally infects
(a) all lymphocytes (b) activator B cells
(c) cytotoxic T cells (d) $T_4$ lymphocytes

**288.** Which one of the following depresses brain activity and produces feelings of calmness, relaxation and drowsiness?
(a) Morphine (b) Valium
(c) Amphetamines (d) Hashish

**289.** Which one of the following is not correctly matched?
(a) *Glossina palpalis* – Sleeping sickness
(b) *Culex pipiens* – Filariasis
(c) *Aedes aegypti* – Yellow fever
(d) *Anopheles culifacies* – Leishmaniasis

**290.** ELISA is used to detect viruses, where
(a) DNA probes are required
(b) Southern blotting is done
(c) Alkaline phosphatase is the key reagent
(d) Catalase is the key reagent

**291.** Short-lived immunity acquired from mother to foetus across placenta or through mother's milk to the infant is categorized as
(a) innate non-specific immunity
(b) active immunity
(c) passive immunity
(d) cellular immunity

**292.** Carcinoma refers to
(a) benign tumours of the connective tissue
(b) malignant tumours of the connective tissue
(c) malignant tumours of the skin or mucous membrane
(d) malignant tumours of the colon

**293.** What is true about T-lymphocytes in mammals?
(a) These are produced in thyroid
(b) There are three main types: cytotoxic T-cells, helper T-cells and suppressor T-cells
(c) These originate in lymphoid tissues
(d) They scavenge damaged cells and cellular debris

**294.** Which one of the following conditions though harmful is also a potential saviour from a mosquito-borne infectious disease?
(a) Leukaemia
(b) Thalassemia
(c) Sickle cell anaemia
(d) Pernicious anaemia

**295.** Cancerous cells can easily be destroyed by radiations due to
(a) rapid cell division
(b) lack of nutrition
(c) fast mutation
(d) lack of oxygen

**296.** L.S.D. is
(a) Hallucinogenic
(b) Sedative
(c) Stimulant
(d) Tranquiliser

**297.** Which one of the following is correctly matched?
(a) Reserpine -Tranquilizer
(b) Cocaine - Opiate narcotic
(c) Morphine - Hallucinogenic
(d) Bhang - Analgesic

**298.** Salmonella is related with
(a) Typhoid (b) Polio
(c) T.B. (d) Tetanus

**299.** Which of the following is the most infectious disease?
(a) Hepatitis-B (b) AIDS
(c) Amoebiosis (d) Malaria

**300.** Small proteins produced by vertebrate cells in response to viral infections inhibiting multiplication are known as
(a) Lipoproteins
(b) Immunoglobulins
(c) Interferons
(d) Antitoxins

**301.** For which of the following disease, there is preventive vaccine?
(a) AIDS (b) Hepatitis B
(c) Syphilis (d) Gonorrhoea

**302.** Vaccines are
(a) treated bacteria or viruses or one of their proteins
(b) MHC (major histocompatibility complex) proteins
(c) curative medicines
(d) monoclonal antibodies

**303.** The cell in the human body invaded by the human immuno-deficiency virus (HIV) is
(a) T-helper cell (b) Erythrocyte
(c) B-cell (d) Macrophage

**304.** It is not possible to apply Koch's postulates to
(a) Diphtheria (b) Cholera
(c) Leprosy (d) Tuberculosis

**305.** During blood typing, agglutination indicates that the
(a) RBC carries certain antigens
(b) Plasma contains certain antigens
(c) RBC carries certain antibodies
(d) Plasma contains certain antibodies

**306.** The gland that regresses with age is
(a) Adrenal (b) Gonad
(c) Thymus (d) Thyroid

**307.** Botulism caused by *Clostridium botulinum* affects the
(a) Intestine
(b) Neuromuscular junction
(c) Spleen
(d) Lymph glands

**308.** Typhoid fever is caused by
(a) Salmonella (b) Shigella
(c) Escherichia (d) Giardia

**309.** Human immuno deficiency virus (HIV) has a protein coat and a genetic material which is
(a) single-stranded DNA
(b) double-stranded DNA
(c) single-stranded RNA
(d) double-stranded RNA

**310.** The use of Cannabis products (bhang, ganja, charas, marijuana or hashish) causes
(a) depression of brain activity and feeling of calmness
(b) alters thoughts, perceptions and feelings
(c) suppresses brain function and relieves pain
(d) stimulates the nervous system and increases alertness and activity

**311.** Which one of the following is an opiate narcotic?
(a) Barbiturates (b) Morphine
(c) Amphetamines (d) LSD

**312.** Which of the following symptoms indicate radiation sickness?
(a) Red and ulcerated skin
(b) Nausea and loss of hair
(c) Nausea and anaemia
(d) Ulcerated skin, nausea, loss of hair and anaemia

**313.** Diphtheria is caused by
(a) poisons released from dead bacterial cells into the host tissue
(b) poisons released by living bacterial cells into the host tissue
(c) excessive immune response by the host's body
(d) poisons released by virus into the host tissues

**314.** Which one of the following diseases is now considered nearly eradicated from India?
(a) Plague
(b) Kala azar
(c) Small pox
(d) Poliomyelitis

**315.** If a certain person shows production of interferons in his body, the chances are that he has got an infection of
(a) typhoid (b) measles
(c) malaria (d) tetanus

**316.** Which one thing is not true about antibiotics?
(a) The term 'antibiotic' was coined by Selman Waksman in 1942.
(b) First antibiotic was discovered by Alexander Fleming.
(c) Each antibiotic is effective only against one particular kind of germ.
(d) Some persons can be allergic to a particular antibiotic.

**317.** Which one of the following is an Indian medicinal plant?
(a) *Saccharum officinarum*
(b) *Rauwolfia serpentina*
(c) *Oryza sativa*
(d) *Solanum melongena*

**318.** Hypersensitivity to an allergen is associated with
(a) aberrant functioning of the immune mechanism
(b) increase in ambient temperature
(c) age of the individual
(d) food habits

**319.** In which one of the following pairs of diseases are caused by viruses?
(a) Tetanus and typhoid
(b) Whooping cough and sleeping sickness
(c) Syphilis and AIDS
(d) Measles and rabies

**320.** Retroviruses are implicated as a cause for cancer in humans, because they
(a) carry gene for reverse transcriptase
(b) may carry cellular proto-oncogenes in their genome
(c) may carry v-oncogenes in their genome
(d) carry single-stranded RNA as their genetic material

**321.** Passive immunity was discovered by
(a) Edward Jenner (b) Emil von Behring
(c) Robert Koch (d) Louis Pasteur

**322.** Chemically an antibody is a
(a) lipid (b) nucleoprotein
(c) protein (d) lipoprotein

**323.** According to the 'immunity theory' of ageing, the process starts with the gradual atrophy and disappearance of
(a) thyroid (b) parathyroid
(c) thymus (d) islets of Langerhans

**324.** Which of the following pair is not correctly matched?
(a) dengue fever – arbovirus
(b) plague – *Yersinia pestis*
(c) syphilis – *Trichuris trichiura*
(d) malaria – *Plasmodium vivax*

**325.** Which of the following diseases is due to an allergic reaction?
(a) goitre (b) skin cancer
(c) hay fever (d) enteric fever

**326.** A cell-coded protein formed in response to infection with most animal viruses is
(a) Antigen (b) Antibody
(c) Interferon (d) Histone

**327.** Obstacle to large-scale transplantation of organs is
(a) Insufficiency of organ donors
(b) Immunological rejection of foreign bodies
(c) Religious or ethnic considerations
(d) Lack of effective surgical techniques

**328.** Which one of the sexually transmitted diseases is correctly matched with its pathogen?
(a) Urethritis – Bacillus anthracis
(b) Syphilis – Treponema pallidum
(c) Gonorrhoea – Entamoeba histolytica
(d) Soft sore – Bacillus brevis

**329.** A sexually transmitted disease caused by bacteria is
(a) Leprosy (b) AIDS
(c) Syphilis (d) Pertussis

**330.** Sarcoma is cancer of
(a) Epithelial tissue
(b) Mesodermal tissues
(c) Blood
(d) Endodermal tissues

**331.** Cells involved in immune mechanism are
(a) Erythrocytes
(b) Lymphocytes
(c) Eosinophils
(d) Thrombocytes

**332.** Opiate narcotic is
(a) Bhang
(b) Charas
(c) Heroin
(d) Nicotine

**333.** Give the correct matching of causative agent/germ and disease
(a) Anopheles – malaria
(b) Leishmania – Sleeping sickness
(c) Glossina – Kala-azar
(d) Wuchereria – Filariasis

**334.** Schizont stage of Plasmodium occurs in human cells
(a) Erythrocytes
(b) Liver cell
(c) Erythrocytes and liver cells
(d) Erythrocytes, liver cells and spleen cells

**335.** The part of life cycle of malarial parasite Plasmodium vivax that is passed in female Anopheles is
(a) Sexual cycle
(b) Pre-erythrocytic schizogony
(c) Exo-erythrocytic schizogony
(d) Post-erythrocytic schizogony

**336.** Who discovered Plasmodium in RBC of human beings?
(a) Ronald Ross (b) Mendel
(c) Laveran (d) Stephens

**337.** Malignant tertian malaria parasite is
(a) Plasmodium falciparum
(b) P. vivax
(c) P.ovale
(d) P.malariae

**338.** In hot summer and cold winter, the number of malaria cases as well as Anopheles declines, reappearance of malaria in humid warm conditions is due to
(a) Surviving malarial parasites in human carriers.
(b) Surviving sporozoites in surviving mosquitoes.
(c) Monkeys
(d) Mosquito larvae in permanent waters.

**339.** Malaria fever coincides with liberation of
(a) Cryptomerozoites
(b) Metacryptomerozoites
(c) Merozoites
(d) Trophozoites

**340.** The infective stage of malarial parasite Plasmodium that enters human body is
(a) Merozoite (b) Sporozoite
(c) Trophozoite (d) Minute form

**341.** Lysozyme that is present in perspiration and tears destroys
(a) Certain types of bacteria
(b) All viruses
(c) Most virus-infected cells
(d) Certain fungi

**342.** Antibodies in our body are complex
(a) steroids (b) prostaglandins
(c) glycoproteins (d) lipoproteins

# A & R and Statement-based Questions

## Assertion and Reason Questions

***Direction for questions 343 to 347:** Read the **assertion** and **reason** carefully to mark the correct option out of the options given below:*

(a) **(A)** is **true** but **(R)** is **false**.
(b) **(A)** is **false** but **(R)** is **true**.
(c) Both **(A)** and **(R)** is **true** and **(R)** is the correct explanation of **(A)**.
(d) Both **(A)** and **(R)** is **true** and **(R)** is not the correct explanation of **(A)**.

**343. Assertion:** Chills and high fever occur in malaria infected patient.
**Reason:** Hemozoin released from ruptured RBCs.

**344. Assertion:** Disease caused by viruses are generally non-infectious.
**Reason:** Cancer is major cause of death among non-infectious diseases.

**345. Assertion:** Saliva in mouth is physiological barrier.
**Reason:** Epithelial line GIT is cellular barrier.

**346. Assertion:** Morphine is given to patient undergone surgery.
**Reason:** Morphine is potent pain killer and sedative.

**347. Assertion:** Colostrum is source of passive immunity.
**Reason:** Colostrum contain antibodies.

## Statement-based Questions:

***Direction for questions 348 to 352:** These type of questions consist of two statement each, printed as **Statement-I** and **Statement-II**. While answering such questions, a student is needed to choose any one of the following four responses.*

(a) **Statement I** is **correct Statement II** is **incorrect**.
(b) **Statement I** is **incorrect Statement II** is **correct**.
(c) Both **Statement I** and **Statement II** are **correct**.
(d) Both **Statement I** and **Statement II** are **incorrect**.

**348. Statement-I:** MALT forms 50% of the lymphoid tissue in human body.
**Statement-II:** AIDS is caused by retrovirus.

**349. Statement-I:** Alpha interferon is biological response modifier.
**Statement-II:** It is used to treat cancer.

**350. Statement-I:** Crack is usually snorted.
**Statement-II:** Coke is hallucinogenic in high dosage.

**351. Statement-I:** Exaggerated immune response to certain antigen is allergy.
**Statement-II:** Adrenalin is use to reduce symptoms of allergy.

**352. Statement-I:** Addiction is physiological attachment.
**Statement-II:** Dependence is the tendency of the body to show withdrawal syndrome if regular doses of drug is abruptly discontinued.

# Matrix-Match Type Questions

**353.** Match the following:

| I (Organism) | II (Disease Caused) | III (Organ Affected) |
|---|---|---|
| 1. Bacteria | (i) Malaria | X. Respiratory passage |
| 2. Virus | (ii) Typhoid | Y. Liver & RBCs |
| 3. Protozoa | (iii) Common cold | Z. Small intestine |

**The correct matching is**

(a) 1 – (ii) – Z, 2 – (iii) – X, 3 – (i) – Y
(b) 1 – (i) – Z, 2 – (iii) – X, 3 – (ii) – Y
(c) 1 – (iii) – Z, 2 – (ii) – X, 3 – (i) – Y
(d) 1 – (ii) – Z, 2 – (i) – X, 3 – (iii) – Y

**354.** Match the following:

| List-I | List-II |
|---|---|
| 1. *H. influenzae* | (i) Malaria |
| 2. *Rhino virus* | (ii) Pneumonia |
| 3. *P. falciparum* | (iii) Common cold |
| 4. *E. histolytica* | (iv) Amoebiasis |

**The correct matching is**

| | 1 | 2 | 3 | 4 |
|---|---|---|---|---|
| (a) | (ii) | (iii) | (i) | (iv) |
| (b) | (iii) | (iv) | (i) | (ii) |
| (c) | (ii) | (iv) | (iii) | (i) |
| (d) | (iii) | (i) | (ii) | (iv) |

**355.** Match the following:

| I (Organism) | II (Vector) | III (Disease) |
|---|---|---|
| 1. *P. falciparum* | (i) Houseflies | X. Elephantiasis |
| 2. *E. histolytica* | (ii) Mosquitoes | Y. Malaria |
| 3. *W. malayi* | | Z. Amoebiasis |

**The correct matching is**

(a) 1 – (ii) – Y, 2 – (i) – Z, 3 – (ii) – X
(b) 1 – (i) – X, 2 – (ii) – Z, 3 – (ii) – Y
(c) 1 – (ii) – Z, 2 – (i) – X, 3 – (ii) – Y
(d) 1 – (ii) – X, 2 – (i) – Y, 3 – (ii) – Z

**356.** Match the following:

| I (Organism) | II (Vector) | III (Disease) |
|---|---|---|
| A. Worm | 1. *Ascaris* | (i) Amoebiasis |
| B. Protozoa | 2. *Wuchereria* | (ii) Typhoid |
| C. Virus | 3. *E. histolytica* | (iii) Ringworms |
| D. Bacteria | 4. *Rhino* | (iv) Elephantiasis |
| E. Fungi | 5. *P. falciparum* | (v) Ascariasis |
| | 6. *Salmonella* | (vi) Common cold |
| | 7. *S. pneumonia* | (vii) Pneumonia |
| | 8. *Microsporum* | (viii) Malaria |
| | 9. *Trichophyton* | |
| | 10. *Epidermophyton* | |

(a) 1 – A – (v), 2 – A – (iv), 3 – B – (i), 4 – C – (vi), 5 – B – (viii), 6 – D – (ii), 7 – D – (vii), 8 – E – (iii), 9 – E – (iii), 10 – E – (iii)
(b) 1 – A – (v), 2 – A – (iv), 3 – C – (vi), 4 – B – (i), 5 – B – (vii), 6 – D – (vii), 7 – D – (ii), 8 – E – (iii), 9 – E – (iii), 10 – E – (iii)
(c) 1 – A – (iv), 2 – A – (v), 3 – B – (i), 4 – B – (vi), 5 – C – (vii), 6 – D – (ii), 7 – D – (iii), 8 – E – (vii), 9 – E – (iii), 10 – E – (iii)
(d) 1 – B – (i), 2 – A – (iv), 3 – A – (v), 4 – C – (vi), 5 – B – (ii), 6 – D – (vii), 7 – D – (vii), 8 – E – (iii), 9 – E – (iii), 10 – E – (iii)

(Note: Any 4 of these can be used for a question.)

**357.** Match the following:

| List-I (Disease Transmitted Through) | List-II (Disease) |
|---|---|
| 1. Food & water borne | (i) Typhoid |
| 2. Air borne | (ii) Pneumonia |
| 3. Insect vector | (iii) Elephantiasis |
| | (iv) Amoebiasis |
| | (v) Common cold |
| | (vi) Malaria |
| | (vii) Ascariasis |

**The correct matching is**

| | 1 | 2 | 3 |
|---|---|---|---|
| (a) | (i),(ii),(vii) | (iv),(iii) | (v),(vi) |
| (b) | (i),(iv),(vii) | (ii),(v) | (iii),(vi) |
| (c) | (i),(ii),(iv) | (iii),(vi) | (v),(vii) |
| (d) | (i),(vi),(iv) | (ii),(iii) | (v),(vii) |

## NCERT Exemplar Questions

**1.** The term 'Health' is defined in many ways. The most accurate definition of the term health would be
(a) Health is the state of body and mind in a balanced condition.
(b) Health is the reflection of a smiling face.
(c) Health is a state of complete physical, mental and social well-being.
(d) Health is the symbol of economic prosperity.

**2.** The organisms which cause diseases in plants and animals are called
(a) Pathogens (b) Vectors
(c) Insects (d) Worms

**3.** The clinical test that is used for diagnosis of typhoid is
(a) ELISA (b) ESR
(c) PCR (d) Widal

**4.** Diseases are broadly grouped into infectious and non-infectious diseases. In the list given below, identify the infectious diseases.
i. Cancer
ii. Influenza
iii. Allergy
iv. Small pox
(a) i and ii (b) ii and iii
(c) iii and iv (d) ii and iv

**5.** The sporozoites that cause infection, when a female *Anopheles* mosquito bites a person are formed in
(a) Liver of person
(b) RBCs of mosquito
(c) Salivary glands of mosquito
(d) Gut of mosquito

6. The disease chikungunya is transmitted by
(a) House fly (b) *Aedes* mosquito
(c) Cockroach (d) Female *Anopheles*

7. Many diseases can be diagnosed by observing the symptoms in the patient. Which group of symptoms are indicative of pneumonia?
(a) Difficulty in respiration, fever, chills, cough, headache.
(b) Constipation, abdominal pain, cramps, blood clots.
(c) Nasal congestion and discharge, cough, constipation, headache.
(d) High fever, weakness, stomach pain, loss of appetite and constipation.

8. Cancer causing genes are called
(a) Structural genes
(b) Expressor genes
(c) Oncogenes
(d) Regulatory genes

9. In malignant tumours, the cells proliferate, grow rapidly and move to other parts of the body to form new tumours. This stage of disease is called
(a) Metagenesis (b) Metastasis
(c) Teratogenesis (d) Mitosis

10. When an apparently healthy person is diagnosed as unhealthy by a psychiatrist, the reason could be that
(a) The patient was not efficient at his work.
(b) The patient was not economically prosperous.
(c) The patient shows behavioural and social maladjustment.
(d) He does not take interest in sports

11. Which of the following are the reason(s) for Rheumatoid arthritis? Choose the correct option.
i. The ability to differentiate pathogens or foreign molecules from self-cells increases.
ii. Body attacks self-cells.
iii. More antibodies are produced in the body.
iv. The ability to differentiate pathogens or foreign molecules from self-cells is lost.
(a) i and ii (b) ii and iv
(c) iii and iv (d) i and iii

12. AIDS is caused by HIV. Among the following, which one is not a mode of transmission of HIV?
(a) Transfusion of contaminated blood
(b) Sharing the infected needles
(c) Shaking hands with infected persons
(d) Sexual contact with infected persons

13. 'Smack' is a drug obtained from the
(a) Latex of *Papaver somniferum*
(b) Leaves of *Cannabis sativa*
(c) Flowers of *Datura*
(d) Fruits of *Erythroxylum coca*

14. The substance produced by a cell in viral infection that can protect other cells from further infection is
(a) Serotonin
(b) Colostrum
(c) Interferon
(d) Histamine

15. Transplantation of tissues/organs to save certain patients often fails due to the rejection of such tissues/organs by the patient. Which type of immune response is responsible for such rejections?
(a) Auto-immune response
(b) Humoral immune response
(c) Physiological immune response
(d) Cell-mediated immune response

16. Antibodies present in colostrum which protect the new born from certain diseases is of
(a) Ig G type (b) Ig A type
(c) Ig D type (d) Ig E type

17. Tobacco consumption is known to stimulate the secretion of adrenaline and nor-adrenaline. The component causing this could be
(a) Nicotine
(b) Tannic acid
(c) Curamin
(d) Catechin

18. Antivenom against snake poison contains
(a) Antigens
(b) Antigen-antibody complexes
(c) Antibodies
(d) Enzymes

19. Which of the following is not a lymphoid tissue?
(a) Spleen (b) Tonsils
(c) Pancreas (d) Thymus

20. Which of the following glands is large sized at birth but reduces in size with ageing?
(a) Pineal (b) Pituitary
(c) Thymus (d) Thyroid

21. Hemozoin is a
(a) Precursor of haemoglobin.
(b) Toxin released from *Streptococcus* infected cells.
(c) Toxin released from *Plasmodium* infected cells.
(d) Toxin released from *Haemophilus* infected cells.

22. Which of the following is not the causal organism for ringworm?
(a) *Microsporum*
(b) *Trichophyton*
(c) *Epidermophyton*
(d) *Macrosporum*

23. A person with sickle cell anaemia is
(a) More prone to malaria
(b) More prone to typhoid
(c) Less prone to malaria
(d) Less prone to typhoid

## Previous Years' Questions

1. Consider the following four statements (1–4) regarding kidney transplant and select the two correct ones out of these. [AIPMT 2010 PRE]
(A) Even if a kidney transplant is proper, the recipient may need to take immune suppressants for a long time
(B) The cell-mediated immune response is responsible for the graft rejection
(C) The B-lymphocytes are responsible for rejection of graft
(D) The acceptance of rejection of a kidney transplant depends on specific interferons
The two correct statements are
(a) (b) and (c)
(b) (c) and (d)
(c) (a) and (c)
(d) (a) and (b)

2. Which one of the following statements is correct with respect to AIDS? [AIPMT 2010 PRE]
(a) HIV can be transmitted through eating food together with an infected person.
(b) Drug addicts are least susceptible to HIV infection.
(c) AIDS patients are being fully cured with proper care and nutrition.
(d) The causative HIV retrovirus enters helper T-lymphocytes thus reducing their numbers.

3. Widal test is used for diagnosis of: [AIPMT 2010 PRE]
(a) Malaria
(b) Pneumonia
(c) Tuberculosis
(d) Typhoid

4. Ringworm in humans is caused by [AIPMT 2010 PRE]
(a) Bacteria
(b) Fungi
(c) Nematodes
(d) Viruses

5. Select the correct statement from the ones given below [AIPMT 2010 PRE]
(a) Barbiturates when given to criminals make them tell the truth.
(b) Morphine is often given to persons who have undergone surgery, as a pain killer.
(c) Chewing tobacco lowers blood pressure and heart rate.
(d) Cocaine is given to patients after surgery as it stimulates recovery.

6. A person suffering from a disease caused by Plasmodium experiences recurring chill and fever at the time when? [AIPMT 2010 MAINS]
(a) The sporozoites released from RBCs are being rapidly killed and broken down inside the spleen.
(b) The trophozoites reach maximum growth and give out certain toxins.
(c) The parasite after its rapid multiplication inside RBCs ruptures them, releasing the stage to enter fresh RBCs.
(d) The microgametocytes and megagametocytes are being destroyed by the WBCs.

7. Which one of the following techniques is safest for detection of cancers? [AIPMT 2010 MAINS]
(a) Magnetic resonance imaging (MRI)
(b) Radiography (X-ray)
(c) Computed tomography (CT)
(d) Histopathological studies

8. Fastest distribution of some injectable material/medicine and with no risk of any kind can be achieved by injecting it into the [AIPMT 2010 MAINS]
(a) Muscles
(b) Arteries
(c) Veins
(d) Lymph vessels

9. Select the correct statement with respect to diseases and immunization. [AIPMT 2011 MAINS]
(a) If due to some reason B and T lymphocytes are damaged, the body will not produce antibodies against a pathogen.
(b) Injection of dead/inactivated pathogens causes passive immunity.
(c) Certain protozoans have been used in mass production of hepatitis B vaccine.
(d) Injection of snake antivenom against snake bite is an example of active immunization.

**10.** Common cold is not cured by antibiotics, because it is [AIPMT 2011 MAINS]
(a) caused by a virus
(b) caused by a gram-positive bacterium
(c) caused by a gram-negative bacterium
(d) not an infectious disease

**11.** Which one of the following options gives the correct matching of a disease with its causative organism and mode of infection? (A: Typhoid, B: Causative organism, C: Mode of infection) [AIPMT 2011 MAINS]
(a) A: Typhoid, B: *Salmonella typhi*, C: With inspired air
(b) A: Pneumonia, B: *Streptococcus pneumonia*, C: Droplet infection
(c) A: Elephantiasis, B: *Wuchereria bancrofti*, C: With infected water and food
(d) A: Malaria, B: *Plasmodium vivax*, C: Bite of male Anopheles mosquito

**12.** The pathogen Microsporum responsible for ringworm disease in humans belongs to the same kingdom of organisms as that of [AIPMT 2011 MAINS]
(a) Taenia, a tapeworm
(b) Wuchereria, a filarial worm
(c) Rhizopus, a mould
(d) Ascaris, a round worm

**13.** Common cold is not cured by antibiotics because it is [AIPMT 2011 MAINS]
(a) Caused by a virus.
(b) Caused by a gram-positive bacterium.
(c) Caused by a gram-negative bacterium.
(d) Not an infectious disease.

**14.** Where will you look for the sporozoites of the malarial parasite? [AIPMT 2011 PRE]
(a) Red blood corpuscles of humans suffering from malaria
(b) Spleen of infected humans
(c) Salivary glands of freshly moulted female anopheles mosquito
(d) Saliva of infected female Anopheles Mosquito

**15.** Which one of the following acts as a physiological barrier to the entry of microorganisms in human body? [AIPMT 2011 PRE]
(a) Tears
(b) Monocytes
(c) Skin
(d) Epithelium of urogenital tract

**16.** At which stage of HIV infection does one usually shows symptoms of AIDS? [AIPMT 2011 PRE]
(a) When viral DNA is produced by reverse transcriptase.
(b) When HIV replicates rapidly in helper T-lymphocytes and damages large number of these.
(c) With 15 days of sexual contact with an infected person.
(d) When the infecting retrovirus enters host cells.

**17.** A certain patient is suspected to be suffering from acquired immunodeficiency syndrome. Which diagnostic technique will you recommend for its detection? [AIPMT 2011 PRE]
(a) MRI (b) Ultra sound
(c) WIDAL (d) ELISA

**18.** In which one of the following options the two examples are correctly matched particular type of immunity? [AIPMT 2012 PRE]

| Examples | Type of immunity |
|---|---|
| (a) Polymorpho nuclear leukocytes and monocytes | Cellular barriers |
| (b) Anti-tetanus and anti-snake bite injections | Active immunity |
| (c) Saliva in mouth and tears in eyes | Physical barriers |
| (d) Mucus coating of epithelium lining the urinogenital tract and the HCl in stomach | Physiological barriers |

**19.** Cirrhosis of liver is caused by chronic intake of: [AIPMT 2012 PRE]
(a) Opium
(b) Alcohol
(c) Tobacco (chewing)
(d) Cocaine

**20.** Which one of the following in not a property of cancerous cells, whereas the remaining three are? [AIPMT 2012 PRE]
(a) They compete with normal cells for vital nutrients
(b) They do not remain confined in the area of formation
(c) They divide in an uncontrolled manner
(d) They show contact inhibition

**21.** Common cold differs from pneumonia, in that: [AIPMT 2012 PRE]

(a) pneumonia is a communicable disease, whereas the common cold is a nutritional deficiency disease.
(b) pneumonia can be prevented by a live attenuated bacterial vaccine, whereas common cold has no effective vaccine.
(c) pneumonia is caused by a virus, while common cold is caused by the bacterium Haemophilus influenza.
(d) pneumonia pathogen infects alveoli, whereas common cold affects nose and respiratory passage but not the lungs.

**22.** Widal test is carried out to test: [AIPMT 2012 PRE]
(a) Malaria
(b) Diabetes mellitus
(c) HIV/AIDS
(d) Typhoid fever

**23.** Motile zygote of *Plasmodium* occurs in: [AIPMT 2012 PRE]
(a) Gut of female Anopheles
(b) Salivary glands of Anopheles
(c) Human RBCs
(d) Human liver

**24.** Which one of the following statements is correct with respect to immunity? [AIPMT 2012 MAINS]
(a) The antibodies against small pox pathogen are produced by T-lymphocytes.
(b) Antibodies are protein molecules each of which has four light chains.
(c) Rejection of a kidney graft is the function of B-lymphocytes.
(d) Preformed antibodies need to be injected to treat the bite by a viper snake.

**25.** Which one of the following organisms is scientifically correctly named, correctly printed according to the International rules of nomenclature and correctly described? [AIPMT 2012 MAINS]
(a) *Plasmodium falciparum* – a protozoan pathogen causing the most serious type of malaria
(b) *Felis tigris* – The Indian tiger, well protected in Gir forests
(c) *E.Coli* – Full name Entamoeba coli, a commonly occurring bacterium in human intestine
(d) *Musca domestica* – The common house lizards, a reptile

**26.** Identify the molecules (a) and (b) shown below and select the right option giving their source and use. [AIPMT 2012 MAINS]

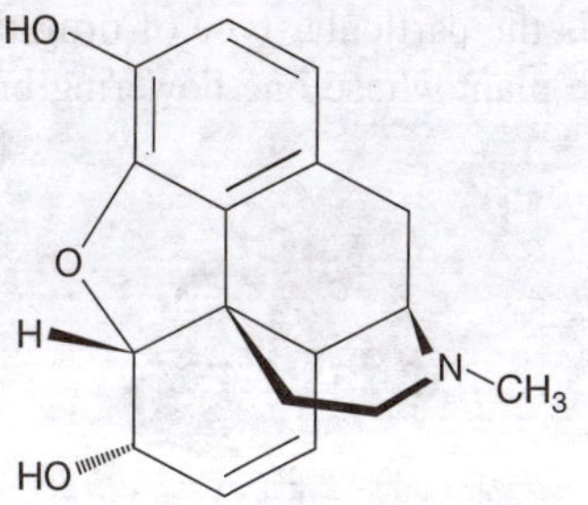

(a)

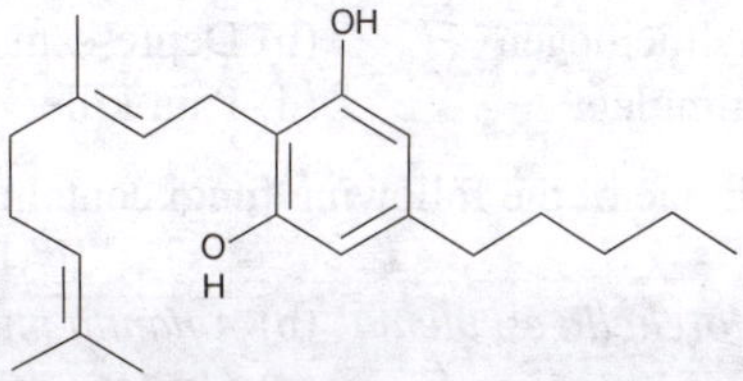

(b)

**Options:**

| Molecule | Source | Use |
|---|---|---|
| (a) (b) Heroin | Cannabis sativa | Depressant and slows down body functions |
| (b) (b) Cannabinoid | Atropa belladonna | Produces hallucinations |
| (c) (a) Morphine | Papaver somniferum | Sedative and pain killer |
| (d) (a) Cocaine | Erythroxylum coca | Accelerates the transport of dopamine |

**27.** The cell-mediated immunity inside the human body is carried out by? [AIPMT 2013]
(a) T-lymphocytes (b) B-lymphocytes
(c) Thrombocytes (d) Erythrocytes

**28.** Infection of Ascaris usually occurs by: [AIPMT 2013]
(a) Drinking water containing eggs of Ascaris
(b) Eating imperfectly cooked pork
(c) Tse-tse fly
(d) Mosquito bite

**29.** At which stage of HIV infection does one usually show symptoms of AIDS? [AIPMT 2014]
(a) Within 15 days of sexual contact with an infected person
(b) When the infected retro virus enters host cells
(c) When HIV damages large number of helper T-Lymphocytes
(d) When the viral DNA is produced by reverse transcriptase

**30.** Which is the particular type of drug that is obtained from the plant whose one flowering branch is shown below? [AIPMT 2014]

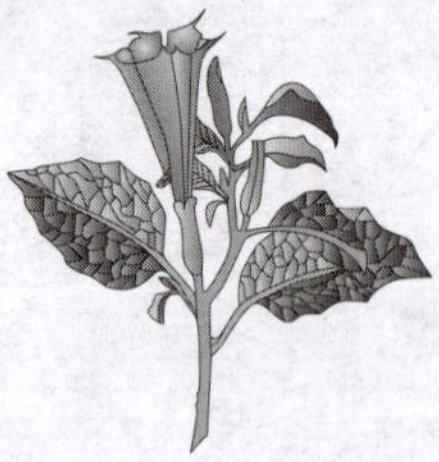

(a) Hallucinogen (b) Depressant
(c) Stimulant (d) Pain-killer

**31.** Which one of the following fungi contains hallucinogens? [AIPMT 2014]
(a) *Morchella esculenta* (b) *Amanita muscaria*
(c) *Neurospora sp.* (d) *Ustilago sp.*

**32.** Grafted kidney may be rejected in a patient due to [RE-AIPMT 2015]
(a) Cell-mediated immune response
(b) Passive immune response
(c) Innate immune response
(d) Humoral immune response

**33.** If you suspect major deficiency of antibodies in a person, to which of the following would you look for confirmatory evidence? [RE-AIPMT 2015]
(a) Serum albumins (b) Haemocytes
(c) Serum globulins (d) Fibrinogen in plasma

**34.** Which of the following immunoglobulins constitute the largest percentage in human milk? [RE-AIPMT 2015]
(a) Ig M (b) Ig A
(c) Ig G (d) Ig D

**35.** The active form of *Entamoeba histolytica* feeds upon: [AIPMT 2015]
(a) Erythrocytes, mucosa and submucosa of colon
(b) Mucosa and submucosa colon only
(c) food in intestine
(d) blood only

**36.** HIV that causes AIDS first starts destroying: [AIPMT 2015]
(a) B-Lymphocytes
(b) Leucocytes
(c) Helper T-Lymphocytes
(d) Thrombocytes

**37.** Match each disease with its correct type of vaccine: [AIPMT 2015]

| | |
|---|---|
| (a) tuberculosis | (1) harmless virus |
| (b) whooping cough | (2) inactivated toxin |
| (c) diphtheria | (3) killed bacteria |
| (d) polio | (4) harmless bacteria |

(a) A:2, B:1, C:3, D:4 (b) A:3, B:2, C:4, D:1
(c) A:4, B:3, C:2, D:1 (d) A:1, B:2, C:4, D:2

**38.** Which of the following endoparasites of humans show viviparity? [AIPMT 2015]
(a) *Ancylostoma duodenale*
(b) *Enterobius vermicularis*
(c) *Trichinella spiralis*
(d) *Ascaris lumbricoides*

**39.** Which of the following sets of disease is caused by bacteria? [NEET 2016 – PHASE II]
(a) Typhoid and smallpox
(b) Tetanus and mumps
(c) Herpes and influenza
(d) Cholera and tetanus

**40.** Which of the following is correct regarding AIDS causative agent HIV? [NEET 2016 – PHASE II]
(a) HIV is enveloped virus that contains two identical molecules of single-stranded RNA and two molecules of reverse transcriptase
(b) HIV is unenveloped retrovirus
(c) HIV does not escape but attacks the acquired immune response
(d) HIV is enveloped virus containing one molecule of single-stranded RNA and one molecule of reverse transcriptase

**41.** Which of the following statements is not true for cancer cells in relation to mutations? [NEET 2016 – PHASE I]
(a) Mutations in proto-oncogenes accelerate the cell cycle
(b) Mutations destroy telomerase inhibitor
(c) Mutations inactivate the cell control
(d) Mutations inhibit production of telomerase

**42.** Antivenom injection contains preformed antibodies while polio drops that are administered into the body contain [NEET 2016 – PHASE I]
(a) Activate pathogens
(b) Harvested antibodies
(c) Gamma globulin
(d) Attenuated pathogens

**43.** In higher vertebrates, the immune system can distinguish self-cells and non-self. If this property is lost due to genetic abnormality and it attacks self-cells, then it leads to: [NEET 2016 – PHASE I]
(a) Allergic response (b) Graft rejection
(c) Auto-immune disease (d) Active immunity

**44.** Asthma may be attributed by: [NEET 2016 – PHASE I]
(a) Bacterial infection of the lungs
(b) Allergic reaction of the mast cells in the lungs
(c) Inflammation of the trachea
(d) Accumulation of fluid in the lungs

**45.** Which of the following statements is correct? [NEET Regional 2017]
(a) AIDS is caused by a group of viruses called rhinovirus.
(b) Acquired immunity is pathogen specific.
(c) The exaggerated response of the immune system to certain antigens present in the environment is called Auto-immunity.
(d) Bone marrow acts as a filter of the blood by trapping blood-borne micro-organisms.

**46.** Match List–I with List–II and select the correct option. [NEET Regional 2017]

| List–I | | List–II | |
|---|---|---|---|
| (A) | *Plasmodium* | (i) | Ringworm |
| (B) | *Wuchereria* | (ii) | Amoebiasis |
| (C) | *Entamoeba* | (iii) | Elephantiasis |
| (D) | *Microsporum* | (iv) | Malaria |

| | (A) | (B) | (C) | (D) |
|---|---|---|---|---|
| (a) | (iv) | (iii) | (ii) | (i) |
| (b) | (iv) | (i) | (ii) | (iii) |
| (c) | (iv) | (iii) | (i) | (ii) |
| (d) | (i) | (iii) | (ii) | (iv) |

**47.** Transplantation of tissues/organs fails often due to non-acceptance by the patient's body. Which type of immune is responsible for such rejections? [NEET 2017]
(a) Cell-mediated immune response
(b) Hormonal immune response
(c) Physiological immune response
(d) Autoimmune response

**48.** MALT constitutes about ______ present of the lymphoid tissue in human body. [NEET 2017]
(a) 20% (b) 70%
(c) 10% (d) 50%

**49.** Which of the following is not an autoimmune disease? [NEET 2018]
(a) Psoriasis (b) Alzheimer's disease
(c) Rheumatoid arthritis (d) Vitiligo

**50.** In which disease does mosquito-transmitted pathogens cause chronic inflammation of lymphatic vessels? [NEET 2018]
(a) Elephantiasis (b) Ringworm disease
(c) Ascariasis (d) Amoebiasis

**51.** Which part of poppy plant is used to obtain the drug 'Smack'? [NEET 2018]
(a) Flowers (b) Roots
(c) Latex (d) Leaves

**52.** Colostrum, the yellowish fluid, secreted by mother during the initial days of lactation is very essential to impart immunity to the new-born infants because it contains: [NEET 2019]
(a) Monocytes
(b) Macrophages
(c) Immunoglobulin A
(d) Natural killer cells

**53.** Identify the correct pair representing the causative agent of typhoid fever and the confirmatory test for typhoid. [NEET 2019]
(a) *Streptococcus pneumonia* / Widal test
(b) *Salmonella typhi* / Anthrone test
(c) *Salmonella typhi* / Widal test
(d) Plasmodium vivax / UTI test

**54.** Which of the following immune responses is responsible for rejection of kidney graft? [NEET 2019]
(a) Humoral immune response
(b) Inflammatory immune response
(c) Cell-mediated immune response
(d) Auto-immune response

**55.** Drug called 'Heroin' is synthesized by: [NEET 2019]
(a) Acetylation of morphine
(b) Glycosylation of morphine
(c) Nitration of morphine
(d) Methylation of morphine

**56.** Identify the **wrong** statement with reference to immunity. [NEET 2020]
(a) When exposed to antigen (living or dead) antibodies are produced in the host's body. It is called 'Active immunity'.
(b) When ready- made antibodies are directly given, it is called 'Passive immunity'.
(c) Active immunity is quick and gives full response.
(d) Foetus receives some antibodies from mother, it is an example for passive immunity.

**57.** The infection stage of *Plasmodium* that enters the human body is: [NEET 2020]
(a) Trophozoites (b) Sporozoites
(c) Female gametocytes (d) Male gametocytes

**58.** Match the following diseases with the causative organism and select the **correct** option.

| List-I | List-II |
|---|---|
| (A) Typhoid | (i) Wuchereria |
| (B) Pneumonia | (ii) Plasmodium |
| (C) Filariasis | (iii) Salmonella |
| (D) Malaria | (iv) Haemophilus |

[NEET 2020]

| | (A) | (B) | (C) | (D) |
|---|---|---|---|---|
| (a) | (i) | (iii) | (ii) | (iv) |
| (b) | (iii) | (iv) | (i) | (ii) |
| (c) | (ii) | (i) | (iii) | (iv) |
| (d) | (iv) | (i) | (ii) | (iii) |

**59.** Match the following:

| List-I | List-II |
|---|---|
| 1. Filariasis | (i) Haemophilus influenzae |
| 2. Amoebiasis | (ii) Trichophyton |
| 3. Pneumonia | (iii) Wuchereria banchofti |
| 4. Ringworm | (iv) Entamoeba histolytica |

**The correct matching is** [NEET 2021]

| | 1 | 2 | 3 | 4 |
|---|---|---|---|---|
| (a) | (ii) | (iii) | (i) | (iv) |
| (b) | (iv) | (i) | (iii) | (ii) |
| (c) | (iii) | (iv) | (i) | (ii) |
| (d) | (i) | (ii) | (iv) | (iii) |

**60.** Given below are two statements: [NEET 2022]

**Statement I:** Autoimmune disorder is a condition where body defence mechanism recognizes its own cells as foreign bodies.

**Statement II:** Rheumatoid arthritis is a condition where body does not attack self cells.

In the light of the above statements, chose the **most appropriate** answer from the options given below:

(a) Both **Statement I** and **Statement II** are incorrect.
(b) **Statement I** is correct but **Statement II** is incorrect.
(c) **Statement I** is incorrect but **Statement II** is correct.
(d) Both **Statement I** and **Statement II** are correct.

**61.** Select the **incorrect** statement with respect to acquired immunity. [NEET 2022]

(a) Anamnestic response is elicited on subsequent encounters with the same pathogen.
(b) Anamnestic response is due to memory of first encounter.
(c) Acquired immunity is non-specific type of defence present at the time of birth.
(d) Primary response is produced when our body encounters a pathogen for the first time.

**62.** In which blood corpuscles, the HIV undergoes replication and produces progeny viruses? [NEET 2023]

(a) B-lymphocytes (b) Basophils
(c) Eosinophils (d) $T_H$ cells

**63.** Match List I with List II. [NEET 2023]

| List I | List II |
|---|---|
| A. Heroin | I. Effect on cardiovascular system |
| B. Marijuana | II. Slow down body functions |
| C. Cocaine | III. Pain killer |
| D. Morphine | IV. Interfere with transport of dopamine |

Choose the correct answer from the options given below:

(a) A - I, B - II, C - III, D - IV
(b) A - IV, B - III, C - II, D - I
(c) A - III, B - IV, C - I, D - II
(d) A - II, B - I, C - IV, D - III

**64.** Match List I with List II. [NEET 2023]

| List I | List II |
|---|---|
| A. Ringworm | I. *Haemophilus influenzae* |
| B. Filariasis | II. *Trichophyton* |
| C. Malaria | III. *Wuchereria bancrofti* |
| D. Pneumonia | IV. *Plasmodium vivax* |

Choose the correct answer from the options given below:

(a) A - II, B - III, C - I, D - IV
(b) A - III, B - II, C - I, D - IV
(c) A - III, B - II, C - IV, D - I
(d) A - II, B - III, C - IV, D - I

**65.** Match List-I with List-II: [NEET 2024]

| List-I | List-II |
|---|---|
| (A) Common cold | (i) *Plasmodium* |
| (B) Haemozoin | (ii) Typhoid |
| (C) Widal test | (iii) Rhinoviruses |
| (D) Allergy | (iv) Dust mites |

Choose the correct answer from the options given below:
(a) (A)-(ii), (B)-(iv), (C)-(iii), (D)-(i)
(b) (A)-(i), (B)-(iii), (C)-(ii), (D)-(iv)
(c) (A)-(iii), (B)-(i), (C)-(ii), (D)-(iv)
(d) (A)-(iv), (B)-(ii), (C)-(iii), (D)-(i)

**66.** Match List-I with List-II [NEET 2024]

| List-I | List-II |
|---|---|
| (A) Typhoid | (i) Fungus |
| (B) Leishmaniasis | (ii) Nematode |
| (C) Ringworm | (iii) Protozoa |
| (D) Filariasis | (iv) Bacteria |

Choose the correct answer from the options given below:
(a) (A)-(i), (B)-(iii), (C)-(ii), (D)-(iv)
(b) (A)-(iv), (B)-(iii), (C)-(i), (D)-(ii)
(c) (A)-(iii), (B)-(i), (C)-(iv), (D)-(ii)
(d) (A)-(ii), (B)-(iv), (C)-(iii), (D)-(i)

**67.** Which of the following are Autoimmune disorders? [NEET 2024]

A Myasthenia gravis
B Rheumatoid arthritis
C Gout
D Muscular dystrophy
E Systemic Lupus Erythematosus (SLE)

Choose the most appropriate answer from the options given below:
(a) A, B and D only (b) A, B, and E only
(c) B, C and E only (d) C, D and E only

**68.** Match List-I with List-II: [NEET 2024]

| List-I | List-II |
|---|---|
| (A) Cocaine | (i) Effective sedative in surgery |
| (B) Heroin | (ii) *Cannabis sativa* |
| (C) Morphine | (iii) *Erythroxylum* |
| (D) Marijuana | (iv) *Papaver somniferum* |

Choose the correct answer from the options given below:
(a) (A)-(iv), (B)-(iii), (C)-(i), (D)-(ii)
(b) (A)-(i), (B)-(iii), (C)-(ii), (D)-(iv)
(c) (A)-(ii), (B)-(i), (C)-(iii), (D)-(iv)
(d) (A)-(iii), (B)-(iv), (C)-(i), (D)-(ii)

**69.** Given below are two statements: [NEET 2024]
**Statement I:** Bone marrow is the main lymphoid organ where all blood cells including lymphocytes are produced.
**Statement II:** Both bone marrow and thymus provide micro environments for the development and maturation of T-lymphocytes.
In the light of the above statements, choose the most appropriate answer from options given below:
(a) Both statement I and statement II are correct.
(b) Both statement I and statement II are incorrect.
(c) Statement I is correct but statement II is incorrect.
(d) Statement I is incorrect but statement II is correct.

## Answer Key

### Multiple Choice Questions: Level I

| | | | | | | | | | |
|---|---|---|---|---|---|---|---|---|---|
| **1.** (b) | **2.** (b) | **3.** (c) | **4.** (a) | **5.** (c) | **6.** (d) | **7.** (d) | **8.** (c) | **9.** (d) | **10.** (c) |
| **11.** (c) | **12.** (c) | **13.** (b) | **14.** (b) | **15.** (c) | **16.** (c) | **17.** (b) | **18.** (b) | **19.** (b) | **20.** (d) |
| **21.** (a) | **22.** (b) | **23.** (c) | **24.** (a) | **25.** (b) | **26.** (d) | **27.** (a) | **28.** (d) | **29.** (c) | **30.** (d) |
| **31.** (a) | **32.** (c) | **33.** (b) | **34.** (d) | **35.** (c) | **36.** (a) | **37.** (b) | **38.** (d) | **39.** (c) | **40.** (c) |
| **41.** (b) | **42.** (a) | **43.** (c) | **44.** (c) | **45.** (d) | **46.** (c) | **47.** (a) | **48.** (d) | **49.** (b) | **50.** (c) |
| **51.** (c) | **52.** (a) | **53.** (d) | **54.** (b) | **55.** (b) | **56.** (b) | **57.** (c) | **58.** (a) | **59.** (c) | **60.** (b) |
| **61.** (b) | **62.** (b) | **63.** (b) | **64.** (b) | **65.** (b) | **66.** (c) | **67.** (c) | **68.** (a) | **69.** (b) | **70.** (d) |
| **71.** (d) | **72.** (c) | **73.** (c) | **74.** (b) | **75.** (b) | **76.** (b) | **77.** (c) | **78.** (b) | **79.** (c) | **80.** (b) |
| **81.** (d) | **82.** (c) | **83.** (c) | **84.** (a) | **85.** (b) | **86.** (a) | **87.** (c) | **88.** (a) | **89.** (b) | **90.** (c) |
| **91.** (b) | **92.** (b) | **93.** (d) | **94.** (b) | **95.** (a) | **96.** (b) | **97.** (d) | **88.** (c) | **89.** (c) | **100.** (d) |
| **101.** (c) | **102.** (a) | **103.** (b) | **104.** (c) | **105.** (b) | **106.** (b) | **107.** (d) | **108.** (d) | **109.** (c) | **110.** (c) |
| **111.** (c) | **112.** (b) | **113.** (c) | **114.** (c) | **115.** (c) | **116.** (b) | **117.** (a) | **118.** (c) | **119.** (a) | **120.** (b) |

| | | | | | | | | | |
|---|---|---|---|---|---|---|---|---|---|
| **121.** (d) | **122.** (a) | **123.** (a) | **124.** (b) | **125.** (c) | **126.** (c) | **127.** (d) | **128.** (c) | **129.** (b) | **130.** (b) |
| **131.** (c) | **132.** (b) | **133.** (b) | **134.** (c) | **135.** (b) | **136.** (d) | **137.** (d) | **138.** (a) | **139.** (a) | **140.** (d) |
| **141.** (c) | **142.** (c) | **143.** (a) | **144.** (c) | **145.** (b) | **146.** (d) | **147.** (b) | **148.** (c) | **149.** (a) | **150.** (c) |
| **151.** (c) | **152.** (d) | **153.** (d) | **154.** (b) | **155.** (b) | **156.** (b) | **157.** (b) | **158.** (a) | **159.** (b) | **160.** (b) |
| **161.** (d) | **162.** (b) | **163.** (d) | **164.** (b) | **165.** (c) | **166.** (b) | **167.** (b) | **168.** (d) | **169.** (d) | **170.** (a) |
| **171.** (b) | **172.** (b) | **173.** (c) | **174.** (a) | **175.** (b) | **176.** (b) | **177.** (a) | **178.** (b) | **179.** (c) | **180.** (c) |
| **181.** (a) | **182.** (b) | **183.** (b) | **184.** (c) | **185.** (b) | **186.** (b) | **187.** (b) | **188.** (a) | **189.** (c) | **190.** (a) |
| **191.** (c) | **192.** (c) | **193.** (d) | **194.** (c) | **195.** (b) | **196.** (a) | **197.** (d) | **198.** (a) | **199.** (c) | **200.** (d) |
| **201.** (b) | **202.** (b) | **203.** (a) | **204.** (b) | **205.** (b) | **206.** (b) | **207.** (d) | **208.** (c) | **209.** (b) | **210.** (b) |
| **211.** (d) | **212.** (d) | **213.** (c) | **214.** (d) | **215.** (d) | **216.** (c) | **217.** (b) | **218.** (b) | **219.** (b) | **220.** (d) |
| **221.** (b) | **222.** (b) | **223.** (b) | **224.** (a) | **225.** (b) | **226.** (a) | **227.** (b) | **228.** (d) | **229.** (b) | **230.** (b) |
| **231.** (b) | **232.** (c) | **233.** (a) | **234.** (b) | **235.** (a) | **236.** (b) | **237.** (d) | **238.** (a) | **239.** (b) | **240.** (b) |
| **241.** (c) | **242.** (c) | **243.** (b) | **244.** (b) | **245.** (c) | **246.** (c) | **247.** (d) | **248.** (c) | **249.** (d) | **250.** (c) |
| **251.** (d) | **252.** (c) | **253.** (b) | **254.** (b) | **255.** (b) | **256.** (b) | **257.** (b) | **258.** (d) | **259.** (a) | **260.** (c) |
| **261.** (b) | **262.** (d) | **263.** (b) | **264.** (d) | **265.** (d) | **266.** (c) | **267.** (c) | **268.** (d) | **269.** (d) | **270.** (c) |
| **271.** (d) | **272.** (b) | **273.** (c) | **274.** (b) | **275.** (b) | | | | | |

## Multiple Choice Questions: Level II

| | | | | | | | | | |
|---|---|---|---|---|---|---|---|---|---|
| **276.** (c) | **277.** (c) | **278.** (a) | **279.** (c) | **280.** (d) | **281.** (d) | **282.** (b) | **283.** (a) | **284.** (c) | **285.** (a) |
| **286.** (b) | **287.** (d) | **288.** (b) | **289.** (d) | **290.** (c) | **291.** (c) | **292.** (c) | **293.** (c) | **294.** (c) | **295.** (a) |
| **296.** (a) | **297.** (a) | **298.** (a) | **299.** (a) | **300.** (c) | **301.** (b) | **302.** (a) | **303.** (a) | **304.** (c) | **305.** (a) |
| **306.** (c) | **307.** (b) | **308.** (a) | **309.** (c) | **310.** (b) | **311.** (b) | **312.** (d) | **313.** (a) | **314.** (c, d) | **315.** (b) |
| **316.** (c) | **317.** (b) | **318.** (a) | **319.** (d) | **320.** (b) | **321.** (b) | **322.** (c) | **323.** (c) | **324.** (c) | **325.** (c) |
| **326.** (c) | **327.** (b) | **328.** (b) | **329.** (c) | **330.** (b) | **331.** (b) | **332.** (c) | **333.** (d) | **334.** (c) | **335.** (a) |
| **336.** (c) | **337.** (a) | **338.** (b) | **339.** (c) | **340.** (b) | **341.** (a) | **342.** (c) | | | |

## A & R and Statement-based Questions

| | | | | | | | | | |
|---|---|---|---|---|---|---|---|---|---|
| **343.** (c) | **344.** (b) | **345.** (a) | **346.** (c) | **347.** (c) | **348.** (c) | **349.** (c) | **350.** (c) | **351.** (c) | **352.** (c) |

## Matrix-Match Type Questions

| | | | | |
|---|---|---|---|---|
| **353.** (a) | **354.** (a) | **355.** (a) | **356.** (a) | **357.** (b) |

## NCERT Exemplar Questions

| | | | | | | | | | |
|---|---|---|---|---|---|---|---|---|---|
| **1.** (c) | **2.** (a) | **3.** (d) | **4.** (d) | **5.** (d) | **6.** (b) | **7.** (a) | **8.** (c) | **9.** (b) | **10.** (c) |
| **11.** (b) | **12.** (c) | **13.** (a) | **14.** (c) | **15.** (d) | **16.** (b) | **17.** (a) | **18.** (c) | **19.** (c) | **20.** (c) |
| **21.** (c) | **22.** (d) | **23.** (c) | | | | | | | |

## Previous Years' Questions

| | | | | | | | | | |
|---|---|---|---|---|---|---|---|---|---|
| **1.** (d) | **2.** (d) | **3.** (d) | **4.** (b) | **5.** (b) | **6.** (c) | **7.** (a) | **8.** (c) | **9.** (a) | **10.** (a) |
| **11.** (b) | **12.** (c) | **13.** (a) | **14.** (d) | **15.** (a) | **16.** (b) | **17.** (d) | **18.** (a) | **19.** (b) | **20.** (d) |
| **21.** (d) | **22.** (d) | **23.** (a) | **24.** (d) | **25.** (a) | **26.** (c) | **27.** (a) | **28.** (a) | **29.** (c) | **30.** (a) |
| **31.** (b) | **32.** (a) | **33.** (c) | **34.** (b) | **35.** (a) | **36.** (c) | **37.** (c) | **38.** (c) | **39.** (d) | **40.** (a) |
| **41.** (d) | **42.** (d) | **43.** (c) | **44.** (b) | **45.** (b) | **46.** (a) | **47.** (a) | **48.** (d) | **49.** (b) | **50.** (a) |
| **51.** (c) | **52.** (c) | **53.** (c) | **54.** (c) | **55.** (a) | **56.** (c) | **57.** (b) | **58.** (b) | **59.** (c) | **60.** (b) |
| **61.** (c) | **62.** (d) | **63.** (d) | **64.** (d) | **65.** (c) | **66.** (b) | **67.** (a) | **68.** (b) | **69.** (d) | |

# HINTS AND EXPLANATION

## Multiple Choice Questions: Level II

**276.** Tetanus toxoid is a vaccine consisting of growth products of *Clostridium tetani* treated with formal aldehyde serving as an active immunizing agent. Hence, it is weakened germs. The first tetanus toxoid (inactivated toxin) was produced in 1924 and was used successfully to prevent tetanus in the armed services during World War II. In the mid-1940s, tetanus vaccine was combined with diphtheria toxoid and inactivated pertussis vaccine to make the combination DTP vaccine for routine childhood immunization.

**277.** The letter T in T-lymphocyte refers to thymus. In human anatomy, the thymus is an organ located in the upper anterior portion of the chest cavity just behind the sternum.

**278.** Common Cold, AIDS is a pair of viral diseases. Viruses are a very common type of infectious disease. Typhoid is a bacterial disease.

**279.** Malignant tumours may exhibit metastasis. Cancer (medical term: malignant neoplasm) is a class of disease, in which a group of cells display uncontrolled growth (division beyond the normal limits), invasion (intrusion on and destruction of adjacent tissues), and sometimes metastasis spread to other locations in the body via lymph or blood.

**280.** The use of anti-histamines and steroids gives quick relief from allergy. Antihistamines are drugs that block the action of histamine (a compound released in allergic inflammatory reactions) at the H1 receptor sites, responsible for immediate hypersensitivity reactions such as sneezing and itching.

**281.** Cornea transplant in humans is almost never rejected. This is because it has no blood supply. Cornea is a transparent layer of tissue, continuous with the sclerotic that forms the front part of the vertebrate eye, over the iris and lens.

**282.**

| Column I | Column II |
|---|---|
| (1) Amoebiasis | Use only sterilized food and water |
| (2) Diphtheria | DPT vaccine |
| (3) Cholera | Use oral rehydration therapy |
| (4) Syphilis | *Treponema pallidum* |

**283.** **Physiological barriers:** Acid in the stomach, saliva in the mouth, tears from eyes–all prevent microbial growth.

**284.** Hashish causes after-thought perceptions and hallucinations. Hashish is a prepared from *Cannabis* composed of the compressed trichomes collected from cannabis plant. Psychoactive effects vary between types of Hashish but are usually the same as those of other cannabis preparations such as marijuana.

**285.** Serum globulins → It makes 2–3% of plasma proteins.

**286.** Pollen grains of many species are responsible for some of the severe allergies and bronchial affliction in some people often lead to chronic respiratory disorders: asthma, bronchitis.

**287.** They mainly affect T4 lymphocyte.

**288.** Amphetamines bring about increased alertness and sleeplessness. Hashish is a hallucinogen. Valium is a tranquilizer. Morphine is an opiate narcotic.

**289.** Leishmaniasis is transmitted by sand fly *Phlebotomus argentipes*, Anopheles transmits malaria.

**290.** ELISA test is a technique used to detect and quantitate extremely small amount of a protein, antibody or antigen with the help of enzyme. The commonly used enzymes are peroxidase and alkaline phosphatase. Southern blotting and DNA probes are used in molecular analysis of DNA. Catalase is not involved in ELISA.

**291.** Mother's milk is very essential for the new-born infant because **colostrum** (yellowish fluid secreted by mother during the initial days of lactation) has **abundant antibodies (Ig A)** for its protection. During pregnancy, some antibodies are transferred from mother to foetus through the placenta. These are also examples of **passive immunity**.

**292.** Carcinomas are malignant growths of the epithelial tissue that cover or line body organs.

**293.** The lymphocytes which differentiate in thymus are known as T-lymphocytes. T-Lymphocytes are responsible for cellular immune response.

**294.** A sickle cell anaemia affected person is more resistant to mosquito-borne infectious disease because the sickle-cell-shaped RBCs are hostile to the protozoa Plasmodium.

**295.** The ability of radiations to kill cells is highest in the tissue with the highest number of dividing cells. Tumour cells proliferate rapidly. Hence, tumours are killed more rapidly by radiations.

**296.** LSD or (Lysergic acid diethylamide) is an extract of ergot of fungus *Claviceps purpurea.* It is most powerful hallucinogen which causes horrible dreams, chronic psychosis, etc.

**297.** Morphine is an opiate narcotic, Bhang is a hallucinogen, Reserpine derived from *Rauwolfia* is used as tranquilizer, cocaine is a stimulant.

**298.** Tetanus is caused by *Clostridium tetani*. Tuberculosis is caused by *Mycobacterium tuberculosis*. Polio is caused by virus.

**299.** We know that HBV causes serum hepatitis. It is most frequently transmitted by blood or by blood-contaminated instruments.

**300.** Interferons are glycoprotein produced by vertebrate cells against viral infection.

**301.** Hepatitis is a viral disease; two subgroups are hepatitis type A virus (HAV) and hepatitis type B virus (HBV). HBV causes serum hepatitis; it is most frequently transmitted by blood, products of blood or blood-contaminated instruments. Since only adults are susceptible to HBV, but vaccines are available. While children and young adults are susceptible to HAV, no vaccines are acceptable.

**302.** Vaccine contains dead, attenuated form or antigen of a pathogen which can be injected to provide immunity towards that pathogen. Monoclonal antibodies are homogenous immunological reagents of defined specificity so that these can be utilized for diagnosis and screening with certainty

**303.** They are helper T–cells.

**304.** Koch's postulates are not applicable to the bacteria causing leprosy and syphilis. *Mycobacterium leprae* causing leprosy produces endospores on which Koch's postulates are not applicable.

**305.** Antibodies bind to specific antigens to produce large insoluble complexes which render them harmless and facilitate their destruction by other cells of the immune system; this process is called agglutination.

**306.** Thymus gland is present in children with maximum development at puberty and thereafter it begins to shrink and atrophies with the development of sex glands.

**307.** Botulism is caused by ingestion of food containing toxins of *Clostridium botulinum*. Before the introduction of a strict canning code, the food canning industry was responsible for many deaths each year from botulism (Food poisoning). Botulism is a rare, but serious paralytic process caused by a nerve toxin is produced by the bacterium *Clostridium botulinum*.

**308.** Typhoid fever is caused by Salmonella typhi.

**309.** HIV is a spherical, enveloped virus of about 90–120 nm diameter. Its nucleocapsid is icosahedral and its genome consists of a single-stranded RNA filament segmented into two identical filaments and associated with two 'reverse transcriptase enzyme'.

**310.** Tranquilizers bring about depression of brain activity and feeling of calmness. Stimulants stimulate the nervous system and increase alertness and activity. Hallucinogens *(Cannabis* products) alter thoughts, perceptions and feelings.

**311.** Opiate narcotics are opium and its derivatives which suppress brain activity and relieve pain. Also called painkillers. These are extracted from unripe capsules of poppy plant *(Papaver somniferum)*. E.g. Morphin, Heroin.

**312.** Exposure to radiation results in the following immediate effects:
- (i) Change in cell metabolism
- (ii) Crystallization of haemoglobin
- (iii) Breakdown of RBCs
- (iv) Loss of hair and nails
- (v) Impairment of vision and damage of different tissues

**313.** Diptheria is a highly infectious disease caused by *Cornybacterium diptheriae* which liberates soluble toxin. The toxin affects nerves and cause double vision, difficulty in swallowing and paralysis of breathing muscles and limbs.

**314.** Small pox, caused by Variola virus, is acute highly communicable disease which has been eradicated not only from India but from the whole world. Polio is completely eradicated in 2016.

**315.** Interferons are produced in response to viral infections. Typhoid and tetanus bacterial diseases. Malaria is caused by a protozoan. Measles is a viral disease.

**316.** 'Each antibiotic is effective only against one particular kind of germ' is not correct.

**317.** *Rauwolfia serpentina* belong to family *Apocynaceae,* its roots yield a chemical useful for high blood pressure.

**318.** Allergy means all kinds of untoward reactions manifested in the body due to hypersensitivity of substances called allergens. Allergy reactions occur due to liberation of histamine by tissue cells.

**319.** Tetanus and typhoid are caused by bacteria.

Whooping cough is caused by bacteria. Sleeping sickness is caused by parasitic flees. Syphilis is caused by bacteria while AIDS is final stage of HIV viral disease.

Measles and Rabies are caused by virus.

**320.** Cancer is initiated when the inactive proto oncogenes are activated to cellular oncogenes which trigger uncontrolled cell multiplication.

**321.** In 1980 the anti-toxin based immunity to diphtheria was discovered by Von Behring. He received Nobel prize in physiology/medicine in 1901 for his discovery of diphtheria antitoxin.

**322.** Antibodies are specific proteins synthesized by the host in response to an antigen. All antibody molecules are immunoglobulins.

**323.** According to the immunity theory, ageing occurs due to loss of power of defence against invasion of germs and pathogens. The process starts with the gradual atrophy and disappearance of the thymus gland during middle age.

**324.** 'Syphilis–Trichuris tichiura' is not correctly matched, because syphilis is caused by Treponema palladium bacteria. Methaemoglobin is denatured haemoglobin.

**325.** Hay fever is due to some fungal spores sensitivity, which is an allergic disease with symptoms of bronchial asthma and skin rash and also with increase in eosinophil (white cells) of blood.

**326.** A special defence system works specially against viral infection. It has no effect on micro-organism. Cells invaded by a virus produce an antiviral protein called interferon (lFN). The latter in released from the infected cell and on reaching the nearby non-infected cells it makes them resistant to the virus infection.

**327.** The major obstacle in transplantation of organs is that the recipient body does not accept the donor's organ. The body defence mechanism rejects and treats the transplanted organ as a foreign particle and reacts actively.

**328.** Syphilis – *T. pallidum*

**329.** Syphilis – *T. pallidum* is STD caused by bacteria

**330.** **Sarcoma** is cancer of the connective or supportive tissue (bone, cartilage, fat, muscle, blood vessels) and soft tissue obtained from mesoderm

**331.** Lymphocytes are the part of specific defence system called immune system.

**332.** Heroin is an opiate narcotic (opium derivative) chemically it is Diacetylmorphine (for this purpose acetic anhydride is used)

**333.** *Wuchereria*–Filariasis

**334.** Schizont or asexual stage occurs in human erythrocytes and liver cells.

**335.** Plasmodium vivax completes sexual cycle or Gamogony in female Anopheles mosquito. Asexual cycle is passed in man (Schizogony).

**336.** Laveran discovered Plasmodium in RBC of human beings.

**337.** In human beings, different types of malaria are caused by 4 different species of Plasmodium. They are:

(1) Benign Tertian Malaria – *Plasmodium vivax*

(2) Malignant (Pernicious or cerebral) Tertian Malaria – *Plasmodium falciparum*

(3) Quartan Malaria - *Plasmodium malariae*

(4) Mild Tertian Malaria – *Plasmodium ovale*

**338.** It is due to surviving sporozoites in surviving mosquitoes.

**339.** Malarial parasite *(Plasmodium vivax),* Protist of class Sporozoa, digenetic parasite causes malarial fever in human. The malarial parasite was discovered by Laveran (1880). Sir Ronald Ross (1898) discovered that Malaria disease is spread by mosquitoes. Its life cycle completes in two organisms: Primary host, female *Anopheles* mosquito and man (Intermediate or Secondary host). It enters human blood through sporozoites. Malarial fever begins with the release of merozoites in the liver cells, from RBC of human.

**340.** The infective stage of *Plasmodium* that enters human blood is sporozoite.

**341.** Lysozyme is an antibacterial agent which is secreted by the major salivary glands.

**342.** Whenever our body gets attacked by some foreign invaders, our body's immune system produces some chemicals to kill or to react against the invader. These chemicals are made up of carbohydrates and proteins, i.e. glycoproteins called antibody.

## NCERT Exemplar Questions

1. Health is not just the absence of disease. It is a state of complete physical, mental, social and psychological well-being.
2. A wide range of organisms belonging to bacteria, viruses, fungi protozoans, helminthes, etc., could cause diseases in man. Such disease causing organisms are called pathogens.
3. The chemical test that is used for diagnosis of typhoid is Widal test.
4.

| Non-infectious diseases | Infectious diseases |
|---|---|
| Cancer | Influenza |
| Allergy | Small pox |

5. The sporozoites that cause infection, when a female *Anopheles* mosquito bites a person are formed in intestine of mosquito.
6. Dengue and chikunguniya are transmitted by *Aedes* mosquitoes.
7. • Difficulty in respiration, fever, chills, cough, headache: *Pneumonia*
   • Constipation, abdominal pain, cramps, blood clots: *Amoebiasis*
   • Nasal congestion and discharge, cough, sore throat, headache: *Common cold.*
   • High fever, weakness, stomach pain, loss of appetite and constipation: *Typhoid*
8. Oncogenes are cancer causing genes.
9. In malignant tumours, the cells proliferate, grow rapidly and move to other parts of the body to form new tumours. This stage of disease is called metastasis.
10. When an apparently healthy person is diagnosed as unhealthy by a psychiatrist, the reason could be that the patient shows behavioural and social maladjustment.
11. Rheumatoid arthritis is an autoimmune disease in which
    • Body attacks self-cells
    • The ability to differentiate pathogens or foreign molecules from self-cells is lost.
12. Mode of transmission of HIV:
    • Transfusion of contaminated blood
    • Sharing of infected needles
    • Sexual contact with infected persons
13. • 'Smack' is a drug obtained from the latex of *Papaver somniferum.*
    • Smack are brown sugar, the common name of Heroin.
    • Heroin is obtained by acetylation of morphine.
14. The substance produced by a cell in viral infection that can protect other cells from further infection is interferon.
15. Transplantation of tissues/organs to save certain patients often fails due to rejection of such tissues/organs by the patient. **Cell-mediated immune response** is responsible for such rejections.
16. Antibodies present in colostrum which protect the new-born from certain diseases is of **IgA type.**
17. Tobacco consumption is known to stimulate secretion of adrenaline and nor-adrenaline. The component causing this could be **nicotine.** Morphine, cocaine, codeine and nicotine are all alkaloids.
18. Anti-venom against snake poison contains **antibodies.**
19. Spleen, Tonsils and Thymus are lymphoid tissues while pancreas is a mixed gland.
20. **Thymus** glands is large sized at birth but reduces in size with ageing.
21. Haemozoin is a toxin released from *Plasmodium* infected cells.
22. *Microsporum, Trichophyton and Epidermophytonare* the causal organism for ringworm while *Macrosporum* is a brown alga.
23. A person with sickle cell anemia is **less prone to malaria.**

## Previous Years' Questions

1. To prevent graft (kidney transplant) rejection, the principle is to use chemicals, which inhibit the entire activity of the immune system. When this occurs graft rejection is delayed, it has been shown that immunosuppression may make patients more prone to develop cancers. One way of overcoming the problems of radiation and, immunosuppression is to suppress only the cells responsible for rejection, normally the killer T-cells. In this way, the rest of the patient's immune system would continue to function normally. The most promising approach is to

treat the patient with monoclonal antibodies that recognize and destroy the killer T-cells. A monoclonal antibody has been developed, which is a very effective at preventing rejection of transplanted kidneys.

2. AIDS (Acquired Immuno Deficiency Syndrome) is a viral disease of immune system. It is caused by virus Human Immunodeficiency Virus (HIV). In AIDS patients, the virus homes on $CD_4$ + T-cells (helper T-lymphocytes), infecting and killing them until none are left. Without their crucial immune system cells, the body cannot mount a defence against invading bacteria or viruses. AIDS patient die off infections that a healthy person could fight off.

3. Widal test is bacterial agglutination test, originally introduced by Widal for diagnosis of typhoid fever. Widal test is based upon antigen–antibody serological interactions. Typhoid or enteric fever is caused by a Gram-negative bacterium salmonella commonly found in the human intestine. Infection of typhoid bacteria stimulates production of immune-specific agglutinins, which are released in blood plasma.

4. Ringworm refers to fungal infections that are on the surface of the skin. Although the world is full of yeasts, moulds and fungi, only a few cause skin problems. These agents are called dermatophytes.

5. Morphine exerts its principal pharmacological effect on the central nervous system and gastrointestinal tract. Its primary actions of therapeutic value are analgesic and sedation.

6. In malaria, chill and fever is due to release of a toxic substance haemozoin, formed by breakdown of haemoglobin present in RBCs. It will be released after the rupture of RBCs in erythrocytic schizogony,

7. Magnetic Resonance Imaging (MRI) is a non-invasive technique, which uses strong magnetic field and provides information about chemistry, metabolic and biochemical data of tissue without time-consuming chemical analysis. It is the safest technique for detection of cancer since it does not utilize radiations and therefore does not cause any side-effect. Histopathological study is not safe as it is an invasive technique while radiography and Computed Tomography (CT) use harmful X-rays.

8. Intravenous therapy or IV therapy is providing the liquid substances (or medicine) through drip, directly into the vein. The word intravenous simply means ‘within a vein’. Compared with other routes of administration, the intravenous root is the fastest way to deliver fluids and medications throughout the body.

9. The primary and secondary immune responses are carried out with the help of two special types of lymphocytes present in our blood, i.e., B-lymphocytes and T-lymphocytes. The B-lymphocytes produce an array (a range) of proteins in response to pathogens into our blood to fight with them. These proteins are called antibodies. The T-cells themselves do not secrete antibodies but help B-cells to produce them.

10. Common cold is not cured by antibiotics because it is caused by a virus called rhinovirus.

11. Bacteria like *Streptococcus pneumoniae* and *Haemophilus influenzae* are responsible for the disease pneumonia in humans which infect alveoli (air filled sacs) of the lungs. As a result of infection, the alveoli get filled with fluid leading to severe problem in respiration. A healthy person acquires infection by inhaling the droplets/aerosols released by an infected person or even by sharing glasses and utensils with an infected person.

12. Many fungi belonging to the generus Microsporum, Trichophyton and Epidermophyton are responsible for ringworms which is one of the most common infectious disease in man. Microsporum is a member of class-Deuteromycetes (Fungi Imperfecti) of Kingdom-fungi. Rhizopus (bread mould) is a member of class-Zygomycetes (Conjugation fungi) of Kingdom-Fungi.

13. Antibiotics work mainly against bacteria.

14. Sporozoite are the infective stage of malarial parasite. They are present in the saliva of infected female Anopheles mosquito.

15. Physiological barriers to the entry of microorganisms in human body are tears in eyes, saliva in mouth and HCl in stomach. The enzyme lysozyme is found in tears and saliva and inhibits the synthesis of peptidoglycan present in the cell wall of microorganisms, especially eubacteria.

16. AIDS symptoms appear in most advanced stage of HIV disease. Some people show HIV symptom shortly but it usually take more than 10 years. HIV attacks T-helper cells which regulate both hormonal and cellular immunity. This causes their depletion due to which patient’s immune system become very weak.

17. ELISA (Enzyme-linked Immunosorbent Assay), also known as an enzyme immunoassay (EIA), is a biochemical technique used mainly in immunology to detect the presence of an antibody or an antigen in a sample. It is a useful tool for determining serum antibody concentrations (such as with HIV test). ELISA was the first screening test widely used for HIV because of its high sensitivity.

**18.** Innate immunity is non-specific type of defence that is present at the time of birth. This is accomplished by providing different types of barriers to the entry of foreign agents into our body. Innate immunity consists of four types of barriers. These are —

**(i) Physical barriers:** Skin on our body is the main barrier which prevents entry of micro-organisms. Mucus coating of the epithelium lining the respiratory, gastrointestinal and urogenital tracts also help in trapping microbes entering our body.

**(ii) Physiological barriers:** Acid in the stomach, saliva in the mouth, tears from eyes–all prevent microbial growth.

**(iii) Cellular barriers:** Certain types of leukocytes (WBC) of our body like polymorpho-nuclear leukocytes (PMNL-neutrophils) and monocytes and natural killer (type of lymphocytes) in the blood as well as macrophages in tissues can phagocytose and destroy microbes.

**(iv) Cytokine barriers:** Virus-infected cells secrete proteins called interferons which protect non-infected cells from further viral infection.

**19.** Excess alcohol intake for a long term(chronic) → Alcoholic hepatitis → Fatty liver → Cirrhosis.

**20.** In our body, cell growth and differentiation is highly controlled and regulated. In cancer cells, there is breakdown of these regulatory mechanisms. Normal cells show a property called contact inhibition by virtue of which contact with other cells inhibits their uncontrolled growth. Cancer cells appear to have lost this property. As a result, cancerous cells just continue to divide giving rise to masses of cells called tumours.

**21.** Bacteria like Streptococcus pneumoniae and Haemophilus influenza are responsible for the disease pneumonia in humans which infects the alveoli (air filled sacs) of the lungs. As a result of the infection, the alveoli get filled with fluid leading to severe problems in respiration. The symptoms of pneumonia include fever, chills, cough and headache.

Many viruses also cause diseases in human beings. Rhino viruses represent one such group of viruses which cause one of the most infectious human ailments – the common cold. They infect the nose and respiratory passage but not the lungs. Common cold is characterized by nasal congestion and discharge, sore throat, hoarseness, cough, headache, tiredness, etc., which usually last for 3–7 days.

**22.** Typhoid fever could be confirmed by Widal test.

**23.**

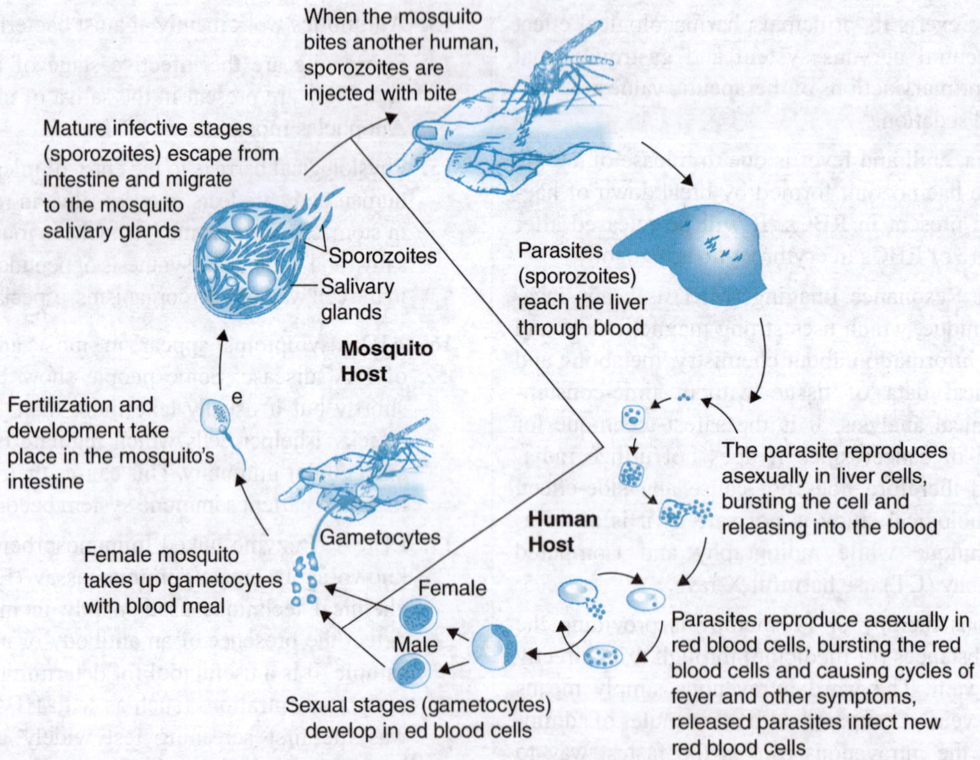


Because fertilization and development take place in the mosquito's intestine.

**24.** Preformed antibodies need to be injected to treat the bite of a viper snake. It is also a type of immunization which is called passive immunization.

**25.** (a) ***Plasmodium falciparum*** – A protozoan pathogen causes the most serious type of malaria, that is, falciparum malaria.

(b) ***Panthera tigris*** – Indian tiger but not protected in Gir forest.

(c) *E.Coli* is *Escherichia coli* commonly occurring bacteria in human intestine as symbiont.

(d) **Musca domestica** – House fly.

**26.**

| Type of Drug | Examples |
|---|---|
| Sedatives and tranquil-lizers (depressant) | Benozodiazepines (e.g., Bar-biturates, Valium), Re-serpine |
| Opiate narcotics (Seda-tive and pain killer) | Opium, Pethidine, Metha-done, Morphine, Heroine |
| Stimulants | Caffeine, Cocaine, Amphet-amines |
| Hallucinogens | LSD, Mescalin, psilocybin, Charas, Marijuana, Bhang Hashish, Ganja |

**27.** T-lymphocytes mediate C.M.I. (cell-mediated immunity)

**28.** Contaminated water and soil (with eggs of *Ascaris*) is the source of infection with *Ascaris*.

**29. Life cycle of HIV:**

HIV enters the body of the person → HIV's RNA genome enters the macrophages → RNA genome replicates to form viral DNA by the help of enzyme reverse transcriptase → Incorporation of viral DNA into host cell's DNA and starts producing virus particles (**Macrophages now act as HIV factory**) → Simultaneous entry of HIV into **Helper T-lymphocytes ($T_H$)**, replicates and release more virus particles after lysis of Helper T-lymphocytes → Progressive decrease in the number of helper T-lymphocytes → Person acquires an immune-deficient condition and starts suffering from various infections that usually do not occur do not occur in a healthy individual, e.g. bacteria especially **Mycobacterium, viruses, fungi** and even parasites like **Toxoplasma** → Death.

**30.**

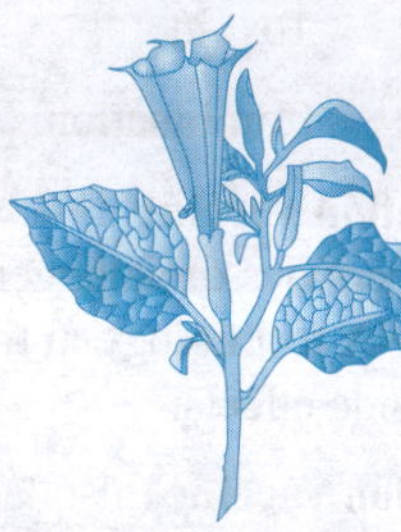

Datura produces hallucinogens.

**31.** Several mushrooms such as *Amanita muscaria*, *Psilocybe mexicana* and *Panaeolus* spp. secretes hallucinogenic substances like psilocybin and psilocin. These substances may destroy brain cells and the power of perception in human beings.

**32.** Grafted kidney may be rejected in a patient due to the cell-mediated immune response that is mediated by T-lymphocytes. The body is able to differentiate 'self' and 'non-self'. Therefore, tissue matching, blood group matching are essential before undertaking any graft/transplant and even after this the patient has to take immunosuppressants all his/her life.

**33.** Serum globulins test provides confirmatory evidence measuring the deficiency of antibodies (γ-globulin) in a person.

**34.** Colostrum has high levels of IgA (secretory antibodies), which provide passive immunity to foetus.

**35.** *Entamoeba histolytica* is found in the colon. It feeds on mucosa, submucosa as well as phagocytose RBCs.

**36.** HIV enters into helper T-lymphocytes ($T_H$), replicates and produce progeny viruses. The progeny viruses released in the blood attack other helper T-lymphocytes. This is repeated leading to progressive decrease in the number of helper T-lymphocytes in the body of the infected person.

**37.** Tuberculosis vaccine (BCG) has inactivated bacteria. In whooping cough vaccine, there are killed pathogens of *Bordetella pertussis* which cause whooping cough. In DPT, diphtheria toxoid is present. Sabin polio vaccine contains inactivated virus.

| | | |
|---|---|---|
| **First-generation vaccine** (inactivation of whole pathogen) | Live attenuated | OPV, BCG, Small pox, Influenza |
| | Killed | Typhoid, Salk, Cholera, Rabies, Plague |
| | Toxoid | Diphtheria, Tetanus |
| | Combination | DPT, MMR |
| **Second-generation vaccine** Antigenic polypeptides of pathogens are produced with recombinant DNA technology in transgenic organisms. These have no side effects. | | 1. Hepatitis B vaccine (produced from transgenic yeast)<br>2. Meningococcal<br>3. Pneumococcal |
| **Third-generation vaccine** (also known as **DNA vaccine**) | | Leukaemia virus vaccine |

**38.** *Trichinella spiralis* is an endoparasite found in human intestine. It is the smallest nematode producing larvae in large number (viviparous). Other nematode which shows viviparity is *Wuchereria.*

**39.** Cholera is caused by *Vibrio cholerae* and tetanus is caused by *Clostridium tetanii.* mumps, small pox, herpes and influenza are viral diseases.

**40.**

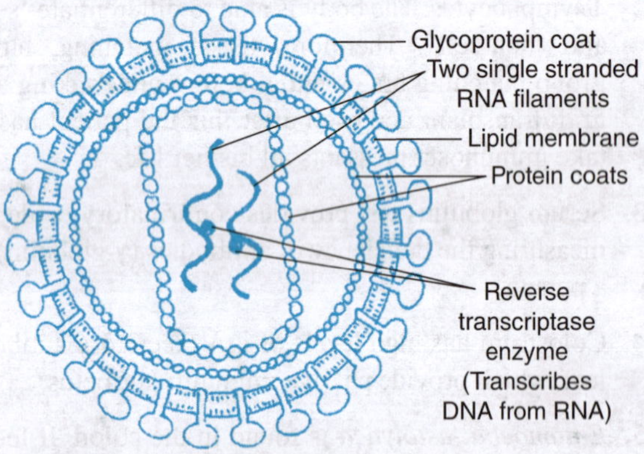


Diagrammatic representation of HIV

AIDS is caused by retrovirus human immunodeficiency virus (HIV). It consists of an outer coat known as viral envelope and inner core known as viral core. The viral core consists of viral RNA (single standard) and enzymes, i.e. reverse transcriptase, protease and integrase.

**41.** The progressive shortening of telomeres (DNA sequences at chromosomal ends) is prevented by telomerase. This enzyme is an attractive target for cancer therapy.

**42.** Polio drop contains live attenuated pathogens.

**43.** In higher vertebrates, the immune system can distinguish self-cells and non-self. If this property is lost due to genetic abnormality and it attacks self-cells, then it leads to auto-immune diseases.

Graft rejection is because of CMI (cell-mediated immunity).

Active immunity is developed due to vaccine.

**44.** Asthma is an allergic disease caused by allergic reaction of mast cell in response to allergen.

**45.** (a) AIDS is caused by retrovirus.

(b) **Acquired immunity** is pathogen-specific and not present since birth.

(c) The exaggerated response of the immune system to certain antigens present in the environment is called Allergy.

(d) Spleen traps the blood-borne micro-organisms and acts as a filter of the blood.

**46.**

| Disease | Causative agent |
|---|---|
| Ringworm | *Microsporum fungus* |
| Elephantiasis | *Wuchereria* |
| Malaria | *Plasmodium* |
| Amoebiasis | *Entamoeba* |

**47.** Cell-mediated immune response causes non-acceptance or rejection of graft or transplanted tissues/organs.

**48.** MALT or Mucosa Associated Lymphoid Tissue constitutes about 50 percent of the lymphoid tissue in human body. It is scattered along mucosal lining in the human body.

**49.** • Alzheimer's disease is chronic neurodegenerative disorder.

• Autoimmune skin diseases is Psoriasis and Vitiligo.

• Rheumatoid arthritis is non-organ-specific autoimmune disease.

**50.** *Wuchereria (W. bancrofti* and *W. malayi),* the filarial worms cause a slowly developing chronic inflammation of the organs in which they live for many years, usually the lymphatic vessels of the lower limbs and the disease is called **elephantiasis** or **filariasis.** The genital organs are also often affected, resulting in gross deformities. The pathogens are transmitted to a healthy person through the bite of female mosquito vectors.

**51.** *Smack* is chemically diacetylmorphine which is a white, odourless, bitter crystalline compound. This is obtained by acetylation of morphine, which is extracted from the latex of poppy plant *Papaver somniferum.*

**52.** The yellowish fluid colostrum secreted by mother during the initial days of lactation has abundant antibodies (IgA) to protect the infant. It is an example of passive immunity.

**53.** *Salmonella typhi* is a pathogenic bacterium which causes typhoid fever in human beings, and confirmatory test for typhoid is Widal test.

**54.** The body is able to differentiate 'self' and 'non-self', and the cell-mediated immune response is responsible for the graft rejection.

**55.** Heroin, commonly called *smack* is chemically diacetylmorphine which is a white, odourless, bitter crystalline compound. This is obtained by acetylation of morphine, which is extracted from the latex of poppy plant *Papaver somniferum*.

**56.** The correct option is (c) because active immunity is slow and takes time to give its full effective response in comparison to passive immunity where pre-formed antibodies are administered.

**57.** *Plasmodium* enters the human body as sporozoites (Infectious stage) through the bite of Infected Female *Anopheles* mosquito.

**58.** Typhoid fever in humans is caused by pathogenic bacterium *Salmonella typhi.* Pneumonia is caused by Streptococcus *Pneumoniae* and *Haemophilus influenzae.* Filariasis or elephantiasis is caused by the filarial worm, *Wuchereria bancrofti* and *Wuchereria malayi.* Malaria is caused by different species of *Plasmodium.*

**59.**

| | |
|---|---|
| Filariasis | Filariasis is the disease caused by Wuchereria bancrofti, filarial worm. |
| Amoebiasis | Amoebiasis/Amoebic dysentery is caused by a protozoan parasite. *Entamoeba histolytica* in the large intestine of human. |
| Pneumonia | Pneumonia is caused by bacteria like *Streptococcus pneumoniae* and *Haemophilus influenzae.* |
| Ringworm | Ringworm is caused by fungi belonging to genera Microsporum, Trichophyton and Epidermophyton. |

**60.** Statement I is correct but Statement II is incorrect.

So, the option (b) is the correct answer as autoimmune disorder is a condition where body defense mechanism recognises its own cells as foreign bodies. Sometimes, due to genetic and other unknown reasons, the body attacks self- cells.

Rheumatoid arthritis is an autoimmune disease where body attacks self-cells, therefore this statement is incorrect.

**61.** Anamnestic response or secondary immune response is a highly intensified response due to memory of first encounter. When our body encounters a pathogen for the first time then the body elicits the primary immune response. When there is a subsequent encounter with the same pathogen, secondary or anamnestic immune response is elicited.

Option (c) is the correct answer as acquired immunity is a specific type of defence which is not present at the time of birth.

Option (a), (b) and (d) are true statements and hence cannot be the answer.

**62.** HIV enters into helper T-lymphocytes ($T_H$), replicates and produce progeny viruses. The progeny viruses released in the blood attack other helper T-lymphocytes.

**63.**

| | |
|---|---|
| Heroin | Slow down body functions |
| Marijuana | Effect on cardiovascular system |
| Cocaine | Interfere with transport of dopamine |
| Morphine | Pain killer |

**64.**

| | |
|---|---|
| Ringworm | *Trichophyton* |
| Filariasis | *Wuchereria bancrofti* |
| Malaria | *Plasmodium vivax* |
| Pneumonia | *Haemophilus influenzae* |

**65.** Correct answer is option (c) because
- Common cold is caused by Rhinoviruses.
- Haemozoin is released in blood due to ruptured RBCs after *Plasmodium* infection.
- Widal test is used to confirm the typhoid fever.
- Allergy is caused due to dust mites.

**66.** The correct answer is option (b) as
- Typhoid – Caused by *Salmonella typhimurium* (Bacteria)
- Leishmaniasis – Caused by protozoan *i.e., Leishmania donovani*
- Ringworm – Caused by fungi belonging to the genera *Microsporum, Trichophyton* and *Epidermophyton*
- Filariasis – Caused by *Wuchereria bancrofti* and *Wuchereria malayi* (Nematode)

**67.** The correct answer is option (b) as Myasthenia Gravis, Rheumatoid Arthritis and Systemic Lupus Erythematosus (SLE) are autoimmune disorders.
- Muscular dystrophy is a genetic disorder which progressively affects the skeletal muscles.
- Gout is the inflammation of joints, occurs due to deposition of uric acid crystals. Uric acid is formed by metabolism of purines.

**68.** The correct option is (d) as

A. Cocaine – Obtained from plant *Erythroxylum coca*, stimulating action on CNS.

B. Heroin – Formed by the acetylation of morphine which is obtained from plant *Papaver somniferum*.

C. Morphine – Obtained from *Papaver somniferum*, is an effective sedative in surgery.

D. Marijuana – Obtained from *Cannabis sativa*, produces hallucinogenic effect and affects cardiovascular system of the body.

**69.** Both statements are true. Bone marrow is main lymphoid organ. Both thymus and bone marrow provide micro-environment for development and maturation of T- lymphocyte.

# Biotechnology: Principles and Processes

# 12

## LEARNING OBJECTIVES

- Understand the concepts of genetic engineering
- Know more about the complete mechanism of recombinant DNA technology
- Learn the principle and process of gel electrophoresis
- Know more about cloning vectors
- Know more about the genetically modified organisms, its importance and safety
- Discuss about bio-safety and patents in biotechnology

## Chapter Overview

- According to **European Federation of Biotechnology (EFB),** biotechnology is **'the integration of natural science and organisms, cells, parts thereof and molecular analogues for products and services.'**
- Few examples of biotechnology:
  1. Use of IVF (In Vitro Fertilization) technique to obtain a test-tube baby
  2. Synthesis of a gene and its use
  3. Correction of a defective gene
  4. Developing a DNA vaccine
- There are two basic or core techniques that helped in origin of biotechnology: **Genetic engineering and maintenance of sterile (microbial contamination free) ambience in chemical engineering processes.**
- **Benefit of asexual reproduction:** It preserves and maintains the genetic information without introducing variations.
- **Benefit of sexual reproduction:** It introduces variations and results information of various genetic set-up out of which few may be beneficial to the organism and population too.
- In sexual reproduction many undesirable genes are also introduced along with the desired genes and these cannot be restricted from the process by traditional hybridization. Processes used in plant and animal breeding.
- By the techniques of genetic engineering, it is possible to introduce the one or set of desired genes only into the target organism. Such techniques involve-creation of recombinant DNA, use of gene cloning and gene transfer.
- **Origin of replication:** It is the specific DNA on a chromosome which is responsible for initiating replication. Alien DNA is linked up with origin of replication and ensures its replication and multiplication. This can also be termed as cloning as the DNA is making copies of itself.
- **First artificial recombinant DNA molecule was formed** by **Stanley Cohen** and **Herbert Boyer** in 1972. They join antibiotic resistance gene with plasmid of ***Salmonella typhimurium*** by the use of restriction endonucleases (molecular scissors) and DNA ligase and transfer of recombinant DNA into a host like *E.coli*.
- **Three basic steps in genetically modifying an organism: 1.** Identification of the DNA segment with desired gene. **2.** Transfer of the identified DNA into the host. **3.** Maintenance of transferred DNA in the host and ensuring its introduction in its progeny.

---

Refer NCERT Ch 9: Biotechnology : Principles and Process

- **Tools of Recombinant DNA Technology**: Restriction enzymes, cloning vectors and competent host **(Fig. 12.1)**
- In **1963,** it was found that two enzymes were responsible to restrict the growth of the bacteriophage in *E.coli* **(defense mechanism of bacteria or immune system of bacteria against viruses)** one added methyl group to the DNA and other enzyme can cuts DNA at specific sites. This was later termed as restriction endonuclease.
- Nucleases are the enzymes that cut DNA. These are of two types **Endonucleases:** These cut DNA in between. **Exonucleases:** These remove nucleotides form the ends of the DNA.

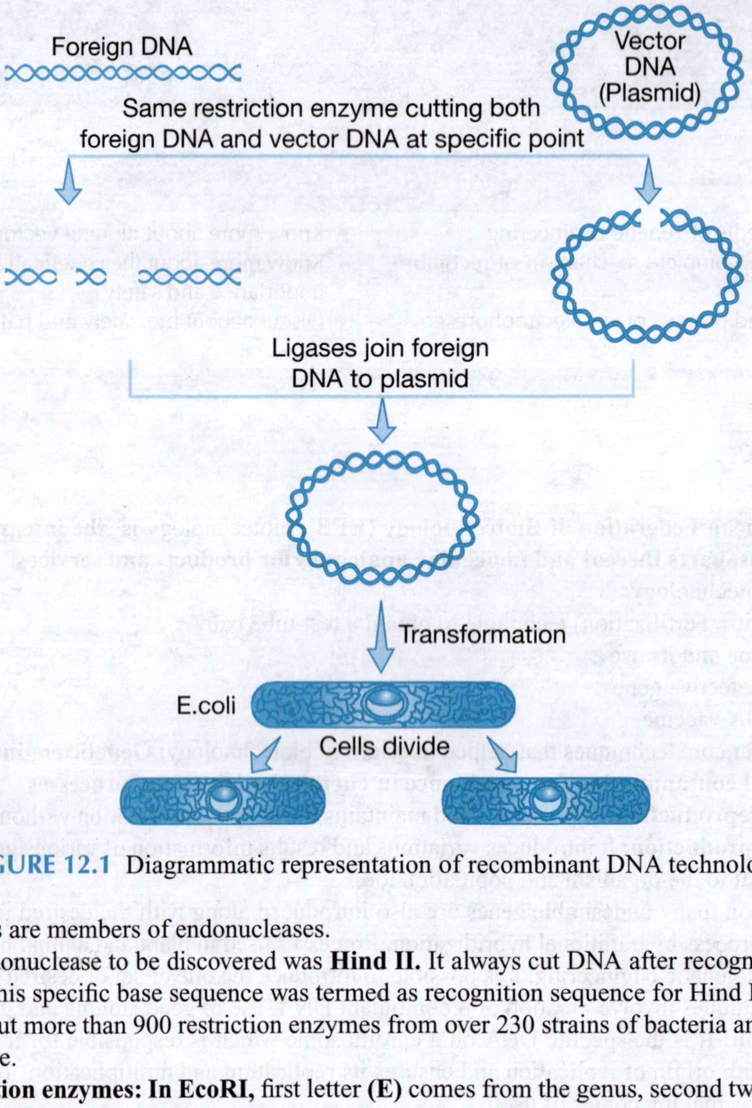


**FIGURE 12.1** Diagrammatic representation of recombinant DNA technology

- Restriction enzymes are members of endonucleases.
- **First** restriction endonuclease to be discovered was **Hind II.** It always cut DNA after recognizing a specific sequence of **six base pairs**. This specific base sequence was termed as recognition sequence for Hind II.
- Today we know about more than 900 restriction enzymes from over 230 strains of bacteria and each with own specific recognition sequence.
- **Naming of Restriction enzymes: In EcoRI,** first letter **(E)** comes from the genus, second two letters **(co)** comes from the species, **R** is derived from the name of strain, roman number following **(I)** is the order indicated in which the enzymes were isolated.
- Each restriction enzyme recognize a **specific DNA sequence – pallindromic DNA** (as given in **Fig. 12.2).** Pallindromic DNA sequence reads same on the two strands of DNA if the orientation of the reading is kept same.
  Example: 5′ -------- GAATTC ------- 3′
  3′ -------- CTTAAG ------- 5′
- Restriction enzyme cut the pallindromic DNA sequences and can produce **sticky or blunt end.**

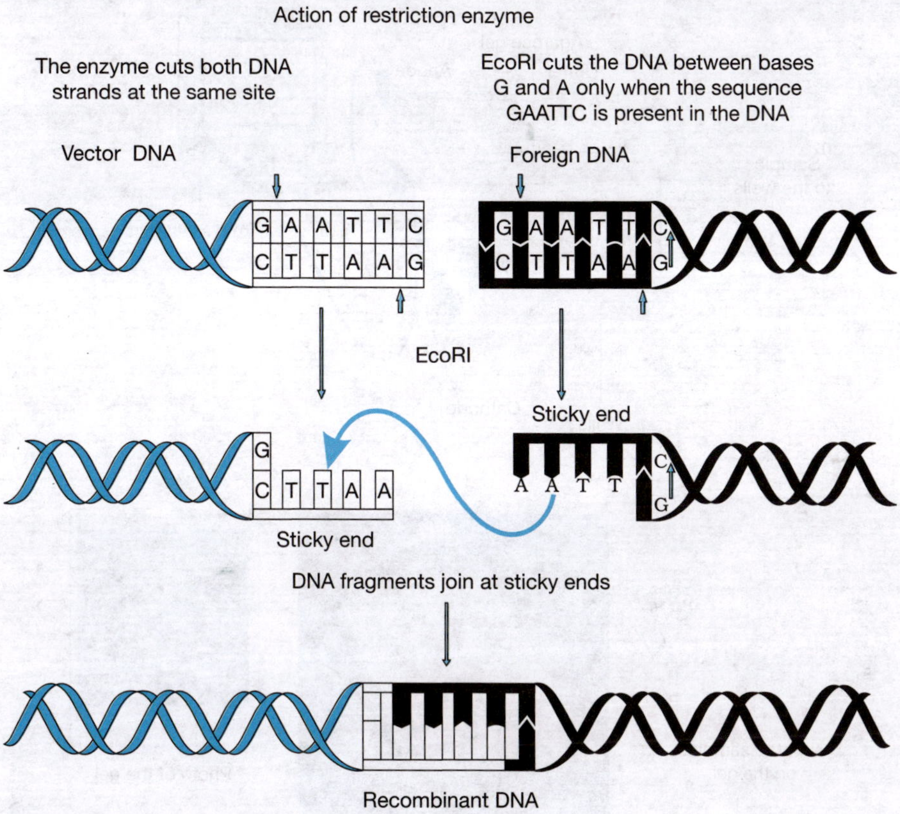


**FIGURE 12.2** Steps in formation of recombinant DNA by action of restriction endonuclease enzyme–EcoRI

- When only one type of restriction enzyme is being used, same kind of sticky ends can be produced in foreign DNA and vector like plasmid which can be later on joined by **DNA ligase** enzyme.
- Fragments of DNA generated by restriction enzyme are separated by **gel electrophoresis** in which the **negatively charged DNA fragments (Fig. 12.3)** are forced to move towards the anode under an electrical field through a medium (**usually agarose gel extracted from sea weed**). DNA fragments move according to their size-smaller the fragment more distance it will travel.
- DNA fragments are first stained with **Ethidium bromide** and then observed under **UV-rays**. DNA fragments which occur **bright orange coloured bands**.
- **Elution:** The separated bands of DNA are cut out of the agarose gel and extracted from the gel piece **(Fig. 12.3)**.
- **Cloning Vectors:** Plasmids **(double stranded circular DNA capable of independent replication)** and Bacteriophages are most commonly used vectors for cloning.

**Transposon-Based Vectors:** Transposons, or "jumping genes," can be used as vectors to insert genetic material into various locations within a genome. They are valuable for creating insertional mutagenesis libraries.

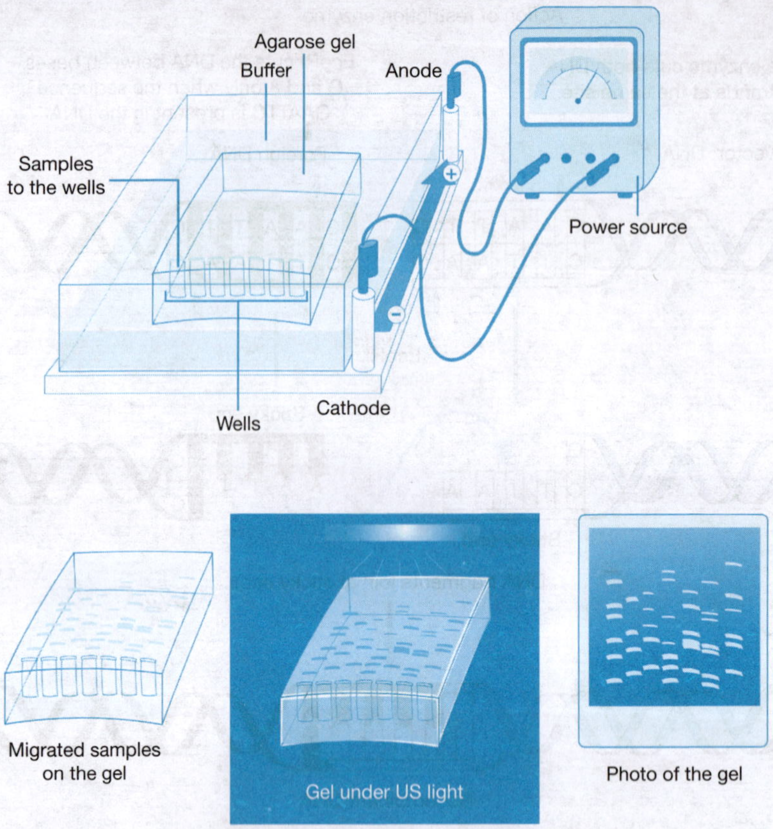


**FIGURE 12.3** A typical agarose gel electrophoresis showing migration of undigested and digested set of DNA fragments

- **Features required to facilitate cloning into a vector**: (i) Origin of replication (ori) ,(ii) Selectable marker and (iii) Cloning sites
  - (i) **Origin of replication (ori):** It initiate replication and decide the copy number (we choose high copy no.)
  - (ii) **Selectable marker**: This selectable marker ensures: Selective growth of transformants and identification and elimination of non-transformants. **Examples of selectable markers:** Antibiotic resistance gene for **chloramphenicol, ampicillin, tetracycline** and **kanamycin** are useful selectable markers for **E.coli.** Normally E.coli do not contain any resistance against the above mentioned antibiotics.
  - (iii) **Cloning sites**: Vector should have very few (preferably 1) recognition sites for the commonly used restriction enzymes.
- **Selection of recombinants can be done by:**

**(a) Inactivation of antibiotics**

**Example: Vector pBR322** (a plasmid) has two antibiotic resistance genes-**amp$^R$** (ampicillin resistance gene) and **tet$^R$** (tetracycline resistance gene). If a foreign DNA is ligated at the **BamHI site** of the tetracycline resistance gene **(Fig. 12.4)**, then the resistance against the tetracycline will be lost by the recombinant plasmid. Such recombinants can be selected out from the

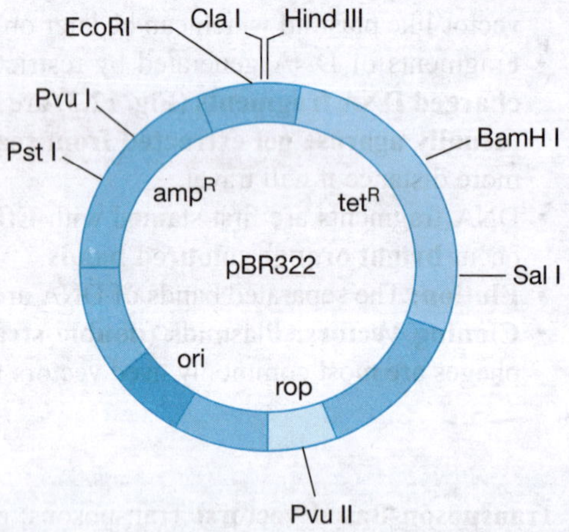


**FIGURE 12.4** E. coli cloning vector pBR322 showing restriction sites (Hind III, EcoR I, BamH I, Sal I, Pvu II, Pst I, Cla I). ori and antibiotic resistance genes (amp$^R$ and tet$^R$). rop codes for the proteins involved in the replication of the plasmid

non-recombinants by growing them in tetracycline containing medium. Non-recombinants grow in medium with both types of antibiotics but the recombinants can grow in ampicillin containing medium only. This is a **cumbersome** process as it involves simultaneous plating of two plates with different antibiotics.

**(b) Insertional activation**

In this process, **chromogenic substrates** are being used as alternative selectable markers.

Recombinants and non-recombinants give different colours in the presence of chromogenic substrate.

**Example:** A recombinant DNA was inserted into the **coding sequence of the β - galactosidase enzyme** in the plasmid of *E.coli*. This results in inactivation of the gene for β-galactosidase enzyme. In presence of chromogenic substrate: Non-recombinants give blue colour and recombinants give no colour.

- **Vectors for cloning genes in plants and animals (eukaryotic cell):** Modified Tumor inducing (Ti) plasmid of *Agrobacterium tumifaciens* used for the plant cell and **retroviruses** are used for animal cells.
- **Competent Host:** DNA is a hydrophilic molecule and it cannot pass through the plasma membrane. Process of making the bacterial cells competent so that they can take up plasmid DNA: **(i)** Treatment of bacterial cells with specific concentrations of divalent cations like calcium. This increases the chances or efficiency of recombinant DNA entry into the bacterial cell wall through the pores. **(ii)** Incubation of bacterial cells with recombinant DNA on ice. There after these are placed briefly at 42°C (also known as heat shock) after which it will again transferred on ice. This process enables the bacteria to take up recombinant DNA. **(iii)** Lipofaction. **(iv)** elctroduction **(v) Microinjection:** Direct injection of recombinant DNA into the nucleus of the animal cell. **(vi) Biolistics or Gene gun:** High velocity micro particles of **Gold or Tungsten** coated with recombinant DNA are bombarded on **plant cells. (vii)** Use of **disarmed pathogen vectors**.
- **Isolation of the Genetic Material:** First step is lysis of the cell from which the DNA has to be obtained. For this purpose various enzymes are being used: (i) **Lysozyme** for bacteria. (ii) **Cellulase** for plant cell. (iii) **Chitinase** for fungal cell.
- **Chilled ethanol** is added to precipitate DNA threads in the suspension. Thus DNA is obtained in pure form **(Fig. 12.5)**.

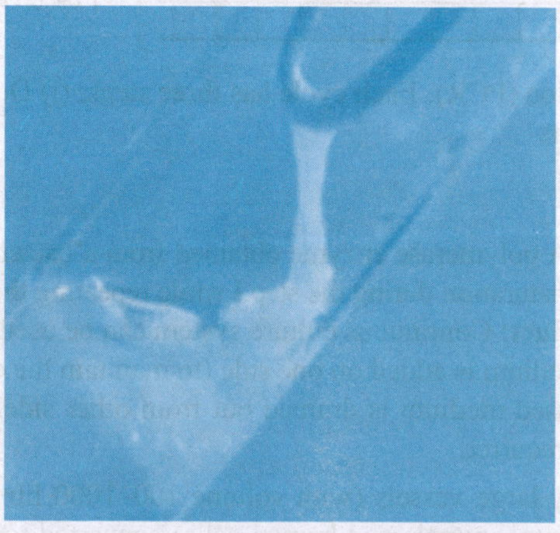

FIGURE 12.5 Collection of fine thread of DNA by spooling

- **Amplification of Gene of Interest using PCR (Fig. 12.6)** (Polymerase Chain Reaction) **2.** By this reaction, many copies of the 'gene of interest' are being formed in vitro. Each cycle of PCR is having three steps:

**(a) Denaturation of DNA:** Separation of DNA strands by exposing them to high temperature (high temperature induced denaturation).

**(b) Primer Annealing:** Addition of primers to the separated DNA strands. Primers are the small chemically synthesized oligonucleotides that are complimentary to the DNA.

**(c) Extension of Primers:** This step is mediated by **DNA polymerase (or Taq polymerase)** enzyme. This enzyme uses the genomic DNA as a template and extends the oligonucleotide primer to obtain another strand of DNA.

- **In PCR cycle (Fig. 12.6) $2^n$ copies of DNA is produced (where 'n'is number of cycle).**

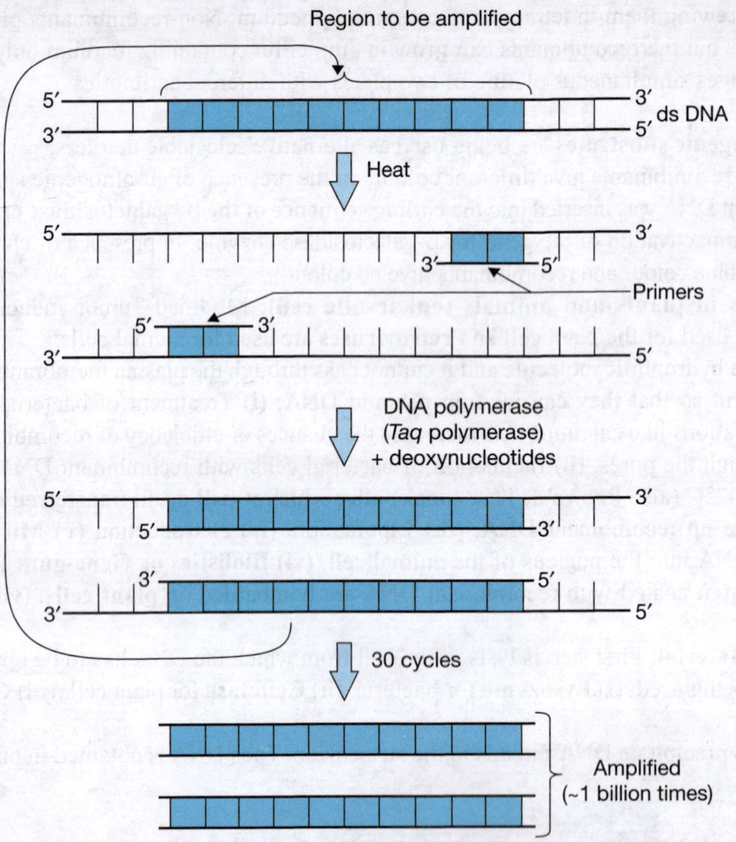


**FIGURE 12.6** Polymerase chain reaction (PCR): Each cycle has three steps: (i) Denaturation, (ii) Primer annealing and (iii) Extension of primers

- **Taq polymerase** enzyme is a DNA polymerase enzyme obtained from a bacterium *Thermus aquaticus*. This enzyme is **thermally stable** and can resist denaturation during the step I while repeating the replication of DNA.
- **Obtaining the Foreign gene product:** Continuous culture system can be used for producing higher yields of required proteins. In such systems, fresh medium is added on one side (to maintain the cells in their most physiologically active or exponential phase) while the used medium is drained out from other side. For producing very high yields of the desired proteins, **bioreactors** are required.
- **Bioreactors:** Bioreactors are very large vessels (with volume 100–1000 litres) in which the raw materials are biologically (by use of microbial plants, animals and human cells) converted to products like enzymes. In a bioreactor optimum conditions (temperature, pH, oxygen, salts, minerals, vitamins, substrate, etc.) are maintained for maximum growth **(Fig. 12.7)**. Most common type of bioreactor is 'stirring type' (or stirring tank bioreactor).
- **'Stirring type' (or stirring tank) bioreactor**: It is usually cylindrical or with a curved base so that the contents in the reactor should mix properly. The stirrer performs mixing and ensures the availability of oxygen throughout the reactor. Instead of stirring, air can also be bubbled into the reactor. Components of a 'stirring type' bioreactor are the following: An agitator system, An oxygen delivery system, A foam control system, A temperature control system, pH control system, Sampling ports: To extract small volumes of culture periodically.
- **Downstream processing**: It includes **separation, purification and preservation**. Clinical trials are also done in case of drugs. Downstream processing and quality control testing depends upon the type of product.

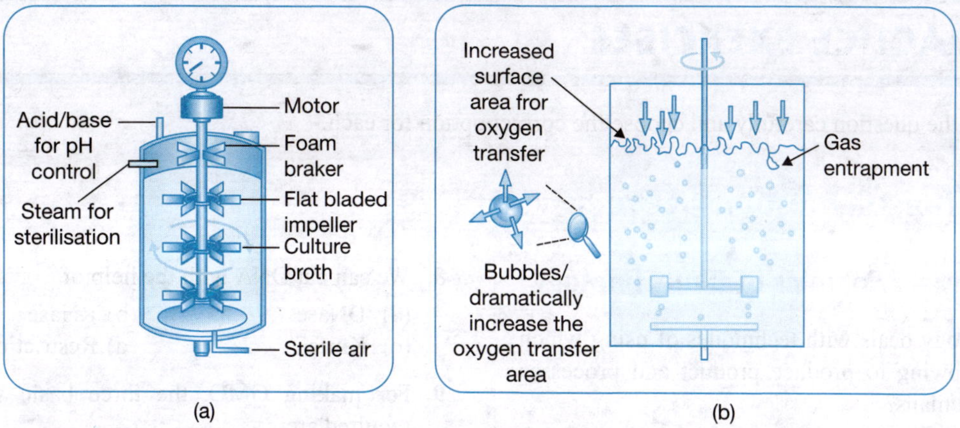


**FIGURE 12.7** (a) Simple stirred-tank bioreactor, (b) Sparged stirred-tank bioreactor through which sterile air bubbles are sparged

| Restriction | Source (Organism and Strain) | Sequence Recognized |
|---|---|---|
| 1. Pvu II | *Proteus vulgaris* | 5′CAG↓CTG3′ |
| | | 3′GTC↑GAC5′ |
| 2. Pvu I | *Proteus vulgaris* | 5′CGAT↓CG3′ |
| | | 3′GC↑TAGC5′ |
| 3. Bam HI | *Bacillus amyloliquefaciens* H | 5′G↓GA TCC3′ |
| | | 3′CCTAG↑G5′ |
| 4. Eco RI | *Escherichia coli* RY 13 | 5′G↓AATTC3′ |
| | | 3′CTTAA↑G5′ |
| 5. Eco R II | *E. coli* R 245 | 5′C↓CA(T)GG3′ |
| | | 3′GGT(A)C↑C5′ |
| 6. Hind II | *Haemophilus influenzae* Rd | 5′GTPy↓PuAC3′ |
| | | 3′CAPu↑PyTG5′ |
| 7. Hind III | *H. influenza* Rd | 5′A↓AGCTT3′ |
| | | 3′TTCGA↑A5′ |
| 8. Sal I | *Streptomyces albus* G | 5′G↓TCGAC3′ |
| | | 3′CAGCT↑G5′ |
| 9. Cla I | *Caryophanom latum* L | 5′AT↓CGAT3′ |
| | | 3′TAGC↑TA5′ |
| 10. Pst I | *Providencia stuartii* | 5′CTGCA↓G3′ |
| | | 3′G↑ACGTC5′ |

# PRACTICE EXERCISES

**Direction:** Read the question carefully and choose the correct option for each.

## Multiple Choice Questions: Level I

### Biotechnology – Principles of Biotechnology

**1.** Biotechnology deals with techniques of using which of the following to produce product and processes useful to humans?
(a) Enzyme from organism (b) Live organism
(c) Vitamins (d) Both (a) and (b)

**2.** Biotechnology mainly uses
(a) GMO (b) Bacteria
(c) Virus (d) Animals

**3.** Select the process/technique included under biotechnology.
(a) IVF (test tube baby)
(b) Gene synthesis
(c) Developing DNA vaccine
(d) All of these

**4.** Which of the following is true about EFB definition of biotechnology?
(a) It includes traditional view.
(b) It includes modern molecular biotechnology.
(c) Definition is the integration of natural science and organisms, cells, parts thereof, and molecular analogues for products and services.
(d) All the above

**5.** Which of the following can be biotechnological products?
(a) Antibiotics (b) Vaccine
(c) Enzymes (d) All of these

**6.** Select the false statement from the following.
(a) Genetic engineering includes techniques to alter chemistry of genetic material (DNA and RNA).
(b) Sexual reproduction is more advantageous than asexual reproduction.
(c) Genetic engineering allows us to introduce desirable set of genes without the undesirable gene into the target organism.
(d) Plasmid is autonomously replicating linear extra chromosomal DNA.

**7.** Multiplication of alien DNA in organism requires
(a) ROP (b) ORI
(c) Stop codon (d) TATA box

**8.** We can cut DNA with the help of
(a) DNase (b) RNase
(c) Knife (d) Restriction enzyme

**9.** For making GMO, the three basic steps that are required are
(a) Identification of DNA with desirable gene.
(b) Introduction of identified DNA into the host.
(c) Maintenance of introduced DNA in the host and transfer of the DNA to its progeny.
(d) All the above

**10.** Who isolated antibiotic resistance gene from salmonella typhimurium in 1972?
(a) Jacob and Monod
(b) Stanley Cohen and Herbert Boyer
(c) Osborn
(d) Boliver

**11.** Genetic engineering means
(a) Gene manipulation
(b) Tissue culture
(c) Utilization of microbes in industries
(d) Somatic hybridization

**12.** Biotechnology helps in synthesizing
(a) New generation antibiotics
(b) New vaccines
(c) MAB (monoclonal antibodies)
(d) All of these

**13.** Genetic engineering is possible because of the discovery of
(a) Transduction
(b) Transformation
(c) Restriction enzyme and DNA ligase
(d) Electron microscopy

**14.** Biotechnology reveals the use of
(a) Microorganisms in industrial processes
(b) rDNA
(c) Engineered bacteria for the production of antibiotics and antibodies
(d) All the above

**15.** Manipulation in gene has been made possible because of
(a) Discovery of restriction endonuclease
(b) Development of method for production of r-DNA
(c) Discovery of producing desired genes
(d) All the above

**16.** Transgenic plants are the ones
(a) Grown in artificial medium after hybridization in the field.
(b) Produced by a somatic embryo in artificial medium.
(c) Generated by introducing foreign DNA into a cell and regenerating a plant from the cell.
(d) Produced after protoplast fusion in an artificial medium.

**17.** The below figure represents

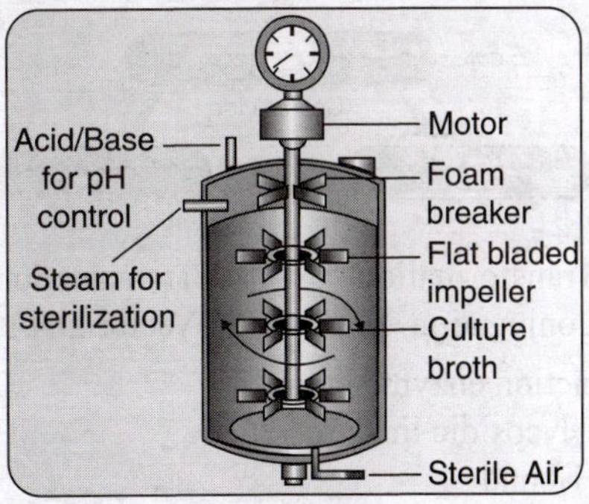


(a) Sparged stirred-tank bioreactor
(b) Simple stirred-tank bioreactor
(c) Thermo regulator
(d) Power generator

**18.** Genetic engineering Techniques are used to alter:
(a) DNA (b) RNA
(c) Proteins (d) Both 1 & 2

**19.** Select correct statements for bioprocess engineering
(a) It involves maintenance of sterile ambience
(b) It enables growth of only desired microbes
(c) Antibiotics, vaccines & enzymes are some example of biotechnological products.
(d) All are correct

**20** Sexual reproduction
(A) Provide scope for variations.
(B) Allow unique combination of gene setup
(C) Preserves genetic information
(D) Beneficial to organism as well as population.

Select correct set of statements.
(a) A, B and C (b) B, C and D
(c) A, B and D (d) A, B, C and D

**21.** Read the following sentences about construction of 1st artificial rDNA molecule.
(A) It was formed by Cohen & Boyer in 1982.
(B) Plasmid of S. typhimurium was used by cutting out antibiotic resistance gene.
(a) Statement I is incorrect but statement II is true.
(b) Both Statements I and II are true
(c) Both Statements I and II are false
(d) Statement I is correct but statement II is false

**22.** Match the Colum

| I | II |
|---|---|
| 1. Restriction enzymes | A. Vector |
| 2. Mosquito | B. Identical copies |
| 3. ORI | C. Molecular Scissors |
| 4. Cloning | D. Initiation of replication |

(a) 1-C, 2-A, 3-D, 4-B
(b) 1-B, 2-C, 3-A, 4-D
(c) 1-B, 2-D, 3-A, 4-C
(d) 1-C, 2-B, 3-D, 4-A

**23.** The ability to make exact, multiple copies of gene is called
(a) Manipulation (b) Recombination
(c) Cloning (d) Hybridization

## Tools of Recombinant DNA Technology

### *A. Restriction Enzyme*

**24.** Which diagram correctly represents the cutting of both strands of DNA by EcoRI?

(a)
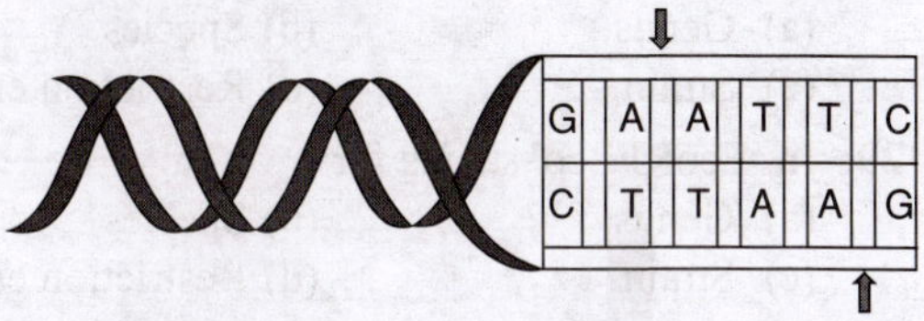


(b)
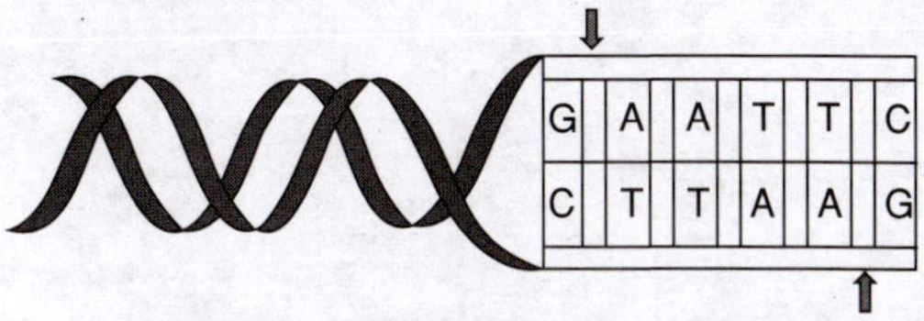


(c)
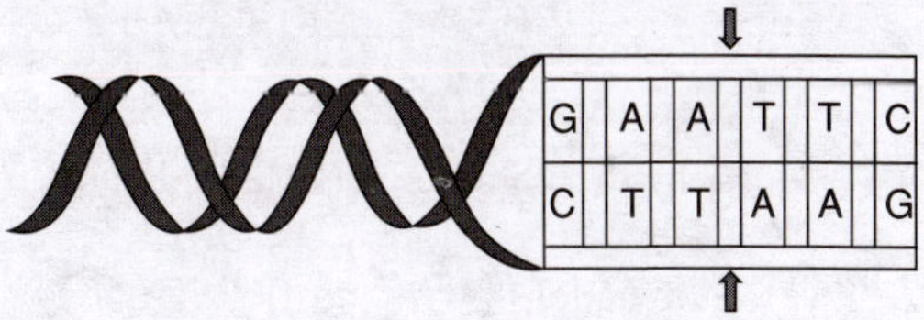

(d) 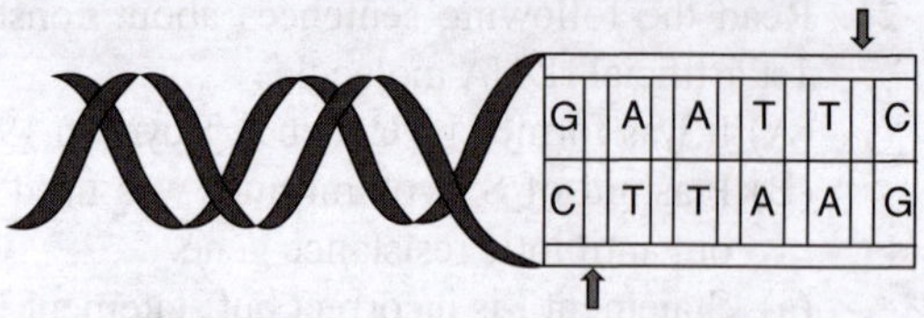


**25.** Hind II recognizes a specific sequence of how many base pairs?

(a) 4 (b) 6
(c) 8 (d) 10

**26.** The sequence recognized by restriction endonucleases

(a) ORI
(b) Recognition sequence
(c) Palindrome sequence
(d) Both (b) and (c)

**27.** Select the incorrect statement.

(a) More than 900 restriction enzymes have been isolated from over 230 strains of bacteria.
(b) In the year 1963, the two enzymes responsible for restricting the growth of bacteriophage in Escherichia coli were isolated.
(c) Some key tools for recombinant DNA technology are restriction enzyme, polymerase enzyme, ligase, vectors and host root organisms.
(d) EcoRI cut the DNA between bases A and T only when the sequence GAATTC is present in the DNA.

**28.** In 'EcoRI' R stands for

(a) Genus (b) Species
(c) Strain (d) Restriction enzyme

**29.** In 'EcoRI' 'co' stands for

(a) Genus (b) Species
(c) Strain (d) Restriction enzyme

**30.** What is 'B' in the figure?

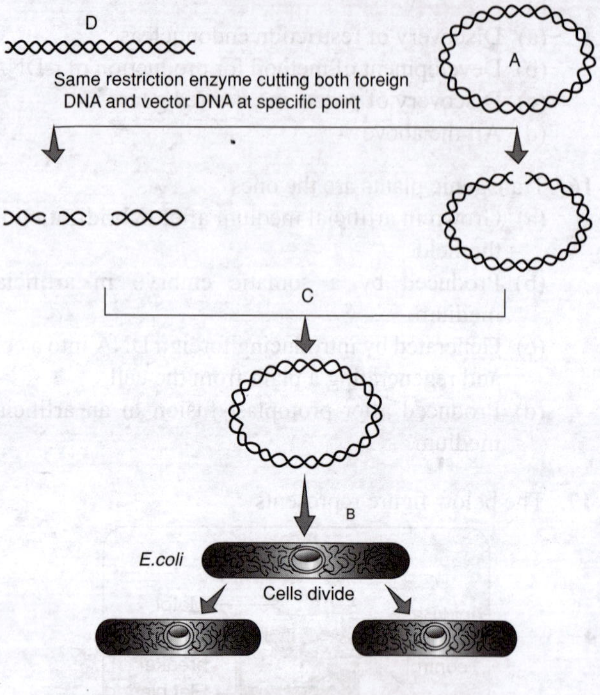


(a) Transformation (b) Transduction
(c) Conjugation (d) Vector DNA

**31.** Restriction enzyme breaks

(a) Glycosidic linkage
(b) H-bond
(c) Sugar–phosphate linkage
(d) All of these

**32.** The sequence recognized by EcoRI is

(a) 5′-GAATTC-3′ 3′-CTTAAG-5′
(b) 5′-CCAATG-3′ 3′-GAATCC-5′
(c) 5′-GATACC-3′ 3′-CCTAAG-5′
(d) 5′-CATTAG-3′ 3′-GATAAC-5′

**33.** EcoRI cuts palindrome sequence which produces overhanging stretches called sticky ends on each strand. These are named sticky because

(a) They can combine with any DNA.
(b) They form hydrogen bonds with their complementary cut counterpart.
(c) They facilitate the action of the enzyme DNA ligase.
(d) Both (b) and (c)

**34.** Restriction enzymes recognize specific

(a) Palindromic region (b) Exons
(c) Introns (d) None of these

**35.** The first restriction enzyme type II was discovered from

(a) *E. coli* (b) *Haemophilus influenzae*
(c) *Pseudomonas* (d) *Xanthomonas*

**36.** Restriction endonuclease is a
(a) Enzyme for transcription
(b) Molecular blade
(c) Enzyme for replication
(d) Enzyme for transduction

**37.** Restriction enzymes of *E. coli* are
(a) HindIII (b) BamHI
(c) EcoRI, EcoRII (d) All of these

**38.** Bacteria possessing restriction endonuclease enzymes remain
(a) Affected by bacteriophages
(b) Unaffected by bacteriophages
(c) Resistant to drugs and heat
(d) None of these

**39.** Restriction endonuclease type II cuts
(a) Both the strands dsDNA
(b) ssDNA
(c) Single strand of dsDNA
(d) Both (b) and (c)

**40.** Bacteria protects themselves from viral attack by producing
(a) Exonuclease (b) Endonuclease
(c) DNA ligase (d) Gyrase

**41.** Restriction endonuclease
(a) Cuts DNA molecule at random
(b) Cuts DNA from specific palindromic site
(c) Restricts DNA synthesis
(d) Synthesize DNA

**42.** Molecular scissor is
(a) Restriction endonuclease
(b) Helicase
(c) Urease
(d) Peptidase

**43.** Which of the following bacteria is not a source of restriction endonuclease?
(a) *Haemophilus influenzae*
(b) *Escherichia coli*
(c) *Agrobacterium tumefaciens*
(d) *Bacillus amyloliquefaciens*

**44.** Which of the following cuts the DNA at a specific place?
(a) Restriction endonuclease
(b) DNA ligase
(c) Exonuclease
(d) Alkaline phosphatase

**45.** Broken ends of two DNA strands are joined by
(a) Exonuclease (b) Endonuclease
(c) DNA ligase (d) Gyrases

**46.** Which of the following statements does not hold true for restriction enzyme?
(a) It recognizes a palindromic nucleotide sequence.
(b) It is an endonuclease.
(c) It is isolated from viruses.
(d) It produces the same kind of sticky ends in different DNA molecules.

**47.** Select set of correct statements:
(a) The first restriction endonuclease discovered was Hind II
(b) Hind II was isolated & characterised five years later
(c) Hind II recognises specific sequence of eight base pairs
(d) Hind II is isolated from Haemophilus influenza.
(a) a, b and d only (b) a, b and c only
(c) b, c and d only (d) b and d only

**48.** First Restriction enzymes recognised was
(a) Bam HI (b) Hind II
(c) Eco RI (d) Ham I

**49.** Today, more than ________ Restriction enzymes have been isolated from over ________ strains of bacteria.
(a) 230, 900 (b) 230, 600
(c) 900, 230 (d) 900, 200

**50.** Bacteria protecting themselves from bacteriophages were
(a) Able to add methyl group to DNA
(b) Able to cut DNA
(c) Resistant to drugs & heat
(d) Both a & b

**51.** Select incorrect statements about EcoRI.
(A) First letter in name of enzyme comes from genus.
(B) Second two letters come from variety.
(C) R comes from species.
(D) I indicates the order of isolation.
(a) A, B, & C only (b) B, C & D only
(c) B & C only (d) A & D only

**52.** Select correct statements.
(A) RE belong to class of enzymes called nucleases.
(B) Each RE functions by inspecting the length of DNA Sequence.
(C) RE cuts each of two strands of double helix by breaking glycosidic bonds.
(D) Each RE recognises specific palindromic nucleotide sequences in DNA.
(a) A, B & C only (b) A, B & D only
(c) B, C & D only (d) A, B, C & D

**53.** **Assertion:** Single stranded portions left on DNA by the action of action of RE are called sticky ends.
**Reason:** These single strands form hydrogen bonds with their complementary cut counterparts.

(a) (A) is false but (R) is true
(b) Both (A) and (R) are true and (R) is the correct explanation of (A)
(c) Both (A) and (R) are true but (R) is not the correct explanation of (A)
(d) (A) is true but (R) is false.

**54.** When cut by same RE, resultant DNA fragments
(A) Have same kind of sticky ends
(B) Sticky ends may differ.
(C) Can be joined by using DNA ligases
(D) Are used to create recombinant molecules of DNA
Select correct statements
(a) A, C & D (b) A & D Only
(c) A, B & D (d) B & D Only

**55.** In gel electrophoresis of DNA
(A) Separation of DNA fragments occur according to their size & length
(B) DNA fragments move towards cathode under electric field.
(C) Commonly used matrix is agarose from sea weeds.
(D) Main aim is to separate DNA fragments.
(E) DNA fragments are visualised by staining with ethidium bromide, under visible light
Select correct statements.
(a) A, C, D & E only (b) A, C & D only
(c) A, B, D & E only (d) B, D & E only

**56.** Vector are engineered so that
(A) They help easy linking of foreign DNA
(B) They help in selection of recombination from non – recombinants.
(a) Both A & B are correct
(b) Both A & B are incorrect
(c) A is correct, B is incorrect
(d) A is incorrect, B is correct

**57.** Select correct statements.
(A) Replication of plasmids & bacteriophages is dependent on control of chromosomal DNA in bacterial cells.
(B) & bacteriophages have high copy numbers of their genomes within bacterial cells.
(C) Certain plasmids have 15-100 copies per cell
(D) Alien piece of DNA is linked to plasmid DNA to get equal copy number as that of plasmid.
(a) A, B, D are correct (b) A, C, D are correct
(c) B, C, D are correct (d) A, B, C are correct

**58.** Features required to facilitate cloning in vector is/are
(a) Ori site (b) Selectable marker
(c) Cloning sites (d) All of these

**59.** Select correct statements about Ori.
(A) It is sequence where transcription starts
(B) Alien DNA linked to Ori site can be made to replicate in host.
(C) It controls copy number of linked DNA
(a) A & D only (b) A & B only
(c) B & C only (d) A & C only

**60.** Select correct statement about selectable markers.
(A) They help to identify and eliminate non transformants.
(B) They help to permit growth of transformants.
(C) Antibiotic resistant genes serve as useful selectable markers.
(a) A & B only (b) B & C only
(c) A & C only (d) A, B & C

**61.** The process through which a piece of DNA is introduced in host bacterium is called.
(a) Transcription (b) Translation
(c) Transformation (d) Replication

**Direction for Q62–63:** Choose the correct option:
(a) (A) is false but (R) is true
(b) Both (A) and (R) are true and (R) is the correct explanation of (A)
(c) Both (A) and (R) are true but (R) is not the correct explanation of (A)
(d) (A) is true but (R) is false.

**62.** **Assertion:** Vector needs to have few recognition sites for restriction enzyme.
**Reason:** Presence of more than one restriction enzyme sites will generate several fragments and thus complicate process.

**63.** **Assertion:** Selection of recombinants due to inactivation of antibiotics is tedious process.
**Reason:** It requires simultaneous plating of transformants on two plates with different antibiotics

**64.** Selection of recombinants can be done with
(a) Inactivation of antibiotics
(b) Insertional inactivation
(c) Use of chromogenic substrates
(d) All of these

**65.** When insertional inactivation occurs in B galactosidase gene,
(A) Recombinant colonies give blue colour.
(B) Recombinant colonies do not give any colour.
(C) Recombinant colonies produce B galactosidase enzyme
(D) Recombinant colonies don't produce B galactosidase enzyme

(a) Both A & C are correct
(b) Both B & D are correct
(c) Both A & D are correct
(d) Both B & C are correct

**66.** Select incorrect statements
(A) A. tumifaciens is pathogen of monocot plant.
(B) A. tumifaciens is able to transform normal cells in to tumour.
(C) Retroviruses have ability to transform normal cells in cancerous cells, in both plants & animals.
(D) Disarmed retroviruses and Ti plasmid of A. tumifaciens are used to deliver foreign DNA.
(A) A, B & C only (B) A & C only
(C) B & C only (D) B, C & D only

## B. Electrophoresis

**67.** The extraction of DNA from a gel piece is known as
(a) Spooling (b) Elution
(c) AGE (d) Annealing

**68.** The fragmented DNA can be visualized by staining DNA with
(a) NaCl (b) Ethidium bromide
(c) Ethylene bromide (d) NaBr

**69.** Which of the following DNA is undigested by restriction endonuclease in this diagram?

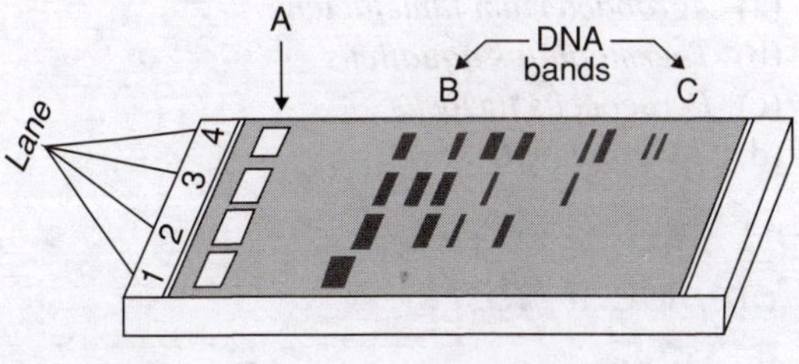


(a) Lane 1 (b) Lane 2
(c) Lane 3 (d) Lane 4

**70.** Gel electrophoresis is used for
(a) Construction of rDNA
(b) Isolation of DNA
(c) Cutting of DNA
(d) Separation of DNA fragments according to their size or length

**71.** During electrophoresis, DNA fragments move towards the
(a) Anode (b) Cathode
(c) Both the poles (d) None of these

## C. Cloning Vector

**72.** For cloning of foreign DNA it is attached with *ori* gene of vector which controls
(a) Replication
(b) Copy number of replicating DNA
(c) Both (a) and (b)
(d) None of these

**73.** Find the true statement.
(a) *Ori* means origin of transcription.
(b) Some bacterial cell may have copy number of plasmid that varies from 15–100.
(c) Vector should have many recognition sites for commonly used restriction enzymes so that alien DNA can attach to any one of the sites easily.
(d) TetR gene in pBR322 can be cleaved by PvuI and PstI.

**74.** Which of the following antibiotic resistance genes are used as selectable marker for *E. coli*?
(a) Chloramphenicol
(b) Tetracycline
(c) Kanamycin
(d) All of these

**75.** If alien DNA is introduced using SalI in pBR322 then transformant will grow on
(a) Ampicillin (b) Tetracycline
(c) Both (a) and (b) (d) None of these

**76.** Select the incorrect matching.

| | |
|---|---|
| (a) pBR322 | – *E. coli* cloning vector |
| (b) EcoRI, Cla I, Hind III | – Restriction enzyme |
| (c) ROP | – Protein involved in the replication of the plasmid |
| (d) PCR | – Technique in which multiple copies of the gene (or DNA) of interest is synthesized in vitro |

**77.** Select the incorrect statement.
(a) Selection of recombinants due to inactivation of antibiotic is a cumbersome procedure.
(b) Insertional inactivation of β-galactosidase leads to colourless colonies.
(c) Insertional inactivation of β-galactosidase leads to blue color colonies.
(d) In insertional inactivation, the rDNA is inserted within the coding sequence of an enzyme β-galactosidase.

**78.** Which vector is use to deliver gene in animal cell?
(a) Retroviruses (b) Disarmed retroviruses
(c) Ti-plasmid (d) *E. coli*

**79.** Lable A and B in the below Figure:

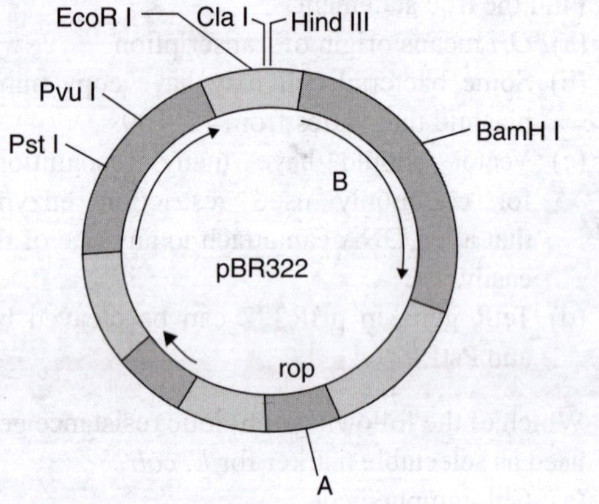


(a) A: PvuII, B: BamHI
(b) A: PvuII, B: $tet^R$ gene
(c) A: EcoR gene, B: $tet^R$ gene
(d) A: PvuII, B: $Amp^R$ gene

**80.** pBR322 is the most extensively studied
(a) Plasmid DNA of *E. coli*
(b) Foreign gene
(c) rDNA
(d) Clone

**81.** Plasmids are
(a) Extranuclear genes of bacteria
(b) Endosymbiont of bacterial cells
(c) Best vector DNA
(d) All of these

**82.** Plasmids are suitable vector for gene cloning because
(a) They are smaller circular DNA
(b) They are linear DNA
(c) They can shuttle between prokaryotes and eukaryotes
(d) None of the above

**83.** $T_i$ plasmid used in plant genetic engineering is a plasmid of
(a) *Azotobacter* (b) *Rhizobium*
(c) *Agrobacterium* (d) *Saccharomyces*

**84.** Which one of the following is commonly used in the transfer of foreign DNA to crop plants?
(a) *Penicillium expansum*
(b) *Trichoderma harzianum*
(c) *Meloidogyne incognita*
(d) *Agrobacterium tumefaciens*

**85.** Which of the following is a plasmid?
(a) pBR322 (b) BamHI
(c) SalI (d) EcoRII

**86.** Bacteriophages are used in biotechnology as
(a) Vector or vehicle DNA
(b) Cloning organism
(c) Restriction enzyme synthesizers
(d) None of these

**87.** The ability to form tumours is found in plasmids of
(a) *E. coli* (b) *Pseudomonas*
(c) *Agrobacterium* (d) *Pneumococcus*

**88.** Oncogenic character is seen in
(a) *E. coli* (b) pBR322
(c) $T_i$ plasmids (d) $R_i$ plasmids

**89.** Transgenic plants are produced by inserting desired genes in
(a) pBR322 (b) $T_i$ plasmids
(c) Lambda phage (d) None of these

**90.** Which is not a vector for rDNA technology?
(a) Plasmids (b) Cosmids
(c) Phages (d) Mosquitoes

**91.** What is the source of Ti plasmid which is modified and used as a cloning vector to deliver the desired genes into plant cells?
(a) *Agrobacterium tumefaciens*
(b) *Thermophilus aquaticus*
(c) *Pyrococcus furiosus*
(d) *Aedes aegypti*

## D. Competent Host

**92.** To make bacterium competent (Transformation with recombinant DNA) we use
(a) Specific concentration of $Ca^{2+}$ ion
(b) Heat shock (42°C)
(c) Both (a) and (b)
(d) None of these

**93.** By which method is rDNA directly placed in nucleus of animal cell?
(a) Gene gun (biolistics) (b) Heat shock
(c) $CaCl_2$ (d) Micro-injection

**94.** The way to introduce alien DNA into host cell includes
(a) Disarmed pathogens
(b) Biolistics or gene gun
(c) Micro-injection
(d) All of these

**95.** Which method is suitable for transferring an alien DNA into a plant cell?
(a) $CaCl_2$ (b) Biolistics or gene gun
(c) Micro-infection (d) Heat shock

**96.** Electroporation involves
(a) Promotion of seed germination by induced inhibition of water with electric current.
(b) Making transient pores in cell membrane to facilitate entry of gene constructs.
(c) Purification of saline water with the help of an artificial membrane.
(d) Passage of sucrose through sieve pores by electro-osmosis.

**97.** Significance of the 'heat shock' method in bacterial transformation is to facilitate
(a) Binding of DNA to the cell wall.
(b) Uptake of DNA through membrane transport proteins.
(c) Uptake of DNA through transient pores in the bacterial cell wall.
(d) Expression of antibiotic resistance gene.

**98.** Cancer is generally caused due to the activation/conversion of ________ to ________ and/or inactivation of ________.
(a) Oncogene, tumour suppressor gene, proto-oncogene
(b) Tumour suppressor gene, oncogene, proto-oncogene
(c) Proto-oncogene, oncogene, tumour suppressor gene
(d) Oncogene, proto-oncogene, tumour suppressor gene

**99.** DNA cannot pass the cell membrane, since
(a) It is hydrophilic molecule
(b) It is hydrophobic molecule
(c) It is negatively charged
(d) It is macromolecule.

**100.** Competence in case of bacterial cells is related to
(a) Force bacteria to take plasmid
(b) Treatment of $Ca^{++}$ and heat shock
(c) Removing cell wall of bacterial cells
(d) Both a & b

**101.** Read following sentences.
**Statement I:** Treating cells with calcium ions in specific concentration increases the efficiency of entry of DNA through pores in cell wall
**Statement II:** Heat shock treatment to cells enables them to take up recombinant DNA
(a) Statement I is incorrect but statement II is true.
(b) Both Statements I and II are true
(c) Both Statements I and II are false
(d) Statement I is correct but statement II is false

**102.** Biolistics or gene gun method is efficiently used for
(a) Animal cells (b) Plant cells
(c) Bacterial cells (d) All of these

**103.** Microinjection method, to introduce foreign DNA into hosts, is used more commonly for
(a) Animal cells (b) Plant cells
(c) Bacterial cells (d) All of these

## Processes of Recombinant DNA Technology

**104.** Arrange the following process in the sequence used in rDNA technology.
(1) Isolation of DNA
(2) Fragmentation of DNA by RE
(3) Isolation of desired DNA fragment
(4) Ligation of DNA fragment into vector
(5) Transferring rDNA into host
(6) Culturing host cells in a medium at large scale
(7) Extraction of the desired product
(a) 1, 2, 3, 4, 5, 6, 7 (b) 1, 2, 3, 4, 6, 5, 7
(c) 2, 1, 3, 4, 5, 6, 7 (d) 1, 2, 3, 5, 4, 6, 7

**105.** In majority of organisms the genetic material is
(a) DNA (b) RNA
(c) mRNA (d) Protein

**106.** Which match is correct for the enzyme which is used to extract DNA in following organism?
(a) Plant cell–Cellulase (b) Fungus–Chitinase
(c) Bacteria–Lysozyme (d) All are correct

**107.** In isolation of genetic material (DNA) from nucleus, the RNA can be removed by ribonuclease and protein by protease. The purified DNA then precipitates after the addition of ________.
(a) $CaCl_2$ (b) Ether
(c) Chilled ethanol (d) Acetic acid

**108.** Which of the following is used to check the progression of restriction enzyme digestion?
(a) PCR (b) ROP
(c) AGE (d) All

**109.** PCR stands for
(a) Polymer chain reaction
(b) Polymerase chain reactor
(c) Polymerase chain reaction
(d) Polymerization, combination, recognition

**110.** PCR includes
(a) Denaturation (b) Annealing
(c) Extension (d) All of these

**111.** 30 cycles of PCR amplified DNA approximately is how many times?
(a) 1 billion times (b) 1 million times
(c) 100 times (d) 1000 times

**112.** If any protein encoding gene is expressed in a ________ host, it is called a ________ protein.
(a) Homologous host, recombinant
(b) Heterologous host, recombinant
(c) Heterologous host, non-recombinant
(d) Homologous host, non-recombinant

**113.** What is the maximum volume of culture that can be processed in bioreactors?
(a) 10–100 litres (b) 100–1000 litres
(c) 1–10 litres (d) 1000–1,00,000 litres

**114.** The host cultured in a continuous culture system where inside the used medium is drained out from one side while fresh medium is added from the other to maintain cells in their physiologically ________ phase.
(a) Lag (b) Log
(c) Stationary (d) Declining

**115.** Bioreactors have
(a) Foam control system, temperature control system
(b) Oxygen delivery system
(c) pH control system
(d) All the above

**116.** Which of the following will be done with product formed by rDNA technology?
(a) Product has to be formulated with suitable preservation.
(b) Formulation has to undergo clinical trials.
(c) Strict quality control testing is done.
(d) All the above

**117.** rDNA is a
(a) Chimeric DNA
(b) Hybrid DNA-RNA
(c) Recombinant of vector DNA and desired gene/s
(d) Both (a) and (c)

**118.** Plasmids are
(a) ssDNA (b) dsDNA (linear)
(c) dsDNA (circular) (d) denatured-DNA

**119.** The best cloning organism for genetic engineering and biotechnology is
(a) *Agrobacterium* (b) *Pseudomonas*
(c) *E. coli* (d) Lambda phage

**120.** Engineered bacterium carries
(a) Plasmids (b) rDNA
(c) cDNA (d) ssDNA

**121.** Engineered bacteria are reproduced by inserting
(a) Plasmids DNA
(b) Desired DNA (gene/s) loaded on vector DNA
(c) Vehicle DNA
(d) Phage DNA

**122.** Which of the following is a correct matching?

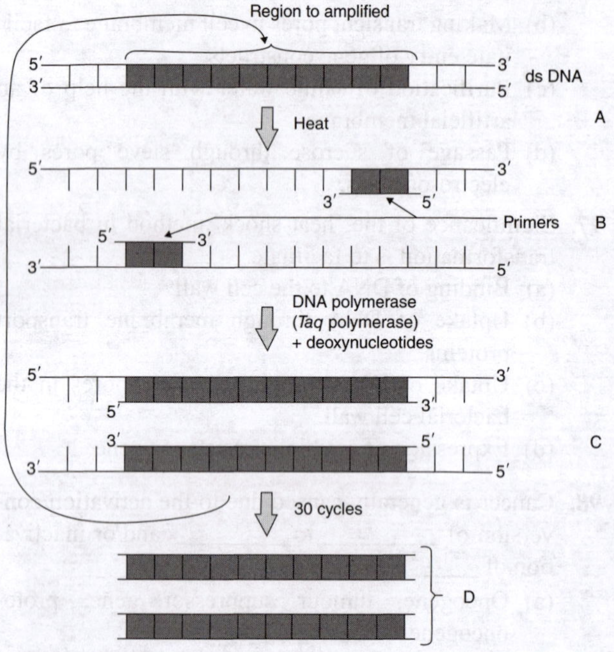


| | |
|---|---|
| (a) Denaturation | Occurs at room temperature |
| (b) Annealing | DNA polymerase is required for this process |
| (c) Extension | Taq polymerase and deoxynucleotides are required |
| (d) Amplification | 1 billion times in 10 cycles |

**123.** Electrophoresis and Southern blotting techniques are used in
(a) DNA fingerprinting (b) Gene synthesis
(c) Gene cloning (d) All of these

**124.** PCR technique was discovered by
(a) Hamilton Smith (b) Mullis
(c) E. Southern (d) Milstein

**125.** Genes for antibiotic resistance are located on
(a) Bacterial genome (b) Plasmids
(c) Mesosomes (d) Plasma membrane

**126.** The specific DNA sequence in which EcoRI cuts is
(a) GATTCG (b) GAATTC
(c) GTTCAA (d) TTCCAA

**127.** PCR is related to
(a) DNA cloning
(b) DNA amplification
(c) DNA selective replication
(d) All of these

**128.** ________ is the use of biology in industrial process and improvement of quality of life.
(a) Genetic engineering (b) Biotechnology
(c) Eugenics (d) Microbiology

**129.** PCR technique is considered as best for
(a) DNA synthesis (b) DNA amplification
(c) Protein synthesis (d) Amino acid synthesis

**130.** The enzyme used in PCR technology is
(a) DNA polymerase (b) Taq polymerase
(c) Reverse transcriptase (d) Both (a) and (b)

**131.** In the PCR technology, the DNA segment is replicated over a billion times. This repeated replication is catalyzed by the enzyme
(a) RNA polymerase
(b) Taq DNA polymerase
(c) DNA dependent RNA polymerase
(d) Primase

**132.** An antibiotic resistance gene in a vector usually helps in the selection of
(a) Competent cells (b) Transformed cells
(c) non-competent cells (d) None of these

**133.** The role of DNA ligase in the construction of a recombinant DNA molecule is
(a) Formation of phosphodiester bond between two DNA fragments.
(b) Formation of hydrogen bonds between sticky ends of DNA fragments.
(c) Ligation of all purine and pyrimidine bases.
(d) None of the above

**134.** Which of the following steps are catalysed by Taq polymerase in a PCR reaction?
(a) Denaturation of template DNA
(b) Annealing of primers to template DNA
(c) Extension of primer end on the template DNA
(d) All the above

**135.** A bacterial cell was transformed with a recombinant DNA that was generated using a human gene. However, the transformed cells did not produce the desired protein. Reasons could be
(a) Human gene may have intron which bacteria cannot process.
(b) Amino acid codons for humans and bacteria are different.
(c) Human protein is formed but degraded by bacteria.
(d) All the above

**136.** Which of the following should be chosen for best yield if one were to produce a recombinant protein in large amounts?
(a) Laboratory flask of largest capacity
(b) A stirred-tank bioreactor without inlets and outlets
(c) A continuous culture system
(d) Any of the above

**137.** Who among the following was awarded the Nobel Prize for the development of PCR technique?
(a) Herbert Boyer (b) Hargovind Khurana
(c) Kary Mullis (d) Arthur Kornberg

**138.** Which process is represented in following diagram?

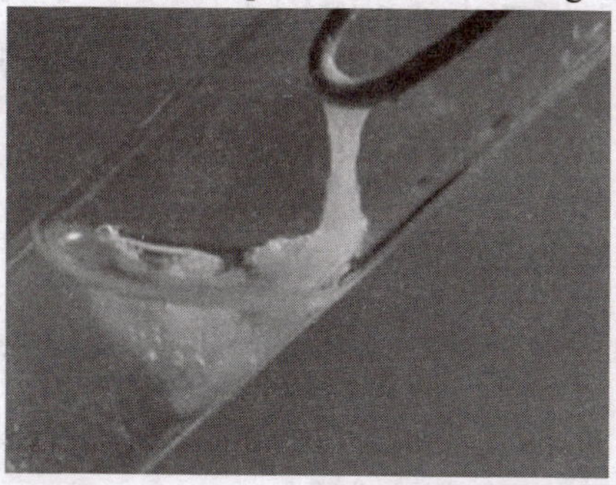

(a) PCR (b) DNA fingerprinting
(c) CTAB (d) DNA spooling

**139.** The source of Taq polymerase used in PCR technique is a
(a) Thermophilic fungus
(b) Mesophilic fungus
(c) Thermophilic bacteria
(d) Halophilic bacteria

**140.** The thermostable enzyme 'Taq' and 'Pfu' isolated from thermophilic bacteria are
(a) RNA polymerase
(b) DNA polymerase
(c) Restriction endonuclease
(d) DNA ligase

**141.** The process of removing DNA after precipitation by chilled ethanol is called
(a) Elusion
(b) Spooling
(c) Downstream processing
(d) Upstream processing

**142.** AGE is used
(a) To check progression of restriction enzyme digestion
(b) To separate DNA fragments
(c) To purity fragments of DNA
(d) All of these

**143.** To check the progression of restriction enzyme digestion of DNA, the technique used is
(a) AGE (b) PAGE
(c) Southern blotting (d) Northern blotting

**144.** Small chemically synthesized oligonucleotides which are complementary to regions of DNA and used in PCR, are called
(a) Probes
(b) Primers
(c) Initiation sequences
(d) Termination sequences

**145.** The mixture of PCR reaction contains
(a) ds DNA + DNA polymerase + One set of primers
(b) ds DNA + DNA polymerase + One set of primers + deoxyoligonucleotides
(c) ds DNA + DNA polymerase + two sets of primers
(d) ds DNA + DNA polymerase + two sets of primers + deoxyoligonucleotides

**146.** Assertion: The expression of recombination DNA in host cells in of utmost importance.
Reason: The ultimate aim of almost all recombinant technologies is to produce the desirable protein.
(a) (A) is false but (R) is true
(b) Both (A) and (R) are true and (R) is the correct explanation of (A)
(c) Both (A) and (R) are true but (R) is not the correct explanation of (A)
(d) (A) is true but (R) is false.

**147.** The cells harbouring cloned genes of interest can be obtained by
(a) Growing on small scale in laboratory
(b) Using bioreactors to produce large volumes
(c) Continuous culture system to maintain cells in log phase
(d) All of these

**148.** Higher yields of desired protein is possible with
(a) Small scale production in laboratory
(b) Continuous culture system
(c) Use of large scale bioreactors
(d) Both b & c

**149.** The speciality of a stirred type reactor is
(a) to maintain optimum temperature
(b) to facilitate even mixing
(c) to facilitate oxygen availability in reactor
(d) Both b & c

**150.** Sampling ports on bioreactors are used
(a) To add raw materials
(b) To maintain temperature
(c) To withdraw small volumes of cultures
(d) To control foam

**151.** After completion of synthesis of desired product, it should undergo,
(a) Separation and purification
(b) Formulation with preservatives
(c) Quality control testing
(d) All of these

**152.** In biotechnological applications, what is the role of downstream processing?
(A) Purification of desired products.
(B) Isolation of genetic material.
(C) Introduction of foreign genes.
(D) Amplification of DNA.
(a) A only (b) B and D only
(c) A and C only (d) A and B only

**153.** What is the role of restriction enzymes in genetic engineering?
(A) Amplification of DNA.
(B) Cutting DNA at specific recognition sites.
(C) Introduction of foreign genes into plasmids.
(D) Purification of DNA fragments.
(a) A and C only (b) B and D only
(c) B and C only (d) B only

## Multiple Choice Questions: Level II

**154.** Transgenic plants are the ones
(a) generated by introducing foreign DNA into a cell and regenerating a plant from that cell
(b) produced after protoplast fusion in artificial medium
(c) grown in artificial medium after hybridization in the field
(d) produced by a somatic embryo in artificial medium

**155.** The linking of antibiotic resistance gene with the plasmid vector became possible with
(a) DNA polymerase (b) exonucleases
(c) DNA ligase (d) endonucleases

**156.** Restriction endonuclease
(a) cuts the DNA molecule at specific sites
(b) restricts the synthesis of DNA inside the nucleus
(c) synthesizes DNA
(d) cuts the DNA molecules randomly

**157.** Two microbes found to be very useful in genetic engineering are
(a) *Vibrio cholerae* and a tailed bacteriophage
(b) *Diplococcus sp.* and *Pseudomonas sp.*
(c) Crown gall bacterium and *Caenorhabditis elegans*
(d) *Escherichia coli* and *Agrobacterium tumefaciens*

**158.** Production of human protein in bacteria by genetic engineering is possible because
(a) the human chromosome can replicate in bacterial cell
(b) the mechanism of gene regulation is identical in human and bacteria
(c) bacterial cell can carry out the RNA splicing reactions
(d) the genetic code is universal

**159.** The Ti plasmid is often used for making transgenic plants. This plasmid is found in
(a) Azotobacter
(b) Rhizobium of the roots of leguminous plants
(c) Agrobacterium
(d) Yeast as a 2 μm plasmid

**160.** Which of the following enzymes are used to join bits of DNA?
(a) ligase (b) primase
(c) DNA polymerase (d) endonuclease

**161.** Manipulation of DNA in genetic engineering became possible due to the discovery of
(a) restriction endonuclease
(b) DNA ligase
(c) transcriptase
(d) primase

**162.** Which of the following cuts DNA at specific sites?
(a) Restriction endonuclease (*E.coli*)
(b) Ligase
(c) Exonuclease
(d) Alkaline phosphate

**163.** Which of the following properties make plasmids suitable vectors for gene cloning?
(a) Plasmids often carry antibiotic resistance gene
(b) Plasmids can shuttle between prokaryotic and eukaryotic cells
(c) plasmids are small circular DNA molecules with their own replication origin site
(d) Plasmids are small circular DNA molecules that can integrate with chromosomal DNA

**164.** One bacterium which is extensively used in genetic engineering work in plants is
(a) *Agrobacterium tumefaciens*
(b) *Bacillus coagulens*
(c) *Xanthomonas citri*
(d) *Clostridium septicum*

**165.** Introduction of one or more genes into an organism which normally does not possess them or their deletion by using artificial means (not by breeding) comes under
(a) molecular biology
(b) cytogenetics
(c) genetic hybridization
(d) genetic engineering

**166.** Which of the following is related to genetic engineering?
(a) Plastid (b) Plasmid
(c) Heterosis (d) Heterocyst

**167.** The chemical knives of DNA are
(a) Polymerases
(b) Endonucleases
(c) Transcriptase
(d) Ligases

**168.** Recombinant DNA is achieved by cleaving the pro DNAs by
(a) Exonucleases
(b) Ligase
(c) Restriction endonuclease
(d) Primase

**169.** Restriction endonucleases are
(a) synthesized by bacteria as part of their defence mechanism
(b) use for in vitro DNA synthesis
(c) used in genetic engineering for ligating two DNA molecules
(d) present in mammalian cells for degradation of DNA when the cell dies

**170.** Genetic engineering is possible because
(a) we can see DNA by electron microscope
(b) we can cut DNA at specific sites by endonucleases like DNase I
(c) restriction endonucleases purified from bacteria can be used in vitro
(d) the phenomenon of transduction in bacteria is well understood

**171.** An enzyme that joins the ends of two strands of nucleic acid is a
(a) polymerase (b) synthetase
(c) helicase (d) ligase

# A & R and Statement-based Questions

## Assertion and Reason Questions

***Direction for questions 172 to 176:** Read the **assertion** and **reason** carefully to mark the correct option out of the options given below:*

(a) **(A)** is **true** but **(R)** is **false**.
(b) **(A)** is **false** but **(R)** is **true**.
(c) Both **(A)** and **(R)** is **true** and **(R)** is the correct explanation of **(A)**.
(d) Both **(A)** and **(R)** is **true** and **(R)** is not the correct explanation of **(A)**.

**172. Assertion:** Plasmid can be used as vector for recombinant DNA technology.
**Reason:** Plasmid is autonomously replicating DNA.

**173. Assertion:** During electrophoresis DNA moves towards cathode.
**Reason:** DNA is negatively charged molecule.

**174. Assertion:** Retrovirus have ability to transform normal animal cell into cancerous cell.
**Reason:** Retrovirus can convert protooncogene into oncogene in normal cell.

**175. Assertion:** In Eco RI, the latter 'co' is derived from the species of bacteria from which it is obtained.
**Reason:** Eco RI is the name of bacteria that can infect virus.

**176. Assertion:** Restrictions endonuclease are known as molecular scissors.
**Reason:** They can cut DNA (biomolecule) at specific site.

## Statement-based Questions:

***Direction for questions 177 to 178:** These type of questions consist of two statement each, printed as **Statement-I** and **Statement-II**. While answering such questions, a student is needed to choose any one of the following four responses.*

(a) **Statement I** is **correct Statement II** is **incorrect**.
(b) **Statement I** is **incorrect Statement II** is **correct**.
(c) Both **Statement I** and **Statement II** are **correct**.
(d) Both **Statement I** and **Statement II** are **incorrect**.

**177. Statement-I:** Two enzyme responsible for restricting the growth of bacteriophages in E coli were isolated in 1963.
**Statement-II:** The one which add methyl group to DNA is known as restriction endonuclease.

**178. Statement-I:** Presence of more than one restriction site in vector will ease the process of gene cloning.
**Statement-II:** Fragments of DNA can be separated by electrophoresis.

**179. Statement-I:** Extraction of electrophoresed DNA from agar gel piece is known as elution.
**Statement-II:** Purified DNA is finally precipitated out by using chilled ethanol.

**180. Statement-I:** By microinjection process, rDNA is directly injected into animal cell nucleus.
**Statement-II:** Disarmed pathogen vector can be used to transfer r DNA to host cell.

**181. Statement-I:** Large scale production of biotechnological products require bioreactor.
**Statement-II:** Downstream processing include separation and purification of products.

# Matrix-Match Type Questions

**182.** Match the following:

| List-I (Enzymes) | List-II (Action) |
|---|---|
| 1. Restriction enzymes | (i) Enzymes removing nucleotides from the ends of the DNA |
| 2. Exonucleases | (ii) Enzymes responsible for cutting DNA at specific locations |
| 3. Endonucleases | (iii) Enzymes responsible for joining cut ends of DNA |
| 4. Ligase | (iv) Enzymes making cuts at specific positions within DNA |

**The correct matching is**

| | 1 | 2 | 3 | 4 |
|---|---|---|---|---|
| (a) | (ii) | (i) | (iv) | (iii) |
| (b) | (i) | (ii) | (iv) | (iii) |
| (c) | (iv) | (i) | (iii) | (ii) |
| (d) | (iii) | (i) | (iv) | (ii) |

**183.** Match the following:

| I (Name of Restriction Enzymes ex. EcoRI) | II (Convention for Naming) |
|---|---|
| 1. E | (i) First letter of the name of strain |
| 2. co | (ii) Order in which enzymes were isolated from the strain of bacteria |
| 3. R | (iii) First letter of the name of genus |
| 4. I | (iv) Two letters of the name of species |

**The correct matching is**

| | 1 | 2 | 3 | 4 |
|---|---|---|---|---|
| (a) | (iii) | (iv) | (i) | (ii) |
| (b) | (i) | (ii) | (iv) | (iii) |
| (c) | (iv) | (i) | (iii) | (ii) |
| (d) | (iii) | (i) | (iv) | (ii) |

**184.** Match the following:

| List-I (Sequence) | List-II (Site) |
|---|---|
| 1. ORI sequence | (i) Sequence of DNA base pairs reads same on the two strands |
| 2. Recognition sequence | (ii) Specific DNA sequence for initiation of DNA replication |
| 3. Palindrome sequence | (iii) Specific base sequence on DNA where restriction enzyme cuts DNA |

**The correct matching is**

| | 1 | 2 | 3 |
|---|---|---|---|
| (a) | (ii) | (iii) | (i) |
| (b) | (iii) | (i) | (ii) |
| (c) | (ii) | (i) | (iii) |
| (d) | (i) | (iii) | (ii) |

**185.** Match the following:

| List-I | List-II |
|---|---|
| 1. Elution | (i) Autonomously replicating circular extra-chromosomal DNA |
| 2. Cloning | (ii) Introduction of foreign DNA into a host |
| 3. Plasmid | (iii) Process for separation of DNA fragments |
| 4. Electrophoresis | (iv) Extraction of DNA fragments from gel |
| 5. Transformation | (v) Process of making multiple identical copies of template DNA |

**The correct matching is**

| | 1 | 2 | 3 | 4 | 5 |
|---|---|---|---|---|---|
| (a) | (iv) | (v) | (i) | (iii) | (ii) |
| (b) | (ii) | (iii) | (v) | (i) | (iv) |
| (c) | (iv) | (v) | (iii) | (i) | (ii) |
| (d) | (ii) | (v) | (i) | (iii) | (iv) |

**186.** Match the following:

| List-I (Technique) | List-II (Use) |
|---|---|
| 1. Bioreactor | (i) Selection of transformed cells |
| 2. Downstream Processing | (ii) In vitro synthesis of multiple copies of gene of interest |
| 3. Selectable marker | (iii) Separation & purification of desired product |
| 4. PCR | (iv) Production of desired recombinant protein on larger scale |

**The correct matching is**

| | 1 | 2 | 3 | 4 |
|---|---|---|---|---|
| (a) | (iv) | (iii) | (i) | (ii) |
| (b) | (i) | (iii) | (iv) | (ii) |
| (c) | (iv) | (i) | (iii) | (ii) |
| (d) | (iii) | (i) | (iv) | (ii) |

## NCERT Exemplar Questions

1. Which of the following enzyme catalyze the removal of nucleotides from the ends of DNA?
(a) Endonuclease (b) Exonuclease
(c) DNA ligase (d) Hind-II

2. The transfer of genetic material from one bacterium to another through the mediation of a viral vector is termed as
(a) Transduction (b) Conjugation
(c) Transformation (d) Translation

3. Which of the given statement is correct in the context of visualizing DNA molecules separated by agarose gel electrophoresis?
(a) DNA can be seen in visible light.
(b) DNA can be seen without staining in visible light.
(c) Ethidium bromide stained DNA can be seen in visible light.
(d) Ethidium bromide stained DNA can be seen under exposure to UV light.

4. 'Restriction' in restriction enzyme refers to
(a) Cleaving of phosphodiester bond in DNA by the enzyme.
(b) Cutting of DNA at specific position only.
(c) Prevention of the multiplication of bacteriophage in bacteria.
(d) All of the above

5. Which of the following is not required in the preparation of recombinant DNA molecule?
(a) Restriction endonuclease
(b) DNA ligase
(c) DNA fragments
(d) *E. coli*

6. In agarose gel electrophoresis, DNA molecules are separated on the basis of their
(a) Charge only (b) Size only
(c) Charge to size ratio (d) All of the above

7. The important feature in a plasmid to serve as a vector in gene cloning programme is
(a) Origin of replication (ori)
(b) Presence of a selectable marker
(c) Presence of sites for restriction endonuclease
(d) All of the above

8. While isolating DNA from bacteria, which of the following enzymes is not used?
(a) Lysozyme (b) Ribonuclease
(c) Deoxyribonuclease (d) Protease

9. Which of the following contributed in popularizing the PCR (Polymerase Chain Reactions) technique?
(a) Easy availability of DNA template
(b) Availability of synthetic primers
(c) Availability of cheap deoxyribonucleotides
(d) Availability of 'Thermostable' DNA polymerase

10. Significance of 'heat shock' method in bacterial transformation is to facilitate
(a) Binding of DNA to the cell wall.
(b) Uptake of DNA through membrane transport proteins.
(c) Uptake of DNA through transient pores in the bacterial cell wall.
(d) Expression of antibiotic resistance gene.

11. The role of DNA ligase in the construction of a recombinant DNA molecule is
(a) Formation of phosphodiester bond between two DNA fragments.
(b) Formation of hydrogen bonds between sticky ends of DNA fragments.
(c) Ligation of all purine and pyrimidine bases.
(d) None of the above

12. Which of the following bacteria is not a source of restriction endonuclease?
(a) *Haemophilus influenzae*
(b) *Escherichia coli*
(c) *Agrobacterium tumefaciens*
(d) *Bacillius amyloli quefaciens*

13. Which of the following steps are catalysed by *Taq* DNA polymerase in a PCR reaction?
(a) Denaturation of template DNA
(b) Annealing of primers to template DNA
(c) Extension of primer end on the template DNA
(d) All of the above

14. Which of the following statements does not hold true for restriction enzyme?
(a) It recognizes a palindromic nucleotide sequence
(b) It is an endonuclease
(c) It is isolated from viruses
(d) It produces the same kind of sticky ends in different DNA molecules

## Previous Years' Questions

1. Stirred-tank bioreactors have been designed for [AIPMT 2010 PRE]
   (a) Addition of preservatives of the product
   (b) Purification of the product
   (c) Ensuring anaerobic conditions in the culture vessel
   (d) Availability of oxygen throughout the process

2. Restriction endonucleases are enzymes which [AIPMT 2010 PRE]
   (a) Make cuts at specific positions within the DNA molecule
   (b) Recognize a specific nucleotide sequence for binding of DNA ligase
   (c) Restrict the action of the enzyme DNA polymerase
   (d) Remove nucleotides from the ends of the DNA molecule

3. Which one of the following palindromic base sequences in DNA can be easily cut at the middle by some particular restriction enzyme? [AIPMT 2010 PRE]
   (a) 5′–CGTTCG –3′
   3′–ATGGTA–5′
   (b) 5′-GATATG–3′
   3′–CTACTA–5′
   (c) 5′–GAATTC–3′
   3′–CTTAAG–5′
   (d) 5′–CACGTA–3′
   3′–CTCAGT– 5′

4. In genetic engineering, a DNA segment (gene) of interest is transferred to the host cell through a vector. Consider the following four agents (A–D) in this regard and select the correct option about which one or more of these can be used as a vector/vectors
   (a) A Bacterium (b) Plasmid
   (c) Plasmodium (d) Bacteriophage
   [AIPMT 2010 MAINS]
   (a) (A), (B) & (D) only (b) (A) only
   (c) (A) & (C) only (d) (B) & (D) only

5. Which of the following are used in gene cloning? [AIPMT 2010 MAINS]
   (a) Nucleosides (b) Lomasomes
   (c) Mesosomes (d) Plasmids

6. Which one of the following is now being commercially produced by biotechnological procedures? [AIPMT 2010 MAINS]
   (a) Nicotine (b) Morphine
   (c) Quinine (d) Insulin

7. Agarose extracted from sea weeds finds use in [AIPMT 2011 PRE]
   (a) Tissue culture
   (b) PCR
   (c) Gel electrophoresis
   (d) Spectrophotometry

8. There is a restriction endonuclease called Eco RI. What does 'co' part in it stand for? [AIPMT 2011 PRE]
   (a) Coelom (b) Coenzyme
   (c) coli (d) Colon

9. Given below is a sample portion of DNA strand giving the base sequence on the opposite strands. What is so special shown in it? [AIPMT 2011 PRE]
   5′_GAATTC_3′
   3′_CTTAAG_5′
   (a) Deletion mutation
   (b) Start codon at the 5′ end
   (c) Palindromic sequence of base pairs
   (d) Replication completed

10. Which one of the following techniques made it possible to genetically engineer living organisms? [AIPMT 2011 MAINS]
    (a) Recombinant DNA techniques
    (b) X-ray diffraction
    (c) Heavier isotope labelling
    (d) Hybridization

11. For transformation, micro-particles coated with DNA to be bombarded with gene gun are made up of: [AIPMT 2012 PRE]
    (a) Silver or Platinum
    (b) Platinum or Zinc
    (c) Silicon or Platinum
    (d) Gold or Tungsten

12. Which one is a true statement regarding DNA polymerase used in PCR? [AIPMT 2012 PRE]
    (a) It is used to ligate introduced DNA in recipient cells
    (b) It serves as a selectable marker
    (c) It is isolated from a virus
    (d) It remains active at high temperature

13. The figure below is the diagrammatic representation of the *E. coli* vector pBR 322. Which one of the given options correctly identifies its certain component(s)?

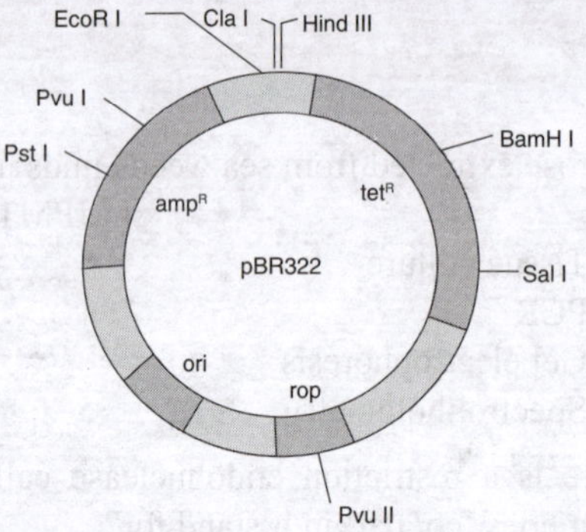


[AIPMT 2012 PRE]

(a) Ori-original restriction enzyme
(b) Rop-reduced osmotic pressure
(c) Hind III, EcoRI-selectable markers
(d) amp$^R$, tet$^R$-antibiotic resistance genes

**14.** Biolistics (gene-gun) is suitable for: [AIPMT 2012 MAINS]

(a) Transformation of plant cells
(b) Constructing recombinant DNA by joining with vectors
(c) DNA fingerprinting
(d) Disarming pathogen vectors

**15.** Which one of the following represents a palindromic sequence in DNA cut by Eco RI? [AIPMT 2012 MAINS]

(a) 5′–CCAATG–3′
3′–GAATCC–5′
(b) 5′–CATTAG–3′
3′–GATAAC–5′
(c) 5′–GATACC–3′
3′–CCTAAG–5′
(d) 5′–GAATTC–3′
3′–CTTAAG–5′

**16.** The figure below shows three steps (A, B, C) of Polymerase Chain Reaction (PCR). Select the option giving correct identification together with what it represents? [AIPMT 2012 MAINS]

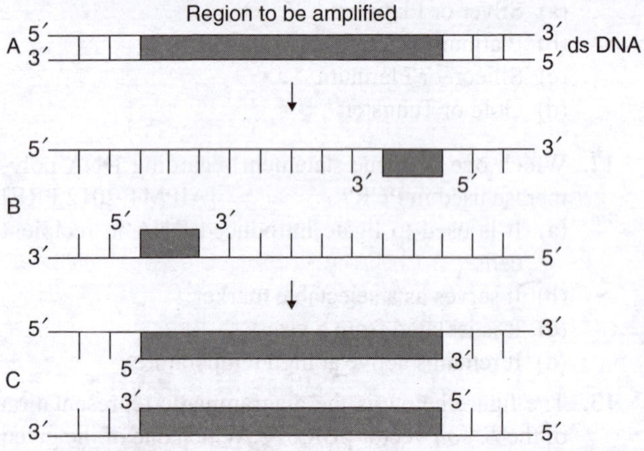


**Options**:

(a) A: Denaturation at a temperature of about 50ºC
(b) C: Extension in the presence of heat stable DNA polymerase
(c) A: Annealing with two sets of primers
(d) B: Denaturation at a temperature of about 98ºC separating the two DNA strands

**17.** In genetic engineering, the antibiotics are used: [AIPMT 2012 MAINS]

(a) To select healthy vectors
(b) As sequences from where replication starts
(c) To keep the cultures free of infection
(d) As selectable markers

**18.** Which of the following is not correctly matched for the organism and its cell wall degrading enzyme? [AIPMT 2013]

(a) Bacteria – Lysozyme
(b) Plant cells – Cellulase
(c) Algae – Methylase
(d) Fungi – Chitinase

**19.** DNA fragments generated by the restriction endonucleases in a chemical reaction can be separated by: [AIPMT 2013]

(a) Centrifugation
(b) Polymerase chain reaction
(c) Electrophoresis
(d) Restriction mapping

**20.** Which vector can be cloned only a small fragment of DNA? [AIPMT 2014]

(a) Bacteria artificial chromosome
(b) Yeast artificial chromosome
(c) Plasmid
(d) Cosmid

**21.** The DNA molecule to which the gene of interest is integrated for cloning is called: [RE-AIPMT 2015]

(a) Vector (b) Template
(c) Carrier (d) Transformer

**22.** The cutting of DNA at specific locations is possible with the discovery of: [RE-AIPMT 2015]

(a) Probes (b) Selectable markers
(c) Ligases (d) Restriction enzymes

**23.** Which of the following restriction enzymes produce blunt ends? [NEET 2016 – PHASE II]

(a) *Eco RV* (b) *Xho I*
(c) *Hind III* (d) *Sal I*

**24.** Which of the following is not a component of downstream processing? [NEET 2016 – PHASE II]

(a) Purification (b) Preservation
(c) Expression (d) Separation

**25.** A foreign DNA and plasmid cut by the same restriction end nuclease can be joined to form a recombinant plasmid using [NEET 2016 – PHASE II]
(a) *Taq polymerase* (b) *Polymerase III*
(c) *Ligase* (d) *Eco RI*

**26.** Stirred-tank bioreactors have been designed for [NEET 2016 – PHASE II]
(a) Addition of preservatives to the product.
(b) Availability of oxygen throughout the process.
(c) Ensuring anaerobic conditions in the culture vessel.
(d) Purification of the product.

**27.** Which of the following is a restriction endonuclease? [NEET 2016 – PHASE I]
(a) Hind II (b) Protease
(c) DNase I (d) RNase

**28.** The taq polymerase enzyme is obtained from: [NEET 2016 – PHASE I]
(a) *Thermus aquaticus*
(b) *Thiobacillus ferroxidans*
(c) *Bacillus subtilis*
(d) *Pseudomonas putida*

**29.** Which of the following is not a feature of the plasmids? [NEET 2016 – PHASE I]
(a) Independent replication
(b) Circular structure
(c) Transferable
(d) Single-stranded

**30.** Restriction endonucleases are : [NEET Regionl 2017]
(a) Used in genetic engineering for ligating two DNA molecules.
(b) Used for in vitro DNA synthesis.
(c) Synthesized by bacteria as part of their defense mechanism.
(d) Present in mammalian cell for degradation of DNA when the cells dies.

**31.** What is the criterion for DNA fragments movement on agarose gel during gel electrophoresis? [NEET 2017]
(a) The smaller the fragment size, the farther it moves.
(b) Positively charged fragments move to farther end.
(c) Negatively charged fragments do not move.
(d) The larger the fragment size, the farther it moves.

**32.** A gene whose expression helps to identify transformed cell is known as: [NEET 2017]
(a) Vector (b) Plasmid
(c) Structural gene (d) Selectable marker

**33.** The process of separation and purification of expressed protein before marketing is called [NEET 2017]
(a) Downstream processing
(b) Bioprocessing
(c) Postproduction processing
(d) Upstream processing

**34.** The DNA fragments separated on an agarose gel can be visualized after staining with: [NEET 2017]
(a) Acetocarmine (b) Aniline blue
(c) Ethidium bromide (d) Bromophenol blue

**35.** DNA fragments are: [NEET 2017]
(a) Negatively charged
(b) Neutral
(c) Either positively or negatively charged depending on their size
(d) Positively charged

**36.** The correct order of steps in Polymerase Chain Reaction (PCR) is [NEET 2018]
(a) Extension, Denaturation, Annealing
(b) Denaturation, Extension, Annealing
(c) Annealing, Extension, Denaturation
(d) Denaturation, Annealing, Extension

**37.** DNA precipitation out of a mixture of biomolecules can be achieved by treatment with: [NEET 2019]
(a) Chilled ethanol
(b) Methanol at room temperature
(c) Chilled chloroform
(d) Isopropanol

**38.** Following statements describe the characteristics of the enzyme Restriction Endonuclease. Identify the **incorrect** statement. [NEET 2019]
(a) The enzyme binds DNA at specific sites and cuts only one of the two strands.
(b) The enzyme cuts the sugar-phosphate backbone at specific sites on each strand.
(c) The enzyme recognizes a specific palindromic nucleotide sequence in the DNA.
(d) The enzyme cuts DNA molecule at identified position within the DNA.

**39.** Which one of the following equipment is essentially required for growing microbes on a large scale for industrial production of enzymes? [NEET 2019]
(a) Sludge digester (b) Industrial oven
(c) Bioreactor (d) BOD incubator

**40.** In gel electrophoresis, separated DNA fragments can be visualized with the help of: [NEET 2020]
(a) Acetocarmine in bright blue light

(b) Ethidium bromide UV radiation
(c) Acetocarmine in UV radiation
(d) Ethidium bromide in infrared radiation

**41.** Identify the **wrong** statement with regard to Restriction Enzymes [NEET 2020]
(a) Each restriction enzyme functions by inspecting the length of a DNA sequence.
(b) They cut the strand of DNA at palindrome sites.
(c) They are useful in genetic engineering.
(d) Sticky ends can be joined by using DNA ligases.

**42.** Choose the **correct** pair from the following: [NEET 2020]

| | | |
|---|---|---|
| (a) Ligases | – | Join the two DNA molecules |
| (b) Polymerases | – | Break the DNA into fragments |
| (c) Nucleases | – | Separate the two strands of DNA |
| (d) Exonucleases | – | Make cuts at specific positions within DNA |

**43.** The sequence that controls the copy number of the linked DNA in the vector, is termed : [NEET 2020]
(a) Selectable marker (b) Ori site
(c) Palindromic sequence (d) Recognition site

**44.** The specific palindromic sequence which is recognized by EcoRI is: [NEET 2020]
(a) 5′ - GAATTC - 3′ 3′ - CTTAAG - 5′
(b) 5′ - GGAACC - 3′ 3′ - CCTTGG - 5′
(c) 5′ - CTTAAG - 3′ 3′ - GAATTC - 5′
(d) 5′ - GGATCC - 3′ 3′ - CCTAGG - 5′

**45.** DNA strands on a gel stained with ethidium bromide when viewed under UV radiation, appear as: [NEET 2021]
(a) Bright blue bands (b) Yellow bands
(c) Bright orange bands (d) Dark red bands

**46.** During the process of gene amplification using PCR, if very high temperature is not maintained in the beginning, then which of the following steps of PCR will be affected first? [NEET 2021]
(a) Ligation (b) Annealing
(c) Extension (d) Denaturation

**47.** A specific recognition sequence identified by endonucleases to make cuts at specific positions within the DNA is [NEET 2021]
(a) Poly(A) tail sequences
(b) Degenerate primer sequence
(c) Okazaki sequences
(d) Palindromic Nucleotide sequences

**48.** During the purification process for recombinant DNA technology, addition of chilled ethanol precipitates out: [NEET 2021]
(a) Polysaccharides
(b) RNA
(c) DNA
(d) Histones

**49.** Plasmid pBR322 has Pst 1 restriction enzyme site within gene $amp^R$ that confers ampicillin resistance. If this enzyme is used for inserting a gene for β-galactosidase production and the recombinant plasmid is inserted in an *E.coli* strain [NEET 2021]
(a) it will be able to produce a novel protein with dual ability.
(b) it will not be able to confer ampicillin resistance to the host cell.
(c) the transformed cells will have the ability to resist ampicillin as well as produce β-galactoside.
(d) it will lead to lysis of host cell.

**50.** Which one of the following statement is **not true** regarding gel electrophoresis technique? [NEET 2022]
(a) The separated DNA fragments are stained by using ethidium bromide.
(b) The presence of chromogenic substrate gives blue coloured DNA bands on the gel.
(c) Bright orange coloured bands of DNA can be observed in the gel when exposed to UV light.
(d) The process of extraction of separated DNA strands from gel is called elution.

**51.** Given below are two statements: one is labelled as **Assertion (A)** and the other is labelled as **Reason (R)**. [NEET 2022]

**Assertion (A):** Polymerase chain reaction is used in DNA amplification.

**Reason (R):** The ampicillin resistant gene is used as a selectable marker to check transformation.

In the light of the above statements, choose the **correct** answer from the options given below:
(a) Both **(A)** and **(R)** are correct but **(R)** is not the correct explanation of **(A)**.
(b) **(A)** is correct but **(R)** is not correct.
(c) **(A)** is not correct but **(R)** is correct.
(d) Both **(A)** and **(R)** are correct and **(R)** is the correct explanation of **(A)**.

**52.** In the following palindromic base sequences of DNA, which one can be cut easily by particular restriction enzyme? [NEET 2022]

(a) 5′ G A A T T C 3′, 3′ C T T A A G 5′
(b) 5′ C T C A G T 3′, 3′ G A G T C A 5′
(c) 5′ G T A T T C 3′, 3′ C A T A A G 5′
(d) 5′ G A T A C T 3′, 3′ C T A T G A 5′

**53.** Given below are two statements: [NEET 2022]

**Statement I:** Restriction endonucleases recognise specific sequence to cut DNA known as palindromic nucleotide sequence.

**Statement II:** Restriction endonucleases cut the DNA strand a little away from the centre of the palindromic site.

In the light of the above statements, choose the **most appropriate** answer from the options given below:
(a) Both **Statement I** and **Statement II** are incorrect.
(b) **Statement I** is correct but **Statement II** is incorrect.
(c) **Statement I** is incorrect but **Statement II** is correct.
(d) Both **Statement I** and **Statement II** are correct.

**54.** Which of the following is **not** a desirable feature of a cloning vector? [NEET 2022]
(a) Presence of a marker gene.
(b) Presence of single restriction enzyme site.
(c) Presence of two or more recognition sites.
(d) Presence of origin of replication.

**55.** During the purification process for recombinant DNA technology, addition of chilled ethanol precipitates out: [NEET 2023]
(a) DNA (b) Histones
(c) Polysaccharides (d) RNA

**56.** In gene gun method used to introduce alien DNA into host cells, microparticles of ________ metal are used. [NEET 2023]
(a) Zinc (b) Tungsten or gold
(c) Silver (d) Copper

**57.** Upon exposure to UV radiation, DNA stained with ethidium bromide will show: [NEET 2023]
(a) Bright blue colour
(b) Bright yellow colour
(c) Bright orange colour
(d) Bright red colour

**58.** Main steps in the formation of Recombinant DNA are given below. Arrange these steps in a correct sequence. [NEET 2023]
A. Insertion of recombinants DNA into host cell.
B. Cutting of DNA at specific location by restriction enzyme.
C. Isolation of desired DNA fragment.
D. Amplification of gene of interests using PCR.

Choose the correct answer from the options given below:
(a) C, A, B, D (b) C, B, D, A
(c) B, D, A, C (d) B, C, D, A

**59.** What is the fate of a piece of DAN carrying only gene of interest which is transferred into an alien organism? [NEET 2024]
A The piece of DNA would be able to multiply itself independently in the progeny cells of the organism.
B It may get integrated into the genome of the recipient.
C In may multiply and be inherited along with the host DNA.
D The alien piece of DNA is not an integral part of chromosome.
E It shows ability to replicate.

Choose the correct answer from the options given below:
(a) A and B only (b) D and E only
(c) B and C only (d) A and E only

**60.** Hind II always cuts DNA molecules at a particular point called recognition sequence and it consists of: [NEET 2024]
(a) 8 bp (b) 6 bp
(c) 4 bp (d) 10 bp

**61.** The capacity to generate a whole plant from any cell of the plant is called: [NEET 2024]
(a) Totipotency (b) Micropropagation
(c) Differentation (d) Somatic hybridization

**62.** Which of the following are fused in somatic hybridization involving two varieties of plants? [NEET 2024]
(a) Callus (b) Somatic embryos
(c) Protoplasts (d) Pollens

**63.** Which of the following statements is incorrect? [NEET 2024]
(a) A bio-reactor provides optimal growth conditions for achieving the desired product.
(b) Most commonly used bio-reactors are of stirring type.
(c) Bio-reactors are used to produce small scale bactcrial cultures.
(d) Bio-reactors have an agitator system, an oxygen delivery system and foam control system.

**64.** The following diagram showing restriction sites in *E.coli* cloning vector pBR322. Find the role of 'X' and 'Y' genes. [NEET 2024]

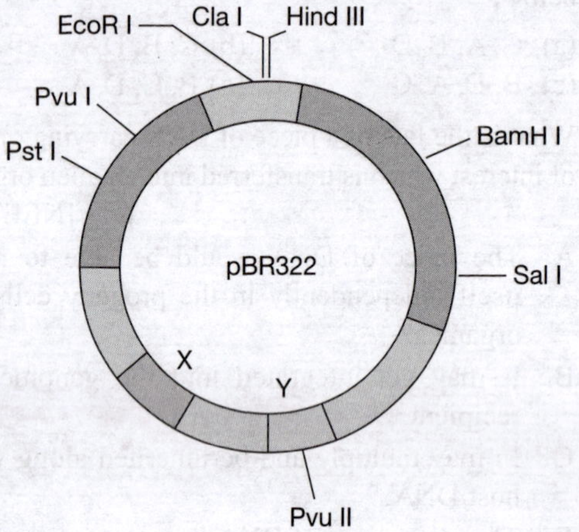


(a) The gene 'X' is responsible for resistance to antibiotics and 'Y' for protein involved in the replication of Plasmid.
(b) The gene 'X' is responsible for controlling the copy number of the linked DNA and 'Y' for protein involved in the replication of Plasmid.
(c) The gene 'X' is for protein involved in replication of Plasmid and 'Y' for resistance to antibiotics.
(d) Gene 'X' is responsible for recognition sites and 'Y' is responsible for antibiotic resistance.

**65.** The "Ti plasmid" of *Agrobacterium tumefaciens* stands for [NEET 2024]
(a) Tumour inhibiting plasmid.
(b) Tumour independent plasmid.
(c) Tumour inducing plasmid.
(d) Temperature independent plasmid.

## Answer Key

### Multiple Choice Questions: Level I

| | | | | | | | | | |
|---|---|---|---|---|---|---|---|---|---|
| 1. (d) | 2. (a) | 3. (d) | 4. (d) | 5. (d) | 6. (d) | 7. (b) | 8. (d) | 9. (d) | 10. (b) |
| 11. (a) | 12. (d) | 13. (c) | 14. (d) | 15. (d) | 16. (c) | 17. (b) | 18. (d) | 19. (d) | 20. (c) |
| 21. (a) | 22. (a) | 23. (c) | 24. (b) | 25. (b) | 26. (d) | 27. (d) | 28. (c) | 29. (b) | 30. (a) |
| 31. (c) | 32. (a) | 33. (b) | 34. (a) | 35. (b) | 36. (b) | 37. (c) | 38. (b) | 39. (a) | 40. (b) |
| 41. (b) | 42. (a) | 43. (c) | 44. (a) | 45. (c) | 46. (c) | 47. (a) | 48. (b) | 49. (c) | 50. (d) |
| 51. (c) | 52. (b) | 53. (b) | 54. (a) | 55. (b) | 56. (a) | 57. (c) | 58. (d) | 59. (c) | 60. (d) |
| 61. (c) | 62. (b) | 63. (b) | 64. (d) | 65. (b) | 66. (b) | 67. (b) | 68. (b) | 69. (a) | 70. (d) |
| 71. (a) | 72. (c) | 73. (b) | 74. (d) | 75. (a) | 76. (c) | 77. (c) | 78. (b) | 79. (b) | 80. (a) |
| 81. (d) | 82. (d) | 83. (c) | 84. (d) | 85. (a) | 86. (a) | 87. (c) | 88. (c) | 89. (b) | 90. (d) |
| 91. (a) | 92. (c) | 93. (d) | 94. (d) | 95. (b) | 96. (b) | 97. (c) | 98. (c) | 99. (a) | 100. (d) |
| 101. (b) | 102. (b) | 103. (a) | 104. (a) | 105. (a) | 106. (d) | 107. (c) | 108. (c) | 109. (c) | 110. (d) |
| 111. (a) | 112. (b) | 113. (b) | 114. (b) | 115. (d) | 116. (d) | 117. (d) | 118. (c) | 119. (c) | 120. (b) |
| 121. (b) | 122. (c) | 123. (a) | 124. (b) | 125. (b) | 126. (b) | 127. (b) | 128. (b) | 129. (b) | 130. (d) |
| 131. (b) | 132. (b) | 133. (a) | 134. (c) | 135. (a) | 136. (c) | 137. (c) | 138. (d) | 139. (c) | 140. (b) |
| 141. (b) | 142. (d) | 143. (a) | 144. (b) | 145. (d) | 146. (b) | 147. (d) | 148. (d) | 149. (d) | 150. (c) |
| 151. (d) | 152. (a) | 153. (d) | | | | | | | |

### Multiple Choice Questions: Level II

| | | | | | | | | | |
|---|---|---|---|---|---|---|---|---|---|
| 154. (a) | 155. (c) | 156. (a) | 157. (d) | 158. (d) | 159. (c) | 160. (a) | 161. (a) | 162. (a) | 163. (c) |
| 164. (a) | 165. (d) | 166. (b) | 167. (b) | 168. (c) | 169. (a) | 170. (c) | 171. (d) | | |

### A & R and Statement-based Questions

| | | | | | | | | | |
|---|---|---|---|---|---|---|---|---|---|
| 172. (c) | 173. (b) | 174. (c) | 175. (a) | 176. (c) | 177. (a) | 178. (b) | 179. (c) | 180. (c) | 181. (c) |

### Matrix-Match Type Questions

| | | | | |
|---|---|---|---|---|
| 182. (a) | 183. (a) | 184. (a) | 185. (a) | 186. (a) |

### NCERT Exemplar Questions

| | | | | | | | | | |
|---|---|---|---|---|---|---|---|---|---|
| 1. (b) | 2. (a) | 3. (d) | 4. (c) | 5. (d) | 6. (b) | 7. (d) | 8. (c) | 9. (d) | 10. (c) |
| 11. (a) | 12. (c) | 13. (c) | 14. (c) | | | | | | |

### Previous Years' Questions

| | | | | | | | | | |
|---|---|---|---|---|---|---|---|---|---|
| 1. (d) | 2. (a) | 3. (c) | 4. (d) | 5. (d) | 6. (d) | 7. (c) | 8. (c) | 9. (c) | 10. (a) |
| 11. (d) | 12. (d) | 13. (d) | 14. (a) | 15. (d) | 16. (b) | 17. (d) | 18. (c) | 19. (c) | 20. (c) |
| 21. (a) | 22. (d) | 23. (a) | 24. (c) | 25. (c) | 26. (b) | 27. (a) | 28. (a) | 29. (d) | 30. (c) |
| 31. (a) | 32. (d) | 33. (a) | 34. (c) | 35. (a) | 36. (d) | 37. (a) | 38. (a) | 39. (c) | 40. (b) |
| 41. (d) | 42. (a) | 43. (b) | 44. (a) | 45. (c) | 46. (d) | 47. (d) | 48. (c) | 49. (b) | 50. (b) |
| 51. (a) | 52. (a) | 53. (d) | 54. (c) | 55. (a) | 56. (b) | 57. (c) | 58. (d) | 59. (c) | 60. (b) |
| 61. (a) | 62. (c) | 63. (d) | 64. (a) | 65. (d) | | | | | |

# HINTS AND EXPLANATION

## Multiple Choice Questions: Level II

**154.** Transgenic plants are the ones generated by introducing foreign DNA into a cell and regenerating a plant from that cell.

**155.** The linking of antibiotic resistance gene with the plasmid vector became possible with DNA ligase. DNA ligase is an enzyme that is able to join together two portions of DNA and therefore plays an important role in DNA repair. DNA ligase is also used in recombinant DNA technology as it ensures that the foreign DNA is bound to the plasmid into which it is incorporated.

**156.** Restriction endonuclease cuts the DNA molecule at some specific sites, works from inside the DNA molecule and opens it up as a zipper.

**157.** *Escherichia coli* is a bacterium found in human colon. On this bacterium, scientists have made extensive genetic experiments to make some vital chemicals like insulin. Another bacterium is *Agrobacterium tumefaciens* which causes crown gall in plants is extensively used for genetic experiments.

**158.** The genetic code is universal. This means that a given triplet codon codes for the same amino acid in all organisms with a few exceptions in eukaryotic mitochondria.

**159.** *Azotobacter* is a free living nitrogen fixing bacteria. *Rhizobium* is a symbiotic bacterium fixing atmospheric nitrogen. Ti plasmid is found in *Agro bacterium.*

**160.** Ligase enzymes catalyses condensation of two molecules involving hydrolysis of ATP or any other such triphosphate. DNA ligase is used to join bits of DNA.

**161.** Restriction endonucleases are enzymes which identify specific sequences and cleave at specific sites on the DNA. DNA ligase fuses isolated DNA segments. Primase synthesizes the primer before replication.

**162.** Restriction endonuclease cut DNA act at specific site.

**163.** Cloning vectors are carriers or vehicle of passenger DNA. Plasmids are small extranuclear circular DNAs carrying extrachromosomal genes in bacteria and some fungi. They replicate independently. So can be used as vectors.

**164.** Agrobacterium is considered natural agent of genetic engineering. Agrobacterium is a genus of bacteria that causes tumours in plants. *Agrobacterium tumefaciens* is the most common studied species in this genus. Agrobacterium is well known for its ability to transfer DNA between itself and plants, and for this reason it has become an important tool for plant improvement by genetic engineering.

**165.** Genetic engineering in the science of gene manipulation. Genetic engineering, genetic modification (GM) and gene splicing are terms for the process of manipulating genes, generally implying that the process is outside the *organism's* natural *reproductive process.* It involves the isolation, manipulation, transfer, and reintroduction of *DNA* into *cells* or *model organisms* usually to express a *protein*.

**166.** The word plasmid was used by Lederberg (1952) for any extrachromosomal autonomous element. They are present as accessory DNA circles in bacteria. They are also regarded as extranuclear genetic material. Plasmids are used in genetic engineering.

**167.** Polymerases synthesizes new DNA strands Ligases ligate (join) DNA segments. Transcriptases are involved in transcription. Endonuclease recognizes specific DNA sequences and cleaves at specific sites.

**168.** Ligase binds two segments of DNA Primase initiates synthesis of RNA primer. Exonucleases cleaves DNAs from terminal ends.

**169.** Restriction endonucleases is synthesized by bacteria as part of their defence mechanism

**170.** Genetic engineering is DNA manipulation technology that produces and modifies DNA sequences. Restriction endonucleases identify specific DNA sequences and cleave at those sites.

**171.** Enzyme helicase unwinds the DNA helix and unzips the two strands of DNA. Polymerase synthesizes the new DNA strand. DNA ligase joins two strand of nucleic acid.

## NCERT Exemplar Questions

1. Exonucleases remove nucleotides from the ends of the DNA, whereas endonucleases make cuts at specific positions within the DNA.
2. The transfer of genetic material from one bacterium to another through the mediation of a vector like virus is termed as transduction.
3. The separated DNA fragments can be visualized only after staining the DNA with a compound known as ethidium bromide followed by exposure to ultraviolet radiation (we cannot see pure DNA fragments in the visible light and without staining).
4. 'Restriction' in Restriction enzyme refers to prevention of the multiplication of bacteriophage in bacteria.
5. (1) Restriction enzymes
   (2) Polymerase enzymes
   (3) Ligases
   (4) Vectors
   (5) Host organism
6. The differential mobility of DNA depends upon size of DNA.
7. The most important feature in a plasmid to be used as a vector is origin of replication (ori).
8. While isolating DNA from bacteria lysozyme, ribonuclease and protease, enzymes is used.
9. If the process of replication of DNA is repeated many times, the segment of DNA can be amplified to approximately billion times i.e., 1 billion copies are made. Such repeated amplification is achieved by the use of a thermostable DNA polymerase (isolated from a thermophilic bacterium ***Thermus aquaticus***), which is active during the high temperature induced denaturation of double-stranded DNA.
10. Significance of 'heat shock' method in bacterial transformation is to facilitate uptake of DNA through transient pores in the bacterial cell wall.
11. The role of DNA ligase in the construction of a recombinant DNA molecule is formation of phosphodiester bond between two DNA fragments.
12. *Haemophilus injluenzae, Escherichia coli* and *Bacillius quifacieus* are source of restriction endonuclease.
13. *Taq polymerase* is used between annealing and extension, helps in extension of primer end on the template DNA.
14. **Restriction enzyme:**
    - recognizes a palindromic nucleotide sequence
    - is an endonuclease isolated from bacteria
    - produces the same kind of sticky ends in different DNA molecules

## Previous Years' Questions

1. The most common type of aerobic bioreactor in use today is the stirred-tank reactor, which features a specific internal configuration designed to provide a specific circulation pattern. The stirred-tank bioreactors have been designed for availability of oxygen throughout the processes.
2. Restriction enzymes are degradative enzymes which recognize and cut up DNA that is foreign to a cell. These enzymes protect bacteria against intruding DNA from other organisms such as virus or other bacterial cells.
3. The palindromic base sequence is a sequence in double-stranded nucleic acids that reads the same on both strands when reading one strand from left to right and the other from right to lcft (i.e., both strands are read 5′– 3′).

   Out of the given options:

   5′–GAATTC–3′ 3′–CTTAAG–5′ is a palindromic sequence that can be cut at about the middle by particular restriction enzyme.
4. Plasmids are the extrachromosomal DNA found in bacterial cells. These are commonly used as vectors in genetic engineering programmes because they have the capacity of binding with eukaryotic DNA.

   Bacteriophage is a virus that is parasitic within a bacterium. These also are the important tools in genetic engineering as cloning
5. Plasmids are used as vector in gene cloning.
6. Now-a-days, genetically cngineered insulin is being produced at commercial level. The biotechnological procedure involves synthesis of two DNA sequences corresponding to A and B insulin chains. The two

DNA sequences or genes are made to fuse with plasmids and later allowed to form insulin chains.

**7.** Electrophoresis is used to separate DNA fragments of various lengths. Gel electrophoresis is a method for separation and analysis of macromolecules (DNA, RNA and proteins) and their fragments, based on their size and charge. Now-a-days, the most commonly used matrix is agarose which is a natural polymer extracted from seaweeds (e.g., Gelidium, Gracilaria, Gigartina, etc.).

**8.** Restriction endonuclease recognizes a particular palindromic sequence and degrades the same. It was so called because it restricts the growth of bacteriophase in the bacterium (e.g., E. coli). The convention for naming these enzymes is that the first letter of the name comes from the bacterial genus; the second two letter come from the species, and the fourth letter from strain, e.g., E**co**RI comes from Escherichia **co**li RY13. Roman numbers following the names indicate the order in which the enzymes were isolated.

**9.** Palindromic DNA is a base sequence of DNA, which reads the same forward or backward. It has similar sequence in both the strands. Different types of palindromic sequences are recognized by restriction endonucleases.

**10.** Recombinant DNA technology is joining together of DNA molecules from two different species that are inserted into a host organism to produce new genetic combinations.

**11.** For gene transfer into the host cell without using vector microparticles made of Tungsten and Gold coated with foreign DNA are bombarded into target cells at a very high velocity.

**12.** The name of this DNA polymerase is *Taq* polymerase extracted from a thermophilic bacteria. It is a relatively thermostable enzyme which is used in PCR during denaturation, which requires high temperature.

**13.**

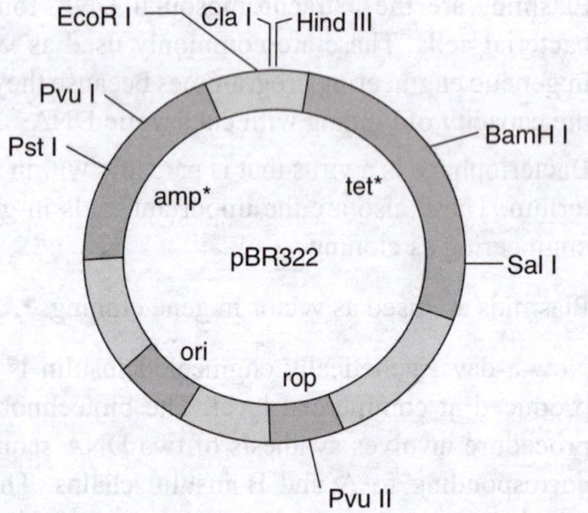


E. coli cloning vector pBR322 showing restriction sites (Hind III, EcoR I, BamH I, Sal I, Pvu II, Pst I, Cla I), ori and antibiotic resistance genes (amp$^R$ and tet$^R$). Rop codes for the proteins involved in the replication of the plasmid.

**14.** **Biolistics or Gene gun:** High velocity particles of Gold or Tungsten coated with recombinant DNA are bombarded on plant cells.

**15.** 5′ – GAATTC – 3′
3′ – CTTAAG – 5′
It is a palindromic sequence of DNA cut by restriction enzyme ECoRI.

**16.** Expansion proceeds at 72ºC in the presence of Taq DNA polymerase in PCR

**17.** In genetic engineering, the antibiotics are used as selectable markers.

**18.** Methylase enzyme is used for methylation. Bacterial cell wall degraded by lysozyme, plant cell wall degraded by cellulase and fungi cell wall degraded by chitinase.

**19.** Electrophoresis is used to separate DNA fragments of various lengths generated by the sequence selective cleaving action of restriction endonucleases, with the smallest DNA fragments traveling the farthest, and the largest DNA fragments traveling the smallest distance from the wells where the DNA fragments are introduced onto the separating medium, i.e. the agarose gel matrix.

**20.** You know that plasmids and bacteriophages have the ability to replicate within bacterial cells independent of the control of chromosomal DNA. Bacteriophages, because of their high number per cell, have very high copy numbers of their genome within the bacterial cells. Some plasmids may have only one or two copies per cell, whereas others may have 15-100 copies per cell. It can carry small fragment of DNA.

**21.** Plasmid DNA act as **vectors/vehicle** to transfer the piece of DNA (gene of interest) attached to it.

**22.** Restriction endonuclease enzyme cuts the DNA at specific site (paliandronic sequence).

**23.** *Eco RV* creates blunt ends. The enzyme recognizes palindromic 6-base DNA sequence 5′-GAT↓ATC-3′ and make a cut at arrow. The complementary sequence is then 3′-CTA↓TAG-5′. The ends are blunt and lighted into blunt cloning site easily but with lower efficiency than sticky ends. The restriction site of other enzymes are flowy and all produces sticky ends.

| Restriction enzyme | Restriction site |
|---|---|
| *Sal I* | 5′ G↓TCGAC3′<br>3′CAGCT↑G5′ |
| *Hind III* | 5′ A↓AGCTT3′<br>3′TTCGA↑A5′ |
| *Xho I* | 5′ C↓TCGAG3′<br>3′GAGCT↑C5′ |

**24.** Downstream process is the process of separation and purification of products synthesized in bioreactors. After the completion of biosynthetic stage, the product has to be subjected through a series of processes before it is ready for marketing as a finished product. The processes include separation and purification, collectively referred to as downstream processing.

**25.** The joining of DNA involves several processes. After having cut the source DNA as well as the vector DNA with a specific restriction enzyme, the cut out 'gene of interest' from the source DNA and the cut vector with space are mixed and ligase is added. This results in the preparation of recombinant DNA.

**26.** A stirred-tank reactor is usually cylindrical or with a curved base to facilitate the mixing of the reactor contents. The stirrer facilitates even mixing and oxygen availability throughout the bioreactor. Alternatively air can be bubbled through the reactor.

**27.** Following are examples of Restriction endonuclease Hind II, BamH I, Sal I, Pvu II, Pst I, Pvu I, EcoR I, Cla I, Hind III

**28.** Taq polymerase enzyme is obtained from bacteria thermus aquaticus.Thiobacillus ferroxidans metabolizing iron and sulphur and producing sulphuric acid. Bacullus subtilis is used to produce enzyme such as amylase and proteases used in laundry detergents. It also used to produce hyaluronic acid. Pseudomonal putida used for bioremediation (removal of oil spills).

**29.** Plasmid is extra chromosomal doubled-stranded circular DNA found in bacteria (prokaryote) generally used for vector in biotechnology.

**30.** Restriction endonuclease are synthesized by bacteria as part of their defense mechanism (to restrict the growth of bacteriophage virus inside them). It cuts DNA at specific sites called restriction site (paliandronic sequence).

**31.** DNA fragments during gel electrophoresis, separate (resolve) according to their size due to sieving effect provided by agarose gel (obtained from sea weeds like gracilleria and gelidium).

**32.** Selectable markers in recombination DNA technology helps in identification and elimination of non-transformants and selectively permits the growth of the transformants.

**33.** The various stages of processing that occur after the completion of fermentation or biosynthetic stage which include separation and purification and preservation of product is called downstream processing.

**34.** Ethidium bromide (Et Br) is used to stain the DNA fragments and will appear as orange-coloured bands when kept under UV light.

**35.** As DNA contains phosphoric acid, they are negatively charged.

**36.** Polymerase chain reaction (PCR) is used to amplify gene of interest. Each cycle has three steps in correct order is: (i) Denaturation; (ii) Primer annealing; and (iii) Extension of primers

**37.** Other biomolecules from mixture can be removed by appropriate treatments and purified DNA ultimately precipitates out after the addition of chilled ethanol.

**38.** Each restriction endonuclease functions by 'inspecting' the length of a DNA sequence. Once it finds its specific recognition sequence, it will bind to the DNA and **cut each of the two strands** of the double helix at specific points in their sugar-phosphate backbones. Each restriction endonuclease recognizes a specific **palindromic nucleotide sequence** in the DNA.

**39.** Bioreactors can be thought of as vessels in which raw materials are biologically converted into specific products, individual enzymes, on large scale, etc., using microbial plant, animal or human cells. A bioreactor provides the optimal conditions for achieving the desired product by providing optimum growth conditions (temperature, pH, substrate, salts, vitamins, oxygen).

**40.** The separated DNA fragments can be visualised only after staining the DNA with Ethidium bromide followed by exposure to UV radiation.

**41.** Restriction endonucleases make cuts at specific positions within the DNA.

They function by inspecting the length of a DNA sequence.

Restriction endonuclease bind to the DNA and cut the two strands of double helix at specific points in their sugar-phosphate backbones.

They are used in genetic engineering to form recombinant molecules of DNA.

DNA ligases join the DNA fragments.

**42.** Ligases join the two DNA molecules.

**43.** The correct option is (b) because *Ori* sequence is responsible for controlling the copy number of the linked DNA in the vector. *Ori i.e.* origin of replication is responsible for initiation of replication.

**44.** The correct option is (a) because the specific palindromic sequence which is recognised by EcoRI is

5′ - GAATTC - 3′
3′ - CTTAAG - 5′

**45.** The separated DNA fragments can be visualised only after staining the DNA with a compound known as ethidium bromide followed by exposure to UV radiation. You can see bright orange coloured bands of DNA in a ethidium bromide stained gel exposed to UV light.

**46.** High temperature about 94°C is required for the process of denaturation which is the first step of PCR.

**47.** Each restriction endonuclease recognizes a specific palondromic nucleotide sequence in the DNA. Once it finds its specific recognition sequence it bind to DNA and cuts each of the two strands of DNA.

**48.** Various enzymes like protease, RNase, etc. are added to break down substances like proteins, RNA, etc. Once all these substances are broken down, DNA is left which is precipitated out by adding chilled ethanol.

**49.** pBR322 is a commonly used cloning vector. When the gene for β-galactosidase is inserted in the ampicillin resistance gene by using Pst I, the recombinant E.coli will lose ampicillin resistance due to insertional inactivation of the antibiotic resistance gene.

**50.** Separation and isolation of DNA fragments-

(i) Restriction endonuclease enzymes cut the DNA in fragments.

(ii) Fragments of DNA are separated by **gel electrophoresis** in which the negatively charged DNA fragments are forced to move towards the anode under an electrical field through a medium (usually agarose gel). DNA fragments move according to their size-smaller the fragment more distance it will travel.

(iii) **Visualization of DNA fragments:** DNA fragments are first stained with **Ethidium bromide** and then observed under **UV-rays**. DNA fragments occur **bright orange-colored bands.**

(iv) **Elution:** The separated bands of DNA are cut out of the agarose gel and extracted from the gel piece.

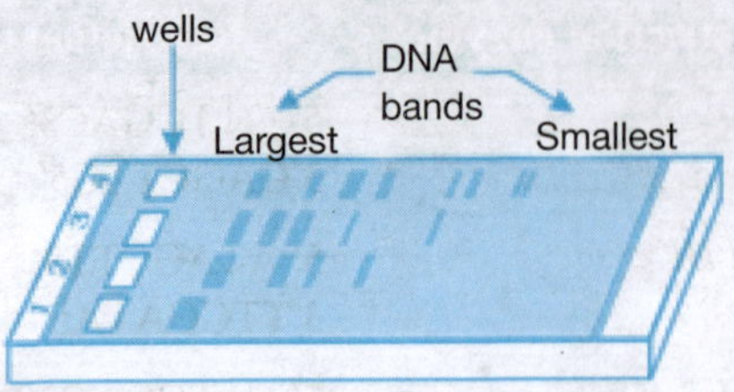


**51.** Polymerase chain reaction is used in DNA amplification.

Ampicillin resistance gene is a selectable marker that helps to check transformation by selection of transformants.

Here, given reason is irrelevant so, the option (a) is the correct answer.

**52.** Option (a) is the correct answer as a palindromic DNA sequence is a DNA sequence of base pairs that reads same on the two strands when orientation of reading is kept the same.

Out of the four options, option (a) is the only palindromic sequence.

5′GAATTC3′
3′CTTAAG5′

**53.** Both Statement I and Statement II are correct.

So the option (d) is the correct answer.

Each restriction endonuclease recognises a specific palindromic nucleotide sequences in the DNA. It will bind to the DNA and cut each of the two strands of double helix at specific points.

Restriction enzymes cut the strand of DNA a little away from the centre of the palindrome site; but between the same two bases on the opposite strands. Thus produces sticky ends.

**54.** Cloning vectors are the carriers of the desired gene in the host cell. The features are:

(a) Presence of origin of replication
(b) Presence of marker genes
(c) Presence of very few, preferably single recognition site for the commonly used restriction enzymes

**55.** During the purification process for recombinant DNA technology, addition of chilled ethanol precipitates out DNA as collection of fine threads in suspension which can be removed by spooling.

**56.** In gene gun method used to introduce alien DNA into host cells, microparticles of Tungsten or gold metal are used to coat foreign DNA

**57.** After Gel electrophoresis, visualization of DNA occurs with ethidium bromide after exposure to UV radiation showing bright orange colour fluorescent bands of DNA.

**58.** For Recombinant DNA technology correct sequence for the process is:

1. Isolation of desired DNA fragment.
2. Cutting of DNA at specific location by restriction enzyme.
3. Amplification of gene of interests using PCR
4. Insertion of recombinants DNA into host cell.

**59.** Correct answer is option (c) because

The fate of a piece of DNA carrying only gene of interest which is transferred into an alien organism are:

(B) It may get integrated into the genome of the recipient.

(C) It may multiply and be inherited along with the host DNA.

- This piece of DNA would not be able to multiply itself in the progeny cells of the organism but when gets integrated into the genome of the recipient, it may multiply and be inherited along with the host DNA.

**60.** The correct answer is option (b).

The first restriction endonuclease – *Hin*d II, whose functioning depends on a specific DNA nucleotide sequence was isolated. It was found that *Hin*d II always cut DNA molecules at a particular point by recognising sequence of six base pairs.

Option (a), (c) and (d) are incorrect.

**61.** Totipotency is defined as the capacity to generate a whole plant from any cell of the plant.

**62.** Protoplast of two varieties of plants are fused in somatic hybridization.

**63.** Correct answer is option (c).

The statement (3) is incorrect because bioreactors are used for processing of large volumes (100 –1000 litres) of culture, produce biological products at large levels.

**64.** Correct answer is option (b) because

'*X*' in the given diagram is *ori* while '*Y*' is *rop*.

'*X*' which is *ori* is responsible for controlling the copy number of the linked DNA and also the point from where process of replication starts and '*Y*' which is *rop* codes for protein involved in the replication of plasmid.

Options (a), (c) and (d) are incorrect as '*X*' and '*Y*' are not related to these functions.

**65.** The correct answer is option (c) as Ti-plasmid of *Agrobacterium tumefaciens* is tumor inducing plasmid, containing T-DNA which causes tumor in several dicot plants.

Options (a), (b) and (d) are not correct.

# 13 Biotechnology and Its Application

## LEARNING OBJECTIVES

- Discuss the various biotechnological application in the field of agriculture
- Describe how biotechnology proves a boon in the medicinal field
- Explain how biotechnology include therapeutics, diagnostics, processed food, bioremediation, waste treatment, and energy production
- Discuss tissue culture and somatic hybridization
- Learn more about the ethical issues in the biotechnological field

## Chapter Overview

- Biotechnology involves industrial scale production of biopharmaceuticals and biologicals with use of GMOs.
- Therapeutics, genetically modified crops, diagnostics, processed food, waste treatment and energy productions are among the various applications of biotechnology.
- During green revolution, food production was tripled (although not enough for the growing population).
- Agrochemicals cause environmental pollution. Use of genetically modified crops provide a solution for this problem.
- **GMOs (Genetically Modified Organisms):** Any organism (e.g., bacterial fungi, plant, animal, etc.) whose genes are altered by manipulation is termed as Genetically Modified Organism (GMO).
- **Use of genetic modification in plants are following:**
  (1) Crops are made more tolerant to unfavourable conditions or abiotic stresses e.g., cold, salt, heat, drought, etc.
  (2) Development of pest-resistant crops (this reduces the use of pesticides in field).
  (3) Post-harvest losses are reduced.
  (4) Mineral usage efficiency of plants is increased (exhaustion of fertility of soil is delayed).
  (5) **Nutritional value of food is increased, e.g., Vitamin A enriched rice (Golden Rice).**
  (6) GMs are also being used to develop the tailor-made plants to supply alternative resources to industries in the form of starches, fuels and pharmaceuticals.
- **Bt toxin gene:** This gene is found in bacterium *Bacillus thuringiensis* and it produces Bt toxin. This gene has been expressed in plants to make them insect-resistant. Thus, there will be no requirement of pesticides. Examples of crops with Bt toxin gene: Bt cotton, Bt corn, rice, tomato, potato and soyabean.
- **Bt cotton**: Some strains of a bacterium-*Bacillus thuringiensis*, produce some proteins that are capable of killing. some insects like: Lepidopterans - Tobacco budworm, Armyworm, etc. Coleopterans – Beetles Dipterans - Flies, Mosquitoes, etc. This crop is first Bt crop grown by Indian farmers.
- **Mechanism of action of Bt toxin:** During a particular phase of their development, *Bacillus thuringiensis* form protein crystals which contain an insecticidal protein called **Bt toxin protein**. This protein is in **inactive protoxin** form because of which the bacteria itself is not affected. But when this toxin is ingested by any insect, the crystals are solubilized by

Refer NCERT Ch 10: Biotechnology and Its Applications

the **alkaline pH** of the gut releasing the toxin. The toxin gets activated and binds to the surface of midgut epithelial cells creating the pores. The cells swell and undergo lysis gradually leading to the death of insect.

- **Cry gene:** These are the various types of genes that code for the Bt toxins. **Example:** (I) cryIAc and cryIIAb code for proteins that control the cotton bollworms. (II) cryIAb code for proteins that control the corn borers.
- **Pest Resistant Plants:** In **tobacco plants**, yield is greatly reduced due to the infection of ***Meloidegyne incognitia*** in **roots**. This infection was prevented by a strategy based on **RNA interference (RNAi)**.
- **RNA interference (RNAi):** It is a method of cellular defence in all eukaryotic organisms. Addition of a complementary dsRNA molecule → It binds to mRNA → Prevention of translation **(Silencing of mRNA).** Source of this complementary dsRNA molecule may be from an infection by viruses having RNA genomes or mobile genetic elements like transposons that replicate via an RNA intermediate.
- Nematode specific genes were introduced into the host plant by using the *Agrobacterium* vectors. This introduced DNA produced both sense and anti-sense RNA in the host cells because of which these two strands form a double stranded RNA (both are complementary to each other). This initiated RNAi and causes silencing of specific mRNA of nematode. As a result, the parasite is unable to survive in a transgenic host.
- In this world, about **thirty recombinant therapeutics** have been approved for human use, out of which about twelve are being marketed in India at present.

**(I) Genetically Engineered Insulin:** In 1983, an American company—**Eli Lilly**, produced Chain A and Chain B separately by introducing two DNA sequences in plasmids of *E.coli*. These chains were extracted and joined together by two **disulphide bonds** to form the human insulin.

- Earlier, insulin was isolated from the pancreas of the slaughtered cattle and pigs. This insulin from animal source caused allergy and **other immunological responses** (allergic reactions) in some patients.
- Insulin consists of two chains called, Chain A and Chain B, which are linked to each other by disulphide bond. In human, insulin is synthesized as a pro-hormone having C peptide as an extra chain and removal of C peptide from the structure make the insulin mature and functional.

**(II) Gene therapy:** It refers to all those methods that allow the correction of a gene defect that has been diagnosed in a child or embryo.

- In 1990, first clinical gene therapy was given to a four year old girl suffering from **ADA (Adenosine Deaminase) deficiency**. In such patients the gene for **Adenosine Deaminase** is deleted. There are two approaches for the treatment (although both are not completely curative):
  1. Bone marrow transplantation in some children.
  2. Enzyme replacement therapy (Functional ADA is injected into the patient).
- Introduction of a functional ADA cDNA into the lymphocytes by using a **retroviral vector**. Genetically engineered lymphocytes are returned into the body of patient. It requires frequent treatment.
- If the gene (for producing ADA) isolated from the bone marrow is introduced into the cells of early embryo, ADA deficiency can be permanently cured.

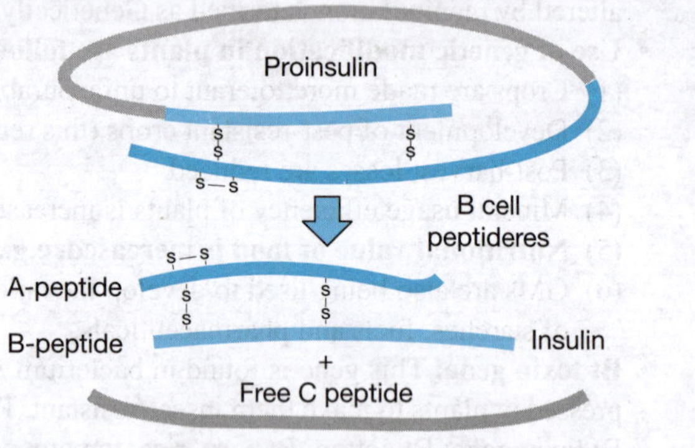

FIGURE 13.1 Maturation of pro-insulin into insulin

**(III) Molecular Diagnosis:** Techniques that can help in early detection of disease are:

**(a) Recombinant DNA technology (RDT):** A probe (ssRNA or DNA tagged with a radioactive molecule) can hybridize with its complimentary DNA in a clone of cells. This is followed by detection with autoradiography. If the gene is mutated, it will not be complimentary to the probe and hence, it will not appear on the photographic film.

**(b) Polymerase Chain Reaction (PCR):** PCR can detect the pathogens (bacteria or virus) at very low concentrations by the amplification of nucleic acids even before the development of the symptoms. PCR can detect HN in suspected patients of AIDS. and also PCR can detect mutations in genes in suspected patients of cancer.

**(c) Enzyme Linked Immuno-sorbent Assay (ELISA):** ELISA is based on the principle of antigen - antibody reaction. Presence of a pathogen in body can be detected by the presence of either the antigens (proteins, glycoproteins, etc.) or antibodies formed against it.

**(d) Transgenic Animals:** Those animals in which their DNA is modified to have and express an extra (foreign) gene are termed as transgenic animals.

- Many transgenic animals have been developed e.g., transgenic mice, rabbits, pigs, sheep, cows, fishes, etc. More than 95 per cent of existing transgenic animals are **mice**.
- **Transgenic animals are used to** study normal physiology development Insulin-like growth factor. By introducing the genes from other species that alter the formation and function of this factor, we can have more information regarding the biological role of Insulin—like growth factor.
- Many transgenic animals are designed in a way that they make us understand how the genes contribute to a disease and also we can work on new possible treatments. Diseases for which the transgenic models exist: Cancer, Cystic fibrosis, Rheumatoid arthritis and Alzheimer's disease.
- **Transgenic animals are used for biological products as:**
  - Production of α-1-Antitrypsin (used to treat emphysema).
  - Treatment of phenylketonuria (PKU) and cystic fibrosis.
  - Production of Human protein-enriched milk by the **first transgenic cow-Rosie in 1997**. This milk possesses human protein-alpha-lactalbumin and was nutritionally more balanced than natural cow milk for human babies (2.4 gms proteins/L).

**(e) Vaccine safety:** Transgenic mice are used to test the safety of polio vaccine.

**(f) Chemical safety testing (Toxicity or safety testing):** Transgenic animals are made more sensitive to the toxins than non-transgenic animals so that the effects of toxins can be obtained in less time.

**Ethical Issues**

- **GEAC (Genetic Engineering Approval Committee)** is an Indian Government organization which is authorized to make decisions on the validity of the research and the safety issues regarding the introduction of the genetically modified organisms for the public services (as food, medicine, etc.)
- **Biopiracy:** It is the use of biological resources (bio-resources) by the multinational companies and other organizations without proper authorization from the concerned countries and people without compensatory payment.
- **Rice:** In India itself, there are more than 2,00,000 varieties of rice (one of the richest rice biodiversity of the world). Twenty seven varieties of the Basmati rice (grown for its aroma and flavour) are grown in India. In 1997, an American company got patent rights on a new variety of Basmati rice (Indian Basmati X Semi-dwarf varieties) through the US Patent and Trademark Office.
- **Turmeric** and **Neem** were also attempted to be patented for their uses, products and processes in which they were involved.
- Recently Indian Parliament has cleared the Second amendment of the Indian Patents Bill to take various issues under consideration like-patent terms, emergency provisions and research, and development related issues.

**Tissue Culture**

- **Tissue culture** is an in vitro technique of regeneration of a whole plant from any part of a plant by growing it on culture medium under aseptic conditions.
- The capacity of a cell explant to grow into a whole plant is called **totipotency**.
- The part of the plant taken for tissue culture is called **explant**.
- The method of growing or producing thousands of plants through tissue culture is called **micropropagation**.
- The nutrient medium for tissue culture should have following components:

  1. Carbon source – sucrose
  2. Inorganic salts
  3. Growth regulators – auxins, cytokinins, etc.
  4. Vitamins
  5. Amino acids

- The plants produced from tissue culture are genetically identical to the original plant from which they are grown, and so they are called **somaclones**.
- Advantages of tissue culture:
  1. Large number of plants can be grown in short time.
  2. Disease-free plants can be developed from diseased plants.
  3. Seedless plants can be multiplied.
  4. The plants where sexual reproduction is absent may undergo somatic hybridization.

**Somatic Hybridization**

- The process of fusion of protoplast of somatic cells obtained from different varieties or species of plant on a suitable nutrient medium in vitro to develop a somatic hybrid is called **somatic hybridization.** It is carried out by the following steps:
  1. Single cells from selected plants are isolated.
  2. The cell walls of cells are digested by enzymes like pectinase and cellulase, to expose the naked protoplasts.
  3. Naked protoplasts surrounded only by plasma membranes are isolated.
  4. The isolated protoplasts are fused to obtain hybrid protoplasts under sterile conditions in special nutrient media by **sodium nitrate and polyethylene glycol** or by a very brief high voltage electric current.
  5. The hybrid protoplasts are cultured in a suitable media to form new plants.
- Somatic hybrids in plants were first obtained between two species of tobacco (Nicotiana glauca and N. langsdorfi) by **Carlson** et. al.
- In 1972. Somatic hybrids from different species of Brassica, Petunia and Solanum have been developed successfully.
- **Pomato** is a somatic hybrid between potato and tomato that belong to two different genera. This plant did not have all desired combination of characteristic for its commercial utilization. Similarly, somatic hybrids were produced between rice and carrot.

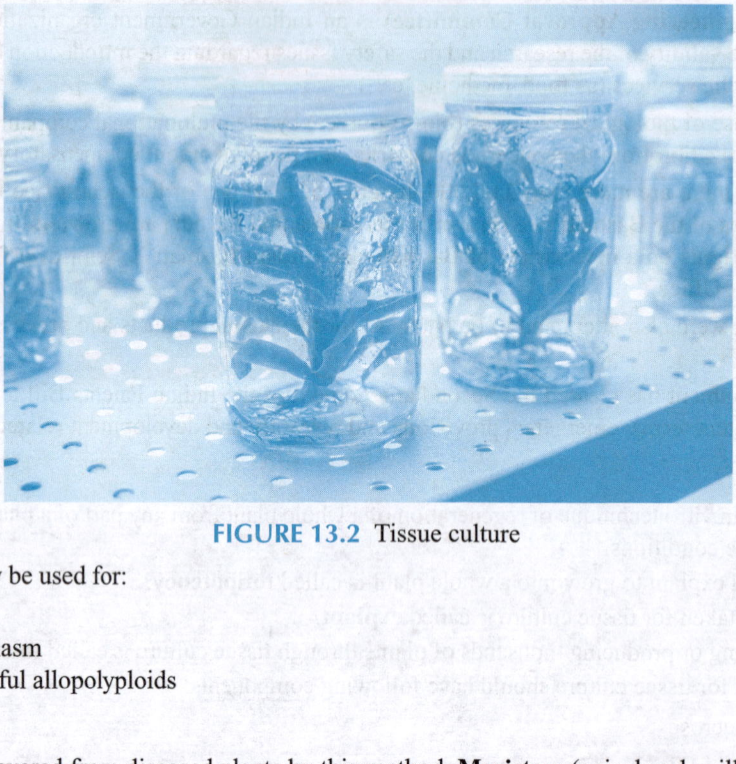

FIGURE 13.2 Tissue culture

- Somatic hybrids may be used for:
  1. Gene transfer
  2. Transfer of cytoplasm
  3. Production of useful allopolyploids

**Meristem Culture**

Healthy plants can be recovered from diseased plants by this method. **Meristem** (apical and axillary) is the only virus-free part of a virus-infected plant. By removing the meristem and growing it in vitro, virus-free plants can be obtained. Some plants developed by meristem culture are banana, sugarcane, potato, etc.

# PRACTICE EXERCISES

**Direction:** Read the question carefully and choose the correct option for each.

## Multiple Choice Questions: Level I

### Introduction

**1.** The applications of Biotechnology include
(A) Therapeutics
(B) Diagnostics
(C) GM crops for agriculture
(D) Processed food
(E) Bioremediation
(F) Waste treatment
(G) Energy production
(a) A, B, C, E only (b) C only
(c) B, C, D, E only (d) All of these

**2.** Golden rice is a
(a) Hybrid (b) GM plant
(c) Transgenic plant (d) Both (b) and (c)

**3.** Which of the GMO is used by biotechnology?
(a) Microbes and fungi (b) Plants
(c) Animals (d) All of these

**4.** Critical research areas of biotechnology are
(a) Providing the best catalyst in the form of improved organism usually a microbe or pure enzyme.
(b) Creating optimal condition through engineering for a catalyst to act.
(c) Downstream processing technologies to purify the protein organic compound.
(d) All the above

### Application in Agriculture

**5.** Transgenic plants (genetically modified or GM plants) are produced by inserting desired genes in the plasmid of
(a) *E. coli* (b) *Pseudomonas*
(c) *Bacillus subtilis* (d) *Agrobacterium*

**6.** Salt stress, disease resistance and cold stress in plants can be introduced by
(a) Genetic engineering
(b) Tissue culture
(c) Hybridoma technology
(d) None of these

**7.** Food production can be increased by
(a) Agrochemical based agriculture
(b) Organic agriculture
(c) Genetically engineered based agriculture
(d) All of these

**8.** After Green Revolution how many times does food supply has been increased?
(a) 2 (b) 3
(c) 4 (d) 5

**9.** Genetic engineering is useful for
(a) Agriculture
(b) Medical research
(c) Treatment and diagnosis of diseases
(d) All of these

**10.** Increased yield in Green Revolution is due to
(a) Use of agrochemicals (fertilizers and pesticides)
(b) Use of improved crop varieties
(c) Use of better management practice
(d) All of these

**11.** The following are the advantages of GM crops except
(a) They reduce reliance on chemical pesticides
(b) Increase efficiency of mineral usage
(c) Enhanced nutritional value of food
(d) Post harvest losses are more

**12.** Bt stands for
(a) Bacterial toxin
(b) Botulinum toxin
(c) *Bacillus thuringiensis*
(d) Bacillus toxin

**13.** Which of the following crops are now genetically modified by Bt-toxin gene?
(A) Cotton (B) Corn
(C) Rice (D) Tomato
(E) Potato (F) Soyabean
(a) A, B and C only (b) D and E only
(c) A and F only (d) All of these

**14.** Some strains of *Bacillus thuringiensis* produce proteins that kill certain insects like
(a) Lepidopterans (b) Coleopterans
(c) Dipterans (d) All of these

**15.** Select the correct matching.

| | |
|---|---|
| (a) Lepidopterans | Tobacco bud worm, armyworm |
| (b) Coleopterans | Beetles and bud worm |
| (c) Dipterans | Flies, mosquitoes, spiders |
| (d) Aves | Lady bird, hummingbird |

**16.** Antisense transcription is like carrying genes as much as
(a) On sense strand of DNA
(b) On Antisense strand of DNA
(c) On genetic RNA
(d) On tRNA

**17.** Bt-toxin is insecticidal because
(a) Activated toxin binds to the surface of midgut epithelial cells and creates pores that causes swelling and lysis and eventually cause death of the insect.
(b) It decreases the growth of the nervous system of the insect.
(c) It makes the insects unable to fly
(d) It kills insects by affecting its blood flow.

**18.** Bt-crops are not affected by Bt-toxin because
(a) Toxin exist as inactive protoxin.
(b) It has special antibodies against toxin.
(c) Its intracellular medium is alkaline so toxin remains inactive.
(d) All the above

**19.** Select the correct statement.
A. Most Bt-toxins are insect group non-specific.
B. Bt-toxin gene is coded with the name 'CRY'.
C. Genes cryIAc and cryIIAb form protein that control cotton bollworms.
D. cryIAb gene forms protein that control corn borer.
(a) A and B (b) D only
(c) C and D (d) C only

**20.** The following are all genes except
(a) cryIAc (b) cryIAb
(c) ROP (d) SalI

**21.** Protein encoded gene cryIAb controls
(a) Cotton bollworm
(b) Beetles
(c) Corn borer
(d) Flies

**22.** Golden rice is enriched in
(a) Beta carotene (b) Lysine
(c) Vitamin C (d) Iron

**23.** Bt-toxin is obtained from
(a) Bacilli (b) Cocci
(c) Vibrio (d) Spirillum

**24.** A nematode ________ infects the roots of tobacco plants and causes great reduction in yield.
(a) Ancylostoma
(b) Hookworm
(c) *Meloidogyne incognita*
(d) Wuchereria

**25.** The first transgenic crop plant was
(a) Cotton (b) Cereals
(c) Tobacco (d) Pea

**26.** RNAi process takes place in
(a) Prokaryotes
(b) Unicellular eukaryotes only
(c) Multicellular eukaryote only
(d) All eukaryotes

**27.** Which of the following is true about RNAi process?
(a) It is a method of cellular defense.
(b) It involves silencing of a specific mRNA due to a complementary dsRNA molecule.
(c) Source of complementary RNA in this process may be infection by viruses having RNA genomes.
(d) All are true

**28.** The most commonly used bacterium in plant genetic engineering is
(a) *E. coli* (b) *Rhizobium*
(c) *Klebsiella* (d) *Agrobacterium*

**29.** Identify A and B in the diagram.

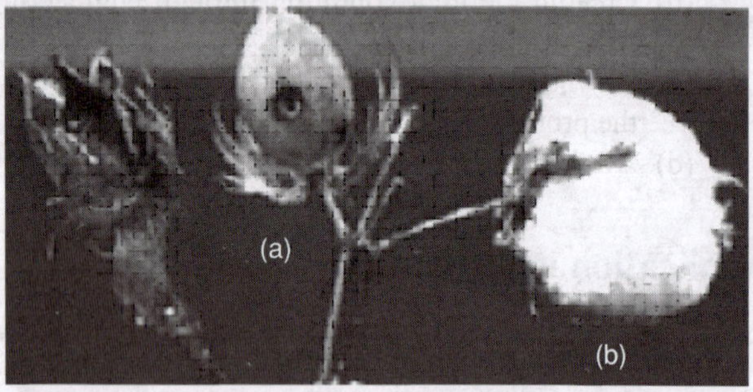


(a) A: A fully mature cotton boll, B: Destroyed by bollworms
(b) A: Destroyed by bollworms, B: Fully mature cotton boll
(c) A: Destroyed by virus, B: Immature cotton boll
(d) A: Immature normal cotton boll, B: Destroyed by virus

**30.** In which of the processes is both the DNA strands transcribed?
(a) PCR (b) DNA replication
(c) RNAi (d) Southern blotting

**31.** Which of the following vector is used to transfer nematode specific gene in host plant?
(a) Virus (b) Rhizobium
(c) Agrobacterium (d) Cosmid

**32.** What is true about Bt-toxin?
(a) The concerned bacillus has antitoxins.
(b) The inactive protoxin gets converted into active form in the insect gut.
(c) Bt-protein exists as active toxin in the bacillus.
(d) The activated toxin enters the ovary of pest to sterilize it and thus prevent its multiplication.

**33.** RNAi stands for
(a) RNA infection (b) RNA induction
(c) RNA interference (d) RNA inhibition

**34.** The abbreviation 'B' in Bt-toxin stands for
(a) Biotechnology
(b) Biotoxin
(c) Bacillus
(d) Toxin released by bacterium

**35.** Which of the following is the source of complementary strand in mRNA silencing?
(a) An infection by viruses having RNA genome
(b) Mobile genetic elements (Transposons)
(c) Both (a) and (b)
(d) Proteins

**36.** Some of the characteristics of Bt-cotton are
(a) Long fibre and resistance of aphids.
(b) Maximum yield, long fibre and resistance to beetle pests.
(c) High yield and production of toxin protein crystal which kills dipteran pests only.
(d) High yield and resistance to bollworms.

**37.** Golden rice is
(a) A variety of rice grown along the yellow river in China.
(b) Long stored rice having yellow colour tint.
(c) A transgenic rice having gene for β-carotene.
(d) Wild variety of rice with yellow coloured grains.

**38.** In RNAi, genes are silenced using
(a) ssDNA (b) dsDNA
(c) dsRNA (d) ssRNA

**39.** Crystals of Bt-toxin produced by some bacteria do not kill the bacteria themselves because
(a) Bacteria are resistant to the toxin
(b) Toxin is immature
(c) Toxin is inactive
(d) Bacteria encloses toxin in a special sac

**40.** Silencing of a gene could be achieved through the use of
(a) Short interfering RNA (RNAi)
(b) Antisense RNA
(c) By both
(d) None of these

**41.** In tissue culture, any part of a plant is taken out and grown in a test tube under sterile conditions in a special nutrient medium to regenerate whole plant. The part of plant used for this purpose is known as
(a) Somaclone (b) Embryo
(c) Explant (d) Zygote

**42.** The capacity to regenerate whole plant from plant cell or explant is known as
(a) Totipotency (b) Pluripotency
(c) Metaplasia (d) Atrophy

**43.** The method of producing thousands of plants through tissue culture is called
(a) Explant
(b) Totipotency
(c) Somaclone
(d) Micro-propagation

**44.** Which of the following plants have been produced by tissue culture method on commercial scale?
(a) Tomato (b) Banana
(c) Apple (d) All of these

**45.** The scientists have succeeded in culturing meristems of which of the following plants?
(a) Banana (b) Sugarcane
(c) Potato (d) All of these

**46.** The part of virus infected plant used for tissue culture, free from viruses is
(a) Flower (b) Leaf
(c) Apical meristem (d) All of these

**47.** Protoplast from two different varieties of plants, each having a desirable character, can be fused by a process known as
(a) Somatic hybridization
(b) Monohybrid cross
(c) Tissue culture
(d) Embryo culture

**48.** Tomato and potato protoplast is fused to form
(a) Topoto (b) Pomato
(c) Totato (d) Tomapo

**49.** Find out the incorrect statement.
(a) Virus free plant can be obtained by meristem culture.
(b) In micro-propagation soma clones are produced.
(c) Plant cell without cell wall is known as protoplast.
(d) Pomato (Somatic hybrid) has all the desired combinations of characteristics for its commercial utilization.

**50.** In tissue culture, the nutrient medium should contain
(a) Carbon source, eg., Sucrose
(b) Inorganic salt, vitamin and amino acid
(c) Growth regulators like auxins and cytokinins
(d) All the above

**51.** Which of the following are the advantages of SCP?
(a) Rich in high quality protein and poor in fat content.
(b) Production is based on industrial effluents so it helps to minimize the environmental pollution.
(c) It can be produced in laboratories throughout the year.
(d) All the above

**52.** Somatic hybridization is a technique of
(a) Natural breeding
(b) Natural pollination
(c) Artificial pollination
(d) Somatic cell hybridization

**53.** Somaclonal variations appear in plants
(a) Growing in polluted soil or water
(b) Exposed to gamma rays
(c) Raised in tissue culture
(d) Transformed by recombinant DNA technology

**54.** In crop improvement programme, virus free clones can be obtained through
(a) Embryo culture (b) Shoot apex culture
(c) Grafting (d) Hybridization

**55.** Pollen grains of a plant, where $2n = 28$ are cultured to get callus by tissue culture method. What would be the number of chromosomes in the cells of the callus?
(a) 14 (b) 56
(c) 28 (d) 21

**56.** A transgenic food crop which may help in solving the problem of night blindness in developing countries is
(a) Bt soybean (b) Golden rice
(c) Flavr Savr tomatoes (d) Star link maize

**57.** Main objective of production/use of herbicide-resistant GM crops is to
(a) Encourage eco-friendly herbicides
(b) Reduce herbicide accumulation in food articles for health safety
(c) Eliminate weeds from the field without the use of manual labour
(d) Eliminate weeds from the field without the use of herbicides

## Application in Medicine

**58.** How many recombinant therapeutics have been approved for human use all over the world?
(a) 10 (b) 20
(c) 30 (d) 90

**59.** Which of the following is produced by genetically engineered bacterium?
(a) Tyrosine (b) Insulin
(c) Glycogen (d) ADH

**60.** How many recombinant products are presently being marketed in India?
(a) 10 (b) 20
(c) 12 (d) 30

**61.** Which of the following is not used as a bioweapon?
(a) *Bacillus anthracis*
(b) Botulinum toxin
(c) *Bacillus thuringiensis*
(d) Small pox

**62.** The main challenge for the production of insulin using rDNA technique is
(a) Production of A peptide
(b) Production of B peptide
(c) Getting insulin assembled into a mature form
(d) All the above

**63.** Transgenic plants are produced by
(a) Inducing gene mutation
(b) Arresting spindle fibre formation
(c) Deleting sex chromosome
(d) Introducing foreign genes

**64.** Peptide A and peptide B is linked by how many disulphide in proinsulin?
(a) 1 (b) 2 (c) 3 (d) 4

**65.** Some of the steps involved in the production of humulin are given below. Choose the correct sequence.
(1) Purification of humulin.
(2) Extraction of recombinant gene product from *E. coli*.
(3) Culturing recombinant *E. coli* in bioreactors.
(4) Introduction of recombinant plasmid into *E. coli*.
(5) Synthesis of gene for human insulin artificially.
(6) Insertion of human insulin gene into plasmid.
(a) 2, 1, 4, 3, 5, 6 (b) 1, 3, 5, 6, 2, 4
(c) 5, 6, 4, 3, 2, 1 (d) 3, 5, 2, 1, 6, 4

**66.** Which American company in 1983 prepared humulin?
(a) Eli Lilly (b) Ranbaxy
(c) Sun pharma (d) Glaxosmithkline

**67.** During the process of prohormone 'proinsulin' into mature insulin synthesis
(a) C-peptide is added to proinsulin
(b) C-peptide is removed from proinsulin
(c) β-peptide is added to proinsulin
(d) β-peptide is removed from proinsulin

**68.** Select the true statements from the following.
(1) Insulin from animal source, may develop allergy in some patients.
(2) C-peptide is not present in mature insulin.
(3) Recombinant therapeutics do not induce unwanted immunological response.
(4) Insulin can be administered orally to diabetic patients
(a) 1 and 3 only (b) 1 and 2 only
(c) 3 and 4 only (d) 1, 2 and 3 only

**69.** Which of the following peptide chain is removed during maturation of pro-insulin into insulin?
(a) A-peptide (b) B-peptide
(c) C-peptide (d) B and C peptide

**70.** The Bt-toxin is not toxic to human beings because
(a) The pro Bt-toxin inactivation requires above human body temperature.
(b) The Bt-toxin recognizes only insect specific target.
(c) The Bt-toxin formation from pro Bt-toxin requires pH lower than that present in the human stomach.
(d) Conversion of pro Bt-toxin to Bt-toxin takes place only in highly alkaline conditions.

**71.** Which micro-organism is use to produce Insulin?
(a) Yeast (b) Algae
(c) Bacteria (d) Virus

**72.** Why is insulin not administered orally to diabetic patients?
(a) Insulin is bitter in taste.
(b) Insulin is a peptide.
(c) Insulin will lead to sudden decrease in blood sugar if given orally.
(d) Insulin leads to peptic ulcer if given orally.

**73.** Pro-insulin contains
(a) A-peptide (b) B-peptide
(c) C-peptide (d) All of these

**74.** The first clinical gene therapy was given in
(a) 1992 (b) 1990
(c) 1995 (d) 1997

**75.** Select the incorrect matching.
(a) ADA → Adenosine Deaminase
(b) ELISA → Enzyme Linked Immunosorbent Assay
(c) PCR → Polymers Chain Reaction
(d) PKU → Phenyl Ketonuria

**76.** The term 'molecular scissor' generally refers to
(a) DNA polymerase
(b) RNA polymerase
(c) Restriction endonuclease
(d) DNA ligase

**77.** ADA deficiency is due to
(a) Insertion of gene (b) Deletion of gene
(c) Duplication of gene (d) Translocation of gene

**78.** Permanent cure for ADA deficiency is
(a) Genetically engineered lymphocyte
(b) Bone marrow transplantation
(c) Enzyme replacement therapy
(d) ADA gene introduced in early embryonic stages

**79.** The first clinical gene therapy was given to a ______ old girl.
(a) 2 year (b) 6 year
(c) 4 year (d) 8 year

**80.** The conventional method of diagnosis involves
(a) Urine analysis (b) ELISA
(c) PCR (d) rDNA technology

**81.** PCR is used in the detection of
(a) HIV (AIDS) (b) Cancer
(c) Genetic disorder (d) All of these

**82.** When a patient with defective ADA is treated, which of the following steps are performed for gene therapy?
(A) Lymphocytes are obtained from the patients.
(B) Lymphocytes are transferred to culture dishes.
(C) Lymphocytes are transected with normal ADA genes.
(D) The transected cells are returned to the patients.
(a) All the above (b) Only C and D
(c) Only D (d) SCID cannot be treated

**83.** Which of the following is a benefit to have insulin produced by biotechnology?
(a) It is just as effective and is less expensive
(b) It can be produced in large quantity
(c) It is non-allergic
(d) All of these

**84.** Which one of the following genes is defective in patients suffering from serve combined immunodeficiency syndrome (SCID)?
(a) RNase (b) ADA
(c) Carbonic anhydrase (d) DNase

**85.** A functional ADA cDNA can be introduced into cells of the patients receiving gene therapy by using vector constituted by
(a) *E. coli* (b) Reovirus
(c) Retrovirus (d) Agrobacterium

**86.** Which of the following is used as probe?
(a) Single stranded DNA
(b) dsDNA tagged with a radioactive molecule.
(c) Single stranded RNA tagged with a radioactive molecule.
(d) dsRNA

**87.** Which gene does not appear in photographic film in autoradiography?
(a) Housekeeping gene
(b) Structural gene
(c) Mutated gene
(d) Transcriptionally active gene

**88.** Which of the following is based on antigen-antibody reaction?
(a) PCR
(b) ELISA
(c) Serum analysis
(d) Southern blotting

**89.** Which of the following can be detected in ELISA?
(a) Protein antigen
(b) Glycoprotein antigen
(c) Antibodies synthesized against pathogen
(d) Any of these

**90.** The first clinical gene therapy was done for the treatment of
(a) AIDS
(b) Cancer
(c) Cystic fibrosis
(d) SCID (Servere Combined Immuno Deficiency resulting from the deficiency of ADA)

**91.** ADA is an enzyme which is deficient in the genetic disorder SCID. What is the full form of ADA?
(a) Adenosine deoxyaminase
(b) Adenosine deaminase
(c) Aspartate deaminase
(d) Arginine dearginase

**92.** Identify A, B and C in the diagram.

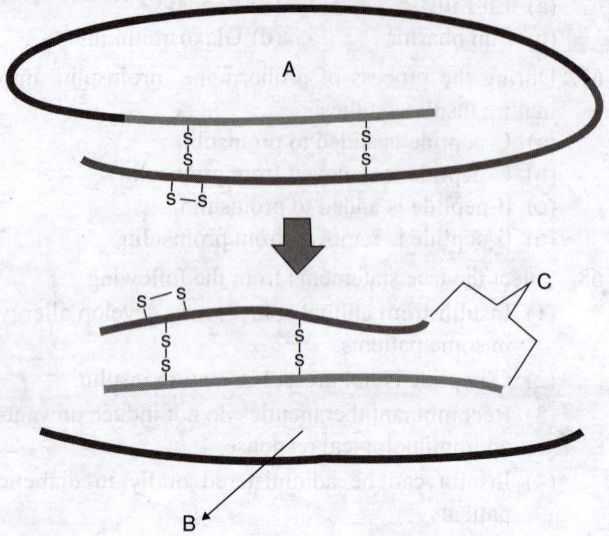


(a) A Proinsulin, B Free C peptide, C Insulin
(b) A Free C peptide, B Proinsulin, C Insulin
(c) A Insulin, B Proinsulin, C Free C peptide
(d) A Free C peptide, B Insulin, D Proinsulin

**93.** Humulin is a
(a) Natural insulin
(b) Human insulin synthesized by genetically engineered *E. coli*
(c) Human insulin synthesized by pancreas
(d) Chemically synthesized insulin

**94.** Humulin was first marketed by
(a) Eli Lilly (b) Sun pharma
(c) Nova Industry (d) May and Baker

**95.** Engineered bacteria have successfully been used for the commercial production of
(a) Human insulin (b) Melatonine
(c) Thyrosine (d) Testosterone

## Application of Transgenic Animals

**96.** Over 95 per cent of all existing transgenic animals are
(a) Pig (b) Mice
(c) Sheep (d) Cow

**97.** Transgenic organisms are used
(a) To study disease
(b) To produce biological product
(c) To test vaccine safety
(d) All of these

**98.** Match the columns

| Column-I | Column-II |
|---|---|
| A. Emphysema | 1. Test to detect antigen or antibody |
| B. Rosie | 2. α-1 antitrypsin |
| C. ELISA | 3. Protein enriched milk |
| D. ROP | 4. Codes for proteins involved in plasmid replication |

(a) A-2, B-3, C-1, D-4 (b) A-1, B-3, C-4, D-2
(c) A-1, B-2, C-3, D-4 (d) A-4, B-3, C-2, D-1

**99.** Transgenic animals are prepared for the following disease analysis except
(a) Cancer
(b) Cystic fibrosis and Alzheimer's
(c) Rheumatoid arthritis
(d) AIDS

**100.** 'Rosie' a transgenic cow known to produce a type of milk which has all the following characteristics except
(a) Protein content of 2.4 gm/litre
(b) Has human α-lactalbumin
(c) More balance diet than normal milk for babies
(d) Rich in cholesterol

**101.** Rosie was produced in the year
(a) 2000 (b) 1999
(c) 1997 (d) 2007

**102.** GMO/transgenic animal are used in testing safety of polio vaccine before they are used on human?
(a) Transgenic sheep
(b) Transgenic cow
(c) Transgenic viruses
(d) Transgenic mice

**103.** DNA or RNA segment tagged with radioactive molecules is called
(a) Vector (b) Probe
(c) Clone (d) Plasmid

**104.** The transgenic animals are those which have
(a) foreign DNA in some of its cells
(b) foreign DNA in all its cells
(c) foreign RNA in all its cells
(d) DNA and RNA both in the cells

## Ethical Issues in Gene Manipulation

**105.** How many varieties of rice have been estimated to be present in India?
(a) 200 (b) 20,000
(c) 200,000 (d) 2,000,000

**106.** The use of bioresources by multinational companies and other organizations, without proper authorization from the countries and people concerned without compensatory payment, is called
(a) Bioethics (b) Biopiracy
(c) Bioterror (d) Bioweapon

**107.** Which variety or rice was patented by a US company even though the highest number of varieties of this rice is found in India?
(a) Sharbati Sonora (b) Co-667
(c) Basmati (d) Lerma Roja

**108.** The Government of India took what step to cater to the requirement of patent terms and other emergency provisions with regard to biopiracy?
(a) Biopiracy act
(b) India Patents Bill
(c) RTI Act
(d) Negotiable Instruments Act

**109.** Which Indian plants have either been patented or attempts have been made to patent them by western nations for their commercial use?
(a) Basmati rice
(b) Turmeric
(c) Neem
(d) All of these have been targeted

## Multiple Choice Questions: Level II

**110.** Which one of the following is commonly used in transfer of foreign DNA into crop plants?
(a) *Meloidogyne incognita*
(b) *Agrobacterium tumefaciens*
(c) *Penicillium expansum*
(d) *Trichoderma harzianum*

**111.** What is true about Bt toxin?
(a) Bt protein exists as active toxin in the Bacillus.
(b) the activated toxin enters the ovaries of the pest to sterilize it and thus prevent its multiplication.
(c) the concerned Bacillus has antitoxins.
(d) the inactive protoxin gets converted into active form in the insect gut.

**112.** The genetic defect-adenosine deaminase (ADA) deficiency may be cured permanently by
(a) administering adenosine deaminase activators.
(b) introducing bone marrow cells producing ADA into cells at early embryonic stages.
(c) enzyme replacement therapy.
(d) periodic infusion of genetically engineered lymphocytes having functional ADAcDNA.

**113.** The bacterium *Bacillus thuringiensis* is widely used in contemporary biology as
(a) insecticide
(b) agent for production of dairy products
(c) source of industrial enzyme
(d) indicator of water pollution

**114.** Human insulin is being commercially produced from transgenic species of
(a) Rhizobium (b) Saccharomyces
(c) Escherichia (d) Mycobacterium

**115.** What is antisense technology?
(a) When a piece of RNA that is complementary in sequence is used to stop expression of a specific gene.
(b) RNA polymerase producing DNA.
(c) A cell displaying a foreign antigen used for synthesis of antigens.
(d) Production of somaclonal variants in tissue cultures.

**116.** Cry endotoxins obtained from Bacillus thuringiensis are effective against
(a) Nematodes (b) Boll worms
(c) Mosquitoes (d) Flies

**117** A genetically engineered micro-organism is used successfully in bioremediation of oils spills is a species of
(a) Trichoderma (b) Xanthomonas
(c) Bacillus (d) Pseudomonas

**118.** Introduction of food plants developed by genetic engineering is not desirable because
(a) economy of developing countries may suffer.
(b) these products are less tasty as compared to the already existing products.
(c) this method is costly.
(d) there is danger of entry of virus and toxins with introduced crop.

**119.** The first transgenic crop was
(a) Pea (b) Flax
(c) Tobacco (d) Cotton

## A & R and Statement-based Questions

### Assertion and Reason Questions

***Direction for questions 120 to 124:** Read the **assertion** and **reason** carefully to mark the correct option out of the options given below:*

**(a)** **(A)** is **true** but **(R)** is **false**.
**(b)** **(A)** is **false** but **(R)** is **true**.
**(c)** Both **(A)** and **(R)** is **true** and **(R)** is the correct explanation of **(A)**.
**(d)** Both **(A)** and **(R)** is **true** and **(R)** is not the correct explanation of **(A)**.

**120.** **Assertion:** ELISA can detect antigen or antibodies.
**Reason:** ELISA is method of molecular diagnosis based on antigen-antibody reaction.

**121.** **Assertion:** Bt toxin doesn't harm bacteria itself.
**Reason:** It is found as inactive protoxin in bacteria.

**122.** **Assertion:** Oral insulin is not given to diabetic patients.
**Reason:** Insulin is digested by our enzymes.

**123.** **Assertion:** Bt toxin is produced by fungus.
**Reason:** Bt toxin is toxic insecticidal protein.

**124. Assertion:** GEAC makes decision regarding the validity of GM research.

**Reason:** GEAC is genetic engineering approval committee.

## Statement-based Questions:

***Direction for questions 125 to 129:*** *These type of questions consist of two statement each, printed as* **Statement-I** *and* **Statement-II.** *While answering such questions, a student is needed to choose any one of the following four responses.*

**(a) Statement I** is **correct Statement II** is **incorrect**.
**(b) Statement I** is **incorrect Statement II** is **correct**.
**(c)** Both **Statement I** and **Statement II** are **correct**.
**(d)** Both **Statement I** and **Statement II** are **incorrect**.

**125. Statement-I:** Gene therapy is generally use to treat genetic diseases.

**Statement-II:** First clinical gene therapy is given in year 1997.

**126. Statement-I:** PCR and ELISA are more sensitive diagnostic tests.

**Statement-II:** They are useful for early detection of diseases.

**127. Statement-I:** Transgenic mice are used to detect safety of polio vaccine.

**Statement-II:** $\alpha$-1- antitrypsin is recombinant protein use to treat asthma.

**128. Statement-I:** Meloidegyne incognita infects root of tobacco.

**Statement-II:** RNAi is adopted to prevent this infestation.

**129. Statement-I:** Genetic modification is use to enhance nutritional value of food.

**Statement-II:** Vitamin A enriched rice is GMO.

## Matrix-Match Type Questions

**130.** Match the following:

| List-I (Enzymes) | List-II (Action) |
|---|---|
| 1. Biofortified plant | (i) Mobile genetic elements |
| 2. Bt toxin | (ii) mRNA silencing |
| 3. RNAi | (iii) Pest resistant plants |
| 4. Transposons | (iv) Golden rice |

**The correct matching is**

| | 1 | 2 | 3 | 4 |
|---|---|---|---|---|
| (a) | (iv) | (iii) | (ii) | (i) |
| (b) | (iv) | (ii) | (iii) | (i) |
| (c) | (ii) | (iii) | (i) | (iv) |
| (d) | (iii) | (ii) | (iv) | (i) |

**131.** Match the following:

| List-I | List-II | List-III | List-IV |
|---|---|---|---|
| 1. Cotton | A. RNA interference | X. B. thuringiensis | i. Nematode |
| 2. Tobacco | B. Insecticidal protein. | Y. Agrobacterium sp. | ii. Ballworm |

**The correct matching is**

(a) 1 – B – X – ii, 2 – A – Y – i
(b) 1 – A – X – ii, 2 – B – Y – i
(c) 1 – B – X – i, 2 – A – Y – ii
(d) 1 – A – Y – ii, 2 – B – X – i

**132.** Match the following:

| List-I | List-II (Example) |
|---|---|
| 1. Pest resistant crops | (i) Rosie |
| 2. Enhanced nutritional value crops | (ii) ELISA |
| 3. Molecular Diagnosis of disease | (iii) Golden rice |
| 4. Human protein enriched milk | (iv) Bt cotton |

**The correct matching is**

| | 1 | 2 | 3 | 4 |
|---|---|---|---|---|
| (a) | (iv) | (iii) | (ii) | (i) |
| (b) | (i) | (iv) | (ii) | (iii) |
| (c) | (ii) | (iii) | (iv) | (i) |
| (d) | (iv) | (iii) | (i) | (ii) |

**133.** Match the following:

| List-I (Application) | List-II (Tools) |
|---|---|
| 1. Vaccine safety | (i) PCR, ELISA |
| 2. Molecular diagnosis of disease | (ii) RNA interference |
| 3. Pest resistant crops | (iii) Transgenic mice |

**The correct matching is**

| | 1 | 2 | 3 |
|---|---|---|---|
| (a) | (ii) | (iii) | (i) |
| (b) | (ii) | (i) | (iii) |
| (c) | (iii) | (i) | (ii) |
| (d) | (iii) | (ii) | (i) |

**134.** Match the following:

| List-I (Use of GM Plant) | List-II (Use) |
|---|---|
| 1. Increasing crop-yield | (i) B. thuringiensis |
| 2. Improved nutritional value of crops | (ii) Green revolution |
| 3. Pest resistant crops | (iii) Golden rice |
| 4. Crops tolerant to obiotic stress | (iv) Resistance to cold, drought, salt, heat etc |

**The correct matching is**

| | 1 | 2 | 3 | 4 |
|---|---|---|---|---|
| (a) | (ii) | (iii) | (i) | (iv) |
| (b) | (iii) | (ii) | (i) | (iv) |
| (c) | (ii) | (iv) | (i) | (iii) |
| (d) | (ii) | (i) | (iii) | (iv) |

## NCERT Exemplar Questions

**1.** Bt cotton is not
(a) A GM plant
(b) Insect resistant
(c) A bacterial gene expressing system
(d) Resistant to all pesticides

**2.** C-peptide of human insulin is
(a) A part of mature insulin molecule.
(b) Responsible for the formation of disulphide bridges.
(c) Removed during the maturation of pro-insulin to insulin.
(d) Responsible for its biological activity.

**3.** GEAC stands for
(a) Genome Engineering Action Committee
(b) Ground Environment Action Committee
(c) Genetic Engineering Approval Committee
(d) Genetic and Environment Approval Committee

**4.** α-l antitrypsin is
(a) An antacid
(b) An enzyme
(c) Used to treat arthritis
(d) Used to treat emphysema

**5.** A probe which is a molecule is used to locate homologous sequence in a mixture of DNA or RNA molecules, it could be
(a) A single stranded RNA
(b) A single stranded DNA
(c) Either RNA or DNA
(d) Can be ssDNA but not ssRNA

**6.** Choose the correct option regarding Retrovirus:
(a) An RNA virus that can synthesize DNA during infection
(b) A DNA virus that can synthesize RNA during infection
(c) An ssDNA virus
(d) A dsRNA virus

**7.** The site of production of ADA in the body is
(a) Erythrocytes (b) Lymphocytes
(c) Blood plasma (d) Osteocytes

**8.** A protoxin is
(a) A primitive toxin
(b) A denatured toxin
(c) Toxin produced by protozoa
(d) Inactive toxin

**9.** The trigger for activation of toxin of *Bacillus thuringiensis* is
(a) Acidic pH of stomach
(b) High temperature
(c) Alkaline pH of gut
(d) Mechanical action in the insect gut

**10.** In RNAi, the genes are silenced using
(a) ssDNA (b) dsDNA
(c) dsRNA (d) ssRNA

## Previous Years' Questions

**1.** Some of the characteristics of Bt cotton are [AIPMT 2010 PRE]
(a) Long fibre and resistance to aphids.
(b) Medium yield, long fibre and resistance to beetle pests.
(c) High yield and production of toxic protein crystals which kill dipteran pests.
(d) High yield and resistance to bollworms.

**2.** Genetic engineering has been successfully used for producing [AIPMT 2010 PRE]
(a) Transgenic mice for testing safety of polio vaccine before use in humans.
(b) Transgenic models for studying new treatments for certain cardiac diseases.
(c) Transgenic cow Rosie which produces high fat milk for making ghee.
(d) Animals like bulls are used in farm work as they have super power.

**3.** DNA or RNA segment tagged with a radioactive molecule is called [AIPMT 2010 PRE]
(a) Vector (b) Probe
(c) Clone (d) Plasmid

**4.** Which one of the following is used as vector for cloning genes into higher organisms? [AIPMT 2010 PRE]
(a) Baculovirus
(b) *Salmonella typhemurium*
(c) *Rhizopus nigricans*
(d) Retrovirus

**5.** An improved variety of transgenic basmati rice [AIPMT 2010 PRE]
(a) Does not require chemical fertilizers and growth hormones.
(b) Gives high yield and is rich in vitamin-A.
(c) Is completely resistant to all insects, pests and diseases of paddy.
(d) Gives high yield but has no characteristic aroma.

**6.** The process of RNA interference has been used in the development of plants resistant to: [AIPMT 2011 PRE]
(a) Fungi (b) Viruses
(c) Insects (d) Nematodes

**7.** Read the following four statements (A-D) about certain mistakes in two of them.
(A) The first transgenic buffalo, Rosie produced milk which was human alpha-lactalbumin enriched.
(B) Restriction enzymes are used in isolation of DNA from other macromolecules.
(C) Downstream processing is one of the steps of rDNA technology.
(D) Disarmed pathogen vectors are also used in transfer of rDNA into the host. [AIPMT 2011 MAINS]

Which of the two statements have mistakes?
(a) B and C (b) C and D
(c) A and C (d) A and B

**8.** Silencing of mRNA has been used in producing transgenic plants resistant to [AIPMT 2011 MAINS]
(a) Bollworms (b) Nematodes
(c) White rusts (d) Bacterial blights

**9.** *Bacillus thuringiensis* forms protein crystals which contain insecticidal protein. This protein [AIPMT 2011 MAINS]
(a) Binds with epithelial cells of midgut of the insect pest ultimately killing it.
(b) Is coded by several genes including the gene cry.
(c) Is activated by acid pH of the foregut of the insect pest.
(d) Does not kill the carrier bacterium which is itself resistant to this toxin.

**10.** Consider the following statements (A–D) about organic farming: [AIPMT 2011 MAINS]
(A) Utilizes genetically modified crops like Bt cotton.
(B) Uses only naturally produced inputs like compost.
(C) Does not use pesticides and urea.
(D) Produces vegetables rich in vitamins and minerals.
(a) B, C, and D
(b) C and D only
(c) B and C only
(d) A and B only

**11.** Maximum number of existing transgenic animals is of: [AIPMT 2011 PRE]
(a) Mice (b) Cow
(c) Pig (d) Fish

**12.** Tobacco plants resistant to a nematode have been developed by the introduction of DNA that produced (in the host cells): [AIPMT 2012 MAINS]
(a) A particular hormone
(b) An antioxidant
(c) A toxic protein
(d) Both sense and anti-sense RNA

**13.** The first clinical gene therapy was given for treating: [AIPMT 2012 MAINS]
(a) Chicken pox
(b) Rheumatoid arthritis
(c) Adenosine deaminase deficiency
(d) Diabetes mellitus

**14.** Consumption of which one of the following foods can prevent the kind of blindness associated with vitamin 'A' deficiency? [AIPMT 2012 PRE]
(a) 'Flaver Savr' tomato (b) Canolla
(c) Golden rice (d) Bt-Brinjal

**15.** Which of the following Bt crops is being grown in India by the farmers? [AIPMT 2013]
(a) Maize (b) Cotton
(c) Brinjal (d) Soybean

**16.** The colonies of recombinant bacteria appear white in contrast to blue colonies of non-recombinant bacteria because of: [AIPMT 2013]
(a) Non-recombinant bacteria containing beta galactosidase.
(b) Insertional inactivation of alpha galactosidase in non-recombinant bacteria.
(c) Insertional inactivation of alpha galactosidase in recombinant bacteria.
(d) Inactivation of glycosidase enzyme in recombinant bacteria.

**17.** The first human hormone produced by recombinant DNA technology is [AIPMT 2014]
(a) Insulin (b) Estrogen
(c) Thyroxin (d) Progesterone

**18.** The introduction of t-DNA into plants involves: [RE-AIPMT 2015]
(a) Altering the pH of soil, then heat-socking the plants.
(b) Exposing the plants to cold for a brief period.
(c) Allowing the plant roots to stand in water.
(d) Infection of the plant by Agrobacterium tumefaciens.

**19.** In Bt cotton, the Bt toxin present in plant tissue as pro-toxin is converted into active toxin due to [AIPMT 2015]
(a) Alkaline pH of the insect gut.
(b) Acidic pH of the insect gut.
(c) Action of gut micro-organisms.
(d) Presence of conversion factors in insect gut.

**20.** Which body of the Government of India regulates GM research and safety of introducing GM organism for public services? [AIPMT 2015]
(a) Bio-safety committee
(b) Indian Council of Agricultural Research
(c) Genetic Engineering Approval Committee
(d) Research Committee on Genetic Manipulation

**21.** Which kind of therapy was given in 1990 to a four-year-old girl with adenosine deaminase (ADA) deficiency? [NEET 2016 – PHASE II]
(a) Chemotherapy (b) Immunotherapy
(c) Radiation therapy (d) Gene therapy

**22.** Which part of the tobacco plant is infected by *Meloidogyne incognita*? [NEET 2016 – PHASE I]
(a) Flower (b) Leaf
(c) Stem (d) Root

**23.** The two polypeptides of human insulin are linked together by: [NEET 2016 – PHASE I]
(a) Hydrogen bonds (b) Phosphodiester bond
(c) Covalent bond (d) Disulphide bridges

**24.** A genetically engineered bacterium first used for cleaning the oil spills was a species of: [NEET Regional 2017]
(a) *Rhizobium* (b) *Escherichia*
(c) *Pseudomonas* (d) *Bacillus*

**25.** In gene therapy, to treat adenosine deaminase deficiency disorder, which of the patients blood cells are used? [NEET Regional 2017]
(a) Thrombocytes
(b) Erythrocytes
(c) Lymphocytes
(d) Both Erythrocytes and Lymphocytes

**26.** What is the meaning of Bt in Bt cotton? [NEET Regional 2017]
(a) Cotton seeds carrying and endotoxin gene from Bacillus thuringiensis against pink boll – worm
(b) Baculovirus treated cotton seeds against pink boll – worm
(c) Bigger thread of disease-resistant cotton with better tensile strength
(d) Cotton produced by biotechnology using restriction Enzyme and Ligases to resist microbial infection.

**27.** Which technique helps to identify a bacterial or viral pathogen in a human body even when its concentration is very low and clinical symptoms are not yet visible? [NEET Regional 2017]
(a) Differential leucocyte count
(b) ELISA
(c) Total leucocyte count
(d) PCR

**28.** Which of the following is commonly used as a vector for introducing a DNA fragment in human lymphocytes? [NEET 2018]
(a) Retrovirus (b) $\lambda$ phage
(c) Ti plasmid (d) pBR 322

**29.** In India, the organization responsible for assessing the safety of introducing genetically modified organisms for public use is [NEET 2018]
(a) Indian Council of Medical Research (ICMR)
(b) Research Committee on Genetic Manipulation (RCGM)
(c) Council for Scientific and Industrial Research (CSIR)
(d) Genetic Engineering Appraisal Committee (GEAC)

**30.** Use of bioresources by multinational companies and organizations without authorization from the concerned country and its people is called [NEET 2018]
(a) Bio-infringement (b) Biodegradation
(c) Biopiracy (d) Bio exploitation

**31.** A 'new' variety of rice was patented by a foreign company, though such varieties have been present in India for a long time. This is related to [NEET 2018]
(a) Co-667 (b) Lerma Rojo
(c) Sharbati Sonora (d) Basmati

**32.** Which of the following is **true** for Golden rice? [NEET 2019]
(a) It is pest resistant, with a gene from *Bacillus thuringiensis.*
(b) It is drought tolerant, developed using *Agrobacterium* vector.
(c) It has yellow grains, because of a gene introduced from a primitive variety of rice.
(d) It is Vitamin A enriched, with a gene from daffodil.

**33.** What triggers activation of protoxin to active Bt toxin of *Bacillus thuringiensis* in bollworm? [NEET 2019]
(a) Moist surface of midgut
(b) Alkaline pH of gut
(c) Acidic pH of stomach
(d) Body temperature

**34.** Match the following columns and select the **correct** option: [NEET 2020]

| Column - I | Column – II |
|---|---|
| (A) Bt cotton | (i) Gene therapy |
| (B) Adenosine deaminase deficiency | (ii) Cellular defence |
| (C) RNAi | (iii) Detection of HIV infection |
| (D) PCR | (iv) Bacillus thuringiensis |

| | (A) | (B) | (C) | (D) |
|---|---|---|---|---|
| (a) | (iv) | (i) | (ii) | (iii) |
| (b) | (iii) | (ii) | (i) | (iv) |
| (c) | (ii) | (iii) | (iv) | (i) |
| (d) | (i) | (ii) | (iii) | (iv) |

**35.** Which of the following statements is **not correct**? [NEET 2020]
(a) In man insulin is synthesised as a proinsulin.
(b) The proinsulin has an extra peptide called C-peptide.
(c) The functional insulin has A and B chains linked together by hydrogen bonds.
(d) Genetically engineered insulin is produced in *E-Coli.*

**36.** Match the organism with its use in biotechnology. [NEET 2020]

| Column - I | Column - II |
|---|---|
| (A) Bacillus thuringiensis | (i) Cloning vector |
| (B) Thermus aquaticus | (ii) Construction of first rDNA molecule |
| (C) Agrobacterium tumerfaciens | (iii) DNA polymerase |
| (D) *Salmonella thphimurium* | (iv) Cry proteins |

Choose the **correct** option from the following :

| | (A) | (B) | (C) | (D) |
|---|---|---|---|---|
| (a) | (ii) | (iv) | (iii) | (i) |
| (b) | (iv) | (iii) | (i) | (ii) |
| (c) | (iii) | (ii) | (iv) | (i) |
| (d) | (iii) | (iv) | (i) | (ii) |

**37.** Bt cotton variety that was developed by the introduction of toxin gene of *Bacillus thuringiensis* (Bt) is resistant to : [NEET 2020]
(a) Insect pests (b) Fungal diseases
(c) Plant nematodes (d) Insect predators

**38.** Which of the following is not an application of PCR (Polymerase Chain Reaction)? [NEET 2021]
(a) Detection of gene mutation
(b) Molecular diagnosis
(c) Gene amplification
(d) Purification of isolated protein

**39.** Now a days it is possible to detect the mutated gene causing cancer by allowing radioactive probe to hybridise its complimentary DNA in a clone of cells, followed by its detection using autoradiography because: [NEET 2021]

(a) mutated gene does not appear on photographic film as the probe has complimentarity with it.
(b) mutated gene partially appears on a photographic film.
(c) mutated gene completely and clearly appears on a photographic film.
(d) mutated gene does not appear on a photographic film as the probe has no complimentarity with it.

**40.** For effective treatment of the disease, early diagnosis and understanding its pathophysiology is very important. Which of the following molecular diagnostic techniques is very useful for early detection? [NEET 2021]

(a) Hybridization Technique
(b) Western Blotting Technique
(c) Southern Blotting Technique
(d) ELISA Technique

**41.** With regard to insulin choose correct options.

(A) C-peptide is not present in mature insulin.
(B) The insulin produced by rDNA technology had C-peptide.
(C) The pro-insulin has C-peptide.
(D) A-peptide and B-peptide of insulin are interconnected by disulphide bridges.

Choose the correct answer from the options given below : [NEET 2021]

(a) (A) and (D) only (b) (B) and (D) only
(c) (B) and (C) only (d) (A), (C) and (D) only

**42.** The Adenosine deaminase deficiency results into: [NEET 2021]

(a) Addison's disease
(b) Dysfunction of Immune system
(c) Parkinson's disease
(d) Digestive disorder

**43.** Transposons can be used during which one of the following? [NEET 2022]

(a) Gene silencing
(b) Autoradiography
(c) Gene sequencing
(d) Polymerase Chain Reaction

**44.** In gene therapy of Adenosine Deaminase (ADA) deficiency, the patient requires periodic infusion of genetically engineered lymphocytes because: [NEET 2022]

(a) Gene isolated from marrow cells producing ADA is introduced into cells at embryonic stages.
(b) Lymphocytes from patient's blood are grown in culture, outside the body.
(c) Genetically engineered lymphocytes are not immortal cells.
(d) Retroviral vector is introduced into these lymphocytes.

**45.** Statements related to human insulin are given below. [NEET 2022]

Which statement(s) is/are **correct** about genetically engineered insulin?

(a) Pro-hormone insulin contain extra stretch of C-peptide.
(b) A-peptide and B-peptide chains of insulin were produced separately in *E.coli*, extracted and combined by creating disulphide bond between them.
(c) Insulin used for treating diabetes was extracted from cattles and pigs.
(d) Pro-hormone insulin needs to be processed for converting into a mature and functional hormone.
(e) Some patients develop allergic reactions to the foreign insulin.

Choose the **most appropriate** answer from the options given below:

(a) (B) only
(b) (C) and (D) only
(c) (C), (D) and (E) only
(d) (A), (B) and (D) only

**46.** Which one of the following techniques does not serve the purpose of early diagnosis of a disease for its early treatment? [NEET 2023]

(a) Serum and Urine analysis
(b) Polymerase Chain Reaction (PCR) technique
(c) Enzyme Linked Immuno - Sorbent Assay (ELISA) Technology
(d) Recombinant DNA Technology

**47.** Give below are two statements: [NEET 2024]

**Statement I:** Bt toxins are insect group specific and coded by a gene cry IAc

**Statement II:** Bt toxin exists as inactive protoxin in *B. thuringiensis*. However, after ingestion by the insect the inactive protoxin gets converted into active from due to acidic pH of the insect gut.

In the light of the above statements, choose the correct answer from the options given below:

(a) Both Statement I and Statement II are true.
(b) Both Statement I and Statement II are false.
(c) Statement I is true but Statement II is false.
(d) Statement I is false but Statement II is true.

**48.** Match List-I with List-II: [NEET 2024]

| List-I | List-II |
|---|---|
| (A) $\alpha$-1 antitrypsin | (i) Cotton bollworm |
| (B) Cry IAb | (ii) ADA deficiency |
| (C) Cry IAc | (iii) Emphysema |
| (D) Enzyme replacement therapy | (iv) Corn borer |

Choose the correct answer from the options given below:

(a) (A)-(ii), (B)-(i), (C)-(iv), (D)-(iii)
(b) (A)-(iii), (B)-(i), (C)-(ii), (D)-(iv)
(c) (A)-(iii), (B)-(iv), (C)-(i), (D)-(ii)
(d) (A)-(ii), (B)-(iv), (C)-(i), (D)-(iii)

## Answer Key

### Multiple Choice Questions: Level I

| | | | | | | | | | |
|---|---|---|---|---|---|---|---|---|---|
| **1.** (d) | **2.** (d) | **3.** (d) | **4.** (d) | **5.** (d) | **6.** (a) | **7.** (d) | **8.** (b) | **9.** (d) | **10.** (d) |
| **11.** (d) | **12.** (c) | **13.** (d) | **14.** (d) | **15.** (a) | **16.** (b) | **17.** (a) | **18.** (a) | **19.** (c) | **20.** (d) |
| **21.** (c) | **22.** (a) | **23.** (a) | **24.** (c) | **25.** (c) | **26.** (d) | **27.** (d) | **28.** (d) | **29.** (b) | **30.** (c) |
| **31.** (c) | **32.** (b) | **33.** (c) | **34.** (c) | **35.** (c) | **36.** (d) | **37.** (c) | **38.** (c) | **39.** (c) | **40.** (c) |
| **41.** (c) | **42.** (a) | **43.** (d) | **44.** (d) | **45.** (d) | **46.** (c) | **47.** (a) | **48.** (b) | **49.** (d) | **50.** (d) |
| **51.** (d) | **52.** (d) | **53.** (c) | **54.** (b) | **55.** (a) | **56.** (b) | **57.** (c) | **58.** (c) | **59.** (b) | **60.** (c) |
| **61.** (c) | **62.** (c) | **63.** (d) | **64.** (b) | **65.** (c) | **66.** (a) | **67.** (b) | **68.** (d) | **69.** (c) | **70.** (d) |
| **71.** (c) | **72.** (b) | **73.** (d) | **74.** (b) | **75.** (c) | **76.** (c) | **77.** (b) | **78.** (d) | **79.** (c) | **80.** (a) |
| **81.** (d) | **82.** (a) | **83.** (d) | **84.** (b) | **85.** (c) | **86.** (c) | **87.** (c) | **88.** (b) | **89.** (d) | **90.** (d) |
| **91.** (b) | **92.** (a) | **93.** (b) | **94.** (a) | **95.** (a) | **96.** (b) | **97.** (d) | **98.** (a) | **99.** (d) | **100.** (d) |
| **101.** (c) | **102.** (d) | **103.** (b) | **104.** (b) | **105.** (c) | **106.** (b) | **107.** (c) | **109.** (b) | **109.** (d) | |

### Multiple Choice Questions: Level II

| | | | | | | | | | |
|---|---|---|---|---|---|---|---|---|---|
| **110.** (b) | **111.** (d) | **112.** (b) | **113.** (a) | **114.** (c) | **115.** (a) | **116.** (b) | **117.** (d) | **118.** (d) | **119.** (c) |

### A & R and Statement-based Questions

| | | | | | | | | | |
|---|---|---|---|---|---|---|---|---|---|
| **120.** (c) | **121.** (c) | **122.** (c) | **123.** (b) | **124.** (c) | **125.** (a) | **126.** (c) | **127.** (a) | **128.** (c) | **129.** (c) |

### Matrix-Match Type Questions

| | | | | |
|---|---|---|---|---|
| **130.** (a) | **131.** (a) | **132.** (a) | **133.** (c) | **134.** (a) |

### NCERT Exemplar Questions

| | | | | | | | | | |
|---|---|---|---|---|---|---|---|---|---|
| **1.** (d) | **2.** (c) | **3.** (c) | **4.** (d) | **5.** (c) | **6.** (a) | **7.** (b) | **8.** (d) | **9.** (c) | **10.** (c) |

### Previous Years' Questions

| | | | | | | | | | |
|---|---|---|---|---|---|---|---|---|---|
| **1.** (d) | **2.** (a) | **3.** (b) | **4.** (d) | **5.** (b) | **6.** (d) | **7.** (d) | **8.** (b) | **9.** (a) | **10.** (c) |
| **11.** (a) | **12.** (d) | **13.** (c) | **14.** (c) | **15.** (b) | **16.** (a) | **17.** (a) | **18.** (d) | **19.** (a) | **20.** (c) |
| **21.** (d) | **22.** (d) | **23.** (d) | **24.** (c) | **25.** (c) | **26.** (a) | **27.** (d) | **28.** (a) | **29.** (d) | **30.** (c) |
| **31.** (d) | **32.** (d) | **33.** (b) | **34.** (a) | **35.** (c) | **36.** (b) | **37.** (a) | **38.** (d) | **39.** (d) | **40.** (d) |
| **41.** (d) | **42.** (b) | **43.** (a) | **44.** (c) | **45.** (a) | **46.** (a) | **47.** (c) | **48.** (c) | | |

# HINTS AND EXPLANATION

## Multiple Choice Questions: Level II

**110.** *Agrobacterium tumefaciens* is commonly used for transfer of foreign DNA into crop plants.

**111.** Inactive protoxin gets converted into active form in the insect gut because of alkaline pH

**112.** By introducing bone marrow cells producing ADA into cells at, early embryonic stages, the genetic defect adenosine deaminase (ADA) deficiency may be cured permanently. It is due to mutation.

**113.** The bacterium *Bacillus thuringiensis* is widely used in contemporary biology as insecticide. Bacillus thuringiensis (also known as Bt) is a gram-positive soil-dwelling bacterium of the genus Bacillus. *Bacillus thuringiensis* produces a parasporal insecticidal crystal protein.

**114.** It is commercial produced by *E.Coli*

**115.** The process of RNA interference (RNA i) has been used in the development of plants resistant to nematodes like *Meloidogyne incognita*, which infects the **roots** of tobacco plants and causes great reduction in yield. RNAi takes place in all eukaryotic organisms as a method of cellular defense. This method involves silencing of a specific mRNA due to a complementary dsRNA molecule that binds and prevents translation of the mRNA (silencing).

**116.** There are number of them, for example, the proteins encoded by the genes cry lAc and cry II Ab control the cotton bollworms, that of cry lAb control corn borers.

**117.** *Pseudomonas putida* is used for bioremediation of oil spills.

**118.** Plants developed by genetic engineering are called transgenic plants or genetically modified crops from which genetically modified food is produced. For their production, micro-organisms (bacteria, virus) are used. So, by consuming them, there is a danger of entry of viruses and toxins causing different types of allergies and other health hazards to human beings.

**119.** The first transgenic crop was tobacco developed in USA in 1986, it was herbicide resistant.

## NCERT Exemplar Questions

**1.** Bt cotton is a GM plant, insect resistant and a bacterial gene expressing system.

**2.** C-peptide of human insulin is removed during maturation of pro-insulin to insulin.

**3.** GEAC stands for Genetic Engineering Approval Committee.

**4.** a-I antitrypsin is used to treat emphysema.

**5.** A single stranded DNA or RNA, tagged with a radioactive molecule is called Probe.

**6.** Retrovirus is an RNA virus that can synthesize DNA during infection.

**7.** The site of production of ADA in the body is lymphocytes.

**8.** Bt toxin is a protein. This toxin does not kill *Bacillus* because the Bt toxin protein exists as inactive protoxins but once an insect ingest the inactive toxin, it is converted into an active form of toxin due to the alkaline **pH** of the gut which solubilizes the crystals.

**9.** The trigger for activation of toxin of *Bacillus thuringiensis* is alkaline pH of gut.

**10.** RNAi takes place in all eukaryotic organisms as a method of cellular defense. This method involves silencing of a specific mRNA due to the complementary dsRNA molecule that binds to and prevents translation of the mRNA (silencing).

## Previous Years' Questions

1. Specific Bt toxin genes were isolated from B. thuringiensis and incorporated into several plants such as cotton. The toxin is coded by a gene named cry. There are a number of them, e.g., the proteins encoded by the genes cry lAc and cry II Ab control the cotton bollworms, that of cry lAb control corn borers.
2. Transgenic mice are being developed for use in testing the safety of vaccines before they are used on humans. Transgenic mice are being used for testing toxicity of drugs. Transgenic animals are made to carry genes which make them more sensitive to toxic substances than non-transgenic animals. They are then exposed to toxic substances and the effects studied. Toxicity testing in such animals will allow us to obtain results in less time.
3. Probe is a defined nucleic acid molecule that can be used in molecular hybridization procedures to identify specific nucleic acid sequences that are complementary to it, by virtue of a label carried by the probe. The label may be radioactive or non-radioactive.
4. Retroviruses are RNA containing animal viruses that replicate through a DNA intermediate. Retroviruses in animals have the ability to transform normal cells into cancerous cells. A better understanding of the act, of delivering genes by pathogen in these eukaryotic hosts has generated knowledge to transform these tools of pathogen into useful vectors for delivering genes of interest to humans. Retroviruses have been disarmed and are now used to deliver desirable genes into animal cells.
5. Golden rice is a variety of *Oryza sativa* produced through genetic engineering to biosynthesize beta-carotene, a precursors of pro-vitamin-A in the edible parts of rice. The research that led to golden rice was conducted with the goal of helping children who suffer from vitamin-A deficiency in poor countries. Golden rice has been bred to be especially disease-resistant, resulting in better crop yields.
6. The process of RNA interference (RNA i) has been used in the development of plants resistant to nematodes like *Moloidegyne incognitia*, which infects the **roots** of tobacco plants and causes a great reduction in yield. RNAi takes place in all eukaryotic organisms as a method of cellular defense. This method involves silencing of a specific mRNA due to a complementary dsRNA molecule that binds to and prevents translation of the mRNA (silencing).
7. Transgenic Rosiae is actually cow. It was the first transgenic cow produced in 1997. Restriction enzymes cut the DNA at specific site. The separation of DNA is performed by gel electrophoresis.
8. The process of RNA interference (RNA i) has been used in the development of plants resistant to nematodes like *Moloidegyne incognitia*, which infects **roots** of tobacco plants and causes great reduction in yield.
9. Soil bacterium Bacillus thuringiensis (Bt) possesses is a gene family cry gene (1-40) over its plasmid, which forms an endotoxic proteins, cry protein (protein crystals) during a particular phase of its growth. These crystals contain a toxic insecticidal protein. This toxin, however, does not kill the Bacillus. Actually, the Bt toxin protein exists as inactive protoxins but once an insect ingests the inactive toxin, it is converted into an active form of toxin due to the alkaline Ph of the gut which solubilizes the crystals. The activated toxin binds to the surface of midgut epithelial cells and creates pores that cause cell swelling and lysis and eventually cause death of the insect.
10. Organic farming is the form of agriculture that relies on techniques such as crop rotation, green manure, compost and biological pest control to maintain soil productivity. It excludes use of manufactured fertilizers, pesticides, plant growth regulators, genetically modified organisms, livestock antibiotics, etc. It uses only naturally produced inputs like composts.
11. Animals that have had their DNA manipulated to possess and express an extra (foreign) gene are known as transgenic animals, e.g., rats, rabbits, pig, sheep, cows, fish, etc. Over 95% of all existing transgenic animals are mice.
12. RNA interference technique, sense and antisense RNA fused to form ds RNA that silence the expression of m-RNA of nematode.
13. **Gene therapy** is the use of DNA as a pharmaceutical agent to treat disease. It derives its name from the idea to treat disease. The most common form of gene therapy involves using DNA that encodes a functional, therapeutic gene to replace a mutated gene.
14. Golden rice is a variety of *Oryza sativa* rice produced through genetic engineering to biosynthesize beta-carotene, a precursor of vitamin-A in the edible part of rice (i.e. endosperm). The research that led

to golden rice was conducted with the goal of helping children who suffer from vitamin-A deficiency. Because many children in countries where there is a dietary deficiency in vitamin-A rely on rice as a staple food, the genetic modification of rice to produce the vitamin-A precursor beta-carotene is seen as a simple and less expensive alternative to vitamin supplements.

**15.** Bt cotton is commonly grown Bt crop of India.

**16.** Lac operon Z–gene produce beta *galactosidase* that convert X–gal chromogen into blue colour in non-recombinant bacteria. If this gene is affected by insertion inactivation, this reaction does not take place and bacteria appear white. But this inactivation takes place in beta-galactosidase gene not in α-galactosidase gene in recombinant bacteria. so right answer is non-recombinant bacteria containing beta galactosidase enzyme that cause blue colour colonies of bacteria.

**17.** Insulin used for diabetes was earlier extracted from pancreas of slaughtered cattle and pigs. Insulin from an animal source, though caused some patients to develop allergy or other types of reactions to the foreign protein. Insulin consists of two short polypeptide chains: chain A and chain B, that are linked together by disulphide bridges. In mammals, including humans, insulin is synthesized as a prohormone (like a pro-enzyme, the pro-hormone also needs to be processed before it becomes a fully mature and functional hormone) which contains an extra stretch called the C peptide. This C peptide is not present in the mature insulin and is removed during maturation into insulin. The main challenge for production of insulin using rDNA techniques was getting insulin assembled into a mature form. In 1983, Eli Lilly an American company prepared two DNA sequences corresponding to A and B, chains of human insulin and introduced them in plasmids of *E. coli* to produce insulin chains. Chains A and B were produced separately, extracted and combined by creating disulphide bonds to form human insulin.

**18.** Tumour-inducing (Ti) plasmid of Agrobacterium tumifaciens.

- *Agrobacterium tumifaciens* is pathogenic to various dicot plants. It can transfer a piece of DNA known as T-DNA which can convert normal plant cells into a tumour. These tumour cells direct the synthesis of chemicals required by bacteria.
- Tumour-inducing (Ti) plasmid of Agrobacterium tumifaciens is now modified into a cloning vector which is no more pathogenic to plants but still can deliver the target genes into various plants.

**19.** The Bt toxin protein exist as inactive protoxins but once an insect ingest the inactive toxin, it is converted into an active form of toxin due to the alkaline pH of the gut which solubilizes the crystals.

**20.** The Indian Government has set up organizations such as **GEAC** (Genetic Engineering Approval Committee), which will make decisions regarding the validity of GM research and the safety of introducing GM organisms for public services.

**21.** The first clinical gene therapy was given in 1990 to a 4-year old girl with adenosine deaminase (ADA) deficiency. This enzyme is crucial for the immune system to function. The disorder is caused due to deletion of the gene for adenosine deaminase. In some children, ADA deficiency can be cured by bone marrow transplantation; in others, it can be treated by enzyme replacement therapy, in which functional ADA is given to the patient by injection.

**22.** *Meloidegyne incognitia* is a nematode, which infects roots of tobacco plant and results in root knot disease.

**23.** Insulin consists of two short polypeptide chains: chain A and chain B that are linked together by two disulphide bridges.

**24.** *Pseudomonas putida* carries some plasmids capable of hydrolysing hydrocarbons found in crude petroleum such as xylene, toluene, naphthalene, camphor, etc. These genes are found on plasmids of different strains. Through genetic recombination and hybridization, all these plasmids were introduced in a single cell of *Pseudomonas putida* and this genetically modified bacterium had shown its ability to feed on wide varieties of hydrocarbons. It was named as **super bug** or oil feeding bug and was successfully used in controlling crude oil pollution in ocean due to leakage of crude petroleum from oil tankers. It was fast developed by Dr. Anand Mohan Chakraborty. This is known as **bioremediation.**

**25.** Gene therapy for the ADA-deficient patients:

(1) Lymphocytes of patient are obtained and grown in a culture.

(2) Introduction of functional ADA cDNA into the lymphocytes by using a retroviral vector.

(3) Genetically engineered lymphocytes are returned into the body of patient.

**26.** Bt (Bt stand for *Bacillus thuringeinesis*) toxin gene: This gene is found in a bacterium *Bacillus thuringiensis* and it produces Bt toxin (endotoxin). This gene has been expressed in plants to make them insect-resistant. Thus, there will be no requirement of pesticides.

**27.** Polymerase Chain Reaction can detect the pathogens (bacteria or virus) at very low concentrations by the amplification of nucleic acids even before development of the symptoms. Few uses of PCR:

- PCR can detect HIV in suspected patients of AIDS.
- PCR can detect mutations in genes in suspected patients of cancer.

**28.** **Disarmed** retroviruses are most commonly used to deliver genes into animal cells. Modified Ti plasmid is used to deliver genes of our interest into variety of plants.

**29.** The Indian Government has set up organizations such as GEAC (Genetic Engineering Approval Committee), which will make decisions regarding the validity of GM research and the safety of introducing GM organisms for public services.

**30.**
- **Bio-piracy** is the term used to refer to the use of bio-resources by multinational companies and other organizations without proper authorization from the countries and people concerned without compensatory payment.
- **Bioexploitation** is exploitation of natural resources.
- **Biodegradation** is breakdown of organic matter by microorganism.
- **Infringement** refers to the violation of law or a right.

**31.** It is related to Basmati rice. Basmati rice is distinct for its unique aroma and flavour and 27 documented varieties of Basmati are grown in India. Sharbati Sonara, Kalyan sona and Larma rojo are varieties of wheat. Co-667 is variety of rice.

**32.** Enhanced nutritional value of food, e.g., golden rice, i.e., Vitamin 'A' enriched rice.

**33.** Bt toxin protein exist as inactive *protoxins* but once an insect ingest the inactive toxin, it is converted into an active form of toxin due to the **alkaline pH** of the gut which solubilize the crystals. The activated toxin binds to the surface of midgut epithelial cells and creates pores that cause cell swelling and lysis and eventually cause death of the insect.

**34.** The correct option is (a) because

(A) In Bt cotton the specific Bt toxin gene was isolated from *Bacillus thuringiensis.*

(B) The first clinical gene therapy was given in 1990 to a 4-year old girl with adenosine deaminase (ADA) deficiency.

(C) RNAi (RNA interference) takes place in all eukaryotic organisms as a method of cellular defense.

(D) PCR is now routinely used to detect HIV in suspected AIDS patients.

**35.** The correct option is (c) because functional insulin has A and B chains linked together by disulphide bridges.

**36.** (A) *Bacillus thuringiensis* is a source of Cryproteins.

(B) *Thermus aquaticus* is a source of thermostable DNA polymerase (Taq polymerase) used in PCR.

(C) *Agrobacterium tumefaciens* is a cloning vector.

(D) The construction of 1st recombinant DNA molecule was performed using native plasmid of *Salmonella typhimurium.*

**37.** Bt cotton is resistant to cotton bollworm (Insect pest). *cry* I Ac and *cry* II Ab genes have been introduced in cotton to protect it from cotton bollworm. This makes Bt cotton as bio pesticide.
Ammonia and Hydrogen.

**38.**
- It is used for making multiple copies of the gene. Hence, PCR is used for gene amplification.
- PCR-based assays have been developed that detect the presence of gene sequences of the infectious agents.
- It is also used in detecting mutations.

**39.**
- Autoradiography allows the detection/localisation of radioactive isotope within a biological sample.
- Probe is a radio labelled ssDNA or ssRNA depending on the technique. To identify the mutated gene probe is allowed to hybridise to its complementary DNA in a clone of cells followed by detection using autoradiography. The mutated gene will not appear on the photographic film, because the probe does not have complementarity with the mutated gene.

**40.** ELISA can be used for early detection of an infection either by detecting the presence of pathogenic antigen or by detecting the antibodies synthesized against the pathogen.

**41.**

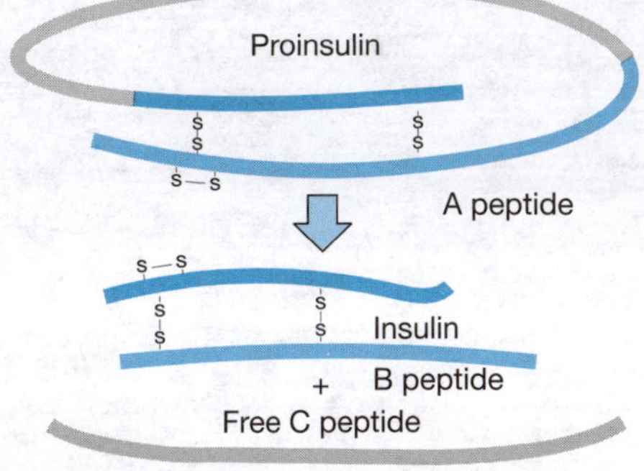


Maturation of pro-insulin into insulin

- Insulin is synthesized as a pro-hormone which contains A-chain, B-chain and an extra stretch called the C-peptide.
- C-peptide is not present in mature insulin called humulin.
- Chains A and B are connected by interchain disulphide bridges.

**42.** **Adenosine deaminase** (ADA) enzyme is crucial for the immune system to function. Hence, its deficiency results in the dysfunction of immune system.

**43.** The source of the complementary RNA for RNAi could be **mobile genetic elements (transposons)** that replicate via an RNA intermediate. It is used in silencing of specific mRNA produced by gene.

**44.** ADA enzyme is crucial for immune system to function.

Gene therapy steps:

(a) Lymphocytes from patient blood are grown in culture outside body.

(b) A function ADA CDNA using a retroviral vector is introduced in lymphocytes.

So, option (b) & (d) are steps.

Gene isolated from marrow cells producing ADA is introduced into cells at embryonic stages gives permanent cure of disorder. Thus, if does not require periodic infusion of lymphocytes.

Since, genetically engineered lymphocyte are not immortals, the patient requires periodic infusion of these cells.

**45.** Option (a) is the correct answer as genetically engineered insulin has A-peptide and B-peptide chains of insulin which are produced separately in *E.coli*, then they are extracted and combined by creating disulphide bond between them.

Statement (A) is incorrect as genetically engineered insulin does not have an extra stretch of C-peptide.

Statement (C) is incorrect as insulin obtained from cattles and pigs is not genetically engineered insulin.

Statement (D) is incorrect because conversion of pro-insulin to insulin is not required during production of insulin by genetic engineering as A-peptide and B-peptide chains are produced separately.

Statement (E) is incorrect as allergic reactions to insulin are mostly seen when the insulin is obtained from animals.

**46.** Using conventional methods of diagnosis (serum and urine analysis, etc.) early detection is not possible. Recombinant DNA technology, Polymerase Chain Reaction (PCR) and Enzyme Linked Immuno-sorbent Assay (ELISA) are some of the techniques that serve the purpose of early diagnosis.

**47.** The correct answer is option (c) as specific Bt toxin genes were isolated from *Bacillus thuringiensis* and incorporated into the several crop plants such as cotton. The choice of genes depends upon the crop and the targeted pest as most Bt toxins are insect-group specific. The toxin is coded by a gene named *cry*. There are a number of them, for example, the proteins encoded by the genes *cry* IAc and *cry* IIAb control the cotton bollworms, that of *cry* IAb controls corn borer. Bt toxin protein exist as inactive *protoxins* but once an insect ingest the inactive toxin, it is converted into an active form of toxin due to the **alkaline** pH of the gut which solubilise the crystals. So activated by alkaline pH not acidic pH.

**48.** The correct answer is option (c) as
$\alpha$–1 antitrypsin $\rightarrow$ is used for treatment of Emphysema
*Cry* I Ab gene $\rightarrow$ controls corn borer
*Cry* I Ac gene $\rightarrow$ controls cotton bollworms
Enzyme replacement therapy $\rightarrow$ can be used as treatment option in ADA deficiency, which is also an autoimmune disease.

# MOCK TEST-1

## Botany

1. What would happen if in a gene encoding a polypeptide of 50 amino acids, 25th codon (UAU) is mutated to UAA?
   (a) A polypeptide of 24 amino acids will be formed.
   (b) Two polypeptide 24 and 25 amino acids will be formed.
   (c) A polypeptide of 49 amino acids will be formed.
   (d) A polypeptide of 25 amino acids will be formed.

2. The RNA polymerase holoenzyme transcribes:
   (a) The promoter, structural gene and the terminator region.
   (b) The promoter, and the terminator region.
   (c) The structural gene and the promoter region.
   (d) The structural gene only.

3. Match The Following.

| List–I (Part of nucleus) | List–II (Function) |
|---|---|
| (A) Perinuclear space | (i) Holds two chromatids of chromosome |
| (B) Nucleolus | (ii) Barrier between nucleus & cytoplasm |
| (C) Centromere | (iii) Site for active ribosomal RNA synthesis |
| (D) Nuclea pore | (iv) Passages for movement of molecules between nucleus & cytoplasm |
| (E) Satellite | (v) Secondary constriction on chromosome present at a constant location |

   (a) A – (iii), B – (iv), C – (ii), D – (i), E – (v)
   (b) A – (iii), B – (i), C – (iv), D – (ii), E – (v)
   (c) A – (ii), B – (iv), C – (i), D – (iii), E – (v)
   (d) A – (ii), B – (iii), C – (i), D – (iv), E – (v)

4. Refer the given statements and select the correct option:
   (i) Percentage of homozygous dominant individuals obtained by selfing Aa individuals is 25%.
   (ii) Types of genetically different gametes produced by genotype AABbcc are 2.
   (iii) Phenotypic ratio on monohybrid F2 progeny in case of *Mirbilis jalapa* is 3 : 1
   (a) All the statements are true
   (b) Statements (i) and (ii) are true, but statement (iii) is false.
   (c) Statements (i) and (ii) and true, but statement (iii) is false.
   (d) Statements (ii) and (iii) are true, but statement (i) is true.

5. Which of the following is incorrect regarding ZW-ZZ type of sex determination?
   (a) It occurs in birds and some reptiles.
   (b) Females are homogametic and males are heterogametic.
   (c) 1 : 1 sex ratio is produced in the offspring.
   (d) All of these

6. **Assertion:** Fungi are saprophytes, parasites and symbionts.

   **Reason :** Most fungi are absorb soluble organic matter from dead substrates, some depend on living plants and animals and they can also live in association with algae and with roots of higher plants.

(a) (A) is false but (R) is true.
(b) Both (A) and (R) are true and (R) is the correct explanation of (A).
(c) Both (A) and (R) are true but (R) is not the correct explanation of (A).
(d) (A) is true but (R) is false.

**7.** Mendel's Law of independent assortment holds good for genes situated on the
(a) Non-homologous chromosomes
(b) Homologous chromosomes
(c) Extra nuclear genetic element
(d) Same chromosome

**8.** Blue eye colour in humans is an autosomal recessive trait. Black eyed son of a blue eyed mother marries a blue eyed girl. If the first child is blue eyed, what is the probability of the second child also being blue eyed?
(a) 0% (b) 25%
(c) 50% (d) 100%

**9.** Blood smear of African person shows some abnormal elongated RBCs and he also shows resistant against certain type of malaria, then which of the following may not be correct?
(a) He might be a carrier of some autosomal recessive disease.
(b) His haemoglobin chain may show polymerisation at high $O_2$ concentration.
(c) There may be some point mutation.
(d) He may have better chance of survival in population.

**10.** Single shield-shaped cotyledon of monocot seed is called:
(a) Coleorhiza (b) Coleoptile
(c) Scutellum (d) Epiblast

**11.** Many pulses of daily use belong to one of the families below:
(a) Solanaceae (b) Fabaceae
(c) Liliaceae (d) Poaceae

**12.** Superior ovary with oblique septa having swollen placenta with many ovules are characteristic features of:
(a) Solanaceae (b) Asteraceae
(c) Liliaceae (d) Labiatae

**13.** Match The Following.

| List–I (Plant) | | List–II (Stem modification) | | List–III (Function) |
|---|---|---|---|---|
| 1. Turmeric | (A) | Thorns | (i) | Photosynthesis |
| 2. Pumpkin | (B) | Flattened green structure | (ii) | Help in climbing |
| 3. Citrus | (C) | Underground stem | (iii) | Protection from browsing animals |
| 4. Opuntia | (D) | Stem tendrils | (iv) | Storage & perennation |

(a) 1 – C – iv, 2 – D – ii, 3 – A – iii, 4 – B – i
(b) 1 – A – iv, 2 – D – ii, 3 – C – iii, 4 – B – i
(c) 1 – C – ii, 2 – D – iii, 3 – A – iv, 4 – B – i
(d) 1 – A – iv, 2 – D – ii, 3 – B – i, 4 – C – iii

**14.** *Claviceps* and *Neurospora* belongs to
(a) Deuteromycetes (b) Basidiomycetes
(c) Phycomycetes (d) Ascomycetes

**15.** Select odd one with respect to viral diseases.
(a) Mosaic formation (b) Vein clearing
(c) Stunted growth (d) Citrus canker

**16.** **Statement I:** Photosynthetically $C_4$-plants are less efficient than $C_3$-plants.
**Statement II:** The operation of $C_4$-pathway requires the involvement of only bundle sheath cells.
Mark the correct choice from given options :
(a) Statement I is incorrect but Statement II is true.
(b) Both Statement I and Statement II are true.
(c) Both Statement I and Statement II are false.
(d) Statement I is correct but Statement II is false.

**17.** Inferior ovary and cypsella fruit are found in
(a) Compositae
(b) Ranunculaceae
(c) Malvaceae
(d) Liliaceae

**18.** Basal placentation is found in
(a) Compositae
(b) Cruciferae
(c) Malvaceae
(d) Solanaceae

**19.** The placentation in Leguminosae is
(a) Axile
(b) Parietal
(c) Free-central
(d) Marginal

**20.** Read the following statements and choose the incorrect statements for pollen grain:

(i) The vegetative cell is bigger, has abundant food reserve and a large irregularly shaped nucleus.

(ii) The generative cell is small and floats in the cytoplasm of the vegetative cell.

(iii) In over 60 percent of angiosperms, pollen grains are shed at 3-celled stage.

(iv) The period for which pollen grains remain viable is highly variable and to some extent depends on the prevailing temperature and humidity.

(v) In some cereals such as rice and wheat, pollen grains maintain viability for months.

(vi) In some members of Rosasceae, Leguminosae and Solanaceae, pollen grains lose viability within 30 minutes of their release.

(vii) It is not possible to store pollen grains of a large number of species for years in liquid nitrogen (-196°C).

(a) (iii), (iv), (v) and (vi)
(b) (i), (ii) and (iv)
(c) (iii), (v), (vi) and (vii)
(d) None of these

**21.** Consider the following events:

A. Two nuclear divisions.
B. One cycle of DNA replication.
C. Formation of four haploid cells in the end.
D. Genetically identical daughter cells.

How many are incorrect for meiosis?

(a) A, B and C
(b) B and C
(c) Only D
(d) C and D

**22.** Select the incorrect statement with respect to the $G_0$-phase of the cells cycle.

(a) Cells do not proliferate
(b) Also called quiescent stage
(c) Cells remain metabolically inactive
(d) Heart cells exited $G_1$ phase to enter this phase during development process.

**23.** Match the following.

| List–I | List–II |
|---|---|
| (A) Phenyl ketonuria | (i) Dominance |
| (B) Skin colour in humans | (ii) Polygenic inheritance |
| (C) Centromere | (iii) Codominance |
| (D) Flower position in pea plant | (iv) Pleiotropy |

(a) A – (iv), B – (ii), C – (i), D – (iii)
(b) A – (iv), B – (iii), C – (i), D – (ii)
(c) A – (ii), B – (i), C – (iii), D – (iv)
(d) A – (ii), B – (iii), C – (i), D – (iv)

**24.** Natural ecosystem in an area

(a) has self-regulation by positive and negative feedback.
(b) always has unidirectional flow of minerals.
(c) cannot overcome resilience.
(d) may be small or large but not capable of self-existence.

**25.** Organisms which are restricted to a narrow range of salinity are called:

(a) Euryhaline
(b) Stenohaline
(c) Stenothermal
(d) Eurythermal

**26.** Competition is more acute when

(a) resource is unlimited.
(b) resource is in limit and competing individuals is different.
(c) the niche of competeting individuals is different.
(d) resource partitioning and coexistence between competing individuals are observed.

**27.** Match the following.

| List–I (Molecule) | List–II (bond) |
|---|---|
| (A) Nucleoside | (i) 3-5 phosphodiester bond |
| (B) Nucleotide | (ii) N-glycosidic bond |
| (C) Dinucleotide | (iii) Phosphodiester bond |

(a) A – (ii), B – (iii), 3 – (i)
(b) A – (iii), B – (ii), 3 – (i)
(c) A – (i), B – (ii), 3 – (iii)
(d) A – (ii), B – (i), 3 – (iii)

**28.** Choose odd one out with respect to functional aspect of ecosystem

(a) Mineral cycling
(b) Stratification
(c) Productivity
(d) Decomposition

**29.** Ecosystem functions like productivity and degradation represent ___ and ____ of energy

(a) input, Output
(b) transfer, Input
(c) output, Input
(d) output, Transfer

**30.** Age pyramid of a population

(a) is urn shaped if the reproductive age group individuals are more than the pre-reproductive group but less than the post-reproductive group.
(b) upright for the growing population.

(c) is bell like when reproductive individuals are equal to post-reproductive group.
(d) may be urn shaped for stable population.

**31.** The high diversity shown by a single species due to allelic variations over its distributional range is called
(a) Species Diversity
(b) Ecological Diversity
(c) Genetic Diversity
(d) Ecosystem diversity

**32.** Select the mis-match
(a) A.V. Humboldt : Species-area relationship
(b) David Tilman : Ecological pyramids
(c) Robert May : Global species Diversity
(d) Paul Ehrlich : Rivet popper hypothesis

**33.** Match the following.

| List–I Microbes | | List–II Product | | List–III |
|---|---|---|---|---|
| A. | S. cerevisiae | (i) | Citric acid | Y. Yeast |
| B. | Aspergillus niger | (ii) | Statin | Z. Fungus |
| C. | Penicillium notatum | (iii) | Cyclosporin A | |
| D. | Trichoderma polysporum. | (iv) | Penicillin | |
| E. | Monascus purpereus | (v) | Ethanol | |

(a) A – 5 – Y, B – 1 – Z, C – 4 – Z, D – 3 – Z, E – 2 – Y,
(b) A – 3 – Y, B – 1 – Z, C – 4 – Z, D – 5 – Z, E – 2 – Y,
(c) A – 5 – Y, B – 1 – Z, C – 2 – Z, D – 3 – Z, E – 4 – Y,
(d) A – 2 – Y, B – 5 – Z, C – 4 – Z, D – 3 – Z, E – 1 – Y,

**34.** Egg plant belongs to
(a) Solanaceae (b) Cruciferae
(c) Gramineae (d) Liliaceae

**35.** What percent of PAR is captured by transducers to sustain the entire living world?
(a) 1 – 5% (b) 2 – 10%
(c) 0.2 – 1% (d) 0.8 – 1.6%

**36.** What does the filiform apparatus do at the entrance into ovule?
(a) It guides pollen tube from a synergid to egg
(b) It helps in the entry of pollen tube into a synergid
(c) It prevents entry of more than one pollen tube into the embryo sac
(d) It brings about opening of the pollen tube

**37.** The functional megaspore undergoes
(a) 2 meiotic divisions to form mature embryo sac
(b) 3 mitotic divisions to form mature embryo sac
(c) 2 mitotic divisions to form mature embryo sac
(d) 3 meiotic divisions to form mature embryo sac

**38.** Product of sexual reproduction generally generates
(a) Longer viability of seeds
(b) Prolonged dormancy
(c) New genetic combination leading to variation
(d) Large biomass

**39.** Match the List and select the correct answer-

| List–I | List–II |
|---|---|
| (P) Zn | (W) NAD |
| (Q) Haem | (X) Peroxidase |
| (R) Niacin | (Y) Phosphodiester bond |
| | (Z) Carboxypeptidase |

(a) P – W, Q – X, R – Z and Y
(b) P – Z, Q – X and Y, R – W
(c) P – Y and Z, Q – X, R – W
(d) P – X Q – W, R – Y and Z

**40.** Match the List I and II & chose the correct combination:

| List–I | List–II |
|---|---|
| (A) Protein content | (i) Maize |
| (B) Vitamin content | (ii) Carrot |
| (C) Micronutrient content | (iii) Spinach |
| (D) Amino acid content | (iv) Atlas-66 |

(a) A – (iv), B – (ii), C – (iii), D – (i)
(b) A – (iv), B – (ii), C – (i) D – (iii)
(c) A – (iii), B – (i), C – (ii), D – (iv)
(d) A – (ii), B – (iv), C – (iii), D – (i)

**41.** Which of the following is not an advantage of mycorrhiza?
(a) Nitrogen fixation
(b) Resistant to root borne pathogen
(c) Tolerance to salinity and drought
(d) Phosphorus absorption

**42.** Which of the following statements are correct about enzymes?

(a) Enzymes increase the rate of a reaction by increasing the energy of substrate molecules.

(b) Enzymes generally have similar temperature optimum but different pH optimum.

(c) Lower is the value of $K_m$ for an enzyme higher is the substrate binding affinity of enzyme.

(d) Enzymes are biomolecule and they are functional only inside cells.

(a) a, b and c (b) b and c
(c) a and c (d) a, b, c and d

**43.** Edible part of tomato is

(a) epicarp (b) pericarp & placenta
(c) mesocarp (d) thalamus

**44.** Choose correct option for given statements:

(i) A population has certain attributes that an individual organism does not, like birth rates, death rates and sex ratio.

(ii) An individual may have births and deaths, but a population has birth rates and death rates.

(iii) In a population birth rates and death rates refer to per capita births and deaths, respectively.

(iv) The birth rates and death rates expressed is change in numbers (increase or decrease) with respect to members of the population.

(v) An individual is either a male or a female but a population has a sex ratio (per cent females and males).

(vi) The tiger census in our national parks and tiger reserves is often based on pug marks and faecal pellets.

(vii) For instance, if a new habitat is just being colonised, immigration may contribute more significantly to population growth than birth rates.

(a) Two incorrect
(b) More than four correct
(c) Less than five correct
(d) One incorrect

**45.** Only source of energy in RBCs is

(a) Kreb's cycle
(b) Glycolysis
(c) Hexose monophosphate shunt
(d) ETS

# Zoology

**46.** **Assertion :** Starch can hold iodine molecules in the helical portion.

**Reason :** Starch is present as a store house of energy in plant tissues.

(a) (A) is false but (R) is true.
(b) Both (A) and (R) are true and (R) is the correct explanation of (A).
(c) Both (A) and (R) are true but (R) is not the correct explanation of (A).
(d) (A) is true but (R) is false.

**47.** The continued state of contraction caused by rapid succession of many stimuli is called

(a) muscle twitch (b) tetanus
(c) fatigue (d) cramp

**48.** External fertilization is found in:

(a) Amphiuma (b) Trygon
(c) Catla (d) Salamander

**49.** Match the List – I with List – II and choose the correct option:

| List–I (Molecule) | List–II (Bond) |
|---|---|
| (A) Porifera | (i) Canal system |
| (B) Aschelminthes | (ii) Water-vascular system |
| (C) Annelida | (iii) Muscular pharynx |
| (D) Arthropoda | (iv) Jointed appendages |
| (E) Echinodermata | (v) Metameres |

Options

(a) A - ii, B - iii, C - v, D - iv, E - i
(b) A - ii, B - v, C - iii, D - iv, E - i
(c) A - i, B - iii, C - v, D - iv, E - ii
(d) A - i, B - v, C - iii, D - iv, E - ii

**50.** Which of the following substances is totally reabsorbed through renal tubules?

(a) Na (b) $H_2O$
(c) K (d) $C_6H_{12}O_6$

**51.** Match the column I with column II.

| I | II |
|---|---|
| 1. Muscular Dystrphy | A. Auto-Immune Disorder |
| 2. Myasthenia Gravis | B. Genetic Disorder |
| 3. Arthritis | C. Accumulation of Uric Acid |
| 4. Gout | D. Inflammation of Joints |

(a) 1-A, 2-B, 3- C, 4-D
(b) 1-D, 2-C, 3- B, 4-A
(c) 1-B, 2-A, 3- D, 4-C
(d) 1-C, 2-D, 3- A, 4-B

**52.** The figure shows four animals (A), (B), (C) and (D). Select the correct answer with respect to a common characteristics of two of these animals.

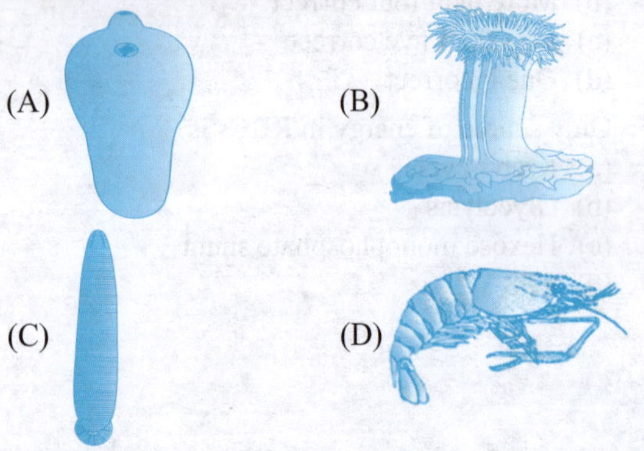

Options:

(a) (C) and (D) have a true coelom
(b) (A) and (D) respire mainly through body wall
(c) (B) and (C) show radial symmetry
(d) (A) and (B) have cnidoblasts for self defence

**53.** Fill in the blanks:-

(i) _A ___can cause vasodilation and there by decrease the blood pressure.
(ii) _B ___is also capable of reabsorption of $HCO_3^-$

Options

(a) A → ANF, B → Henle's loop
(b) A → ADH, B → DCT
(c) A → ADH, B → PCT
(d) A → ANF, B → DCT

**54.** Which one of these animals is not a homeotherm?

(a) Psittacula (b) Macropus
(c) Camelus (d) Chelone

**55.** Figure shows human urinary system with structures labelled A to D select the option which correctly identifies them and gives their characteristics and/or functions.

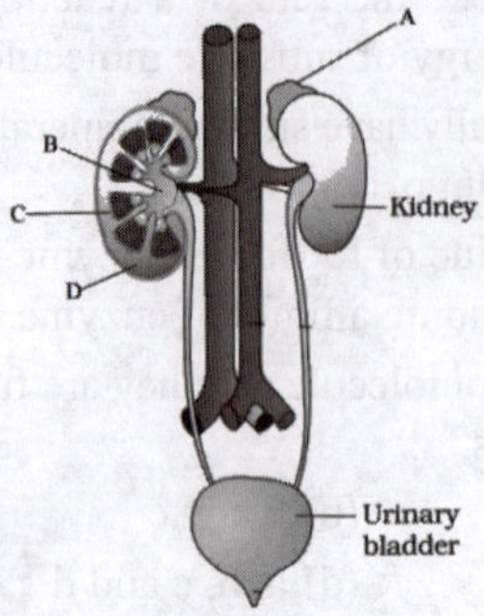


Options:

(a) D-Cortex : Outer part of kidney and do not contain any part of nephrons.
(b) A-Adrenal gland: Located at the anterior part of kidney. Secrete Catecholamines which stimulate glycogen breakdown.
(c) B-Pelvis: Broad funnel shaped space inner to hilum, directly connected to loops of Henle.
(d) C-Medulla- Inner zone of kidney and contains complete nephrons.

**56.** Which characters for reproduction in living organisms are correct from given characters ?

(i) Fungi multiply and spread easily due to the millions of asexual spores
(ii) Lower organisms like yeast and hydra reproduce by budding
(iii) In Planaria (flat worms) regeneration not present
(iv) The fungi, the filamentous algae, the protonema of mosses, all easily multiply by fragmentation
(v) Unicellular organisms like bacteria, unicellular algae and Amoeba, reproduction is synonymous with growth, i.e., increase in number of cells.

(a) (i), (ii) and (iii)
(b) (i), (ii), (iv) and (v)
(c) (ii), (iii) and (iv)
(d) (i) and (v) only

**57.** **Statement I:** Diabetes Insipidus is featured by excessive urination and too much thirst.

**Statement II:** The anterior lobe of pituitary gland secretes Anti-Diuretic Hormone (ADH).

(a) Statement I is incorrect but statement II is true.
(b) Both Statements I and II are true.
(c) Both Statements I and II are false.
(d) Statement I is correct but statement II is false

**58.** All of the following hormones shows following mechanism except one:

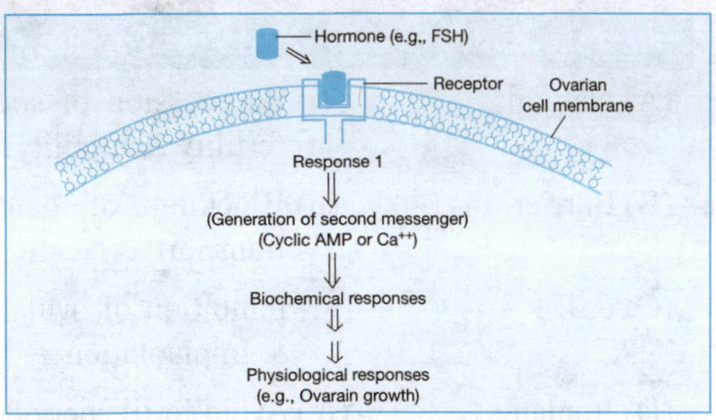


(a) Hypothalamic and Pituitary hormones
(b) Thyroxin and Steroid hormones
(c) Pineal hormone
(s) Adrenal medulla hormones

**59.** Which is the following hormone is related with physical, mental and sexual growth of a baby. It is the main calorigenic hormone which also regulates BMR:
(a) GH (b) Thyroxine
(c) Cortisol (d) Insulin

**60.** In frog, mesorchium is a thin fold of membrane extending between:
(a) Two testes (b) Liver and kidneys
(c) Two kidneys (d) Kidneys and testes

**61.** Read the following statements and find out how many of these are correct for the given figure:

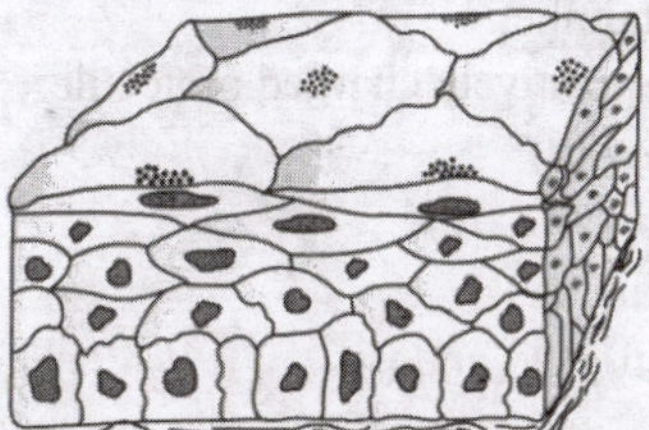

A. Multi-layered epithelium
B. Limited role in secretion and absorption
C. Main function is to provide protection against chemical and mechanical stresses
D. They cover the dry surface of skin, moist surface of buccal cavity and pharynx.

(a) Four (b) Three
(c) Two (d) One

**62. Statement I:** Diaphragm helps in human respiration.

**Statement II:** Contraction of diaphragm decreases volume of thoracic chamber.
(a) Statement I is incorrect but Statement II is true.
(b) Both Statement I and Statement II are true.
(c) Both Statement I and Statement II are false.
(c) Statement I is correct but Statement II is false

**63.** Appearance of dark-coloured peppered moth among the light-coloured ones as a result of increased industrial pollution is an example of:
(a) Disruptive selection
(b) Stabilising selection
(c) Directional selection
(d) None of these

**64.** What was the most significant trend in the evolution of modern man (*Homo sapiens*) from his ancestors?
(a) Increasing cranial capacity
(b) Upright posture
(c) Shortening of jaws
(d) Binocular vision

**65. Statement I:** Passage of ova through the female reproductive tract is facilitated by amoeboid movement of fallopian tube.

**Statement II:** Cilliary movement in trachea help in removing dust particles & foreign substances inhaled along the atmospheric air.
(a) Statement I is incorrect but Statement II is true.
(b) Both Statement I and Statement II are true.
(c) Both Statement I and Statement II are false.
(d) Statement I is correct but Statement II is false

**66.** During pulmonary circulation:
(a) deoxygenated blood is pumped into the pulmonary artery.
(b) deoxygenated blood is pumped into pulmonary vein.
(c) both (A) and (B).
(d) oxygenated blood is carried by the pulmonary veins into right atrium.

**67.** *Entamoeba histolytica* is a ____A____ parasite in the ____B____ of humans which causes amoebiasisis or amoebic dysentery.
(a) A - Bacterial; B - Large intestine
(b) A - Protozoan; B - Small intestine
(c) A - Bacterial; B - Oesophagus
(d) A - Protozoan; B - Large intestine

**68.** An antibody is represented as:
(a) $H_2L_4$ (b) $H_3L_3$
(c) $H_4L_4$ (d) $H_2L_2$

**69.** Which of the following statement(s) is/are true for menstrual cycle?
(i) It occurs in female of all mammals.
(ii) In human non-pregnant normal females, menstruation is repeated at an average interval of about 28/29 days.

(iii) In human beings, ovulation cycles ceases around 50 years of age; that is termed as menopause.
(iv) Lack of menstruation is always an indicator of pregnancy.
(v) Menstruation only occurs if the released ovum is fertilised.
(vi) Menarche is the last menstruation.
(a) (i), (iii), (iv), (v), and (vi)
(b) (iii), (iv) and (v)
(c) (ii) and (vi) only
(d) Only (ii) and (iii)

**70.** LSD is obtained from:
(a) *Claviceps* (b) *Trichoderma*
(c) *Ephedra* (d) *Penicillium*

**71.** Fibrosis of lungs that causes serious lung damage is a characteristic feature of
(a) Bronchial asthma
(b) Emphysema
(c) Asbestosis
(d) Pertussis

**72.** Binding of oxygen with haemoglobin is primarily related to:
(a) Partial pressure of $CO_2$
(b) $H^+$ concentration
(c) pH and temperature
(d) Partial pressure $O_2$

**73.** Which of the given statements are correct?
(i) Innate immunity is a specific type of defence, that is present at the time of birth.
(ii) Malignant malaria is caused by *Plasmodium falciparum*.
(iii) Malaria could be confirmed by Widal test.
(iv) Active immunity is slow and takes time to give its full effective response.
(v) Saliva in the mouth acts as physiological barrier for pathogens.
(a) (ii), (iv) and (v)
(b) (i) and (iii)
(c) (i) and (v)
(d) (ii), (iii) and (v)

**74.** If mammalian ovum fails to get fertilized, which one of the following is unlikely?
(a) Estrogen secretion further decreases
(b) Progesterone secretion rapidly declines
(c) Corpus luteum will disintegrate
(d) Primary follicle starts developing

**75.** Match the following.

| List–I (Method) | List–II (Mode of action) |
|---|---|
| (A) Natural | (i) Suppression of sperm fertility & motility |
| (B) Barrier | (ii) Blocking of gamete transport |
| (C) IUD | (iii) Inhibition of ovulation & Implantation |
| (D) Implants | (iv) Avoid fertile period |
| (E) Surgical | (v) Prevent physical meeting of sperm & ovum |

(a) A – (iv), B – (v), C – (i), D – (iii), E – (ii)
(b) A – (iii), B – (ii), C – (i), D – (iv), E – (v)
(c) A – (ii), B – (iii), C – (i), D – (v), E – (iv)
(d) A – (ii), B – (i), C – (iii), D – (iv), E – (v)

**76.** Which of the following statements are correct?
(i) Ti plasmid of Agrobacteriun tumefaciens is used to deliver desirable gene into plant cells.
(ii) Hind II always cuts DNA molecules at a particular point by recognising a specific sequence of six base pairs.
(iii) Separated DNA fragments cannot be visualised without staining on an agarose gel electrophoresis.
(iv) 'Ori' is the sequence responsible for controlling the copy number.
(v) DNA is a positively charged molecule.
(a) (i), (iii) and (v)
(b) (i), (ii), (iii) and (iv)
(c) (iii), (iv) and (v)
(d) (i), (ii), (iii), (iv) and (v)

**77.** The main objective of production/use herbicide resistant GM crops is to:
(a) eliminate weeds from the field without the use of herbicides
(b) encourage eco-friendly herbicides
(c) Both (A) and (B)
(d) eliminate weeds from the field without the use of manual labour

**78.** Which of the following is not applicable to *Agrobacterium tumefaciens*?
(a) Pathogen of several dicot plants
(b) Has ability to transform cells
(c) Delivers gene of our interest
(d) Ti plasmid of it is always pathogenic to plants without any exception

**79.** Which statement is true about bioreactor?

(A) Bioreactor provides the optimal conditions for obtaining the desired products.

(B) Raw materials are biologically converted into specific products.

(C) Commonly stirring is required.

(D) Large volume of cultures cannot be processed.

(a) A, B (b) B, C

(c) C, D (d) A, B, C, D

**80.** Name the factors of steps indicated with numbers (i), (ii) and (iii):

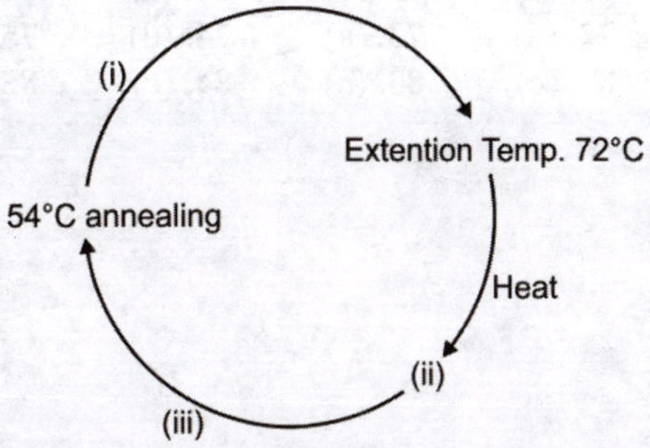


(a) (i) Taq polymerase (ii) Denaturation at 94° C (iii) Primer

(b) (i) Denaturation at 94°C (ii) Taq polymerase (iii) Primer

(c) (i) Primer (ii) Denaturation at 94°C (iii) Taq polymerase

(d) (i) Ligation (ii) Extension (iii) Taq polymerase

**81.** Different peaks are observed during density gradient centrifugation of human DNA. The bulk DNA forms a major peak and the other small peaks are referred to as:

(a) Non-Repetitive DNA (b) SNPs (Snips)

(c) Taq-DNA (d) Satellite DNA

**82.** Use of certain chemicals and radiation to change the base sequences of genes of crop plants is termed.

(a) Recombinant DNA technology

(b) Transgenic mechanism

(c) Mutation breeding

(d) Gene therapy

**83.** Match the following.

| List–I | List–II | List–III | List–IV |
|---|---|---|---|
| 1. Cotton | (A) RNA interference | (X) *B. thuringiensis* | (i) Nematode |
| 2. Barrier | (B) Insecticidal protein | (Y) *Agrobacterium sp.* | (ii) Ballworm |

(a) 1 – B – X – ii, 2 – A – Y – i

(b) 1 – A – X – ii, 2 – B – Y – i

(c) 1 – B – X – i, 2 – A – Y – ii

(d) 1 – A – Y – ii, 2 – B – X – i

**84.** If 'X' is a hormone which controls the carbohydrate metabolism in the body and 'Y' is a hormone which controls the secretion of 'X', then 'X' and 'Y' are

(a) Insulin and somatotrophin

(b) Aldosterone and growth hormone

(c) Glucocorticoid and ACTH respectively

(d) Glucocorticoid and GHRH

**85.** The receptors of neurotransmitters are present on/in the:

(a) Pre-synaptic membrane

(b) Synaptic cleft

(c) Post-synaptic membrane

(d) Ion channels

**86.** Select the true statement.

(a) A band is present in the middle of sarcomere

(b) H zone is present in the middle of A - band

(c) M line is present in the middle of H - zone

(d) All of these

**87.** Which one is the vasoconstrictor?

(a) ANF

(b) Renin

(c) Angiotensin-II

(d) Histamine

**88.** Amino acids are transported from the intestine to liver by:

(a) Hepatic artery

(b) Hepatic portal vein

(c) Pulmonary vein

(d) Hepatic vein

**89.** Diaphragm is a dome-shaped muscular structure which separates:

(a) Coelomic cavity from pelvic cavity

(b) Pleural cavity from thoracic cavity

(c) Thoracic cavity from abdominal cavity

(d) Pelvic cavity from abdominal cavity

**90.** The breakdown of biomolecules i.e. dipeptides, lactose, maltose and sucrose etc. occur mainly in the:

(a) Ilium

(b) Pyloric region of stomach

(c) Duodenum region of small intestine

(d) Caecum region of large intestine

## Answer Key

### Botany

| | | | | | | | | | |
|---|---|---|---|---|---|---|---|---|---|
| **1.** (a) | **2.** (d) | **3.** (d) | **4.** (b) | **5.** (b) | **6.** (b) | **7.** (a) | **8.** (c) | **9.** (b) | **10.** (c) |
| **11.** (b) | **12.** (a) | **13.** (a) | **14.** (d) | **15.** (d) | **16.** (c) | **17.** (a) | **18.** (a) | **19.** (d) | **20.** (c) |
| **21.** (c) | **22.** (c) | **23.** (a) | **24.** (a) | **25.** (b) | **26.** (b) | **27.** (a) | **28.** (b) | **29.** (a) | **30.** (b) |
| **31.** (c) | **32.** (b) | **33.** (a) | **34.** (a) | **35.** (b) | **36.** (b) | **37.** (b) | **38.** (c) | **39.** (b) | **40.** (a) |
| **41.** (a) | **42.** (b) | **43.** (b) | **44.** (b) | **45.** (b) | | | | | |

### Zoology

| | | | | | | | | | |
|---|---|---|---|---|---|---|---|---|---|
| **46.** (c) | **47.** (b) | **48.** (c) | **49.** (c) | **50.** (d) | **51.** (c) | **52.** (a) | **53.** (d) | **54.** (d) | **55.** (b) |
| **56.** (b) | **57.** (d) | **58.** (b) | **59.** (b) | **60.** (d) | **61.** (a) | **62.** (d) | **63.** (c) | **64.** (a) | **65.** (a) |
| **66.** (a) | **67.** (d) | **68.** (d) | **69.** (d) | **70.** (a) | **71.** (c) | **72.** (d) | **73.** (a) | **74.** (d) | **75.** (a) |
| **76.** (b) | **77.** (d) | **78.** (d) | **79.** (a) | **80.** (a) | **81.** (d) | **82.** (c) | **83.** (a) | **84.** (c) | **85.** (c) |
| **86.** (d) | **87.** (c) | **88.** (b) | **89.** (c) | **90.** (c) | | | | | |

## Hints and Explanations

## BOTANY

**1** For 50 amino acid the codons (triplet) required are 150. If 25TH codon converted to stop codon amino acid, translation stops. Therefore a polypeptide of 24 amino acid will be formed.

**2.** RNA polymerase transcribe only structural gene.

**3.**

| List–I (Part of nucleus) | List–II (Function) |
|---|---|
| (A) Perinuclear space | (i) Barrier between nucleus & cytoplasm |
| (B) Nucleolus | (ii) Site for active ribosomal RNA synthesis |
| (C) Centromere | (iii) Holds two chromatids of chromosome |
| (D) Nuclea pore | (iv) Passages for movement of molecules between nucleus & cytoplasm |
| (E) Satellite | (v) Secondary constriction on chromosome present at a constant location |

**4.** (i)

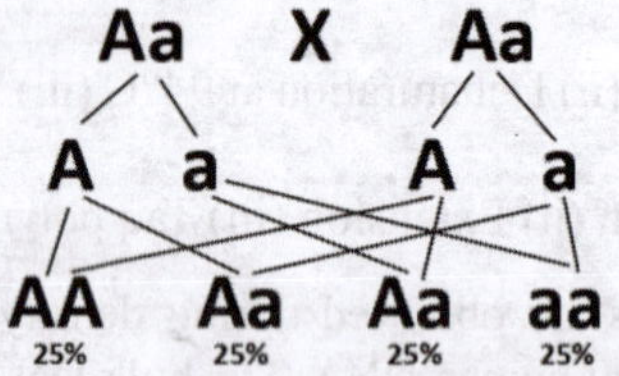


AA = Homozygous dominant probability is 25%.

(ii) Type of gametes = $2^n$ ; n = no. of heterozygous pair AA Bb cc, $2^1 = 2$; only two type of gametes are formed.

(iii) *Mirabilis jalapa* is example of incomplete dominance therefore ratio of $F_2$ progeny in both genotypic and phenotypic is 1 : 2 : 1.

**5.** Male heterogamety: In some organisms, e.g., birds and some reptiles a different mechanism of sex determination is observed in this case the total number of chromosomes is same in both males and females. But two different types of gametes in terms of the sex chromosomes, are produced by females, i.e., female heterogametic. In order to have a distinction with the mechanism of sex determination described earlier, the two different sex chromosomes of a female bird has been designated to be the Z and W chromosomes.

In these organisms the females have one Z and one W chromosome, whereas males have a pair of Z-chromosomes besides the autosomes. 1:1 sex ratio is produced in offspring.

**6.** Fungi are either saprophytic (they feed on dead plant and animal material), parasitic (they feed off a living host) or symbiotic (they share a mutually beneficial relationship with another organism). Saprophytic fungi release enzymes to soften the dead plant or animal.

**7.** The law of independent assortment is applicable to those factors or genes which are either located distantly on the same chromosome or occur on different (homologous) chromosomes.

**8.** Black eye is dominant over blue eye

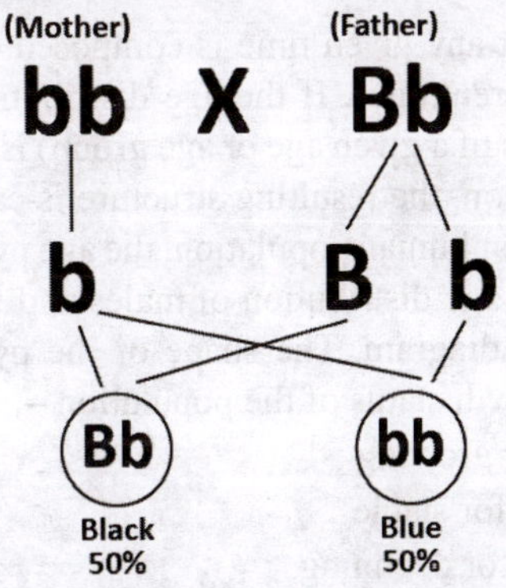


In any chance their probability is 50% only.

**9.** His haemoglobin chain may show polymerisation at low oxygen concentration. Malarial parasite can not enter in cell having Hbs haemoglobin.

**10.** The outer covering of endosperm separates the embryo by a proteinous layer called aleurone layer. The embryo is small and situated in a groove at one end of the endosperm. It consists of one large and shield shaped cotyledon known as scutellum and a short axis with a plumule and a radicle. The plumule and radical are enclosed in sheaths which are called coleoptile and coleorhizae respectively.

**11.** Many pulses of daily use belong to one of the family fabaceae. Examples—Gram, arhar, sem, moong, soyabean.

Solanaceae (potato family)

Liliaceae (lily family)

Poaceae (cereal or grass family)

**12.** Solanaceae Gynoecium: bicarpellary, syncarpous; ovary superior, bilocular, placenta swollen with many ovules

**13.**

| | | |
|---|---|---|
| Turmeric | Underground | Storage & perennation |
| Pumpkin | Stem tendrils | Help in climbing |
| Citrus | Thorns | Protection from browsing animals |
| Opuntia | Flattened green structure | Photosynthesis |

**14.** Examples of Ascomycetes is *Aspergillus, Claviceps* and *Neurospora.* Many members like morels and truffles are edible and are considered delicacies.

**15.** Citrus canker caused by bacteria

**16.** Photosynthetically $C_4$-plants are more efficient than $C_3$-plants.

Photosynthesis in $C_4$ plants takes place in mesophyll and bundle sheath cells.

**17.** The compositae family has an inferior ovary with cypsela fruit that has hair-like projections thereon called the pappus.

**18.** Basal placentation is observed in the Asteraceae family, which stands out as one of the largest and the most geographically widespread families of plant species. Within this family, various flowers, such as marigold and sunflower, are included.

**19.** Marginal placentation is a feature of the Leguminosae family. The flowers exhibit a monocarpellary unilocular ovary, and the ovules are situated in rows near the margin on the placenta formed along the ventral suture.

**20.** (iii) In over 60 percent of angiosperms, pollen grains are shed at 2-celled stage.

(v) In some cereals such as rice and wheat, pollen grains lose viability within 30 minute of their release.

(vi) In some members of Rosasceae, Leguminosae and Solanaceae, pollen grains maintain viability for months.

(vii) It is possible to store pollen grains of a large number of species for years in liquid nitrogen (-196°C) and used as pollen bank.

**21.** Meiosis involves two sequential cycles of nuclear and cell division called meiosis I and meiosis II but only a single cycle of DNA replication.

Meiosis I is initiated after the parental chromosomes have replicated to produce identical sister chromatids at the S phase.

Meiosis involves pairing of homologous chromosomes and recombination between them. Therefore daughter cells are not genetically identical.

Four haploid cells are formed at the end of meiosis II.

**22.** Some cells in the adult animals do not appear to exhibit division (e.g.,heart cells) and many other cells divide only occasionally, as needed to replace cells that have been lost because of injury or cell death. These cells that do not divide further exit $G_1$ phase to enter an inactive stage called quiescent stage ($G_0$) of the cell cycle. Cells in this stage remain metabolically active but no longer proliferate unless called on to do so, depending on the requirement of the organism.

**23.**

| | |
|---|---|
| (A) Phenyl ketonuria | (i) Pleiotropy |
| (B) Skin colour in humans | (ii) Polygenic inheritance |
| (C) Flower position in pea plant | (iii) Dominance |
| (D) Blood group in humans | (iv) Codominance |

**24.** The ecosystems which develop in nature without human support or interference are called natural ecosystems. This ecosystem is self-regulated by positive and negative feedback.

**25.** A few organisms can tolerate and thrive in a wide range of temperatures (they are called eury thermal), but, a vast majority of them are restricted to a narrow range of temperatures (such organisms are called stenothermal).

**Euryhaline:** Organisms tolerant to wide range of salinities.

**Stenohaline:** Organisms tolerant to a narrow of salinities.

**26.** It is generally believed that competition occurs when closely related species compete for the same resources that are limiting, but this is not entirely true. Firstly, totally unrelated species could also compete for the same resource.

**27.**

| | |
|---|---|
| (A) Nucleoside | (i) N-glycosidic bond |
| (B) Nucleotide | (ii) Phosphodiester bond |
| (C) Dinucleotide | (iii) 3-5 phosphodiester bond |

**28.** The components of the ecosystem are seen to function as a unit when you consider the following aspects:

(i) productivity;
(ii) decomposition;
(iii) energy flow; and
(iv) nutrient (mineral) cycling.

**29.** The ecosystem, in order to appreciate the input (productivity), transfer of energy (food chain/web, nutrient cycling) and the output (degradation and energy loss).

**30.** A population at any given time is composed of individuals of different ages. If the age distribution (per cent individuals of a given age or age group) is plotted for the population, the resulting structure is called an age pyramid. For human population, the age pyramids generally show age distribution of males and females in a combined diagram. The shape of the pyramids reflects the growth status of the population –

(a) Upright for growing
(b) Bell shape for stable
(c) Urn shape for declining.

**31.** Genetic diversity: A single species might show high diversity at the genetic level over its distributional range. The genetic variation shown by the medicinal plant *Rauwolfia vomitoria* growing indifferent Himalayan ranges might be in terms of the potency and concentration of the active chemical (reserpine) that the plant produces. India has more than 50,000 genetically different strains of rice, and 1,000 varieties of mango.

**32.** Robert May places the global species diversity at about 7 million.

German naturalist and geographer **Alexander von Humboldt:** Species-Area relationships

The 'rivet popper hypothesis used by Stanford ecologist :Paul Ehrlich.

**David Tilman's:** Long term ecosystem experiment shows property of stable community.

**33.**

| | | |
|---|---|---|
| *S. cerevisiae* | Ethanol | Yeast |
| *Aspergillus niger* | Citric acid | Fungus |
| *Penicillium notatum* | Penicillin | Fungus |
| *Trichoderma polysporum.* | Cyclosporin A | Fungus |
| *Monascus purpereus* | Statin | Yeast |

**34.** Eggplant (*Solanum melongena*), commonly known as brinjal, belongs to the Solanaceae family and is included under the genus Solanum.

**35.** Plants capture only 2-10 per cent of the PAR and this small amount of energy sustains the entire living world.

**36.** The synergids have special cellular thickenings at the micropylar tip called filiform apparatus, which play an important role in guiding the pollen tubes into the synergid.

**37.** Functional megaspore ---- (Mitosis) → 2 Nuclei are formed which move to the opposite poles ---- (Mitosis) → 4 nucleated stage ---- (Mitosis) → 8 Nucleated stage.

These mitotic divisions are free nuclear type and cell wall formation occur after attaining the 8-nucleate stage. 6 of the 8 nuclei develop cell wall while the remaining 2 nuclei (called polar nuclei) are enclosed in a common cell wall making a central large cell, situated below the egg apparatus.

**38.** Inheritance is the process by which characters are passed on from parent to progeny; it is the basis of heredity. Sexual reproduction produces new recombination leading to variation. Variation is the degree by which progeny differ from their parents.

**39.** Zinc is a cofactor for the proteolytic enzyme carboxy peptidase.

Coenzyme nicotinamide adenine dinucleotide (NAD) and NADP contain the vitamin niacin.

Heme is iron containing prosthetic group in cytochromes, haemoglobin, myoglobin, catalase and peroxides.

**40.** Maize hybrids that had twice the amount of the amino acids, lysine and tryptophan, compared to existing maize hybrids were developed. Wheat variety, Atlas 66, having a high protein content, has been used as a donor for improving cultivated wheat. It has been possible to develop an iron-fortified rice variety containing over five times as much iron as in commonly consumed varieties.

**41.** Fungi like those belonging to the genus *Glomus* form mycorrhiza with roots of higher plants. Fungal partner absorbs phosphorus from the soil and provide it to the plant. In addition plants also receives other benefits - Resistance to root-borne pathogens, tolerance to salinity and drought and increased growth and development of plants.

**42.** Enzyme does not have any effect on energy of substrate. Michaelis Constant (Michaelis Menten Constant, $k_m$) Machaelis constant or $k_m$ of an enzyme is the substrate concentration at which the reaction catalysed by the enzyme attains half its maximum velocity. It indicates the affinity of the enzyme to its substrate. A low $k_m$ indicates strong affinity, while a high $k_m$ shows low affinity. If an enzyme acts on more than one substrate, it shows different $k_m$ values for them.

Enzyme are biomolecule but they are functions outside cell also, therefore they use in invitro reactions. Therefore statement (b) and (c) are correct.

**43.**

| | |
|---|---|
| Tomato | *Lycopersicum esculentum* (botanical name) |
| Berry fruit | Pericarp and Placenta (edible part) |

**44.** A population has certain attributes that an individual organism does not. An individual may have births and deaths, but a population has birth rates and death rates. In a population these rates refer to per capita births and deaths, respectively. The rates, hence, expressed is change in numbers (increase or decrease) with respect to members of the population. Another attribute characteristic of a population is sex ratio. An individual is either a male or a female but a population has a sex ratio.

**45.** RBCs lack nucleus. Glycolysis occurring in cytoplasm is the only source of energy in RBCs.

# ZOOLOGY

**46.** Starch forms helical secondary structures and can hold iodine molecules in the helical portion. Cellulose is also homopolymer found in plants, but cannot hold iodine molecules as it does not contain complex helices.

**47.** Tetanus is a disease in which there is a lack of relaxation among successive stimuli in sustained muscle contraction.

**48.** Most Amphibian (exception showing internal fertilization - Amphiuma, salamander) and Osteichthyes (Catla) shows external fertilization whereas Chondrichthyes (eg-trygon) show internal fertilization.

**49.** **Porifera:** Sponges have a water transport or canal system. Water enters through minute pores (ostia) in the body wall into a central cavity, spongocoel.

**Aschelminthes:** They are bilaterally symmetrical, triploblastic and pseudocoelomate animals. Alimentary canal is complete with a well-developed muscular pharynx.

**Annelida:** Their body surface is distinctly marked out into segments ormetameres.

**Arthropoda:** The body of arthropods is covered by chitinous exoskeleton. The body consists of head, thorax and abdomen. They have jointed appendages (arthros-joint, poda-appendages).

**Echinodermata:** The most distinctive feature of echinoderms is the presence of water vascular system which helps in locomotion, capture and transport of food and respiration. An excretory system is absent.

**50.** Glucose($C_6H_{12}O_6$) is completely reabsorbed in PCT (part of renal tubules).

**51.** (c) 1-B, 2-A, 3- D, 4-C.

**52.** (a) Liver fluke (Platyhelminthes)

(b) Adamsia (Cnidaria) have cnidoblasts and show radial symmetry.

(c) Hirudinaria (Annelida) have true coelom

(d) Prawn (Arthropoda) have true coelom

**53.** Increase in blood flow to the atria of the heart → Atria releases Atrial Natriuretic Factor (ANF) → Vasodilation (dilation of blood vessels) → Decrease in blood pressure → GFR decreases. ANF mechanism works as a check on the renin-angiotensin mechanism.

**Functions of DCT:** Conditional reabsorption of $Na^+$ and water. Reabsorption of $HCO_3^-$ and selective secretion of $H^+$, $K^+$ and $NH_3$ for maintaining the pH and sodium-potassium balance in blood.

**54.** They are warm-blooded (homeotherms) animals, i.e., they are able to maintain a constant body temperature. Example Birds: Psittacula (Parrot) and Mammals: Macropus (Kangaroo) and Camelus (camel)

Chelone is reptile and poikilotherm (cold blooded)

**55.**

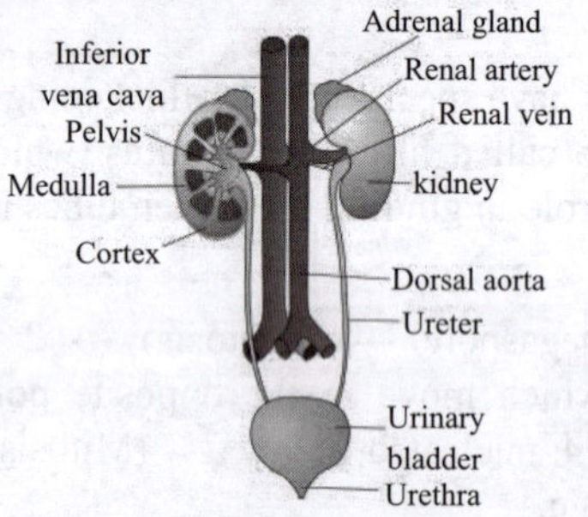


Cortex contain part of nephron and medulla does not contain whole nephron but part of it. Pelvis not connected directly with loop of Henle. C is cortex

**56.** (iii) In Planaria (flat worms), true regeneration is observed i.e. a fragmented organisms re-generate the lost part of its body and becomes a new organisms

**57.** The Anti-Diuretic Hormone (ADH) is secreted from posterior pituitary gland.

**58.**

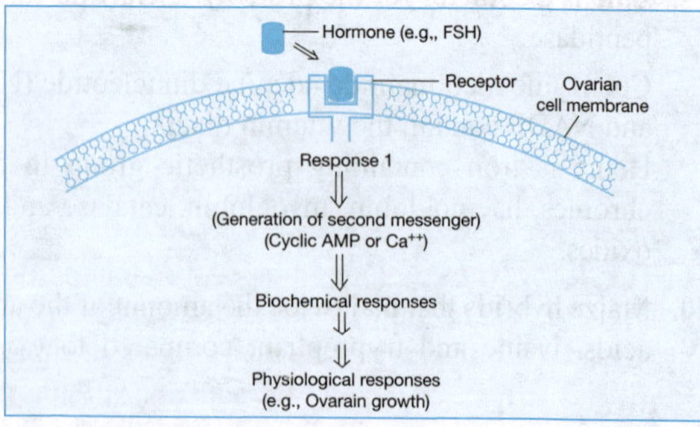


Thyroxin (intranuclear) and Steroid hormone (cytoplasmic) have intracellular receptor whereas all other have receptor situated on cell membrane.

**59.** Functions of Thyroid gland / hormones:
(a) Regulation of the basal metabolic rate (BMR).
(b) Regulate the process of red blood cell formation.
(c) Controlling the metabolism of carbohydrates, proteins and fats.
(d) Maintenance of water and electrolyte balance.
(e) It also help in mental, physical and sexual growth of baby.

**60.** In frogs, a cylindrical testis is located near each kidney, suspended by the mesorchium. Multiple vasa efferentia originate from each testis, passing through the mesorchium to connect with the uriniferous tubules in the posterior region of the kidney. These vasa efferentia then open into Bidder's canal, which, in turn, communicates with the ureter.

**61.** Compound epithelium is made of more than one layer (multi-layered) of cells and thus has a limited role in secretion and absorption. Their main function is to provide protection against chemical and mechanical stresses. They cover the dry surface of the skin, the moist surface of buccal cavity, pharynx, inner lining of ducts of salivary glands and of pancreatic ducts.

**62.** Contraction of diaphragm increases volume of thoracic chamber in the anterio-posterior axis.

**63.** Directional selection: In such selection the longest or the shortest individuals are selected by nature and increase in frequency in the forth-coming generations. In directional selection it is always the 'extreme' which is favored. Evolution of DDT resistant mosquitoes, evolution of giraffe, and industrial melanism in peppered moth are the examples of directional selection.

**64.** Among the stories of evolution of individual species, the story of evolution of modern man is most interesting and appears to parallel evolution of human brain (increasing cranial capacity) and language.

**65.** Passage of ova through the female reproductive tract is facilitated by cilliary movement of fallopian tube.

**66.** The blood pumped by the right ventricle enters the pulmonary artery, whereas the left ventricle pumps blood into the aorta.
The deoxygenated blood pumped into the pulmonary artery is passed onto the lungs from where the oxygenated blood is carried by the pulmonary veins into the left atrium. This pathway constitutes the pulmonary circulation.

**67.** *Entamoeba histolytica* is a protozoan parasite in the large intestine of human which causes amoebiasisis (amoebic dysentery). Houseflies act as mechanical carriers and serve to transmit the parasite from faeces of infected person to food and food products, thereby contaminating them. Drinking water and contaminated food by the faecal matter are the main source of infection.

**68.** Each antibody molecule has four peptide chains, two small called light chains and two longer called heavy chains. Hence, an antibody is represented as $H_2L_2$.

**69.** (i) It occurs in female primates (monkey, apps, human).
(iv) Lack of menstruation is not always an indicator of pregnancy. It may also be due to stress, poor health, etc.
(v) Menstruation only occurs if the released ovum is not fertilised.
(vi) The first menstruation begins at puberty and is called menarche.

**70.** LSD is a crystalline amidated alkaloid obtained from ergot, an extract obtained from fruiting body of fungus *Claviceps purpurea* (parasite on Rye plant). It is the most powerful hallucinogen. It is usually smoked. LSD causes nightmares (horrible dreams), hallucination, floating sensation, chronic psychosis and severe damage to the CNS. It may cause unconsciousness and even death. It brings about chromosomal aberrations and foetal abnormalities. An LSD addict can be easily recognized from incoherence in writing and drawing.

**71.** Occupational Respiratory Disorders: In certain industries, especially those involving grinding or stone-breaking (asbestosis), so much dust is produced that the defense mechanism of the body cannot fully cope with the situation. Long exposure can give rise to inflammation leading to fibrosis (proliferation of fibrous tissues) and thus causing serious lung damage. Workers in such industries should wear protective masks.

**72.** Binding of oxygen with hemoglobin is primarily related to partial pressure of $O_2$. Partial pressure of $CO_2$, hydrogen ion concentration and temperature are the other factors which can interfere with this binding.

**73.** (i) Innate immunity is a non-specific type of defence that is present at the time of birth.
(iii) Typhoid could be confirmed by Widal test.

**74.** In the absence of fertilization, the corpus luteum degenerates so there is rapid decline in progesterone secretion. This causes disintegration of the endometrium leading to menstruation, marking a new cycle.

**75.**

| | |
|---|---|
| Natural | Avoid fertile period |
| Barrier | Prevent physical meeting of sperm & ovum |
| IUD | Suppression of sperm fertility & motility |
| Implants | Inhibition of ovulation & Implantation |
| Surgical | Blocking of gamete transport |

**76.** (v) DNA is a negatively charged molecule.

**77.** These types of plants were developed to help farmers control weeds without the use of manual labour that competes with crops for soil, space, water, and sunlight. So, the correct option is 'Eliminate weeds from the field without the use of manual labour'.

**78.** *Agrobacterium tumefaciens*, a pathogen of several dicot plants (not all plants) is able to deliver a piece of DNA known as 'T-DNA' to transform normal plant cells into a tumor and direct these tumor cells to produce the chemicals required by the pathogen. Similarly, retroviruses in animals have the ability to transform normal cells into cancerous cells. And disarmed Ti plasmid is no more pathogenic.

**79.** Small volume cultures cannot yield appreciable quantities of products. To produce in large quantities, the development of bioreactors, where large volumes (100-1000 liters) of culture can be processed, was required. Thus, bioreactors can be thought of as vessels in which raw materials are biologically converted into specific products, individual enzymes, etc., using microbial plant, animal or human cells. A bioreactor provides the optimal conditions for achieving the desired product by providing optimum growth conditions (temperature, pH, substrate, salts, vitamins, oxygen). Most commonly used bioreactor are of stirring type. So statement A, B and C are correct.

**80.** The PCR amplification cycle involves following three steps.

(i) **Denaturation**
The target DNA is heated to a high temperature (usually 94°C). It results in separation of the two strands. Each single strand of the target DNA acts as a template for DNA synthesis.
(ii) **Annealing**
In this step, two small chemically synthesized oligonucleotides (that are complementary to the regions of DNA) primers anneal (or hybridize) to each of the single stranded template DNA. This step occur at temperature usually 40 - 60 $_0$C.
(iii) **Primer Extension (Polymerization).**
In this step a thermo stable enzyme Taq DNA Polymerase (isolated from a bacterium, Thermus aquaticus) is used to extend primers using the nucleotides and the genomic DNA as template. Synthesis of new DNA strand begins in between the primers, using deoxyribonucleotide triphosphates and $Mg^{2+}$.
The optimum temperature for this polymerization is kept at 72°C. The Taq DNA Polymerase remain active during the high temperature induced denaturation of double stranded DNA. If the process of replication of DNA is repeated many times, the segment of DNA can be amplified to approximately billion times (i.e., 1 billion copies are made).

**81.** When density gradient centrifugation is done, bulk DNA is represented by a major peak while the repetitive DNA is represented by other small peaks. These small peaks are also referred as satellite DNA.
On the basis of base composition (A : T rich or G : C rich), length of segment and the number of repetitive segments, satellite DNA is classified into many categories-micro satellites, mini satellites, etc.

**82.** Use of certain chemicals and radiation to change the base sequences of genes of crop plants is termed as mutation breeding. Mutation is induced artificially through use of chemicals or radiations like gamma radiations. In moong bean, resistance to yellow mosaic virus and powdery mildew were induced by mutations.

**83.**

| | | | |
|---|---|---|---|
| Cotton | Insecticidal protein. | *B. thuringiensis* | Ballworm |
| Tobacco | RNA interference | *Agrobacterium sp.* | Nematode |

**84.** Carbohydrate metabolism is regulated by glucocorticoid released by adrenal cortex of adrenal gland and secretion of glucocorticoid is stimulated by ACTH. Somatotrophin regulates the release of GH.
Aldosterone regulates the water and electrolyte balance in the body.
GHRH secreted by hypothalamus stimulates the release of growth hormone from the pituitary gland.

**85.** The neurotransmitters that are released by pre–synaptic membrane and attaches to the receptors that are present on the post-synaptic membrane

**86.**

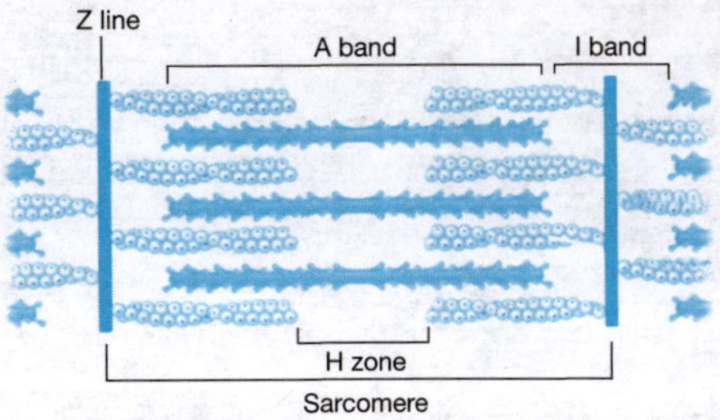


- A band is present in the middle of the sarcomere.
- H-zone is present in the middle of the A-band
- M-line is present in the middle of H-zone.

**87.** Vasoconstrictors : Angiotensin II
Vasodilators : ANF, histamine
Renin is also known as angiotensinogenase which catalyses the conversion of inactive angiotensinogen to angiotensin-II ultimately.

**88.** Hepatic artery carries oxygenated blood to the liver.
Hepatic vein carries deoxygenated blood from the liver to heart.
Hepatic portal vein carries blood from digestive system to liver.

**89.** Thoracic cavity is closed below by the diaphragm which is a dome-shaped structure made up of muscles and separates thoracic cavity from abdominal cavity (containing most of the digestive organs).

**90.** Duodenum region of small intestine. Because the enzyme requires the breakdown of biomolecules i.e. dipeptides, lactose, maltose and sucrose are present in the succus entericus (intestinal juice).

# MOCK TEST-2

## Botany

**1.** Match the following.

| List–I (Organelle) | List–II (Function) |
|---|---|
| (A) ER | (i) Synthesis of glycoprotein & glycolipid |
| (B) Golgi complex | (ii) Synthesis of protein & lipids |
| (C) Lysosomes | (iii) Contain water / sap/ food/ excretory product |
| (D) Vacuoles | (iv) Storage of hydrolytic enzymes |

(a) A – (iii), B – (iv), C – (ii), D – (i)
(b) A – (ii), B – (i), C – (iv), D – (iii)
(c) A – (ii), B – (iv), C – (iii), D – (i)
(d) A – (iii), B – (i), C – (iv), D – (ii)

**2.** *Rhizophora* produces pneumatophores for:
(a) rapid absorption
(b) mechanical support
(c) anchoring
(d) gaseous exchange

**3.** Food is stored in adventitious roots in:
(a) carrots (b) sweet potato
(c) sugar beets (d) all of these

**4.** In dorsiventral leaf, the locations of the phloem and palisade tissue, respectively, are:
(a) Abaxial and Adaxial
(b) Adaxial and Abaxial
(c) Abaxial and Abaxial
(d) Adaxial and Adaxial

**5.** Casparian strips are present on which wall of the endodermal cells?
(a) Tangential walls (b) Radial walls
(c) Both (A) and (B) (d) None of these

**6.** Match the following.

| List–I (Term) | List–II (Part of plant) |
|---|---|
| (A) Pulvinus | (i) Swollen end of pedicel bearing flower whorls |
| (B) Rachis | (ii) Common axis on which leaflets are arranged in pinnately compound leaf |
| (C) Receptacle | (iii) Swollen leaflets in leguminous plants |

(a) A – (iii), B – (i), C – (ii)
(b) A – (ii), B – (iii), C – (i)
(c) A – (ii), B – (i), C – (iii)
(d) A – (iii), B – (ii), C – (i)

**7.** Which of the following characters for algae are incorrect from given characters?
(i) At least a half of the total carbon dioxide fixation on earth is carried out by algae through photosynthesis.
(ii) Being photosynthetic they decrease the level of dissolved oxygen in their immediate environment.
(iii) Many species of *Porphyra, Laminaria* and *Sargassum*, are fresh water algae
(iv) Certain freshwater brown and red algae produce large amounts of Pyrenoids, used as water holding substances
(v) Agar obtained from *Gelidium* and *Gracilaria*
(vi) *Chlorella* and *Spirulina* are used as food supplements by space travellers.

(a) (i), (ii), (v) and (vi)
(b) (i), (ii) (iii) and (iv)
(c) (ii), (iii) and (v)
(d) (ii), (iii) and (iv)

**8.** Isotopes used for proving semiconservative replication of DNA were:
(a) $^{14}N$ and $^{31}P$
(b) $^{14}N$ and $^{14}C$
(c) $^{14}N$ and $^{15}N$
(d) $^{14}C$ and $^{31}P$

**9.** Find the wrongly matched pair:

| | |
|---|---|
| (a) Har Gobind Khorana | - Synthesised RNA molecules chemically |
| (b) George Gamow | - Codon is triplet |
| (c) Meselson and Stahl | - Regulation of gene expression |
| (d) Frederick Sanger | - Amino acid sequencing |

**10.** Which one of the following statements is incorrect?
(a) DNA chemically is less reactive and structurally more stable when compared to RNA.
(b) A nitrogenous base is linked to the pentose sugar through a Phosphodiester linkage to form a nucleoside
(c) The presence of thymine at the place of Uracil confers additional stability to DNA.
(d) Meselson and Stahl provided experimental evidence for semiconservative DNA replication.

**11.** **Statement I:** Presence of photorespiration is considered as a wasteful and energy consuming process in crop plants, ultimately leads to reduction in yield.

**Statement II:** In photorespiration, there is synthesis of sugar with utilization of ATP.
(a) Statement I is incorrect but Statement II is true.
(b) Both Statement I and Statement II are true.
(c) Both Statement I and Statement II are false.
(d) Statement I is correct but Statement II is false

**12.** Which of the following is a correct match?

| | |
|---|---|
| (a) Haemophilia | - Y-chromosome |
| (b) Sickle-cell anaemia | - X-chromosome |
| (c) Down syndrome | - 21$^{st}$ chromosome |
| (d) Parkinson's disease | - X- and Y- chromosome |

**13.** Which of the following organisms breed only once in lifetime?
(a) Birds
(b) Bamboo
(c) Oysters
(d) Mammals

**14.** Sporopollenin is found in:
(a) outer wall of pollens
(b) inner wall of pollens
(c) pollen tube
(d) male gametes

**15.** Both the zebra and African lion live in the tropical grasslands but occupy different:
(a) habitats
(b) biospheres
(c) environments
(d) ecological niches

**16.** First common intermediate formed by the oxidation of fat, carbohydrates and deamination of Proteins is:
(a) Acetyl-CoA
(b) Pyruvic acid
(c) PHAP
(d) $\alpha$-ketoglutarate

**17.** Self-incompatibility:
(i) is a device to prevent inbreeding.
(ii) provides cross pollination.
(iii) ensures cross fertilization.
(iv) is governed by pollen- pistil interaction.
(v) is governed by series of multiple alleles.
(vi) prevents self-pollen (from the same flower or other flowers of the same plant) from fertilization or pollen tube growth in the pistil.
(a) All are correct
(b) All are wrong
(c) (i), (ii), (iii) are correct
(d) (iv) and (v) are wrong

**18.** Natality is the characteristic of population which means:
(a) The total number of individuals present per unit area at a given time.
(b) The increase in number of individuals in a population under given environmental conditions.
(c) Loss of individuals due to death in a population under given environmental conditions.
(d) The movement of individuals into and out of population.

**19.** Tasmanian wolf is a marsupial while wolf is a placental mammal. This shows:
(a) Genetic drift
(b) Parallel evolution
(c) Divergent evolution
(d) Inheritance of acquired characters

**20.** Which kind of ecological pyramid is represented by the table given below:

| | |
|---|---|
| Carnivores | 12 gm/m² |
| Herbivores | 8 gm/m² |
| Producers | 4 gm/m² |

(a) Inverted pyramid of numbers
(b) Inverted pyramid of biomass
(c) Inverted pyramid of energy
(d) Upright pyramid of numbers

**21.** In light reaction of photosynthesis, which of the following phenomenon is observed during cyclic as well as non-cyclic photophosphorylation?
(a) Formation of ATP
(b) Release of $O_2$
(c) Involvement of both pigment system-I and pigment system – II
(d) Formation of $NADPH_2$

**22.** Which does not belong to kingdom Monera?
(a) Mycoplasma (b) Archaebacteria
(c) Slime moulds (d) Eubacteria

**23.** When stomata close, which of the following events does not occur?
(a) Guard cells become flaccid
(b) Sugar is converted to starch
(c) O.P. of guard cells decreases
(d) Accumulation of oxygen takes place

**24.** Nucleolus in eukaryotic cells is:
(a) Visible in metaphase
(b) Bounded by a membrane
(c) The site for synthesis of RNA polymerase
(d) The site for packaging of r-RNAs with ribosomal proteins

**25.** Match the following.

| List–I (Scientist) | List–II (Material used in experiment) |
|---|---|
| (A) Meselson & Stahl | (i) R & S strains of *S. pneumoniae* |
| (B) Hershey & Chasc | (ii) Heavy isotope of nitrogen |
| (C) F. Griffith | (iii) Radioactive photosphorus & sulphur |

(a) A – (ii), B – (iii), C – (i)
(b) A – (iii), B – (i), C – (ii)
(c) A – (ii), B – (i), C – (iii)
(d) A – (iii), B – (ii), C – (i)

**26.** During meiosis I, the bivalent chromosomes clearly appear as tetrads during:
(a) Diakinesis (b) Diplotene
(c) Leptotene (d) Pachytene

**27.** Guard cells help in:
(a) fighting against infection
(b) protection against grazing
(c) transpiration
(d) guttation

**28.** Floral rewards to a moth providing safe places to lay eggs occur in ____________ and none of the two can complete its life cycle without the other.
(a) Hibiscus (b) Yucca
(c) Both (a) and (b) (d) None of these

**29.** In cryopreservation, germplasm is maintained at
(a) -196° F (b) 0° F
(c) -100° F (d) None

**30.** In bacterial photosynthesis and chemosynthesis, oxygen is not evolved because on these processes:
(a) $CO_2$ is not used
(b) $H_2S$ is not used
(c) $H_2O$ is not used
(d) Carbohydrate is not synthesized

**31.** Which of the following is correct about light reaction?
(a) Light is required.
(b) ATPs are produced during reaction.
(c) NADPH is produce during reaction.
(d) All of the above

**32.** Match the following.

| List–I (Microbes) | List–II (Byproducts) |
|---|---|
| (A) *Clostridium sp.* | (i) $C_6H_8O_7$ |
| (B) *Methanobacterium sp.* | (ii) $C_3H_6O_3$ |
| (C) *Acetobacter sp.* | (iii) $CH_4$ |
| (D) *Aspergillus sp.* | (iv) $C_4H_8O_2$ |
| (E) *Lactobacillus sp.* | (v) $CH_3$ COOH ($C_2H_4O_2$) |

(a) A – (iv), B – (iii), C – (v), D – (i), D – (ii)
(b) A – (iii), B – (ii), C – (iv), D – (i), D – (v)
(c) A – (i), B – (iv), C – (v), D – (ii), D – (iii)
(d) A – (ii), B – (iii), C – (i), D – (v), D – (v)

**33.** Pollination in Cycasis by:
(a) Insects
(b) Birds
(c) Wind
(d) Water

**34.** Which one of the following is used in making of bread?
(a) *Rhizopus stolonifer*
(b) *Saccharomyces cerevisiae*
(c) Zygosaccharomyces sp.
(d) *Saccharomyces ludwigii*

**35.** Which is the common organelle that is found in both eukaryotes and prokaryote?
(a) Lysosome
(b) Ribosome
(c) Vacuole
(d) Mitochondria

**36.** When the organisms live together in such a manner that one organism is benefited while others have no effects, it is termed as:
(a) Parasitism
(b) Mutualism
(c) Tautomerism
(d) Commensalism

**37.** Match the following.

| List–I | List–II |
|---|---|
| (A) Haemophilia | (i) Reduction in rate of synthesis of globin chains of Haemoglobin |
| (B) Sickle-cell anemia | (ii) Substitution of Glu-acid by Valine in B globin chain of haemoglobin |
| (C) Phenyl ketonuria | (iii) Protein in cascade of blood clotting is affected |
| (D) Thalassemia | (iv) Lack of enzyme for conversion of phenylalanine to tyrosine |

(a) A – (iii), B – (ii), C – (iv), D – (i)
(b) A – (iii), B – (i), C – (ii), D – (iv)
(c) A – (ii), B – (i), C – (iii), D – (iv)
(d) A – (ii), B – (i), C – (iv), D – (iii)

**38.** In-situ conservation of natural genetic resources can be achieved by establishing:
(a) National Parks
(b) Wildlife sanctuaries
(c) Biosphere reserves
(d) All of these

**39.** Identify the correct statements.
1. Respiratory pathway includes anabolism and catabolism.
2. In fermentation, there is net gain of only 2 molecule of ATP for each molecule of glucose.
3. The NADH synthesized in glycolysis is transferred to mitochondria and undergoes reductive phosphorylation.

(a) 1, 2 and 3
(b) 1 and 2 only
(c) 2 and 3 only
(d) 1 and 3 only

**40.** In order for the human population to achieve zero population growth which of the following must occur?
(a) There must be more post reproductive individuals than reproductive individuals.
(b) There must be more prereproductive than reproductive individuals.
(c) There must be the same number or fewer prereproductive individuals as there are reproductive individuals.
(d) All of the above

**41.** All of the following processes occur in the endoplasmic reticulum except:
(a) urea cycle
(b) Protein glycosylation
(c) Fatty acid elongation
(d) Fatty acid desaturation

**42.** Which of the following statement regarding pyruvate during aerobic respiration is incorrect?
(a) Pyruvate is formed by the glycolytic catabolism carbohydrates in the mitochondrial matrix.
(b) It enters mitochondrial matrix & undergoes oxidative decarboxylation.
(c) The conversion of pyruvic acid to acetyl CoA is catalysed by pyruvic dehydrogenase.
(d) Two molecules of NADH are produced from the metabolism of two molecules of pyruvic acid.

**43.** Select the correct match :

| List–I | List–II |
|---|---|
| (A) Lamp brush chromosomes | (i) Oocytes of amphibians |
| (B) Allosomes | (ii) X & Y chromosomes |
| (C) Polytone chromosomes | (iii) Salivary glands of Drosophila |

(D) All of the above

**44.** Group of ribosomes jointed with each other by m-RNA is called:
(a) Lysosome
(b) Polysome
(c) Microsome
(d) Spherosome

**45.** In lac operon structural gene 'Z' is responsible for the synthesis of the enzyme:
(a) Galactosidase transacetylase
(b) Galactosidase permease
(c) β-galactosidase
(d) None of the above

## Zoology

**46.** A transgenic food crop which may help in solving the problem of night blindness in developing countries is:
(a) Golden rice (b) BtSoyabean
(c) Starlink maize (d) FlavrSavr tomato

**47.** Which of the following steps are catalysed by Taq polymerase in a PCR reaction?
(a) Extension of primer end on the template DNA
(b) Annealing of primers to template DNA
(c) Denaturation of template DNA
(d) All of the above

**48.** GEAC stands for:
(a) Genome Engineering Action Committee
(b) Ground Environment Action Committee
(c) Genetic Engineering Approval Committee
(d) Genetic and Environment Approval committee

**49.** Illegal and unlawful development of biomaterials without payment to inhabitants of their region is called:
(a) Biowar
(b) Biopiracy
(c) Biopatent
(d) Biotechnology

**50.** Identify the plasmid:
(a) *AluI* (c) *Hind III*
(c) Eco RI (d) pBR322

**51.** Which is true?
(a) Coenzyme = Holoenzyme + Apoenzyme
(b) Holoenzyme = Coenzyme + Apoenzyme
(c) Apoenzyme = Holoenzyme + Exoenzyme
(d) Holoenzyme = Apoenzyme + Endoenzyme

**52.** Besides giving out secretory vesicles, Golgi apparatus is also concerned with formation of:
(a) Plastids
(b) Lysosomes
(c) Grana of chloroplasts
(d) Cell plates after cell division in plants

**53.** Match the following.

| List–I | List–II |
|---|---|
| (A) Pest resistant crops | (i) Rosie |
| (B) Enhanced nutritional value crops | (ii) ELISA |
| (C) Molecular Diagnosis of disease | (iii) Golden rice |
| (D) Human protein enriched milk | (iv) Bt cotton |

(a) A – (iv), B – (iii), C – (ii), D – (i)
(b) A – (i), B – (iv), C – (ii), D – (iii)
(c) A – (ii), B – (iii), C – (iv), D – (i)
(d) A – (iv), B – (iii), C – (i), D – (ii)

**54.** NAD and FAD used as H-acceptor in aerobic respiration are:
(a) Nucleosides (b) Nucleotides
(c) Dinucleotides (d) Oligonucleotides

**55.** Mechanism of muscle contraction occurs when:
(a) Thick and thin filaments slide over each other.
(b) Thin filament slides over thick filament.
(c) Thick filaments slide over thin filament.
(d) Both filaments slide in same direction.

**56.** Which of the following is not a steroid hormone?
(a) Estrogen (b) Androgen
(c) Thyroxine (d) Aldosterone

**57.** Read the given statements and select the correct option.

**Statement I:** The tumour inducing plasmid (Ti plasmid) acts as a cloning vector in recombinant DNA technology.

**Statement II:** The Ti plasmid which is used in the mechanisms of delivering genes to a cell remains pathogenic.

(a) Statement I is incorrect but Statement II is true.
(b) Both Statement I and Statement II are true.
(c) Both Statement I and Statement II are false.
(d) Statement I is correct but Statement II is false

**58.** Why the presence or absence of hymen is not a reliable indicator of virginity or sexual experience?
(a) Hymen is only broken by coitus.
(b) Hymen can also be ruptured by a sudden fall.
(c) Hymen may be either presence or absent in female.
(d) All of the above

**59.** Decreased levels of estrogen is a common cause for:
(a) Gout (b) Tetany
(c) Arthritis (d) Osteoporosis

**60.** Which of the following is an autoimmune disease?
(a) Cancer
(b) Asthma
(c) Erythroblastosis foetalis
(d) Rheumatoid heart disease

**61.** The most popularly known blood grouping is the ABO grouping. It is named ABO and not ABC, because "O" in it refers to having:
(a) No antigens A and B on RBCs
(b) Other antigens besides A and B on RBCs
(c) Over dominance of this type on the genes for A and B types
(d) One antibody only-either anti –A or anti-B on the RBCs

**62.** Filaria, malaria, dengue fever, sleeping sickness, yellow fever, etc., are transmitted by:
(a) Insects (b) Bacteria
(c) Houseflies (d) Mosquitoes

**63.** Match the following.

| List–I | List–II |
|---|---|
| (A) Non-medicated IUD | (i) Suppress sperm motility and fertility |
| (B) Copper releasing IUD | (ii) Make uterus unsuitable for implantation |
| (C) Hormone releasing IUD | (iii) Phagocytosis of sperms in uterus |

(a) A – (iii), B – (i), C – (ii)
(b) A – (ii), B – (i), C – (iii)
(c) A – (i), B – (iii), C – (ii)
(d) A – (iii), B – (ii), C – (i)

**64.** **Assertion:** *Papaver somniferum* is cultivated to obtain drugs.
**Reason:** Morphine is obtained from its latex.
(a) Both Assertion and Reason are correct and Reason is the correct explanation for Assertion.
(b) Both Assertion and Reason are correct but Reason is not the correct explanation for Assertion.
(c) Assertion is correct but Reason is incorrect.
(d) Both Assertion and Reason are incorrect.

**65.** Smack is obtained by:
(a) alkylation of cocaine
(b) acetylation of morphine
(c) hydroxylation of morphine
(d) methylation of benzodiazepines

**66.** The best description for neurons found usually in embryonic stage is:
(a) One axon and two or more dendrites
(b) One axon and one dendrite
(c) No axon and no dendrite
(d) One axon only

**67.** Signals from fully developed foetus and placenta ultimately lead to parturition which requires the release of:
(a) Estrogen from placenta
(b) Oxytocin from maternal pituitary
(c) Oxytocin from foetal pituitary
(d) Relaxin from placenta

**68.** 'Saheli' is:
(a) A diaphragm for females
(b) A diaphragm used by males
(c) An oral contraceptive for females
(d) A surgical method of sterilization in males

**69.** In spermatogenesis, the phase of maturation involves:
(a) The growth of spermatogonia into primary spermatocyte.
(b) The formation of spermatogonia from gonocytes through mitosis.
(c) The formation of spermatids from primary spermatocytes through meiosis.
(d) The formation of oogonia from the spermatocytes through meiosis.

**70.** Emphysema is a:
(a) Renal disease (b) Neural disease
(c) Pulmonary disease (d) Cardiovascular disease

**71.** Match the terms given under List 'A' with their functions given under List 'B' and select the answer from the options given below:

| List–A | List–B |
|---|---|
| (A) Lymphatic system | (i) Carries oxygenated blood |
| (B) Pulmonary vein | (ii) Immune response |

| List–A | List–B |
|---|---|
| (C) Thrombocytes | (iii) To drain back the tissue fluid to the circulatory |
| (D) Lymphocytes | (iv) Coagulation of blood |

(a) A – (ii), B – (i), C – (iii), D – (iv)
(b) A – (iii), B – (i), C – (iv), D – (ii)
(c) A – (iii), B – (i), C – (iii), D – (iv)
(d) A – (ii), B – (i), C – (iii), D – (iv)

**72.** Which of the given statements are not correct regarding cancer?
(i) Cancer causing viruses have genes called viral oncogenes.
(ii) Malignant tumours remain confined to their original location.
(iii) Cancer cells do not exhibit contact inhibition.
(iv) X-rays and UV rays are not potent carcinogens.
(v) Cancer detection is based on biopsy.
(a) (iii) and (v) (b) (ii) and (iv)
(c) (iii) and (v) (d) (ii), (iv) and (v)

**73.** Match the terms given in List I with their physiological processes given in List II and choose the correct answer:

| List–I | List–II |
|---|---|
| (A) Proximal convoluted tubule | (i) Formation of concentrated urine |
| (B) Distal convoluted tubule | (ii) Filtration of blood |
| (C) Henle's loop | (iii) Reabsorption of 70-80% of electrolytes |
| (D) Counter-current mechanism | (iv) Ionic balance |
| (E) Renal corpuscle | (v) Maintenance of concentration gradient in medulla |

(a) A – iii, B – v, C – iv, D – ii, E – i
(b) A – iii, B – iv, C – i, D – v, E – ii
(c) A – i, B – iii, C – ii, D – v, E – iv
(d) A – iii, B – i, C – iv, D – v, E – ii

**74.** Nissl's granules are present in ________ and their work is to:
(a) Blood and help in coagulation
(b) Sarcoplasm and help in contraction
(c) Neuron and help in protein synthesis
(d) Neuron and help in nutrition and excretion

**75.** Characteristic of hormones are:
(a) Non-nutritive chemicals
(b) Inner-cellular messenger
(c) Trace amount production
(d) All of the above

**76.** Mutation theory explaining organic evolution was proposed by:
(a) E. Darwin (b) W. Harvey
(c) Hugo de Vries (d) Louis Pasteur

**77.** Match the following and choose the correct options:

| List–I | List–II |
|---|---|
| (A) Trophoblast | (i) Embedding of blastocyst in the endometrium |
| (B) Cleavage | (ii) Group of cells that would differentiate as embryo |
| (C) Inner cell mass | (iii) Outer layer of blastocyst attached to the endometrium |
| (D) Implantation | (iv) Mitotic division of zygote |

(a) A – ii, B – i, C – iii, D – iv
(b) A – iii, B – iv, C – ii, D – i
(c) A – iii, B – i, C – ii, D – iv
(d) A – ii, B – iv, C – iii, D – i

**78.** Which one of the following is called milk ejection hormone and birth hormone?
(a) Vasopressin
(b) Oxytocin
(c) Somatotropic hormone
(d) Prolactin

**79.** The organs which look different but have the same basic structure and origin are known as:
(a) Homologous (b) Vestigial
(c) Heterologous (d) Analogous

**80.** Match the following:

| List–I | List–II |
|---|---|
| (A) Basophils | (i) Phagocytosis |
| (B) Neutrophils | (ii) Inflammation |
| (C) Plasma cells | (iii) Blood clotting |
| (D) Thrombocytes | (iv) Antibodies |

(a) A - (ii), B - (i), C - (iv), D - (iii)
(b) A - (ii), B - (ii), C - (iii), D - (iv)
(c) A - (i), B - (ii), C - (iv), D - (iii)
(d) A - (iv), B - (i), C - (ii), D - (iii)

**81.** **Assertion:** The testes are situated outside the abdominal cavity within a pouch called scrotum.

**Reason:** The scrotum helps in maintaining the low temperature which is necessary for spermatogenesis.

(a) (A) is false but (R) is true.
(b) Both (A) and (R) are true and (R) is the correct explanation of (A).
(c) Both (A) and (R) are true but (R) is not the correct explanation of (A).
(d) (A) is true but (R) is false.

**82.** According to the sliding filament theory of muscle contraction,

(a) Actin binds ATP ad breaks it apart as actin pulls against myosin.
(b) Calcium ions are released from myosin as the filaments slide by.
(c) The thick and thin filaments do not change length during this process.
(d) All are correct

**83.** Birds and mammals share one of the following characteristics as a common feature:

(a) Viviparity
(b) Pigmented skin
(c) Warm blooded nature
(d) Alimentary canal with some modification

**84.** **Assertion:** The amount of $CO_2$ that can diffuse through diffusion membrane per unit difference in partial pressure is much higher compared to that of $O_2$.

**Reason:** Solubility of $CO_2$ is 20-25 times higher than that of $O_2$.

(a) (A) is false but (R) is true.
(b) Both (A) and (R) are true and (R) is the correct explanation of (A).
(c) Both (A) and (R) are true but (R) is not the correct explanation of (A).
(d) (A) is true but (R) is false.

**85.** Which of following main nitrogenous waste eliminated through saliva?

(a) Urea (b) Creatine
(c) $HCO_3^-$ (d) Uric acid

**86.** Part of nephron impermeable to salt is:

(a) Descending limb of loop of henle
(b) Ascending limb of henle
(c) Distal convoluted tubule
(d) Collecting ducts

**87.** Match List I and List II, and select the correct answer using the codes given below the lists:

| List–I (Animals) | List–II (Organs of locomotion) |
|---|---|
| (A) Paramecium | (i) Parapodia |
| (B) Pila | (ii) Flagellum |
| (C) Trypanosoma | (iii) Foot |
| (D) Neries | (iv) Cilia |
| | (v) Tube feet |

(a) A - (iv), B - (iii), C - (ii), D - (i)
(b) A - (ii), B - (iii), C - (i), D - (v)
(c) A - (i), B - (v), C - (ii), D - (iv)
(d) A - (v), B - (i), C - (iv), D - (iii)

**88.** The source of Taq polymerase used in PCR technique is a

(a) Thermophilic fungus
(b) Mesophilic fungus
(c) Thermophilic bacteria
(d) Halophilic bacteria

**89.** First restriction enzyme was isolated from:

(a) *E. coli*
(b) *Haemophilus influenza*
(c) *Pseudomonas*
(d) *Xanthomonas*

**90.** **Assertion:** Nucleotide has three chemically distinct components.

**Reason:** Nucleotide is made of a homocyclic compounds, a monosaccharide & a sulphate group.

(a) (A) is false but (R) is true.
(b) Both (A) and (R) are true and (R) is the correct explanation of (A).
(c) Both (A) and (R) are true but (R) is not the correct explanation of (A).
(d) (A) is true but (R) is false.

## Answer Keys

### Botany

| | | | | | | | | | |
|---|---|---|---|---|---|---|---|---|---|
| **1.** (b) | **2.** (d) | **3.** (b) | **4.** (a) | **5.** (c) | **6.** (d) | **7.** (d) | **8.** (c) | **9.** (c) | **10.** (b) |
| **11.** (d) | **12.** (c) | **13.** (b) | **14.** (a) | **15.** (d) | **16.** (a) | **17.** (a) | **18.** (b) | **19.** (b) | **20.** (b) |
| **21.** (a) | **22.** (c) | **23.** (d) | **24.** (d) | **25.** (a) | **26.** (d) | **27.** (c) | **28.** (b) | **29.** (d) | **30.** (c) |
| **31.** (d) | **32.** (a) | **33.** (c) | **34.** (b) | **35.** (b) | **36.** (d) | **37.** (a) | **38.** (d) | **39.** (b) | **40.** (c) |
| **41.** (a) | **42.** (a) | **43.** (d) | **44.** (b) | **45.** (c) | | | | | |

### Zoology

| | | | | | | | | | |
|---|---|---|---|---|---|---|---|---|---|
| **46.** (a) | **47.** (a) | **48.** (c) | **49.** (b) | **50.** (d) | **51.** (b) | **52.** (b) | **53.** (a) | **54.** (c) | **55.** (b) |
| **56.** (c) | **57.** (d) | **58.** (d) | **59.** (d) | **60.** (d) | **61.** (a) | **62.** (a) | **63.** (a) | **64.** (a) | **65.** (b) |
| **66.** (d) | **67.** (b) | **68.** (c) | **69.** (c) | **70.** (c) | **71.** (b) | **72.** (b) | **73.** (b) | **74.** (c) | **75.** (d) |
| **76.** (c) | **77.** (b) | **78.** (b) | **79.** (a) | **80.** (a) | **81.** (b) | **82.** (c) | **83.** (c) | **84.** (b) | **85.** (a) |
| **86.** (a) | **87.** (a) | **88.** (c) | **89.** (b) | **90.** (d) | | | | | |

## Hints and Explanations

### BOTANY

**1.**

| | |
|---|---|
| (A) ER | (i) Synthesis of protein & lipids |
| (B) Golgi complex | (ii) Synthesis of glycoprotein & glycolipid |
| (C) Lysosomes | (iii) Storage of hydrolytic enzymest |
| (D) Vacuoles | (iv) Contain water / sap/ food/ excretory product |

**2.** *Rhizophora* growing in swampy areas, many roots come out of the ground and grow vertically upwards. Such roots, called pneumatophores, help to get oxygen for respiration.

**3.** Tap roots of carrot, turnip and adventitious roots of sweet potato, get swollen and store food.

**4.** In a dicot leaf, the palisade parenchyma is positioned on the adaxial side, while the phloem is located on the abaxial side.

**5.** The tangential as well as radial walls of the endodermal cells have a deposition of water impermeable, waxy material-suberin-in the form of casparian strips.

**6.**

| | |
|---|---|
| (A) Pulvinus | (i) Swollen leaflets in leguminous plants |
| (B) Rachis | (ii) Common axis on which leaflets are arranged in pinnately compound leaf |
| (C) Receptacle | (iii) Swollen end of pedicel bearing flower whorls |

**7.** (ii) Being photosynthetic they increase the level of dissolved oxygen in their immediate environment.

(iii) Many species of Porphyra, Laminaria and Sargassum, are marine algae

(iv) Certain freshwater brown and red algae produce large amounts of Hydrocolloids, used as water holding substances and are produced by marine algae

**8.** *E. coli* in a medium containing $^{15}NH_4Cl$ ($^{15}N$ is the heavy isotope of nitrogen) as the only nitrogen source for many generations. The result was that $^{15}N$ was incorporated into newly synthesized DNA (as well as other nitrogen containing compounds).

This heavy DNA molecule could be distinguished from the normal DNA by centrifugation in a cesium chloride (CsCl) density gradient (Please note that $^{15}N$ is not a radioactive isotope, and it can be separated from $^{14}N$ only based on densities).

**9.** It is now proven that DNA replicates semiconservative. It was shown first in *Escherichia coli* and subsequently in higher organisms, such as plants and human cells. Matthew Meselson and Franklin Stahl performed the following experiment in 1958.

**10.** A nitrogenous base is linked to the pentose sugar through a N-glycosidic linkage.

**11.** In photorespiration pathway, there is neither synthesis of sugar, nor of ATP. It result in the release of $CO_2$ with utilization of ATP.

**12.** Down's Syndrome: The cause of this genetic disorder is the presence of an additional copy of the chromosome number 21 (trisomy of 21).

**13.** Some organisms breed only once in their lifetime: Pacific salmon fish, bamboo

**14.** The hard outer layer called the exine is made up of sporopollenin which is one of the most resistant organic material known.

**15.** Zebra and African lion live in same habitat, environment and biosphere but their ecological niche is different means their function, role and position is different.

**16.** The generation of ATP through the oxidation of fatty acids and carbohydrates involves a common intermediate, namely Acetyl CoA. This shared metabolic pathway underscores the fundamental role of Acetyl CoA in energy production. Acetyl CoA is synthesized in mitochondria by a number of reactions: oxidative decarboxylation of pyruvate, beta oxidation of fatty acids.

**17.** All the statements are correct.

**18.** *Natality* refers to the number of births during a given period in the population that are added to the initial density.

**19.** Placental mammals in Australia also exhibit adaptive radiation in evolving into varieties of such placental mammals each of which appears to be 'similar' to a corresponding marsupial (e.g., Placental wolf and Tasmanian wolf-marsupial).

Parallel evolution is the evolution of geographically separated groups in such a way that they show morphological resemblance.

**20.**

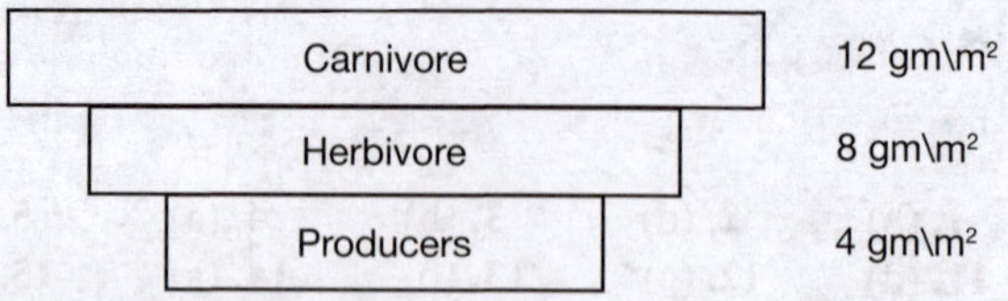


**21.** Photophosphorylation is the synthesis of ATP from ADP and inorganic phosphate in the presence of light. When the two photosystems work in a series, first PS II and then the PS I, a process called non-cyclic photo-phosphorylation occurs. The two photosystems are connected through an electron transport chain, as seen earlier – in the Z scheme. Both ATP and NADPH + $H^+$

**22.** Slime moulds belong to kingdom Protista.

**23.** Guard cells help in opening and closing of stomata. When guard cell becomes flaccid, stomata closes due to flaccidity. O.P. decreases and sugar is converted to starch. Accumulation of $O_2$ in guard cell is not related with opening and closing.

**24.** The content of nucleolus is continuous with the rest of the nucleoplasm as it is not a membrane bound structure. It is a site for active ribosomal RNA synthesis. Larger and more numerous nucleoli are present in cells actively carrying out protein synthesis.

**25.**

| | |
|---|---|
| (A) Meselson & Stahl | (i) Heavy isotope of nitrogen |
| (B) Hershey & Chase | (ii) Radioactive phosphorus & sulphur |
| (C) F. Griffith | (iii) R & S strains of *S. pneumoniae* |

**26.** During this stage bivalent chromosome clearly appears as tetrads.

**27.** Transpiration is the evaporative loss of water by plants. It occurs mainly through the stomata in the leaves. Besides the loss of water vapor in transpiration, exchange of oxygen and carbon dioxide in the leaf also occurs through pores called stomata (sing. : stoma). Normally stomata are open in the day time and close during the night. The immediate cause of the opening or closing of the stomata is a change in the turgidity of the guard cells.

**28.** In some species floral rewards are in providing safe places to lay eggs; an example is that of the tallest flower of *Amorphophallus* (the flower itself is about 6 feet in height). A similar relationship exists between a species of moth and the plant *Yucca* where both species – moth and the plant – cannot complete their life cycles without each other. The moth deposits its eggs in the locule of the ovary and the flower, in turn, gets pollinated by the moth. The larvae of the moth come out of the eggs as the seeds start developing.

**29.** Cryopreservation is done at -196° C

**30.** In green plants $H_2O$ is the hydrogen donor and is oxidized to $O_2$. Some organisms do not release $O_2$ during photosynthesis. When $H_2S$, instead is the hydrogen donor for purple and green sulphur bacteria, the 'oxidation' product is sulphur or sulphate depending on the organism and not $O_2$.

**31.** All the given statements are correct regarding light reaction.

**32.**

| | |
|---|---|
| (A) *Clostridium sp.* | (i) $C_6H_8O_7$ |
| (B) *Methanobacterium sp.* | (ii) $CH_4$ |
| (C) *Acetobacter sp.* | (iii) $CH_3COOH$ ($C_2H_4O_2$) |
| (D) *Aspergillus sp.* | (iv) $C_4H_8O_2$ |
| (E) *Lactobacillus sp.* | (v) $C_3H_6O_3$ |

**33.** Pollination in gymnosperms is carried out by wind.

**34.** *Saccharomyces cerevisiae is* used for bread-making and commonly called brewer's yeast.

**35.** Prokaryotic cells lack membrane-bound organelles, excluding structures like mitochondria, plastids, and lysosomes, all of which are membrane-bound. However, prokaryotic cells do contain ribosomes.

**36.** *Commensalism:* This is the interaction in which one species benefits and the other is neither harmed nor benefited.

**37.**

| | |
|---|---|
| (A) Haemophilia | (i) Protein in cascade of blood clotting is affected |
| (B) Sickle-cell anemia | (ii) Substitution of Glu-acid by Valine in B globin chain of haemoglobin |
| (C) Phenyl ketonuria | (iii) Lack of enzyme for conversion of phenylalanine to tyrosine |
| (D) Thalassemia | (iv) Reduction in rate of synthesis of globin chains of Haemoglobin |

**38.** *In situ* conservation– Faced with the conflict between development and conservation, many nations find it unrealistic and economically not feasible to conserve all their biological wealth. Invariably, the number of species waiting to be saved from extinction far exceeds the conservation resources available. On a global basis, this problem has been addressed by eminent conservationists.

**39.** NADH produced during glycolysis is transported into the mitochondria, where it participates in oxidative phosphorylation.

**40.** Zero population means birth rate = Death rate which results in stable population. Pre-reproductive cannot give birth as well as post reproductive cannot give birth.

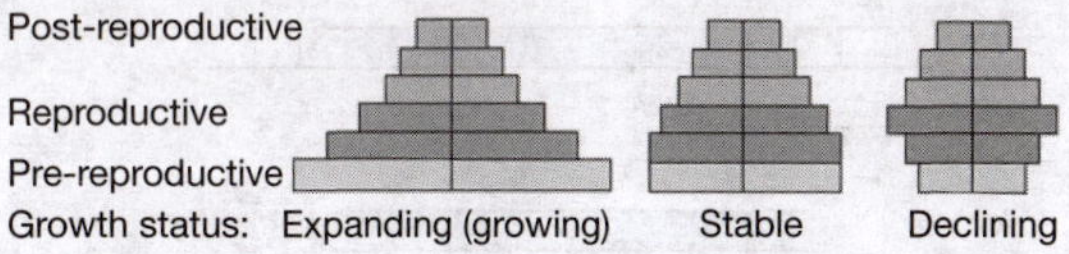


**41.** Urea cycle takes place in liver.

**42.** Glycolysis: The term glycolysis has originated from the Greek words, *glycos* for sugar, and *lysis* for splitting. The scheme of glycolysis was given by Gustav Embden, Otto Meyerhof, and J. Parnas, and is often referred to as the EMP pathway. In anaerobic organisms, it is the only process in respiration. Glycolysis occurs in the cytoplasm of the cell and is present in all living organisms.

**43.** (a) Lamp brush chromosomes can be seen oocytes of amphibians.

(b) Allosomes are sex chromosomes (X and Y)

(c) Polytene chromosomes can be seen in salivary glands of drosophila.

**44.** Several ribosomes may attach to a single mRNA and form a chain called polyribosomes or polysome. The ribosomes of a polysome translate the mRNA into proteins.

**45.** The *z* gene codes for $\beta$-galactosidase ($\beta$-gal), which is primarily responsible for the hydrolysis of the disaccharide, lactose into its monomeric units, galactose and glucose.

## Zoology

**46.** Enhanced nutritional value of food, e.g., Vitamin 'A' enriched rice.

**47.**

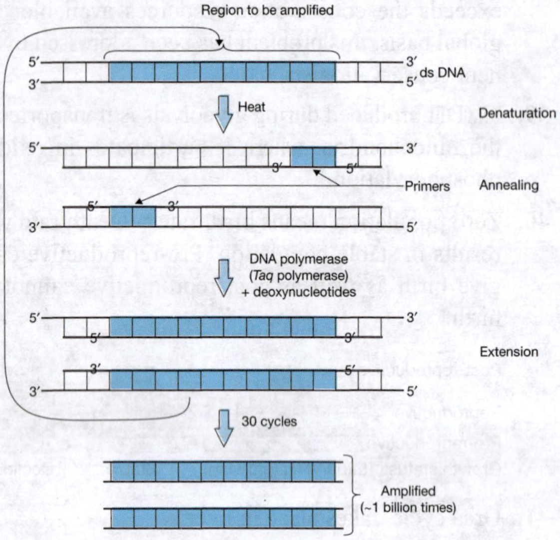


**48.** GEAC (Genetic Engineering Approval Committee)

**49.** Biopiracy is the term used to refer to the use of bio-resources by multinational companies and other organizations without proper authorization from the countries and people concerned without compensatory payment.

**50.**

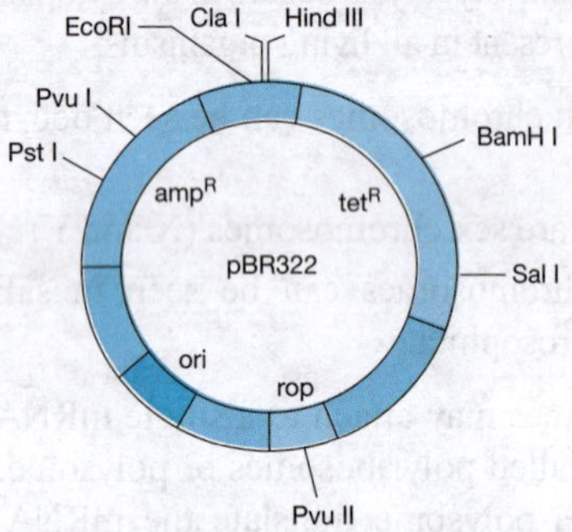


**51.** Holoezyme is complete functional enzyme made up of apoenzyme (protein part) and coenzyme (like cofactor, prosthetic group.)

**52.** Lysosomes are membrane bound vesicular structures formed by the process of packaging in the golgi apparatus.

**53.**

| List–I | List–II |
|---|---|
| (A) Pest resistant crops | (i) Bt cotton |
| (B) Enhanced nutritional value crops | (ii) Golden rice |
| (C) Molecular Diagnosis of disease | (iii) ELISA |
| (D) Human protein enriched milk | (iv) Rosie |

**54.** NAD is nicotinamide adenine Dinucleotide.

FAD is flavin adenine Dinucleotide.

**55.** The mechanism of muscle contraction is most effectively described by the sliding filament theory. According to this theory, the contraction of a muscle fiber occurs through the sliding movement of thin filaments over thick filaments. This process involves the actin filaments sliding over the myosin filaments, leading to a reduction in the length of the sarcomere and, consequently, the contraction of the muscle fiber.

**56.** On the basis of their chemical nature, hormones can be divided into groups:

(i) peptide, polypeptide, protein hormones (e.g., insulin, glucagon, pituitary hormones, hypothalamic hormones, etc.)

(ii) steroids (e.g., cortisol, testosterone, estradiol and progesterone)

(iii) iodothyronines (thyroid hormones)

(iv) amino-acid derivatives (e.g., epinephrine).

**57.** The tumour inducing (Ti) plasmid of *Agrobacterium tumefaciens* has been modified into cloning vector which is not pathogenic to the plants, however it is still able to use its mechanism to deliver genes of our interest into various plants.

**58.** The vaginal opening is partially covered by a membrane known as the hymen. This membrane may be torn during the first instance of sexual intercourse, but it can also be disrupted by other activities such as a sudden fall or jolt, the insertion of a vaginal tampon, or active participation in sports like horseback riding or cycling. Additionally, in certain cases, the hymen may persist even after sexual intercourse. Consequently, the presence or absence of the hymen cannot be considered a dependable indicator of a person's virginity or sexual experience.

**59.** Osteoporosis: Age-related disorder characterized by decreased bone mass and increased chances of fractures. Decreased levels of estrogen is a common cause.

**60.** Rheumatoid arthritis which affects many people in our society is an auto-immune disease.

**61.**

| Blood Group | Antigens on RBCs | Antibodies in Plasma | Donor's Group |
|---|---|---|---|
| A | A | anti-B | A, O |
| B | B | anti-A | B, O |
| AB | A, B | nil | AB, A, B, O |
| O | nil | anti-A, B | O |

**62.** Malaria, dengue, Filaria-- spreads via mosquito while Tse – Tse fly spreads sleeping sickness.

**63.**

| | |
|---|---|
| (A) Non-medicated IUD | (i) Phagocytosis of sperms in uterus |
| (B) Copper releasing IUD | (ii) Suppress sperm motility and fertility |
| (C) Hormone releasing IUD | (iii) Make uterus unsuitable for implantation |

**64.** Both Assertion and Reason are correct and Reason is the correct explanation for Assertion.

**65.** Smack is obtained by acetylation of morphine which is extracted from the latex of poppy plant *Papaver somniferum*.

**66.** Neurons are categorized into three types based on the number of axons and dendrites they possess. These types include multipolar neurons, which have one axon and two or more dendrites and are commonly found in the cerebral cortex; bipolar neurons, characterized by one axon and one dendrite, typically found in the retina of the eye; and unipolar neurons, where the cell body has only one axon and is commonly found, especially in the embryonic stage.

**67.** The signals for parturition originate from the fully developed foetus and the placenta which induce mild uterine contractions called foetal ejection reflex. These triggers release of oxytocin from the maternal pituitary.

**68.** *Saheli*–the new oral contraceptive for the females contains a non-steroidal preparation.

**69.** A primary spermatocyte completes the first meiotic division (reduction division) leading to formation of two equal, haploid cells called secondary spermatocytes, which have only 23 chromosomes each. The secondary spermatocytes undergo the second meiotic division to produce four equal, haploid spermatids.

**70.** Emphysema is a chronic disorder in which alveolar walls are damaged due to which respiratory surface is decreased. One of the major causes of this is cigarette smoking.

**71.** (A) Lymphatic system is involved in immune response.

(B) Pulmonary in originates from lungs and transports oxygenated blood.

(C) Thrombocytes helps in coagulation of blood

(D) Lymphocytes help to drain back the tissue fluid to circulatory system.

**72.** (ii) Benign tumours remain confined to their original location.

(iv) X-rays and UV-rays are carcinogenic.

**73.** (A) Proximal Convoluted Tubule (PCT): PCT is lined by simple cuboidal brush border epithelium which increases the surface area for reabsorption. Nearly all of the essential nutrients, and 70-80 per cent of electrolytes and water are reabsorbed by this segment.

(B) Distal Convoluted Tubule (DCT): Conditional reabsorption of $Na^+$ and water takes place in this segment. DCT is also capable of reabsorption of $HCO_3^-$ and selective secretion of hydrogen and potassium ions and $NH_3$ to maintain the pH and sodium-potassium balance in blood.

(C) Henle's Loop: Reabsorption is minimum in its ascending limb. However, this region plays a significant role in the maintenance of high osmolarity of medullary interstitial fluid.

(D) The flow of filtrate in the two limbs of Henle's loop is in opposite directions and thus forms a counter current. The flow of blood through the two limbs of *vasa recta* is also in a counter current pattern.

(E) Renal corpuscle is responsible for filtration of blood.

**74.** The cell body contains cytoplasm with typical cell organelles and certain granular bodies called Nissl's granules. Short fibres which branch repeatedly and project out of the cell body also contain Nissl's granules and are called dendrites.

**75.** All the statements are correct regarding hormones.

**76.** Hugo de Vries proposed mutation theory on evening primrose.

**77.** The mitotic division starts as the zygote moves through the isthmus of the oviduct called cleavage towards the uterus and forms 2, 4, 8, 16 daughter cells called blastomeres. The embryo with 8 to 16 blastomeres is called a morula. The morula continues to divide and transforms into blastocyst as it moves further into the uterus. The blastomeres in the blastocyst are arranged into an outer layer called trophoblast and an inner group of cells attached to trophoblast called the inner cell mass. The trophoblast layer then gets attached to the endometrium and the inner cell mass gets differentiated as the embryo. After attachment, the uterine cells divide rapidly and covers the blastocyst. As a result, the blastocyst becomes embedded in the endometrium of the uterus. This is called implantation and it leads to pregnancy.

**78.** The release of the hormone oxytocin from maternal pituitary leads to the milk ejection. Oxytocin stimulates the muscle contraction surrounding the breast to squeeze out the milk.

**79.** Whales, bats, Cheetah and human (all mammals) share similarities in the pattern of bones of forelimbs. Though these forelimbs perform different functions in these animals, they have similar anatomical structure – all of them have humerus, radius, ulna, carpals, metacarpals and phalanges in their forelimbs. Hence, in these animals, the same structure developed along different directions due to adaptations to different needs. This is divergent evolution and these structures are homologous. Homology indicates common ancestry.

**80.** Neutrophils, eosinophils and basophils are different types of granulocytes, while lymphocytes and monocytes are the agranulocytes. Neutrophils are the most abundant cells (60-65 per cent) of the total WBCs and basophils are the least (0.5-1 per cent) among them. Neutrophils and monocytes (6-8 per cent) are phagocytic cells which destroy foreign organisms entering the body. Basophils secrete histamine, serotonin, heparin, etc., and are involved in inflammatory reactions.

**81.** The process of spermatogenesis requires lower temperature (2-2.5°C) than the body and hence testes (site of spermatogenesis) are present outside the abdominal cavity. The pouch is known as the scrotum or scrotal sac.

**82.** Contraction is best explained by the sliding filament theory which states that contraction of a muscle fiber takes place by the sliding of the thin filaments over the thick filaments.

**83.** Birds & mammals are homo- thermal animals.

**84.** As the solubility of $CO_2$ is 20-25 times higher than that of $O_2$, the amount of $CO_2$ that can diffuse through the diffusion membrane per unit difference in partial pressure is much higher compared to that of $O_2$.

**85.** Urea is a nitrogenous waste product that can be eliminated from the body through various means, one of which is in the form of saliva. Urea is the final product that is broken down in the amino acid breakdown of the body.

**86.** The descending limb of the loop of Henle is impermeable to salts.

**87.** (a) Paramecium moves by cilia

(b) Pila belongs to mollusc, moves by foot

(c) Trypanosoma is protozoa moves by flagellum

(d) Nereis is annelid moves by parapodium

**88.** Repeated amplification in PCR is achieved by the use of a thermostable DNA polymerase, isolated from bacteria *Thermus aquaticus*, which remain active during the high temperature induced denaturation of ds DNA.

**89.** First restriction enzyme Hind – II was isolated from *Haemophilus influenza* by Smith Hamilton.

**90.** Nucleotide is made of a heterocyclic compound, a monosaccharide & a sulphate group.

# Credits

## Chapter 1

**Page 1.3**—nobeastsofierce / Shutterstock

## Chapter 2

**Page 2.1**—nobeastsofierce / Shutterstock

## Chapter 3

**Page 3.1**—nobeastsofierce / Shutterstock

## Chapter 4

**Page 4.1**—nobeastsofierce / Shutterstock; **Page 4.1**—Jun MT. Shutterstock / Brian Maudsley. Shutterstock; **Page 4.3**—Kletr / Shutterstock

## Chapter 5

**Page 5.1**—nobeastsofierce / Shutterstock

## Chapter 6

**Page 6.1**—nobeastsofierce / Shutterstock

## Chapter 7

**Page 7.1**—nobeastsofierce / Shutterstock

## Chapter 8

**Page 8.3**—nobeastsofierce / Shutterstock

## Chapter 9

**Page 9.1**—nobeastsofierce / Shutterstock

## Chapter 10

**Page 10.1**—nobeastsofierce / Shutterstock

## Chapter 11

**Page 11.1**—nobeastsofierce / Shutterstock; **Page 11.4**—Moonnoon. Shutterstock; **Page 11.6**—schankz. Shutterstock; **Page 11.12**—designua. 123rf.com

## Chapter 12

**Page 12.1**—nobeastsofierce / Shutterstock; **Page 12.5**—Soleil Nordic. Shutterstock

## Chapter 13

**Page 13.1**—nobeastsofierce / Shutterstock; **Page 13.4**—KentaStudio/Shutterstock